CW01370818

Cosmetic Dermatology
Products and Procedures

Cosmetic Dermatology

Products and Procedures

Edited by

Zoe Diana Draelos MD
Consulting Professor
Department of Dermatology
Duke University School of Medicine
Durham, North Carolina
USA

Second Edition

WILEY Blackwell

This edition first published 2016
© 2016 by John Wiley & Sons, Ltd
© 2010 by Blackwell Publishing, Ltd

Registered office: John Wiley & Sons, Ltd, The Atrium, Southern Gate, Chichester, West Sussex, PO19 8SQ, UK

Editorial offices: 9600 Garsington Road, Oxford, OX4 2DQ, UK
The Atrium, Southern Gate, Chichester, West Sussex, PO19 8SQ, UK
111 River Street, Hoboken, NJ 07030-5774, USA

For details of our global editorial offices, for customer services and for information about how to apply for permission to reuse the copyright material in this book please see our website at www.wiley.com/wiley-blackwell

The right of the author to be identified as the author of this work has been asserted in accordance with the UK Copyright, Designs and Patents Act 1988.

All rights reserved. No part of this publication may be reproduced, stored in a retrieval system, or transmitted, in any form or by any means, electronic, mechanical, photocopying, recording or otherwise, except as permitted by the UK Copyright, Designs and Patents Act 1988, without the prior permission of the publisher.

Designations used by companies to distinguish their products are often claimed as trademarks. All brand names and product names used in this book are trade names, service marks, trademarks or registered trademarks of their respective owners. The publisher is not associated with any product or vendor mentioned in this book. It is sold on the understanding that the publisher is not engaged in rendering professional services. If professional advice or other expert assistance is required, the services of a competent professional should be sought.

The contents of this work are intended to further general scientific research, understanding, and discussion only and are not intended and should not be relied upon as recommending or promoting a specific method, diagnosis, or treatment by health science practitioners for any particular patient. The publisher and the author make no representations or warranties with respect to the accuracy or completeness of the contents of this work and specifically disclaim all warranties, including without limitation any implied warranties of fitness for a particular purpose. In view of ongoing research, equipment modifications, changes in governmental regulations, and the constant flow of information relating to the use of medicines, equipment, and devices, the reader is urged to review and evaluate the information provided in the package insert or instructions for each medicine, equipment, or device for, among other things, any changes in the instructions or indication of usage and for added warnings and precautions. Readers should consult with a specialist where appropriate. The fact that an organization or Website is referred to in this work as a citation and/or a potential source of further information does not mean that the author or the publisher endorses the information the organization or Website may provide or recommendations it may make. Further, readers should be aware that Internet Websites listed in this work may have changed or disappeared between when this work was written and when it is read. No warranty may be created or extended by any promotional statements for this work. Neither the publisher nor the author shall be liable for any damages arising herefrom.

Library of Congress Cataloging-in-Publication Data

Cosmetic dermatology (Draelos)
  Cosmetic dermatology : products and procedures / edited by Zoe Diana Draelos.—Second edition.
    p. ; cm.
  Includes bibliographical references and index.
  ISBN 978-1-118-65558-0 (cloth)
  I. Draelos, Zoe Kececioglu, editor. II. Title.
  [DNLM: 1. Cosmetics.   2. Dermatologic Agents.   3. Cosmetic Techniques.   4. Dermatologic Surgical Procedures.
  5. Skin Care—methods. QV 60]
  RL87
  646.7′2—dc23

2015030110

A catalogue record for this book is available from the British Library.

Wiley also publishes its books in a variety of electronic formats. Some content that appears in print may not be available in electronic books.

Cover images: background © Getty Images/Ian Hooton/SPL; middle © Getty Images/Renee Keith

Set in 9.5/12pt Minion Pro by Aptara Inc., New Delhi, India
Printed and bound in Singapore by Markono Print Media Pte Ltd

2   2017

Contents

Contributors, viii

Foreword, xii

Preface, xiii

Part I: Basic Concepts, 1

Section 1: Skin Physiology Pertinent to Cosmetic Dermatology, 3

1. Epidermal Barrier, 3
   Sreekumar Pillai, Megan Manco, and Christian Oresajo

2. Photoaging, 13
   Kira Minkis, Jillian Havey Swary, and Murad Alam

3. Pigmentation and Skin of Color, 23
   Jasmine C. Hollinger, Chesahna Kindred, and Rebat M. Halder

4. Sensitive Skin and the Somatosensory System, 33
   Francis McGlone and David Reilly

5. Novel, Compelling, Non-invasive Techniques for Evaluating Cosmetic Products, 42
   Thomas J. Stephens, Christian Oresajo, Lily I. Jiang, and Robert Goodman

6. Contact Dermatitis and Topical Agents, 52
   David E. Cohen, Alexandra Price, and Sarika Ramachandran

Section 2: Delivery of Cosmetic Skin Actives, 65

7. Percutaneous Delivery of Cosmetic Actives to the Skin, 65
   Sreekumar Pillai, Surabhi Singh, and Christian Oresajo

8. Creams and Ointments, 75
   Irwin Palefsky

Part II: Hygiene Products, 81

Section 1: Cleansers, 83

9. Bar Cleansers, 83
   Anthony W. Johnson, K.P. Ananthapadmanabhan, Stacy Hawkins, and Greg Nole

10. Personal Cleansers: Body Washes, 96
    Keith Ertel and Heather Focht

11. Facial Cleansers and Cleansing Cloths, 103
    Thomas Barlage, Susan Griffiths-Brophy, and Erik J. Hasenoehrl

12. Hand Cleansers and Sanitizers, 110
    Duane Charbonneau

13. Shampoos for Normal Scalp Hygiene and Dandruff, 124
    James R. Schwartz, Eric S. Johnson, and Thomas L. Dawson, Jr.

Section 2: Moisturizers, 132

14. Facial Moisturizers, 132
    Yohini Appa

15. Hand and Foot Moisturizers, 139
    Teresa M. Weber, Andrea M. Schoelermann, Ute Breitenbach, Ulrich Scherdin, and Alexandra Kowcz

16. Sunless Tanning Products, 148
    Angelike Galdi, Peter Foltis, and Christian Oresajo

17. Sunscreens, 153
    Dominique Moyal, Angelike Galdi, and Christian Oresajo

Section 3: Personal Care Products, 160

18. Antiperspirants and Deodorants, 160
    Eric S. Abrutyn

19. Blade Shaving, 166
    Kevin Cowley, Kristina Vanoosthuyze, Gillian McFeat, and Keith Ertel

Part III: Adornment, 175

Section 1: Colored Facial Cosmetics, 175

20. Facial Foundation, 177
    Sylvie Guichard and Véronique Roulier

21. Camouflage Techniques, 186
    Anne Bouloc

22. Lips and Lipsticks, 193
    Catherine Heusèle, Hervé Cantin, and Frédéric Bonté

23 Eye Cosmetics, 199
Sarah A. Vickery, Robyn Kolas, and Fatima Dicko

Section 2: Nail Cosmetics, 207

24 Nail Physiology and Grooming, 207
Anna Hare and Phoebe Rich

25 Colored Nail Cosmetics and Hardeners, 217
Paul H. Bryson and Sunil J. Sirdesai

26 Cosmetic Prostheses as Artificial Nail Enhancements, 226
Douglas Schoon

Section 3: Hair Cosmetics, 234

27 Hair Physiology and Grooming, 234
Maria Hordinsky, Ana Paula Avancini Caramori, and Jeff C. Donovan

28 Hair Dyes, 239
Rene C. Rust and Harald Schlatter

29 Permanent Hair Waving, 251
Annette Schwan-Jonczyk, Gerhard Sendelbach, Andreas Flohr, and Rene C. Rust

30 Hair Straightening, 262
Harold Bryant, Felicia Dixon, Angela Ellington, and Crystal Porter

31 Hair Styling: Technology and Formulations, 270
Thomas Krause and Rene C. Rust

Part IV: Anti-aging, 281

Section 1: Cosmeceuticals, 283

32 Botanicals, 283
Carl R. Thornfeldt

33 Antioxidants and Anti-inflammatories, 295
Bryan B. Fuller

34 Peptides and Proteins, 308
Karl Lintner

35 Cellular Growth Factors, 318
Rahul C. Mehta and Richard E. Fitzpatrick

36 Topical Cosmeceutical Retinoids, 325
Olivier Sorg, Gürkan Kaya, and Jean H. Saurat

37 Topical Vitamins, 336
Donald L. Bissett, John E. Oblong, and Laura J. Goodman

38 Clinical Uses of Hydroxyacids, 346
Barbara A. Green, Eugene J. Van Scott, and Ruey J. Yu

39 The Contribution of Dietary Nutrients and Supplements to Skin Health, 357
Helen Knaggs, Steve Wood, Doug Burke, Jan Lephart, and Jin Namkoong

Section 2: Injectable Anti-aging Techniques, 364

40 Botulinum Toxins, 364
J. Daniel Jensen, Scott R. Freeman, and Joel L. Cohen

41 Hyaluronic Acid Fillers, 375
Mark S. Nestor, Emily L. Kollmann, and Nicole Swenson

42 Calcium Hydroxylapatite for Soft Tissue Augmentation, 380
Stephen Mandy

43 Autologous Skin Fillers, 385
Amer H. Nassar, Andrew S. Dorizas, and Neil S. Sadick

44 Polylactic Acid Fillers, 390
Kenneth R. Beer and Jacob Beer

Section 3: Resurfacing Techniques, 395

45 Superficial Chemical Peels, 395
M. Amanda Jacobs and Randall Roenigk

46 Medium Depth Chemical Peels, 402
Gary D. Monheit and Virginia A. Koubek

47 CO_2 Laser Resurfacing: Confluent and Fractionated, 412
Mitchel P. Goldman and Ana Marie Liolios

48 Nonablative Lasers, 429
Adam S. Nabatian and David J. Goldberg

49 Dermabrasion, 437
Christopher B. Harmon and Daniel P. Skinner

Section 4: Skin Modulation Techniques, 445

50 Laser-assisted Hair Removal, 445
Keyvan Nouri, Voraphol Vejjabhinanta, Nidhi Avashia, and Jinda Rojanamatin

51 Radiofrequency Devices, 451
Vic Narurkar

52 LED Photomodulation for Reversal of Photoaging and Reduction of Inflammation, 456
David McDaniel, Robert Weiss, Roy Geronemus, Corinne Granger, and Leila Kanoun-Copy

Section 5: Skin Contouring Techniques, 463

53 Liposuction: Manual, Mechanical, and Laser Assisted, 463
Anne Goldsberry, Emily Tierney, and C. William Hanke

54 Liposuction of the Neck, 476
Kimberly J. Butterwick

55 Hand Recontouring with Calcium Hydroxylapatite, 485
Kenneth L. Edelson

Section 6: Implementation of Cosmetic Dermatology into Therapeutics, 492

56 Anti-aging Regimens, 492
Karen E. Burke

57 Over-the-counter Acne Treatments, 501
Emmy M. Graber and Diane Thiboutot

58 Rosacea Regimens, 509
Joseph Bikowski

59 Eczema Regimens, 517
Zoe D. Draelos

60 Psoriasis Regimens, 522
Laura F. Sandoval, Karen E. Huang, and Steven R. Feldman

Index, 529

Contributors

Eric S. Abrutyn
TPC2 Advisors Inc., Boquete, Chiriqui, Republic of Panama

Murad Alam
Feinberg School of Medicine, Northwestern University, Chicago, IL, USA

K.P. Ananthapadmanabhan
Unilever HPC R&D, Trumbull, CT, USA

Yohini Appa
Johnson & Johnson, New Brunswick, NJ, USA

Nidhi Avashia
Boston University School of Medicine, Boston, MA, USA

Thomas Barlage
Procter & Gamble Company, Sharon Woods Technical Center, Cincinnati, OH, USA

Jacob Beer
Department of Dermatology, University of Pennsylvania, PA, USA

Kenneth R. Beer
General, Surgical and Esthetic Dermatology, West Palm Beach, FL, USA

Joseph Bikowski
Bikowski Skin Care Center, Sewickley, PA, USA

Donald L. Bissett
Procter & Gamble Beauty Science, The Procter & Gamble Co., Sharon Woods Innovation Center, Cincinnati, OH, USA

Frédéric Bonté
LVMH Recherche, Saint Jean de Braye, France

Anne Bouloc
Vichy Laboratoires, Cosmétique Active International, Asnières, France

Ute Breitenbach
Beiersdorf AG, Hamburg, Germany

Harold Bryant
L'Oréal Institute for Ethnic Hair and Skin Research, Chicago, IL, USA

Paul H. Bryson
OPI Products Inc., Los Angeles, CA, USA

Doug Burke
Nu Skin and Pharmanex Global Research and Development, Provo, UT, USA

Karen E. Burke
The Mount Sinai Medical Center, New York, NY, USA

Kimberly J. Butterwick
Cosmetic Laser Dermatology, San Diego, CA, USA

Hervé Cantin
LVMH Recherche, Saint Jean de Braye, France

Ana Paula Avancini Caramori
Department of Dermatology, Complexo Hospitalar Santa Casa de Porto Alegre, Porto Alegre, Brazil

Duane Charbonneau
Procter and Gamble Company, Health Sciences Institute, Mason, OH, USA

David E. Cohen
The Ronald O. Perelman Department of Dermatology, New York University School of Medicine, New York, NY, USA

Joel L. Cohen
AboutSkin Dermatology and DermSurgery, Englewood, and Department of Dermatology, University of Colorado at Denver, Aurora, CO, USA

Kevin Cowley
Gillette Innovation Centre, Reading, UK

Thomas L. Dawson, Jr.
Agency for Science, Technology and Research (A*STAR), Institute for Medical Biology, Singapore

Fatima Dicko
Procter & Gamble Cosmetics, Hunt Valley, MD, USA

Felicia Dixon
L'Oréal Institute for Ethnic Hair and Skin Research, Chicago, IL, USA

Jeff C. Donovan
Division of Dermatology, University of Toronto, Toronto, Canada

Andrew S. Dorizas
Sadick Dermatology, New York, NY, USA

Kenneth L. Edelson
Icahn School of Medicine at Mount Sinai and Private Practice, New York, NY, USA

Angela Ellington
L'Oréal Institute for Ethnic Hair and Skin Research, Chicago, IL, USA

Keith Ertel
Procter & Gamble Co., Cincinnati, OH, USA

Steven R. Feldman
Center for Dermatology Research, Wake Forest University School of Medicine, Winston-Salem, NC, USA

Richard E. Fitzpatrick (deceased)
Department of Dermatology, UCSD School of Medicine, San Diego, CA, USA

Andreas Flohr
Wella/Procter & Gamble Service GmbH, Darmstadt, Germany

Heather Focht
Procter & Gamble Co, Cincinnati, OH, USA

Peter Foltis
L'Oréal Research, Clark, NJ, USA

Scott R. Freeman
Sunrise Dermatology, Mobile, AL, USA

Bryan B. Fuller
DermaMedics LLC, Oklahoma City, OK, USA

Angelike Galdi
L'Oréal Research and Innovation, Clark, NJ, USA

Roy Geronemus
Maryland Laser Skin and Vein Institute, Hunt Valley, MD, and Johns Hopkins University School of Medicine, Baltimore, MD, USA

David J. Goldberg
Mount Sinai School of Medicine, New York, NY, and Skin Laser and Surgery Specialists of New York and New Jersey, USA

Mitchel P. Goldman
Cosmetic Laser Dermatology and Volunteer Clinical Professor of Dermatology at the University of California, San Diego, CA, USA

Anne Goldsberry
Laser and Skin Surgery Center of Indiana, Carmel, IN, USA

Laura J. Goodman
Procter & Gamble Beauty Science, The Procter & Gamble Co., Sharon Woods Innovation Center, Cincinnati, OH, USA

Robert Goodman
Thomas J. Stephens & Associates Inc., Texas Research Center, Carrollton, TX, USA

Emmy M. Graber
Boston University School of Medicine, Boston, MA, USA

Corinne Granger
Director of Instrumental Cosmetics, L'Oreal Research, Asnieres, France

Barbara A. Green
NeoStrata Company, Inc., Princeton, NJ, USA

Susan Griffiths-Brophy
Procter & Gamble Company, Sharon Woods Technical Center, Cincinnati, OH, USA

Sylvie Guichard
L'Oréal Research, Chevilly-Larue, France

Rebat M. Halder
Howard University College of Medicine, Washington, DC, USA

C. William Hanke
Laser and Skin Surgery Center of Indiana, Carmel, IN, USA

Anna Hare
Emory School of Medicine, Atlanta, GA, USA

Christopher B. Harmon
Surgical Dermatology Group, Birmingham, AL, USA

Erik J. Hasenoehrl
Procter & Gamble Company, Ivorydale Technical Center, Cincinnati, OH, USA

Jillian Havey Swary
Feinberg School of Medicine, Northwestern University, Chicago, IL, USA

Stacy Hawkins
Unilever HPC R&D, Trumbull, CT, USA

Catherine Heusèle
LVMH Recherche, Saint Jean de Braye, France

Jasmine C. Hollinger
Howard University College of Medicine, Washington, DC, USA

Maria Hordinsky
Department of Dermatology, University of Minnesota, Minneapolis, MN, USA

Karen E. Huang
Center for Dermatology Research, Wake Forest University School of Medicine; Winston-Salem, NC, USA

M. Amanda Jacobs
Division of Dermatology, Geisinger Health Systems, Danville, PA, USA

J. Daniel Jensen
Scripps Clinic, Bighorn Mohs Surgery and Dermatology Center, La Jolla, CA, USA

Lily I. Jiang
Thomas J. Stephens & Associates Inc., Texas Research Center, Richardson, TX, USA

Anthony W. Johnson
Unilever HPC R&D, Trumbull, CT, USA

Eric S. Johnson
Procter & Gamble Beauty Science, Cincinnati, OH, USA

Leila Kanoun-Copy
L'Oréal Research, Chevilly Larue, France

Gürkan Kaya
Department of Dermatology, Geneva University Hospital, Geneva, Switzerland

Chesahna Kindred
Howard University College of Medicine, Washington, DC, USA

Helen Knaggs
Nu Skin and Pharmanex Global Research and Development, Provo, UT, USA

Robyn Kolas
Procter & Gamble Cosmetics, Hunt Valley, MD, USA

Emily L. Kollmann
Center for Clinical and Cosmetic Research, Aventura, FL, USA

Virginia A. Koubek
Total Skin and Beauty Dermatology Center, PC, and Departments of Dermatology and Ophthalmology, University of Alabama, Birmingham, AL, USA

Alexandra Kowcz
Beiersdorf Inc, Wilton, CT, USA

Thomas Krause
Wella/Procter & Gamble Service GmbH, Darmstadt, Germany

Jan Lephart
Nu Skin and Pharmanex Global Research and Development, Provo, UT, USA

Karl Lintner
KAL'IDEES SAS, Paris, France

Ana Marie Liolios
Private Practice, Fairway, Kansas, MO, USA

Megan Manco
L'Oréal Recherche, Clark, NJ, USA

Stephen Mandy
Volunteer Professor of Dermatology, University of Miami, Miami, FL, and Private Practice, Miami Beach, FL, USA

David McDaniel
McDaniel Institute of Anti Aging Research, Virginia Beach, VA, Eastern Virginia Medical School, Norfolk VA and Old Dominion University Norfolk VA, USA

Gillian McFeat
Gillette Innovation Centre, Reading, UK

Francis McGlone
School of Natural Sciences and Psychology, Liverpool John Moores University, Liverpool, UK

Rahul C. Mehta
SkinMedica, Inc, An Allergan Company, Carlsbad, CA, USA

Kira Minkis
Department of Dermatology, Weill Cornell Medical College, New York, NY, USA

Gary D. Monheit
Total Skin and Beauty Dermatology Center, PC, and Departments of Dermatology and Ophthalmology, University of Alabama, Birmingham, AL, USA

Dominique Moyal
La Roche-Posay Laboratoire Dermatologique, Asnières sur Seine, France

Adam S. Nabatian
Albert Einstein College of Medicine, Bronx, NY, USA

Jin Namkoong
Nu Skin and Pharmanex Global Research and Development, Provo, UT, USA

Vic Narurkar
Bay Area Laser Institute, San Francisco, CA, and University of California Davis Medical School, Sacramento, CA, USA

Amer H. Nassar
Sadick Dermatology, New York, NY, USA

Mark S. Nestor
Center for Clinical and Cosmetic Research, Aventura, FL, USA

Greg Nole
Unilever HPC R&D, Trumbull, CT, USA

Keyvan Nouri
University of Miami Miller School of Medicine, Miami, FL, USA

John E. Oblong
Procter & Gamble Beauty Science, The Procter & Gamble Co., Sharon Woods Innovation Center, Cincinnati, OH, USA

Christian Oresajo
L'Oréal Research, Clark, NJ, USA

Irwin Palefsky
Cosmetech Laboratories, Inc., Fairfield, NJ, USA

Sreekumar Pillai
L'Oréal Research, Clark, NJ, USA

Crystal Porter
L'Oréal Institute for Ethnic Hair and Skin Research, Chicago, IL, USA

Alexandra Price
The Ronald O. Perelman Department of Dermatology, New York University School of Medicine, New York, NY, USA

Sarika Ramachandran
The Ronald O. Perelman Department of Dermatology, New York University School of Medicine, New York, NY, USA

David Reilly
Unilever Research, Colworth Science Park, Sharnbrook, Bedford, UK

Phoebe Rich
Oregon Health and Science University, Portland, OR, USA

Randall Roenigk
Department of Dermatology, Mayo Clinic, Rochester, MN, USA

Jinda Rojanamatin
Institute of Dermatology, Bangkok, Thailand

Véronique Roulier
L'Oréal Research, Chevilly-Larue, France

Rene C. Rust
GSK/Stiefel, Brentford, Middlesex, UK

Neil S. Sadick
Sadick Dermatology, New York, NY and Department of Dermatology, Weill Medical College of Cornell University, New York, NY, USA

Laura F. Sandoval
Center for Dermatology Research, Wake Forest University School of Medicine, Winston-Salem, NC, USA

Jean H. Saurat
Swiss Centre for Applied Human Toxicology, University of Geneva, Geneva, Switzerland

Ulrich Scherdin
Beiersdorf AG, Hamburg, Germany

Harald Schlatter
Procter & Gamble German Innovation Centre, Schwalbach am Taunus, Germany

Andrea M. Schoelermann
Beiersdorf AG, Hamburg, Germany

Douglas Schoon
Schoon Scientific and Regulatory Consulting, Dana Point, CA, USA

Annette Schwan-Jonczyk
Private Practice, Darmstadt, Germany

James R. Schwartz
Procter & Gamble Beauty Science, Cincinnati, OH, USA

Gerhard Sendelbach
Darmstadt, Germany

Surabhi Singh
L'Oréal Research, Clark, NJ, USA

Sunil J. Sirdesai
OPI Products Inc., Los Angeles, CA, USA

Daniel P. Skinner
Surgical Dermatology Group, Birmingham, AL, USA

Olivier Sorg
Swiss Centre for Applied Human Toxicology, University of Geneva, Geneva, Switzerland

Thomas J. Stephens
Thomas J. Stephens & Associates Inc., Texas Research Center, Carrollton, TX, USA

Nicole Swenson
Center for Clinical and Cosmetic Research, Aventura, FL, USA

Diane Thiboutot
Private Practice, Boston, MA, USA

Carl R. Thornfeldt
Episciences, Inc., Boise, ID, USA

Emily Tierney
Department of Dermatology, Tufts University School of Medicine, Boston, MA, USA

Eugene J. Van Scott
Private Practice, Abington, PA, USA

Kristina Vanoosthuyze
Gillette Innovation Centre, Reading, UK

Voraphol Vejjabhinanta
Institute of Dermatology, Bangkok, Thailand

Sarah A. Vickery
Procter & Gamble Cosmetics, Hunt Valley, MD, USA

Teresa M. Weber
Beiersdorf Inc, Wilton, CT, USA

Robert Weiss
Maryland Laser Skin and Vein Institute, Hunt Valley, MD, and Johns Hopkins University School of Medicine, Baltimore, MD, USA

Steve Wood
Nu Skin and Pharmanex Global Research and Development, Provo, UT, USA

Ruey J. Yu
Private Practice, Chalfont, PA, USA

Foreword

Dermatology began as a medical specialty but over the last half century it has evolved to combine medical and surgical aspects of skin care. Mohs skin cancer surgery was the catalyst that propelled dermatology to become a more procedurally based specialty. The combination of an aging population, economic prosperity, and technological breakthroughs has revolutionized cosmetic aspects of dermatology in the past few years. Recent minimally invasive approaches have enhanced our ability to prevent and reverse the signs of photoaging in our patients. Dermatologists have pioneered medications, technologies, and devices in the burgeoning field of cosmetic surgery. Cutaneous lasers, light, and energy sources, the use of botulinum exotoxin, soft tissue augmentation, minimally invasive leg vein treatments, chemical peels, hair transplants, and dilute anesthesia liposuction have all been either developed or improved by dermatologists. Many scientific papers, reviews and textbooks have been published to help disseminate this new knowledge.

Recently it has become abundantly clear that unless photoaging is treated with effective skin care and photoprotection, cosmetic surgical procedures will not have their optimal outcome. Cosmeceuticals are integral to this process but, while some rigorous studies exist, much of the knowledge surrounding cosmeceuticals is hearsay and non-data based marketing information. Given increasing requests by our patients for guidance on the use of cosmeceuticals, understanding this body of information is essential to the practicing dermatologist.

In *Cosmetic Dermatology: Products and Procedures*, Zoe Draelos has compiled a truly comprehensive book that addresses the broad nature of the subspecialty. Unlike prior texts on the subject she has included all the essential topics of skin health. The concept is one that has been long awaited and will be embraced by our dermatologic colleagues and other health care professionals who participate in the diagnosis, and treatment of the skin.

No one is better suited to edit a textbook of this scope than Dr. Zoe Draelos. She is an international authority on Cosmetic Dermatology and she has been instrumental in advancing the field of cosmeceuticals by her extensive research, writing, and teachings. This text brings together experts from industry, manufacturing, research, and dermatology and highlights the best from each of these fields.

Dr. Draelos has divided the book into four different segments. The book opens with *Basic Concepts*, which includes physiology pertinent to cosmetic dermatology, and delivery of cosmetic skin actives. This section is followed by *Hygiene Products*, which include cleansers, moisturizers, and personal care products. The section on *Adornment* includes colored facial products, nail cosmetics, and hair cosmetics. The book concludes with a section on *Anti-aging*, which includes cosmeceuticals, injectable anti-aging techniques, resurfacing techniques, and skin modulation techniques.

You will enjoy dipping into individual chapters or sections depending on your desires, but a full read of the book from start to finish will no doubt enhance your knowledge base and prepare you for the full spectrum of cosmetic dermatology patients.

Enjoy.

Jeffrey S. Dover
August 2009

Addendum

Who better to author and edit a textbook on cosmeceuticals than Zoe Draelos. She is the recognized leader in the field, having done most of the premier studies and written many of the definitive articles on the topic over the last decades.

In her first edition, Dr. Draelos set the standard for comprehensive texts on the subject of cosmeceuticals. With this second edition, she has raised the bar even further, producing a near encyclopedic, comprehensive tome on the subject. It is a treasure trove of information on the subject, without which anyone interested in the topic would be sorely lacking.

Use it as a reference text, dip into chapters or sections from time to time, or if you really want to know this subject, read it from cover to cover.

Enjoy and treasure this work.

Jeffrey S. Dover
Boston, April 2015

Preface

This text is intended to function as a compendium on the field of cosmetic dermatology. Cosmetic dermatology knowledge draws on the insight of the bench researcher, the innovation of the manufacturer, the formulation expertise of the cosmetic chemist, the art of the dermatologic surgeon, and the experience of the clinical dermatologist. These knowledge bases heretofore have been presented in separate textbooks written for specific audiences. This approach to information archival does not provide for the synthesis of knowledge required to advance the science of cosmetic dermatology.

The book begins with a discussion of basic concepts relating to skin physiology. The areas of skin physiology that are relevant to cosmetic dermatology include skin barrier, photoaging, sensitive skin, pigmentation issues, and sensory perceptions. All cosmetic products impact the skin barrier, it is to be hoped in a positive manner, to improve skin health. Failure of the skin to function optimally results in photoaging, sensitive skin, and pigmentation abnormalities. Damage to the skin is ultimately perceived as sensory anomalies. Skin damage can be accelerated by products that induce contact dermatitis. While the dermatologist can assess skin health visually, noninvasive methods are valuable to confirm observations or to detect slight changes in skin health that are imperceptible to the human eye.

An important part of cosmetic dermatology products is the manner in which they are presented to the skin surface. Delivery systems are key to product efficacy and include creams, ointments, aerosols, powders, and nanoparticles. Once delivered to the skin surface, those substances designed to modify the skin must penetrate with aid of penetration enhancers to ensure percutaneous delivery.

The most useful manner to evaluate products used in cosmetic dermatology is by category. The book is organized by product, based on the order in which they are used as part of a daily routine. The first daily activity is cleansing to ensure proper hygiene. A variety of cleansers are available to maintain the biofilm to include bars, liquids, non-foaming, and antibacterial varieties. They can be applied with the hands or with the aid of an implement. Specialized products to cleanse the hair are shampoos, which may be useful in prevention of scalp disease.

Following cleansing, the next step is typically moisturization. There are unique moisturizers for the face, hands, and feet. Extensions of moisturizers that contain other active ingredients include sunscreens. Other products with a unique hygiene purpose include antiperspirants and shaving products. This completes the list of major products used to hygiene and skincare purposes.

The book then turns to colored products for adorning the body. These include colored facial cosmetics, namely facial foundations, lipsticks, and eye cosmetics. It is the artistic use of these cosmetics that can provide camouflaging for skin abnormalities of contour and color. Adornment can also be applied to the nails, in the forms of nail cosmetics and prostheses, and to the hair, in the form of hair dyes, permanent waves, and hair straightening.

From adornment, the book addresses the burgeoning category of cosmeceuticals. Cosmeceuticals can be divided into the broad categories of botanicals, antioxidants, anti-inflammatories, peptides and proteins, cellular growth factors, retinoids, exfoliants, and nutraceuticals. These agents aim to improve the appearance of aging skin through topical applications, but injectable products for rejuvenation are an equally important category in cosmetic dermatology. Injectables can be categorized as neurotoxins and fillers (hyaluronic acid, hydroxyapatite, collagen, and polylactic acid).

Finally, the surgical area of cosmetic dermatology must be addressed in terms of resurfacing techniques, skin modulation techniques, and skin contouring techniques. Resurfacing can be accomplished chemically with superficial and medium depth chemical peels or physically with microdermabrasion and dermabrasion. The newest area of resurfacing involves the use of lasers, both ablative and nonablative. Other rejuvenative devices affecting collagen and pigmentation include intense pulsed light, radiofrequency, and diodes. These techniques can be combined with liposuction of the body and face to recontour the adipose tissue underlying the skin.

The book closes with a discussion of how cosmetic dermatology can be implemented as part of a treatment regimen for aging skin, acne, rosacea, psoriasis, and eczema. In order to allow effective synthesis of the wide range of information included in this text, each chapter has been organized with a template to create a standardized presentation. The chapters open with basic concepts pertinent to each area. From these key points, the authors have developed their information to define the topic, discuss unique attributes, advantages and disadvantages, and indications.

It is my hope that this book will provide a standard textbook for the broad field of cosmetic dermatology. In the past, cosmetic dermatology has been considered a medical and surgical afterthought in dermatology residency programs and continuing medical education sessions. Perhaps this was in part because of the lack of a textbook defining the knowledge base. This is no longer the case. Cosmetic dermatology has become a field unto itself.

Zoe D. Draelos
Durham, NC

PART I
Basic Concepts

SECTION 1: Skin Physiology Pertinent to Cosmetic Dermatology

CHAPTER 1
Epidermal Barrier

Sreekumar Pillai, Megan Manco, and Christian Oresajo
L'Oréal Research, Clark, NJ, USA

> **BASIC CONCEPTS**
> - The outermost structure of the epidermis is the stratum corneum (SC) and it forms the epidermal permeability barrier which prevents the loss of water and electrolytes.
> - Understanding the structure and function of the stratum corneum and the epidermal barrier is vital because it is the key to healthy skin.
> - Novel delivery systems play an increasingly important role in the development of effective skin care products. Delivery technologies such as lipid systems, nanoparticles, microcapsules, polymers and films are being pursued.
> - Cosmetic companies will exploit this new knowledge in developing more efficacious products for strengthening the epidermal barrier and to enhance the functional and aesthetic properties of the skin.

Introduction

Skin is the interface between the body and the environment. There are three major compartments of the skin, the epidermis, dermis and the hypodermis. Epidermis is the outermost structure and it is a multi-layered epithelial tissue divided into several layers. The outermost structure of the epidermis is the stratum corneum (SC) and it forms the epidermal permeability barrier which prevents the loss of water and electrolytes. Other protective/barrier roles for the epidermis include: immune defense, UV protection, and protection from oxidative damage. Changes in the epidermal barrier caused by environmental factors, age or other conditions can alter the appearance as well as the functions of the skin. Understanding the structure and function of the stratum corneum and the epidermal barrier is vital because it is the key to healthy skin and its associated social ramifications.

Structural components of the epidermal barrier

The outer surface of the skin, the epidermis, mostly consists of epidermal cells, known as keratinocytes, that are arranged in several *stratified* layers – the basal cell layer, the spinous cell layer *and* the granular cell layer whose differentiation eventually produces the stratum corneum (SC). Unlike other layers, SC is made of anucleated cells called corneocytes that are derived from keratinocytes. SC forms the major protective barrier of the skin, the epidermal permeability barrier. Figure 1.1 shows the different layers of the epidermis and the components that form the epidermal barrier. SC is a structurally heterogeneous tissue composed of non-nucleated, flat, protein-enriched corneocytes and lipid-enriched intercellular domains [1]. The lipids for barrier function are synthesized in the keratinocytes of the nucleated epidermal layers, stored in the lamellar bodies, and extruded into the intercellular spaces during the transition from the stratum granulosum to the stratum corneum forming a system of continuous membrane bilayers [1,2]. In addition to the lipids, other components such as melanins, proteins of the SC and epidermis, free amino acids and other small molecules also play important roles in the protective barrier of the skin. A list of the different structural as well as functional components of the stratum corneum is shown in Table 1.1.

Corneocytes

Corneocytes are formed by the terminal differentiation of the keratinocytes from the granular layer of the epidermis. The epidermis contains 70% water as do most tissues, yet the SC contains only 15% water. Alongside this change in water content the keratinocyte nuclei and virtually all the subcellular organelles begin to disappear in the granular cell layer

---

Cosmetic Dermatology: Products and Procedures, Second Edition. Edited by Zoe Diana Draelos.
© 2016 John Wiley & Sons, Ltd. Published 2016 by John Wiley & Sons, Ltd.

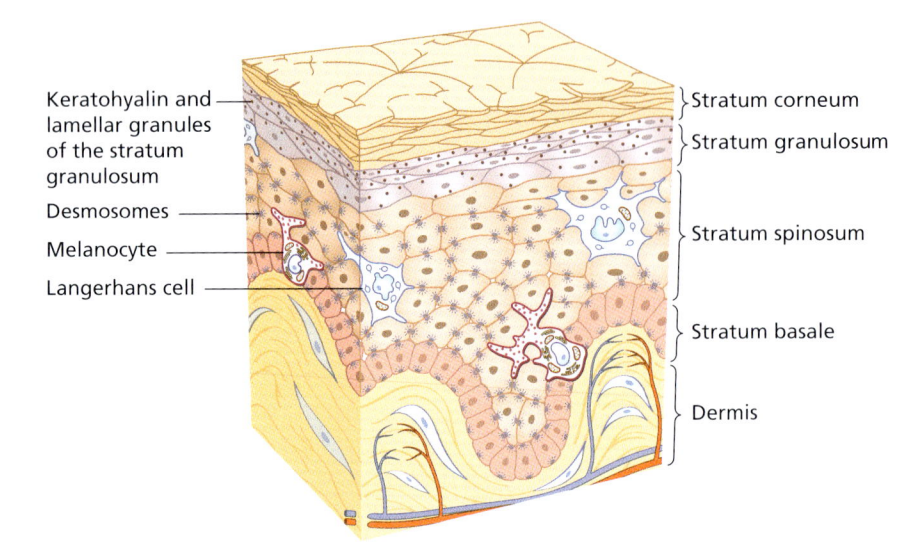

Figure 1.1 Diagram of the epidermis indicating the different layers of the epidermis and other structural components of the epidermal barrier.

leaving a proteinaceous core containing keratins, other structural proteins, free amino acids and amino acid derivatives, and melanin particles that persist throughout the SC. From an oval or polyhedral shape of the viable cells in the spinous layers the keratinocyte starts to flatten off in the granular cell layer and then assumes a spindle shape and finally becomes a flat corneocyte. The corneocyte itself develops a tough chemically resistant protein band at the periphery of the cell, called cornified cell envelope, formed from cross-linked cytoskeletal proteins [3].

Proteins of the cornified envelope

Cornified envelope (CE) contains highly cross-linked proteins formed from special precursor proteins synthesized in the granular cell layer, particularly involucrin, loricrin, and cornifin. In addition to these major protein components, several other minor unique proteins are also cross-linked to the cornified envelope. These include proteins with specific functions such as calcium binding proteins, antimicrobial and immune functional proteins, proteins that provide structural integrity to SC by binding to lipids and desmosomes, and

Table 1.1 Structural and functional components of the stratum corneum

Components	Function	Location
Stratum corneum (SC)	Protection	Topmost layer of epidermis
Cornified envelope (CE)	Resiliency of SC	Outer surface of the SC
Cornified envelope Precursor proteins	Structural proteins that are cross-linked to form CE	Outer surface of the SC
Lamellar granules (LG)	Permeability barrier of skin	Granular cells of epidermis
SC interfacial lipids	Permeability barrier of skin	Lipid bilayers between SC
Lipid-protein cross-links	Scaffold for corneocytes	Between SC and lipid bilayers
Desmosomes and corneodesmosomes	Intercellular adhesion and provide shear resistance	Between keratinocytes and corneocytes
Keratohyalin granules	Formation of keratin "bundles" and NMF precursor proteins	Stratum granulosum
Natural Moisturizing Factor (NMF)	Water holding capacity of SC	Within SC
pH and calcium gradients	Provides differentiation signals and LG secretion signals	All through epidermis
Specialized enzymes (lipases, glycosidases, proteases)	Processing and maturation of SC lipids, desquamation	Within LG and all through epidermis
Melanin granules and "dust"	UV protection of skin	Produced by melanocytes of basal layer, melanin "dust" in SC

protease inhibitors. The cross-linking is promoted by the enzyme transglutaminase that is detectable histochemically in the granular cell layer and lower segments of the stratum corneum. The γ-glutamyl link that results from transglutaminase activity is extremely chemically resistant and this provides the cohesivity and resiliency to the SC.

Lamellar granules and inter-corneocyte lipids
Lamellar granules or bodies (LG or LB) are specialized lipid carrying vesicles formed in suprabasal keratinocytes, destined for delivery of the lipids in the interface between the corneocytes. These lipids form the essential component of the epidermal permeability barrier and provide the "mortar" into which the corneocyte "bricks" are laid for the permeability barrier formation. When the granular keratinocytes mature to the stratum corneum, specific enzymes within the LB process the lipids, releasing the non-polar epidermal permeability barrier lipids, namely, cholesterol, free fatty acids and ceramides, from their polar precursors- phospholipids, glucosyl ceramides, and cholesteryl sulphate, respectively. These enzymes include: lipases, phospholipases, sphingomyelinases, glucosyl ceramidases, and sterol sulphatases [8,9]. The lipids fuse together in the stratum corneum to form a continuous bi layer. It is these lipids along with the corneocytes that constitute the bulk of the water barrier property of the SC [4,21].

Lipid–protein cross-links at the cornified envelope
LG are enriched in a specific lipid unique to the keratinizing epithelia such as the human epidermis. This lipid (a ceramide) has a very long chain omega-hydroxy fatty acid moiety with linoleic acid linked to the omega hydroxyl group in ester form. This lipid is processed within SC to release the omega hydroxy ceramide that gets cross- linked to the amino groups of the cornified envelope proteins. The molecular structure of these components suggests that the glutamine and serine residues of CE envelope proteins such as loricrin and involucrin are covalently linked to the omega hydroxyl ceramides [5,21]. In addition, other free fatty acids (FFA) and ceramides (Cer), may also form protein cross-links on the extracellular side of the CE, providing the scaffold for the corneocytes to the lipid membrane of the SC.

Desmosomes and corneodesmosomes
Desmosomes are specialized cell structures that provide cell-to-cell adhesion (Figure 1.1). They help to resist shearing forces and are present in simple and stratified squamous epithelia as in human epidermis. Desmosomes are molecular complexes of cell adhesion proteins and linking proteins that attach the cell surface adhesion proteins to intracellular keratin cytoskeletal filaments proteins. Some of the specialized proteins present in desmosomes are cadherins, calcium binding proteins, desmogleins and desmocollins. Cross-linking of other additional proteins such as envoplakins and periplakins further stabilizes desmosomes. Corneodesmosomes are remnants of the desmosomal structures that provide the attachment sites between corneocytes and cohesiveness for the corneocytes in the stratum corneum. Corneodesmosomes have to be degraded by specialized proteases and glycosidases, mainly serine proteases, for the skin to shed in a process called desquamation [6].

Keratohyalin granules
Keratohyalin granules are irregularly shaped granules present in the granular cells of the epidermis, thus providing these cells the granular appearance (Figure 1.1). These organelles contains abundant amount of keratins "bundled" together by a variety of other proteins, most important of which is filaggrin (**fil**ament **aggr**egating prote**in**). An important role of this protein, in addition to bundling of the major structural protein, keratin of the epidermis, is to provide the Natural Moisturizing Factor (NMF) for the stratum corneum. Filaggrin contains all the amino acids that are present in the NMF. Filaggrin, under appropriate conditions is dephosphorylated and proteolytically digested during the process when granular cells mature into corneocytes. The amino acids from filaggrin are further converted to the NMF components by enzymatic processing and are retained inside the corneocytes as components of NMF [7,8].

Functions of epidermal barrier

Water evaporation barrier (epidermal permeability barrier)
Perhaps the most studied and the most important function of SC is the formation of the epidermal permeability barrier [1,7,8]. SC limits the transcutaneous movement of water and electrolytes, a function that is essential for terrestrial survival. Lipids, particularly ceramides, cholesterol, and free fatty acids, together form lamellar membranes in the extracellular spaces of the SC that limit the loss of water and electrolytes. Corneocytes are embedded in this lipid-enriched matrix, and the cornified envelope, which surrounds corneocytes, provides a scaffold necessary for the organization of the lamellar membranes. Extensive research, mainly by Peter Elias' group has elucidated the structure, properties and the regulation of the skin barrier by integrated mechanisms [9,11,12]. Barrier disruption triggers a cascade of biochemical processes leading to rapid repair of the epidermal barrier. These steps include increased keratinocyte proliferation and differentiation, increased production of corneocytes and production, processing and secretion of barrier lipids, ultimately leading to the repair of the epidermal permeability barrier. These events are described in more detail in the barrier homeostasis section below. A list of the different functions of human epidermis is shown in Table 1.2.

Table 1.2 Barrier functions of the epidermis

Function	Localization/components involved
Water and electrolyte permeability barrier	SC/corneocyte proteins and extracellular lipids
Mechanical barrier	SC/corneocytes, cornified envelope
Microbial barrier/immune function	SC/lipid components/viable epidermis
Hydration/moisturization	SC/NMF
Protection from environmental toxins/drugs	SC/corneocytes, cornified envelope
Desquamation	SC/epidermis/proteases and glycosidases
UV barrier	SC/melanins of SC/epidermis
Oxidative stress barrier	SC, epidermis/antioxidants

Table 1.3 Antimicrobial components of epidermis and stratum corneum

Component	Class of compound	Localization
Free fatty acids	Lipid	Stratum corneum
Glucosyl ceramides	Lipid	Stratum corneum
Ceramides	Lipid	Stratum corneum
Sphingosine	Lipid	Stratum corneum
Defensins	Peptides	Epidermis
Cathelicidin	Peptides	Epidermis
Psoriasin	Protein	Epidermis
RNAse 7	Nucleic acid	Epidermis
Low pH	Protons	Stratum corneum
"Toll-like" receptors	Protein signaling molecules	Epidermis
Proteases	Proteins	Stratum corneum and epidermis

Mechanical barrier

Cornified envelope provides mechanical strength and rigidity to the epidermis, thereby protecting the host from injury. Specialized protein precursors and their modified amino acid cross-links provide the mechanical strength to the stratum corneum. One such protein, trichohyalin is a multi-functional cross-bridging protein that forms intra and inter protein cross-links between cell envelope structure and cytoplasmic keratin filament network [13]. Special enzymes called transglutaminases, some present exclusively in the epidermis (transglutaminase 3), catalyzes this cross-linking reaction. In addition, adjacent corneocytes are linked by corneodesmosomes, and many of the lipids of the stratum corneum barrier are also chemically cross-linked to the cornified envelope. All these chemical links provide the mechanical strength and rigidity to the SC.

Antimicrobial barrier and immune protection

The epidermal barrier acts as a physical barrier to pathogenic organisms that attempt to penetrate the skin from the outside environment. Secretions such as sebum and sweat and their acid pH provide antimicrobial properties to skin. Microflora that normally inhabit human skin can contribute to the barrier defenses by competing for nutrients and niches that more pathogenic organisms require, by expressing antimicrobial molecules that kill or inhibit the growth of pathogenic microbes and by modulating the inflammatory response [32]. Desquamation that causes the outward movement of corneocytes and their sloughing off at the surface also serves as a built-in mechanism inhibiting pathogens from colonizing the skin. Innate immune function of keratinocytes and other immune cells of the epidermis such as Langerhans cells and phagocytes provide additional immune protection in skin. Epidermis also generates a spectrum of antimicrobial lipids, peptides, nucleic acids, proteases and chemical signals that together forms the antimicrobial barrier (Table 1.3). The antimicrobial peptides are comprised of highly conserved small cysteine rich cationic proteins that are expressed in large amounts in skin. They contain common secondary structures that vary from α helical to β sheets, and their unifying characteristic is the ability to kill microbes or inhibit them from growing. Pathways that generate and regulate the antimicrobial barrier of the skin are closely tied to pathways that modulate the permeability barrier function. Expression of endogenous AMPs coincides with the presence of a number of epidermal structural components that may become part of the permeability barrier. For instance, murine cathelin-related antimicrobial peptide CRAMP and mBD-3 are essential for permeability barrier homeostasis. In addition, acute and chronic skin barrier disruption lead to increased expression of murin β-defensins (mBDs)-1, -3, and -14 and this increase in expression is diminished when the barrier is artificially restored [32].

NMF and skin hydration/moisturization

Natural moisturizing factor (NMF) is a collection of water-soluble compounds that are found in the stratum corneum (Table 1.4). These compounds compose approximately 20–30% of the dry weight of the corneocyte. Many of the components of the NMF are derived from the hydrolysis of filaggrin, a histidine- and glutamine- rich basic protein of the keratohyalin granule. SC hydration level controls the protease that hydrolyze filaggrin and histidase that converts histidine to urocanic acid. As NMF is water soluble and can easily be washed away from SC, the lipid layer surrounding the corneocyte helps seal the corneocyte to prevent loss of NMF.

In addition to preventing water loss from the organism, SC also acts to provide hydration and moisturization to skin. NMF components absorb and hold water allowing the outermost layers of the stratum corneum to stay hydrated despite exposure to the harsh external environment. Glycerol, a major component of the NMF, is an important humectant present in skin that contributes skin hydration. Glycerol is produced

Table 1.4 Approximate composition of skin Natural Moisturizing Factor

Components	% levels
Amino acids and their salts (over a dozen)	30–40
Pyrrolidine carboxylic acid sodium salt (PCA), urocanic acid, ornithine, citruline (derived from filaggrin hydrolysis products)	7–12
Urea	5–7
Glycerol	4–5
Glucosamine, creatinine, ammonia, uric acid	1–2
Cations (sodium, calcium, potassium)	10–11
Anions (phosphates, chlorides)	6–7
Lactate	10–12
Citrate, formate	0.5–1.0

locally within SC by the hydrolysis of triglycerides by lipases, but also taken up into the epidermis from the circulation by specific receptors present in the epidermis called Aquaporins [14]. Other humectants in the NMF include urea, sodium and potassium lactates and PCA [7].

Protection from environmental toxins and topical drugs penetration

The SC also has the important task of preventing toxic substances and topically applied drugs from penetrating the skin. SC acts as a protective wrap due to the highly resilient and cross-linked protein coat of the corneocytes and the lipid enriched intercellular domains. Pharmacologists and topical or "transdermal" drug developers are interested in increasing SC permeation of drugs into the skin. The multiple route(s) of penetration of drugs into the skin can be via hair follicles, interfollicular sites or by penetration through corneocytes and lipid bilayer membranes of the SC. The molecular weight, solubility, and molecular configuration of the toxins and drugs greatly influence the rate of penetration. Different chemical compounds adopt different pathways for skin penetration.

Desquamation and the role of proteolytic enzymes

The process by which individual corneocytes are sloughed off from the top of the SC is called desquamation. Normal desquamation is required to maintain the homeostasis of the epidermis. Corneocyte to corneocyte cohesion is controlled by the intercellular lipids as well as the corneodesmosomes that bind the corneocytes together. The presence of specialized proteolytic enzymes and glycosidases in the SC help in cleavage of desmosomal bonds resulting in release of corneocytes [6]. In addition, SC also contains protease inhibitors that keep these proteases in check and the balance of protease – protease inhibitors play a regulatory role in the control of the desquamatory process. The desquamatory process is also highly regulated by the epidermal barrier function.

The SC contains three families of proteases (serine, cysteine, and aspartate proteases), including the epidermal-specific serine proteases (SP), kallikrein-5 (SC tryptic enzyme, SCTE), and kallikrein 7 (SC chymotryptic enzyme), as well as at least two cysteine proteases, including the SC thiol protease (SCTP), and at least one aspartate protease, cathepsin D. All these proteases play specific roles in the desquamatory process at different layers of the epidermis.

Melanin and UV barrier

Although melanin is not typically considered a functional component of epidermal barrier, its role in the protection of the skin from UV radiation is indisputable. Melanins are formed in specialized dendritic cells called melanocytes in the basal layers of the epidermis. The melanin produced is transferred into keratinocytes in the basal and spinous layers. There are two types of melanin, depending on the composition and the color. The darker eumelanin is most protective to UV than the lighter, high sulphur containing pheomelanin. The keratinocytes carry the melanins through the granular layer and into the SC layer of the epidermis. The melanin "dust" present in the SC is structurally different from the organized melanin granules found in the viable deeper layers of the epidermis. The content and composition of melanins also change in SC depending on sun exposure and skin type of the individual.

Solar ultraviolet radiation is very damaging to proteins, lipids and nucleic acids and cause oxidative damage to these macromolecules. The SC absorbs some ultraviolet energy but it is the melanin particles inside the corneocytes that provide the most protection. Darker skin (higher eumelanin content) is significantly more resistant to the damaging effects of UV on DNA than lighter skin. In addition, UV-induced apoptosis (cell death that results in removal of damaged cells) is significantly greater in darker skin. This combination of decreased DNA damage and more efficient removal of UV-damaged cells play a critical role in the decreased photocarcinogenesis seen in individuals with darker skin [15]. In addition to melanin, trans-urocanic acid (tUCA), a product of histidine deamination produced in the stratum corneum, also acts as an endogenous sunscreen and protects skin from UV damage.

Oxidative stress barrier

The stratum corneum has been recognized as the main cutaneous oxidation target of UV and other atmospheric oxidants such as pollutants and cigarette smoke. Depletion of atmospheric "ozone layer" allows most energetic UV wavelength of sun radiation, i.e. UVC and short UVB to reach earth level. This high energy UV radiation penetrates deep into papillary dermis. UVA radiation in addition to damaging DNA of fibroblasts, also indirectly causes oxidative stress damage of epidermal keratinocytes. The oxidation of lipids and carbonylation of proteins of the SC lead to disruption of epidermal barrier and poor skin condition [16]. In addition to its effects on SC, UV also initiates and activates a complex cascade of biochemical reactions within the epidermis, causing depletion of cellular antioxidants and antioxidant enzymes such as superoxide dismutase (SOD) and catalase. Acute and chronic exposure to UV has been associated with depletion of SOD and catalase in the skin of hairless mice [17]. This lack of antioxidant protection further causes DNA damage, formation of thymine dimers, activation of proinflammatory cytokines and neuroendocrine mediators, leading to inflammation and free radical generation [18]. Skin naturally uses antioxidants to protect itself from photodamage. UV depletes antioxidants from outer stratum corneum. A gradient in the antioxidant levels (alpha-tocopherol, Vitamin C, glutathione and urate) with the lowest concentrations in the outer layers and a steep increase in the deeper layers of the stratum corneum protects the SC from the oxidative stress [19]. Depletion of antioxidant protection leads to UV induced barrier abnormalities. Topical application of antioxidants would support these physiological mechanisms and restore a healthy skin barrier [20,21].

Regulation of barrier homeostasis

Epidermal barrier is constantly challenged by environmental and physiological factors. Since a fully functional epidermal barrier is required for terrestrial life to exist, barrier homeostasis is tightly regulated by a variety of mechanisms.

Desquamation
Integral components of the barrier, corneocytes and the intercellular lipid bilayers are constantly synthesized and secreted by the keratinocytes during the process of terminal differentiation. Continuous renewal process is balanced by desquamation that removes individual corneocytes in a controlled manner by degradation of desmosomal constituent proteins by the stratum corneum proteases. The protease activities are under the control of protease inhibitors that are co-localized with the proteases within the SC. In addition, the activation cascade of the SC proteases is also controlled by the barrier requirement. Lipids and lipid precursors such as cholesterol sulphate also regulate desquamation by controlling the activities of the SC proteases [22].

Corneocyte maturation
Terminal differentiation of keratinocytes to mature corneocytes is controlled by calcium, hormonal factors and by desquamation. High calcium levels in the outer nucleated layers of epidermis stimulate specific protein synthesis and activate the enzymes that induce the formation of corneocytes. Variety of hormones and cytokines control keratinocyte terminal differentiation, thereby regulating barrier formation. Many of the regulators of these hormones are lipids or lipid intermediates that are synthesized by the epidermal keratinocytes for the barrier function, thereby exerting control of barrier homeostasis by affecting the corneocyte maturation. For example, the activators / ligands for the nuclear hormone receptors (example: PPAR – peroxisome proliferation activator receptor and vitamin D receptor) that influence keratinocyte terminal differentiation are endogenous lipids synthesized by the keratinocytes.

Lipid synthesis
Epidermal lipids, the integral components of the permeability barrier, are synthesized and secreted by the keratinocytes in the stratum granulosum after processing and packaging into the LB. Epidermis is a very active site of lipid synthesis under basal conditions and especially under conditions when the barrier is disrupted. Epidermis synthesizes ceramides, cholesterol and free fatty acids (major component of phospholipids and ceramides). These three lipid classes are required in equimolar distribution for proper barrier function. The synthesis, processing and secretion of these lipid classes are under strict control by the permeability barrier requirements. For example, under conditions of barrier disruption, rapid and immediate secretion by already packaged LB occurs as well as transcriptional and translational increases in key enzymes required for new synthesis of these lipids to take place. In addition, as explained in the previous section, many of the hormonal regulators of corneocyte maturation are lipids or lipid intermediates synthesized by the epidermis. Stratum corenum lipid synthesis and lipid content are also altered with various skin conditions such as inflammation and winter xerosis [23,24].

Environmental and physiological factors
Barrier homeostasis is under control of environmental factors such as humidity variations. High humidity (increased SC hydration) downregulates barrier competence (as assessed by barrier recovery after disruption) whereas low humidity enhances barrier homeostasis. Physiological factors can also have influence on barrier function. High stress (chronic as well as acute) increases corticosteroid levels and causes disruption of barrier homeostasis. During periods of psychological stress the cutaneous homeostatic permeability barrier is disturbed, as is the integrity and protective function of the stratum corneum. Many skin diseases, including atopic dermatitis and psoriasis are precipitated or exacerbated by psychological stress [34]. Circadian rhythmicity also applies to skin variables related to skin barrier function. Significant circadian rhythmicity has been observed in transepidermal water loss, skin surface pH, and skin temperature. These observations suggest skin permeability is higher in the evening than in the morning [35]. Conditions that cause skin inflammation can stimulate the secretion of inflammatory cytokines such as interleukins, induce epidermal hyperplasia, cause impaired differentiation and disrupt epidermal barrier functions.

Hormones
Barrier homeostasis/SC integrity, lipid synthesis is all under the control of different hormones, cytokines and calcium. Nuclear Hormone Receptors for both well-known ligands, such as thyroid hormones, retinoic acid, and vitamin D, and "liporeceptors" whose

ligands are endogenous lipids control barrier homeostasis. These liporeceptors include peroxisome proliferator activator receptor (PPAR alpha, beta and gamma) and Liver X receptor (LXR). The activators for these receptors are endogenous lipids and lipid intermediates or metabolites such as certain free fatty acids, leukotrienes, prostanoids and oxygenated sterols. These hormones mediated by their receptors control barrier at the level of epidermal cell maturation (corneocyte formation), transcriptional regulation of terminal differentiation proteins and enzymes required for lipid processing, lipid transport and secretion into LB.

pH and calcium

Outermost stratum corneum pH is maintained in the acidic range, typically in the range of 4.5–5.0 by a variety of different mechanisms. This acidity is maintained by formation of free fatty acids from phospholipids; sodium proton exchangers in the SC and by the conversion of histidine of the NMF to urocanic acid by histidase enzyme in the SC. In addition, lactic acid, a major component of the NMF, plays a major role in maintaining the acid pH of the stratum corneum. Maintenance of an acidic pH in the stratum corneum is important for the integrity/cohesion of the SC as well as the maintenance of the normal skin microflora. The growth of normal skin microflora is supported by acidic pH while a more neutral pH supports pathogenic microbes invasion of the skin.

This acidic pH is optimal for processing of precursor lipids to mature barrier forming lipids and for initiating the desquamatory process. The desquamatory proteases present in the outer stratum corneum such as the thiol proteases and cathepsins are more active in the acidic pH, whereas the SCCE and SCTE present in the lower stratum corneum are more active at the neutral pH. Under conditions when the pH gradient is disrupted, desquamation is decreased resulting in dry scaly skin and disrupted barrier function.

In the normal epidermis, there is a characteristic intra-epidermal calcium gradient, with peak concentrations of calcium in the granular layer and decreasing all the way up to the stratum corneum [10]. The calcium gradient regulates barrier properties by controlling the maturation of the corneocytes, regulating the enzymes that process lipids and by modulating the desquamatory process. Calcium stimulates a variety of processes including the formation and secretion of lamellar bodies, differentiation of keratinocytes, formation of cornified envelope precursor proteins, and cross-linking of these proteins by the calcium inducible enzyme transglutaminase. Specifically, high levels of calcium stimulate the expression of proteins required for keratinocyte differentiation, including key structural proteins of the cornified envelope, such as loricrin, involucrin, and the enzyme, transglutaminase 1, which catalyzes the cross linking of these proteins into a rigid structure.

Coordinated regulation of multiple barrier functions

Co-localization of many of the barrier functions allows regulation of the functions of the epidermal barrier to be co-ordinated. For example, epidermal permeability barrier, antimicrobial barrier, mechanical protective barrier and UV barrier are all co-localized in the stratum corneum. A disruption of one function can lead to multiple barrier disruptions, and therefore, multiple barrier functions are coordinately regulated. Disruption of permeability barrier leads to activation of cytokine cascade (increased levels of primary cytokines, interleukin-1 and tumor necrosis factor-alpha) which in turn activates the synthesis of antimicrobial peptides of the stratum corneum. Additionally, the cytokines and growth factors released during barrier disruption lead to corneocyte maturation thereby strengthening the mechanical and protective barrier of the skin. Hydration of the skin itself controls barrier function by regulating the activities of the desquamatory proteases (high humidity decreases barrier function and stimulates desquamation). In addition, humidity levels control filaggrin hydrolysis that release the free amino acids that form the NMF (histidine, glutamine arginine and their biproducts) and trans-urocanic acid (deamination of histidine) that serves as UV barrier.

Methods for studying barrier structure and function

Physical methods

Stratum corneum integrity/desquamation can be measured using tape stripping methods. Under dry skin conditions, when barrier is compromised, corneocytes do not separate singly but as "clumps". This can be quantified by using special tapes and visualizing the corneocytes removed by light microscopy. Another harsher tape-stripping method involves stripping of SC using cyanoacrylate glue. These physical methods provide a clue to the binding forces that hold the corneocyte together. The efficacy of treatment with skin moisturizers or emollients that improve skin hydration and reduce scaling can be quantitated using these methods.

Instrumental methods

The flux of water vapor through the skin (transepidermal water loss or TEWL) can be determined using an evaporimeter [25]. This instrument contains two water sensors mounted vertically in a chamber one above the other. When placed on the skin in a stable ambient environment the difference in water vapor values between the two sensors is a measure of the flow of water coming from the skin (TEWL). There are several commercially available evaporimeters [e.g., Tewameter® Courage & Khazaka (Köln, Germany)], which are widely used in clinical practice as well as in investigative skin biology. Recovery of epidermal barrier (TEWL) after barrier disruption using physical methods (e.g.: tape strips) or chemical methods (organic solvent washing) provide valuable information on the epidermal barrier properties [26].

Skin hydration can be measured using Corneometer®. The measurement is based on capacitance of a dielectric medium. Any change in the dielectric constant due to skin surface hydration variation alters the capacitance of a precision measuring capacitor. The measurement can detect even slightest changes in the hydration level. Another important recent development in skin capacitance methodology is using SkinChip®. Skin capacitance imaging of skin surface can be obtained using SkinChip. This method provides information regarding skin microrelief, level of stratum corneum hydration and sweat gland activity. SkinChip technology can be used to quantify regional variation in skin, skin changes with age, effects of hydrating formulations, surfactant effects on corneocytes, acne and skin pore characteristics [27].

Several other recently developed methods for measuring epidermal thickness such as confocal microscopy, dermatoechography and dermatoscopy can provide valuable information on skin morphology and barrier abnormalities [28]. Other more sophisticated (although not easily portable) instrumentation techniques such as ultrasound, optical coherence tomography and the Magnetic Resonance Imaging (MRI) can provide useful information on internal structures of SC/epidermis and its improvements with treatment. MRI has been successfully used to evaluate skin hydration and water behavior in aging skin [29].

Biological methods

Ultrastructural details of SC and the intercellular spaces of the SC can be visualized using transmission electron microscopy (TEM) of thin vertical sections and freeze-fracture replicas, field emission scanning electron microscopy and immunofluorescence confocal laser scanning microscopy [30]. The ultrastructural details of the lipid bilayers within the SC can be visualized by EM after fixation using ruthenium tetroxide. The existence of corneodesmosomes in the SC, and their importance in desquamation can be measured by Scanning electron microscopy (SEM) of skin surface replicas.

The constituent cells of the SC, the corneocytes, can be visualized and quantitated by scraping the skin surface or by use of detergent solution. The suspension so obtained can be analyzed by microscopy, biochemical or immunological techniques.

Punch or shaved biopsy techniques can be combined with immunohistochemistry using specific SC/epidermis specific antibodies to quantify the SC quality. Specific antibodies for keratinocyte differentiation specific proteins, desmosomal proteins or specific proteases can provide answers relating to skin barrier properties.

Relevance of skin barrier to cosmetic product development

Topical products that influence barrier functions

The human skin is constantly exposed to hostile environment. These include changes in relative humidity, extremes of temperature, environmental toxins and daily topically applied products. Daily exposure to soaps and other household chemicals can compromise skin barrier properties and cause unhealthy skin conditions. Prolonged exposure to surfactants removes the epidermal barrier lipids and enhances desquamation leading to impaired barrier properties [7,8]. Allergic reactions to topical products can result in allergic or irritant contact dermatitis, resulting in itchy and, scaly skin and skin redness leading to barrier perturbations.

Cosmetics that restore skin barrier properties

Water is the most important plasticizer of SC. Cracking and fissuring of skin develops as SC hydration declines below a critical threshold. Skin moisturization is a property of the outer SC (also known as stratum disjunctum) as corneocytes of the lower SC (stratum compactum) are hydrated by the body fluids. "Moisturizers" are substances that when applied to skin add water and/or retains water in the SC. Moisturizers affect the SC architecture and barrier homeostatsis, that is, topically applied ingredients are not as inert to the skin as one might expect. A number of different mechanisms behind the barrier-influencing effects of moisturizers have been suggested, such as simple deposition of lipid material outside the skin. Ingredients in the moisturizers may also change the lamellar organization and the packing of the lipid matrix and thereby change skin permeability [33]. The NMF components present in the outer SC act as humectants, absorb moisture from the atmosphere and are sensitive to humidity of the atmosphere. The amino acids and their metabolites, along with other inorganic and organic osmolytes such as urea, lactic acid, taurine and glycerol act as humectants within the outer SC. Secretions from sebaceous glands on the surface of the skin also act as emollients and contribute to skin hydration. A lack of either or any of these components can contribute to dry, scaly skin. Topical application of all of the above components can act as humectants, and can relieve dry skin condition and improve skin moisturization and barrier properties. Film forming polysaccharide materials such as hyaluronic acid, binds and retains water and helps to keep skin supple and soft.

In addition to humectants, emollients such as petroleum jelly, hydrocarbon oils and waxes, mineral and silicone oils and paraffin wax provide an occlusive barrier to the skin, preventing excessive moisture loss from the skin surface.

Topically applied barrier compatible lipids also contribute to skin moisturization and improved skin conditions. Chronologically aged skin exhibits delayed recovery rates after defined barrier insults, with decreased epidermal lipid synthesis. Application of a mixture of cholesterol, ceramides, and essential/nonessential free fatty acids (FFAs) in an equimolar ratio was shown to lead to normal barrier recovery, and a 3:1:1:1 ratio of these four ingredients demonstrated accelerated barrier recovery [31].

Topical application of antioxidants and anti-inflammatory agents also protects skin from UV-induced skin damage by providing protection from oxidative damage to skin proteins and lipids [20,21].

Topically applied substances may penetrate deeper into the skin and interfere with the production of barrier lipids and the maturation of corneocytes. Creams may influence the desquamatory proteases and change the thickness of the SC. The increased understanding of the interactions between topically applied substances and epidermal biochemistry will enhance the possibilities to tailor skin care products for various SC abnormalities [33].

Skin irritation from cosmetics

Thousands of ingredients are used by the cosmetic industry. These include pure compounds, mixtures, plant extracts, oils and waxes, surfactants, detergents, preservatives and polymers. Although all the ingredients used by the cosmetic industry are tested for safety, some consumers may still experience reactions to some of them. Most common reactions are irritant contact reactions while allergic contact reactions are less common. Irritant reactions tend to be more rapid and cause mild discomfort and redness and scaling of skin. Allergic reactions can be delayed, more persistent and sometimes severe. Ingredients previously considered safe can be irritating in a different formulation because of increased skin penetration into skin. More than 50% of the general population perceives their skin as sensitive. It is believed that the perception of sensitive skin is at least in part, related to skin barrier function. People with impaired barrier function may experience higher irritation to a particular ingredient due to its increased penetration into deeper layers of the skin.

Summary and future trends

Major advances have been made in the last several decades in understanding the complexity and functions of the stratum corneum. Extensive research by several groups has elucidated the metabolically active role of the SC and have characterized the major components and their importance in providing protection for the organism from the external environment. New insights into the molecular control mechanisms of desquamation, lipid processing, barrier function and antimicrobial protection have been elucidated in the last decade.

Knowledge of other less well known epithelial organelles such as intercellular junctions, tight junctions, and gap junctions and their role in barrier function in the skin is being elucidated. Intermolecular links that connect intercellular lipids with the corneocytes of the SC and their crucial role for maintaining barrier function is an area being actively researched.

New knowledge in the corneocyte envelope structure and the physical state of the intercellular lipid crystallinity and their interrelationship would lead to development of new lipid actives for improving SC moisturization and for treatment of skin barrier disorders. Further research in the cellular signaling events that control the communication between SC and the viable epidermis will shed more light into barrier homeostasis mechanisms.

Novel delivery systems play an increasingly important role in the development of effective skin care products. Delivery technologies such as lipid systems, nanoparticles, microcapsules, polymers and films are being pursued not only as vehicles for delivering cosmetic actives through skin, but also for improving barrier properties of the skin.

Undoubtedly, skin care and cosmetic companies will exploit this new knowledge in developing novel and more efficacious products for strengthening the epidermal barrier and to improve and enhance the functional and aesthetic properties of the human skin.

References

1. Elias PM. (1983) Epidermal lipids, barrier function, and desquamation. *J Invest Dermatol* **80**, 44s–9s.
2. Menon GK, Feingold KR, Elias PM. (1992) Lamellar body secretory response to barrier disruption. *J Invest Dermatol* **98**, 279–89.
3. Downing DT. (1992) Lipid and protein structures in the permeability barrier of mammalian epidermis. *J Lipid Res* **33**, 301–13.
4. Elias PM. (1996) Stratum corneum architecture, metabolic activity and interactivity with subjacent cell layers. *Exp Dermatol* **5**, 191–201.
5. Uchida Y, Holleran WM. (2008) Omega-O-acylceramide, a lipid essential for mammalian survival. *J Dermatol Sci* **51**, 77–87.
6. Harding CR, Watkinson A, Rawlings AV, Scott IR. (2000) Dry skin, moisturization and corneodesmolysis. *Int J Cosmet Sci* **22**, 21–52.
7. Schaefer H, Redelmeier TE, eds. (1996) *Skin Barrier. Principles of Percutaneous Absorption.* Basel: Karger.
8. Rawlings AV, Matts PJ. (2005) Stratum corneum moisturization at the molecular level: an update in relation to the dry skin cycle. *J Invest Dermatol* **124**, 1099–11.
9. Elias PM (2005). Stratum corneum defensive functions: an integrated view. *J Invest Dermatol* **125**, 183–200.
10. Menon GK, Grayson S, Elias PM. (1985) Ionic calcium reservoirs in mammalian epidermis: Ultrastructural localization by ion-capture cytochemistry. *J Invest Dermatol* **84**, 508–512.
11. Elias PM, Menon GK. (1991) Structural and lipid biochemical correlates of the epidermal permeability barrier. *Adv Lipid Res* **24**, 1–26.
12. Elias PM, Feingold KR. (1992) Lipids and the epidermal water barrier: metabolism, regulation, and pathophysiology. *Semin Dermatol* **11**, 176–82.
13. Steinert PM, Parry DA, Marekov LN. (2003) Trichohyalin mechanically strengthens the hair follicle: multiple cross-bridging roles in the inner root sheath. *J Biol Chem* **278**, 41409–19.
14. Choi EH, Man M-Q, Wang F, Zhang X, Brown BE, Feingold KR, Elias PM. (2005) Is endogenous glycerol a determinant of stratum corneum hydration in humans. *J Invest Dermatol* **125**, 288–93.
15. Yamaguchi Y, Takahashi K, Zmudzka BZ, Kornhauser A, Miller SA, Tadokoro T, Berens W, Beer JZ, Hearing VJ. (2006) Human skin responses to UV radiation: pigment in the upper epidermis protects against DNA damage in the lower epidermis and facilitates apoptosis. *FASEB J* **20**, 1486–8.
16. Sander CS, Chang H, Salzmann S, Muller CSL, Ekanayake-Mudiyanselage S, Elsner P, Thiele JJ. (2002) Photoaging is associated with protein oxidation in human skin in vivo **118**, 618–25.
17. Pence BC, Naylor MF. (1990) Effects of single-dose UV radiation on skin SOD, catalase and xanthine oxidase in hairless mice. *J Invest Dermatol* **95**, 213–16.

18 Pillai S, Oresajo C, Hayward J. (2005) UV radiation and skin aging: roles of reactive oxygen species, inflammation and protease activation, and strategies for prevention of inflammation-induced matrix degradation. *Int J Cosmet Sci* **27**, 17–34.

19 Weber SU, Thiele JJ, Cross CE, Packer L. (1999) Vitamin C, uric acid, and glutathione gradients in murine stratum corneum and their susceptibility to ozone exposure. *J Invest Dermatol* **113**, 1128–32.

20 Pinnell SR. (2003) Cutaneous photodamage, oxidative stress, and topical antioxidant protection. *J Am Acad Dermatol* **48**, 1–19.

21 Lopez-Torres M, Thiele JJ, Shindo Y, Han D, Packer L. (1998) Topical application of alpha-tocopherol modulates the antioxidant network and diminishes UV-induced oxidative damage in murine skin. *Br J Dermatol* **138**, 207–15.

22 Madison KC. (2003) Barrier function of the skin: "La Raison d'Etre" of the epidermis. *J Invest Dermatol* **121**, 231–41.

23 Chatenay F, Corcuff P, Saint-Leger D, Leveque JL. (1990) Alterations in the composition of human stratum corneum lipids induced by inflammation. *Photoderamtol Photoimmunol Photomed* **7**, 119–22.

24 Saint-Leger D, Francois AM, Leveque JL, Stoudemayer TJ, Kligman AM, Grove G. (1989) Stratum corneum lipids in skin xerosis. *Dermatologica* **178**, 151–5.

25 Nilsson GE (1977) Measurement of water exchange through the skin. *Med Biol Eng Comput* **15**, 209.

26 Pinnagoda J, Tupker RA. (1995) Measurement of the transepidermal water loss. In: Serup J, Jemec GBE, eds. *Handbook of Non-Invasive Methods and the Skin*. Boca Raton, Fl: CRC Press, pp. 173–8.

27 Leveque JL, Querleux B. (2003) SkinChip, a new tool for investigating the skin surface in vivo. *Skin Research Technol* **9**, 343–7.

28 Corcuff P, Gonnord G, Pierard GE, Leveque JL. (1996) In vivo confocal microsocopy of human skin: a new design for cosmetology and dermatology. *Scanning* **18**, 351–5.

29 Richard S, Querleux B, Bittoun J, Jolivet O, Idy-Peretti I, de Lacharriere O, Leveque JL. (1993) Characterization of skin in vivo by high resolution magnetic resonance imaging: water behavior and age-related effects. *J Invest Dermatol* **100**, 705–709.

30 Corcuff P, Fiat F, Minondo AM. (2001) Ultrastructure of human stratum corneum. *Skin Pharmacol Appl Skin Physiol* **1**, 4–9.

31 Zettersten EM, Ghadially R, Feingold KR, Crumrine D, Elias PM. (1997) Optimal ratios of topical stratum corneum lipids improve barrier recovery in chronologically aged skin. J Am Acad Dermatol **37**, 403–8.

32 Gallo R, Borkowsk, A. (2011) The coordinated response of the physical and antimicrobial peptide barriers of the skin. *J Invest Dermatol* **131**, 285–7.

33 Loden M. (2012) Effect of moisturizers on epidermal barrier function. *Clin Dermatol* **30**, 286–96.

34 Slominski A. (2007) A nervous breakdown in the skin: stress and the epidermal barrier. *J Clin Invest* **11**, 3166–9.

35 Yosipovitch G, Xiong G, Haus E, Sackett-Lundeen L, Ashkenzai I, Maibach H. (1998) Time-dependent variations of the skin barrier function in humans: transepidermal water loss, stratum corneum hydration, skin surface pH, and skin temperature. *J Invest Dermatol* **1**, 20–23.

CHAPTER 2
Photoaging

Kira Minkis,[1] Jillian Havey Swary,[2] and Murad Alam[2]
[1]Weill Cornell Medical College, New York, NY, USA
[2]Feinberg School of Medicine, Northwestern University, Chicago, IL, USA

> **BASIC CONCEPTS**
> - UV radiation damages human skin connective tissue through several interdependent, but distinct, processes.
> - The normal dermal matrix is maintained through signaling transduction pathways, transcription factors, cell surface receptors, and enzymatic reactions.
> - UV radiation produces reactive oxygen species which inhibit procollagen production, degrade collagen, and damage fibroblasts.

Introduction

Skin, the largest human organ, is chronically exposed to UV radiation from the sun. The skin is at the frontline of defense of the human body against the harmful effects of UV exposure. Chronic absorption of UV radiation leads to potential injuries to the skin which includes photoaging, sunburn, immunosuppression, and carcinogenesis. Photoaging, the most common form of skin damage caused by UV exposure, produces damage to connective tissue, melanocytes, and the microvasculture [1]. Recent advances in understanding photoaging in human skin have identified the physical manifestations, histologic characteristics, and molecular mechanisms of UV exposure.

Definition

Photoaging is the leading form of skin damage caused by sun exposure, occurring more frequently than skin cancer. Photoaging describes clinical, histologic, and functional changes that are characteristic of older, chronically sun-exposed skin. Photoaging culminates from a combination of predominantly chronic UV radiation superimposed on intrinsic aging of the skin. Chronic UV exposure results in premature skin aging, termed cutaneous photoaging, which is marked by fine and coarse wrinkling of the skin, dyspigmentation, sallow color, textural changes, loss of elasticity, and premalignant actinic keratoses. Most of these clinical signs are caused by dermal alterations. Pigmentary disorders such as seborrheic keratoses, lentigines, and diffuse hyperpigmentation are characteristic of epidermal changes [2].

These physical characteristics are confirmed histologically by epidermal thinning and disorganization of the dermal connective tissue. Loss of connective tissue, interstitial collagen fibrils, and accumulation of disorganized connective tissue elastin leads to solar elastosis, a condition characteristic of photoaged skin [3]. Similar alterations in the cellular component and the extracellular matrix of the connective tissue of photoaged skin may affect superficial capillaries, causing surface telangiectasias [4].

The significance of photoaging lies in both the cosmetic and medical repercussions, i.e. in the demand for agents that can prevent or reverse the cutaneous signs associated with photoaging and its strong association with cutaneous malignancies.

Physiology

Photoaged versus chronically aged skin

Skin, like all other organs, ages over time. Aging can be defined as intrinsic and extrinsic. Intrinsic aging is a hallmark of human chronologic aging and occurs in both sun-exposed and non-sun-exposed skin. Extrinsic aging, on the contrary, is affected by exposure to environmental factors such as UV radiation. While sun-protected chronically aged skin and photoaged chronically aged skin share common characteristics, many of the physical characteristics of skin that decline with age show an accelerated decline with photoaging [5]. Compared with photodamaged skin, sun-protected skin is characterized by dryness, fine wrinkles, skin atrophy, homogeneous pigmentation, and seborrheic keratoses [6]. Extrinsically aged skin, on the contrary, is characterized by roughness, dryness, fine as well as coarse wrinkles, atrophy, uneven pigmentation, and superficial vascular abnormalities (e.g. telangiectasias) [6]. It is important to note that these attributes are not absolute and can vary according to Fitzpatrick skin type classification and history of sun exposure.

Cosmetic Dermatology: Products and Procedures, Second Edition. Edited by Zoe Diana Draelos.
© 2016 John Wiley & Sons, Ltd. Published 2016 by John Wiley & Sons, Ltd.

While the pathophysiology of photoaged and photo-protected skin differ, the histologic features of these two entities are distinct. In photo-protected skin, a thin epidermis is present with an intact stratum corneum, the dermoepidermal junction and the dermis are flattened, and dermal fibroblasts produce less collagen. In photoaged skin, the thickness of the epidermis can either increase or decrease, corresponding to areas of keratinocyte atypia. The dermoepidermal junction is atrophied in appearance and the basal membrane thickness is increased, reflecting basal keratinocyte damage.

Changes in the dermis of photoaged skin can vary based on the amount of acquired UV damage. Solar elastosis is the most prominent histologic feature of photoaged skin. The quantity of elastin in the dermis decreases in chronically aged skin, but in UV-exposed skin, elastin increases in proportion to the amount of UV exposure [7,8]. Accumulated elastic fibers occupy areas in the dermal compartment previously inhabited by collagen fibers [9]. This altered elastin deposition is manifest clinically as wrinkles and yellow discoloration of the skin.

Another feature of photoaged skin is collagen fibril disorganization. Mature collagen fibers, which constitute the bulk of the skin's connective tissue, are degenerated and replaced by collagen with a basophilic appearance, termed basophilic degeneration. Additional photoaged skin characteristics include an increase in the deposition of glycosaminoglycans and dermal extracellular matrix proteins [10,11]. In fact, the overall cell population in photodamaged skin increases, leading to hyperplastic fibroblast proliferation and infiltration of inflammatory substrates that cause chronic inflammation (heliodermatitis) [12]. Changes in the microvasculature also occur, as is clinically manifested in surface telangiectasias and other vascular abnormalities.

Photobiology

In order to fully understand the molecular mechanisms responsible for photoaging in human skin, an awareness of the UV spectrum is crucial. The UV spectrum is divided into three main components: UVC (270–290 nm), UVB (290–320 nm), and UVA (320–400 nm). While UVC radiation is filtered by ozone and atmospheric moisture, and consequently never reaches the Earth, UVA and UVB rays do reach the terrestrial surface. Although the ratio of UVA to UVB rays is 20:1 [13] and UVB is greatest during the summer months, both forms of radiation have acute and chronic effects on human skin.

Photoaging is the superposition of UVA and UVB radiation on intrinsic aging. In order to exert biologic effects on human skin, both categories of UV rays must be absorbed by chromophores in the skin. Depending on the wavelength absorbed, UV light interacts with different skin cells at different depths (Figure 2.1). More specifically, energy from UVB rays is mostly absorbed by the epidermis and affects epidermal cells such as the keratinocytes, whereas energy from UVA penetrates deeper into the skin, with ~50% of UVA penetrating into the skin in a fair-skinned individual (versus <10% of UVB photons). UVA therefore affects both epidermal keratinocytes and the deeper dermal fibroblasts. The absorbed energy is converted into varying chemical reactions that cause histologic and clinical changes in the skin. UVA absorption by chromophores mostly acts indirectly by transferring energy to oxygen to generate reactive oxygen species (ROS), which subsequently causes several effects such as transcription factor activation, lipid peroxidation, and DNA-strand breaks. On the contrary, UVB has a more direct effect on the absorbing chromophores and causes cross-linking of adjacent DNA pyrimidines and other DNA-related

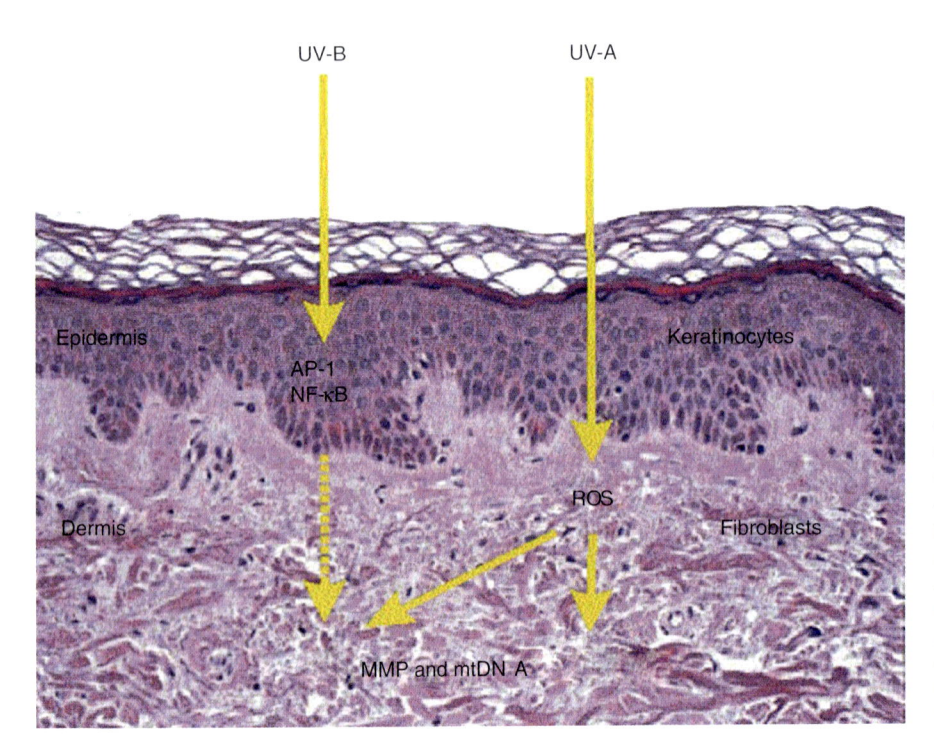

Figure 2.1 Ultraviolet light interacts with different skin cells at different depths. More specifically, energy from UVB rays is mostly absorbed by the epidermis and affects epidermal cells such as the keratinocytes. Energy from UVA rays affects both epidermal keratinocytes and the deeper dermal fibroblasts. AP-1, activator protein 1; NF-κB, nuclear factor κB; MMP, matrix metalloproteinase; mtDNA, mitochondrial DNA; ROS, reactive oxygen species. (Source: Berneburg et al., 2000 [30]. Reproduced with permission of John Wiley & Sons.)

damage [14]. Approximately 50% of UV-induced photodamage is from the formation of free radicals, while mechanisms such as direct cellular injury account for the remainder of UV effects [15]. Thus UVB induced photodamage is implicated as the predominant cause of photoaging. The important role of UVA in photoaging, however, stems from the fact that in distinction to UVB, UVA is also transmitted through glass. This enables exposure indoors, near windows, as well as while driving allowing for significant long-term exposure. Evidence for this includes dramatic unilateral dermatoheliosis as evident in some chronic occupational drivers [16].

Cutaneous microvasculature

Intrinsically aged skin and photodamaged skin share similar cutaneous vasculature characteristics, such as decreased cutaneous temperature, pallor, decreased cutaneous vessel size, reduced erythema, reduced cutaneous nutritional supply, and reduced cutaneous vascular responsiveness [17-19]. However, there are also significant differences in the microvasculature of chronologic sun-protected versus photoaged skin. Studies have reported that the blood vessels in photoaged skin are obliterated and the overall horizontal architecture of the vascular plexuses is disrupted [20]. In contrast to photodamaged skin, intrinsically aged skin does not display a greatly disturbed pattern of horizontal vasculature. Additionally, while cutaneous vessel size has been reported to decrease with age in both scenarios, only photoaged skin exhibits a large reduction in the number of dermal vessels. This reduction is especially highlighted in the upper dermal connective tissue, where it is hypothesized that chronic UV-induced degradation of elastic and collagen fibers is no longer able to provide the physical support required for normal cutaneous vessel maintenance [17].

Furthermore, preliminary studies have reported that the effects of exposure to acute UV radiation differ from chronic exposure. Recent studies have implied that a single exposure to UVB radiation induces skin angiogenesis in human skin *in vivo* [21,22]. The epidermis-derived vascular endothelial growth factor (VEGF) is an angiogenic factor that is significantly upregulated with UV exposure in keratinocytes *in vitro* and in human skin *in vivo*. Chung and Eun [17] have demonstrated, that compared to low VEGF expression in non-UV-irradiated control skin, epidermal VEGF expression increased significantly on days 2 and 3 post-UV-irradiation, consequently inducing cutaneous angiogenesis. Therefore, acute UV exposure has been shown to induce angiogenesis. However, chronic UV-exposed photodamaged skin exhibits a significant reduction in the number of cutaneous blood vessels. The reasons for this discrepancy between the effects of acute and chronic UV exposure on angiogenesis *in vivo* are still under investigation.

Molecular mechanisms of photoaging

Mechanisms of intrinsic aging and extrinsic aging (photoaging) have a significant amount of overlap ultimately culminating in DNA damage as the underlying mechanism. During the last few years substantial progress has been made in exposing the molecular mechanisms accountable for photoaging in human skin. One major theoretical advance that has been elucidated by this work is that UV irradiation damages human skin by at least two interdependent mechanisms:

1. Photochemical generation of ROS; and
2. Activation of cutaneous signal transduction pathways.

These molecular processes and their underlying components are described in detail below. Before these processes are highlighted, however, it is important to consider the structure and function of collagen and its role in maintain the strength and integrity of the skin.

Collagen

Type I collagen accounts for greater than 90% of the protein in the human skin, with type III collagen accounting for a smaller fraction (10%). The unique physical characteristics of collagen fibers are essential for providing strength, structural integrity, and resilience to the skin. Dermal fibroblasts synthesize individual collagen polypeptide chains as precursor molecules called procollagen. These procollagen building blocks are assembled into larger collagen fibers through enzymatic cross-linking and form the three-dimensional dermal network mainly made of collagen types I and III. This intermolecular covalent cross-linking step is essential for maintenance and structural integrity of large collagen fibers, especially type I collagen.

Natural breakdown of type I collagen is a slow process and occurs through enzymatic degradation [23]. Dermal collagen has a half-life of greater than 1 year [23], and this slow rate of type I collagen turnover allows for disorganization and fragmentation of collagen which impair its functions. In fact, fragmentation and dispersion of collagen fibers is a feature of photodamaged skin that is clinically manifest in the changes associated with photodamaged human skin.

The regulation of collagen production is an important mechanism to understand before discussing how this process is impaired. In general, collagen gene expression is regulated by the cytokine, transforming growth factor β (TGF-β), and the transcription factor, activator protein (AP-1), in human skin fibroblasts. When TGF-βs bind to their cell surface receptors (TβRI and TβRII), transcription factors Smad2 and Smad3 are activated, combine with Smad4, and enter the nucleus, where they regulate type I procollagen production. AP-1 has an opposing effect and inhibits collagen gene transcription by either direct suppression of gene transcription or obstructing the Smad complex from binding to the TGF-β target gene (Figure 2.2) [24]. Therefore, in the absence of any inhibiting factors, the TGF-β/Smad signaling pathway results in a net increase in procollagen production.

How does UV irradiation stimulate photoaging?

UV irradiation stimulates photoaging through several molecular mechanisms, discussed in detail below.

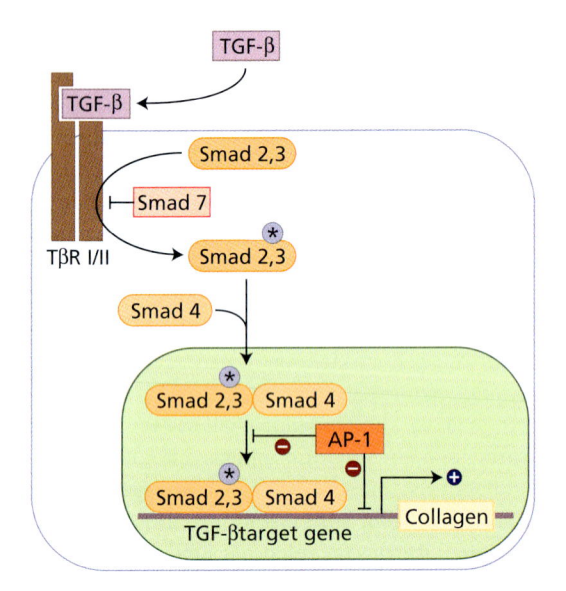

Figure 2.2 The regulation of procollagen production: the TGF-β/Smad signaling pathway. AP-1, activator protein 1; TβR, TGF-β receptor; TGF-β, transforming growth factor β. (Source: Kang et al., 2001 [3]. Reproduced with permission of Elsevier.)

Reactive oxygen species

Approximately 50% of UV-induced photodamage is from the formation of free radicals, while mechanisms such as direct cellular injury account for the remainder of UV effects [15]. Proposed in 1954, the free radical theory of aging suggests that aging is a result of reactions caused by excessive amounts of free radicals, which contain one or more unpaired electrons [25]. Generation of ROS occurs during normal chronologic aging as well as in response to UV light exposure in photoaging [26]. ROS mediate deleterious post-translational effects on aging skin through direct chemical modifications to mitochondrial DNA (mtDNA), cell lipids, deoxyribonucleic acids (DNA), and dermal matrix proteins, including collagens. In fact, a marker of UVA photodamage in human dermal fibroblasts is a 4977 base-pair deletion of mtDNA that is induced by UVA via ROS [27].

The role of ROS in photoaging is not limited to UVA induced photodamage. UVB enhances the levels of NF-κB responsive proteins, such as, inducible nitric oxide synthase (iNOS) and cyclooxygenase-2 (COX-2), and induces the production of nitric oxide (NO). NO is a central player in the regulation of skin cell apoptosis. Furthermore, upon reacting with ROS, NO is transformed into cytotoxic peroxynitrite (ONOO-) which causes lipid peroxidation. Lipid peroxidants are, in part, responsible for the wrinkle formation that is indicative of photoaging [28].

UV radiation inhibits procollagen production: TGF-β/Smad signaling pathway

UV light inhibits procollagen production through two signaling pathways: downregulation of TβRII and inhibition of target gene transcription by AP-1. UV radiation has been reported to disrupt the skin collagen matrix through the TGF-β/Smad pathway [1]. More specifically, UV radiation downregulates the TGF-β type II receptor (TβRII) and results in a 90% reduction of TGF-β cell surface binding, consequently reducing downstream activation of the Smad 2, 3, 4 complex and type I procollagen transcription.

Additionally, UV radiation activates AP-1, which binds factors that are part of the procollagen type I transcriptional complex. This, in turn, reduces TGF-β target gene expression, such as expression of type I procollagen [29].

UV-induced matrix metalloproteinases stimulate collagen degradation

It has been demonstrated that UV irradiation affects the post-translational modification of dermal matrix proteins (through ROS) and also downregulates the transcription of these same proteins (through the TGF-β/Smad signaling pathway). UVA and UVB light also induces a wide variety of matrix metalloproteinases (MMPs) [30]. As their name suggests, MMPs degrade dermal matrix proteins, specifically collagens, through enzymatic activity. UV-induced MMP-1 initiates cleavage of type I and III dermal collagen, followed by further degradation by MMP-3 and MMP-9.

Recall that type I collagen fibrils are stabilized by covalent cross-links. When undergoing degradation by MMPs, collagen molecules can remain cross-linked within the dermal collagen matrix, thereby impairing the structural integrity of the dermis. In the absence of perfect repair mechanisms, MMP-mediated collagen damage can accrue with each UV exposure. This type of collective damage to the dermal matrix collagen is hypothesized to have a direct effect on the physical characteristics of photodamaged skin [14].

In addition to UV induction of MMPs, transcription factors may cause MMP activation. It has been reported that within hours of UV exposure, the transcription factors AP-1 and NF-κB are activated which, in turn, stimulate transcription of MMPs [31].

Fibroblasts regulate their own collagen synthesis

Fibroblasts have evolved to regulate their output of extracellular matrix proteins (including collagen) based on internal mechanical tension [32]. Type I collagen fibrils in the dermis serve as mechanical stabilizers and attachment sites for fibroblasts in sun-protected skin. Surface integrins on the fibroblasts attach to collagen and internal actin–myosin microfilaments provide mechanical resistance by pulling on the intact collagen. In response to this created tension, intracellular scaffolding composed of intermediate filaments and microtubules pushes outward to causing fibroblasts to stretch. This stretch is an essential cue for normal collagen and MMP production by fibroblasts [32].

This mechanical tension model is different in photoaged human skin. Fibroblast–integrin attachments are lost, which prevents collagen fragments from binding to fibroblasts. Collagen–

fibroblast binding is crucial for maintenance of normal mechanical stability. When mechanical tension is reduced, as in photoaged skin, fibroblasts collapse, which causes decreased procollagen production and increased collagenase (COLase) production [32]. Collagen is continually lost as this cycle repeats itself.

Elastosis and cathepsins
One of the histologic hallmarks of photoaging is elastolysis and an accumulation of abnormal elastin in the superficial dermis known as elastosis. One of the most potent enzymes involved in the degradation of elastin is cathepsin K [33]. This enzyme was recently shown to be induced in young fibroblasts in response to UVA irradiation which lead to digestion and clearance of extracellular elastin. This, induction was not seen in fibroblasts from old donors [34]. Thus, cathepsin K appears to play a critical part in clearing MMP-digested elastin in the ECM, a function which is lost with age and leads to the histologic (and corresponding clinical effects) of elastosis [35]. Other studies have also demonstrated the downregulation of cathepsins B, D, and K and upregulation of cathepsin G was seen in photoaged skin and senescent fibroblasts in vitro [36].

UVA induces the aging-associated progerin
Recent data has implicated a protein called progerin as a mechanism of UV induced aging. Patients with Hutchinson–Gilford progeria syndrome (HGPS) have a mutation in LMNA, which encodes an abnormal and truncated form of Lamin A, called progerin [37]. Accumulation of progerin has been shown to result in misshapen nuclei with disrupted nuclear functions, including reduced DNA repair capacity, increased telomere shortening, and increased activation of p53, which ultimately result in a reduced cellular lifespan due to early senescence [38–44].

Progerin has been reported to contribute to aging not only of HPGS cells, but also of normal cells with increasing accumulation of progerin-expressing cells in skin with increasing age [45].

Hirotaka Takeuchi and Thomas M. Rünger recently showed that UVA induced progerin expression in the progerin protein of cultured primary human fibroblasts, specifically in "aged cells," obtained from older donors. These cells had subsequent abnormal nuclear shapes and presumably abnormal nuclear functions, suggesting a novel mechanism by which UV light accelerates aging of the skin [40].

Evolving data
Genetics may also play a role in photoaging. A recent study in France evaluated genetic factors that may affect the severity of skin aging. The authors carried out a genome-wide association study and found a single-nucleotide polymorphism (SNP) that was in significantly associated with global photoaging. This SNP linkage disequilibrium (LD) with two genes which are expressed in the skin, STXBP5L gene and FBXO40 gene, perhaps involved in photoaging [44].

Ethnic skin: photoaging

All races are susceptible to photoaging. However, people with Fitzpatrick skin phototypes IV–VI are less susceptible to the deleterious effects of UV irradiation than people with a lower Fitzpatrick skin type classification. This phenomenon is most likely a result of the protective role of melanin [45]. Studies reporting ethnic skin photoaging are few and far between. However, for the purposes of this discussion, characteristics of photoaging in different ethnic skin categories are briefly highlighted.

In one of the first studies comparing UV absorption amongst different skin types, Kaidbey et al. [46] compared the photoprotective properties of African-American skin with Caucasian skin exposed to UVB irradiation. It was known that only 10% of the total UVB rays penetrated the dermis. However, the mean UVB transmission into the dermis by African-American dermis (5.7%) was found to be significantly less than for Caucasian dermis (29.4%). Similar experiments were performed with UVA irradiation. Although only 50% of the total UVA exposure penetrates into the papillary dermis, UVA transmission into African-American dermis was 17.5% compared to 55% for white epidermis [46]. The physiologic reason behind this difference in black and white skin lies at the site of UV filtration. The malpighian layer (basal cell layer) of African-American skin is the main site of UV filtration, while the stratum corneum absorbs most UV rays in white skin. The malpighian layer of African-American skin removes twice as much UVB radiation as the overlying stratum corneum, thus mitigating the deleterious effects of UV rays in the underlying dermis [47].

In African-Americans, photoaging may not be clinically apparent until the fifth or sixth decade of life and is more common in individuals with a lighter complexion [48]. The features of photoaging in this ethnic skin group manifest as signs of laxity in the malar fat pads sagging toward the nasolabial folds [49]. In patients of Hispanic and European descent, photoaging occurs in the same frequency as Caucasians and clinical signs are primarily wrinkling rather than pigmentary alterations. The skin of East and South-East Asian patients, on the contrary, mainly exhibits pigmentary alterations (seborrheic keratoses, hyperpigmentation, actinic lentigines, sun-induced melasma) and minimal wrinkling as a result of photoaging [50,51]. Finally, very few studies have reported on the signs of photoaging in South Asian (Pakistani, Indian) skin. UV-induced hyperpigmentation, dermatosis papulosa nigra, and seborrheic keratosis are noted [52].

Despite all of these differences, it is important to note that the number of melanocytes per unit area of skin does not vary across ethnicities. Instead, it is the relative amount of melanin packaged into melanocytes that accounts for the physiologic differences between Caucasian skin and ethnic skin [53]. Increasing age leads to senescence of melanocytes. Senescent melanocytes, in turn, can cause greater melanin production that has been observed in some darker-skinned individuals [54]. This may be responsible for the general "bronzing," and darkening, appearing as a "permanent tan" observed in some photoaged individuals of darker skin-tones.

Prevention

Although the effects of the sun's rays appear daunting, there are some ways to avoid the deleterious effects of photoaging. Avoiding photoaging can often prove to be more cost-effective than trying to reverse the signs of photoaging after they have manifested.

Primary prevention
Sun protection

UV rays are especially prevalent during the hours of 10 am–4 pm and sun protection should be encouraged during this time. Sun protection can be offered to patients in the form of sunscreens, sun-protective clothing, and/or sun avoidance. Sun-protective clothing includes any hats, sunglasses, or clothing that would help block the sun's rays. Photoprotective clothing is given a UV protection factor (UPF) rating, which is a measurement of the amount of irradiation that can be transmitted through a specific type of fabric. A UPF of 40–50 is recommended by most dermatologists, as it transmits less than 2.6% of UV irradiation [5].

Traditionally, sunscreens contain one or more chemical filters – those that physically block, reflect, or scatter specific photons of UV irradiation and those that absorb specific UV photons. UVA sunblocks contain the inorganic particulates titanium dioxide or zinc oxide, while UVA-absorbing sunscreens contain terephthalylidene dicamphor sulfonic acid or avobenzene. UVB-absorbing sunscreens can contain salicylates, cinnamates, p-aminobenzoic acid, or a combination of these [55]. The US Food and Drug Administration (FDA) recommended dose of sunscreen application is 2 mg/cm^2 [56].

The sun protection factor (SPF) is an international laboratory measure used to assess the efficacy of sunscreens. The SPF can range from 1 to over 80 and indicates the time that a person can be exposed to UVB rays before getting sunburn with sunscreen application relative to the time a person can be exposed without sunscreen. SPF levels are determined by the minimal amount of UV irradiation that can cause UVB-stimulated erythema and/or pain. The effectiveness of a particular sunscreen depends on several factors, including the initial amount applied, amount reapplied, skin type of the user, amount of sunscreen the skin has absorbed, and the activities of the user (e.g. swimming, sweating).

The sun protection factor is an inadequate determination of skin damage because it does not account for UVA rays. Although UVA rays have an important role in photoaging, their effects are not physically evident as erythema or pain, as are UVB rays. Therefore, it has been suggested that SPF may be an imperfect guide to the ability of a particular sunscreen to shield against photoaging [5]. As a result, combination UVA–UVB sunscreens have been developed and are recommended to protect the human skin from both types of irradiation. Recent changes to labeling of sunscreens in the US require that sunscreens be labeled as broadspectrum if they provide both UVA and UVB protection.

A recent Australian study investigating the effects of daily use of sunscreen (with or without beta-carotene supplementation) found that consistent use of sunscreen had a significant effect on photoaging relative to a matched group of individuals with discretionary sunscreen usage [57]. Thus, individuals should be encouraged to use daily broadspectrum sunscreen in adequate quantity and frequency of application to gain benefit from the photoprotective effects of these agents. The authors saw no effect on aging with β-carotene use, however power was limited.

Secondary prevention
Retinoids

A large number of studies have reported that topical application of 0.025–0.1% all-*trans* retinoic acid (tRA) improves photoaging in human skin [58,59]. Results vary based on treatment duration and applied tRA dose. Retinoids exert their effects by binding to two groups of receptors belonging to the nuclear receptor superfamily: the retinoic acid receptors (RARs) and the retinoid X receptors. Activation of RARs and retinoid X receptors, in turn, results in molecular changes which favor collagen deposition and increasing epidermal thickness. Retinoic acids have been used in an *ex post facto* manner to reverse the signs of photodamage and in a preventative fashion to avoid photoaging.

More specifically, tRA has been shown to induce type I and III procollagen gene expression in photoaged skin [60]. It has been observed that topical tRA induces TGF-β in human skin [61], which stimulates the production of type I and III procollagen.

In addition, tRA has been used in a preventive fashion to avert UV-induced angiogenesis. Kim *et al.* [21] demonstrated that topical application of retinoic acid before UV exposure inhibited UV-induced angiogenesis and increases in blood vessel density. In general, extracellular signal-related kinases (ERKs, or classic MAP kinases) positively regulate epidermally derived VEGF. VEGF stimulates angiogenesis upon UV induction. Retinoic acid inhibits ERKs, which can potentially lead to downregulation of VEGF expression, UV-induced angiogenesis, and angiogenesis-associated photoaging (Figures 2.3 and 2.4) [17].

Finally, tRA has been reported to prevent UV-stimulated MMP expression. The transcription factor, c-Jun, is a key component in forming the AP-1 complex. Recall that the AP-1 complex both inhibits types I and III procollagen and stimulates transcription of MMPs. Retinoic acid blocks the accumulation of c-Jun protein, consequently inhibiting the formation of the AP-1 complex and dermal matrix-associated degradation [62].

Most scientific and clinical evidence in support of topical prescription formulations of retinoids in the treatment of photoaging exist for tretinoin cream (0.02% and 0.05%) and tazarotene cream (0.1%) [63].

These formulations are FDA-approved for the treatment of fine line wrinkles, skin roughness, and mottled hyperpigmentation caused by aging and sun exposure. However, in contrast to clinical signs of photodamage caused by ROS. *In vivo* studies investigating these same antioxidants are ongoing. One such antioxidant, vitamin C, has been shown to mitigate photodamaged keratinocyte formation and erythema post-UV-irradiation [67]. Evidence exists indicating benefit of topical retinols, as well as vitamin C, vitamin B3, and vitamin E in the treatment and prevention of photoaging [68]. Effects of other antioxidants on human skin fibroblasts have also been studied, including green tea antioxidants (green tea polyphenols (GTPs)), caffeine (to a limited degree alone and more so in combination with GTP), and Resveratrol (a phytoalexin, a naturally occurring compound derived from plants). These have been shown to inhibit the generation of free radicals and ROS in human skin fibroblasts *in vitro* [69,70]. However, the effects of antioxidants remains controversial as numerous studies have evaluated the effects of a variety of antioxidants on photoaging with variable effectiveness and *in vitro* studies do not necessarily equate to clinical improvement in randomized controlled clinical trials [71–73].

Inherent defense mechanisms

Although science has developed exogenous mechanisms to prevent and reverse the clinical signs of photoaging, the human skin possesses endogenous machinery built to protect the skin from UV-induced damage. These inherent defense mechanisms include, but are not limited to, increased epidermal thickness, melanin distribution, DNA repair mechanisms and apoptosis of sunburned keratinocytes, MMP tissue inhibitors, and antioxidants [5,46,74-76].

Failure of prevention: immunosuppression

Although photoaging is the most prevalent form of skin damage, local and systemic immunosuppression, leading to skin carcinoma, can result from overexposure to the sun's rays. This immunosuppression is mediated by a combination of DNA damage, epidermal Langerhans' cell depletion, and altered cytokine expression [77,78].

Conclusions

The pathophysiology of photoaging derives from the ability of UV irradiation to exploit established molecular mechanisms which have evolved to maintain the internal milieu of human skin connective tissue. Disruption of the normal skin architecture does not occur through one pathway, but rather is the culmination of several interdependent, but distinct, processes that have gone awry. The integrity of the normal dermal matrix is maintained through signaling transduction pathways, transcription factors, cell surface receptors, and enzymatic reactions that are intertangled and communicate with one another. When UV irradiation is introduced into

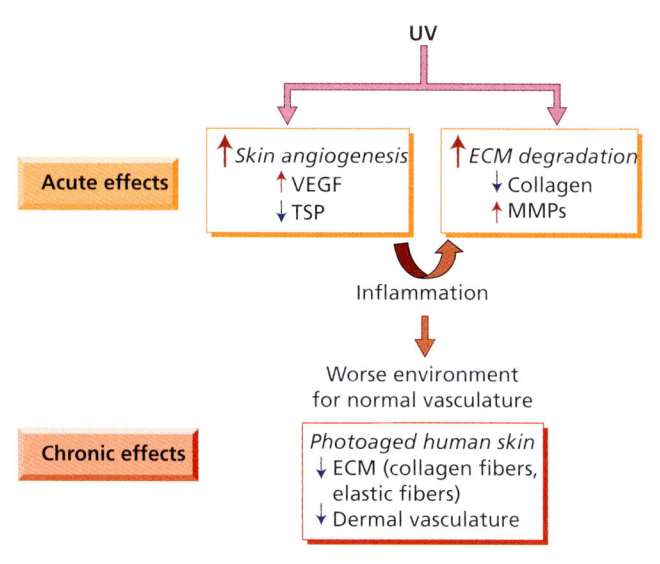

Figure 2.3 Model depicting the acute and chronic effects of UV irradiation on skin angiogenesis and extracellular matrix (ECM) degradation in human skin. MMP, matrix metalloproteinase; TSP, thrombospondin-1 (ECM protein; inhibitor of angiogenesis in epithelial tissues); VEGF, vascular endothelial growth factor. (Source: Chung & Eun, 2007 [17]. Reproduced with permission of John Wiley & Sons.)

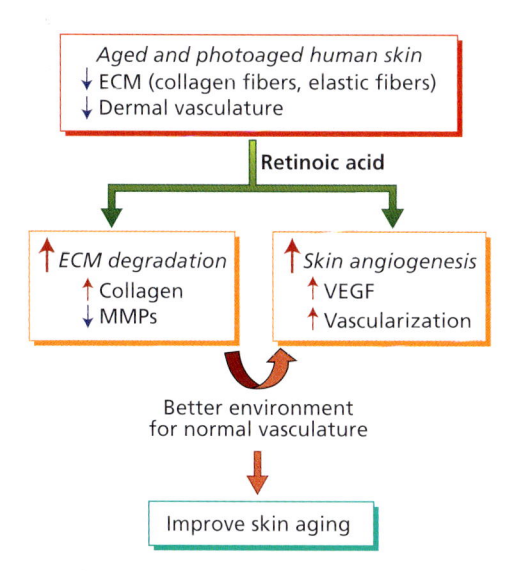

Figure 2.4 Model depicting the effect of topical retinoids on photoaged human skin. ECM, extracellular matrix; MMP, matrix metalloproteinase; VEGF, vascular endothelial growth factor. (Source: Chung and Eun, 2007 [17]. Reproduced with permission of John Wiley & Sons.)

topical retinoids, limited data exists in support of the use of oral retinoids for photoaging [64–66].

Antioxidants

It is important to highlight briefly the role of antioxidants in the reduction of photoaging. *In vitro* studies have discovered a large number of antioxidants that either forestall or reverse the this homeostatic picture, deleterious effects can be implemented. Production of ROS, inhibition of procollagen production, collagen degradation, and fibroblast collapse are only a few known processes amongst the medley of mechanisms still waiting to be discovered that contribute to photoaging. Although human skin is equipped with inherent mechanisms to protect against photoaging and methods of prevention and therapeutics are widely available, these alternatives are not absolute and do not necessarily guarantee a perfect escape from the sun's UV irradiation. Consumer demand for agents capable of preventing or improving the stigmata of photoaging, association of photoaging with malignancies of the skin, as well as incites gained into the process of aging overall provide stimulus to scientists for the continuous study and discover of pathways and molecules involved in extrinsic aging. Novel cutaneous molecular mechanisms affected by UV irradiation are being discovered and consequently, research is underway to discover new solutions to photodamage.

References

1. Quan T, He T, Kang S, Voorhees JJ, Fisher GJ. (2004) Solar ultraviolet irradiation reduces collagen in photoaged human skin by blocking transforming growth factor-beta type II receptor/Smad signaling. *Am J Pathol* **165**, 741–51.
2. Gilchrest B, Rogers G. (1993) Photoaging. In: LimH, SoterN, eds. *Clinical Photomedicine*. New York: Marcel Dekker, pp. 95–111.
3. Kang S, Fisher GJ, Voorhees JJ. (2001) Photoaging: pathogenesis, prevention, and treatment. *Clin Geriatr Med* **17**, 643–59.
4. Weiss RA, Weiss MA, Beasley KL. (2002) Rejuvenation of photoaged skin: 5 years results with intense pulsed light of the face, neck, and chest. *Dermatol Surg* **28**, 1115–9.
5. Rabe JH, Mamelak AJ, McElgunn PJ, Morison WL, Sauder DN. (2006) Photoaging: mechanisms and repair. *J Am Acad Dermatol* **55**, 1–19.
6. Rokhsar CK, Lee S, Fitzpatrick RE. (2005) Review of photorejuvenation: devices, cosmeceuticals, or both? *Dermatol Surg* **31**, 1166–78; discussion 1178.
7. Bernstein E, Brown DB, Urbach F, Forbes D, Del Monaco M, Wu M, et al. (1995) Ultraviolet radiation activates the human elastin promoter in transgenic mice: a novel *in vivo* and *in vitro* model of cutaneous photoaging. *J Invest Dermatol* **105**, 269–73.
8. Lewis KG, Bercovitch L, Dill SW, Robinson-Bostom L. (2004) Acquired disorders of elastic tissue: part I. Increased elastic tissue and solar elastotic syndromes. *J Am Acad Dermatol* **51**, 1–21.
9. El-Domyati M, Attia S, Saleh F, Brown D, Birk DE, Gasparro F, et al. (2002) Intrinsic aging vs photoaging: a comparative histopathological, immunohistochemical, and ultrastructural study of skin. *Exp Dermatol* **11**, 398–405.
10. Mitchell R. (1967) Chronic solar elastosis: a light and electron microscopic study of the dermis. *J Invest Dermatol* **48**, 203–20.
11. Smith JG Jr, Davidson EA, Sams WM Jr, Clark RD. (1962) Alterations in human dermal connective tissue with age and chronic sun damage. *J Invest Dermatol* **39**, 347–50.
12. Lavker R, Kligman A. (1988) Chronic heliodermatitis: a morphologic evaluation of chronic actinic damage with emphasis on the role of mast cells. *J Invest Dermatol* **90**, 325–30.
13. Urbach F. (1992) Ultraviolet A transmission by modern sunscreens: Is there a real risk? *Photodermatol Photoimmunol Photomed* **9**, 237–41.
14. Fisher G, Kang S, Varani J, Bata-Csorgo Z, Wan Y, Datta S, et al. (2002) Mechanisms of photoaging and chronological skin aging. *Arch Dermatol* **138**, 1462–70.
15. Bernstein EF, Brown DB, Schwartz MD, Kaidbey K, Ksenzenko SM. (2004) The polyhydroxy acid gluconolactone protects against ultraviolet radiation in an *in vitro* model of cutaneous photoaging. *Dermatol Surg* **30**, 189–96.
16. Gordon JR, Brieva JC. (2012) Images in clinical medicine. Unilateral dermatoheliosis. *N Engl J Med* **366**(16), e25.
17. Chung JH, Eun HC. (2007) Angiogenesis in skin aging and photoaging. *J Dermatol* **34**, 593–600.
18. Chung JH, Yano K, Lee MK, Youn CS, Seo JY, Kim KH, et al. (2002) Differential effects of photoaging vs intrinsic aging on the vascularization of human skin. *Arch Dermatol* **138**, 1437–42.
19. Kelly RI, Pearse R, Bull RH, Leveque JL, de Riqal J, Mortimer PS. (1995) The effects of aging on the cutaneous microvasculature. *J Am Acad Dermatol* **33**, 749–56.
20. Kligman AM. (1979) Perspectives and problems in cutaneous gerontology. *J Invest Dermatol* **73**, 39–46.
21. Kim MS, Kim YK, Eun HC, Cho KH, Chung JH. (2006) All-*trans* retinoic acid antagonizes UV-induced VEGF production and angiogenesis via the inhibition of ERK activation in human skin keratinocytes. *J Invest Dermatol* **126**, 2697–706.
22. Yano K, Kadova K, Kajiya K, Hong YK, Detmar M. (2005) Ultraviolet B irradiation of human skin induces an angiogenic switch that is mediated by upregulation of vascular endothelial growth factor and by downregulation of thrombospondin-1. *Br J Dermatol* **152**, 115–21.
23. Verzijl N, DeGroot J, Thorpe S. (2000) Effect of collagen turnover on the accumulation of advanced glycation end products. *J Biol Chem* **275**, 39027–31.
24. Massague J. (1998) TGF-β signal transduction. *Annu Rev Biochem* **67**, 753–91.
25. Herman D. (1998) Expanding functional life span. *Exp Geriatr Ontol* **33**, 95–112.
26. Sohal R, Weindruch R. (1996) Oxidative stress, caloric restriction and aging. *Science* **273**, 59–63.
27. Berneburg M, Plettenberg H, Medve-Konig K, Pfahlberg A, Gers-Barlaq H, Gefeler O, et al. (2004) Induction of the photoaging-associated mitochondrial common deletion *in vivo* in normal human skin. *J Invest Dermatol* **122**, 1277–83.
28. Park MH, Park JY, Lee HJ, Kim DH, Chung KW, Park D, et al. (2013) The novel PPAR α/γ dual agonist MHY 966 modulates UVB-induced skin inflammation by inhibiting NF-κB activity. *PLoS One* **8**(10), e76820.
29. Karin M, Liu ZG, Zandi E. (1997) AP-1 function and regulation. *Curr Opin Cell Biol* **9**, 240–6.
30. Berneburg M, Plettenberg H, Krutmann J. (2000) Photoaging of human skin. *Photodermatol Photoimmunol Photomed* **16**, 239–44.
31. Fisher G, Wang ZQ, Datta SC, Varani J, Kang S, Voorhees JJ. (1997) Pathophysiology of premature skin aging induced by ultraviolet light. *N Engl J Med* **337**, 1419–28.

32. Fisher GJ, Varani J, Voorhees JJ. (2008) Looking older: fibroblast collapse and therapeutic implications. *Arch Dermatol* **144**, 666–72.
33. Chapman HA, Riese RJ, Shi GP. (1997) Emerging roles for cysteine proteases in human biology. *Annu Rev Physiol* **59**, 63–88.
34. Codriansky KA, Quintanilla-Dieck MJ, Gan S, Keady M, Bhawan J, Rünger TM. (2009) Intracellular degradation of elastin by cathepsin K in skin fibroblasts – a possible role in photoaging. *Photochem Photobiol* **85**(6), 1356–63.
35. Gilchrest BA. (2013) Photoaging. *J Invest Dermatol* **133**(E1), E2–6. Review.
36. Zheng Y, Lai W, Wan M, Maibach HI. (2011) Expression of cathepsins in human skin photoaging. *Skin Pharmacol Physiol* **24**(1), 10–21.
37. Eriksson M, Brown WT, Gordon LB, Glynn MW, Singer J, Scott L, et al. (2003) Recurrent de novo point mutations in lamin A cause Hutchinson–Gilford progeria syndrome. *Nature* **423**(6937), 293–8.
38. Scaffidi P, Misteli T. Lami. (2006) A-dependent nuclear defects in human aging. *Science.* **312**(5776), 1059–63.
39. Busch A, Kiel T, Heupel WM, Wehnert M, Hübner S. (2009) Nuclear protein import is reduced in cells expressing nuclear envelopathy-causing lamin A mutants. *Exp Cell Res* **315**(14), 2373–85.
40. Decker ML, Chavez E, Vulto I, Lansdorp PM. (2009) Telomere length in Hutchinson–Gilford progeria syndrome. *Mech Ageing Dev* **130**(6):377–83.
41. Musich PR, Zou Y. (2009) Genomic instability and DNA damage responses in progeria arising from defective maturation of prelamin A. *Aging (Albany NY)* **1**(1), 28–37.
42. McClintock D, Ratner D, Lokuge M, Owens DM, Gordon LB, Collins FS, Djabali K. (2007) The mutant form of lamin A that causes Hutchinson–Gilford progeria is a biomarker of cellular aging in human skin. *PLoS One* **2**(12), e1269.
43. Takeuchi H, Rünger TM. (2013) Longwave UV light induces the aging-associated progerin. J Invest Dermatol **133**(7), 1857–62.
44. Le Clerc S, Taing L, Ezzedine K, Latreille J, Delaneau O, Labib T, et al. (2013) A genome wide association study in Caucasian women points out a putative role of the STXBP5L gene in facial photoaging. *J Invest Dermatol* **133**(4), 929–35.
45. Pathak M. (1974) The role of natural photoprotective agents in human skin. In: Fitzpatrick T, Pathak M, eds. *Sunlight and Man.* Toyko: University of Toyko Press.
46. Kaidbey KH, Agin PP, Sayre RM, Kligman AM. (1979) Photoprotection by melanin: a comparison of black and Caucasian skin. *J Am Acad Dermatol* **1**, 249–60.
47. Munavalli GS, Weiss RA, Halder RM. (2005) Photoaging and non-ablative photorejuvenation in ethnic skin. *Dermatol Surg* **31**, 1250–60; discussion 1261.
48. Taylor SC. (2002) Skin of color: biology, structure, function, and implications for dermatologic disease. *J Am Acad Dermatol* **46** (Suppl 2), S41–62.
49. Matory W. (1998) Skin care. In: Matory W, ed. *Ethnic Considerations in Facial Aesthetic Surgery.* Philadelphia: Lippincott-Raven, p. 100.
50. Chung JH, Lee SH, Youn CS, Park BJ, Kim KH, Park KC, et al. (2001) Cutaneous photodamage in Koreans: influence of sex, sun exposure, smoking, and skin color. *Arch Dermatol* **137**, 1043–51.
51. Goh SH. (1990) The treatment of visible signs of senescence: the Asian experience. *Br J Dermatol* **122** (Suppl 35), 105–9.
52. Valia R, ed. (1994) *Textbook and Atlas of Dermatology.* Bombay: Bhalani Publishing House.
53. Szabo G, Gerald AB, Pathak MA, Fitzpatrick TB. (1969) Racial differences in the fate of melanosomes in human epidermis. *Nature* **222**, 1081–2.
54. Bandyopadhyay D, Medrano EE. (2000) Melanin accumulation accelerates melanocyte senescence by a mechanism involving p16INK4a/CDK4/pRB and E2F1. *Ann NY Acad Sci* **908**, 71–84.
55. Seite S, Colige A, Piquemal-Vivenot P, Montastier C, Fourtanier A, Lapiere C, et al. (2000) A full-UV spectrum absorbing daily use cream protects human skin against biological changes occurring in photoaging. *Photodermatol Photoimmunol Photomed* **16**, 147–55.
56. Bowen D. (1998) www.fda.gov/ohrms/dockets/dailys/00/Sep00/090600/c000573_10_Attachment_F.pdf.
57. Hughes MC, Williams GM, Baker P, Green AC. (2013) Sunscreen and prevention of skin aging: a randomized trial. *Ann Intern Med* **158**(11), 781–90.
58. Griffiths CE, Kang S, Ellis CN, Kim KJ, Finkel LJ, Ortiz-Ferrer LC, et al. (1995) Two concentrations of topical tretinoin (retinoic acid) cause similar improvement of photoaging but different degrees of irritation: a double-blind, vehicle-controlled comparison of 0.1% and 0.025% tretinoin creams. *Arch Dermatol* **131**, 1037–44.
59. Kang S, Voorhees JJ. (1998) Photoaging therapy with topical tretinoin: an evidence-based analysis. *J Am Acad Dermatol* **39**, S55–61.
60. Griffiths CE, Russman AN, Majmudar G, Singer RS, Hamilton TA, Voorhees JJ. (1993) Restoration of collagen formation in photodamaged human skin by tretinoin (retinoic acid). *N Engl J Med* **329**, 530–5.
61. Kim HJ, Bogdan NJ, D'Agostaro LJ, Gold LI, Bryce GF. (1992) Effect of topical retinoic acids on the levels of collagen mRNA during the repair of UVB-induced dermal damage in the hairless mouse and the possible role of TGF-beta as a mediator. *J Invest Dermatol* **98**, 359–63.
62. Fisher GJ, Talwar HS, Lin J, Lin P, McPhillips F, Wang Z, et al. (1998) Retinoic acid inhibits induction of c-Jun protein by ultraviolet radiation that occurs subsequent to activation of mitogen-activated protein kinase pathways in human skin in vivo. *J Clin Invest* **101**, 1432–40.
63. Weiss JS, Ellis CN, Headington JT, Tincoff T, Hamilton TA, Voorhees JJ. (1988) Topical tretinoin improves photoaged skin. A double-blind vehicle-controlled study. *JAMA* **259**(4), 527–32.
64. Bagatin E, Parada MO, Miot HA, Hassun KM, Michalany N, Talarico S. (2010) A randomized and controlled trial about the use of oral isotretinoin for photoaging. *Int J Dermatol* **49**(2), 207–14.
65. Hernandez-Perez E, Khawaja HA, Alvarez TY. (2000) Oral isotretinoin as part of the treatment of cutaneous aging. *Dermatol Surg* **26**(7), 649–52.
66. Rabello-Fonseca RM, Azulay DR, Luiz RR, Mandarim-de-Lacerda CA, Cuzzi T, Manela-Azulay M. (2009) Oral isotretinoin in photoaging: clinical and histopathological evidence of efficacy of an off-label indication. *J Eur Acad Dermatol Venereol* **23**(2), 115–23.
67. Lin JY, Selim MA, Shea CR, Grichnik JM, Omar MM, Monteiro-Riviere NA, et al. (2003) UV photoprotection by combination topical antioxidants vitamin C and vitamin E. *J Am Acad Dermatol* **48**, 866–74.
68. Zussman J, Ahdout J, Kim J. (2010) Vitamins and photoaging: do scientific data support their use? *J Am Acad Dermatol* **63**(3), 507–25.
69. Jagdeo J, Brody N. (2011) Complementary antioxidant function of caffeine and green tea polyphenols in normal human skin fibroblasts. *J Drugs Dermatol* **10**(7), 753–61.

70 Jagdeo J, Adams L, Lev-Tov H, Sieminska J, Michl J, Brody N. (2010) Dose-dependent antioxidant function of resveratrol demonstrated via modulation of reactive oxygen species in normal human skin fibroblasts in vitro. *J Drugs Dermatol* **9**(12):1523–6.

71 Janjua R, Munoz C, Gorell E, Rehmus W, Egbert B, Kern D, Chang AL. (2009) A two-year, double-blind, randomized placebo-controlled trial of oral green tea polyphenols on the long-term clinical and histologic appearance of photoaging skin. *Dermatol Surg* **35**(7), 1057–65.

72 Cho S, Lee DH, Won CH, Kim SM, Lee S, Lee MJ, Chung JH. (2010) Differential effects of low-dose and high-dose beta-carotene supplementation on the signs of photoaging and type I procollagen gene expression in human skin in vivo. *Dermatology* **221**(2), 160–71.

73 Zussman J, Ahdout J, Kim J. (2010) Vitamins and photoaging: do scientific data support their use? *J Am Acad Dermatol* **63**(3), 507–25.

74 Huang LC, Clarkin KC, Wahl GM. (1996) Sensitivity and selectivity of the DNA damage sensor responsible for activating p53-dependent G1 arrest. *Proc Natl Acad Sci USA* **93**, 4827–32.

75 Oh JH, Chung AS, Steinbrenner H, Sies H, Brenneisen P. (2004) Thioredoxin secreted upon ultraviolet A irradiation modulates activities of matrix metalloproteinase-2 and tissue inhibitor of metalloproteinase-2 in human dermal fibroblasts. *Arch Biochem Biophys* **423**, 218–26.

76 Soter N. (1995) Sunburn and suntan: immediate manifestations of photodamage. In: Gilchrest B, ed. *Photodamage*. Cambridge, MA: Blackwell Science, pp. 12–25.

77 Vink AA, Moodycliffe AM, Shreedhar V, Ullrich SE, Roza L, Yarosh DB, *et al.* (1997) The inhibition of antigen-presenting activity of dendritic cells resulting from UV irradiation of murine skin is restored by in vitro photorepair of cyclobutane pyrimidine dimers. *Proc Natl Acad Sci USA* **94**, 5255–60.

78 Toews GB, Bergstresser PR, Streilein JW. (1980) Epidermal Langerhans cell density determines whether contact hypersensitivity or unresponsiveness follows skin painting with DNFB. *J Immunol* **124**, 445–53.

CHAPTER 3
Pigmentation and Skin of Color

Jasmine C. Hollinger, Chesahna Kindred, and Rebat M. Halder
Howard University College of Medicine, Washington, DC, USA

> **BASIC CONCEPTS**
> - Differences in the structure, function, and physiology of the hair and skin in individuals of skin of color are important in understanding the structural and physiologic variations that exist and influence disease presentations.
> - Melanin, the major determinant of skin color, absorbs UV light and blocks free radical generation, protecting the skin from sun damage and aging.
> - UV irradiation of keratinocytes induces pigmentation by the upregulation of melanogenic enzymes, DNA damage that induces melanogenesis, increased melanosome transfer to keratinocytes, and increased melanocyte dendricity.
> - Racial differences in hair include the hair type, shape, and bulb.

Introduction

The demographics of the USA reflect a dynamic mixture of people of various ethnic and racial groups. According to the 2010 census, just over one third of the United States population reported their ethnicity and race as something other than non-Hispanic white [1]. Persons of skin of color include Africans, African-Americans, Afro-Caribbeans, Asians, Latinos (Hispanics), Native Americans, Middle Easterners, Alaskan natives, pacific islanders, native Hawaiians and Mediterraneans. The term "black" as in black skin refers to individuals with African ancestry, including Africans, African-Americans, and Afro-Caribbeans. Subgroups exist within each ethnoracial group. The differences in the structure, function, and physiology of the hair and skin in individuals of skin of color are important in understanding the structural and physiologic variations that exist and influence disease presentations. Pigmentation is especially important in patients of skin of color because pigmentary disorder is the most common reason for a visit to a dermatologist in this group [2].

Melanocytes

Melanin, the major determinant of skin color, absorbs UV light and blocks free radical generation, protecting the skin from sun damage and aging. Melanocytes, the cells that produce melanin, synthesize melanin in special organelles, melanosomes. Melanin-filled melanosomes are transferred from one melanocyte to 30–35 adjacent keratinocytes in the basal layer [3]. The number of melanocytes also decreases with age.

There is more than one type of melanin: eumelanin, a dark brown–black pigment; and pheomelanin, a yellow–reddish pigment. Eumelanin is deposited in ellipsoidal melanosomes which contain a fibrillar internal structure. Synthesis of eumelanin increases after UV exposure (tanning). Pheomelanin has a higher sulfur content than eumelanin because of the sulfur-containing amino acid cysteine. Pheomelanin is synthesized in spherical melanosomes and is associated with microvesicles [4]. Although not obvious to the naked eye, most melanin pigments of the hair, skin and, eyes are combinations of eumelanin and pheomelanin [5]. It is generally believed that genetics determine the constitutive levels of pheomelanin and eumelanin. Eumelanin is more important in determining the degree of pigmentation than pheomelanin. Eumelanin, and not pheomelanin, increases with visual pigmentation [5]. Lighter melanocytes have higher pheomelanin content than dark melanocytes. In one study [5], white persons had the least amount of eumelanin, Asian Indians had more, and African-Americans had the highest. Of note, adult melanocytes contain significantly more pheomelanin than cultured neonatal melanocytes.

Melanosomes also differ among different races. In black persons they are mostly in the basal layer, but those of white persons are mostly in the stratum corneum. This is evident in the site of UV filtration: the basal and spinous layers in blacks and the stratum corneum in white persons. Of note, the epidermis of black skin rarely shows atrophied areas [6]. In black skin, melanocytes contain more than 200 melanosomes. The melanosomes are 0.5–0.8 mm in diameter, do not have a limiting membrane, are stuck closely together, and are individually distributed throughout the epidermis. In white skin, the

---

Cosmetic Dermatology: Products and Procedures, Second Edition. Edited by Zoe Diana Draelos.
© 2016 John Wiley & Sons, Ltd. Published 2016 by John Wiley & Sons, Ltd.

melanocytes contain less than 20 melanosomes. The melanosomes are 0.3–0.5 mm in diameter, associated with a limiting membrane, and distributed in clusters with spaces between them. The melanosomes of lighter skin degrade faster than that of dark skin. As a result, there is less melanin content in the upper layers of the stratum corneum. Thus, the melanocytes in black skin are larger, more active in making melanin, and the melanosomes are packaged, distributed, and broken down differently than in white skin.

There is also a difference in melanosomes between individuals within the same race with varying degrees of pigmentation. Despite greater melanin content in darker skins, there is no evidence of major differences in the number of melanocytes [7]. Also, dark Caucasian skin resembles the melanosome distribution observed in black skin [8]. Black persons with dark skin have large, non-aggregated melanosomes and those with lighter skin have a combination of large non-aggregated and smaller aggregated melanosomes [9]. White persons with darker skin have non-aggregated melanosomes when exposed to sunlight and white persons with lighter skin have aggregated melanosomes when not exposed to sunlight [7,8,10]. It has also been shown that the number of melanosomes transferred to keratinocytes is significantly higher in skin of African descent versus white skin [11].

The steps of melanogenesis are as follows. The enzyme tyrosinase hydroxylates tyrosine to dihydroxyphenylalanin (DOPA) and oxidizes DOPA to dopaquinone. Dopaquinone then undergoes one of two pathways. If dopaquinone binds to cysteine, the oxidation of cysteinyldopa produces pheomelanin. In the absence of cysteine, dopaquinone spontaneously converts to dopachrome. Dopachrome is then decarboxylated or tautomerized to eventually yield eumelanin. Melanosomal P-protein is involved in the acidification of the melanosome in melanogenesis [12]. Finally, the tyrosinase activity (not simply the amount of the tyrosinase protein) and cysteine concentration determine the eumelanin–pheomelanin content [5].

Tyrosinase and tyrosinase-related proteins 1 and 2 (TRP-1 and TRP-2) are upregulated when α-melanocyte-stimulating hormone (α-MSH) or adrenocorticotropin binds to melanocortin-1 receptor (MC1R), a transmembrane receptor located on melanocytes [12–15]. The MC1R loss-of-function mutation increases sensitivity to UV-induced DNA damage. Gene expression of tyrosinase is similar between black and white persons despite tyrosinase activity being significantly higher in darker versus lighter skin, but other related genes are expressed differently. The expression of RAB27A, encoding for the melanosome transport molecule, plays an important role in melanocyte melanin content as evident in Griscelli syndrome. In a study by Yoshida-Amano et al., darkly pigmented melanocytes were found to have a substantially higher RAB27A expression and thus able to transfer more to keratinocytes. It was concluded that RAB27A is essential in determining ethnic skin color differences [11]. The MSH cell surface receptor gene for melanosomal P-protein is expressed differently between races. This gene may regulate tyrosinase, TRP-1, and TRP-2 [5].

In addition to the MC1R, protease-activated receptor 2 (PAR-2) is another important receptor that regulates epidermal cells and affect pigmentation [16]. PAR-2 is expressed on many cells and several different organs. Accordingly, the receptor is involved in several physiologic processes, including growth and development, mitogenesis, injury responses, and cutaneous pigmentation. In the skin, PAR-2 is expressed in the keratinocytes of the basal, spinous, and granular layers of the epidermis, endothelial cells, hair follicles, myoepithelial cells of sweat glands, and dermal dendritic-like cells [17,18]. PAR-2 is a seven transmembrane domain G-protein-coupled receptor which undergoes activation via proteolytic cleavage of the NH2 terminus which acts as a tethered ligand which then activates the receptor (autoactivation).

PAR-2 activating protease (PAR-2-AP), endothelial cell-released trypsin, mast cell-released trypsin and chymase, and SLIGKV (Ser-Leu-Ile-Gly-Lys-Val) all irreversibly activate PAR-2 while serine protease inhibitors interfere with the activation of the receptor [19-21]. SLIGKV and trypsin activate PAR-2 to use a Rho-dependent signaling pathway to induce melanosomal phagocytosis by keratinocytes. The result is an increase in pigmentation to the same degree as UV radiation [18-22]. Serine proteases are regulatory proteins involved in tumor growth, inflammation, tissue repair, and apoptosis in various tissues [17]. In the skin, serine protease inhibitors prevent the keratinocytes from phagocytosing melanosomes from the presenting dendritic tip of the melanocyte. This leads to a dose-dependent depigmentation without irritation or adverse events.

PAR-2 also has a proinflammatory effect in the skin [18]. The activation of PAR-2 expressed on endothelial cells by tryptase, trypsin, or PAR-2-AP leads to an increase in proinflammatory cytokines interleukin 6 (IL-6) and IL-8 and also stimulates NF-κB, an intracellular proinflammatory regulator [19]. Mast cells interact with endothelial cells to regulate inflammatory responses, angiogenesis, and wound healing, and PAR-2 has a regulatory role in this cell–cell interaction [18,19].

UV irradiation of keratinocytes induces pigmentation in several ways: upregulation of melanogenic enzymes, DNA damage that induces melanogenesis, increased melanosome transfer to keratinocytes and increased melanocyte dendricity. UV radiation (UVR) increases the secretion of proteases by keratinocytes in a dose-dependent manner. Specifically, UVR directly increases the expression of PAR-2 de novo, upregulates proteases that activate PAR-2, and activates dermal mast cell degranulation [22].

According to the literature, PAR-2 expression is different in skin of color compared to white skin thus, suggesting the involvement of PAR-2 in ethnic skin color phenotypes. One study demonstrated that PAR-2 and its activator trypsin are expressed in higher levels in darker skin. PAR-2 was also found to have higher cleavage ability in highly pigmented skin [23].

Another study did find differences in skin phototypes I, II, and III [22]. UVR increases the expression of PAR-2 in the skin and activated PAR-2 stimulates pigmentation. This study found that the response of PAR-2 to UVR is an important determinant of one's ability to tan. In the non-irradiated skin, PAR-2 expression was confined to the basal layer and just above the basal layer. Irradiated skin showed de novo PAR-2 expression in the entire epidermis or upper two-thirds of the epidermis. Skin phenotype I had a delayed upregulation of PAR-2 expression compared to phenotypes II and III.

Dyspigmentation

After cutaneous trauma or inflammation, melanocytes can react with normal, increased, or decreased melanin production; all of which are normal biologic responses. Increased and decreased production results in postinflammatory hyperpigmentation or hypopigmentation. Postinflammatory hyperpigmentation (PIH) is an increase in melanin production and/or an abnormal distribution of melanin resulting from inflammatory cutaneous disorders or irritation from topical medications [24,25]. Examples include acne, allergic contact dermatitis, lichen planus, bullous pemphigoid, herpes zoster, and treatment with topical retinoids. Often, the PIH resulting from acne is more distressing to darker skinned individuals than the initial acute lesion. The color of the hyperpigmentation in PIH depends on the location of the melanin. Melanin in the epidermis appears brown, while melanin in the dermis appears blue–gray. Wood's lamp examination distinguishes the location of the melanin: the epidermal component is enhanced and the dermal component becomes unapparent [25]. Postinflammatory hypopigmentation shares the same triggers as PIH but instead results from decreased melanin production with clinically apparent light areas [24]. The Wood's lamp examination does not accentuate hypopigmentation in postinflammatory hypopigmentation; it is useful for depigmented disorders such as vitiligo and piebaldism.

The pathogenesis of PIH and postinflammatory hypopigmentation are unknown. It is likely that an inflammatory process in the skin stimulates keratinocytes, melanocytes, and inflammatory cells to release cytokines and inflammatory mediators that lead to the hyperpigmentation or hypopigmentation. The cytokines and inflammatory mediators include leukotriene (LT), prostaglandins (PG), and thromboxane (TXB) [26]. Specifically for PIH, *in vitro* studies revealed that LT-C4, LT-D4, PG-E2, and TXB-2 stimulate human melanocyte enlargement and dendrocyte proliferation. LT-C4 also increases tyrosinase activity and mitogenic activity of melanocytes. Transforming growth factor-α and LT-C4 stimulate movement of melanocytes. In postinflammatory hypopigmentation, the pathogenesis likely involves inflammatory mediators inducing melanocyte cell-surface expression of intercellular adhesion molecule 1 (ICAM-1) which may lead to leukocyte–melanocyte attachments that inadvertently destroy melanocytes. These inflammatory mediators include interferon-gamma, tumor necrosis factor α (TNF-α), TNF-β, IL-6, and IL-7.

Natural sun protective factor in skin of color

It is clear that those who fall within Fitzpatrick skin phototypes IV–VI are less susceptible to photoaging; this is most likely due to the photoprotective role of melanin [27,28]. The epidermis of black skin has a protective factor (PF) for UVB of 13.4 and that of white skin is 3.4 [29]. The mean UVB transmission by black epidermis is 5.7% compared to 29.4% for white epidermis. The PF for UVA in black epidermis is 5.7 and in white epidermis is 1.8 [29]. The mean UVA transmission by black epidermis is 17.5% and 55.5% for white epidermis. Hence, 3–4 times more UVA reaches the upper dermis of white persons than that of black persons.

The main site of UV filtration in white skin is the stratum corneum, whereas in black skin it is the basal layer [29]. The malphigian layer of black skin removes twice as much UVB radiation as the stratum corneum [30]. It is possible that even greater removal of UVA occurs in black skin basal layers [30]. While the above characteristics of natural sun protective factor were studied in black skin, they can probably be extrapolated to most persons of skin phototypes IV–VI.

Skin of color

Epidermis

The epidermal layer of skin is made up of five different layers: stratum basale, stratum spinosum, stratum granulosum, stratum lucidum, and stratum corneum. The stratum basale (also termed the basal layer) is the germinative layer of the epidermis. The time required for a cell to transition from the basal layer through the other epidermal layers to the stratum corneum is 24–40 days. The morphology and structure of the epidermis is very similar among different races, although a few differences do exist.

Stratum corneum

The stratum corneum, the most superficial layer, is the layer responsible for preventing water loss and providing mechanical protection. The cells of the stratum corneum, the corneocytes, are flat cells measuring 50 μm across and 1 μm thick. The corneocytes are arranged in layers; the number of layers varies with anatomic site and race. There are no differences between races in corneocyte surface area, which has a mean size of 900 μm [2,31]. The stratum corneum of black skin is more compact than that of white skin. While the mean thickness of the stratum corneum is the same in black and white skin, black skin contains 20 cell layers while white skin contains 16. The answer to whether or not there are racial differences in spontaneous desquamation is inconclusive [30–32]. It was observed in a study by Wesley *et al.* [32] that blacks have a 2.5 times greater spontaneous desquamation compared with whites and Asians [33]. Parameters for skin barrier function (stratum corneum hydration, sebum secretion, erythema, and laser Doppler flowmetry) are similar, even after an objective epicutaneous test with sodium lauryl sulfate [34].

Transepidermal water loss

Transepidermal water loss (TEWL) is the amount of water vapor loss from the skin, excluding sweat. TEWL increases with the temperature of the skin. Concrete evidence regarding the difference in TEWL between different races has yet to be established. In most studies, TEWL has been found to be greater in black skin compared to white skin but the opposite has also been reported. A study reported no difference in TEWL amongst blacks, whites, and Hispanics [33]. Aside from TEWL, hydration is also a characteristic of skin. One of the ways to measure hydration, or water content, is conductance. Conductance, the opposite of resistance, is increased in hydrated skin because hydrated skin is more sensitive to the electrical field [35]. Skin conductance is higher in black persons and Hispanics than white persons [35]. Lipid content in black skin is higher than that of white skin [36]. However, black skin is more prone to dryness, suggesting that a difference in lipid content has a role. This includes the ratio of ceramide : cholesterol : fatty acids, the type of ceramides, and the type of sphingosine backbone. The total levels of ceramides was approximately 50% lower in the stratum corneum of blacks when compared to whites and Hispanics according to a study [37]. One study suggests that the degree of pigmentation influences lipid differences [39].

Pigmentation affects skin dryness. Skin dryness is greater on sun-exposed (dorsal arm) sites for lighter skin, such as Caucasian and Chinese skin, than sites that are primarily out of the sun (ventral arm) [40]. There is no difference in skin dryness between sites for darker skin, such as African-Americans and Mexicans. For adults less than 51 years of age, skin dryness does not change as a function of ethnicity (African-American, Caucasian, Chinese, and Mexican) for sun-exposed sites and sites that are not primarily sun-exposed. For those 51 years of age and older, skin dryness is higher for African-Americans and Caucasians than for Chinese and Mexicans. As a function of age, skin dryness in African-American skin increases 4% on the dorsal site and 3% on the ventral site; in Caucasian skin, it increases 11% on the dorsal site and 10% on the ventral site. All of the above findings suggest that sun exposure can dry the skin and that melanin provides protection.

Skin reactivity
Mast cells

Sueki *et al.* [41] studied the mast cells of four African-American men and four white men (mean age 29 years) by evaluating punch biopsies of the buttocks with electron microscopy, with the following results. The mast cells of black skin contained larger granules (the authors attributed this to the fusion of granules). Black skin also had 15% more parallel-linear striations and 30% less curved lamellae in mast cells. Tryptase reactivity was localized preferentially over the parallel-linear striations and partially over the dark amorphous subregions within granules of mast cells from black skin, whereas it was confined to the peripheral area of granules, including curved lamellae, in white skin. Cathepsin G reactivity was more intense over the electron-dense amorphous areas in both groups, while parallel-linear striations in black skin and curved lamellae in white skin were negative.

Patch test antigens
Contact dermatits

Irritant contact dermatitis (ICD) is the most common form of dermatitis and loosely defined as non-specific damage to the skin after exposure to an irritant. The various clinical manifestations are influenced by the concentration of chemicals, duration of exposure, temperature, humidity, and anatomic location, and other factors. Acute contact dermatitis presents with the classic findings of localized superficial erythema, edema, and chemosis. Cumulative contact dermatitis presents with similar findings, but with repeated exposure of a less potent irritant [42].

The susceptibility to ICD differs between black and white skin [43]. The structural differences in stratum corneum of black skin (e.g. compact stratum corneum, low ceramide levels) are credited with decreasing the susceptibility to irritants. Reflectance confocal microscopy (RCM) is an imaging tool that permits real-time qualitative and quantitative study of human skin; when used with a near-infrared laser beam, one can create "virtual sections" of live tissue with high resolution, almost comparable with routine histology. Measuring skin reactivity to chemical irritants with RCM and TEWL reveal that white skin had more severe clinical reactions than black skin. The pigmentation in darker skin can make the assessment of erythema difficult and interfere with identification of subclinical degrees of irritancy. Even without clinical evidence of irritation, RCM and histology reveal parakeratosis, spongiosis, perivascular inflammatory infiltrate, and microvesicle formation. Mean TEWL after exposure to irritants is greater for white skin than for black skin. This supports the concept that the stratum corneum of black skin enhances barrier function and resistance to irritants.

There are no differences between white persons and African-Americans in objective and subjective parameters of skin such as dryness, inflammation, overall irritation, burning, stinging, and itching [44]. Acute contact dermatitis with exudation, vesiculation, or frank bullae formation is a more common reaction in white skin whereas dyspigmentation and lichenification is more common in black skin [45].

The response to irritation in Caucasian and African-American skin differs in the degree of severity. Caucasian skin has a lower threshold for cutaneous irritation than African-American skin [46]. Caucasian skin also has more severe stratum corneum disruption, parakeratosis, and detached corneocytes. Both groups have the same degree of intra-epidermal spongiosis epidermal (granular and spinous layer) vesicle formation. The variability in human skin irritation responses sometimes creates difficulty in assessing the differences in skin reactivity between human subpopulations. There are conflicting results in studies comparing the sensitivity to irritants in Asian skin with that in Caucasian skin [34,47–50].

Dermis

The dermis lies deep to the epidermis and is divided into two layers: the papillary and reticular dermis. The papillary dermis is tightly connected to the epidermis via the basement membrane at the dermoepidermal junction. The papillary dermis extends into the epidermis with finger-like projections, hence the name "papillary". The reticular dermis is a relatively avascular, dense, collagenous structure that also contains elastic tissue and glycosaminoglycans. The dermis is made up of collagen fibers, elastic fibers, and an interfibrillar gel of glycosaminoglycans, salt, and water. Collagen makes up 77% of the fat-free dry weight of skin and provides tensile strength. Collagen types I, II, V, and VI are found in the dermis. The elastic fiber network is interwoven between the collagen bundles.

There are differences between the dermis of white and black skin. The dermis of white skin is thinner and less compact than that of black skin [51]. In white skin, the papillary and reticular layers of the dermis are more distinct, contain larger collagen fiber bundles, and the fiber fragments are sparse. The dermis of black skin contains closely stacked, smaller collagen fiber bundles with a surrounding ground substance. The fiber fragments are more prominent in black skin than in white skin. One study showed on histological examinations that African skin type had greater convoluted appearance of the dermal epidermal junction (DEJ) than the Caucasian skin type. This same study also revealed on immunostaining that laminin 332, type IV and VII collagens, and nidogen proteins at the DEJ were lower in African skin compared with Caucasian skin [52]. While the quantity is similar in both black and white skin, the size of melanophages is larger in black skin. Also, the number of fibroblasts and lymphatic vessels are greater in black skin. The fibroblasts are larger, have more biosynthetic organelles, and are more multinucleated in black skin [6]. The lymphatic vessels are dilated and empty with surrounding elastic fibers [51]. No racial differences in the epidermal nerve fiber network have been observed using laser-scanning confocal microscopy, suggesting that there is no difference in sensory perception between races, as suggested by capsaicin response to C-fiber activation [53].

Skin extensibility is how stretchable the skin is. Elastic recovery is the time required for the skin to return to its original state after releasing the stretched skin. Skin elasticity is elastic recovery divided by extensibility. Studies that investigated skin extensibility, elastic recovery, and skin elasticity between races yield conflicting results [32,54]. It is likely that elastic recovery and extensibility vary by anatomic site, race, and age.

Intrinsic skin aging in ethnic skin

The majority of literature regarding facial aging features Caucasian patients. Facial aging is result of the combination of photodamage, fat atrophy, gravitational soft tissue redistribution, and bone remodeling. Figure 3.1 demonstrates the morphologic changes of the face caused by aging. The onset of morphologic aging appears in the upper face during the thirties and gradually progresses to the lower face and neck over the next several decades [55].

Early signs of facial aging occur in the periorbital region. In the late thirties, brow ptosis, upper eyelid skin laxity, and descent of the lateral portion of the eyebrow ("hooding") lead to excess skin of the upper eyelids. During the mid-forties, "bags" under the eyes result from weakening of the inferior orbital septum and prolapse of the underlying intraorbital fat. Lower eyelid fat prolapse may occur as early as the second decade in those with a familial predisposition. Photodamage produces periocular and brow rhytides [55]. The periorbital and midface regions in skin of color tend to have more pronounced signs of facial aging as compared with the upper third of the face. There is also a decreased tendency toward perioral rhytides and radial lip lines in skin of color [56].

Brow ptosis in African-Americans appears to occur to a lesser degree and in the forties opposed to the thirties compared to that in whites [57]. Prolapse of the lacrimal gland may masquerade as lateral upper eyelid fullness in African-Americans [58]. For Hispanics, the brow facial soft tissues sag at an earlier age [59]. In Asians, the descent of thick juxtabrow tissues in the lateral orbit coupled with the absences of a supratarsal fold may create a prematurely tired eye [55].

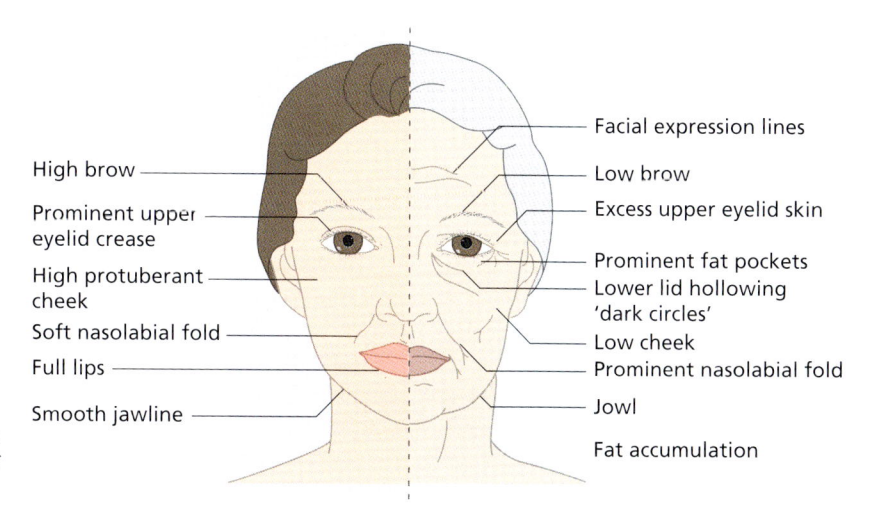

Figure 3.1 Morphologic signs of aging. (Source: Halder, 2006 [55]. Adapted with permission of Taylor & Francis.)

The midface show signs of aging during the forties. The malar soft tissue adjacent to the inferior orbital rim descends, accumulating as fullness along the nasolabial fold. The malar soft tissue atrophy and ptosis result in periorbital hollowing and tear trough deformity. Early aging is evident in individuals of African, Asian, and Hispanic origin in the midface region more so than the upper or lower regions. Signs include tear trough deformity, infraorbital hollowing, malar fat ptosis, nasojugal groove prominence, and deepening of the nasolabial fold. This predisposition to midface aging is likely the result of the relationship of the eyes to the infraorbital rim, basic midface skeletal morphology, and skin thickness [55].

The soft tissue of the lower face is supported in a youthful anatomic position by a series of retaining ligaments within the superficial musculo-aponeurotic system (SMAS) [60]. The SMAS is a discrete fascial layer that envelops the face and forms the basis for resuspending sagging facial tissues [15]. The SMAS fascia envelope maintains tension on facial muscles and offsets soft tissue sagging. In the late thirties, gradual ptosis of the SMAS and skin elastosis sets the stage for jowl formation. Accumulation of submandibular fat and a sagging submandibular gland may have a role in interrupting the smooth contour of a youthful jaw line. Changes in the lower face lead to changes in the neck because the SMAS is anatomically continuous with the platysma muscle. Sagging of the SMAS–platysma unit and submandibular fat redistribution gradually blunts the junction between the jaw and neck. A "double chin" appears at any age as a result of cervicomental laxity with excess submental fat deposits. During the fifties, diastasis and hypertrophy of the anterior edge of the platysma muscle may produce vertical banding in the cervicomental area. During the sixth, seventh, and eighth decades, progressive soft tissue atrophy and bony remodeling of the maxilla and mandible create a relative excess of sagging skin, further exaggerating facial aging. Jowling is a sign of lower facial aging in black persons [55]. In some cases, a bony chin underprojection make create excess localized submental fatty deposits despite a smoothly contoured jaw line. However, in Asians, jowl formation may result from fat accumulation in the buccal space [55]. The "double chin" is more common in Caucasians under 40 years of age than Asians of the same age group, but more common in Asians over 40 years of age because of redundant cervical skin [61].

Extrinsic aging (photoaging) of ethnic skin

Sunlight is a major factor for the appearance of premature aging, independent of facial wrinkling, skin color, and skin elasticity. By the late forties, individuals with greater sun exposure appear older than those with less sun exposure. However, the perceived age of individuals in their late twenties is unaffected by sun exposure. Solar exposure greatly increases the total wrinkle length by the late forties. The extent of dermal degenerative change seen by the late forties correlates with premature aging. There is a high correlation between perceived age and facial wrinkles; perceived age and elastosis; and perceived age and the quantity of collagen. The grenz zone is a subepidermal band of normal dermis consisting of normal collagen fibers and thought to be a site of continual dermal repair. The grenz zone becomes visually apparent only after there is sufficient elastotic damage. With progressive elastosis, the grenz zone becomes thinner [62].

Histopathology
Epidermis

The absolute number of Langerhans cells vary from person to person but chronic sun exposure decreases their number or depletes them [63]. The severely sun-damaged skin has many vacuolated cells in the spinous layer, excessively vacuolated basal keratinocytes and melananocytes, cellular atypia, and loss of cellular polarity. Apoptosis in the basal layer is increased. A faulty stratum lucidum and horny layer result from intracellular vesicles in the cells of the basal and spinous layers (sunburn cells), apoptosis, and dyskeratosis. There is focal necrobiosis in the epidermis and dermis in sun-exposed skin. While histologic findings of photoaging in white sun-exposed skin include a distorted, swollen, and distinctly cellular stratum lucidum, the stratum lucidum of African-American sun-exposed skin remains compact and unaltered [6]. The stratum lucidum in black skin is not altered by sunlight exposure [6].

With age, the dermoepidermal junction becomes flattened with multiple zones of basal lamina and anchoring fibril reduplication. Microfibrils in the papillary dermis become more irregularly oriented. Compact elastic fibers show cystic changes and separation of skeleton fibers with age. The area occupied by the superficial vascular plexus in specimens of equal epidermal surface length decreases from the infant to young adult (21–29 years) to adult (39–52 years) age groups, then increased in the elderly adult (73–75 years) age group [64]. With the exception of the vascularity in the elderly adult group, the above features are similar to those seen in aging white skin, and suggest that chronologic aging in white and black skin is similar. Oxytalan fibers are found in the papillary dermis of sun-exposed skin of white individuals in their twenties and early thirties but disappear in the forties. In black skin, the oxytalan fibers are still found in the dermis of individuals in their fifties. No solar elastosis is seen in specimens of black sun-exposed skin. Older black subjects have an increased number and thickness of elastic fibers that separate the collagenous fiber layer in the reticular dermis. The sun-exposed skin of a 45-year-old light- complexioned black female shared the same amount and distribution of elastic fibers as those in white sun-exposed skin [6].

The grenz zone consists of small fibers oriented horizontally and replaces the papillary dermis. When elastotic material accumulates in the dermis, it crowds out all the collagenous fibers, which are resorbed. As the elastic material is resorbed, wisps of collagenous fibers form in its place. Widely spaced, larger collagenous fiber bundles lie between the waning elastotic masses. The total volume of the dermis gradually diminishes as the spaces between the remaining collagenous and elastic fibers are reduced. When the epidermis rests directly on top of the horizontally oriented, medium-sized collagenous fiber bundles of the intermediate dermis, the dermis lacks a papillary and grenz zone and the dermis cannot sufficiently support the epidermis. As a result, the shrinking dermis crinkles and small wrinkles form. This may be the reason for the absence of a structural basis in secondary wrinkles and may explain why wrinkles flatten out when fluids are injected into the skin or when edema occurs [63].

Photoaging in skin of color has variable presentations. Wrinkling is not as common a manifestation of photoaging in black persons, South Asians, or darker complexioned Hispanics as in white persons because of the photoprotective effects of melanin. All racial groups are eventually subjected to photoaging. Within most racial groups, the lighter complexioned individuals show evidence of photodamaged skin. Caucasian skin has an earlier onset and greater skin wrinkling and sagging signs than darker skin types. Visual photoaging assessments reveal that white skin has more severe fine lines, rhytides, laxity, and overall photodamage than African-American skin [45].

Photoaging is uncommon in black persons but is more often seen in African-Americans than in Africans or Afro-Caribbeans. The reason may be the heterogeneous mixture of African, Caucasian, and Native American ancestry often seen in African-Americans. In African-Americans, photoaging appears primarily in lighter complexioned individuals and may not be apparent until the late fifth or sixth decades of life [65]. Photoaging in this group appears as fine wrinkling and mottled pigmentation. In spite of the photoprotective effects of melanin, persons of skin of color are still prone to photoaging, but the reason is not completely known. Infrared radiation may also contribute to photodamage. There is evidence that chronic exposure to natural or artificial heat sources can lead to histologic changes resembling that of UV-induced changes, such as elastosis and carcinoma [66]. The pigmentary manifestations of photoaging common in skin of color include seborrheic keratoses, actinic lentigines, mottled hyperpigmentation, and solar-induced facial melasma [67]. However, African-American skin has greater dyspigmentation, with increased hyperpigmentation and unevenness of skin tone [44].

Hair

There are two types of hair fibers: terminal and vellus. Terminal hair is found on the scalp and trunk. Vellus hair is fine and shorter and softer than terminal hair. The hair fiber grows from the epithelial follicle, which is an invagination of the epidermis from which the hair shaft develops via mitotic activity and into which sebaceous glands open. The hair follicle is one of the most proliferative cell types in the body and undergoes growth cycles. The cycles include anagen (active growth), catagen (regression), and telogen (rest). Each follicle follows a growth pattern independent of the rest. The hair follicle is lined by a cellular inner and outer root sheath of epidermal origin and is invested with a fibrous sheath derived from the dermis. Each hair fiber is made up of an outer cortex and a central medulla. Enclosing the hair shaft is a layer of overlapping keratinized scales, the hair cuticle that serves as protective layers.

Racial differences in hair include the hair type, shape, and bulb. There are four types of hair: helical, spiral, straight, and wavy. The spectrum of curliness is displayed in Figure 3.2. The vast majority of black persons have spiral hair [68]. The hair of black persons is naturally more brittle and more susceptible to breakage and spontaneous knotting than that of white persons. The kinky form of black hair, the weak intercellular cohesion between cortical cells, and the specific hair grooming practices among black persons account for the accentuation of these findings [68]. The shape of the hair is different between races: black hair has an elliptical shape, Asian hair is round-shaped straight hair, and Caucasian hair is intermediate [69,70]. The bulb determines the shape of the hair shaft, indicating a genetic difference in hair follicle structure [31]. The cross-section of black hair has a longer major axis, a flattened elliptical shape, and curved follicles. Asian hair has the largest cross-sectional area and Western European hair has the smallest [70,71]. Black persons have fewer elastic fibers anchoring the hair follicles to the dermis than white subjects. Melanosomes were in the outer root sheath and in the bulb of vellus hairs in black, but not in white persons. Black hair also has more pigment and on microscopy has larger melanin granules than hair from light-skinned and Asian individuals. Similarities between white and black hair include: cuticle thickness, scale size and shape, and cortical cells [71].

While the curly nature of black hair is believed to result from the shape of the hair follicle [71], research has shown that the curliness of hair correlates with the distribution of cortical cells independent of ethnoracial origin [72]. Black hair follicles have a helical form, whereas the Asian follicle is completely straight and the Caucasian hair form is intermediate [71]. Mesocortical, orthocortical, and paracortical cells are the three cell types in the hair cortex. In straight hair, mesocortical cells predominate [72]. In wavy hair, the orthocortical and mesocortical cells are interlaced around

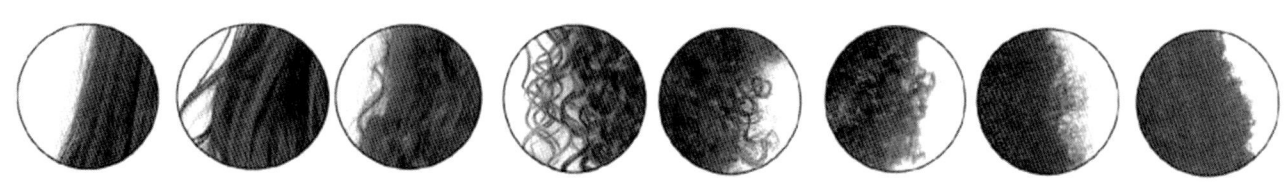

Figure 3.2 The spectrum of curliness in human hair. (Source: Loussouarn et al., 2007 [*Int J Dermatol* **46** (Suppl 1), 2-6.] Reproduced with permission of John Wiley & Sons.)

paracortical cells. In tightly curled hair, the mesocortex disappears, making orthocortical cells the majority. Distinct cortical cells express the acidic hair keratin K38. Figure 3.3 displays the distribution of K38 cells in straight, wavy, and tightly curled hair. Straight hair has a patchy but homogenous pattern of positively charged K38 cells surrounding a core of negatively charged cells. As the degree of curl decreases, the K38 pattern becomes asymmetric, independent of ethnic origin. In tightly curled hair, K38 accumulates on the concave side of the hair fiber and the medulla compartment disappears.

There are no differences in keratin types between hair from different races and no differences in amino acid composition of hair from different races [73]. Among Caucasian, Asian, and Africans, there are no differences in the intimate structures of fibers, whereas geometry, mechanical properties, and water swelling differed according to ethnic origin [74]. One study [75] in 1941 did find variation in the levels of some amino acids between black and white hair. Black subjects had significantly greater levels of tyrosine, phenylalanine, and ammonia in the hair, but were deficient in serine and threonine.

The morphologic features of African hair were examined using the transmission and scanning electron microscopic (SEM) techniques in an unpublished study. The cuticle cells of African hair

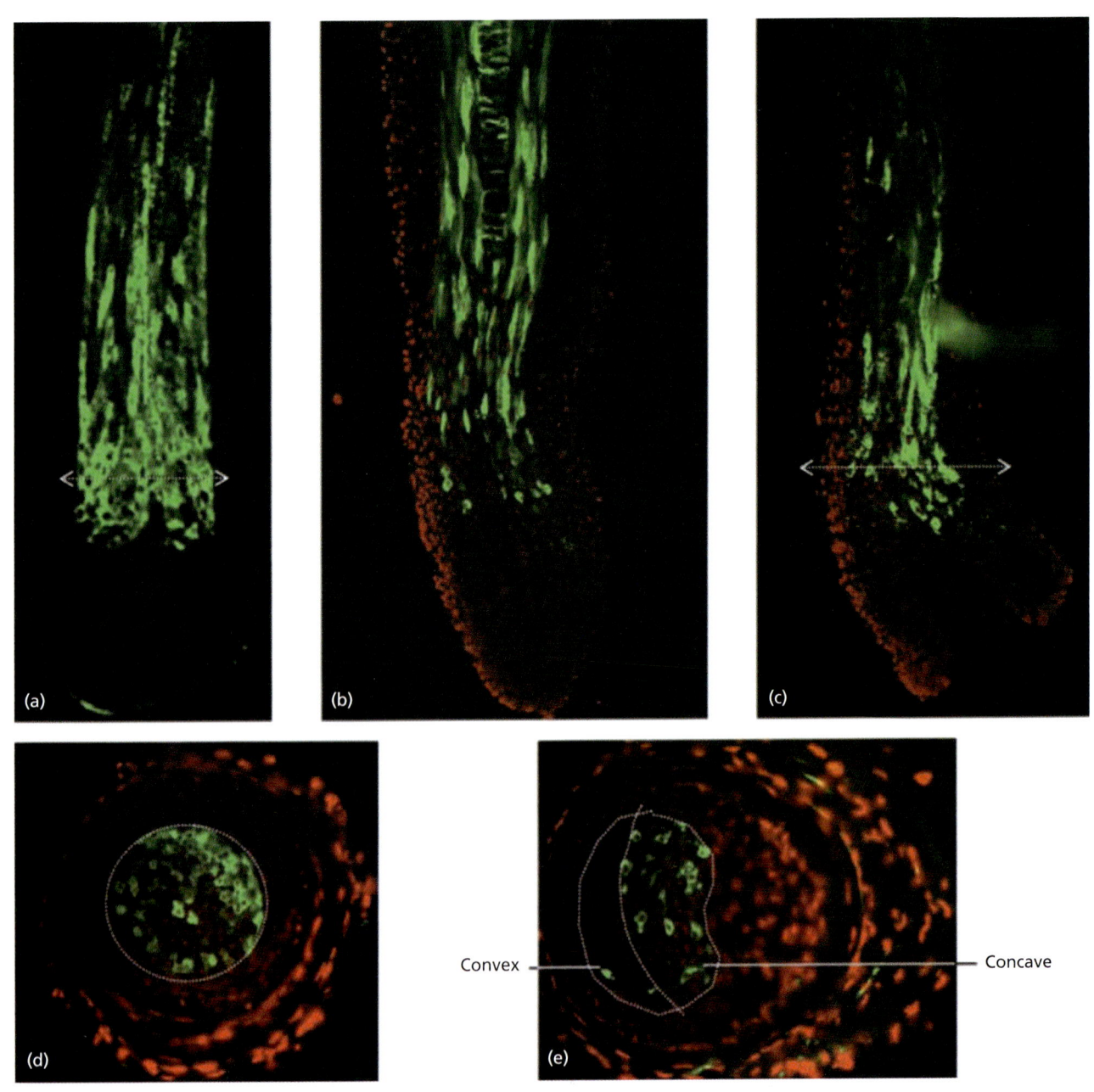

Figure 3.3 K38 hair keratin distribution in hair follicles. K38 pattern in (a) straight, (b) wavy, and (c) curly hair longitudinal sections. K38 pattern in (d) straight and (e) curly hair cross-sections. (Source: Thibaut et al., 2007 [72]. Reproduced with permission of John Wiley & Sons.)

were compared with those of Caucasian hair. Two different electronic density layers were shown. The denser exocuticle is derived from the aggregation of protein granules that first appear when the scale cells leave the bulb region. The endocuticle is derived from the zone that contains the nucleus and cellular organites. The cuticle of Caucasian hair is usually 6–8 layers thick and constant in the hair perimeter, covering the entire length of each fiber. However, black hair has variable thickness; the ends of the minor axis of fibers are 6–8 layers thick, and the thickness diminishes to 1–2 layers at the ends of the major axis. The weakened endocuticle is subject to numerous fractures (Handjur C, Fiat, Huart M, Tang D, Leory F, unpublished data).

References

1. US Census Bureau. (2010) Overview of Race and Hispanic Origin: 2010: 2010 Census Briefs. March 2011 online at: www.census.gov/prod/cen2010/briefs/c2010br-02.pdf. Accessed 24 May 2015.
2. Halder RM, Nandedkar MA, Neal KW. (2003) Pigmentary disorders in ethnic skin. *Dermatol Clin* **21**, 617–28.
3. Fitzpatrick TB, Szabo G. (1959) The melanocytes: cytology and cytochemistry. *J Invest Dermatol* **32**, 197–209.
4. Jimbow K, Oikawa O, Sugiyama S, Takeuchi T. (1979) Comparison of eumelanogenesis and pheomelanogenesis in retinal and follicular melanocytes: role of vesiculo-globular bodies in melanosome differentiation. *J Invest Dermatol* **73**, 278–84.
5. Wakamatsu K, Kavanagh R, Kadekaro AL, Terzieva S, Sturm RA, Leachman S, *et al.* (2006) Diversity of pigmentation in cultured human melanocytes is due to differences in the type as well as quantity of melanin. *Pigment Cell Res* **19**, 154–62.
6. Montagna W, Carlisle K. (1991) The architecture of black and white facial skin. *J Am Acad Dermatol* **24**, 929–37.
7. Taylor SC. (2002) Skin of color; biology, structure, function, implications for dermatologic disease. *J Am Acad Dermatol* **46**, S41–62.
8. Toda K, Fatnak MK, Parrish A, Fitzpatrick TB. (1972) Alteration of racial differences in melanosome distribution in human epidermis after exposure to ultraviolet light. *Nat New Biol* **236**, 143–4.
9. Olson RL, Gaylor J, Everett MA. (1973) Skin color, melanin, and erythema. *Arch Dermatol* **108**, 541–4.
10. Jimbow M, Jimbow K. (1989) Pigmentary disorders in Oriental skin. *Clin Dermatol* **7**, 11–27.
11. Yoshida-Amano Y, Hachiya A, Ohuchi A, Kobinger GP, Kitahara T, Takema Y, *et al.* (2012) Essential role of RAB27A in determining constitutive human skin color. *PLoSOne* **7**, e41160.
12. Abdel-Malek Z, Swope VB, Suzuki I, Akcali C, Harriger MD, Boyce ST, *et al.* (1995) Mitogenic and melanogenic stimulation of normal human melanocytes by melanotropic peptides. *Proc Natl Acad Sci USA* **92**, 1789–93.
13. Sturm RA, Teasdale RD, Box NF. (2001) Human pigmentation genes: identification, structure and consequences of polymorphic variation. *Gene* **277**, 49–62.
14. Rees JL. (2003) Genetics of hair and skin color. *Annu Rev Genet* **37**, 67–90.
15. Suzuki I, Cone RD, Im S, Nordlund J, Abdel-Malek ZA. (1996) Binding of melanotropic hormones to the melanocortin receptor MC1R on human melanocytes stimulates proliferation and melanogenesis. *Endocrinology* **137**, 1627–33.
16. Hou L, Kapas S, Cruchley AT, Macey MG, Harriott P, Chinni C, *et al.* (1998) Immunolocalization of protease-activated receptor-2 in skin: receptor activation stimulates interleukin-8 secretion by keratinocytes *in vitro*. *Immunology* **94**, 356–62.
17. Steinhoff M, Neisius U, Ikoma A, Fartasch M, Heyer Gisela, Skov PS, *et al.* (2003) Proteinase-activated receptor-1 mediates itch: a novel pathway for pruritus in human skin. *J Neurosci* **23**, 6176–80.
18. Shpacovitch VM, Brzoska T, Buddenkotte J, Stroh C, Sommerhoff CP, Ansel JC, *et al.* (2002) Agonists of proteinase-activated receptor 2 induce cytokine release and activation of nuclear transcription factor κB in human dermal microvascular endothelial cells. *J Invest Dermtol* **118**, 380–5.
19. Seiberg M, Paine C, Sharlow E, Andrade-Gordon P, Constanzo M, Eisinger M, *et al.* (2000) Inhibition of melanosome transfer results in skin light-ening. *J Invest Dermatol* **115**, 162–7.
20. Nystedt S, Ramakrishnan V, Sundelin J. (1996) The proteinase-activated receptor 2 is induced by inflammatory mediators in human endothelial cells: comparison with the thrombin receptor. *J Biol Chem* **271**, 14910–5.
21. Bohm SK, Kong W, Bromme D, Smeekens SP, Anderson DC, Connolly A, *et al.* (1996) Molecular cloning, expression and potential functions of the human proteinase-activated receptor-2. *Biochem J* **314**, 1009–16.
22. Scott G, Deng A, Rodriguez-Burford C, Seiberg M, Han R, Babiarz L, *et al.* (2001) Protease-activated receptor 2, a receptor involved in melanosome transfer, is upregulated in human skin by ultraviolet irradiation. *J Invest Dermatol* **117**, 1412–20.
23. Babiarz-Magee L, Chen N, Seiberg M, Lin CB. (2004) The expression and activation of protease-activated receptor-2 correlate with skin color. *Pigment Cell Res* **17**, 241–51.
24. Gilchrest BA. (1977) Localization of melanin pigmentation in skin with Wood's lamp. *Br J Dermatol* **96**, 245–7.
25. Morelli JG, Norris DA. (1993) Influence of inflammatory mediators and cytokines on human melanocyte function (Review). *J Invest Dermatol* **100** (2 Suppl), 191S–5S.
26. Grover R, Morgan BDG. (1996) Management of hypopigmentation following burn injury. *Burns* **22**, 727–30.
27. Johnston GA, Svukabd KS, McLelland J. (1998) Melasma of the arms associated with hormone replacement therapy (letter). *Br J Dermatol* **139**, 932.
28. Pathak MA, Fitzpatrick TB. (1974) The role of natural photoprotective agents in human skin. In: FitzpatrickTB, PathakMA, HarberLC, SeijiM, KukitaA, eds. *Sunlight and Man*. Tokyo: University of Tokyo Press, pp. 725–50.
29. Kligman AM. (1974) Solar elastosis in relation to pigmentation. In: FitzpatrickTB, PathakMA, HarberLC, SeijiM, KukitaA, eds. *Sunlight and Man*. Tokyo: University of Tokyo Press, pp. 157–63.
30. Kaidbey KH, Agin PP, Sayre RM, Kligman AM. (1979) Photoprotection by melanin: a comparison of black and Caucasian skin. *J Am Acad Dermatol* **1**, 249–60.
31. Manuskiatti W, Schwindt DA, Maibach HI. (1998) Influence of age, anatomic site and race on skin roughness and scaliness. *Dermatology* **196**, 401–7.
32. Courcuff P, Lotte C, Rougier A, Maibach HI. (1991) Racial differences in corneocytes: a comparison between black, white, and Oriental skin. *Acta Dermatol Venereol* **71**, 146–8.

33. Warrier AG, Kligman AM, Harper RA, Bowman J, Wickett RR. (1996) A comparison of black and white skin using noninvasive methods. *J Soc Cosmet Chem* **47**, 229–40.
34. Wesley NO, Maibach HI. (2003) Racial (ethnic) differences in skin properties: The objective data. *Am J Clin Dermatol* **4**, 843–60.
35. Aramaki J, Kawana S, Effendy I, Happle R, Löffler H. (2002) Differences of skin irritation between Japanese and European women. *Br J Dermatol* **146**, 1052–6.
36. Triebskorn A, Gloor M. (1993) Noninvasive methods for the determination of skin hydration. In: Forsch PJ, Kligman AM, eds. *Noninvasive Methods for the Quantification of Skin Functions*. Berlin; New York (NY): Springer-Verlag, pp. 42–55.
37. La Ruche G, Cesarini JP. (1992) Histology and physiology of black skin. *Ann Dermatovenereologica* **119**, 567–74.
38. Rawlings AV. (2006) Ethnic skin types: Are there differences in skin structure and function? *Int J Cosmet Sci* **28**, 79–93.
39. Reed JT, Ghadially R, Elias MM. (1995) Skin type but neither race nor gender, influence epidermal permeability barrier function. *Arch Dermatol* **131**, 1134–8.
40. Diridollou S, de Rigal J, Querleux B, Leroy F, Holloway Barbosa V. (2007) Comparative study of the hydration of the stratum corneum between four ethnic groups: influence of age. *Int J Dermatol* **46** (Suppl 1), 11–4.
41. Sueki H, Whitaker-Menezes D, Kligman AM. (2001) Structural diversity of mast cell granules in black and white skin. *Br J Dermatol* **144**, 85–93.
42. Modjtahedi SP, Maibach HI. (2002) Ethnicity as a possible endogenous factor in irritant contact dermatitis: comparing the irritant response among Caucasians, blacks, and Asians. *Contact Dermatitis* **47**, 272–8.
43. Hicks SP, Swindells KJ, Middelkamp-Hup MA, Sifakis MA, González E, González S. (2003) Confocal histopathology of irritant contact dermatitis *in vivo* and the impact of skin color (black vs white). *J Am Acad Dermatol* **48**, 727–34.
44. Grimes P, Edison BL, Green BA, Wildnauer RH. (2004) Evaluation of inherent differences between African-American and white skin surface properties using subjective and objective measures. *Cutis* **73**, 392–6.
45. Berardesca F, Maibach H. (1996) Racial differences in skin pathophysiology. *J Am Acad Dermatol* **34**, 667–72.
46. Galindo, GR, Mayer JA, Slymen D, Almaguer DD, Clapp E, *et al.* (2007) Sun sensitivity in 5 US ethnoracial groups. *Cutis* **80**, 25–30.
47. Robinson MK. (2002) Population differences in acute skin irritation responses. Race, sex, age, sensitive skin and repeat subject comparisons. *Contact Dermatitis* **46**, 86–93.
48. Foy V, Weinkauf R, Whittle E, Basketter DA. (2001) Ethnic variation in the skin irritation response. *Contact Dermatitis* **45**, 346–9.
49. Robinson MK. (2000) Racial differences in acute and cumulative skin irritation responses between Caucasian and Asian populations. *Contact Dermatitis* **42**, 134–43.
50. Tadaki T, Watanabe M, Kumasaka K, Tanita Y, Kato T, Tagami H, *et al.* (1993) The effect of tretinoin on the photodamaged skin of the Japanese. *Tohoku J Exp Med* **169**, 131–9.
51. Montagna W, Giusseppe P, Kenney JA. (1993) The structure of black skin. In: Montagna W, Giusseppe P, Kenney JA, eds. *Black Skin Structure and Function*. Academic Press, pp. 37–49.
52. Girardeau-Hubert S, Pageon H, Asselineau D. (2012) *In vivo* and *in vitro* approaches in understanding the differences between Caucasian and African skin types: Specific involvement of the papillary dermis. *Int J Dermatol* **51** Suppl 1, 1–4.
53. Reilly DM, Ferdinando D, Johnston C, Shaw C, Buchanan KD, Green MR. (1997) The epidermal nerve fiber network: characterization of nerve fibers in human skin by confocal microscopy and assessment of racial variations. *Br J Dermatol* **137**, 163–70.
54. Berardesca E, Rigal J, Leveque JL, *et al.* (1991) *In vivo* biophysical characterization of skin physiological differences in races. *Dermatologica* **182**, 89–93.
55. Harris MO. (2006) Intrinsic skin aging in pigmented races. In: Halder RM, ed. *Dermatology and Dermatological Therapy of Pigmented Skins*. Taylor & Francis Group, pp. 197–209.
56. Alexis AF, Alam M. (2012) Racial and ethnic differences in skin aging: Implications for treatment with soft tissue fillers. *J Drugs Dermatol* **11**, s30; discussion s32.
57. Matory WE. (1998) Aging in people of color. In: Matory WE, ed. *Ethnic Considerations in Facial Aesthetic Surgery*. Philadelphia: Lippincott-Raven, 151–70.
58. Bosniak SL, Zillkha MC. (1999) *Cosmetic Blepharoplasty and Facial Rejuvenation*. New York: Lippincott-Raven.
59. Ramirez OM. (1998) Facial surgery in the Hispano-American patient. In: Matory WE, ed. *Ethnic Considerations in Facial Aesthetic Surgery*. Philadelphia: Lippincott-Raven, pp. 307–20.
60. Stuzin JM, Baker TJ, Gordon HL. (1992) The relationship of the superficial and deep facial fascias: relevance to rhytidectomy and aging. *Plast Reconstr Surg* **89**, 441–9.
61. Shirakable Y. (1988) The Oriental aging face: an evaluation of a decade of experience with the triangular SMAS flap technique. *Aesthetic Plast Surg* **12**, 25–32.
62. Warren R, Garstein V, Kligman AM, Montagna W, Allendorf RA, Ridder GM. (1991) Age, sunlight, and facial skin: a histologic and quantitative study. *J Am Acad Dermatol* **25**, 751–60.
63. Montagna W, Kirchner S, Carlisle K. (1989) Histology of sun-damaged human skin. *J Am Acad Dermatol* **12**, 907–18.
64. Herzberg AJ, Dinehart SM. (1989) Chronologic aging in black skin. *Am J Dermatopathol* **11**, 319–28.
65. Halder RM. (1998) The role of retinoids in the management of cutaneous conditions in blacks. *J Am Acad Dermatol* **39** (Part 3), S98–103.
66. Kligman LH. (1982) Intensification of ultraviolet-induced dermal damage by infrared radiation. *Arch Dermatol* **272**, 229–38.
67. Halder RM, Richards GM. (2006) Photoaging in pigmented skins. In: Halder RM, ed. *Dermatology and Dermatological Therapy of Pigmented Skins*. Taylor & Francis Group, pp. 211–20.
68. Halder RM. (1983) Hair and scalp disorders in blacks. *Cutis* **32**, 378–80.
69. Bernard BA. (2003) Hair shape of curly hair. *J Am Acad Dermatol* **48** (6 Suppl), S120–6.
70. Vernall DO. (1961) Study of the size and shape of hair from four races of men. *Am J Phys Anthropol* **19**, 345.
71. Brooks O, Lewis A. (1983) Treatment regimens for "styled" black hair. *Cosmet Toiletries* **98**, 59–68.
72. Thibaut S, Barbarat P, Leroy F, Bernard BA. (2007) Human hair keratin network and curvature. *Int J Dermatol* **46** (Suppl 1), 7–10.
73. Gold RJ, Scriver CG. (1971) The amino acid composition of hair from different racial origins. *Clin Chim Acta* **33**, 465–6.
74. Franbourg A, Hallegot P, Baltenneck F, Toutain C, Leroy F. (2003) Current research on ethnic hair. *J Am Acad Dermatol* **48** (6 Suppl), S115–9.
75. Menkart J, Wolfram L, Mao I. (1966) Caucasian hair, Negro hair and wool: similarities and differences. *J Soc Cosmet Chem* **17**, 769–87.

CHAPTER 4
Sensitive Skin and the Somatosensory System

Francis McGlone[1] and David Reilly[2]

[1] School of Natural Sciences & Psychology, Liverpool John Moores University, Liverpool, UK
[2] Unilever Research, Colworth Science Park, Sharnbrook, Bedford, UK

> **BASIC CONCEPTS**
> - The primary sensory modality subserving the body senses is collectively described as the somatosensory system and comprises all those peripheral afferent nerve fibers, and specialized receptors, subserving cutaneous, and proprioceptive sensitivity.
> - Individuals with sensitive skin demonstrate heightened reactivity of the cutaneous somatosensory system.
> - A separate set of neurons mediates itch and pain. The afferent neurons responsible for histamine-induced itch in humans are unmyelinated C-fibers.
> - Low threshold mechanoreceptors are responsible for the sensation of touch, a wide range of receptor systems code for temperature, and as the skin's integrity is critical for survival, there are an even larger number of sensory receptors and nerves that warn us of damage to the skin.
> - With the recent discovery of a class of neurones that respond optimally to gentle stroking touch (sharing commonality with the itch and pain nerves) our understanding of the skin's sensitivity is entering a new chapter.

Introduction

The primary sensory modality subserving the body senses is collectively described as the somatosensory system, and comprises all those peripheral afferent nerve fibers, and specialized receptors, subserving cutaneous and proprioceptive sensitivity. The latter processes information about limb position and muscle forces which the central nervous system uses to monitor and control limb movements and, via elegant feedback and feedforward mechanisms, ensure that a planned action or movement is executed fluently. This chapter focuses on sensory inputs arising from the skin surface – cutaneous sensibility – and describes the neurobiological processes that enable the skin to "sense." Skin sensations are multimodal and are classically described as sensing the four submodalities of touch, temperature, itch and pain. We also consider the growing evidence for a fifth submodality, present only in hairy skin, which is preferentially activated by slowly moving, low force, mechanical stimuli.

This brief introduction to somatosensation starts with the discriminative touch system. Sensation enters the peripheral nervous system via sensory axons that have their cell bodies sitting just outside the spinal cord in the dorsal root ganglia, with one ganglion for each spinal nerve root. Neurons are the building blocks of the nervous system and somatosensory neurons are unique in that, unlike most neurons, the electrical signal does not pass through the cell body but the cell body sits off to one side, without dendrites. The signal passes directly from the distal axon process to the proximal process which enters the dorsal half of the spinal cord, and immediately turns up the spinal cord forming a white matter column, the dorsal columns, which relay information to the first brain relay nucleus in the medulla. These axons are called the primary afferents, because they are the same axons that carry the signal into the spinal cord. Sensory input from the face does not enter the spinal cord, but instead enters the brainstem via the trigeminal nerve (one of the cranial nerves). Just as with inputs from the body, there are four modalities of touch, temperature, itch and pain, with each modality having different receptors traveling along different tracts projecting to different targets in the brainstem. Once the pathways synapse in the brainstem, they join those from the body on their way up to a relay in the thalamus and then on to higher cortical structures. Sensory information arising from the skin is represented in the brain in the primary and secondary somatosensory cortex, where the contralateral body surfaces are mapped in each hemisphere.

Peripheral nervous system

The skin is the most extensive and versatile organ of the body and in a fully grown adult covers a surface area approaching $2\,m^2$. This surface is far more than a just a passive barrier. It

---

Cosmetic Dermatology: Products and Procedures, Second Edition. Edited by Zoe Diana Draelos.
© 2016 John Wiley & Sons, Ltd. Published 2016 by John Wiley & Sons, Ltd.

contains in excess of 2 million sweat glands and 5 million hairs covering all surfaces, apart from the soles of the feet and the palms of the hands (glabrous skin). Evidence is also emerging that non-glabrous skin contains a system of nerves that code specifically for the pleasant properties of touch. Skin consists of an outer, waterproof, stratified squamous epithelium of ectodermal origin – the epidermis – plus an inner, thicker, supporting layer of connective tissue of mesodermal origin – the dermis. The thickness of this layer varies from 0.5mm over the eyelid to >5.0 mm over the palm and sole of the foot.

Touch

Of the four "classic" submodalities of the somatosensory system, discriminative touch subserves the perception of pressure, vibration, and texture and relies upon four different receptors in the digit skin:
1. Meissner corpuscles;
2. Pacinian corpuscles;
3. Merkel disks; and
4. Ruffini endings.

These are collectively known as low threshold mechanoreceptors (LTMs), a class of cutaneous receptors that are specialized to transduce mechanical forces impinging the skin into nerve impulses. The first two are classified as fast adapting (FA) as they only respond to the initial and final contact of a mechanical stimulus on the skin, and the second two are classified as slowly adapting (SA) as they continue firing during a constant mechanical stimulus. A further classification relates to the LTM's receptive field (RF; i.e. the surface area of skin to which they are sensitive). The RF is determined by the LTM's anatomic location within the skin, with those near the surface at the dermal–epidermal boundary, Meissner corpuscles and Merkel disks, having small RFs, and those lying deeper within the dermis, Pacinian corpuscles and Ruffini endings, having large RFs (Figure 4.1).

Psychophysical procedures have been traditionally employed to study the sense of touch where differing frequencies of vibrotactile stimulation are used to quantify the response properties of this sensory system. Von Bekesy [1] was the first to use vibratory stimuli as an extension of his research interests in audition. In a typical experiment participants were asked to respond with a simple button-press when they could just detect the presence of a vibration presented to a digit, within one of two time periods. This two alternative force choice paradigm (2-AFC) provides a threshold-tuning curve, the slopes of which provide information about a particular class of LTM's response properties.

Bolanowski et al. [2] proposed that there are four distinct psychophysical channels mediating tactile perception in the glabrous skin of the hand. Each psychophysically determined channel is represented by one of the four anatomic end organs and nerve fiber subtypes, with frequencies in the 40–500 Hz range providing a sense of "vibration," transmitted by Pacinian corpuscles (PC channel or FAI); Meissner corpuscles being responsible for the sense of "flutter" in the 2–40 Hz range (NPI channel or FAII); the sense of "pressure" being mediated by Merkel disks in the 0.4–2.0 Hz range (NPIII or SAI); and Ruffini end organs producing a "buzzing" sensation in the 100–500 Hz range (NPII or SAII). Neurophysiologic studies support this model, but there is still some way to go to link the anatomy with perception (Table 4.1).

There have been relatively few studies of tactile sensitivity on hairy skin, the cat being the animal of choice for most of these studies. Mechanoreceptive afferents (Aβ fibers) have been described that are analogous to those found in human glabrous skin (FAI, FAII, SAI, SAII), and Essick and Edin [3] have described sensory fibers with these properties in human facial skin. The relationship between these sensory fibers and tactile perception is still uncertain.

Sensory axons are classified according to their degree of myelination, the fatty sheath that surrounds the nerve fiber. The degree of myelination determines the speed with which the axon can conduct nerve impulses and hence the nerves conduction velocity. The largest and fastest axons are called Aα and include some of the proprioceptive neurons, such as the muscle stretch

Table 4.1 Main characteristics of primary sensory afferents innervating human skin

Class	Modality	Axonal diameter (μm)	Conduction velocity (m s^{-1})
Myelinated			
Aα	Proprioceptors from muscles and tendons	20	120
Aβ	Low threshold mechanoreceptors	10	80
Aδ	Cold, noxious, thermal	2.5	12
Unmyelinated			
C-pain	Noxious, heat, thermal	1	<1
C-tactile	Light stroking, gentle touch	1	<1
C-tutonomic	Autonomic, sweat glands, vasculature	1	<1

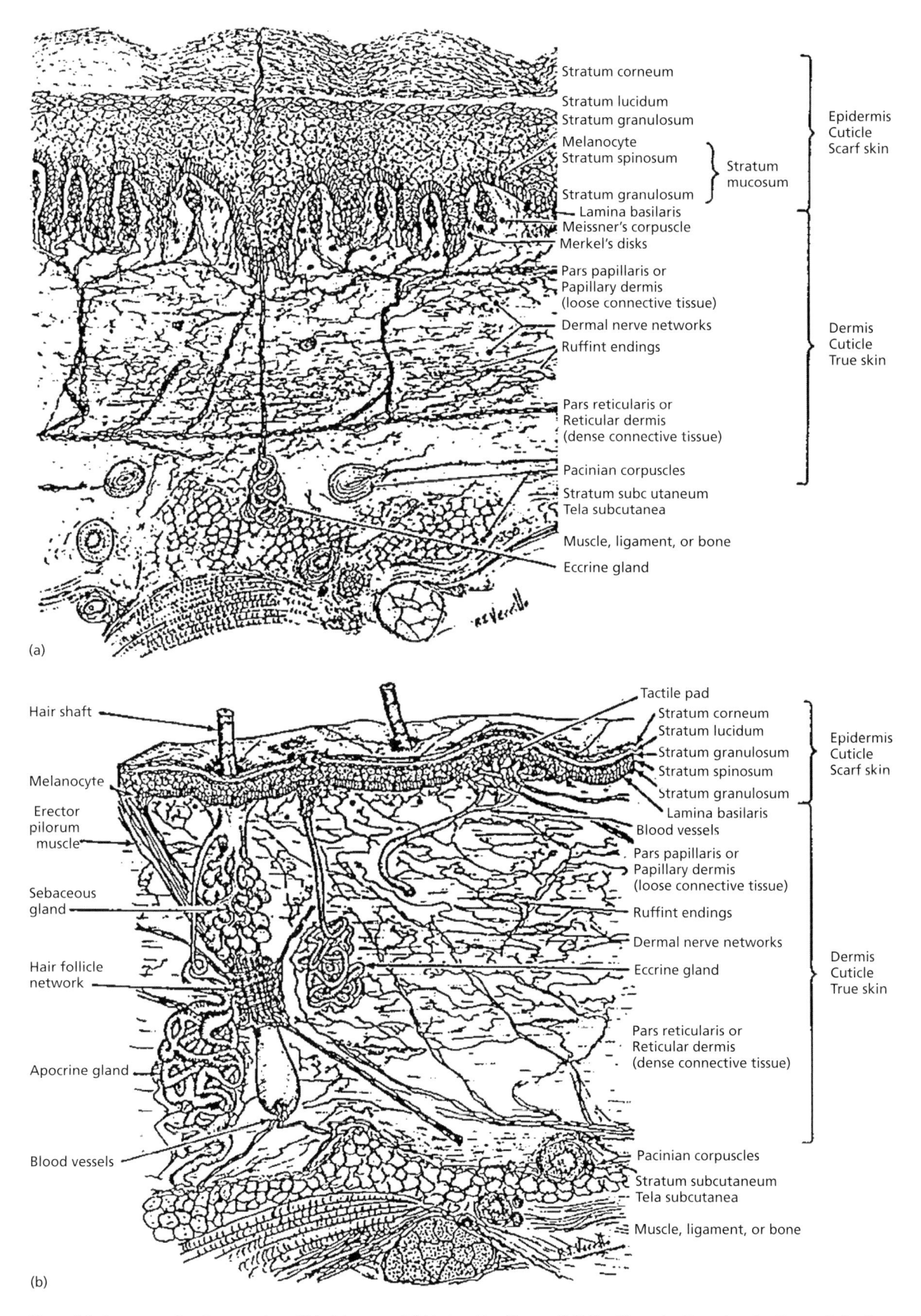

Figure 4.1 A cross-sectional perspective of (a) glabrous and (b) hairy skin. (Source: R.T. Verrillo, artist. Reproduced with permission.)

receptors. The second largest group, called Aβ, includes all of the discriminative touch receptors being described here. Pain, itch and temperature include the third fourth and fifth groups, Aδ and C-fibers.

Electrophysiological studies on single peripheral nerve fibers innervating the human hand have provided a generally accepted model of touch that relates the four anatomically defined types of cutaneous or subcutaneous sense organs to their neural response patterns [4]. The technique used in these studies is called microneurography and involves inserting a fine tungsten microelectrode, tip diameter <5 μm, through the skin and into the underlying median nerve which innervates the thumb and first two digits (Figure 4.2).

Temperature

The cutaneous somatosensory system detects changes in ambient temperature over an impressive range, initiated when thermal stimuli that differ from a homeostatic set-point excite temperature specific sensory nerves in the skin, and relay this information to the spinal cord and brain. It is important to recognize that these nerves code for temperature change, not absolute temperature, as a thermometer does. The system does not have specialized receptor end organs such as those found with LTMs but uses free nerve endings throughout skin to sense changes in temperature. Within the innocuous thermal sensing range there are two populations of thermosensory fibers, one that responds to warmth (warm receptors) and one that responds to cold (cold receptors), and include fibers from the Aδ and C range. Specific cutaneous cold and warm receptors have been defined as slowly conducting units that exhibit a steady-state discharge at constant skin temperature and a dynamic response to temperature changes [5,6]. Cold-specific and warm-specific receptors can be distinguished from nociceptors that respond to noxious low and high temperatures <20°C and >45°C) [7,8], and also from thermosensitive mechanoreceptors [5,9]. Standard medical textbooks describe the cutaneous cold sense in humans as being mediated by myelinated A-fibers with CVs in the range 12–30 ms^{-1} [10], but recent work concludes that either human cold-specific afferent fibers are incompletely myelinated "BC" fibers, or else there are C as well as A cold fibers, with the C-fiber group contributing little to sensation (Figure 4.3) [11].

The free nerve endings for cold-sensitive or warm-sensitive nerve fibers are located just beneath the skin surface. The terminals of an individual temperature-sensitive fiber do not branch profusely or widely. Rather, the endings of each fiber form a small, discretely sensitive point, which is separate from the sensitive points of neighboring fibers. The total area of skin occupied by the receptor endings of a single temperature-sensitive nerve fiber is relatively small (approximately 1 mm in diameter), with the density of these thermosensitive points varying in different body regions. In most areas of the body there are 3–10 times as many cold-sensitive points as warm-sensitive points. It is well-established from physiologic and psychologic testing that warm-sensitive and cold-sensitive fibers are distinctively different from one another in both structure and function.

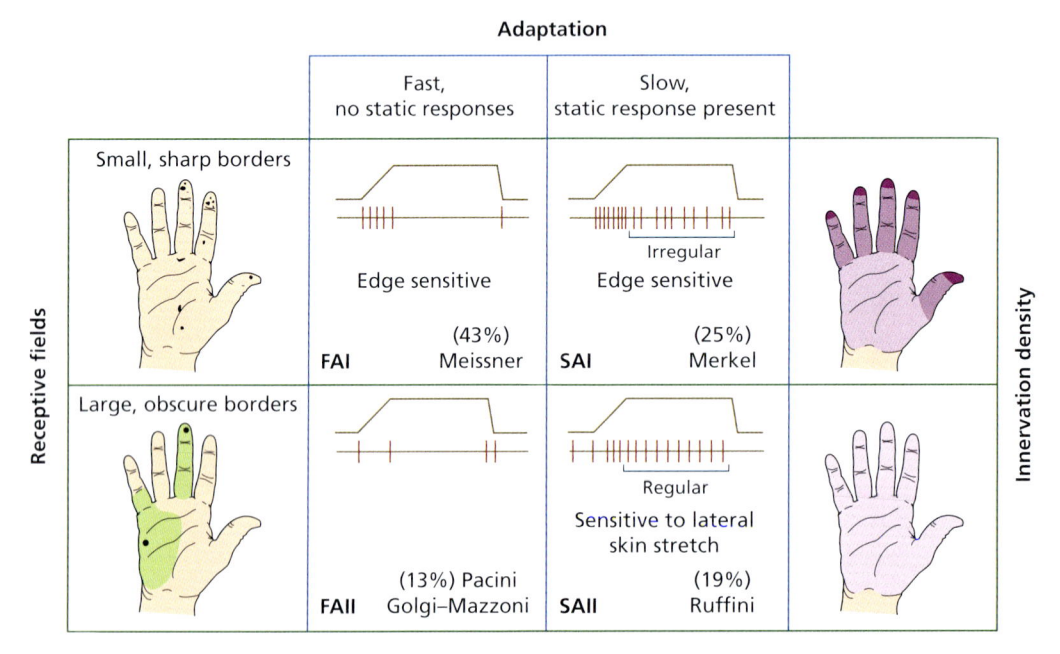

Figure 4.2 The four types of low threshold mechanoreceptors in human glabrous skin are depicted. The four panels in the center show the nerve firing responses to a ramp and hold indentation and the frequency of occurrence (%) and putative morphologic correlate. The black dots in the left panel show the receptive fields of type I (top) and type II (bottom) afferents. The right panel shows the average density of type I (top) and type II (bottom) afferents with darker area depicting higher densities. (Source: Westling, 1986 [29]. Reproduced with permission.)

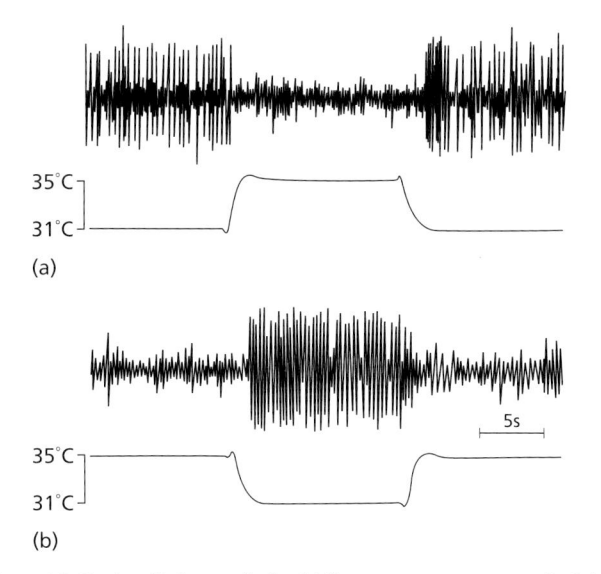

Figure 4.3 Resting discharge of a C cold fiber at room temperature [11]. (a) The resting discharge is suppressed by warming of the receptive field (RF) from 31°C to 35°C. (b) From a holding temperature of 35°C, at which the unit is silent, activity is initiated by cooling the RF to 31°C. (Time bar: 5 s.)

Pain

Here we consider a system of peripheral sensory nerves that innervate all cutaneous structures and whose sole purpose is to protect the skin against potential or actual damage. These primary afferents include Aδ and C-fibers which respond selectively and linearly to levels of thermal, mechanical, and chemical stimuli that are tissue-threatening. This encoding mechanism is termed nociception and describes the sensory process detecting any overt, or impending, tissue damage. The term pain describes the perception of irritation, stinging, burning, soreness, or painful sensations arising from the skin. It is important to recognize that the perception of pain not only depends on nociceptor input, but also on other processes and pathways giving information about emotional or contextual components. Pain is therefore described in terms of an "experience" rather than just a simple sensation. There are again submodalities within the nociceptive system (Aδ and C) subserving nociception. Aδ fibers are thin (1–5 µm), poorly myelinated axons of mechanical nociceptors, thermal receptors, and mechanoreceptors with axon potential conduction velocities of approximately 12 ms^{-1}. C-fibers are very thin (<1 µm) unmyelinated slowly conducting axons of <1 ms^{-1}. Mechanical nociceptors are in the Aδ range and possess receptive fields distributed as 5–20 small sensitive spots over an area approximately 2–3 mm in diameter. In many cases activation of these spots depends upon stimuli intense enough to produce tissue damage, such as a pinprick. Aδ units with a short latency response to intense thermal stimulation in the range 40–50°C have been described as well as other units excited by heat after a long latency – usually with thresholds in excess of 50°C.

Over 50% of the unmyelinated axons (C-fibers) of a peripheral nerve respond, not only to intense mechanical stimulation, but also to heat and noxious chemicals, and are therefore classified as polymodal nociceptors [12] or C-mechano-heat (CMH) nociceptors [13]. Receptive fields consist of single zones with distinct borders and in this respect they differ from Aδ nociceptors that have multipoint fields. Innervation densities are high and responses have been reported to a number of irritant chemicals such as dilute acids, histamine, bradykinin, and capsaicin. Following inflammation some units can acquire responsiveness to stimuli to which they were previously unresponsive. Recruitment of these "silent nociceptors" implies spatial summation to the nociceptive afferent barrage at central levels, and may therefore contribute to primary hyperalgesia after chemical irritation and to secondary hyperalgesia as a consequence of central sensitization.

Nociceptors do not show the kinds of adaptation response found with rapidly adapting LTMs (i.e. they fire continuously to tissue damage), but pain sensation may come and go and pain may be felt in the absence of any nociceptor discharge. They rely on chemical mediators around the nerve ending which are released from nerve terminals and skin cells in response to tissue damage. The axon terminals of nociceptive axons possess no specialized end organ structure and for that reason are referred to as free nerve endings. This absence of any encapsulation renders them sensitive to chemical agents, both intrinsic and extrinsic, and inflammatory mediators released at a site of injury can initiate or modulate activity in surrounding nociceptors over an area of several millimeters leading to two kinds of sensory responses termed hyperalgesia – the phenomenon of increased sensitivity of damaged areas to painful stimuli. Primary hyperalgesia occurs within the damaged area; secondary hyperalgesia occurs in undamaged tissues surrounding this area.

Itch

One further sensation mediated by afferent C-fibers is that of itch. The sensation of itch has, in the past, been thought to be generated by the weak activation of pain nerves, but with the recent finding of primary afferent neurons in humans [14] and spinal projection neurons in cats [15], which have response properties that match those subjectively experienced after histamine application to the skin, it is now recognized that separate sets of neurons mediate itch and pain, and that the afferent neurons responsible for histamine-induced itch in humans are unmyelinated C-fibers. Until relatively recently it was thought that histamine was the final common mediator of itch, but clinical observations where itch can be induced mechanically, or is not found with an accompanying flare reaction, cannot be explained by histamine-sensitive pruriceptors leading to evidence for the existence of histamine-independent types of itch nerves [16] in which itch is generated without a flare reaction by cowhage spicules. As with the existence of multiple types of pain afferents, different classes of itch nerves are also likely to account for the various experiences of itch reported by patients [17].

Pleasure

In recent years a growing body of evidence has been accumulating, from anatomical, psychophysical, electrophysiological, and neuroimaging studies, that a further submodality of afferent, slowly conducting, unmyelinated C-fibers exists in human hairy skin that are neither nociceptive nor pruritic, but that respond preferentially to low force, slowly moving mechanical stimuli. These nerve fibers have been classified as C-tactile afferents (CT-afferents) and were first described by Nordin [18] and Johansson et al. [19]. Evidence of a more general distribution of CT-afferents have subsequently been found in the arm and the leg, but never in glabrous skin sites such as the palms of the hands or the soles of the feet [20]. It is well known that mechanoreceptive innervation of the skin of many mammals is subserved by A and C afferents, but until the observations of Nordin and Vallbo C-mechanoreceptive afferents in human skin appeared to be lacking entirely.

The functional role of CT-afferents is not fully known, but their neurophysiological response properties, fiber class, and slow conduction velocities preclude their role in any rapid mechanical discriminative or cognitive tasks, and point to a more limbic function, particularly the emotional aspects of tactile perception [21]. However, the central neural identification of low-threshold C mechanoreceptors, responding specifically to light touch, and the assignment of a functional role in human skin has only recently been achieved. In a study on a unique patient lacking large myelinated Ab-fibers, it was discovered that activation of CT-afferents produced a faint sensation of pleasant touch, and functional neuroimaging showed activation in the insular cortex but no activation the primary sensory cortex, identifying CT-afferents as a system for limbic touch that might underlie emotional, hormonal, and affiliative responses to skin–skin contacts between individuals engaged in grooming and bonding behaviors – pleasant touch [22]. If pain is elicited via sensory C- and Aδ-fibers then it is reasonable to speculate that the same system may be alternatively modulated to deliver a sensation of pleasure. A study employing the pan-neuronal marker PGP9.5 and confocal laser microscopy has identified a population of free nerve endings in the epidermis that may be the putative anatomic substrate for this submodality [23].

Sympathetic nerves

Although this chapter deals with sensory aspects of skin innervation it is important to acknowledge the role of a class of efferent (motor) nerves that innervate various skin structures: (a) blood vessels; (b) cutaneous glands; and (c) unstriated muscle in the skin (e.g. the erectors of the hairs). In sensitive skin conditions, and some painful neuropathic states, sympathetic nerves have a role in exacerbating inflammation and irritation (for review see Roosterman et al. [24]).

The central projections

The submodalties of skin sensory receptors and nerves that convey information to the brain about mechanical, thermal, pruritic and painful stimulation of the skin are grouped into three different pathways in the spinal cord and project to different target areas in the brain. They differ in their receptors, pathways, and targets, and also in the level of decussation (crossing over) within the CNS. Most sensory systems *en route* to the cerebral cortex decussate at some point, as projections are mapped contralaterally. The discriminative touch system crosses in the medulla, where the spinal cord joins the brain, the pain/itch/pleasure system crosses at the point of entry into the spinal cord.

Spinal cord

All the primary sensory neurons have their cell bodies situated outside the spinal cord in the dorsal root ganglion, there being one ganglion for every spinal nerve root.

Tactile primary afferents, or first order neurons, immediately turn up the spinal cord towards the brain, ascending in the dorsal white matter and forming the dorsal columns. In a cross-section of the spinal cord at cervical levels, two separate tracts can be seen: the midline tracts comprise the gracile fasciculus conveying information from the lower half of the body (legs and trunk), and the outer tracts comprise the cuneate fasciculus conveying information from the upper half of the body (arms and trunk). At the medulla, situated at the top of spinal cord, the primary tactile afferents make their first synapse with second order neurons where fibers from each tract synapses in a nucleus of the same name – the gracile fasciculus axons synapse in the gracile nucleus, and the cuneate axons synapse in the cuneate nucleus. The neurons receiving the synapse provide the secondary afferents and cross immediately to form a new tract on the contralateral side of the brainstem – the medial lemniscus – which ascends through the brainstem to the next relay station in the midbrain, the thalamus.

As with the tactile system, pain, itch, CTs and thermal primary afferents synapse ipsilaterally and then the secondary afferents cross, but the crossings occur at different levels. Pain and temperature afferents enter the dorsal horn of the spinal and synapse within one or two segments, forming the Lissauer tract as they do so. The dorsal horn is a radially laminar structure. The two types of pain fibers, C and Aδ, enter different layers of the dorsal horn. Aδ fibers enter the posterior marginalis and the nucleus proprius, and synapse on a second set of neurons. These are the secondary afferents which will relay the signal to the thalamus. The secondary afferents from both layers cross to the opposite side of the spinal cord and ascend in the spinothalamic tract. The C-fibers enter the substantia gelatinosa and synapse, but they do not synapse on secondary afferents. Instead they synapse on interneurons – neurons that do not project out of the immediate area but relay the signal to the secondary afferents in either the posterior marginalis or the nucleus proprius. The spinothalamic tract ascends the entire length of the cord and the entire brainstem and by the time it reaches the midbrain appears to be continuous with the medial lemniscus. These tracts enter the thalamus together.

It is important to note that although the bulk of afferent input adheres to the plan outlined above there is a degree of mixing that goes on between the tracts.

We have concentrated on somatosensory inputs from the body thus far, but as facial skin is often the source of sensitive reactions to topical applications, its peripheral and central anatomy and neurophysiology is briefly summarized here. The trigeminal nerve innervates all facial skin structures (including the oral mucosa) and, just as with the spinal afferents, these neurons have their cell bodies outside of the CNS in the trigeminal ganglion with their proximal processes entering the brainstem. Just as in the spinal cord, the three modalities of touch, temperature, and pain have different receptors in the facial skin, travel along different tracts, and have different targets in the brainstem – the trigeminal nucleus – a relatively large structure that extends from the midbrain to the medulla.

The large diameter (Aβ) fibers enter directly into the main sensory nucleus of the trigeminal and, as with the somatosensory neurons of the body, synapse and then decussate, the secondary afferents joining the medial lemniscus as it projects to the thalamus. The small diameter fibers conveying pain and temperature enter midbrain with the main Vth cranial nerve, but then descend down the brainstem to the caudal medulla where they synapse and cross. These descending axons form a tract, the spinal tract of V, and synapse in the spinal nucleus of V, so called because it reaches as far down as the upper cervical spinal cord. The spinal nucleus of V comprises three regions along its length: the subnucleus oralis, the subnucleus interpolaris, and the subnucleus caudalis. The secondary afferents from the subnucleus caudalis cross to the opposite side and join the spinothalamic tract where the somatosensory information from the face joins that from the body, entering the thalamus in a separate nucleus, the ventroposterior medial (VPM) nucleus.

Brain

The third order thalamocortical afferents (from thalamus to cortex) travel up through the internal capsule to reach the primary somatosensory cortex, located in the post-central gyrus, a fold of cortex just posterior to the central sulcus (Figure 4.4a).

The thalamocortical afferents convey all of the signals, whether from the ventroposterior lateral (VPL) or VPM nucleus,

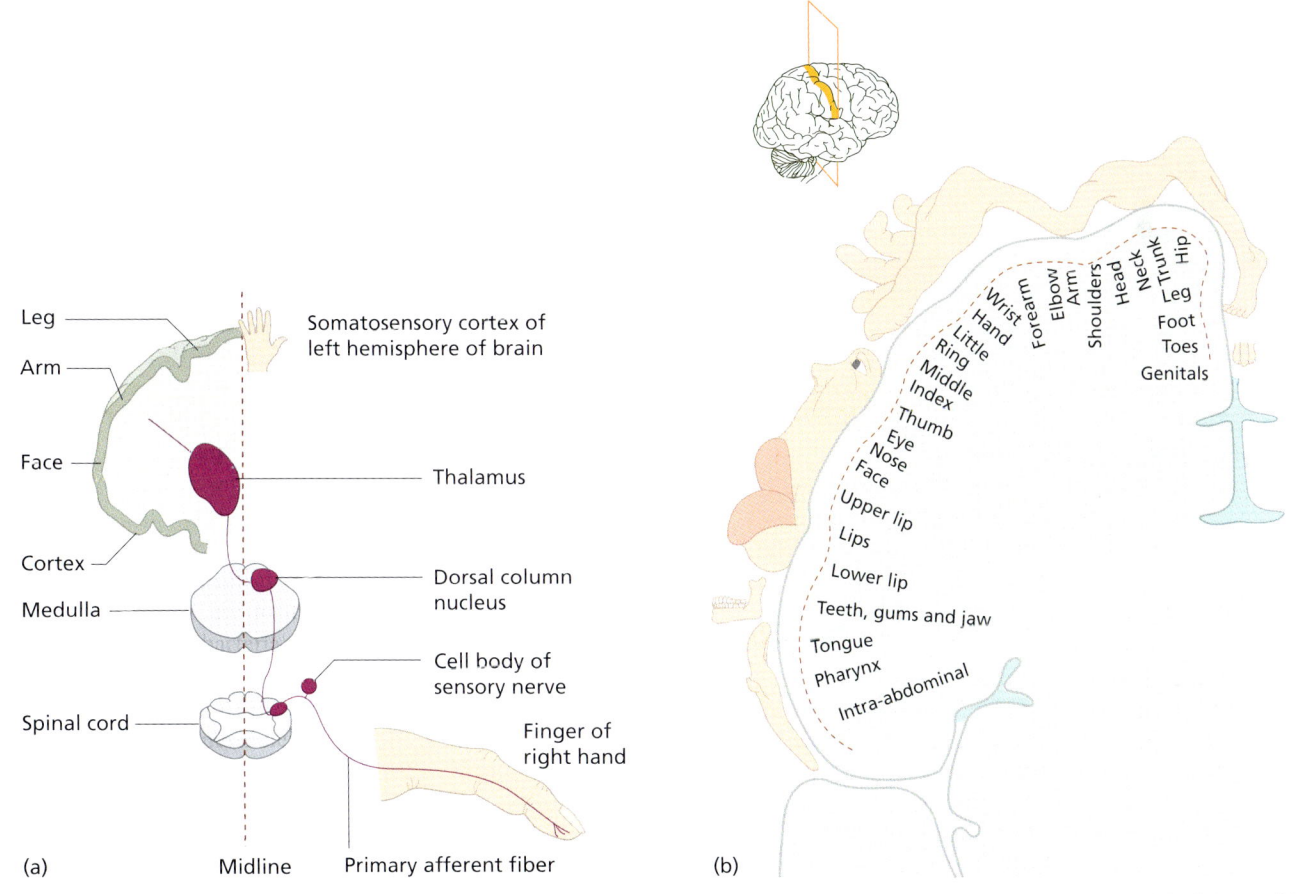

Figure 4.4 (a) Outline of the somatosensory pathways from the digit tip to primary somatosensory cortex, via the dorsal column nuclei and the thalamus. (b) Penfield's somatosensory homunculus. Note the relative overrepresentation of the hands and lips, and the relative underrepresentation of the trunk and arms.

to primary somatosensory cortex where the sensory information from all body surfaces is mapped in a somatotopic (body-mapped) manner [25], with the legs represented medially, at the top of the head, and the face represented laterally (Figure 4.4b). Within the cortex there are thought to be eight separate areas primarily subserving somatosensation: primary somatosensory cortex, SI, comprised of four subregions (2, 1, 3a and 3b); secondary somatosensory cortex, SII, located along the superior bank of the lateral sulcus [26]; the insular cortex; and the posterior parietal cortex, areas 5 and 7b (Figure 4.5).

As with studies of the peripheral nervous system, outlined above, the technique of microneurography has again been used, in this case to study the relationship between skin sensory nerves and their central projections, as evidenced by the use of concurrent functional magnetic resonance imaging (fMRI). Microstimulation of individual LTM afferents, projecting to RFs on the digit, produces robust, focal, and orderly (somatotopic) hemodynamic (BOLD) responses in both primary and secondary somatosensory cortices [27]. It is expected that this technique will permit the study of many different topics in somatosensory neurophysiology, such as sampling from FA and SA mechanoreceptors and C-fibers with neighboring or overlapping RFs on the skin, quantifying their spatial and temporal profiles in response to electrical chemical and/or mechanical stimulation of the skin areas they innervate, as well as perceptual responses to microstimulation.

Finally, the forward projections from these primary somatosensory areas to limbic and prefrontal structures has been studied with fMRI in order to understand the affective representations of skin stimulation for both pain and pleasure [28] and it is hoped that studies of this nature will help us to understand better the emotional aspects of both negative and positive skin sensations.

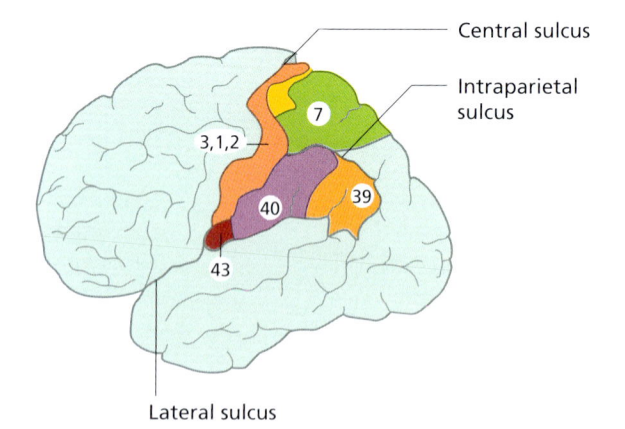

Figure 4.5 Cortical areas subserving somatosensation. Primary somatosensory cortex is located in the posterior bank of the central sulcus and the posterior gyrus and comprises areas 2, 1, 3a and 3b, secondary somatosensory cortex is located in the upper bank of the lateral sulcus with two further somatosensory regions in the posterior parietal cortex, areas 5 and 7b.

Conclusions

In this chapter we describe the neural architecture of the skin senses, where it has been shown that the skin surfaces we groom when applying cosmetic agents are receptive to a wide variety of physicochemical forms of stimulation. Low threshold mechanoreceptors are responsible for the sensation of touch, a wide range of receptor systems code for temperature, and, as the skin's integrity is critical for survival, there are an even larger number of sensory receptors and nerves that warn us of damage to the skin – the pain and itch systems. In addition to this "classic" description of the skin senses, we also provide recent evidence for the existence of another skin receptor system which shares many of the same characteristics as the pain system with one important distinction – this system of sensory nerves is excited by low force, slowly moving tactile stimulation – such as that employed when grooming the body surfaces. This C-fiber-based system of peripheral mechanosensitive cutaneous sensory nerves is therefore serving both a protective and hedonic role in body grooming behaviours and may well provide the neural substrate driving the rewarding (pleasant) sensations experienced during grooming – if personal care of the skin were not pleasant why would we do it?

References

1 von Bekesy G. (1939) Uber die Vibrationsempfindung. [On the vibration sense.] *Akust Z* **4**, 315–34.
2 Bolanowski SJ, Gescheider GA, Verrillo RT, Checkosky CM. (1988) Four channels mediate the mechanical aspects of touch. *J Acoust Soc Am* **84**, 1680–94.
3 Essick GK, Edin BB. (1995) Receptor encoding of moving tactile stimuli in humans: the mean response of individual low-threshold mechanoreceptors to motion across the receptive field. *J Neurosci* **15**, 848–64.
4 Valbo AB, Johansson RS. (1978) The tactile sensory innervation of the glabrous skin of the human hand. In: GordonG, ed. *Active Touch*. New York: Pergamon, pp. 29–54.
5 Hensel H, Boman KKA. (1960) Afferent impulses in cutaneous sensory nerves in human subjects. *J Neurophysiol* **23**, 564–78.
6 Hensel H. (1973) Cutaneous thermoreceptors. In: IggoA, ed. *Somatosensory System*. Berlin: Springer-Verlag, pp. 79–110.
7 Torebjörk H. (1976) A new method for classification of C-unit activity in intact human skin nerves. In: BonicaJJ, Albe-FessardD, eds. *Advances in Pain Research and Therapy*. New York: Raven, pp. 29–34.
8 Campero M, Serra J, Ochoa, JL. (1966) C-polymodal nociceptors activated by noxious low temperature in human skin. *J Physiol* **497**, 565–72.
9 Konietzny F. (1984) Peripheral neural correlates of temperature sensations in man. *Hum Neurobiol* **3**, 21–32.
10. Darian-Smith I. (1984) Thermal sensibility. In: Darian-SmithI, ed. *Handbook of Physiology, Vol. 3, Sensory Processes*. Bethesda, MD: American Physiological Society, pp. 879–913.

11. Campero M, Serra J, Bostock H, Ochoa JL. (2001) Slowly conducting afferents activated by innocuous low temperature in human skin. *J Physiol* **535**, 855–65.
12. Bessou M, Perl ER. (1969) Response of cutaneous sensory units with unmyelinated fibres to noxious stimuli. *J Neurophysiol* **32**, 1025–43.
13. Campbell JN, Raja SN, Cohen RH, Manning DC, Khan AA, Meyer RA. (1989) Peripheral neural mechanisms of nociception. In: WallPD, MelzackR. eds. *Textbook of Pain*. Edinburgh: Churchill Livingstone, pp. 22–45.
14. Schmelz M, Schmidt R, Bickel A, Handwerker HO, Torebjörk HE. (1997) Specific C-receptors for itch in human skin. *J Neurosci* **17**, 8003–8.
15. Andrew D, Craig AD. (2001) Spinothalamic lamina 1 neurons selectively sensitive to histamine: a central neural pathway for itch. *Nat Neurosci* **4**, 72–7.
16. Ikoma A, Handwerker H, Miyachi Y, Schmelz M. (2005) Electrically evoked itch in humans. *Pain* **113**, 148–54.
17. Yosipovitch G, Goon ATJ, Wee J, Chan YH, Zucker I, Goh CL. (2002) Itch characteristics in Chinese patients with atopic dermatitis using a new questionnaire for the assessment of pruritus. *Int J Dermatol* **41**, 212–6.
18. Nordin M. (1990) Low threshold mechanoreceptive and nociceptive units with unmyelinated (C) fibres in the human supraorbital nerve. *J Physiol* **426**, 229–40.
19. Johansson RS, Trulsson M, Olsson KA, Westberg KG. (1988) Mechanoreceptor activity from the human face and oral mucosa. *Exp Brain Res* **72**, 204–8.
20. Valbo AB, Hagbarth K-E, Torebjork HE, Wallin BG. (1979) Somatosensory, proprioceptive and sympathetic activity in human peripheral nerves. *Physiol Rev* **59**, 919–57.
21. Essick G, James A, McGlone FP. (1999) Psychophysical assessment of the affective components of non-painful touch. *Neuroreport* **10**, 2083–7.
22. Olausson H, Lamarre Y, Backlund H, Morin C, Wallin BG, Starck S, et al. (2002) Unmyelinated tactile afferents signal touch and project to the insular cortex. *Nat Neurosci* **5**, 900–4.
23. Reilly DM, Ferdinando D, Johnston C, Shaw C, Buchanan KD, Green M. (1997) The epidermal nerve fibre network: characterization of nerve fibres in human skin by confocal microscopy and assessment of racial variations. *Br J Dermatol* **137**, 163–70.
24. Roosterman D, Goerge T, Schneider SW, Bunnett NW, Steinhoff M. (2006) Neuronal control of skin function: the skin as a neuroimmunoendocrine organ. *Physiol Rev* **86**, 1309–79.
25. Maldjian JA, Gotschalk A, Patel RS, Detre, JA, Alsop DC. (1999) The sensory somatotopic map of the human hand demonstrated at 4T. *Neuroimage* **10**, 55–62.
26. Maeda K, Kakigi R, Hoshiyama M, Koyama S. (1999) Topography of the secondary somatosensory cortex in humans: a magentoencephalographic study. *Neuroreport* **10**, 301–6.
27. Trulsson M, Francis ST, Kelly EF, Westling G, Bowtell R, McGlone FP. (2001) Cortical responses to single mechanoreceptive afferent microstimulation revealed with fMRI. *Neuroimage* **13**, 613–22.
28. Rolls E, O'Doherty J, Kringelbach M, Francis S, Bowtell R, McGlone F. (2003) Representation of pleasant and painful touch in the human orbitofrontal cortex. *Cereb Cortex* **10**, 284–94.
29. Westling GK. (1986) Sensori-motor mechanisms during precision grip in man. Umea University medical dissertation. New Series 171, Umea, Sweden.

CHAPTER 5

Novel, Compelling, Non-invasive Techniques for Evaluating Cosmetic Products

Thomas J. Stephens,[1] Christian Oresajo,[2] Lily I. Jiang,[1] and Robert Goodman[1]
[1] Thomas J. Stephens & Associates Inc., Texas Research Center, Richardson, TX, USA
[2] L'Oréal Research, Clark, NJ, USA

BASIC CONCEPTS

- Skin care products must be studied for safety and efficacy.
- Non-invasive techniques were developed to assess the skin without a biopsy.
- Non-invasive techniques are used to evaluate visual appearance, moisturization, barrier integrity, oiliness, elasticity, firmness, erythema, and skin color.
- New photography techniques have been developed to detect photoaging features of the skin.

Introduction

Clinical trials for substantiation of cosmetic claims should be designed with good scientific rigor. In 1999, Rizer *et al.* [1] described an integrated, multidimensional approach for achieving this goal. The multistep process consisted of the following: careful subject selection, subject self-assessment of product performance, clinical grading, documentation photography, non-invasive bioengineering methods, and statistical analysis.

Clinical expert grading has been the key endpoint for many clinical trials. Many grading scales and atlases have been developed over the years that provided guidance for clinical grading [2,3,4,5]. Although it takes rigorous training and cumulative experience to achieve a level of consistency, expert graders are able to provide accurate assessment of skin conditions that no other bioinstrumentation or device could match. This is because during in-clinic live grading, experts can feel, touch and observe the skin's response from various angles.

Multiple bioinstrumentation devices have been developed over the years to assess the skin's physical and mechanical properties [6]. These devices provide an objective and quantitative assessment of the skin condition. Additionally, bioinstrumentation studies can provide valuable information about the mechanism of action of cosmetics on skin. Use of the bioinstrumentation does have limitations in certain clinical situations. Most bioinstrumentation devices focus on a very small area of the skin which may not be representative of changes in other areas of the face. In some trials products are applied to the surface of the skin prior to a measurement which results in poor surface contact with the device and/or false readings. It is for these reasons that bioinstrumentation data may not provide the needed evidence to substantiate a product performance claim.

Digital photography has been widely used to document of changes before and after product applications. In recent years, the development of specialized digital photography and image analysis tools, has provided clinical investigators with a new objective and quantitative tools for assessing changes in skin. Digital photography of skin when combined with image analysis can be a powerful tool for quantifying improvements in wrinkles, hyperpigmentation, pore size, skin tone evenness and skin tone brightness. Unlike bioinstrumentation, digital photography and image analysis can capture changes on the face or area of interest globally, providing a more comprehensive and realistic assessment; this is especially true in the case of colorimetry.

This chapter was written to introduce dermatologists, cosmetic surgeons and clinical researchers to the cost-effective, non-invasive methods for substantiating cosmetic claims. The chapter will include an overview of commonly used non-invasive bioinstrumentation methods in cosmetic studies and a description of various types of high resolution digital photography and their application for evaluating changes in skin. Emerging technologies for skin imaging will be discussed at the end.

Cosmetic Dermatology: Products and Procedures, Second Edition. Edited by Zoe Diana Draelos.
© 2016 John Wiley & Sons, Ltd. Published 2016 by John Wiley & Sons, Ltd.

Commonly used non-invasive bioinstrumentation methods in cosmetic studies

Approximately 90% or more of the cosmetic studies performed today are designed to support claims relating to improvements of fine lines or wrinkles, uneven skin pigmentation associated with sun exposure and/or hormonal changes, enlarged pores, skin radiance, skin roughness, skin tone, and skin dryness. Table 5.1 provides a listing of commonly used, non-invasive techniques that are used to help support these specific claims. For the reader who would like to learn more about these techniques or other non-invasive methods, there are a number of excellent books and articles available in the chapter's reference list [6–12].

Ideally, an investigator would like to see agreement between the clinical grading, non-invasive bioinstrumentation measurements and subject self-perception questionnaires. Occasionally, investigators get good concordance between clinical grading and self-perception questionnaires, but discordance with the more "objective" non-invasive technique. There are two main reasons for this discordance. First, most bioinstrumentation devices focus on a small area of a few millimetres in diameter. Going back to the exact same location during post baseline assessment is tricky and changes in that particular spot may not reflect changes on the face or area of interest globally. Second, most of those devices do not directly assess the features of photodamage, such as wrinkles, pores, and pigmentation, the same way as the graders see. However, these two issues can be overcome using the combined digital photography and image analysis approach discussed in the following sections of this chapter.

Use of digital photography as a non-invasive technique for assessing skin features

Unlike bioinstrumentation devices, digital photography has the advantage of capturing the changes before and after product usage of the whole assessment area, thus allowing comprehensive global analysis similar to the assessment done by expert graders.

The challenge for clinical documentation photography is twofold: to choose the best photographic technique relative to the aims of the study and to maximize consistency of the imaging at each clinic visit throughout the trial. The key to successful photography in clinical trials is the application of standardization, which includes the control subject's positioning, dress, lighting conditions, depth of field, background, and facial expression from visit to visit. The goal is to have images that accurately show treatment effects for use in medical and scientific journals. There is no place for misrepresenting clinical outcomes by changing viewing angles, altering lighting conditions, or having the subject apply facial makeup after using a product [13,14].

The first step to successful photography is to create the appropriate lighting and other photographic techniques specific to the skin conditions of interest in the clinical study. A study involving a product designed to reduce the appearance of fine lines and wrinkles demands significantly different lighting than would trials involving acne, photoaging skin, skin dryness or flakiness, scars, wound healing, postinflammatory hyperpigmentation (PIH), or pseudofolliculitis barbae. In order to ensure a high degree of color consistency in photographic technique, the photographer should include color standard chips in each documentation image. Typically, these standards include small reference chips of white, 18% reflectance gray, black, red, green, and blue, as well as a millimeter scale for size confirmation. In addition, a more comprehensive color chart such as a ColorChecker® (X-Rite America Inc., Grand Rapids, MI, USA) should be photographed under the exact standard lighting immediately before starting each photo visit.

Equally crucial is the careful and detailed recording of all aspects of lighting, camera, and lens settings in order to achieve maximum consistency of documentation photographs. Photographing each different photographic set-up provides more certainty that photographs at subsequent sessions are identical to the images made at baseline visit.

Prior to photography, all makeup and jewelry must be removed, and hair kept clear of the subject's face by use of a neutral-color headband. Clothing should be covered by a gray or black cloth drape to prevent errors caused by color reflected from colored clothing. Subject must adopt a neutral facial

Table 5.1 Commonly used bioinstruments and non-invasive procedures.

Name	Use
NOVA Meter	Moisturization
SKICON	Moisturization
Corneometer	Moisturization
TEWA Meter	Skin barrier function assessment
Derma Lab	Skin barrier function assessment
AquaFlux® Closed System	Skin barrier function assessment
Delfin VapoMeter® Closed System	Skin barrier function assessment
Cutometer	Firmness and elasticity
ChromaMeter	Skin tone, erythema, skin lightening, brightness
Mexameter	Skin tone, erythema, skin lightening
Sebumeter	Oiliness (sebum)
Sebutapes	Oiliness
D-Squames	Scaling, exfoliation, and cell renewal
Silicone replica impressions	Skin texture, wrinkling
Ultrasound	Skin density, skin thickness
Optical Coherence Tomography (OCT)	Visualizing the fine structures of skin
Confocal imaging	Visualizing cell structures of skin

expression, no smiling, frowning, or squinting during the photo shoot. Subject's body position, such as seat height, orientation of legs, position of head and neck, will also be marked since body position often affects the positioning of the face. At each subsequent visit in the study, it is essential to use image ghosting software to match post baseline images with baseline images. Subject's position and facial expression need to be maintained the same way as baseline images. Only under these conditions we can be assured that changes in the skin are due to product effect, and are not artifacts caused by careless photographic technique. When the study is over, the sequence of images should look almost like a time-lapse video; the only difference from one image to another is the condition of the subject's skin.

At Stephens & Associates, Inc. we have designed fully equipped photographic studios within our clinics so that subjects can be photographed under standardized conditions from visit to visit (Figure 5.1). These studios are manned by experienced medical photographers who have been trained in the basic science of conducting a clinical trial. While it is not possible for many clinics to have fully equipped studios with medical photographers in their office, there are other off-the-shelf alternatives which will allow them to control the quality of the images in clinical research.

Canfield's VISIA CR and VISIA CR2 are standardized camera systems that have been designed for use in clinical research. VISIA systems are composed of an oval shaped plastic shell containing a digital camera and lighting system. Subject positioning is controlled by forehead and chin rests. The unit is controlled by Mirror software. Multiple lighting modes are equipped and a series of pictures under different lighting modes can be taken quickly. Image ghosting is also included to allow position alignment at post baseline visits. VISIA systems can be operated by individuals with little to no experience in photography.

VISIA systems, while easy to use, have limitations in certain situations. The chin and head rests are sometimes too small for individuals with large faces, resulting in "jammed in" appearance. The chin rest also interferes with the assessment of jaw-lines and facial sagging. Because of the close proximity of the subject's face and the flash and camera, images can only be taken with the subject's eyes closed. Pictures with the eyes closed do not capture effectively conditions such as dark circles and under-eye puffiness; therefore they are not suitable for clinical studies testing an eye treatment. In addition, the VISIA systems are limited to capture the face only.

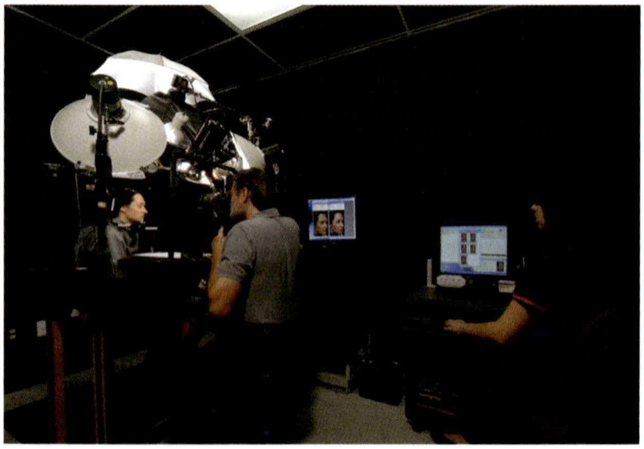

Review of terminology in clinical photography

As mentioned earlier, it is important to create the appropriate lighting and other photographic techniques specific to the skin conditions of interest in the clinical study. Individuals incorporating digital photography into a clinical trial are often faced with the difficult task of understating the vocabulary used by staff at clinical research organizations (CROs). This section provides a concise description of commonly used terms and techniques in clinical photography.

Visible light photography

This refers to images made with unfiltered full-spectrum (white) light. It is the most common type of photography used in clinical trials. Proper positioning of the strobe flashes is a critical step for capturing various skin conditions in cosmetic clinical trials. Clinical studies involving evenness of color and skin tone require a more generalized, evenly distributed, visible lighting method while the imaging of fine lines, wrinkles, under eye bags, skin texture, and scaling is best achieved by placing the flashes in an off-axis direction. Off-axis lighting refers to lighting that is placed somewhat above and to the side to create small shadows and highlights on the skin thereby giving a three-dimensional quality to the image. Once the lighting conditions have been optimized, it is imperative that the photographer uses documentation notes, setup photographs, light metering and color charts to prevent lighting changes from visit to visit.

Visible light photography is recommended for all clinical studies as all clinical grading and subject self-assessments are done under visible light. Photos taken under visible light serve as good documentation and communication/advertising tools for demonstrating changes occurring before and after product usage.

Raking light photography

This refers to images taken with unfiltered full-spectrum (white) light at a scant angle (~20–45 degrees, depending on condition) relative to the surface of interest. This kind of lighting casts certain features as shadows, such as facial wrinkles and cellulite dimples, thus enhancing those features. A comparison of photos taken under regular visible light vs. raking light is shown in Figure 5.2.

Figure 5.1 An example of a Stephens & Associates, Inc. photographic studio. The studio is equipped for taking photographs using standard lighting, parallel and polarized lighting, cross polarized lighting and raking light.

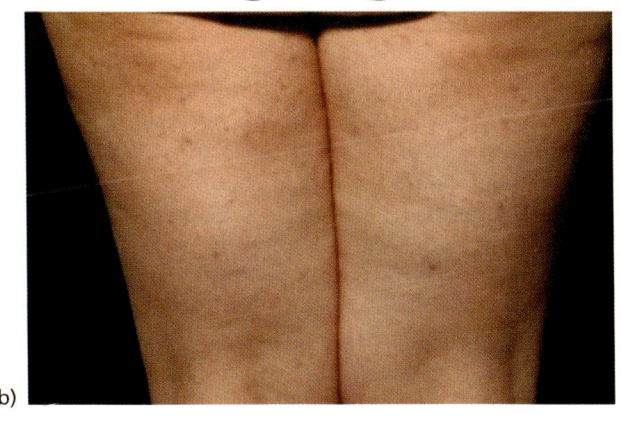

5. Novel, Compelling, Non-invasive Techniques for Evaluating Cosmetic Products   45

Figure 5.2 An example of raking light photography technique accentuating cellulite condition on the back of the thighs. (a) Standard light; (b) raking light.

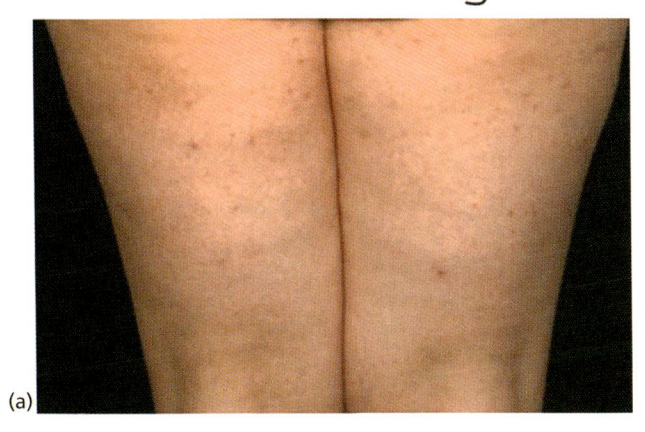

Polarized photography

This involves the placement of linear polarizing filters on both the lighting flash head(s) and in front of the lens of the digital camera. This allows the documentation of skin in two different ways [15].

The parallel-polarized lighting technique accentuates the reflection of light from the skin and tends to obscure fine topical detail because of strong reflections from the lighting source(s). Parallel-polarized light minimizes subsurface details, such as erythema and pigmentation, while allowing for enhanced viewing of the surface features of the skin, such as sweat, oily skin, and pores.

The cross-polarized lighting technique involves fixing the transmission axis of the lens polarizer 90° to the axis of the lighting polarizer. This virtually eliminates the reflection of light (glare) from the surface of the skin and accentuates the color element of the skin, such as pigmentation, the appearance of inflammation from acne lesions, erythema, rosacea, and telangiectasia. Photodamaged skin becomes somewhat more apparent, and some subsurface vascular features are made visible. Cross-polarized photography is useful for evaluating products designed to mitigate the appearance of dyschromic lesions, erythema, acne, and postinflammatory pigmentation (PIH) resulting from acne. This technique is highly recommended for acne studies [16].

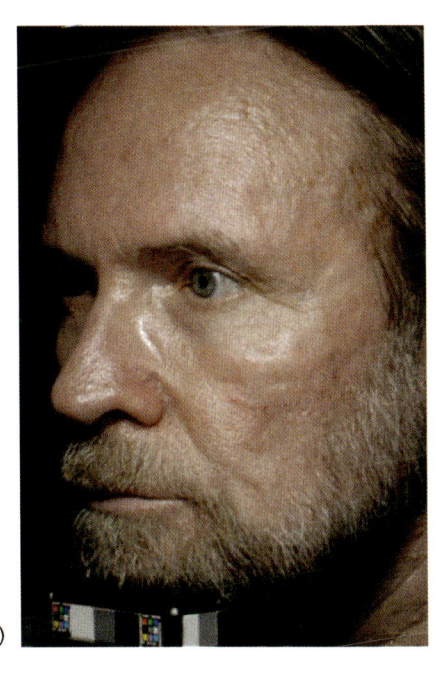

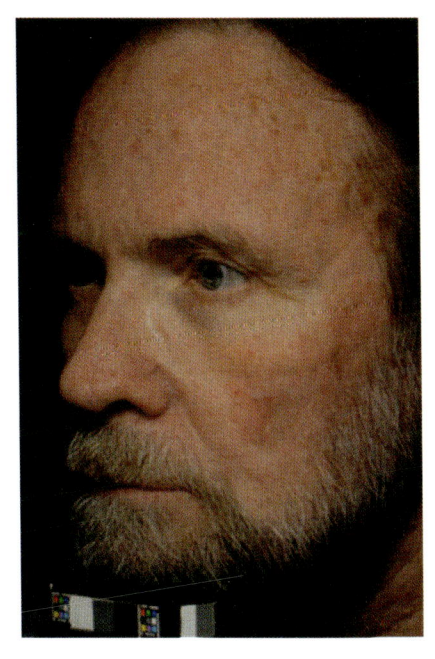

Examples of a parallel-polarized lighting technique and cross-polarized lighting technique can be found in Figure 5.3.

UV reflectance photography

This is a technique designed to highlight or enhance hyperpigmentation on the face. This is accomplished through filtering a flash source to only allow UV light to pass on to the subject's skin allowing visualization of subsurface melanin distribution.

Figure 5.3 Examples of a parallel-polarized lighting technique (a) and cross-polarized lighting technique (b).

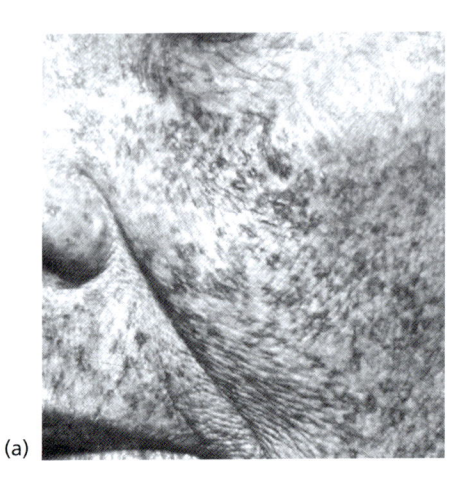

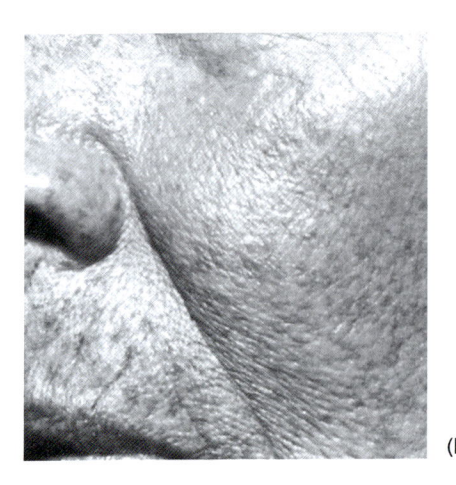

Figure 5.4 Before and after UV reflectance photographs of a subject treated with a skin lightening product. (a) Ultraviolet reflectance at baseline. (b) Ultraviolet reflectance at 12 weeks.

Figure 5.4 shows before and after UV reflectance photographs of a subject treated with a skin lightening product. A UV-blocking filter is placed in front of the lens of the digital camera. Note the improvement in the appearance and distribution of mottled and diffuse hyperpigmentation in the photograph on the right.

UV fluorescence photography

This is primarily used to visualize the locations of *Propionibacterium acnes* in the pores of subjects with acne. Porphyrins produced by *P. acnes* exhibit an orange–red fluorescence under UVA light. Excitation of *P. acnes* on skin is achieved using a xenon flash lamp equipped with an UVA bandpass filter. The resulting fluorescence can be recorded using a high-resolution digital camera equipped with an UV barrier filter. An example of this technique can be found in Figure 5.5.

Researchers have reported that UV fluorescence photography is a reliable, fast, and easy screening technique to demonstrate the suppressive effect of topical antibacterial agents on *P. acnes* [17]. Investigators need to be aware of a problem that can occur with using this technique to monitor *P. acnes* on the face. Many soaps, cosmetics, or sunscreen products contain quenching agents that can interfere with the accuracy of this imaging process. This can lead to an erroneous conclusion about the elimination of P. acnes from the face.

Digital fluorescence photography has other applications in dermatologic research. The technique can be used to detect salicylic acid in the skin and follicles of subjects participating in claim studies, as well as follow the migration of sunscreen products over the surface of face. Following the migration of sunscreen products over the surface can help explain why some sunscreen products find their way into the eyes producing stinging, burning, and ocular discomfort.

Guide photographs refer to photographs taken of mock subjects before the clinical trial begins to provide the sponsor and investigator with choices of techniques to best capture the dermatologic condition being studied. The chosen image becomes the guide, or standard, for photographing all subjects in the trial.

Use of raking light optical profilometry (RLOP) to detect improvements in periocular fine lines and wrinkles

Optical profilometry refers to a technique in which photographic images of silicone rubber impressions taken of facial skin can be analyzed for changes in lines and wrinkles. Grove *et al.* [18] reported that optical profilometry provides an element of objectivity that can complement clinical assessment in the study of agents that are useful for treating photodamaged skin.

While no one would argue that optical profilometry is a time proven method for assessing textural changes, preparing quality silicone replicas can be quite challenging even for

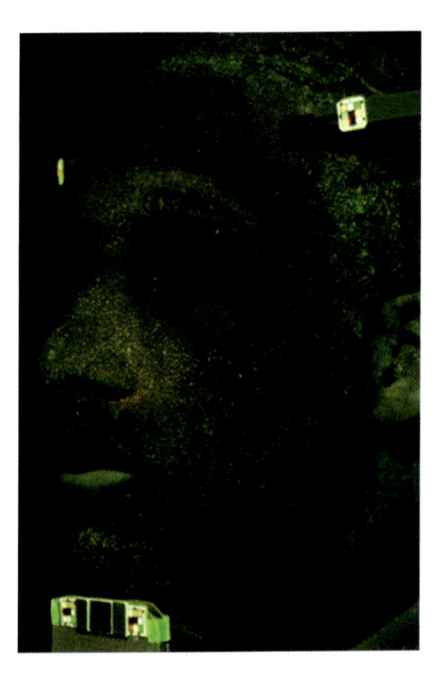

Figure 5.5 Ultraviolet fluorescence technique.

veteran clinicians. Making skin replicas is labor intensive, highly variable due to the procedure, and is typically done on a small area. Common problems include replicating positioning errors, air bubbles in the replica impression, and controlling the polymerization process. Slight variations in temperature, humidity, and body temperature can produce unsuitable replica impressions.

In an effort to reduce the frustration level associated with preparing silicone replicas, we began investigations into using high-resolution digital photographs for quantifying changes in fine line and wrinkles on the face. Off-axial lighting, a common lighting technique used for clinical photography, could be used to create small shadows and highlights that could help define the surface texture of skin. Flash lighting can be placed above and at a 45° angle to the side of the face to create a three-dimensional effect of texture in a two-dimensional plane. The raw image files can be analyzed for fine lines and wrinkles on the face. The term to describe this technique is RLOP.

This method was further improved and automated by Dr. Jiang at Stephens & Associates, Inc. We named the method SWIRL (**S**tephens **W**rinkle **I**maging using **R**aking **L**ight) [19]. The SWIRL method reports five wrinkle parameters, wrinkle count, length, width, area, and relative depth. Importantly, the SWIRL method has been fully validated through clinical studies and all five wrinkle parameters show excellent correlation with clinical grading scores for wrinkle severity [19]. An example of this method is shown in Figure 5.6.

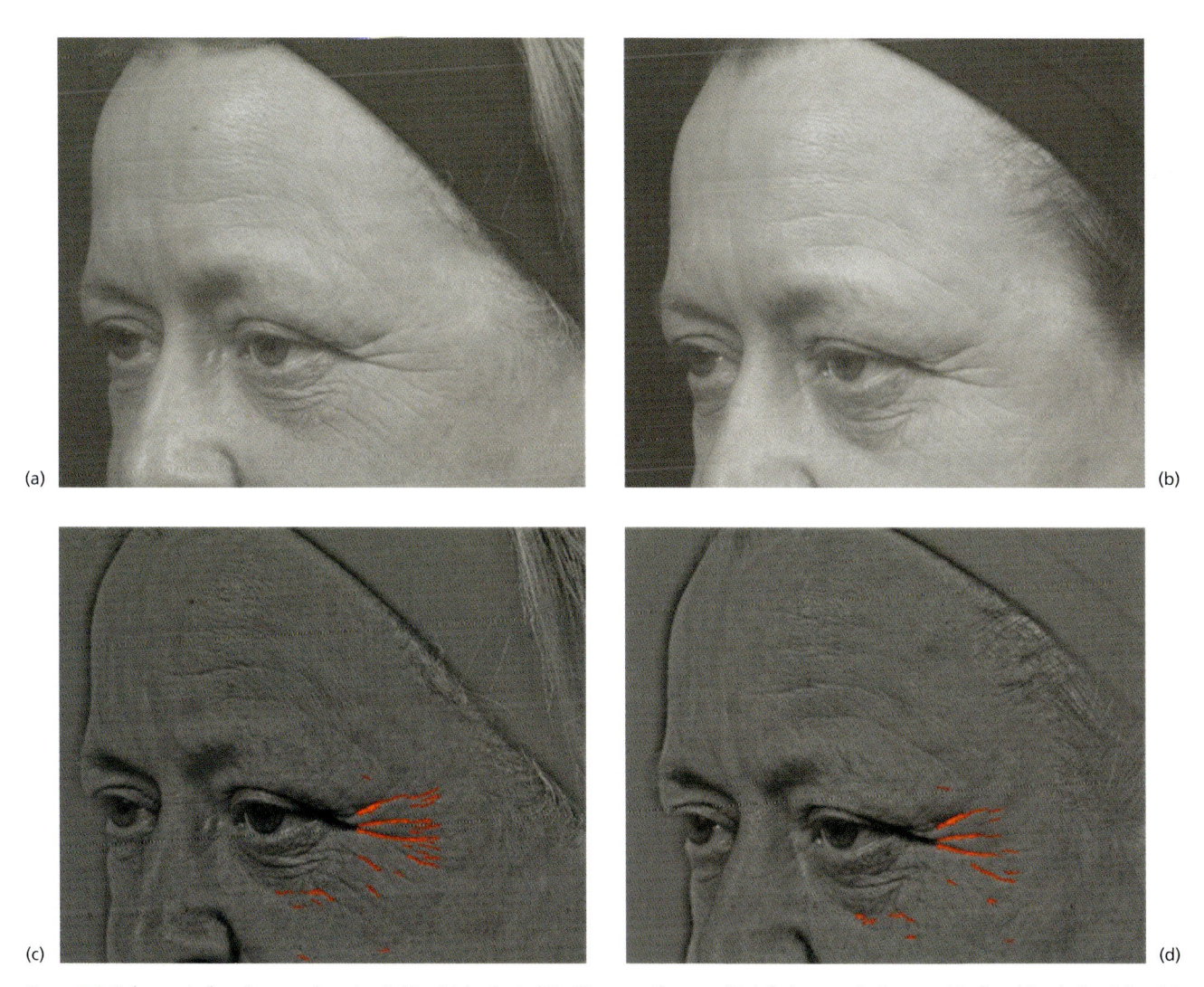

Figure 5.6 Before and after photographs using Raking Light Optical Profilometry. Top row: Digital photographs from a trial of a subject before (a) and 8 weeks after (b) treatment. Note the improvement in the appearance of wrinkling under the eye. Bottom row: Photographs shows wrinkles and fine lines highlighted in red after SWIRL analysis. (c) Baseline. (d) Eight weeks after. The area of interest (AOIs) were + located in each digital image by using anatomic landmarks as anchors.

RLOP technology and SWIRL method complement and support the results of clinical grading of fine line and wrinkles. They have several advantages over traditional optical profilometry on silicone replicas.

These advantages include:
- RLOP and SWIRL can be performed on multiple sites on the face using a single digital photograph.
- RLOP technology and SWIRL method allow for precise location of the area of interest in each digital photograph through imaging software.
- Digital images can be archived electronically for an indefinite period of time.
- Results are expressed in meaningful units and endpoints.
- The area of interest is significantly larger than can be captured in a replica impression.
- RLOP and SWIRL can measure the full length of a wrinkle unlike traditional optical profilometry which limits the measured area to the size of the replica impression.

A non-invasive method for assessing the antioxidant protection of topical formulations in humans

It is well-documented that the addition of antioxidants such as vitamins C, E, and A to skin care formulation can be beneficial in preventing and minimizing skin damage associated with UV light [20–22]. Manufacturers often face a difficult task when formulating with antioxidants, because they are easily destroyed or altered by oxidation which can occur during product manufacturing, filling, or storage.

To address these concerns, Pinnell and colleagues developed a human antioxidant assay which assesses the potential of topical antioxidants to enter into the skin and provide adequate protection against UV damage generated by a solar simulator. Antioxidants provide protection from UVR-induced damage by diminishing or blocking the formation of reactive oxygen species which is clinically manifested by erythema [22].

The technique involves the open applications of antioxidant products and a vehicle control to the demarcated areas on the lower back of subjects for four consecutive days. On day 3 the minimal erythema dose (MED) is determined for each subject. This is the dose of UV light that produces slight redness on fair-skinned individuals.

On day 4, the demarcated sites treated with the antioxidant product, vehicle control, and an untreated site receive solar-simulated UV irritation of 1–5X MED at 1X MED intervals. On day 5, the erythema level of each site can be assessed and the investigator has the option of collecting punch biopsies at the treatment sites and analyzing the tissues for multiple biomarkers such as thymine dimers, interleukins, metaloproteins, Langerhans cells (CD1a), p53, and sunburn cells [17,18]. Traditionally, erythema level can be qualitatively graded or quantitatively measured using the Minolta Chromameter or Mexameter. To maintain accuracy of the measurements, both instruments must be appropriately calibrated and care must be taken to measurement same anatomical location with the light pressure of the instrument to the skin surface so as not to cause skin blanching. Both instruments can only sample a small area of the skin which sometimes may not be representative of the total required assessment area. In order to avoid these issues, Pinnell and colleagues adopted using digital images taken using cross-polarized photography to assess the erythema level.

Figure 5.7 shows a pattern of UV responses for a site treated with an antioxidant and a site treated with a vehicle control. Using image analysis, the regular RGB photos can be converted to Lab color space, allowing accurate determination of the "a*" (degree of redness according to the CIE color standard) value of each irradiated spot. The result can then be used to calculate a protection factor for the antioxidant product (Table 5.2).

Using this technique, Pinnell and associates have been able to formulate a third generation antioxidant product that provides protection against the damaging effects of UV light. The formulation containing 15% ascorbic acid, 1% alfa-tocopherol, and 0.5% ferulic acid was found to be effective in reducing thymine dimers known to be associated with skin cancer [23,24].

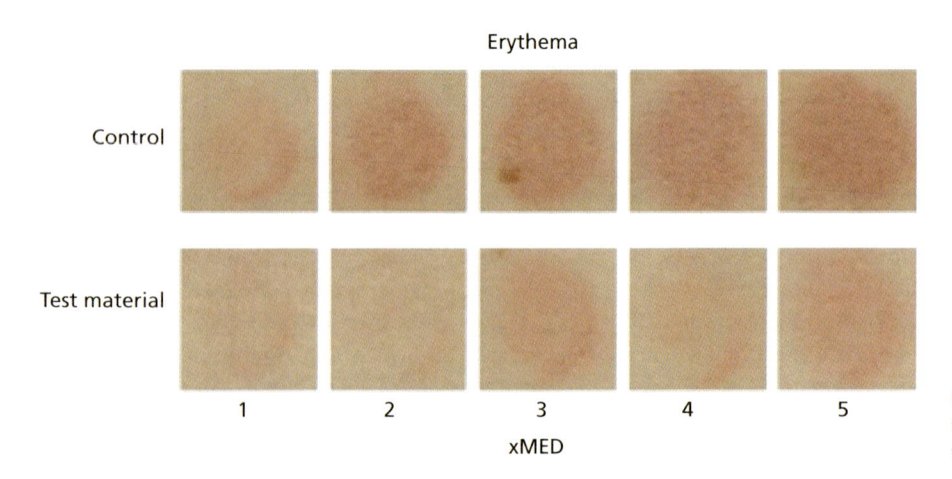

Figure 5.7 Pattern of UV responses for a site treated with an antioxidant and a site treated with a vehicle control.

Table 5.2 Results of theoretical antioxidant protection factor calculations.

	Increase from unexposed (adjusted for MED)	Protection factor (%)
No treatment (control)	10.50	0.0
Antioxidant	6.30	40.0
Vehicle control	10.23	2.6

MED, minimal erythema dose.

Use of image analysis for assessing a variety of skin conditions

At Stephens & Associates, Inc. we have combined the various photography techniques with image analysis methods to provide objective and quantitative analyses for assessing a variety of skin conditions and supporting a wide range of clinical claims. Table 5.3 lists the image analysis tools we have developed so far.

Various other methods of image analysis for photoaging and other skin features have been developed in recent years by many research companies including P&G and Amway. In order for these methods to work well in support of clinical claims, correct photography technique and high precision digital photos are a must. In addition, these methods need to be tested and validated through large clinical trials.

Emerging technology for skin imaging and assessment

Clinical studies demand more objective, quantitative, and non-invasive tools for skin assessments. There are three areas that are of particular interest. First, devices that allow visualization of skin structure underneath the skin surface. Second, imaging of the skin in 3-dimensions. Third, quantitative assessment of skin radiance. In this section of the chapter we highlight several emerging technologies and methodologies.

SIAScope (MedX Health) is a device based on the spectrophotometric intracutaneous analysis method pioneered by Dr. Cotton [25]. The light can penetrate about 2 millimeters deep into the skin and remitted light is analyzed to differentiate chromophores and assess the quantity of melanin, hemoglobin, and collagen (Figure 5.8). This device has been used for diagnostic of melanomas but its application in clinical trials is at the beginning stage.

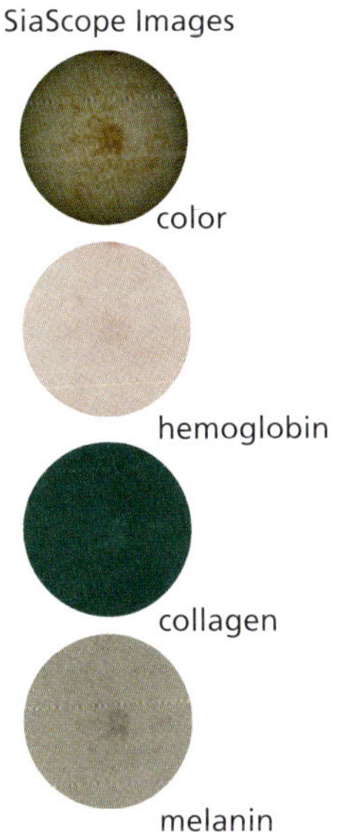

Figure 5.8 An example of images captured using SiaScope.

Table 5.3 Image analysis tools developed by Stephens & Associates, Inc.

Feature of interest	Photography lighting	Analysis and output parameters
Wrinkles/fine lines	Raking	SWIRL: wrinkle count, length, width, area, relative depth
Hyperpigmentation	Cross polarized, UV	Hyperpigmentation: count of pigmented spots, area, and average size UV damage: number of damaged area and total area covered by UV damage
Skin tone evenness	Cross polarized	Skin tone evenness index
Skin brightness	Cross polarized	Skin brightness index L*
Pore	Cross polarized Parallel polarized	Pores: number of pores, area, and relative depth
Oily skin	Parallel polarized	Oily skin: percentage of area with oily skin
Makeup removal	UV	Bare face: percentage of makeup removed
Acne	Cross polarized	Erythema: a*
UV protection	Cross polarized	Erythema: a* and protection factor
Eczema	Cross polarized	Erythema: a*
Lip	Visible	Lip wrinkle analysis: wrinkle count, length, width, area, and relative depth

Note: L* and a* are coordinates in the CIELAB colorimetric system where L* is the total quantity of light reflected or skin brightness (described as light, dark, etc.) and a* represents color ranging from red (positive values) to green (negative values).

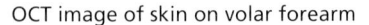

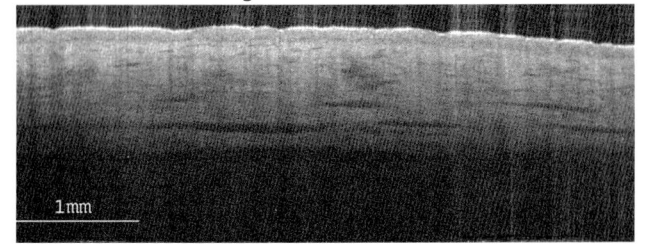

Figure 5.9 An example of images taken using VivoSight.

A non-invasive method for reviewing sub-layers or the cellular structure of the skin would be helpful to reveal changes happening underneath the surface of the skin and provide insight on product functions. VivoSight (Michelson Diagnostics) is a device based on optical coherence tomography (OCT) technology. It converts reflected light from a laser beam into images of skin layers with axial resolution less than 7.5 micrometers (Figure 5.9). VivaScope (Caliber ID) is a confocal laser scanning microscope that reveals the cellular structure underneath the skin with axial resolution of less than 5 micrometers. Both devices are great research tools; however, image analysis and result interpretation is convoluted at current stage.

To capture skin sagging conditions and wrinkle depth it is best to use a 3D imaging system. There are several 3D imaging systems on the market, such as PRIMOS (Canfield), Antera 3D (Miravex), and Clarity Research 3D (BPBT). The PRIMOS and Clarity Research 3D systems utilize photo booths designed for the face, while Antera 3D is a handheld device with flexibility on the target area. As with 2D imaging, subject positioning is the key for consistent assessment using the 3D imaging system.

Skin radiance is an important attribute for photoaging; however it is also the most difficult attribute to quantify. There are two papers aimed at dissecting the definition of skin radiance and proposing different ways to quantify skin radiance [26,27]. This is definitely an area which deserves further research and exploration.

Conclusions

Photography and other non-invasive techniques are important to assess the efficacy and safety of cosmetic products. Often, the non-invasive assessments provide confirmation of the expert grader assessments. It is reassuring to see consistency within the data sets to confirm a positive effect of cosmetics and skin care products. This validation technique is necessary to truly evaluate products. This chapter presents several cutaneous research tools.

References

1 Rizer RL, Sigler ML, Miller DL. (1999) Evaluating performance benefits of conditioning formulations on human skin. In: SchuellerR, RomanowskiP, eds. *Conditioning Agents for Hair and Skin*, pp. 345–51.
2 Carruthers A, Carruthers J, Hardas B, Kaur M, Goertelmeyer R, et al. (2008) A validated grading scale for crow's feet. *Dermatol Surg* **34** Suppl 2, S173–8.
3 Fitzpatrick RE, Goldman MP, Satur NM, Tope WD. (1996) Pulsed carbon dioxide laser resurfacing of photo-aged facial skin. *Arch Dermatol* **132**(4), 395–402.
4 Griffiths CEM, Wang TS, Hamilton TA, Voorhees JJ, Ellis CN. (1992) A photonumeric scale for the assessment of cutaneous photodamage. *Arch Dermatol* 128(3), 347–51.
5 Kappes UP. (2004) Skin ageing and wrinkles: clinical and photographic scoring. *J Cosmet Dermatol* **3**(1), 23–5.
6 Elsner P, Berardcsa E, Wilhelm KP, Maibach HI. (1995) Bioengineering of the Skin: Methods and Instrumentation. London: Taylor & Francis.
7 Berardesca E. (1997) EEMCO guidance for the assessment of stratum corneum hydration: electrical methods. *Skin Res Technol* **3**, 126–32.
8 Elsner P, Barel AO, Berardesca B, Gabard B, Serup J. (1998) *Skin Bioengineering*. Basel; New York: Karger.
9 Flosh PJ, Kligman AM. (1993) *Non-Invasive Methods for the Quantification of Skin Functions*. New York: Springler-Verlag.
10 Serup J, Jemec GBE. (1995) *Handbook of Non-Invasive Method and the Skin*. Boca Raton, FL: CRC Press.
11 Elsner P, Berardcsa E, Wilhelm KP, Maibach HI. (2006) *Bioengineering of the Skin: Skin Biomechanics*. Boca Raton, FL: CRC Press.
12 Elsner P, Berardesca E, Wilhelm KP. (2006) *Bioengineering of the Skin: Skin Imaging and Analysis*, 2nd edn. Informaworld (London: Taylor & Francis).
13 Stack LB, Storrow AB, Morris MA, Patton DR. (1999) *Handbook of Medical Photography*. Philadelphia, PA: Hanley & Belfus, pp. 15–20.
14 . Ratner D, Thomas CO, Bickers D. (1999) The use of digital photography in dermatology. *J Am Acad Dermatol* **41**, 749–56.
15 Phillips SB, Kollias N, Gillies R, Muccini A, Drake LA. (1997) Polarized light photography enhances visualization of inflammatory lesions of acne vulgaris. *J Am Acad Dermatol* **37**, 948–52.
16 Rizova E, Kligman A. (2001) New photographic technique for clinical evaluation of acne. *J Eur Acad Dermatol Venereol* **15** (Suppl 3), 13–8.
17 Pagnoni A, Kilgman AM, Kollias N, Goldberg S, Stoudemeyer T. (1999) Digital fluorescence photography can assess the suppressive effect of benzoyl peroxide on Propionibacterium acnes. *J Am Acad Dermatol* **41**, 710–6.
18 Grove GL, Grove MJ, Leyden JJ. (1989) Optical profilometry: an objective method for quantification of facial wrinkles. *J Am Acad Dermatol* **21**, 631–7.
19 Jiang LI, Stephens TJ, Goodman R. (2013) SWIRL, a clinically validated, objective, and quantitative method for facial wrinkle assessment. *Skin Res Technol* **19**(4), 492–8.
20 Rabe JH, Mamelak AJ, EcElgunn JS, Morrison WL, Sauder DN. (2006) Photoaging: mechanisms and repair. *J Am Acad Dermatol* **55**, 1–19.

21 Dreher F, Denig N, Gabard B, Schwindt Da, Maibach MI. (1999) Effect of topical antioxidants on UV-induced erythema formation when administered after exposure. *Dermatology* **198**, 52–5.

22 Pinnell SR. (2003) Cutaneous photodamage, oxidative stress and topical antioxidant protection. *J Am Acad Dermatol* **48**(1), 1–19.

23 Murray JC, Burch JA, Streilein RD, Iannacchione MA, Hall RP, Pinnell SR. (2008) Atopical antioxidant solution containing vitamins C and E stabilized by ferulic acid provides protection for human skin against damage caused by ultraviolet irradiation. *J Am Acad Dermatol* **59**, 418–25.

24 Oresajo C, Stephens T, Hino PD, Law RM, Yatskayer M, Foltis P, et al. (2008) Protective effects of a topical antioxidant mixture containing vitamin C, and phloretin against ultraviolet-induced photodamage in human skin. *J Cosmet Dermatol* **7**, 290–7.

25 Matts PJ, Cotton SD. (2009) Spectrophotometric Intracutaneous Analysis (SIAscopy). In: BarelAO, PayeM and MaibachHI, eds. *Handbook of Cosmetic Science and Technology*, 3rd edn, Chapter 25. Oxford: OUP.

26 Petitjean A, Sainthillier JM, Mac-Mary S, Muret P, Closs B, Gharbi T, Humbert P. (2007) Skin radiance: how to quantify? Validation of an optical method. *Skin Res Technol.* **13**(1), 2–8.

27 Matsubara A, Liang Z, Sato Y, Uchikawa K. (2012) Analysis of human perception of facial skin radiance by means of image histogram parameters of surface and subsurface reflections from the skin. *Skin Res Technol.* **18**(3), 265–71.

CHAPTER 6
Contact Dermatitis and Topical Agents

David E. Cohen, Alexandra Price, and Sarika Ramachandran
The Ronald O. Perelman Department of Dermatology, New York University School of Medicine, New York, NY, USA

> **BASIC CONCEPTS**
> - Hypersensitivity reactions can occur in response to topical agents.
> - Adverse reactions can include irritant contact dermatitis and allergic contact dermatitis.
> - Patch testing is a reliable method for determining the etiology of adverse reactions to topical products.
> - Treatment of hypersensitivity reactions involves prompt recognition with identification and withdrawal of the offending agent.

Introduction

Topical cosmetic medications, cosmeceuticals, and minimally invasive cosmetic procedures play an important role in dermatologic practice. Recent advances have led to a tremendous expansion in the repertory of non-surgical cosmetic treatment modalities. In addition, the wide use of cosmetics and skin care products worldwide increases the possibility of exposure to irritants and contact allergens [1]. Adverse skin reactions to cosmetics include irritant contact dermatitis, allergic contact dermatitis, phototoxic dermatitis, contact urticaria, and foreign body reactions [2,3]. The clinician should be aware of these potential skin reactions and seek to identify the causative agents and other contributing factors. Most of these reactions are treatable without sequelae once the offending agent is recognized and avoided [2].

Approximately 15 million Americans are diagnosed with contact dermatitis [2]. Among patch-tested patients with suspected allergic contact dermatitis, cosmetic agents are implicated in 4% to 9% of cases [4]. Women between 20–55 years of age are most affected by cosmetic contact dermatitis [4–6]. The US Food and Drug Administration (FDA) regulations on cosmetics are based on two important laws: the Federal Food, Drug, and Cosmetic Act (FD&C) which prohibits the marketing of adulterated or misbranded cosmetics, and the Fair Packaging and Labeling Act (FPLA) which states that improperly labeled or deceptively packaged products are subject to regulatory action [7]. Ingredient labeling is mandatory in the USA and Europe, and compounds are listed in descending order of amount using the nomenclature format of the International Cosmetic Ingredient Dictionary [8,9]. Currently, listing specific fragrance allergens is voluntary, which allows cosmetic manufacturers to include individual fragrances under a generic "fragrance" listing [10]. With the exception of color additives, cosmetic products and ingredients are not subjected to FDA premarket approval and manufacturers' reporting of adverse reactions is a voluntary process [7]. In order to review the safety of the cosmetic ingredients, the Cosmetic, Toiletries and Fragrance Association (CTFA) sponsors the Cosmetic Ingredient Review (CIR). In 2012, CIR identified eleven ingredients that were unsafe for use in cosmetics [11]. In addition, CIR identified 38 ingredients that were not supported for use in cosmetics [11]. The Safe Cosmetics and Personal Care Products Act introduced to Congress in March of 2013 seeks to greatly expand FDA oversight of chemicals in cosmetic products. This legislation would require companies to report adverse events and demonstrate that cosmetics meet safety standards prior to marketing [12,13]. Reactions to cosmetics can present with a wide range of clinical signs. Therefore, it is important for the clinician to be familiar with the diversity of these presentations to enable prompt diagnosis and treatment.

Pathophysiology and clinical presentation

Irritant contact dermatitis

Most skin reactions to cosmetics are classified as irritant contact dermatitis (ICD) [8]. Irritant contact dermatitis is caused by endogenous and environmental factors and is defined as local inflammation that is not initially mediated by the immune system. The three main pathophysiological changes observed are stratum corneum disruption, epidermal cellular changes, and proinflammatory cytokine release [14]. Ceramides, a major

---

Cosmetic Dermatology: Products and Procedures, Second Edition. Edited by Zoe Diana Draelos.
© 2016 John Wiley & Sons, Ltd. Published 2016 by John Wiley & Sons, Ltd.

component of the stratum corneum, play a key role in the protection against irritants [15]. Repeated exposure to irritants disrupts the epidermal barrier and increases transepidermal water loss [16]. The severity of irritant dermatitis depends on the chemical properties, amount and strength of the agent, and length and frequency of exposure. Repetitive exposures even to mild agents, such as soaps and detergents, can result in irritant dermatitis. In addition, harsh scrubbing with mechanical assistance (brushes, synthetic sponges, or cosmetics containing microabrasive spheres) increases the risk of irritation. Psychiatric disorders leading to obsessive-compulsive skin cleansing can also damage the barrier function of the skin and cause irritant dermatitis [17]. Predisposing factors for the development of irritant dermatitis also include endogenous disorders, such as atopic dermatitis and filaggrin gene defects [18].

Allergic contact dermatitis

Allergic contact dermatitis (ACD) comprises a substantial number of cases of contact dermatitis and represents a true delayed-type (type IV) immune reaction. Previous exposure and sensitization to the causative agent is necessary [2]. Chemical agents act as haptens, which are small electrophilic molecules that bind to carrier proteins and penetrate the stratum corneum barrier of the skin. The antigen-presenting cells (APCs) of the skin (Langerhans cells and/or dermal dendritic cells) digest and display the hapten-protein complex on their surface for presentation to T lymphocytes. The hapten-specific T lymphocytes differentiate into memory T cells, which then undergo clonal expansion. The clinical manifestations of ACD are mediated by the activation of hapten-specific memory T cells in the skin upon re-exposure to the offending allergen.

Sensitization depends on product composition, the potency of the sensitizer, the amount of product applied, the frequency and duration of application, and the physical integrity of the epidermal barrier [19,20]. Filaggrin gene mutation carriers with concurrent atopic dermatitis or hand eczema have an increased risk of developing contact sensitization [21].

While there are no pathognomonic features that unequivocally distinguish ACD and ICD, there are certain clinical features that favor ACD over ICD. While itching can be present in both conditions, it is a key symptom in ACD [22] whereas burning, stinging, soreness, and pain are more characteristic of ICD [22]. ACD occurs upon re-exposure to the allergen following an initial phase of sensitization, whereas ICD is not predicated on prior sensitization and can occur on first exposure to the causative agent [23]. Peak reaction occurs slower in ACD (within 3–4 days) than in acute ICD (within minutes to hours), whereas chronic ICD develops gradually after repeated exposure to milder irritants [22]. The clinical distinction between irritant and allergic dermatitis can be challenging because both conditions can result in eczematous reactions. Clinical manifestations range from mild erythema and scaling with minimal itch to highly pruritic vesicular, bullous, and lichenified plaques. Furthermore, the two conditions can sometimes be superimposed since an irritated and impaired epidermal barrier can facilitate the absorption of haptens that can elicit an immune response in susceptible individuals.

Phototoxic dermatitis

Phytophotodermatitis is a non-immunologic phototoxic skin eruption caused by topical exposure to plant-derived photosensitizing compounds and subsequent exposure to ultraviolet (UV) light. Furocoumarins (psoralens and angelicins) are the most common photosensitizing chemical agents [24]. Plant families that produce these compounds include the Apiaceae (parsley, celery), Rutaceae (citrus fruits), Moraceae (figs), and Fabaceae (peas). Long-wave UVA radiation (340–400 nm) is responsible for the majority of phototoxic reactions resulting in phytophotodermatitis [3]. The skin eruption of phytophotodermatitis occurs on sun-exposed areas in contact with plants containing these photosensitizing compounds [25]. Marked hyperpigmentation, usually in a bizarre configuration or linear pattern, is often the dominant physical finding on clinical presentation. Occasionally, bullous and vesicular lesions can also develop. These phototoxic reactions cause both DNA interstrand crosslinking between UVA activated psoralens and the pyrimidine bases of DNA and cellular membrane damage [26,27].

Contact urticaria

Contact urticaria syndrome is divided into immunologic and non-immunologic subtypes. Non-immunologic contact urticaria is the most common form and occurs in the absence of previous exposure. Localized wheals appear within 30–60 minutes of exposure and are not followed by systemic symptoms. Allergic contact urticaria is an immediate-type (type I) hypersensitivity reaction and occurs in sensitized individuals within minutes to hours following exposure to the allergen. The binding between allergens and immunoglobulin E (IgE) triggers mast cell degranulation and subsequent release of inflammatory products, such as histamine, prostaglandins, leukotrienes, and cytokines. As a consequence, individuals experience erythema, swelling, and pruritus, which may be localized (wheals and fares) or generalized (angioedema, conjunctivitis, bronchoconstriction, hypotension). Severe reactions may be fatal.

Foreign body reactions

Injectable fillers are a group of exogenous substances used for soft tissue augmentation. Fillers are subdivided into agents that are degradable (hyaluronic acid, poly-L-lactic acid, calcium hydroxylapatite) and non-degradable (polymethylmethacrylate and silicone). Some injectable agents such as hyaluronic acids restore volume primarily through their space-filling effects. Others, including silicone, calcium hydroxylapatite, polymethylmethacrylate and poly-L-lactic acid fillers, act as scaffolds for endogenous collagen formation. Adverse immunologic reactions have been reported with practically all the products used. The frequency and degree of these reactions varies based on filler material, injection technique, and host immunologic response.

The normal initial host response to foreign body implantation is the formation of a blood-based matrix on and around the biomaterial, called the provisional matrix. The tissue injury may also lead to activation of the innate immune response and thrombus formation. The provisional matrix is rich in mitogens, chemoattractants, growth factors, and cytokines, providing an excellent medium both for wound healing and foreign body reaction. Acute inflammation is characterized by the presence of neutrophils, mast cell degranulation, and fibrinogen adsorption. The degree of the inflammation is highly dependent upon the injury produced, the site of injection, the material used, and the extent of the provisional matrix formed. The acute phase is followed by a chronic phase inflammatory response, which is characterized by the presence of monocytes, lymphocytes, and plasma cells. After resolution of the acute and chronic phases of inflammation, granulation tissue formation and neovascularization in the new healing tissue ensue [28]. A prolonged inflammatory phase (i.e. longer than 3 weeks) should prompt an investigation to exclude complications, such as infection, allergic reaction, migration, abscess formation, or granulomatous reaction [29]. Foreign body granulomatous reactions have been reported with the use of hyaluronic acid, poly-L-lactic acid, silicone, and other fillers [30]. Biofilm formation, protein impurities, microsphere irregularities have been implicated in causing local granulomatous reactions to fillers [29-31]. Granulomatous reactions are delayed reactions that occur as a result of ineffective phagocytosis. An organized collection of epitheloid macrophages wall off the foreign material with a surrounding infiltrate of lymphocytes. The surrounding lymphocytes secrete a variety of cytokines that cause ongoing macrophage activation and recruitment of inflammatory cells [32]. Clinically, foreign body granulomatous reactions develop over a variable period of time ranging from 5 months to 15 years [33]. Clinical manifestations can include swelling and indurated papules, nodules, or plaques (with or without ulceration). Although rare, granulomatous reactions have been reported to migrate beyond the injection site [34].

Common irritants and allergen groups

Irritants

In the clinical setting, irritant substances are used to treat acne, hyperpigmentation and sun damaged skin. The depth of penetration varies with the agent, the concentration of the agent, and time of exposure. A myriad of "peeling" agents include retinoic, glycolic, trichloroacetic and salicylic acids, resorcinol, and phenol. Irritant reactions and photosensitivity manifested by erythema, scaling and irritation can also occur following the use of topical retinoids. Decreasing the frequency of application and applying a barrier moisturizer along with a sunscreen may improve tolerance [35].

A wide variety of substances can act as irritants given sufficient exposure time and/or concentration (Table 6.1). Mechanical, chemical, and environmental factors can act alone or in combination to produce skin irritation. Mechanical factors include

Table 6.1 List of common skin irritants: mechanical, chemical, and environmental factors known to cause irritant dermatitis. The agents can act alone or in combination to produce contact dermatitis, therefore recognition of all factors involved is crucial for proper management of patients.

Mechanical	Chemical	Environmental
Shaving	Water (wet work)	Excessive heat or sun exposure
Waxing	Alkalis (soaps and cleansers)	Food handling
Laser treatment	Detergents	Saunas andjacuzzis (chlorine)
Abrasive scrubs	Surfactants (sodium lauryl sulfate)	Extreme cold and windburn
Dermabrasion	Whitening agents	Stress
Microdermabrasion	Acids (salicylic, glycolic, tricholoracetic acid)	Dry air
Rubbing of the skin (e.g. when using a soap or scrubbing)	Fragrances and color additives	Hot and/or prolonged showers
Skin cleansing tools (face brushes, synthetic sponges, loofahs)	Sunscreens	Spicy foods, peppers, condiments
Closed-weave face cloths	Oxidizing agents (sodium hypochlorite (bleach) or benzoyl peroxide)	Increased humidity (e.g. sweating from prolonged wearing of occlusive gloves)
Friction (wool, synthetic fibers, or jewelry)	Solvents (benzene, toluene, acetone, alcohol)	Low humidity (air conditioning)
Intense exercise	Vitamin A derivatives (retinoids, retinol)	
Plant parts (thorns, spines, and sharp-edged leaves)		
Microtrauma (fiberglass)		
Pressure (spectacle frames)		
Occlusion tight clothes, rubber/latex gloves		

cosmetic procedures (shaving, waxing, laser therapy, cleansing, dermabrasion), personal habits (excessive rubbing of the skin with soaps, scrubs, wearing tight clothes or shoes, intense exercise), and occupational exposure (latex gloves, microtrauma of the skin). Wet work (i.e. skin exposure to liquids or use of occlusive gloves for longer than two hours per day or frequent hand cleaning) is one of the most common and important causes of skin irritation [36]. Professions at risk include hairdressers, healthcare workers, and food handlers.

The list of the chemical compounds capable of producing irritation of the skin is extensive. Some substances are considered universal irritants. For example, strong acids (hydrofluoric, hydrochloric, sulfuric, nitric acids) and strong caustics (sodium hydroxide, potassium hydroxide) produce severe burns even in brief and small exposures. Solvents, including alcohol, turpentine, ketones, and xylene, remove lipids from the skin, producing direct irritation and facilitating irritant reactions from other substances such as soap and water. Inappropriate skin cleansing with solvents to remove grease, paints, or oils is a common cause of skin irritation. Alkali substances such as soaps are more likely to produce irritation by disrupting the skin barrier, whereas cleansing agents with a pH of approximately 5.5 and alcohol-based hand-cleansing gels are less irritating and preferred for sensitive skin.

Environmental elements such as dry air, extremes of temperature, and weather variations may render the skin more susceptible to cutaneous irritants. Food allergies may cause urticarial reactions; spicy foods and condiments may cause lip and perioral irritant dermatitis. Prolonged exposure to water can cause maceration and desiccation of the skin.

Follicular plugging has been reported secondary to use of isopropyl myristate, an emollient and lubricant used in shaving lotions, shampoos, oils, and deodorants [37]. Sodium lauryl sulfate (SLS), a surfactant found in many topical medications including those for acne, has also been used to study the effects of sequential exposure to irritants on skin barrier function [38].

Subjective irritation, described as a tingling, burning, stinging, or itching sensation without visible skin alteration is also observed following application of topical medications. Propylene glycol, hydroxy acids, and ethanol are capable of eliciting sensory irritation in susceptible individuals. Commonly used medications such as benzoic acid, azelaic acid, lactic acid, benzoyl peroxide, mequinol, and tretinoin can elicit sensory irritation. Sorbic acid is an organic compound used as a preservative in concentrations up to 0.2% in foods, cosmetics, and drugs. Subjective irritation has been demonstrated with 0.5% sorbic acid and to 1% benzoic acid in susceptible individuals [39].

"Sensitive skin" or cosmetic intolerance syndrome is a condition of cutaneous hyperreactivity secondary to substances that are not defined as irritants [40]. The condition encompasses a complex combination of objective and subjective irritative symptoms and may coexist with underlying allergic processes, urticarial reactions, and/or photodermatitis. Endogenous causes include seborrheic dermatitis, psoriasis, rosacea/perioral dermatitis, atopic dermatitis, and body dysmorphobia. Elimination of all cosmetic products for an extended period of time (6–12 months) followed by slow reintroduction (a new product every 2–3 weeks) is helpful when managing cosmetic intolerance syndrome.

Fragrances

Fragrances are a common cause of cosmetic dermatitis. Allergic reactions to fragrances affect 1.7% to 4.1% of the general population [41]. The eruption can be restricted to areas of application (face, neck, hands, axillae) or it can present as a generalized dermatitis. *Myroxylon pereira* (balsam of Peru) should be considered as a potential allergen in patients presenting with a generalized dermatitis [42].

Products containing scents are ubiquitous and include cosmetics, topical medications, toiletries, cleansers, and household cleaning products. The cosmetic products most commonly associated with allergy to fragrances in descending order include deodorants, scented lotions, and fine fragrances [43,44].

In 2005, the European Union mandated that 26 fragrance ingredients known to cause contact allergy be listed individually on the label of cosmetic products sold in Europe [45]. Only eight of these fragrance ingredients are included in fragrance mix I (FM I) and six in fragrance mix II (FM II) (Table 6.2). Patch testing to these 26 fragrances was performed to investigate the frequency of sensitization to these allergens and to assess their importance as screening markers for fragrance hypersensitivity [45]. Patch testing with FM 1, FM 2, balsam of Peru, and hydroxyisohexyl 3-cyclohexene carboxaldehyde (HICC) in the European baseline series failed to detect 12% of those with fragrance hypersensitivity. Non-immunologic contact urticaria reactions can also be triggered by fragrances that contain cinnamaldehyde, a pale yellow, viscous liquid extracted from the oil of cinnamon, or from balsams such as styrax.

According to the North American Contact Dermatitis Group (NACDG), the prevalence of positive patch test reactions to fragrances in the United States is approximately 20%, with positive patch test results to FM I in 8.5% of cases, *Myroxylon pereira* in 7.2% of cases, and FM II in 4.7% of cases [46]. Since FM II has been added to the NACDG standard screening series, the incidence of reactivity to this fragrance screening panel has been increasing while reactivity to FM I and balsam of Peru has been decreasing [46]. Changes in the frequency of sensitization to specific fragrances highlight the importance of continually reviewing and updating patch test screening markers and patch testing with individual fragrance ingredients in suspected cases of fragrance allergy.

Preservatives

Preservative allergy is a common cause of skin care product allergy [47]. Preservatives are low molecular weight, biologically active compounds that prevent product contamination and degradation by microorganisms. The shift from organic solvents and mineral oils to water-based products in the cosmetic

Table 6.2 List of the 26 fragrances that must be specified on the labels of cosmetic products, according to the seventh amendment to the European Directive on Cosmetic Products

International Nomenclature of Cosmetic Ingredients Name
Alpha-isomethyl ionone
Alpha-Amyl cinnamaldehyde[a]
Anisyl alcohol
Benzyl alcohol
Benzyl benzoate
Benzyl cinnamate
Benzyl salicylate
Butylphenylmethylpropional
Cinnamaldehyde[a]
Cinnamylalcohol[a]
Citral[b]
Citronellol[b]
Coumarin[b]
Eugenol[a]
Everniafurfuracea (tree moss)
Everniaprunastri[a] (oak moss)
Farnesol[b]
Geraniol[a]
Hexyl cinnamal[b]
Hydroxycitronellal[a]
Hydroxyisohexyl 3-cyclohexane carboxaldehyde (HICC)[b]
Isoeugenol[a]
Linalool
Limonene
Methyl 2 octynoate

[1]Fragrance ingredients constituting fragrance mix I.
[2]Fragrance ingredients constituting fragrance mix II.

industry has increased the need for preservatives. Allergic contact dermatitis due to preservatives most commonly affects the face, neck, hands, and axillae but also can occur in a generalized distribution.

Formaldehyde allergy is common and is most often caused by formaldehyde-releasing biocides in cosmetics, toiletries, and other products. In the USA, approximately 20% of cosmetics and personal care products contain a formaldehyde-releaser (quaternium-15, imidazolidinyl urea, diazolinyl urea, DMDM-hydantoin, and 2-bromo-2-nitropropane-1,3,-diol) [48]. In Europe, formaldehyde releasers are contained in approximately 8% of cosmetic products, often in combination with other preservatives such as parabens and phenoxyethanol [49]. In a review of 81 formaldehyde-allergic patients, allergic reaction to at least one of the 12 formaldehyde-releasing substances were detected in 79% of the cases and isolated reactions to releasers were rare [50]. Although the role of contact allergy in atopic dermatitis is controversial [51], in one study patients with atopic dermatitis were found to be statistically more likely to have contact hypersensitivity to formaldehyde releasers, but not formaldehyde [52]. Formaldehyde allergy is also reported as a common cause of occupational contact dermatitis. The professions at risk include hairdressers, healthcare workers, painters, photographers, housekeeping personnel, metalworkers, masseurs, and workers dealing with creams, liquid soaps, and detergents [50].

The preservatives methylchloroisothiazolinone (MCI) and methylisothiazolinone (MI) are also important contact allergens. A common preservative in some brands of moist toilet paper (baby wipes and moist towelettes), MCI/MI can cause perianal and perineal allergic contact dermatitis [53]. MCI/MI in fixed combination (MCI/MI at a ratio of 3:1) is widely used for the preservation of aqueous systems in cosmetics, toiletries, and several industrial applications. Despite European restrictions on the use of the mixture of methylchloroisothiazolinone and methylisothiazolinone (MCI/MI) the frequency of positive patch test reactions to MCI/MI has not decreased [54]. Factors that increase the risk of sensitization include chronic dermatitis and the frequent use of leave-on products containing MCI/MI [55]. MI without MCI has also increasingly been used as a preservative in cosmetics and skin care products [56,57]. Standard patch testing screening misses approximately 33% to 60% cases of allergy to MI likely due to the low concentration of MI in the MCI/MI combination patch test [58–60].

Parabens are also one of the most frequently used preservatives in cosmetics. Parabens are present in approximately 40% of European cosmetic products, including make-up, facemasks, hair cleansing products, and liquid soaps [61,62]. Despite their common use, these compounds are weak sensitizers at the usual concentrations of 0.1–0.3% and are uncommon causes of contact dermatitis. Some patients sensitized to paraben-containing medications can use cosmetic products containing parabens with no adverse effects [63]. However, parabens may have a greater sensitization potential when used on previously damaged or broken skin. A multicenter study in patients suffering from chronic leg ulcers suggested paraben sensitivity in 3% of patients [64].

Preservatives are also commonly implicated in allergy to ophthalmic preparations. Phenylmercuric acetate has been implicated as a leading preservative allergen, although it has been suggested that positive patch tests are due to an irritant reaction rather than true contact allergy [65]. In contact lens solutions, previously thimerosal was one of the most frequent positive patch tested preservatives. However, it has been largely replaced by benzalkonium chloride (BAK) [66]. Eyelid dermatitis can be triggered by allergens in ophthalmic products but occurs more commonly as a result of sensitization to environmental allergens [65]. Young females with skin atopy and allergies to cosmetic and skin care products, as well as older subjects with allergy to topical medications are particularly at risk for allergic contact dermatitis in the periorbital area [65]. The thinness of periorbital skin makes it particularly susceptible to allergens.

Botanicals

The widespread use of botanicals in topical cosmetics and therapeutic preparations increases the likelihood of exposure to a variety of potential herbal allergens. Botanicals commonly implicated in cosmetic contact allergy include the Compositae family plants, tea tree oil, propolis (honeybee hive derivative), peppermint, lavender, lichens, henna, among others [67,68]. Some plant-derived compounds have the potential to cause phototoxic effects; for example, bergapten (aka 5-methoxysporalen) is a naturally occurring furanocoumarinin bergamot oil that causes phototoxicity [3]. While the International Fragrance Association has set limits on the amount of bergamot oil allowed in leave on products applied to sun-exposed skin, bergamot essential oil remains one of the most widely used ingredients in modern perfumery and there are no restrictions for bergamot in rinse-off products [69]. Bergapten and psoralens in fig leaves used to prepare a homemade tanning lotion have also been reported to cause phytophotodermatitis [70,71].

Specific cosmetic products

Cleansing agents

Washout products are in contact with the skin for brief periods, making detection of allergy to these agents challenging. Cleansers are applied to remove sebum, desquamated cells, sweat, and microorganisms. Allergens in body-cleansing products and facial cleansers include fragrances, preservatives, surfactants (cocamidopropylbetaine), and vehicle components (lanolin alcohols) [72].

Shampoos contain a combination of cleansing agents and surfactants that act to remove sebum, scales, and microorganisms from the hair and scalp. Conditioner agents neutralize static charge and soften the hair. In a database survey of shampoos, the most common allergens found in order of decreasing prevalence were: fragrances, cocamidopropylbetaine, methylchloroisothiazolone and methylisothiazolone (MCI/MI), formaldehyde releasers, propylene glycol, vitamin E, parabens, benzophenones, iodopropynylbutylcarbamate, and methyldibromolutaronitrile/phenoxyethanol [73]. Allergic reactions are less common compared to leave-on products because of the limited amount of time the substance is in contact with the skin. However, cocamidopropylbetaine (surfactant), formaldehyde, and MCI/MI have been reported as causative agents of allergic contact dermatitis in rinse-off agents.

Moisturizers

Moisturizers are an important source of sensitizing allergens due to their widespread use, distribution over large body areas, repeated exposure, and increased penetration due to their frequent use after cleansing [74]. Common allergens include fragrances, preservatives (formaldehyde releasing and non-formaldehyde releasing), vitamin E, essential oils, benzyl alcohol, propylene glycol, and lanolin [75].

Moisturizers/emollients serve to reduce transepidermal water (TEWL) and increase epidermal water content [76]. Emollients and moisturizers that reduce transepidermal water loss by occlusion may contain lanolin and lanolin derivatives [76]. Inflammatory conditions such as stasis dermatoses can be a predisposing factor for allergic contact dermatitis to common moisturizing ingredients such as lanolin and lanolin derivatives [77]. Although moisturizers are often used in treatment of xerosis and atopic dermatitis, these patients may have a greater risk of sensitization to fragrances and other potential allergens due to impaired skin barrier function [78]. Older individuals are also more likely to react to preservative systems in moisturizers (methyldibromo glutaronitrile, quaternium-15, formaldehyde, diazolidinyl urea, and imidazolidinyl urea) as compared to younger individuals [79].

Skin bleaching agents

Skin lightening products contain a variety of active ingredients including hydroquinone, corticosteroids, mercury and cosmeceutical and botanical skin lighteners such as arbutin, kojic acid, licorice, ascorbic acid, soy and retinoids, among others [80,81]. Hydroquinone is a whitening agent present in up to 2% in over-the-counter creams and 4% in prescription bleaching creams. Irritant and allergic reactions, hypopigmentation and hyperpigmentation, and exogenous ochronosis are known side effects [82]. Contact hypersensitivity to monobenzyl ether of hydroquinone and other hydroquinone derivatives have been reported to cause contact allergy in addition to hydroquinone which is a weak sensitizer [83]. Although the FDA prohibits the use of mercury as an active ingredient in cosmetics and limits mercury as an impurity to 1 ppm, mercury in excess of 1000 ppm can be found in 6% of skin lightening products globally and 3.3% of lightening products purchased in the United States [84].

Topical corticosteroids

Topical corticosteroids are used to treat a broad spectrum of dermatologic disorders. Some skin lightening agents may also contain topical corticosteroids such as hydrocortisone and fluocinolone acetonide. Contact allergy to topical steroids has been reported to occur in between 0.2% and 5% of users [85,86]. Topical corticosteroids can be divided into four groups based on stereochemical structure of the steroid moiety: A (hydrocortisone-tixocortol pivalate type), B (triamcinolone acetonide type), C (betamethasone type), and D (hydrocortisone-17 butyrate type) [87]. Group D is divided into two subgroups, D1 (stable esters) and D2 (labile esters). Intragroup cross-reactivity is reported more frequently than intergroup contact reactivity [88]. Group C corticosteroids have the lowest reported rate of allergenicity, however, are the least studied group to date [89]. Non-halogenated topical steroids (hydrocortisone, budesonide) may be more frequent sensitizers than halogenated steroids. Halogenation reduces the ability of the steroid molecule to bind to arginine, which has been shown to be a factor in the allergenicity of corticosteroids [90]. Contact allergy should be considered in patients with dermatitis that fail to respond to appropriate corticosteroid therapy or when a worsening of their skin condition occurs with treatment. Patients reported at greatest risk include those with stasis dermatitis and chronic leg ulcers, followed by those with hand eczema, atopic dermatitis, anogenital, foot, and facial dermatitis [91]. When patch testing with the comprehensive corticosteroid series, the reactions may be delayed due to the corticosteroid's intrinsic anti-inflammatory effects [92].

Hair dyes and bleaches

Hair dyes are classified as semi-permanent and permanent. Semi-permanent dyes are derived from nitroanilines, nitrophenylenediamines, and nitroaminophenols, which use low molecular weight elements that penetrate the hair cuticle. Permanent dyes act by the means of primary intermediates (*p*-phenylenediamine [PPD] or *p*-aminophenol), which are oxidized by hydrogen peroxide and react with different couplers to produce a wide range of colors. Once oxidized to para-benzo-quinonediamine, PPD is no longer allergenic [93]. The distribution of the reaction is often along the hairline, scalp, and face. Consort dermatitis, the presence of the allergic eruption in the partner of the subject using the allergenic substance, has been described for PPD [93]. Oxidative hair dye products often contain other potent skin sensitizers, such as resorcinol, m-Aminophenol, toluene-2,5,-diamine (PTD), 2-methylresorcinol [94]. While the self-test suggested by hair dye industry may provide valuable information about a patient's potential reactivity, it is dependent on the individual's ability to interpret the test [95,96].

Hair bleaches include hydrogen peroxide solutions that oxidize melanin and ammonium persulfate, a very strong oxidizing agent and a radical initiator, which can be used as a booster supplement in hair dyes. Direct contact with these oxidizing agents can cause irritant dermatitis and rarely, chemical burns [97–99]. Type I and IV hypersensitivity reactions to ammonium persulfate have also been reported [99].

Occupational hand eczema among hairdressers and cosmetologists is a significant health problem and common sensitizers include PPD and glycerylthioglycolate [100]. The use of gloves, mild soaps, and moisturizing creams alleviate the condition but severe refractory cases may require interruption of the occupational activity.

Permanents

A permanent wave is a method of setting the hair in waves or curls followed by treatment with chemicals that can maintain the style for several months. While not as popularly used today as in the past, permanent wave solutions are still used by many consumers. Permanents use mercaptans to cleave disulfide bonds in hair; neutralizers are then added to reshape the configuration. Ammonium thioglycolate (ATG), a cleaving agent in cold permanent wave lotions, can cause extensive hair damage and acute contact irritant dermatitis. Glycerol monothioglycolate (GMTG), also known as an "acid" perm, can cause allergic contact dermatitis and may persist as active allergen in hair shafts in concentrations as low as 0.25% [101]. Cysteamine hydrochloride (CHC), another ingredient in permanent wave solutions preferentially used for color-treated or damaged hair, has also been identified to cause allergic contact dermatitis in hairdressers [102].

Nail products

Nail polish and hardener contain nitrocellulose, resins, plasticizers, solvents and diluents, colors, and suspending agents. Nail product sensitizers include additives, impurities, byproducts that form during polymerization or degradation, and residual monomers [103]. The most common allergen in nail polish and hardeners is tosylamide formaldehyde resin (toluene sulfonamide/formaldehyde resin) closely followed by acrylics (ethy acrylate, 2-hydroxy ethyl acrylate, ethylene glycol dimethacrylate, ethyl cyanoacrylate, methyl methacrylate, and triethylene glycol diacrylate) [46,104]. Copolymers such as phthalic anhydride/trimellitic anhydride/glycols in nail lacquers have also been reported as allergens [103,105–107]. The dermatitis tends to affect places commonly reached by the fingers (e.g. face, eyelids, sides of the neck, mouth), sparing the hands and fingers, a phenomenon known as ectopic contact dermatitis. However, localized dermatitis in the periungal area can occur with acrylic agents, sometimes leading to nail dystrophy [108].

Cosmetic application devices

Sponges, eyelash curlers, and mascara brushes used to apply cosmetic powders and eye makeup can be a potential source of contact allergy in individuals allergic to latex or synthetic rubber [109–111]. Sensitization to thiurams contained in latex or synthetic rubber gloves is often implicated in causing hand dermatitis in hairdressers and healthcare professionals [100]. Nickel containing eyelash curlers and mascara brushes should also be considered as a potential cause of recalcitrant eyelid dermatitis [112].

Contact urticaria to latex is triggered by exposure to the proteins derived from *Hevea brasiliensis* tree. Risk factors include the presence of spina bifida, genitourinary tract abnormalities, previous contact to latex (from multiple surgical procedures, or occupational exposure), hand dermatitis, atopy, and specific food allergies (avocado, banana, chestnut, potato, tomato, kiwi, pineapple, papaya, eggplant, melon, passion fruit, mango, wheat, and cherimoya).

Tattoos

Although relatively uncommon, hypersensitivity reactions to tattoo pigments are clinically relevant because of the increasing popularity and prevalence of tattoos [113]. Tattoo pigments are composed of inorganic metals such as mercury (red), chrome (green), manganese (purple), cobalt (blue), and cadmium (yellow) and of organic preparations such as sandalwood (red) and Brazilwood (red) [114]. These pigments have been implicated in allergic contact dermatitis and eczematous hypersensitivity reactions, as well as photoallergic, lichenoid, granulomatous, sarcoidal and pseudolymphomatous reactions. Allergic contact dermatitis is the most common hypersensitivity reaction to pigments in tattoos, with red pigments representing the most common cause of tattoo related allergic contact dermatitis [115]. ID reaction, also known as autoeczematization or autosensitization reaction, a reaction that develops distant to an initial site of sensitization, has also been associated with contact allergy to tattoo ink [116]. Contact dermatitis has also been reported following temporary henna tattooing. Henna, a natural product derived from the leaves of *Lawsonia inermis*, rarely causes hypersensitivity reactions. However, temporary henna tattoos that also contain PPD have been implicated in allergic contact dermatitis and autosensitization reactions [117,118]. Given the variable and often changing chemical nature of tattoo pigments, and the poor solubility of the ink pigments, it is often difficult to identify the offending agent through patch testing. Further investigation and regulation of these color additives is warranted to better elucidate ink components responsible for these cutaneous allergic reactions.

Local anesthetics

Anesthetic agents can be divided in two groups: esters (benzocaine, tetracaine, and procaine) and amide derivates (lidocaine, mepivacaine, bupivacaine, etidocaine, and prilocaine). Cases of eczematous dermatitis have been reported secondary to the use of topical ester agents and rarely secondary to amide derivates. Contact sensitization to 2.5% lidocaine and 2.5% prilocaine emulsion (EMLA, Astra Zeneca Pharmaceuticals LP, Wilmington, DE, USA) is rare. Uncommon reactions include purpuric eruption, rash, redness, itching, and edema [2].

IgE-mediated reactions to injectable anesthetics represent less than 1% of all adverse events. Delayed-type reactions manifest within 12–48 hours and present as an acute dermatitis (erythema, papules, vesicles and itching) [2,119]. Systemic toxicity occurs when excessive dosage is administered and manifests as light-headedness, tremors, restlessness, seizures, and depressed myocardial contractility. Methemoglobulinemia is an idiosyncratic reaction reported with local injectable anesthetics [119].

A European retrospective study over a 10-year period found that patch testing with a caine mix (benzocaine, tetracaine, and cinchocaine) was more sensitive in detecting contact allergy to local anesthetics than testing to benzocaine alone [120].

Injectables

Hypersensitivity reactions to fillers are reported infrequently. Adverse reactions to soft tissue augmentation include foreign body granulomas, bacterial infections, abscesses, local inflammation, discoloration, ulceration, necrosis, migration, and vascular and neurologic compromise [29,30].

Botulinum toxin is a highly potent neurotoxin that inhibits acetylcholine release at the neuromuscular junction, blocking neuromuscular transmission and reversibly paralyzing striated muscle. Allergic reactions are extremely rare and include generalized pruritus, psoriasiform eruption, urticaria, and erythema multiforme-type reactions [2,121]. The botox formulation also contains human albumin, which can cause rare but severe hypersensitivity reactions including anaphylaxis [122].

Fillers are subdivided into gels that are degradable (hyaluronic acid, poly-L-lactic acid, calcium hydroxylapatite, collagen) and non-degradable (polymethylmethacrylate and silicone). Degradable polymer gels resemble the elements commonly found in the tissues, and therefore are degraded by naturally occurring enzymes, located in the extracellular matrix and/or within macrophages [123]. Hence, fibrous response generated by these hydrophilic gels is minimal. The nonbiodegradable fillers may rarely provoke a chronic granulomatous foreign body reaction that stimulates fibroblastic deposition of collagen around the nonabsorbable filler material. The permanent nature of the nonbiodegradable fillers can make their complications long-lasting and difficult to treat [29].

Hyaluronic acid (HA) is a glucosaminoglycan polysaccharide occurring naturally in skin, connective tissue, and the vitreous humor of the eye. Hyaluronic acid fillers currently available in the United States include Restylane and Restylane L (QMed/Galderma, Uppsala, Sweden; Valeant, Bridgewater, New Jersey, USA), Juvederm Ultra, Ultra Plus, XC, and Voluma (Allergan, Santa Barbara, California, USA), Perlane (QMed/Galderma), Prevelle Silk (Genzyme Corp., Cambridge, Massachusetts, USA) and Belotero (Merz Pharmaceuticals, Greensboro, North Carolina, USA). Hyaluronic acid is not reported to cause allergic contact dermatitis and rarely are hypersensitivity reactions described. Non-inflammatory nodules can occur as a result of superficial injection or uneven distribution of the injected product [30]. Hyaluronidase is a soluble enzyme that can be injected locally at the site of filler placement to break down and hydrolyze HA implants [124,125].

Sculptra (Valeant, Bridgewater, New Jersey, USA) is a poly-L-lactic acid injectable that volumizes the face by stimulating the production of new collagen [126]. This product is indicated for use in HIV-associated lipoatrophy [127]. Like HA, Sculptra can cause superficial skin nodules [128,129]. Early-onset nodules appear gradually 1–3 months after injection and are often palpable but nonvisible. Histologically, early-onset nodules show material surrounded by a scarce cellular reaction [130]. Late-onset inflammatory nodules may appear abruptly 6–36 months after injection and have been reported to wax and wane [130]. These delayed-onset nodules are often visible and accompanied by edema and skin discoloration. Histologically, late-onset nodules typically show a foreign body granulomatous reaction with heavy lymphocytic infiltrate, histiocytes, epitheliod cells, and multinucleated giant cells [131].

Calcium hydroxylapatite (Radiesse, Merz Aesthetics, San Meteo, California, USA) consists of 35% calcium hydroxyapetite (CaHa) microspheres suspended in a 70% gel carrier [126]. The carboxymethylcellulose carrier gel is absorbed and the microspheres remain in the tissue to serve as scaffolding for new collagen formation [126]. Although rare, these CaHa microspheres can elicit a foreign body reaction seen as blue-gray round microspheres in the extracellular matrix or within multinucleated giant cells [30]. Delayed-onset nodules secondary to calcium hydroxylapatite implantation can occur anywhere the substance is injected, but occurs most commonly in the lips [132,133].

Polymethylmethacrylate (Artefill, Suneva Medical Inc., San Diego, CA) is a polymer of microspheres suspended in a bovine collagen and lidocaine. The PPMA microspheres represent the permanent implant whereas the bovine collagen suspension is degradable. Collagen of bovine origin induces allergy reactions in approximately 3% to 4% of the patients and therefore skin testing at least 1 month prior to injection is suggested [30]. Other rare complications include persistent redness, telangiectasia, hypertrophic scarring, nodules, and delayed granulomatous reactions [134].

Silicone refers to a group of compounds derived from silicone-containing synthetics. Polydimethylsiloxanes are the most commonly substances used and contain silicon, oxygen, and methane [135]. The silicone gel is hydrophobic and once introduced in the tissues it is dispersed in vacuoles or droplets, which may be absorbed by macrophages and foreign body giant cells. The cells may then migrate to the reticuloendothelial system and/or evoke a local foreign body reaction in the surrounding tissue. Phagocytes enter and traverse the gel, followed by gradual replacement with connective tissue [123]. Silicone can cause inflammatory and granulomatous reactions at injection sites. Delayed and persistent granulomatous reactions can occur years after injection and can be recalcitrant to treatment [136].

Collagen fillers were voluntarily withdrawn from the US market in 2010 and are currently rarely used in Europe and other parts of the world. Formulations of bovine-derived products previously available included collagen I (Zyderm I and II, Allergan, Irvine, California, USA) and cross-linked collagen (Zyplast, Allergan, Irvine, California, USA). Potential hypersensitivity reactions necessitating prior skin testing limited the usability of the bovine-derived fillers. Human collagen fillers including Cosmoderm I (Allergan), Cosmoderm II (Allergan) and Cosmoplast (Allergan) were also discontinued following the expansion of hyaluronic acid fillers, which have better safety and tolerability profiles [137].

Diagnosis

A thorough history of occupational and environmental exposures is necessary to ascertain potential sources of allergic and irritant contact dermatitis. When history suggests a cause of a reaction, avoidance and observation is informative. When cause and source remain elusive, patch testing may provide additional insight. When the field of potential culprits is wide ranging, patch testing with a comprehensive series of clinically relevant allergens provides a greater opportunity to detect the causative agent(s).

Epicutaneous application of standardized concentrations of allergen chemicals contained in chambers is occluded for 48 hours and then removed. The skin reaction is observed and a second reading is performed in 1–5 days. The presence of induration, erythema, and/or vesicles denotes a positive reaction.

Additionally, prick tests and radio allergo-sorbent tests (RASTs) can be used to detect IgE antibodies to a suspected allergen causing type I hypersensitivity reactions. Very limited data exists regarding the utility of patch testing in chronic idiopathic urticaria [138–140].

Allergy to bovine collagen can be detected by intradermal challenge of 0.1 mL of filler substance on the volar forearm, which is evaluated at 48–72 hours post-implantation. A positive test is defined as induration, erythema, tenderness, or swelling that persists or occurs longer than 6 hours after the injection. Positive subjects must be excluded from the procedure. Repeat testing has been suggested for those with negative reactions [2]. The diagnosis of granulomatous reactions to fillers is often rendered through history and physical examination and may require histologic confirmation and assessment of foreign material [30].

Treatment

Treatment is based on identifying the offending agent with subsequent avoidance. Type I reactions require appropriate interventions with antihistamines, systemic corticosteroids, epinephrine, and supportive therapy based on the severity of the reaction.

Mild allergic and irritant contact dermatitis are treated with avoidance and emollients free of sensitizers. Topical steroids and calcineurin inhibitors may be used to hasten resolution, whereas serious reactions may require addition of systemic immunosuppressant medication. Irritant dermatitis requires proper hygiene including personal protective equipment such as gloves, mild cleansers, and emollients.

The treatment of filler induced granulomatous reactions includes intralesional and systemic corticosteroids and surgical excision in refractory cases [141]. Treatments that have been used for granulomatous reactions secondary to fillers include tetracyclines, tumor necrosis factor inhibitors, topical and systemic calcineurin inhibitors, imiquimod, antimalarials, and isotretinoin [141,142].

Conclusions

Cosmetic products are widely used and reactions to those products are commonly seen in daily dermatologic practice. Prompt recognition with identification and withdrawal of the offending agent are key elements for successful management of such reactions.

References

1. Berne B, Tammela M, Farm G, Inerot A, Lindberg M. (2008) Can the reporting of adverse skin reactions to cosmetics be improved? A prospective clinical study using a structured protocol. *Contact Derm* 58(4), 223–7.
2. Cohen DE, Kaufmann JM. (2003) Hypersensitivity reactions to products and devices in plastic surgery. *Facial Plast Surg Clin North Am* 11(2), 253–65.
3. Pathak MA. (1986) Phytophotodermatitis. *Clin Dermatol* 4(2), 102–21.
4. Warshaw EM, Buchholz HJ, Belsito DV, Maibach HI, Fowler JF, Jr., Rietschel RL, et al. (2009) Allergic patch test reactions associated with cosmetics, retrospective analysis of cross-sectional data from the North American Contact Dermatitis Group, 2001–2004. *J Am Acad Dermatol* 60(1), 23–38.
5. Eiermann HJ, Larsen W, Maibach HI, Taylor JS. (1982) Prospective study of cosmetic reactions, 1977–1980. North American Contact Dermatitis Group. *J Am Acad Dermatol* 6(5), 909–17.
6. Adams RM, Maibach HI. (1985) A five-year study of cosmetic reactions. *J Am Acad Dermatol* 13(6), 1062–9.
7. US Food and Drug Administration. Guidance, Compliance and Regulatory Information – FDA Authority Over Cosmetics [WebContent]. Center for Food Safety and Applied Nutrition (2013) [updated August 3, cited December 19]. Available from: www.fda.gov/cosmetics/guidancecomplianceregulatoryinformation/ucm074162.htm.
8. Engasser PG, Maibach HI. (2003) Cosmetics and skin care in dermatologic practice. In: FreedbergIM, EisenAZ, WolffK, AustenKF, GoldsmithLA, KatzSI, eds. *Fitzpatrick's Dermatology in General Medicine*, 6th edn. New York: McGraw-Hill, pp. 2369–79.
9. Cosmetic Toiletry and Fragrance Association (CFTA). (2010) *International Cosmetic Ingredient Dictionary and Handbook*, 13th edn. Washington, DC: CFTA.
10. American Academy of Dermatology and AAD Association. (1998) Position Statement on The Chemical Identity of Fragrances.
11. Cosmetic Ingredient Review (2012) CIR Annual Report Washington, DC, Cosmetic Ingredient Review; 2013 [cited December 19, 2013]. Available from: www.cir-safety.org/sites/default/files/2012 CIR Annual Report.pdf.
12. H.R. 1385, Safe Cosmetics and Personal Care Products Act of 2013, GovTrack.us; 2013 [cited December 19, 2013]. Available from: www.govtrack.us/congress/bills/113/hr1385.
13. Safe Cosmetics and Personal Care Products Act of 2013: Mirrors TSCA proposals, would greatly expand FDA authority over cosmetics. Washington, DC., Beveridge & Diamond, P.C.; 2013 [updated April 16; cited December 19, 2013].
14. Smith HR, Basketter DA, McFadden JP. (2002) Irritant dermatitis, irritancy and its role in allergic contact dermatitis. *Clin Exp Dermatol* 27(2), 138–46.
15. Heinemann C, Paschold C, Fluhr J, Wigger-Alberti W, Schliemann-Willers S, Farwanah H, et al. (2005) Induction of a hardening phenomenon by repeated application of SLS, analysis of lipid changes in the stratum corneum. *Acta Derm Venereol* 85(4), 290–5.
16. Schliemann S, Schmidt C, Elsner P. (2014) Tandem repeated application of organic solvents and sodium lauryl sulphate enhances cumulative skin irritation. *Skin Pharmacol Physiol* 27(3), 158–63.
17. Shab A, Matterne U, Diepgen TL, Weisshaar E. (2008) Are obsessive-compulsive disorders and personality disorders sufficiently considered in occupational dermatoses? A discussion based on three case reports. *J Germ Soc Dermatol, JDDG* 6(11), 947–51.
18. Visser MJ, Landeck L, Campbell LE, McLean WH, Weidinger S, Calkoen F, et al. (2013) Impact of atopic dermatitis and loss-of-function mutations in the filaggrin gene on the development of occupational irritant contact dermatitis. *Br J Dermatol* 168(2), 326–32.
19. Friedmann PS, Pickard C. (2014) Contact hypersensitivity, quantitative aspects, susceptibility and risk factors. *EXS* 104, 51–71.
20. Park ME, Zippin JH. (2014) Allergic contact dermatitis to cosmetics. *Dermatol Clin* 32(1), 1–11.
21. Thyssen JP, Linneberg A, Ross-Hansen K, Carlsen BC, Meldgaard M, Szecsi PB, et al. (2013) Filaggrin mutations are strongly associated with contact sensitization in individuals with dermatitis. *Contact Derm* 68(5), 273–6.
22. Ale IS, Maibacht HA. (2010) Diagnostic approach in allergic and irritant contact dermatitis. *Expert Rev Clin Immunol* 6(2), 291–310.
23. Section 2. Eczema/Dermatitis. In: WolffK, JohnsonRA, SaavedraAP, eds. (2013) *Fitzpatrick's Color Atlas and Synopsis of Clinical Dermatology*, 7th edn. New York: McGraw-Hill.
24. McGovern, TW. (2012) Dermatoses due to plants. In: BologniaJL, JorizzoJL, SchafferJV, eds. *Dermatology*, 3rd edn. London: Mosby, pp. 273–90.
25. Weber IC, Davis CP, Greeson DM. (1999) Phytophotodermatitis, the other "lime" disease. *J Emerg Med* 17(2), 235–7.
26. Mogi S, Butcher CE, Oh DH. (2008) DNA polymerase eta reduces the gamma-H2AX response to psoralen interstrand crosslinks in human cells. *Exp Cell Res* 314(4), 887–95.
27. Almeida HL, Jr., Sotto MN, Castro LA, Rocha NM. (2008) Transmission electron microscopy of the preclinical phase of experimental phytophotodermatitis. *Clinics (Sao Paulo, Brazil)* 63(3), 371–4.
28. Anderson JM, Rodriguez A, Chang DT. (2008) Foreign body reaction to biomaterials. *Semin Immunol* 20(2), 86–100.
29. Funt D, Pavicic T. (2013) Dermal fillers in aesthetics, an overview of adverse events and treatment approaches. *Clin Cosmet Investig Dermatol* 6, 295–316.
30. Requena L, Requena C, Christensen L, Zimmermann US, Kutzner H, Cerroni L. (2011) Adverse reactions to injectable soft tissue fillers. *J Am Acad Dermatol* 64(1), 1–34; quiz 5–6.
31. Alijotas-Reig J, Miro-Mur F, Planells-Romeu I, Garcia-Aranda N, Garcia-Gimenez V, Vilardell-Tarres M. (2010) Are bacterial growth and/or chemotaxis increased by filler injections? Implications for the pathogenesis and treatment of filler-related granulomas. *Dermatology* 221(4), 356–64.
32. Alijotas-Reig J, Fernandez-Figueras MT, Puig L (2013) Late-onset inflammatory adverse reactions related to soft tissue filler injections. *Clin Rev Allergy Immunol* 45(1), 97–108.
33. Poveda R, Bagan JV, Murillo J, Jimenez Y. (2006) Granulomatous facial reaction to injected cosmetic fillers – a presentation of five cases. *Med Oral Patol Oral Cir Bucal* 11(1), E1–5.
34. Cecchi R, Spota A, Frati P, Muciaccia B. (2014) Migrating granulomatous chronic reaction from hyaluronic Acid skin filler (Restylane), review and histopathological study with histochemical stainings. *Dermatology* 228(1), 14–17.

35 Schorr ES, Sidou F, Kerrouche N. (2012) Adjunctive use of a facial moisturizer SPF 30 containing ceramide precursor improves tolerability of topical tretinoin 0.05%, a randomized, investigator-blinded, split-face study. *J Drugs Dermatol: JDD* **11**(9), 1104–7.

36 Diepgen TL, Kanerva L. (2006) Occupational skin diseases. *Eur J Dermatol* **16**(3), 324–30.

37 Nguyen SH, Dang TP, Maibach HI. (2007) Comedogenicity in rabbit, some cosmetic ingredients/vehicles. *Cutan Ocul Toxicol* **26**(4), 287–92.

38 Kartono F, Maibach HI. (2006) Irritants in combination with a synergistic or additive effect on the skin response, an overview of tandem irritation studies. *Contact Derm* **54**(6), 303–12.

39 Lammintausta K, Maibach HI, Wilson D. (1988) Mechanisms of subjective (sensory) irritation. Propensity to non-immunologic contact urticaria and objective irritation in stingers. *Derm Beruf Umwelt* **36**(2), 45–9.

40 Primavera G, Berardesca E. (2005) Sensitive skin, mechanisms and diagnosis. *Internat J Cosmet Sci* **27**(1), 1–10.

41 Arribas MP, Soro P, Silvestre JF. (2012) Allergic contact dermatitis to fragrances. Part 1. *Actas Dermosifiliogr* **103**(10), 874–9.

42 Zug KA, Rietschel RL, Warshaw EM, Belsito DV, Taylor JS, Maibach HI, *et al.* (2008) The value of patch testing patients with a scattered generalized distribution of dermatitis, retrospective cross-sectional analyses of North American Contact Dermatitis Group data, 2001 to 2004. *J Am Acad Dermatol* **59**(3), 426–31.

43 Heisterberg MV, Menne T, Andersen KE, Avnstorp C, Kristensen B, Kristensen O, *et al.* (2011) Deodorants are the leading cause of allergic contact dermatitis to fragrance ingredients. *Contact Derm* **64**(5), 258–64.

44 Thyssen JP, Linneberg A, Menne T, Nielsen NH, Johansen JD. (2009) The prevalence and morbidity of sensitization to fragrance mix I in the general population. *Br J Dermatol* **161**(1), 95–101.

45 Heisterberg MV, Menne T, Johansen JD. (2011) Contact allergy to the 26 specific fragrance ingredients to be declared on cosmetic products in accordance with the EU cosmetics directive. *Contact Derm* **65**(5), 266–75.

46 Warshaw EM, Belsito DV, Taylor JS, Sasseville D, DeKoven JG, Zirwas MJ, *et al.* (2013) North American Contact Dermatitis Group patch test results, 2009 to 2010. *Dermatitis: Contac Atop Occupat Drug* **24**(2), 50–9.

47 Wetter DA, Yiannias JA, Prakash AV, Davis MD, Farmer SA, el-Azhary RA. (2010) Results of patch testing to personal care product allergens in a standard series and a supplemental cosmetic series: an analysis of 945 patients from the of Clinic Contact Dermatitis Group, 2000-2007. *J Am Acad Dermatol* **63**(5), 789–98.

48 de Groot AC, White IR, Flyvholm MA, Lensen G, Coenraads PJ. (2010) Formaldehyde-releasers in cosmetics, relationship to formaldehyde contact allergy. Part 1. Characterization, frequency and relevance of sensitization, and frequency of use in cosmetics. *Contact Derm* **62**(1), 217.

49 Uter W, Yazar K, Kratz EM, Mildau G, Liden C. (2014) Coupled exposure to ingredients of cosmetic products, II. Preservatives. *Contact Derm* **70**(4), 219–26.

50 Aalto-Korte K, Kuuliala O, Suuronen K, Alanko K. (2008) Occupational contact allergy to formaldehyde and formaldehyde releasers. *Contact Derm* **59**(5), 280–9.

51 Fonacier LS, Aquino MR. (2010) The role of contact allergy in atopic dermatitis. *Immunol Allergy Clin North Am* **30**(3), 337–50.

52 Shaughnessy CN, Malajian D, Belsito DV. (2013) Cutaneous delayed-type hypersensitivity in patients with atopic dermatitis: Reactivity to topical preservatives. *J Am Acad Dermatol* **9**.

53 Gardner KH, Davis MD, Richardson DM, Pittelkow MR. (2010) The hazards of moist toilet paper: allergy to the preservative methylchloroisothiazolinone/methylisothiazolinone. *Arch Dermatol* **146**(8), 886–90.

54 Uter W, Gefeller O, Geier J, Schnuch A. (2012) Methylchloroisothiazolinone/methylisothiazolinone contact sensitization, diverging trends in subgroups of IVDK patients in a period of 19 years. *Contact Derm* **67**(3), 125–9.

55 Maio P, Carvalho R, Amaro C, Santos R, Cardoso J. (2012) Contact allergy to methylchoroisothiazolinone/methylisothiazolinone (MCI/MI), findings from a contact dermatitis unit. *Cutan Ocul Toxicol* **31**(2), 151–3.

56 Geier J, Lessmann H, Schnuch A, Uter W. (2012) Recent increase in allergic reactions to methylchloroisothiazolinone/methylisothiazolinone, is methylisothiazolinone the culprit? *Contact Derm* **67**(6), 334–41.

57 Lundov MD, Opstrup MS, Johansen JD. (2013) Methylisothiazolinone contact allergy – growing epidemic. *Contact Derm* **69**(5), 271–5.

58 Castanedo-Tardana MP, Zug KA. (2013) Methylisothiazolinone. *Dermatitis: Contact Atop Occupat Drug* **24**(1), 2–6.

59 Lundov MD, Thyssen JP, Zachariae C, Johansen JD. (2010) Prevalence and cause of methylisothiazolinone contact allergy. *Contact Derm* **63**(3), 164–7.

60 Ackermann L, Aalto-Korte K, Alanko K, Hasan T, Jolanki R, Lammintausta K, *et al.* (2011) Contact sensitization to methylisothiazolinone in Finland – a multicentre study. *Contact Derm* **64**(1), 49–53.

61 Yazar K, Johnsson S, Lind ML, Boman A, Liden C. (2011) Preservatives and fragrances in selected consumer-available cosmetics and detergents. *Contact Derm* **64**(5), 265–72.

62 Uter W, Yazar K, Kratz EM, Mildau G, Liden C. (2013) Coupled exposure to ingredients of cosmetic products, II. Preservatives. *Contact Derm* **17**.

63 Final amended report on the safety assessment of Methylparaben, Ethylparaben, Propylparaben, Isopropylparaben, Butylparaben, Isobutylparaben, and Benzylparaben as used in cosmetic products (2008) *Int J Toxicol* **27** Suppl 4, 1–82.

64 Barbaud A, Collet E, Le Coz CJ, Meaume S, Gillois P. (2009) Contact allergy in chronic leg ulcers, results of a multicentre study carried out in 423 patients and proposal for an updated series of patch tests. *Contact Derm* **60**(5), 279–87.

65 Landeck L, John SM, Geier J. (2013) Periorbital dermatitis in 4779 patients – patch test results during a 10-year period. *Contact Derm* **11**.

66 Itskaya ES, Dean SJ, Craig JP, Alexandroff AB. (2011) Current dilemmas and controversies in allergic contact dermatitis to ophthalmic medications. *Clin Dermatol* **29**(3), 295–9.

67 Jack AR, Norris PL, Storrs FJ. (2013) Allergic contact dermatitis to plant extracts in cosmetics. *Semin Cutan Med Surg* **32**(3), 140–6.

68 Corazza M, Borghi A, Gallo R, Schena D, Pigatto P, Lauriola MM, *et al.* (2014) Topical botanically derived products, use, skin reactions, and usefulness of patch tests. A multicentre Italian study. *Contact Derm* **70**(2), 90–7.

69 Cosmetic Ingredient Review. (2013) *Safety Assessment of Citrus-Derived Ingredients as Used in Cosmetics*. Washington, DC.

70 Bollero D, Stella M, Rivolin A, Cassano P, Risso D, Vanzetti M. (2001) Fig leaf tanning lotion and sun-related burns: case reports. *Burns* **27**(7), 777–9.

71 Bassioukas K, Stergiopoulou C, Hatzis J. (2004) Erythrodermic phytophotodermatitis after application of aqueous fig-leaf extract as an artificial suntan promoter and sunbathing. *Contact Derm* **51**(2), 94–5.

72 Travassos AR, Claes L, Boey L, Drieghe J, Goossens A. (2011) Non-fragrance allergens in specific cosmetic products. *Contact Derm* **65**(5), 276–85.

73 Zirwas M, Moennich J. (2009) Shampoos. *Dermatitis: Contact Atop Occupat Drug* **20**(2), 106–10.

74 Loden M. (2005) The clinical benefit of moisturizers. *J Eur Acad Dermatol Venereol* **19**(6), 672–88; quiz 86–7.

75 Zirwas MJ, Stechschulte SA. (2008) Moisturizer allergy, diagnosis and management. *J Clin Aesthet Dermatol* **1**(4), 38–44.

76 Draelos ZD. (2013) Modern moisturizer myths, misconceptions, and truths. *Cutis* **91**(6), 308–14.

77 Wilson CL, Cameron J, Powell SM, Cherry G, Ryan TJ. (1991) High incidence of contact dermatitis in leg-ulcer patients–implications for management. *Clin Exp Dermatol* **16**(4), 250–3.

78 Thyssen JP, McFadden JP, Kimber I. (2014) The multiple factors affecting the association between atopic dermatitis and contact sensitization. *Allergy* **69**(1), 28–36.

79 Warshaw EM, Raju SI, Fowler JF, Jr., Maibach HI, Belsito DV, Zug KA, et al. (2012) Positive patch test reactions in older individuals, retrospective analysis from the North American Contact Dermatitis Group, 1994–2008. *J Am Acad Dermatol* **66**(2), 229–40.

80 Ladizinski B, Mistry N, Kundu RV. (2011) Widespread use of toxic skin lightening compounds, medical and psychosocial aspects. *Dermatol Clin* **29**(1), 111–23.

81 Badreshia-Bansal S, Draelos ZD. (2007) Insight into skin lightening cosmeceuticals for women of color. *J Drugs Dermatol: JDD* **6**(1), 32–9.

82 Draelos ZD. (2007) Skin lightening preparations and the hydroquinone controversy. *Dermatol Ther* **20**(5), 308–13.

83 van Ketel WG. (1984) Sensitization to hydroquinone and the monobenzyl ether of hydroquinone. *Contact Dermat* **10**(4), 253.

84 Hamann CR, Boonchai W, Wen L, Sakanashi EN, Chu CY, Hamann K, et al. (2014) Spectrometric analysis of mercury content in 549 skin-lightening products, Is mercury toxicity a hidden global health hazard? *J Am Acad Dermatol* **70**(2), 281–7.

85 Baeck M, Chemelle JA, Terreux R, Drieghe J, Goossens A. (2009) Delayed hypersensitivity to corticosteroids in a series of 315 patients: clinical data and patch test results. *Contact Derm* **61**(3), 163–75.

86 Isaksson M, Bruze M. Corticosteroids. (2005) *Dermatitis: Contact Atop Occupat Drug* **16**(1), 3–5.

87 Coopman S, Degreef H, Dooms-Goossens A. (1989) Identification of cross-reaction patterns in allergic contact dermatitis from topical corticosteroids. *Br J Dermatol* **121**(1), 27–34.

88 Torres MJ, Canto G. (2010) Hypersensitivity reactions to corticosteroids. *Curr Opin Allergy Clin Immunol* **10**(4), 273–9.

89 Davis MD, el-Azhary RA, Farmer SA. (2007) Results of patch testing to a corticosteroid series, a retrospective review of 1188 patients during 6 years at Mayo Clinic. *J Am Acad Dermatol* **56**(6), 921–7.

90 Baeck M, Chemelle JA, Rasse C, Terreux R, Goossens A. (2011) C(16)-methyl corticosteroids are far less allergenic than the non-methylated molecules. *Contact Derm* **64**(6), 305–12.

91 English JS. (2000) Corticosteroid-induced contact dermatitis: a pragmatic approach. *Clin Exp Dermatol* **25**(4), 261–4.

92 Dooms-Goossens A, Andersen KE, Brandao FM, Bruynzeel D, Burrows D, Camarasa J, et al. (1996) Corticosteroid contact allergy: an EECDRG multicentre study. *Contact Derm* **35**(1), 40–4.

93 Veysey EC, Burge S, Cooper S. (2007) Consort contact dermatitis to paraphenylenediamine, with an unusual clinical presentation of tumid plaques. *Contact Derm* **6**(6), 366–7.

94 Yazar K, Boman A, Liden C. (2009) Potent skin sensitizers in oxidative hair dye products on the Swedish market. *Contact Derm* **61**(5), 269–75.

95 Orton D, Basketter D. (2012) Hair dye sensitivity testing, a critical commentary. *Contact Derm* **66**(6), 312–6.

96 Thyssen JP, Sosted H, Uter W, Schnuch A, Gimenez-Arnau AM, Vigan M, et al. (2012) Self-testing for contact sensitization to hair dyes–scientific considerations and clinical concerns of an industry-led screening programme. *Contact Derm* **66**(6), 300–11.

97 Lund JJ, Unwala R, Xia L, Gottlieb V. (2010) Chemical scalp burns secondary to the hair highlighting process, clinical and histopathologic features. *Pediatr Dermatol* **27**(1), 74–8.

98 Chan HP, Maibach HI. (2010) Hair highlights and severe acute irritant dermatitis ("burn") of the scalp. *Cutan Ocul Toxicol* **29**(4), 229–33.

99 Hoekstra M, van der Heide S, Coenraads PJ, Schuttelaar ML. (2012) Anaphylaxis and severe systemic reactions caused by skin contact with persulfates in hair-bleaching products. *Contact Derm* **66**(6), 317–22.

100 Warshaw EM, Wang MZ, Mathias CG, Maibach HI, Belsito DV, Zug KA, et al. (2012) Occupational contact dermatitis in hairdressers/cosmetologists: retrospective analysis of North American Contact Dermatitis Group data, 1994 to 2010. *Dermatitis: Contact Atop Occupat Drug* **23**(6), 258–68.

101 Storrs FJ. (1984) Permanent wave contact dermatitis: contact allergy to glyceryl monothioglycolate. *J Am Acad Dermatol* **11**(1), 74–85.

102 Isaksson M, van der Walle H. (2007) Occupational contact allergy to cysteamine hydrochloride in permanent-wave solutions. *Contact Derm* **56**(5), 295–6.

103 Quartier S, Garmyn M, Becart S, Goossens A. (2006) Allergic contact dermatitis to copolymers in cosmetics–case report and review of the literature. *Contact Derm* **55**(5), 257–67.

104 Drucker AM, Pratt MD. (2011) Acrylate contact allergy, patient characteristics and evaluation of screening allergens. *Dermatitis: Contact Atop Occupat Drug* **22**(2), 98–101.

105 Moffitt DL, Sansom JE. (2002) Allergic contact dermatitis from phthalic anhydride/trimellitic anhydride/glycols copolymer in nail varnish. *Contact Derm* **46**(4), 236.

106 Gach JE, Stone NM, Finch TM. (2005) A series of four cases of allergic contact dermatitis to phthalic anhydride/trimellitic anhydride/glycols copolymer in nail varnish. *Contact Derm* **53**(1), 63–4.

107 Nassif AS, Le Coz CJ, Collet E. (2007) A rare nail polish allergen, phthalic anhydride, trimellitic anhydride and glycols copolymer. *Contact Derm* **56**(3), 172–3.

108 Cruz MJ, Baudrier T, Cunha AP, Ferreira O, Azevedo F. (2011) Severe onychodystrophy caused by allergic contact dermatitis to acrylates in artificial nails. *Cutan Ocul Toxicol* **30**(4), 323–4.

109 Furman D, Fisher AA, Leider M. (1950) Allergic eczematous contact-type dermatitis caused by rubber sponges used for the application of cosmetics. *J Invest Dermatol* **15**(3), 223–31.

110 Vestey JP, Buxton PK, Savin JA. (1985) Eyelash curler dermatitis. *Contact Derm* **13**(4), 274–5.

111 Curtis GH. (1945) Contact dermatitis of eyelids caused by an antioxidant in rubber fillers of eyelash curlers; report of 7 cases. *Arch Dermatol Syphilol* **52**, 262–5.

112 Thyssen JP, Linneberg A, Menne T, Nielsen NH, Johansen JD. (2010) No association between nickel allergy and reporting cosmetic dermatitis from mascara or eye shadow, a cross-sectional general population study. *J Eur Acad Dermatol Venereol* **24**(6), 722–5.

113 Garcovich S, Carbone T, Avitabile S, Nasorri F, Fucci N, Cavani A. (2012) Lichenoid red tattoo reaction, histological and immunological perspectives. *Eur J Dermatol* **22**(1), 93–6.

114 Cruz FA, Lage D, Frigerio RM, Zaniboni MC, Arruda LH. (2010) Reactions to the different pigments in tattoos: a report of two cases. *An Bras Dermatol* **85**(5), 708–11.

115 Mortimer NJ, Chave TA, Johnston GA. (2003) Red tattoo reactions. *Clin Exp Dermatol* **28**(5), 508–10.

116 Litak J, Ke MS, Gutierrez MA, Soriano T, Lask GP. (2007) Generalized lichenoid reaction from tattoo. *Dermatol Surg* **33**(6), 736–40.

117 Evans CC, Fleming JD. (2008) Images in clinical medicine. Allergic contact dermatitis from a henna tattoo. *N Engl J Med* **359**(6), 627.

118 Farrow C. (2002) Hair dye and henna tattoo exposure. *Emerg Nurse* **10**(3), 19–23.

119 Phillips JF, Yates AB, Deshazo RD. (2007) Approach to patients with suspected hypersensitivity to local anesthetics. *Am J Med Sci* **334**(3), 190–6.

120 Brinca A, Cabral R, Goncalo M. (2013) Contact allergy to local anaesthetics-value of patch testing with a caine mix in the baseline series. *Contact Derm* **68**(3), 156–62.

121 Brueggemann N, Doegnitz L, Harms L, Moser A, Hagenah JM. (2008) Skin reactions after intramuscular injection of Botulinum toxin A, a rare side effect. *J Neurol Neurosurg Psychiatr* **79**(2), 231–2.

122 Albumin (Human) 5%. Food and Drug Administration.

123 Christensen L. (2007) Normal and pathologic tissue reactions to soft tissue gel fillers. *Dermatol Surg* **33** Suppl 2, S168–75.

124 Hirsch RJ, Stier M. (2008) Complications of soft tissue augmentation. *J Drugs Dermatol: JDD* **7**(9), 841–5.

125 Brody HJ. (2005) Use of hyaluronidase in the treatment of granulomatous hyaluronic acid reactions or unwanted hyaluronic acid misplacement. *Dermatol Surg* **31**(8 Pt 1), 893–7.

126 Kontis TC. (2013) Contemporary review of injectable facial fillers. *JAMA Facial Plast Surg* **15**(1), 58–64.

127 Keni SP, Sidle DM. (2007) Sculptra (injectable poly-L-lactic acid). *Facial Plast Surg Clin North Am* **15**(1), 91–7, vii.

128 Levy RM, Redbord KP, Hanke CW. (2008) Treatment of HIV lipoatrophy and lipoatrophy of aging with poly-L-lactic acid: a prospective 3-year follow-up study. *J Am Acad Dermatol* **59**(6), 923–33.

129 Palm MD, Woodhall KE, Butterwick KJ, Goldman MP. (2010) Cosmetic use of poly-L-lactic acid: a retrospective study of 130 patients. *Dermatol Surg* **36**(2), 161–70.

130 Hamilton DG, Gauthier N, Robertson BF. (2008) Late-onset, recurrent facial nodules associated with injection of poly-L-lactic acid. *Dermatol Surg* **34**(1), 123–6; discussion 6.

131 Andre P, Lowe NJ, Parc A, Clerici TH, Zimmermann U. (2005) Adverse reactions to dermal fillers, a review of European experiences. *J Cosmet Laser Ther* **7**(3–4), 171–6.

132 Tzikas TL. (2008) A 52-month summary of results using calcium hydroxylapatite for facial soft tissue augmentation. *Dermatol Surg* **34** Suppl 1, S9–15.

133 Sadick NS, Katz BE, Roy D. (2007) A multicenter, 47-month study of safety and efficacy of calcium hydroxylapatite for soft tissue augmentation of nasolabial folds and other areas of the face. *Dermatol Surg* **33** Suppl 2, S122–6; discussion S6–7.

134 Kadouch JA, Kadouch DJ, Fortuin S, van Rozelaar L, Karim RB, Hoekzema R. (2013) Delayed-onset complications of facial soft tissue augmentation with permanent fillers in 85 patients. *Dermatol Surg* **39**(10), 1474–85.

135 Chasan PE. (2007) The history of injectable silicone fluids for soft-tissue augmentation. *Plast Reconstr Surg* **120**(7), 2034–40; discussion 41–3.

136 Ledon JA, Savas JA, Yang S, Franca K, Camacho I, Nouri K. (2013) Inflammatory nodules following soft tissue filler use: a review of causative agents, pathology and treatment options. *Am J Clin Dermatol* **14**(5), 401–11.

137 Sundaram H, Cassuto D. (2013) Biophysical characteristics of hyaluronic acid soft-tissue fillers and their relevance to aesthetic applications. *Plast Reconstr Surg* **132**(4 Suppl 2), 5S–21S.

138 Guerra L, Rogkakou A, Massacane P, Gamalero C, Compalati E, Zanella C, *et al.* (2007) Role of contact sensitization in chronic urticaria. *J Am Acad Dermatol* **56**(1), 88–90.

139 Cancian M, Fortina AB, Peserico A. (1999) Contact urticaria syndrome from constituents of balsam of Peru and fragrance mix in a patient with chronic urticaria. *Contact Derm* **41**(5), 300.

140 Hession MT, Scheinman PL. (2012) The role of contact allergens in chronic idiopathic urticaria. *Dermatitis: Contact Atop Occupat Drug* **23**(3), 110–6.

141 Alijotas-Reig J, Fernandez-Figueras MT, Puig L. (2013) Inflammatory, immune-mediated adverse reactions related to soft tissue dermal fillers. *Semin Arthritis Rheum* **43**(2), 241–58.

142 Lopiccolo MC, Workman BJ, Chaffins ML, Kerr HA. (2011) Silicone granulomas after soft-tissue augmentation of the buttocks, a case report and review of management. *Dermatol Surg* **37**(5), 720–5.

SECTION 2 **Delivery of Cosmetic Skin Actives**

CHAPTER 7

Percutaneous Delivery of Cosmetic Actives to the Skin

Sreekumar Pillai, Surabhi Singh, and Christian Oresajo
L'Oréal Research, Clark, NJ, USA

> **BASIC CONCEPTS**
> - Percutaneous delivery is the penetration of substances into the skin.
> - The goal of effective percutaneous delivery is to provide an effective amount of an active to the skin target site and thereby optimize efficacy while minimizing side effects.
> - The main barrier of the active permeation through the skin is the stratum corneum. The active must cross this skin barrier and permeate transepidermally to be delivered to the target site.
> - Molecules with a molecular weight of less than 500 Daltons penetrate the skin better than molecules with a larger molecular weight. The net charge of a molecule is important in enhancing penetration.

Introduction

Recent developments in new technologies combined with new knowledge in skin biology have advanced innovations in skin availability of actives and novel methods of substance delivery. The goal of this chapter is to review new advances in delivery of actives to the skin and the effects of penetration enhancers. An understanding of the structure of the skin is very important in managing active delivery.

The basics

The goal of percutaneous delivery is to provide an effective amount of an active to the skin target site and thereby optimize efficacy while minimizing side effects. This can be achieved by an understanding of the skin's complex structure and by relying on physical and chemical parameters of vehicles applied to the skin.

Skin physiology

There are defined compartments and biologic structures within the skin that provide opportunities to deliver actives (Figure 7.1). Within these compartments there are many chemical and biologic processes at work that may alter a given active or the physiology of skin target.

The main barrier of active permeation through the skin is the stratum corneum. The active must cross this skin barrier and permeate transepidermally to be delivered to the target site, and the penetration can be moderated by the secretion activity of the appendages. This structure is located at the outermost layer of the epidermis [1]. This transepidermal route can be further subdivided into transcellular and intercellular routes [2]. Delivery of hydrophilic substances can be achieved through sweat gland route; however, this is also minimal in total volume. Therefore, the principal pathway for skin penetration of actives is the transepidermal route (route 1 in Figure 7.1).

Active composition

One of the first steps in understanding the phenomenon of active delivery is to completely characterize the active that is intended for delivery to the skin. There are well-known physical and chemical parameters that are specific to all chemical compounds. The essentials for characterization of actives are typically described in the literature or can be measured in the laboratory. This includes the active's molecular weight, dissociation constant (pK), solubility, and octanol/water [O/W] partition coefficient (log P). These parameters, along with a thorough understanding of the net ionic charge (cationic, anionic, and amphoteric) of the active will help in understanding its penetration profile.

Cosmetic Dermatology: Products and Procedures, Second Edition. Edited by Zoe Diana Draelos.
© 2016 John Wiley & Sons, Ltd. Published 2016 by John Wiley & Sons, Ltd.

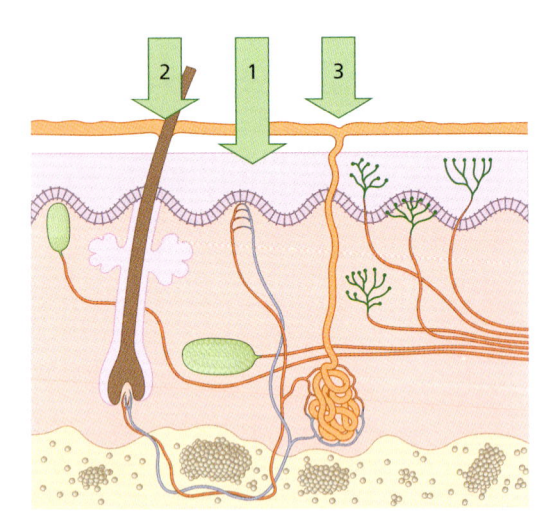

Figure 7.1 Possible pathways for a penetrant to cross the skin barrier. (1) Across the intact horny layer; (2) through the hair follicles with the associated sebaceous glands; or (3) via the sweat glands. (Source: Daniels R. Strategies for skin penetration enhancement. *Skin Care Forum* 37, www.scf-online.com.)

As general rule, molecules with a molecular weight of less than 500 Da penetrate the skin better than molecules with a larger molecular weight. It is also known that the net charge of a molecule is important in enhancing penetration. An un-ionized molecule penetrates the skin better than an ionized molecule. A thorough understanding of the relationship between the dissociation constant and formulation pH is critical. In many cases it is advantageous to keep the pH of a formulation near the pK of the active molecule in an attempt to enhance penetration. When looking at the partition coefficient, molecules showing intermediate partition coefficients (log P O/W of 1–3) have adequate solubility within the lipid domains of the stratum corneum to permit diffusion through this domain while still having sufficient hydrophilic nature to allow partitioning into the viable tissues of the epidermis [3].

Fick's law

The permeation of active across the stratum corneum is a passive process, which can be approximated by Fick's first law:

$$J = \frac{DK}{L}(C) \qquad \text{(equation 7.1)}$$

This defines steady-state flux (J) is related to the diffusion coefficient (D) of the active in the stratum corneum over a diffusional path length or membrane thickness (L), the partition coefficient (K) between the stratum corneum and the vehicle, and the applied drug concentration (C) which is assumed to be constant.

Novel formulation strategies allow for manipulation of the partition coefficient (K) and concentration (C). Skin penetration can be enhanced by the following strategies:

1. Increasing drug diffusion in the skin;
2. Increasing drug solubility in the skin; and/or
3. Increasing the degree of saturation of the drug in the formulation [4].

Equation (7.1) aids in identifying the ideal parameters for the diffusion of the active across the skin. The influence of solubility and partition coefficient on diffusion across the stratum corneum has been extensively studied in the literature [5].

Vehicle effect

Delivery of actives from emulsions

The key for evaluation of the vehicle effect is to understand the dynamics between the vehicle and the active. Based on the physical and chemical nature of the active there are specific formulation strategies that can be designed to enhance delivery of actives.

The primary vector for topical delivery of actives is a semi-solid ointment or emulsion base. The main reason for selection of this dosage form is convenience and cosmetic elegance. Emulsions are convenient because they typically have two phases (hydrophilic and hydrophobic). The bi-phasic nature allows for placement of actives based on solubility and stability. This allows the formulator to bring lipophilic and hydrophilic actives into the dosage form while maintaining the optimized stability profile. The effect of the type of vehicle has been well described in the literature [6]. Numerous references are available for altering the delivery of actives from various emulsion forms (O/W, W/O, multiple emulsions, and nano-emulsions).

Formulation strategies

A basic formulation has many components. Table 7.1 provides an overview of these formula components and also provides a brief summary of the anticipated effect on active delivery. Some of these chemical functions are more clearly defined below in discussion on chemical penetration enhancers.

The ability of vehicles to deliver actives is tied to an understanding of diffusion of actives through various skin compartments (epidermal and dermal). Diffusion of actives across the skin is a passive process. Compounds with low solubility and affinity for the hydrophilic and lipophilic components of the stratum corneum would theoretically partition at a slow rate. These difficulties may be overcome by adding a chemical adjunct to the delivery system that would promote partitioning into the stratum corneum. Partitioning of actives from the dosage form is highly dependent on the relative solubility of the active in the components of the delivery system and in the stratum corneum. Thus, the formulation of the vehicle may markedly influence the degree of

Table 7.1 Formulation components.

Ingredient	Chemical function	Effect on delivery
Water	Carrier/solvent	Hydration
Alcohol	Carrier/solvent	Fluidizes stratum corneum, alters permeability of stratum cornuem
Propylene glycol	Co-solvent/humectant	Alter permeability of stratum corneum. Alter vehicle stratum corneum partition coefficient
Surfactant	Emulsifier/stabilizer	Emulsion particle size reduction, active solubilizer
Emollient	Skin conditioner, active carrier	Alter stratum corneum permeability. Alter vehicle stratum corneum partition coefficient
Delivery system	Protect/target actives	Targeted/enhanced active penetration

penetration of the active. Percutaneous absorption involves the following sequences:
- Partitioning of the molecule into the stratum corneum from the applied vehicle phase;
- Molecular diffusion through the stratum corneum;
- Partitioning from the stratum corneum into the viable epidermis; and
- Diffusion through the epidermis and upper dermis and capillary uptake [7].

One of the most effective formulation techniques to boost active penetration is supersaturation. This chemical process happens when an active's maximum concentration in solution is exceeded by the use of solvents or co-solvents. This type of solution state can happen during the evaporation of an emulsion on the skin. As water evaporates from a cream rubbed on the skin a superconcentrate depot of active forms on the skin. This creates a diffusional concentration gradient across the stratum corneum. One can attempt to boost this effect even further in the formulation by slightly exceeding the maximum solubility of the active in the formula using co-solvents. Supersaturation is an effective technique but the disadvantage is that active recrystallization can take place in this highly concentrated solution state. There are crystallization inhibitors that can be added to supersaturated solution but many experimental data need to be collected on this type of formulation strategy.

Eutectic blends are formulation techniques that can enhance penetration of actives. The melting point of an active influences solubility and hence skin penetration. According to solution theory, the lower the melting point, the greater the solubility of a material in a given solvent, including skin lipids. The melting point can be lowered by formation of a eutectic mixture. This mixture of two components which, at a certain ratio, inhibits the crystalline process of each other such that the melting point of the two components in the mixture is less than that of each component alone. In all cases, the melting point of the active is depressed to around or below skin temperature thereby enhancing solubility. This technique has been used to enhance the penetration of ibuprofen through the skin [8].

Manipulation of the vehicle skin partition coefficient of a formulation can be used as an overall formulation strategy to boost penetration of actives. This can be done by altering the solubility of the active in the vehicle via selection of different excipients. This change in the solubility parameter (δ) of the excipients can be tuned so that the active is more soluble in the stratum corneum than in the vehicle. Hence the diffusional gradient is altered towards the skin and thereby enhancing penetration. It has been shown that a solvent capable of shifting the solubility parameter (δ) of the skin closer to that of the activate will active flux rate [9]. Another strategy is to add a penetration enhancer that alters the membrane permeability of the skin. This strategy is discussed in more detail below.

Skin occlusion can increase stratum corneum hydration, and hence influence percutaneous absorption by altering partitioning between the surface chemical and the skin because of the increasing presence of water, swelling corneocytes, and possibly altering the intercellular lipid phase organization, also by increasing the skin surface temperature, and increasing blood flow [10].

Different substances penetrate different depth levels in the skin for best results. An effective cosmetic is designed so that active substances gets inside the appropriate skin cells, affecting their metabolism in a way that improves their health, yet not damaging overall skin integrity.[30] The ultimate goal of penetration enhancement is to target the active in the stratum corneum and/or epidermis without allowing for systemic absorption. This remains the biggest challenge for active penetration enhancement and it is one of the keys for targeted active delivery.

Penetration enhancers

In this section, the influence of penetration enhancers on the diffusion coefficient and solubility of the active in the stratum corneum is evaluated. The use of topically applied chemical agents (surfactants, solvents, emollients) is a well-known technique to modify the stratum corneum and also modify the chemical potential of selected actives. Collectively, these materials can be referred to as penetration enhancers (PEs). Based on the chemical structure, PEs can be categorized into several groups such as fatty acids, fatty alcohols, terpene fatty acid esters, and pyrrolidone derivatives [11]. PEs commonly used in skin care products have well-known safety profiles but their ability to enhance penetration of an active is challenging because of the manifold ingredients used in many formulations.

Chemical enhancers

They are also known as absorption promoters and accelerants which are "pharmacological inert, nontoxic, non-irritating, non-allergic, rapid onset of action, and suitable duration of action, inexpensive and cosmetically acceptable [32]." A number of solvents (e.g. ethanol, propylene glycol, Transcutol® [Gattefossé, Saint-Priest, France] and N-methyl pyrrolidone) increase permeant partitioning into and solubility within the stratum corneum, hence increasing K_P in Fick's equation (equation 7.1). Ethanol was the first penetration enhancer co-solvent incorporated into transdermal systems [12]. Synergistic effects between enhancers (e.g. Azone® [PI Chemicals, Shanghai, China], fatty acids) and more polar co-solvents (e.g. ethanol, propylene glycol) have also been reported suggesting that the latter facilitates the solubilization of the former within the stratum corneum, thus amplifying the lipid-modulating effect. Similarly, solvents such as Transcutol are proposed to act by improving solubility within the membrane rather than by increasing diffusion. Another solvent, dimethylsulfoxide (DMSO), by contrast, is relatively aggressive and induces significant structural perturbations such as keratin denaturation and the solubilization of membrane components [13]. Table 7.2 is a list of the more commonly utilized chemical penetration enhancers [33].

Table 7.2 Commonly utilized chemical penetration enhancers

Chemical penetration enhancer	Description/function
Pyrrolidones	Permeation enhancer for numerous molecules (hydrophilic and lipophilic). They partition well into human stratum corneum within tissue, act by altering the solvent nature of the membrane, and generate reservoirs which offer potential release of a permeant from the stratum corneum over extended time periods [33].
Oxazolidinones	New class of chemical agents that have the ability to localize co-administered active (i.e. retinoic acid) in skin layers, due to their structural features being closely related to sphingosine and ceramide lipids found in the upper skin layers, resulting in low systemic permeation [31].
Urea	Mechanism may be a consequence of both hydrophilic activity and lipid disruption from these biodegradable and non-toxic molecules consisting of a polar parent moiety and a long chain alkyl-ester group [31].
Azone	Partitions into a bilayer to disrupt their packing arrangement. This non- homogeneous integration of molecules may be dispersed within the barrier lipid or separate domains within the bilayer [31].
Fatty acid	Oleic acid are mono-saturated fatty acids that increase the permeation of lipophilic actives through the skin and buccal mucosa by transdermal cellular pathway [31].
Alcohol, glycol and glycerides	Low molecular weight alkanols solvents enhance the solubility of the active into the matrix of stratum corneum by disrupting its integrity and contributing to enhancing the mass transfer of biochemicals through this tissue [33].
Alkyl-n, n-disubstituted amino acetates	Insoluble in water, but soluble in organic solvents and water-alcohol mixtures with low skin-irritating potential. Skin penetration is increased by the interaction with stratum corneum keratin which results in increasing the hydrating efficiency [31].
Surfactants	Solubilize lipophilic active ingredients and lipids within the stratum corneum. Anionic and cationic surfactants swell the stratum corneum and interact with intercellular keratin. They have the potential to damage human skin as powerful irritants, increasing transepidermal water loss of human skin [31].
Essential oil, terpenes and terpenoids	Operational mechanism modifies the solvent nature of the stratum corneum thereby improving the active partitioning into the tissue. Terpenes and terpenoids are constituents of volatile oils that are considered to be less toxic with low irritancy when compared to surfactants and other synthetic skin penetration enhancers.
Cineole	Natural organic compound (eucalyptol) that promotes the percutaneous absorption of lipophilic actives [31].
Eugenol	Enhances the permeability coefficient of the active with lipid extraction and improvement in the partitioning of the active to the stratum corneum. Slightly soluble in water and soluble in organic solvents. An allylbenzene class of chemical compound (extract of clove oil, nutmeg, cinnamon, and bay leaf) that reduces ability to feel and react to painful stimulation.
Farnesol	Sesquiterpene alcohol (citronella, neroli, lemon grass, tuberose, balsam and tolu) enhances the permeation of diclofenac sodium with its use in perfumery products.
Menthol	Highly effective penetration enhancer used for transdermal delivery of variety of actives and shown to increase the effect when paired with iontophoresis [33]. Used in medical and cosmetic preparations enhancing absorption of desirable molecules to the internal layers of the skin while also functioning as an effective counter- irritant [30].

Physical enhancers

In addition to the chemical penetration enhancers discussed above, there is another class of penetration enhancers known as physical penetration enhancers. These materials stand between chemical enhancers and penetration enhancer devices. This unique classification is because in most cases the materials are particles of chemical origin (polyethylene, salt, sugar, aluminum oxide) but require physical energy to exert an action on the skin. These materials are used to physically débride or excoriate the stratum corneum by abrasive action. This is typically done by rubbing the particles by hand on the skin. New high-tech devices are now available that propel an abrasive against the skin thereby stripping away the stratum corneum.

Penetration enhancement vectors

There are customized carriers (vectors) for delivery of actives to the skin. These vectors are a type of vehicle that allow for enhanced penetration via their small size and unique physical chemical composition. These vectors are known as submicron delivery systems (SDS). Discussion focuses on liposomes, niosomes, lipid particles, and nanocapsules.

Liposomes

Liposomes are colloidal particles formed as concentric biomolecular layers that are capable of encapsulating actives. The lipid bilayer structure of liposomes mimics the barrier properties of biomembranes, and therefore they offer the potential of examining the behavior of membranes of a known composition. Thus, by altering the lipid composition of the bilayer or the material incorporated, it is possible to establish differences in membrane properties. Liposomes store water-soluble substances inside like biologic cells. The phospholipids forming these liposomes enhance the penetration of the encapsulated active agents into the stratum corneum [14].

There is debate on liposome formulations and their mode of action regarding penetration enhancement. Variation in performance may be caused by the variation in formulation and method of manufacture used to prepare this delivery form. Several factors such as size, lamellarity (unilamellar vs. multilamellar), lipid composition, charge on the liposomal surface, mode of application, and total lipid concentration have been proven to influence deposition into the deeper skin layers. It is reported by several authors that the high elasticity of liposome vesicles could result in enhanced transport across the skin as compared to vesicles with rigid membranes.

Liposomes have a heterogeneous lipid composition with several coexisting domains exhibiting different fluidity characteristics in the bi-layers. This property can be used to enhance the penetration of entrapped actives into the skin. It is supposed that once in contact with skin, some budding of liposomal membrane might occur. This could cause a mixing of the liposome bi-layer with intracellular lipids in the stratum corneum which may change the hydration conditions and thereby the structure of lipid lamellae.

This may enhance the permeation of the lipophilic active into the stratum corneum and ease the diffusion of hydrophilic actives into the interlamellar spaces [15].

Niosomes

Niosomes are formed by blending non-ionic surfactants of the alkyl or dialkyl polyglycerol ether class and cholesterol with subsequent hydration in aqueous media. These vesicles can be prepared using a number of manufacturing processes: ether injection, membrane extrusion, microfluidization, and sonication. Niosomes have an infrastructure consisting of hydrophilic, amphiphilic, and lipophilic moieties together and as a result can accommodate active molecules with a wide range of solubilities. They can be expected to target the active to its desired site of action and/or to control its release [16]. Niosomes are similar to liposomes in that they both have a bi-layer structure and their final form depends on the method of manufacture. There are structural similarities between niosomes and liposomes but niosomes do not contain phospholipids. This provides niosomes with a better stability profile because of improved oxidative stability.

Solid lipid nanoparticles

Solid lipid nanoparticles (SLNP) were developed at the beginning of the 1990s as an alternative carrier system to emulsions, liposomes, and polymeric nanoparticles. SLNP have the advantage of requiring no solvents for production processing and of relatively low cost for the excipients. SLNP represents a particle system that can be produced with an established technique of high-pressure homogenization allowing production on an industrial scale. This method also protects the incorporated drug against chemical degradation as there is little or no access for water to enter the inner area core of the lipid particle [17]. Lipid particles can be used as penetration enhancers of encapsulated actives through the skin because of their excellent occlusive and hydrating properties. SLNP have recently been investigated as carriers for enhanced skin delivery of sunscreens, vitamins A and E, triptolide, and glucocorticoids [18].

Nanocapsules

Nanocapsules are a type of submicron delivery system (SDS). This technology can segregate and protect sensitive materials and also control the release of actives. The more obvious opportunity for penetration enhancement of actives is because of their small size (20–1000 nm in diameter). Nanocapsules can be formed by preparing a lipophilic core surrounded by a thin wall of a polymeric material prepared by anionic polymerization of an alkylcyanoacrylate monomer. These very safe types of system have been proposed as vesicular colloidal polymeric drug carriers. Nanocapsules have the ability to enhance penetration but they can also control delivery of actives to the skin.

In a recent study, indomethacin was nano-encapsulated for topical use. This study compared cumulative release of indomethacin dispersed in gel base with indomethacin nano-encapsulated and indomethacin nano-encapsulated in a gel. The highest delivery was achieved with the nanoencapsulated indomethacin (Figure 7.2).

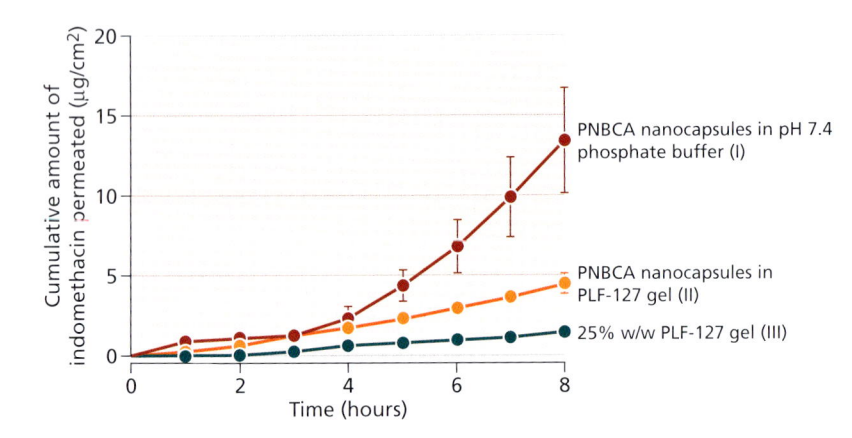

Figure 7.2 Cumulative amount of indomethicin (initial loading 0.5% w/v) per unit area, permeating through excised rat skin when released from PNBCA nanocapsule dispersion in pH 7.4 phosphate buffer, PNBCA nanocapsule dispersion in Pluronic F-127 gel and 25% w/w Pluronic F-127 gel. Each value is the mean ± SE of four determinations. (Source: Miyazaki et al., 2003 [*J Pharm Pharmaceut Sci* **6**, 238–45]. Creative Common license (Attribution-ShareAlike) License.)

Devices for penetration enhancement

Devices for enhancing skin penetration of actives are at the leading edge of skincare technology. When utilizing devices for enhanced penetration of actives it is imperative to look into the regulatory classification of these instruments. The FDA has several guidelines and requirements for medical devices (510K). The 510K regulatory classification is important for safety and efficacy of any consumer device product and an understanding of the regulatory landscape in this area is essential. Four device technologies are reviewed. They range from moderately invasive to mildly invasive in terms of effect on the skin. In all cases, the goal is to reversibly alter the skin barrier function by physical techniques or electro-energetic means. Box 7.1 is a list of the some methods and tools [31]; and further discussion on the more common skin enhancing topics.

Ultrasound waves

Ultrasound waves are sound waves that are above the audible limit (>20 kH). During ultrasound treatment the skin is exposed to mechanical and thermal energy which can alter the skin barrier property. Thermal and non-thermal characteristics of high-frequency sound waves can enhance the diffusion of topically applied actives. Heating from ultrasound increases the kinetic energy of the molecules in the active and in the cell membrane. These physiologic changes enhance the opportunity for active molecules to diffuse through the stratum corneum to the capillary network in the papillary dermis. The mechanical characteristics of the sound wave also enhance active diffusion by oscillating the cells at high speed, changing the resting potential of the cell membrane and potentially disrupting the cell membrane of some of the cells in the area [19].

A recent study on the use of ultrasound and topical skin lightening agents showed the effect of high-frequency ultrasound together with a gel containing skin-lightening agents (ascorbyl glucoside and niacinamide) on facial hyperpigmentation *in vivo* in Japanese women [20].

Patches

Delivery patches have been available for some time. One of the first applications of patch technology was in a transdermal motion sickness (scopolamine) patch. There are commercial products that provide actives in a patch formula. They utilize adhesive technology or a rate-limiting porous membrane to target and localize the actives. Some common patch applications are directed towards reduction of age spots or dark circles under the eye. The key delivery enhancement for patches is a combination of localized delivery and occlusion.

Microneedles

Another type of delivery device is the microneedle. Microneedles are similar to traditional needles, but are fabricated at the micro size. They are generally 1 µm in diameter and range 1–100 µm in length (Figure 7.3). The very first microneedle systems consisted of a reservoir and a range of projections (microneedles 50–100 mm long) extending from the reservoir, which penetrated the stratum corneum and epidermis to deliver the active. The microneedle delivery system is not based on diffusion as in other transdermal drug delivery products but based on the temporary mechanical disruption of the skin and the placement of the active within the epidermis, where it can

Box 7.1 Skin enhancers: physical methods and penetration devices.

Iontophoresis
Ultrasound (phonophoresis and sonophoresis)
Magnetophoresis
Electroporation
Radio frequency
Thermophoresis
Suction ablation
Skin puncture and perforation
Skin stretching
Skin abrasion

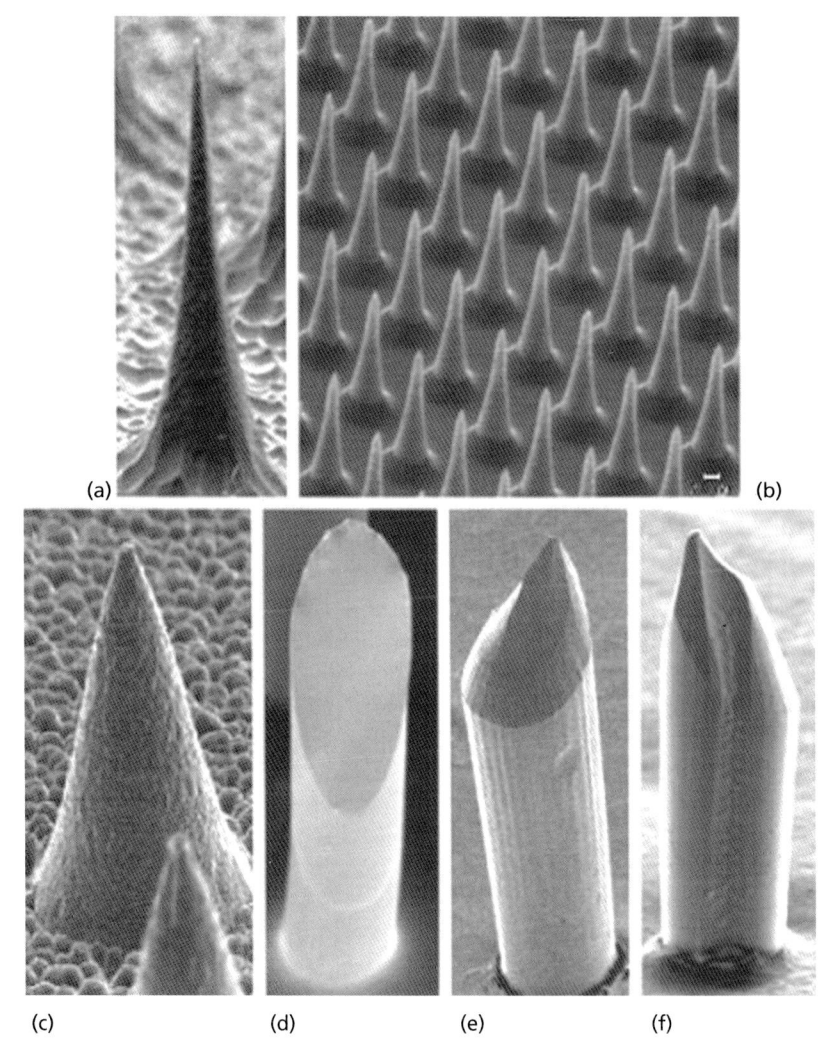

Figure 7.3 Solid microneedles fabricated out of silicon, polymer, and metal, imaged by scanning electron microscopy. (a) Silicon microneedle (150 μm tall) from a 400-needle array etched out of a silicon substrate. (b) Section of an array containing 160 000 silicon microneedles (25 μm tall). (c) Metal microneedle (120 μm tall) from a 400-needle array made by electrodepositing onto a polymeric mold. (d–f) Biodegradable polymer microneedles with beveled tips from 100-needle arrays made by filling polymeric molds. (d) Flat-bevel tip made of polylactic acid (400 μm tall). (e) Curved-bevel tip made of polyglycolic acid (600 μm tall). (f) Curved-bevel tip with a groove etched along the full length of the needle made of polyglycolic acid (400 μm tall). (Source: McAllister et al., 2003 [*Proc Natl Acad Sci USA* **100**, 13755–60]. Reproduced with permission.)

more readily reach its site of action. Microneedles have been fabricated with various materials such as metals, silicon, silicon dioxide, polymers, glass, and other materials. There are already patents granted for these types of moderately invasive delivery system [21].

Iontophoresis

Iontophoresis is a technology that has been brought to the cosmetic industry via the pharmaceutical development field. Iontophoresis passes a small direct current through an active-containing electrode placed in contact with the skin, with a grounding electrode to complete the circuit. Three important mechanisms enhance transport:

1. The driving electrode repels oppositely charged species;
2. The electric current increases skin permeability; and
3. Electro-osmosis moves uncharged molecules and large polar peptides [22].

There are limitations related to this technique. The active ingredient must be water-soluble, ionic, and with a molecular weight below 5000 Da. Even with all of these limitations, reported data show that the drug delivery effectiveness can be increased by one-third through iontophoresis [23].

In vitro and *in vivo* delivery assessment

A key in any evaluation assessment of skin bioavailability of actives is a quantitative measurement of activity by *in vitro* and *in vivo* methods. In early development phases *in vitro* methods provide a quick, reproducible way to identify promising formulations for next phase development studies. There are different techniques for evaluating percutaneous absorption of actives.

Franz cell

A well-known technique for measuring *in vitro* skin permeation is the Franz cell apparatus (Figure 7.4). The test apparatus and technique have been well documented for use within the pharmaceutical and cosmetic industries [24]. The technique utilizes a sampling

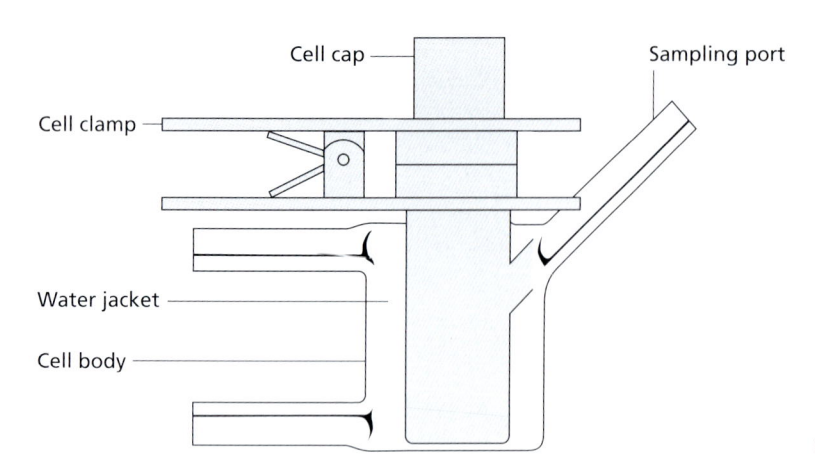

Figure 7.4 The Franz diffusion chamber.

cell which contains a solution reservoir and a sampling port, the top portion of the Franz cell is covered with a biologic membrane or skin substitute. The formulation is added to the top of the cell and periodic samples are taken from the cell reservoir and assays are plotted versus time to develop a time–penetration profile.

Tape stripping

Tape stripping is a technique used for *in vivo* active penetration evaluation. In this procedure, penetration of the active is estimated from the amount recovered in the stratum corneum by adhesive tape stripping at a fixed time point following application [25]. This technique is also recognized by FDA as a viable screening option for dermatologic evaluation [26].

Microdialysis

During the last decade, microdialysis has been shown to be a promising technique for the assessment of *in vivo* and *ex vivo* cutaneous delivery of actives. The technique is based on the passive diffusion of compounds down a concentration gradient across a semi-permeable membrane forming a thin hollow "tube" (typically, a few tenths of a millimeters in diameter), which – at least, in theory – functionally represents a permeable blood vessel (Figure 7.5.). Two kinds of probe are in common use: linear and concentric.

Confocal Raman microspectroscopy

Confocal Raman microspectroscopy (CRS) is a new, non-invasive technique which can be used for *in vivo* skin penetration evaluation. This technique combines Raman spectroscopy with confocal microscopy. CRS is a non-destructive and rapid technique that allows information to be obtained from deep layers under the skin surface, giving the possibility of a real-time tracking of the drug in the skin layers. The specific Raman signature of the active agent enables its identification within the skin [27].

There is a range of techniques of *in vitro* and *in vivo* evaluation for following penetration of actives through the skin. Some are more invasive than others and some are more predictive across various dosage forms utilized on the skin. In Table 7.3 a summary chart shows a good comparison of the techniques based on strengths and weaknesses.

Conclusions and future trends

There are many formulation options available for delivering actives to targets within the skin. Understanding the skin and its interaction with various actives allows the chemist to select delivery options that provide safe and effective properties.

A good understanding of the physicochemical parameters of the active and the desired skin target are needed before deciding on a particular delivery option. Human studies are the "gold standard" against which all methods for measuring percutaneous absorption should be judged. The conduct of human volunteer experiments is well regulated. Study protocols and accompanying toxicologic data must be submitted to an ethics committee for approval [28].

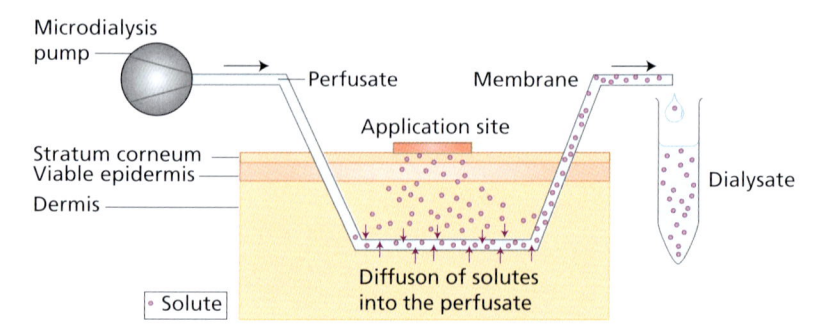

Figure 7.5 The microdialysis apparatus for the evaluation of penetration through the human skin barrier. (Source: Schnetz & Fartasch, 2001 [*Eur J Pharm Sci* **12**, 165–74]. Reproduced with permission of Elsevier.)

Table 7.3 Methods to assess drug penetration into and/or across the skin.

	Method	Measure	Measurement site	Temporal resolution	Technical simplicity
In vitro	Diffusion cell	Q	Transport into and across skin	++	+
In vivo: non- or minimally invasive	Tape stripping	Q	Stratum corneum	0	+
	ATR-FTIR	Q	Stratum corneum	+	+
	Raman	Q/L	Upper skin	+	+
	Microdialysis	Q (free)	Dermis (or subdermis)	++	−
	Vasoconstriction	A	Microcirculation	+	±
In vivo: invasive	Blister	Q	Extracellular fluid	0	±
	Biopsy	Q	Skin	0	+
	Biopsy	Q + L	Skin (depth)	0	±

Q, quantity of drug; A, pharmacological activity of drug; L, drug localization.
Source: Herkenne et al., 2008 [*Pharm Res* **25**, 87–103]. Reproduced with permission of Plenum Publishers.

Next generation delivery technologies are being developed and in some cases are already on the way to the market. Researchers from device and skincare companies are already in collaboration to bring combinations of devices and actives to the field of cosmetic dermatology. The approach can vary from non-invasive LEDs all the way to more invasive, laser-based enhanced penetration of actives. There are many home-use devices coming to the market today. These advances in delivery technology will likely culminate in a commercially available topical product that has its efficacy boosted by some type of chemical or physical delivery device as demonstrated in the delivery of estradiol using either a delivery vesicle (ultra-deformable liposomes) or a device (iontophoresis) [29].

References

1. Chien YW. (1992) *Novel Drug Delivery Systems*, 2nd edn. New York: Marcel Dekker Inc., p. 303.
2. Barry BW. (1987) Penetration enhancers in pharmacology and the skin. In: ShrootB, SchaeferH, eds. *Skin Pharmacokinetics*. Basel: Karger; Vol. 1, pp. 121–37.
3. Heather A, Benson E. (2005) Current drug delivery, penetration enhancement techniques. *Curr Drug Deliv* **2**, 23–33.
4. Moser K, Kriwet K, Naik A, Kalia YN, Guy RH. (2001) Passive skin penetration enhancement and its quantification *in vitro*. *Eur J Pharm Biopharm* **52**, 103–12.
5. Katz M, Poulsen BJ. (1971) Absorption of drugs through the skin. In: Brodie BB, Gilette J, eds. *Handbook of Experimental Pharmacology*. Berlin: Springer Verlag, pp. 103–74.
6. Forster T, Jackwerth B, Pittermann W, Rybinski WM, Schmitt M. (1997) Properties of emulsions: structure and skin penetration. *Cosmet Toiletries* **112**, 73–82.
7. Albery WJ, Hadgraft J. (1979) Percutaneous absorption: theoretical description. *Pharm Pharmacol* **31**, 129–39.
8. Stott PW, Williams AC, Barry BW. (1998) Transdermal delivery from eutectic systems: enhanced permeation of a model drug, ibuprofen. *J Control Release* **50**, 297–308.
9. Sloan KB, ed. (1992) *Prodrugs, Topical and Ocular Drug Delivery Sloan*. New York: Marcel Dekker, pp. 179–220.
10. Bucks D, Guy R, Maibach HI. (1991) Effects of occlusion. In: BronaughRL, MaibachHI, eds. *In Vitro Percutaneous Absorption: Principles, Fundamentals, and Applications*. Boca Raton: CRC Press, pp. 85–114.
11. Osborne DW, Henke JJ. (1997) Skin penetration enhancers. Pharm Technol November, 58–66.
12. Walters KA. (1988) Penetration enhancer techniques. In: HadgraftJ, GuyRH, eds. *Transdermal Drug Delivery*. New York: Marcel Dekker, pp. 197–246.
13. Harrison E, Watkinson AC, Green DM, Hadgraft J, Brain K. (1996) The relative effect of Azone and Transcutol on permeant diffusivity and solubility in human stratum corneum. *Pharm Res* **13**, 542–6.
14. Abeer A, Elzainy W, Gu X, Estelle F, Simons R, Simons KJ. (2003) Hydroxyzine from topical phospholipid liposomal formulations: evaluation of peripheral antihistaminic activity and systemic absorption in a rabbit model. *AAPS PharmSci* **5**, 1–8.
15. Cevc G, Blume G. (1992) Lipid vesicles penetrate into intact skin owing to the transdermal osmotic gradients and hydration force. *Biochim Biophys Acta* **1104**, 226–32.
16. Baillie AJ, Florence AT, Hume LR, Rogerson A, Muirhead GT. (1985) The preparation and properties of niosomes-non-ionic surfactant vesicles. *J Pharm Pharmacol* **37**, 863–8.
17. Kreuter J. (1994) Nanoparticles. In: KreuterJ, ed. *Colloidal Drug Delivery Systems*. New York: Marcel Dekker, pp. 219–342.
18. Müller RH, Mäder K, Gohla S. (2000) Solid lipid nanoparticles (SLN) for controlled drug delivery: a review of the state of the art. *Eur J Pharm Biopharm* **50**, 161–77.
19. Dinno MA, Crum LA, Wu J. (1989) The effect of therapeutic ultrasound on the electrophysiologic parameters of frog skin. *Med Biol* **25**, 461–70.
20. Hakozaki T, Takiwaki H, Miyamot K, Sato Y, Arase S. (2006) Ultrasound enhanced skin-lightening effect of vitamin C and niacinamide. *Skin Res Technol* **12**, 105–13.
21. Yuzhakov VV, Gartstein V, Owens GD. (2003) US Patent 6565532. Micro needle apparatus semi-permanent subcutaneous makeup.
22. Barry BW. (2001) Is transdermal drug delivery research still important today? *Drug Discov Today* **6**, 967–71.

23 Yao N, Gnaegy M, Haas C. (2004) Iontophoresis transdermal drug delivery and its design. *Pharmaceut Form Quality* **6**, 42–4.
24 COLIPA Guidelines for Percutaneous Absorption/Penetration. (1997) European Cosmetic, Toiletry and Perfumery Association.
25 Rougier A, Dupuis D, Lotte C. (1989) Stripping method for measuring percutaneous absorption *in vivo*. In: BronaughRL, MaibachHI, eds. *Percutaneous Absorption: Mechanisms, Methodology, Drug Delivery*, 2nd edn. New York: Marcel Dekker, pp. 415–34.
26 Shah VP, Flynn GL, Yacobi A, Maibach HI, Bon C, Fleischer NM, et al. (1998) Bioequivalence of topical dermatological dosage forms: methods of evaluation of bioequivalence. *Pharm Res* **15**, 167–71.
27 Tfayli A, Piot O, Pitre F, Manfait M. (2007) Follow-up of drug permeation through excised human skin with confocal Raman microspectroscopy. *Eur Biophys J* **36**, 1049–58.
28 World Health Organization (WHO). (1982) *World Medical Association: Proposed International Guidelines for Research Involving Human Subjects*. Geneva: WHO, p. 88.
29 Essa A, Bonner MC, Barry BW. (2002) Iontophoretic estradiol skin delivery and tritium exchange: ultradeformable liposomes. *Int J Pharm* **240**, 55–66.
30 DeHaven C. (2007) Delivery of cosmetic ingredients to the skin. *Science of Skincare*
31 Singla V, Saini S, Singh G, Rana AC, Joshi B. (2011) Penetration enhancers: a novel strategy for enhancing transdermal drug delivery. *Int Res J Pharmacy* **2**(12), 32–36.
32 Vieria R. (2010) Overcoming biological barriers-chemical penetration enhancement. *UK and Ireland Controlled Release Society Newsletter* 14–15.
33 Jungbauer FHW, Coenraods PJ, Kardaun SH. (2001) Toxic hygroscoic contact reaction to N-methyl-2-Pyrrolidone. *Contact Dermatitis* **45**, 303–304.
34 Chun-Ying CUI, Wan-Liang LU. (2005) Sublingual delivery of insulin: Effects of enhancers on the mucosal lipid fluidity and protein conformation, transport, and in vivo hypoglycemic activity. *Biol Pharm Bull* **28**, 2279–88.

CHAPTER 8
Creams and Ointments

Irwin Palefsky
Cosmetech Laboratories, Inc., Fairfield, NJ, USA

> **BASIC CONCEPTS**
> - Creams and ointments are vehicles and delivery systems for dermatological products.
> - Creams (and lotions) are emulsions, either oil-in-water (O/W) or water-in-oil (W/O).
> - Ointments are semisolid preparations used topically for protective emollient effects or as a vehicle for local administration of medicaments.
> - Changes in composition can alter the delivery of active ingredients to the skin as well as change the aesthetics of the product.
> - A big challenge is patient compliance. Users must be happy with the feel/smell/color, etc. of a dermatological cream or ointment.

Definitions of creams (and lotions) and ointments

Creams (and lotions)

Creams (and lotions) are emulsions. While this may seem very basic it is important that we understand what an emulsion is, the different types of emulsions and the role that they play as a vehicle and delivery systems for functional and drug active materials.

In looking for a generally accepted definition I came across the following: "In classic terms, emulsions are colloidal dispersions comprising two immiscible liquids (e.g. oil and water), one of which (the internal or discontinuous phase) is dispersed as droplets within the other (the external phase) [1]". What is missing from this definition is the inclusion of the emulsifier(s) or dispersing agent(s) that are responsible for keeping these two immiscible phases together for an extended period of time. All emulsions are unstable – they will eventually separate into two or more phases. There are no legal definition differences between a cream and a lotion. The determination of what to call an emulsion is usually guided by the viscosity. If an emulsion is thick and can be poured out from a bottle, or pumped out, it is usually described as a lotion. If the emulsion requires a jar or a tube, and does not readily flow it is usually referred to as a cream.

Further in this chapter we will use the term emulsion to refer to creams and lotions.

The other part of a definition of an emulsion is based on the materials that make up the internal phase and the materials that make up the external or continuous phase. The two general categories of emulsions are oil-in-water (O/W) and water-in-oil (W/O) emulsions (Figure 8.1). The names themselves describe the composition of the emulsion.

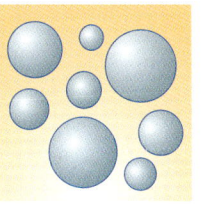

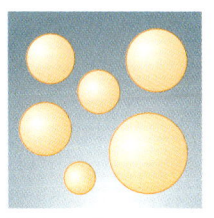

Water in oil   Oil in water

Figure 8.1 Different emulsion types.

Oil-in-water emulsions can also be described by their emulsifier type, i.e. anionic, cationic, nonionic. This terminology refers to the ionic charge (or lack of charge) on the emulsifier system that is predominant in the emulsion.

We also now have oil-in-water emulsions that are based on polymeric emulsifiers and "liquid crystal" emulsifiers. These emulsions hold the two phases together and prevent them from separating by different mechanisms from those seen in traditional emulsions, which use more conventional emulsifying systems.

For more information on this I refer you the chapter on pharmaceutical emulsions and microemulsions in the book *Pharmaceutical Dosage Forms: Disperse Systems*, Volume 2, edited by H.A. Lieberman *et al.* published by Marcel Dekker, Inc., 1996.

Water-in-oil emulsions are becoming increasingly popular as emulsion types for dermatological products. In water-in-oil emulsions the "oil phase" is the external phase and as such these emulsions have become increasingly popular for delivering enhanced skin barrier protection, water resistance and a more effective delivery system for hydrophobic ingredients. In addition, the technology has dramatically improved so that one can now

---

Cosmetic Dermatology: Products and Procedures, Second Edition. Edited by Zoe Diana Draelos.
© 2016 John Wiley & Sons, Ltd. Published 2016 by John Wiley & Sons, Ltd.

develop water-in-oil formulations that have a high degree of consumer/patient acceptance and are not greasy or oily.

Ointments

In searching for a definition of an ointment the best one that I came up with was on the Internet: "Semisolid preparations used topically for protective emollient effects or as a vehicle for local administration of medicaments; ointment bases are various mixtures of fats, waxes, animal and plant oils and solid and liquid hydrocarbons" [2]. This definition is as comprehensive as any I have seen. Ointments are traditionally anhydrous bases and therefore pose less microbial contamination issues than emulsions. In addition, because they are anhydrous in nature and are a combination of water insoluble components, they tend to be more water resistant than emulsions. Ointments tend to have less aesthetic appeal for skin care/dermatology products that need to be used on a regular basis or for an extended period of time. Ointments are frequently described as "oily", "waxy", "greasy", "sticky/tacky", and "heavy". They do however have a more medicinal connotation.

Composition of a cream and an ointment

Oil-in-water cream

The most popular type of emulsion used in everyday skin care products and in "cosmeceutical products" are oil-in-water (O/W emulsions). A generic composition for an O/W emulsion is shown in Table 8.1 [3].

Table 8.1 Composition of an oil-in-water emulsion.

Ingredients	% (weight/weight)
Water phase	
Deionized water	60.0–90.0
Humectant	2.00–7.0
Preservative**	0.05–0.5
Water soluble emulsifier***	0.25–2.5
Thickener(s)	0.1–1.0
Water soluble emollient	0.5–2.0
Chelating agent	0.05–0.20
Oil phase	
Emollient system – oils, esters, silicones etc.	3.0–15.0
Oil soluble emulsifiers	2.0–5.0
"Active ingredients"	As required by regulations
Oil soluble antioxidants	0.05–0.5
Fragrance/essential oil etc.	0.1–2.0
Color	As required
Preservative**	0.05–1.0
pH adjustments	As required

**Preservatives are frequently added in two places in the formulation.
***May also be added into the oil phase.

Each of the components of this formulation has an effect on aesthetics.

Emulsifiers

- The choice of emulsifier will also determine the pH of the emulsion, will affect its application and stability, and affect the delivery of materials into the skin.
- Recently we have seen emulsifier systems focusing around "skin friendly emulsifiers." These are emulsifiers that tend to not adversely affect the barrier properties of the skin and in some cases even help with maintaining its barrier properties. Since the route of delivery into the skin is primarily accomplished through the lipid layer (the mortar in the "bricks and mortar" construction of the skin) the election of emulsifier can determine whether this delivery function disrupts the lipid barrier or is friendly to it. Liquid crystal forming emulsifiers are being used more frequently because of their skin friendly nature. These emulsifiers act like the phospholipids and ceramides found in the skin, and therefore do not disrupt the barrier properties and function because of their compatibility with the skin lipids. Some of the more popular of these liquid crystal forming emulsifiers is lecithin or hydrogenated lecithin. There have been a number of new emulsifiers that have structures similar to lecithin and phospholipids and are therefore very skin friendly [4].
- Another recent trend is the use of emulsifiers that also become part of the emollient system. The most popular of these type of emulsifiers are "cationic" emulsifiers – emulsifiers that have a net positive charge to the skin. Since the skin, because of its amino acid composition has a net "negative charge", a positively charged emulsifier will be attached to the skin and remain on the skin because of electrostatic attraction. Examples of these emulsifiers are behentrimonium methosulfate and dicetyldimonium chloride. Cationic emulsifiers are also very effective when there is a need to formulate low pH emulsions (less than pH 4.5) as cationic emulsifiers are very stable in low pH environments.

Emollients

- The choice of emollient or combination of emollients will have a dramatic effect on feel, application and delivery of the "active" to the skin. Matching solubility of "active" with the oil phase has a great effect in determining the material to be used. Matching the solubility parameter of an organic sunscreen to the solubility parameter of the oil phase has a significant effect on the sunscreen performance.
- The emollient category has been greatly expanded because of the increased use of silicones and the increasing number of "natural" emollients.
- The selection of the emollient combinations is where art and science are combined. Selecting the right combination that provides the proper initial, middle and end feel is one of the biggest challenges affecting the successful development of a cream. Concepts such as "cascading effect" describe this type of change that occurs as you apply an emollient system.

Active ingredients

Examples of active ingredients are sunscreen materials (i.e. octinoxate, titanium dioxide, avobenzone), anti-acne actives (i.e. salicylic acid, benzoyl peroxide) and skin lighteners (hydroquinone) etc.

Humectants

The humectant, usually a glycol or polyol, will have an effect on "skin cushion" and can also be part of the solvent system for an active ingredient. Glycols, such as propylene glycol, butylene glycol etc. are very good solvents for salicylic acid (an FDA approved OTC active ingredient used to treat acne) and are frequently used for this purpose in an emulsion system. In addition they also function to help with freeze/thaw stability.

Thickeners

- The thickener(s) are used to control the viscosity and the rheology of the emulsion and can also help in maintaining the stability or product integrity of the emulsion, especially at elevated temperatures. Even in water-in-oil creams thickeners are used for viscosity control. The viscosity of a cream is primarily determined by the thickener used and the viscosity of the external phase.
- The choice of thickeners, to a large extent, depends upon the compatibility of the thickener with the rest of the ingredients in the formulation, the pH of the formulation and the desired feel that is trying to be achieved.
- The predominant thickeners used in oil-in-water emulsions are acrylic based polymers. The most popular materials are carbomers and their derivatives. Carbomers are a cross-linked polyacrylate polymers and their derivatives which are high molecular weight homopolymers and copolymers of acrylic acid, cross-linked with a polyalkenyl polyether [4]. These polymeric thickeners are very effective in stabilizing emulsions at elevated temperatures. (In water-in-oil emulsions the predominant thickeners for the external phase are waxes – natural or synthetic.)

The composition of a water-in-oil emulsion may not look much different on paper from an oil-in-water emulsion, except that the emulsifier system would be different and would be designed to make a W/O emulsion. The ratio of the two phases is not an indication of the type of emulsion. There are many O/W emulsions in which the oil phase may be at a higher percentage than the water phase and in a W/O emulsion the water phase is frequently at a higher percentage than the oil phase (see Tables 8.2 and 8.3).

Ointments

As with emulsions there can be different ointments. The traditional type of ointment contained very high levels of petrolatum as this material is a very good water resistant film former and serves as a very effective delivery system for "drug actives" on the skin. In Table 8.4 is an example of a traditional petrolatum-based ointment.

In reviewing this formulation you will notice that there is no antimicrobial preservative present. Some ointment formulations put in low levels of antimicrobial preservatives for added protection during consumer use, but anhydrous ointments are hostile environments for bacteria and are generally "self preserving".

The use of an oil soluble emulsifier helps with the application properties of the ointment as well as the ability to wash it off the skin.

Table 8.2 A typical "nonionic" oil-in-water emulsion base.

Ingredients	Function	% weight/weight
Water phase		
Deionized water	External phase vehicle	82.95
Carbomer	Thickener	0.20
Disodium EDTA	Chelating agent	0.10
Butylene glycol	Humectant	2.00
Oil phase		
Cetearyl alcohol (and) ceteareth-20	Emulsifier	2.00
Cyclopentasiloxane	Silicone emollient	4.00
Dimethicone	Silicone emollient	1.00
Caprylic/capric triglyceride	Organic emollient	5.00
Glyceryl stearate (and) PEG100 stearate	Emulsifier	1.25
Triethanolamine (99%)	Neutralizing agent and pH adjuster	0.50
Preservative	Antimicrobial	1.00

The pH of this cream would be 5.5–6.5.
The viscosity would be approx. 15,000-25,000 cps.

Table 8.3 A typical water-in-oil emulsion base that can also be used as a water resistant sunscreen emulsion base.

Ingredients	Function	% weight/weight
Water phase		
Deionized water	External phase vehicle	55.65
Xanthan gum	Water phase thickener/cohesiveness	0.25
Disodium EDTA	Chelating agent	0.10
Butylene glycol	Humectant	2.00
Preservative	Antimicrobial	1.00
Sodium chloride	Emulsion stabilizer	1.00
Oil phase		
Cetyl dimethicone	Oil phase thickener	2.00
Cyclopentasiloxane	Silicone emollient	10.00
Dimethicone	Silicone emollient	3.00
Caprylic/capric triglyceride	Organic emollient	8.00
Cetyl PEG/PPG 10/1 dimethicone	Emulsifier	4.00
Oil soluble actives	Bio-active ingredients	3.00
Jojoba oil	Natural emollient	5.00
C12-15 alkyl benzoate	Solvent/emollient	5.00

The anticipated viscosity of this formulation would be 50,000-80,000 cps.

Table 8.4 A traditional petrolatum-based ointment.

Ingredients	% (weight/weight)
White petrolatum USP	50.0–80.0
Lanolin	1.0–5.0
Natural and/or synthetic waxes	2.0–10.0
Oil soluble emulsifier	1.0–3.0
"Drug actives"	As required
Antioxidants	0.1–0.5
Fragrance/essential oils	0.1–1.0
Skin feel modifiers	1.0–5.0

Table 8.5 A "natural ointment" composition.

Ingredients	% (weight/weight)
Soy bean oil (and) hydrogenated cottonseed oil	50.0–80.0
Lanolin	1.0–5.0
Natural waxes	2.0–10.0
Oil vegetable soluble emulsifier	1.0–3.0
"Drug actives"	As required
Natural antioxidants	0.1–0.5
Natural fragrance/essential oils	0.1–1.0
Natural skin feel modifiers	1.0–5.0

Recently there has been an increased interest in "natural ointments" – ointments that do not use petrochemicals (i.e. petrolatum) and are primarily based on plant derived materials.

The primary difference is in the use of the material that replaces petrolatum in the formulation. There are a number of hydrogenated oil/wax mixtures that are offered and used as "natural petrolatums". In Table 8.5 is a typical "natural ointment" composition.

"Natural ointments" generally do not have the same unctuous, heavy feel that petrolatum-based ointments have and they usually do not leave as much residual feel on the skin. As with petrolatum-based ointments little or no antimicrobial preservative is needed because of the anhydrous nature of the ointment. Antioxidants, however, are a very important components, as these "natural oil-based" ointments have a tendency to turn color and go rancid (similar to what you would see in a vegetable oil) without adequate protection.

While the number of different ingredients that can be used in an emulsion or an ointment can sometimes seem overwhelming, once you break down the product into the attributes and benefits and aesthetics that are desired, the choices become less daunting.

Once the formulations have been put together and evaluated, the next step is the stability testing. This testing is done to determine what happens to the product once it is on the market. The ideal test would be to store the product at ambient temperature for 2–3 years and observe any changes that may occur in product integrity and determine the stability of the "active" ingredient(s) that are present. Since this timeframe is not practical, accelerated stability testing is conducted to predict the long-term stability of the product.

For most pharmaceutical emulsions, this testing involves storage of the finished product at 5°C, 25°C (RT), and 40°C and sometimes at 50°C. Stability at 40°C is traditionally carried out for 3 months [5]. This testing is accepted by the U.S. FDA for expiration dating until a full 2 or 3-year study is complete. Its purpose is to ascertain product integrity and the stability of the drug actives in the product.

Elevated temperature testing (40°C for 3 months) is conducted so that a determination can be made in a reasonable amount of time as to the integrity and stability of the product and to allow the product to be marketed in a reasonable amount of time from the completion of formulation development.

As was mentioned previously in this chapter, the development of the final formulation is a combination of art and science, and both play an important role in the use of the product by the patient or consumer.

Once the type of formulation is determined, the ingredients have been selected, the formulation developed, the appropriate safety, efficacy, preservative testing, and the stability testing completed, the product can now be ready to introduce to the market.

References

1 Block LH. (1996) Pharmaceutical emulsions and microemulsions; emulsions and microemulsion characteristics and attributes. In: LiebermanHA, RiegerMM, BankerGS, eds. *Pharmaceutical Dosage Forms: Disperse Systems*, Vol 2. New York: Marcel Dekker, pp. 47.
2 www.biology-online.org/dictionary/Ointments. Biology on Line; Dictionary-O-Ointments, 2008.
3 "Emulsions" presentation from Cognis Corp, August 2004.
4 www.personalcare.noveon.com/products/carbopol, "Carbopol Rheology Modifiers".
5 Block LH. (1996) Pharmaceutical emulsions and microemulsions; emulsions and microemulsion characteristics and attributes. In: LiebermanHA, RiegerMM, BankerGS, eds. *Pharmaceutical Dosage Forms: Disperse Systems*, Vol 2. New York: Marcel Dekker, pp. 94–95.

PART II

Hygiene Products

SECTION 1 Cleansers

CHAPTER 9
Bar Cleansers

Anthony W. Johnson, K.P. Ananthapadmanabhan, Stacy Hawkins, and Greg Nole
Unilever HPC R&D, Trumbull, CT, USA

> **BASIC CONCEPTS**
> - There are two basic types of cleansing bar – soap bars and synthetic detergent bars.
> - Like all surfactant-based products, cleansing bars can be harsh or mild to skin.
> - Mild cleansing bars have a key role in fundamental skin care.
> - Mild cleansing bars have positive benefits for patients with skin diseases.

Introduction

Cleansing bars – historical perspective

Anecdotally, soap was discovered by prehistoric man, noticing a waxy reside in the ashes of an evening camp fire around a burnt piece of animal carcass. The waxy material was soap. Potash from the ashes (KOH) had hydrolyzed triglyceride from animal fat to produce potassium soap and glycerol. Actual historical records show soap-like materials in use by Sumerians in 2500 BC and there are references to soap in Greek and Roman records and by the Celts in northern Europe. As European civilizations emerged from the Dark Ages in the 9th and 10th centuries soap making was well-established and centered in Marseilles (France), Savona (Italy), and Castilla (Spain). In those days soap was a luxury affordable only by the very rich. Mass manufacture of soap started in the 19th century and was well-established by the turn of the century with individually wrapped and branded bars.

Synthetic detergents emerged in the 20th century, primarily for fabric washing products. While there are many types of synthetic detergent, very few are suitable for making cleansing bars. It is difficult to make a solid product that is able to retain a solid form during multiple encounters with water and at the same time able to resist cracking, crumbling, and hardening when drying between uses. Soap is ideal for making bars but that is not to say that some of the early soap bars did not dry out and develop cracks or become soft and mushy in humid environments. Modern manufacturers are able to formulate soap bars to control the physical behaviour in use and when drying between uses. Despite conversion of many bar uses to liquid format, bars remain an important format in US and even more so globally. Figure 9.1

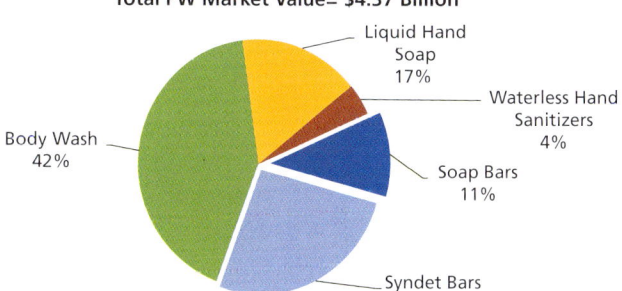

Figure 9.1 Dollar segmentation of U.S. cleanser market shows that bars continue to command significant share. Bars in the U.S. alone have a total value of $1.6 billion of which syndet bars are the majority share. (2013 data.)

shows the segmentation of the US Personal Wash market with all bar cleansers holding 37% share of value. While soap-based bars continue to dominate in total volume, the higher value of synthetic detergent bars command 70% of the dollar share.

The wide range of soap bars available in the skin marketplace today might suggest a wide range of functionality but this is not the case. To develop new claims and gain shelf space in big supermarkets, manufacturers create variants by minor modifications of their basic bar types – the functional properties of soap bar variants are usually very similar – they all lather and they all clean.

Formulation technology of cleansing bars

Cleansing bars are made of surfactants that are solid at room temperature and readily soluble in water. While there are scores

---

Cosmetic Dermatology: Products and Procedures, Second Edition. Edited by Zoe Diana Draelos.
© 2016 John Wiley & Sons, Ltd. Published 2016 by John Wiley & Sons, Ltd.

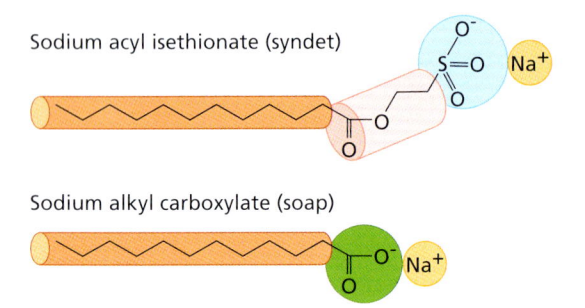

Figure 9.2 Schematic representation of the molecular structures of soap (sodium alkyl carboxylate) and syndet (sodium acyl isethionate) showing the difference in head group structure and size.

of commercially available surfactants only two, alkyl carboxylate (soap) and acyl isethionate (syndet), are used on a large scale for manufacture of cleansing bars (Figure 9.2).

These two surfactant types are quite different, leading to different sensory experiences for the consumer and also differences in their interactions with skin. Soap and syndet have in common that they have the physical properties required to be processed into bars that can withstand the challenges of use in the home. As bars they must have a consistent performance – they must lather easily when new but just as readily as the bar is used up over a period of weeks or months. They should produce lather quickly and easily and should not feel gritty in use. The rate of wear should be optimum, neither too fast nor too slow. They must dry quickly after use but must not crack; they should not break apart if dropped, and should not absorb water and become mushy in a humid environment, like a bathroom. There are not many surfactants that can satisfy this list of seemingly simple practical requirements.

Broadly speaking, there are two types of manufacturing process for making cleansing bars: (a) a continuous process of milling, extrusion, and stamping; and (b) a batch process of melt casting.

Continuous processing

The continuous process starts with synthesis of the basic surfactant, alkyl carboxylate, and then processing this as a solid through various steps during which other ingredients are added until the final composition is attained. After milling and mixing steps to ensure homogeneity, the compounded soap it is extruded as a continuous bar which is chopped and stamped into the individual bar shape of the final product. The technical demands of the continuous process impose constraints on composition and ingredient addition – but it is the fastest and cheapest way to make a cleansing bar.

Batch processing

The essence of the melt cast approach is to make the surfactant and add any desired ingredients to form a hot liquid melt which is poured into individual bar size casts and allowed to set as it cools. This is a much more expensive process but allows for a wider range of additional ingredients in the product formulation. The continuous process is used for most of the mass market bars and the melt cast process for specialist bars often sold in boutiques, custom outlets, and department stores.

Soap bars

There are several major compositional types of soap bar with distinct bar properties and in use behaviors – speed and type of lather, rate of use up, aroma, skin compatibility, tendency for mush, etc. Most bars are either basic or superfatted soap. Basic soaps are blends of medium chain length fatty acid sodium salts (Figure 9.2). Superfatted soaps are similar but with additional fatty acid. There are other categories of soap bars based on the use of specialist ingredients: transparent bars, antibacterial bars, and deodorant bars. There are large numbers of specialist bars that are simply soap containing a wide range of colors, fragrances, and emotive ingredients such as vitamins, aloe, chamomile, and other natural extracts. The emotive ingredients in specialist bars are there to appeal to the senses and emotions with no real expectation that they have any detectable benefit for the skin.

Basic soap

Soap is the sodium salt of a fatty acid. As the salts of weak acids, soaps form alkaline solutions as they dissociate in water. The pH of soap is typically in the pH range 9–11. This is not sufficient to be overtly irritating to skin but is sufficiently high to negatively impact the pH-dependent processes of the stratum corneum which has a natural pH of around 5.5. The fatty acids used in soap making are natural, derived from animal or plant sources, with the most common chain lengths in the range C12 (e.g. coconut fatty acid) to C18 (e.g. tallow/rendered animal fat). C12–14 soaps are soluble and lather easily. C16–18 soaps are less soluble but good for forming solid bars. The plant oils used in soap making are mostly triglycerides and when treated with lye and/or caustic soda they hydrolyze to the fatty acid sodium salts (soap) and glycerol.

Superfatted soap bars

Simple soaps are good cleansers but also drying to skin. Less drying soaps are made by adjusting the soap making process to leave an excess of free fatty acid in the final soap composition (superfatted soaps). This excess fatty acid reduces the lipid stripping and drying effects of a soap bar to a small extent. Beauty soaps are typically superfatted soaps.

Transparent soaps

There are several types of transparent or semi-transparent soap bars. The earliest was a rosin glycerin soap bar developed by Andrew Pears in 1789. The ingredients of Pears patented transparent soap were sodium palmitate, natural rosin, glycerine, water, C12 soap, rosemary extract, thyme extract, and fragrance. The Pears soap of today is made by essentially the same process, which involves dissolving the raw soap and other ingredients in alcohol, pouring into moulds followed by up to 3 months of evaporation and drying.

A different type of transparent bar was introduced in 1955 by Neutrogena based on a patented formulation invented by a Belgian cosmetic chemist, Edmond Fromont. His novel formulation was based on triethanolamine soap (in other words, soap where the neutralizing cation is triethanolamine instead of the usual sodium). The ingredients of the Neutrogena bar are triethanolamine stearate, C12–18 soaps, glycerine, water, and a range of minor ingredients including a little lanolin derivative and fragrance. Triethanolamine forms acid soaps so the pH of the Neutrogena bar at pH 8–9 is lower than a regular soap with sodium as the cation.

Antibacterial and deodorant soap bars

Medicated or antibacterial soaps are a large subcategory of the bar soap market. These products are basic soaps containing one of a limited number of approved antibacterial agents. Some of these products are positioned as deodorant soap to inhibit the odor-producing bacteria of the axilla. However, some are positioned for germ inhibition which has come under increased scrutiny. Washing with any soap is effective for removing and killing the bacteria on skin and the contribution of added antibacterial agents is controversial.

Non-soap detergent bars – syndet bars

Because soap is cheap and easy to manufacture the cleansing bar market has remained predominantly soap bars. However, there has been one non-soap bar technology that has achieved a significant place in the US market over the last 50 years and is now extending its reach to other regions of the world. This product, introduced to the US market in 1957 as the Dove bar, is based on patented acyl isethionate as the surfactant component in combination with stearic acid which has a dual function of providing the physical characteristics for forming a stable bar and also acting as a significant skin protecting and moisturizing ingredient. The high level of stearic acid in the Dove bar is the basis of the one-quarter moisturizing cream in the product. When the patents for this novel technology ran out, several other acyl isethionate bars were introduced in the USA market including Caress, Olay, Cetaphil, and Aveeno.

Interestingly, this mild non-soap technology pioneered in bar with acyl isethionate has only recently been translated in 2009 as a mild and moisturizing surfactant component in liquid cleanser formats. Similar to what was observed in the approach to developing ultra-mild bars, it is expected that this liquid acyl isethionate technology will spread widely where liquid cleansers comprise a large portion of market share, thus reaffirming the value of this "bar technology" for cleansing.

Preservatives

It is of interest that soap bars and syndet bars are self-preserved in the sense that they provide a hostile environment for microorganisms and do not need to contain a preservative to maintain product quality.

Impact of cleansing bars on skin structure and function

Washing with soap removes dirt and grime from skin and is very effective for removing germs and preventing the spread of infection. There is an appreciation that some soaps are harsh and others mild, but washing with soap is so routine and commonplace that most people give no thought to the cleansing process or its impact on skin. This is a mistake. Research over the last few years has revealed several mechanisms by which soap interacts with skin structures to adversely affect normal functioning. It is now clear that mild cleansing has significant benefits for both diseased and healthy skin. Mild cleansing can help reduce the dry skin symptoms of common skin conditions such as eczema, acne, and rosacea simply by eliminating of the aggravations of harsh soap. Mild cleansing can also enhance the attractiveness of normal skin by allowing it to better retain moisture.

Surfactant interaction with the skin–stratum corneum

As described in other chapters of this book, the outer layer of skin, the stratum corneum, is a very effective barrier to the penetration of microorganisms and chemicals unless compromised by damage, disease, or a intrinsic weakness caused by one of the genetic variations now known to impact the functioning of the stratum corneum. Whatever the normal state of the stratum corneum for an individual, the most challenging (i.e. potentially damaging) environmental factor, apart from industrial exposure to solvents and other harsh chemicals, is cleansing. And yet cleansing is a key element of good everyday skincare and there is much variation in the damaging potential of different cleansing products including cleansing bars. Understanding how cleansing products impact skin and knowing the mildest cleansing product technologies is a basic requirement for achieving fundamental skin care.

Soap bar interactions with the stratum corneum

The properties of soap that make it an effective cleanser also determine that it can be drying and irritating to skin. The high charge density of the carboxyl head group of the soap molecule promotes strong protein binding which is bad for skin. Soap binds strongly to stratum corneum proteins and disturbs the water-holding mechanisms of the corneocytes. Soaps also denature stratum corneum enzymes essential for corneocytes maturation and desquamation. The result is an accumulation of corneocytes at the skin surface and the characteristic scaly, flaky, roughness associated with dry skin.

In addition to damaging proteins, soap and other cleansers can disrupt and strip out the lipid bi-layers of the stratum corneum. The bipolar structure of the soap molecule is similar to the bipolar structure of the three major lipid types that make up the lipid bi-layers of the stratum corneum (fatty acids, cholesterol, and ceramides). Soap disrupts the bi-layer structure of these lipids in the stratum corneum and thereby reduces the effectiveness of the stratum corneum water barrier. Transepidermal water loss (TEWL) is increased through the leaky barrier. Also, disruption of the structured lipid matrix around stratum corneum cells (corneocytes) allows the highly soluble components of the skin's natural moisturizing factor (NMF), contained in the protein matrix of the corneocytes, to leach out. Leaching is increased by further cleansing or even simply by contact with water. This process explains the paradox that water is often a major factor for causing dry skin. Effects on the key lipid structures of the stratum corneum add to the damage caused by soap–protein interactions and exacerbate the development of skin dryness – remembering that dry skin is not simply a lack of moisture but a disturbance of normal stratum corneum function with retention and accumulation of superficial corneocytes. The build up of corneocytes at the skin surface is responsible for many symptoms associated with "dry" skin – scaling, flaking, roughness, dull appearance (due to light scattering), tightness, loss of resilience/flexibility/elasticity, and ultimately cracking and irritation.

All soaps have the ability to induce dry and irritated skin and these effects are most evident in challenging environmental condition – cold or hot temperatures with low humidity, excessive exposure to solar UV radiation, and prolonged exposure to wind. The drying potential of soap varies according to composition such as the balance between soluble (C12–14) and less soluble chain lengths (C16–18) of the fatty acids most commonly used to make soap – the higher the soluble component the more drying the soap. Superfatted soaps are a little milder than simple soaps, and triethanolamine soap and glycerol bars the mildest of the commonly available soap bars.

Synthetic detergent bar interactions with the stratum corneum

Synthetic detergent bars (syndet bars) have been available on the US market for 50 years and represent a clear technological difference from soap-based cleansing bars. Nearly all common synthetic detergent bars are based on an anionic surfactant, acyl isethionate. At the time of writing (2015) these bars account for 40% of the cleansing bars sold in the USA. Alkyl glycerol ether sulfonate (AGES) and monoalkyl phosphate (MAPS) are two of a small number of other synthetic detergents that have been tried for manufacture of cleansing bars but none of these have been successful in the US market.

Ironically, because syndet bars are shaped like soap bars and used for cleansing just like a soap bar, most people believe that synthetic detergent bars are just another variety of soap. Most consumers are unaware that there is a fundamental compositional difference between soap and syndet bars that impacts their interactions with skin such that syndet bars are milder than soap bars during cleansing. There is a greater difference between soap and syndet cleansing in terms of healthy and attractive skin than most people realize. It is important for healthcare professionals and dermatologists to appreciate the difference between soap and syndet bars because studies show the difference in mildness is very relevant for their patient groups (see studies described below).

Soap (alkyl carboxylate) and syndet (acyl isethionate) are both anionic surfactants and like all anionic surfactants they interact with skin proteins and skin lipids. But because of the difference in head group physical chemistry soap interactions are more intense leading to a higher potential for inducing dryness and irritation. The carboxylate head group is compact, leading to a high charge density that facilitates binding and denaturing of proteins. By contrast, the isethionate head group is large and diffused, producing a low charge density and less ability to interact with proteins (Figure 9.2).

A second and most important factor contributing to the mildness of the isethionate syndet bar is the ability to formulate acyl isethionate with high levels of stearic acid without losing the ability to lather. In fact, the lather is more dense and creamy than the lather of a typical soap bar. The stearic acid component of the isethionate syndet bar acts as a moisturizing cream and deposits on skin during cleansing, adding to the relative mildness of these types of bar. Superfatting is, in principle, a similar way to reduce the harshness of plain soap but the results are much more modest because the initial harshness of soap is higher than syndet and the upper limit of practical superfatting is closer to 10% compared to the 20–25% fatty acid that can be formulated in an isethionate bar.

The role of pH

Another important difference between soap and syndet bars is pH. Soap has an alkaline pH typically around pH 10–11 whereas isethionate/stearic acid bars are close to pH neutral with a pH of a little over 7. The pH of glycerol bars is in the range pH 8–9. These differences in pH have an effect on the interaction of cleansing bars with the stratum corneum. Skin proteins swell markedly if the cleanser pH is highly alkaline (pH > 8). Optical coherence tomography (OCT) pictures of stratum corneum after exposure to acidic, neutral, and alkaline pH conditions and the corresponding swelling show that there is significantly higher swelling in alkaline pH solutions (Figure 9.3). Strongly binding detergent molecules can increase the swelling further.

High pH also has an impact on stratum corneum lipids. An alkaline pH can ionize fatty acids in the lipid bi-layers making them more like "soap" molecules and destabilizing the highly organized structure of the bi-layers.

These factors contribute to the differences in mildness of soap and syndet bars. Environmental scanning electron microscopy pictures of the skin surface and the corresponding transmission electron microscopy images of the protein-lipid ultrastructure of human skin washed under exaggerated conditions (nine repeat washes) with a syndet and a soap bar are seen in Figure 9.4. It is evident from the micrographs that the syndet bar washed sample exhibits well-preserved cells with intact proteins and lipids compared with the soap washed sample.

More recently, a new class of syndet bars with a combination of syndet surfactants such as acyl isethionate and sulfosuccinate has begun to appear in some of the global markets. These bars have pH values in the range of 5 to 5.5. Since the latter is close to skin's natural pH, "skin friendly" claims are used to imply that the bar being close to skin pH is less damaging to skin. However, it is not clear that a cleanser formulated to match the skin pH is de facto milder because it depends on the harshness of the surfactant under skin pH conditions and how it interacts with the stratum corneum.

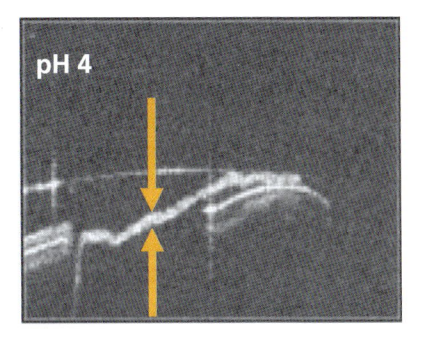

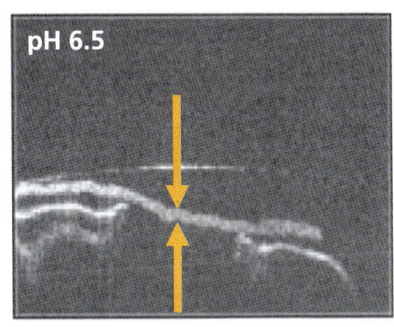

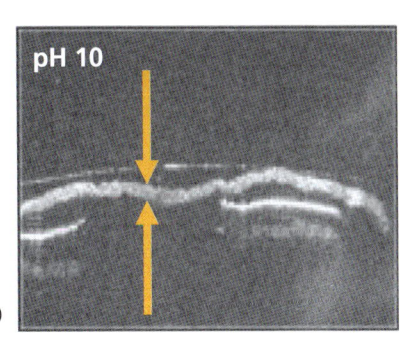

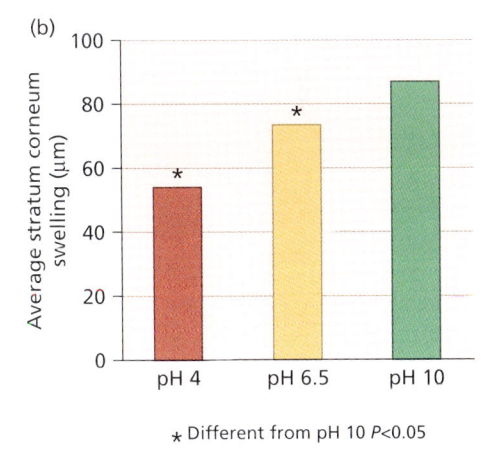

Figure 9.3 Swelling of the stratum corneum in different pH buffer solutions. (a) Optical coherence tomography (OCT) images of *ex vivo* skin treated with different buffer solutions. The arrows show the position and thickness of the stratum corneum. (b) The bar chart provides a graphic representation of the same difference.

* Different from pH 10 $P<0.05$

In order to determine if a commercially available "skin pH" cleansing bar is milder to skin than a neutral pH syndet bar, a forearm controlled application test (FCAT) was carried out. The results for skin dryness and TEWL given in Figure 9.5 shows that the two commercially available pH 5.5 bars were more drying than the pH 7 bar. Since this comparison was made with bars having different surfactants, a further study was designed with prototype bars using the same surfactant composition but at two different pH values. The results given in Figure 9.6 show that here again, the pH 5.5 bar is relatively more drying to skin than the neutral pH bar. These studies clearly show that being at skin pH does not itself result in a milder Bar as compared to a Bar at neutral pH. The drying potential of the bar depends upon the nature of surfactants used in making the Bar and its interaction with the corneum.

The question is why cleansing bars consisting of typical anionic surfactants are more drying and damaging to the barrier at skin pH compared to neutral pH conditions. The answer may be in the interaction of anionic surfactants with the corneum under weak acidic conditions. The isoelectric point (IEP, where the net charge on the surface is zero) of stratum corneum and keratin is around pH 5. As pH is lowered from neutral to acidic pH conditions, net negative charge on the corneum will decrease and will eventually become positive below the IEP. An increase in the number of positively charged sites on the protein with decrease in pH from neutral pH can be thus expected to increase the binding of anionic surfactants to proteins. Results of surfactant binding to human stratum corneum published in the literature and reproduced in Figure 9.7 show that binding of lauroyl isethionate increases with decrease in pH in the acidic range and increases with increase in pH above about pH 9.0. Thus the isethionate binding shows a minimum in the neutral pH region. The binding results do correlate with the increased drying tendency of cleansers with typical anionic surfactant such as isethionate. These results clearly demonstrate that even though pH 5.5 may be "good for skin", it may not be good for a skin cleanser unless the cleanser surfactant is mild under weak-acid conditions.

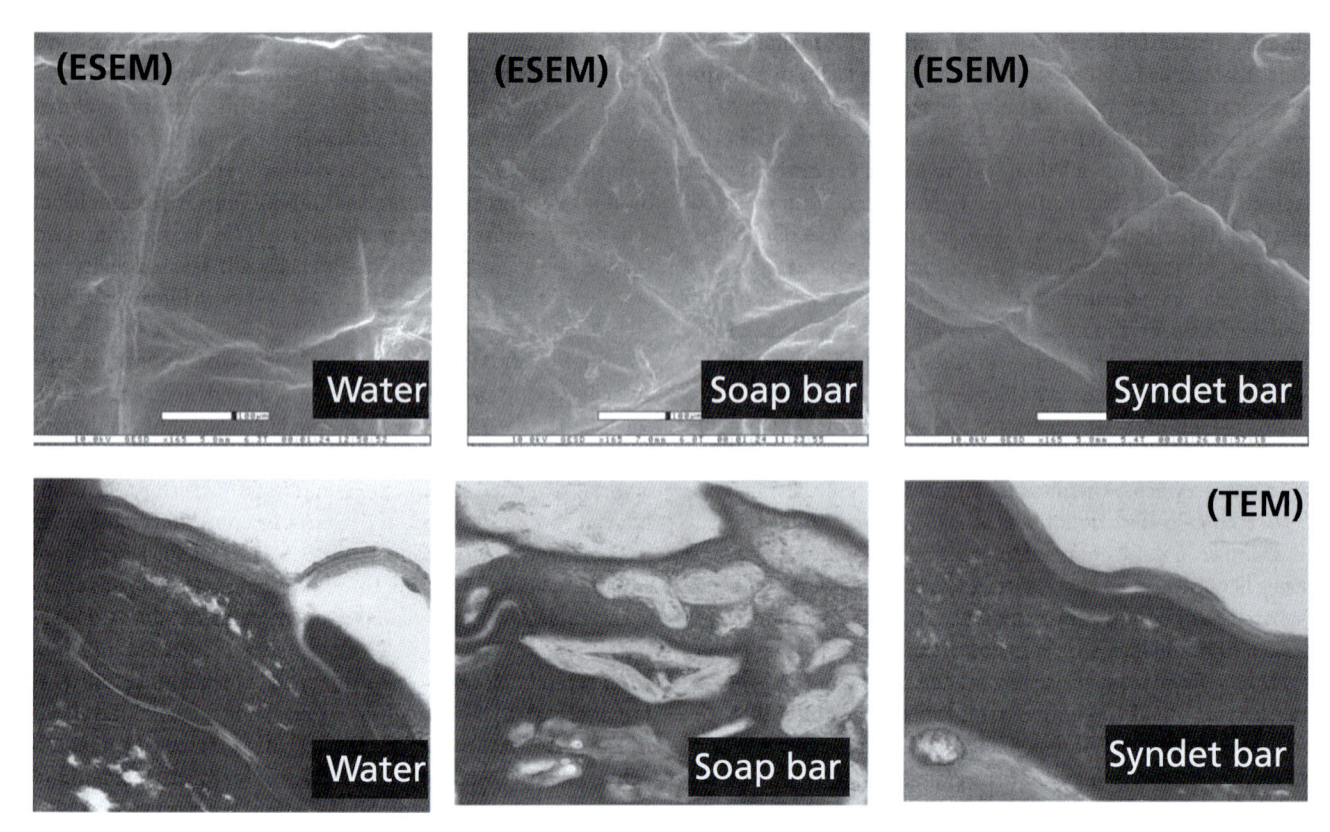

Figure 9.4 Environmental scanning electron micrographs (ESEM) and transmission electron micrographs (TEM) images of human skin washed with water, soap, and a syndet bar (9 repeat washes). Water washed and mild syndet bar washed skin shows well-preserved lipids and plumped (hydrated) corneocytes. By contrast, images of harsh soap-washed skin show significant removal of lipids and damage to proteins.

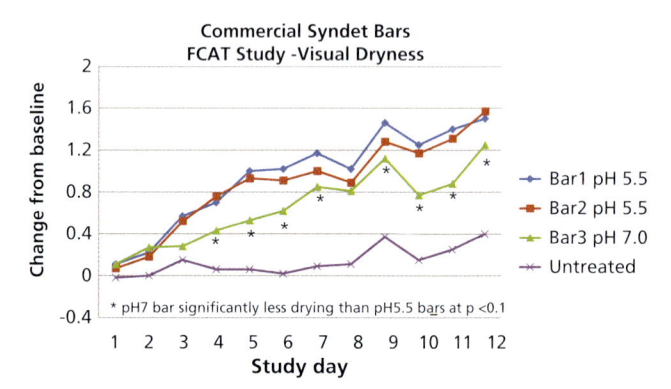

Figure 9.5 Visual dryness change observed in a forearm controlled application test (FCAT) using two commercially available syndet Bars at pH 5.5 based compared to neutral pH syndet bar. Bars at pH 5.5 cause more dryness than the one at pH 7.0.

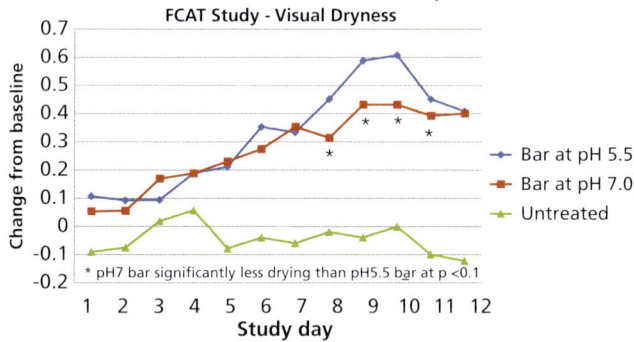

Figure 9.6 Visual dryness change observed in a forearm controlled application test (FCAT) using two syndet bars identical in surfactant composition and differing only in pH. The pH 5.5 bars appears to cause more dryness than the one at pH 7.0.

In summary, high (basic soap) pH cleansing has a number of negative effects such as destabilization of bilayer lipid structure which exist in a naturally weak acid mantle. Under weakly acidic conditions, on the other hand, there is an increase in the positively charged sites on the keratin proteins leading to increased anionic surfactant binding. This evidence suggests that neutral pH cleansing is the ideal point for minimizing damage with conventional cleansers.

Cycle of dryness

Many consumers are not aware of the differences in drying and irritation potential between soap bars and synthetic detergent bars. In

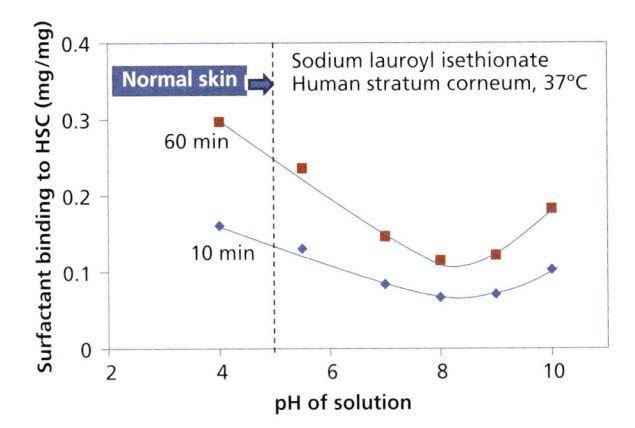

Figure 9.7 Binding of anionic surfactant, sodium lauroyl isethionate, increases with decrease in pH from neutral pH region. Binding shows a minimum around the neutral pH region. Increase in binding with decrease in pH in the acidic region is thought to be due to increase in the number of positive sites and reduction in the negative sites. IEP (isoelectric point of keratin is around pH 5)

practice, most cleansing products are not drying to an extent that is readily perceivable and under normal conditions of use cleansing bars seldom produce irritation and inflammation. However, in other circumstances, particularly drying environmental conditions or with compromised diseased skin, some cleansing bars can cause severe dryness and irritation. Why is this?

Under normal conditions it is likely that the skin is superficially dried by most cleansers but is rapidly able to restore its ability to hold moisture and maintain healthy functioning. However, under challenging environmental conditions, particularly the harsh cold winters of Canada and the northern USA and the hot dry summers of the central plains and western desert areas of the USA, recovery after washing is likely to be less rapid. Without supplemental moisturization, a vicious cycle of damage and inadequate recovery is quickly established, leading initially to dry skin but quickly progressing to deeper damage with fissuring of the stratum corneum (cracking), deeper penetration of the surfactant, irritation, and ultimately full-thickness cracking of the stratum corneum leading to chapping and bleeding. This may sound extreme but anyone with a tendency to develop dry skin will recognize this scenario of rapid deterioration to more severe irritation when the weather is drying – particularly for hand washing.

While we have described the various interactions of soap and syndet surfactants with skin proteins and lipids, these effects are never in isolation. They are cumulative and mutually reinforcing for inducing skin dryness. To better understand how they work in concert, it is helpful to see them as a sequence of events in the cycle of dryness (Figure 9.8).

Beginning with intact skin, soap is used to remove surface dirt and oils, however, it will also solubilize and remove lipids at the surface of which the smaller fatty acids (C18–20) are most readily depleted. The loss of these protective lipids increase the exposure of corneocytes to water.

Within corneocytes is Natural Moisturizing Factor, a mixture of hydrophilic materials that help hold water within the corneocyte. The increased exposure due to lipid loss allows water to more easily penetrate the corneocyte and wash away the water-loving NMF. Excess water exposure overhydrates exposed corneocytes and coupled with high pH of soap causes the corneocytes to swell. Rapid deswelling as they lose their excess moisture after washing causes a drying-stress that can cause detachment of corneocytes from the

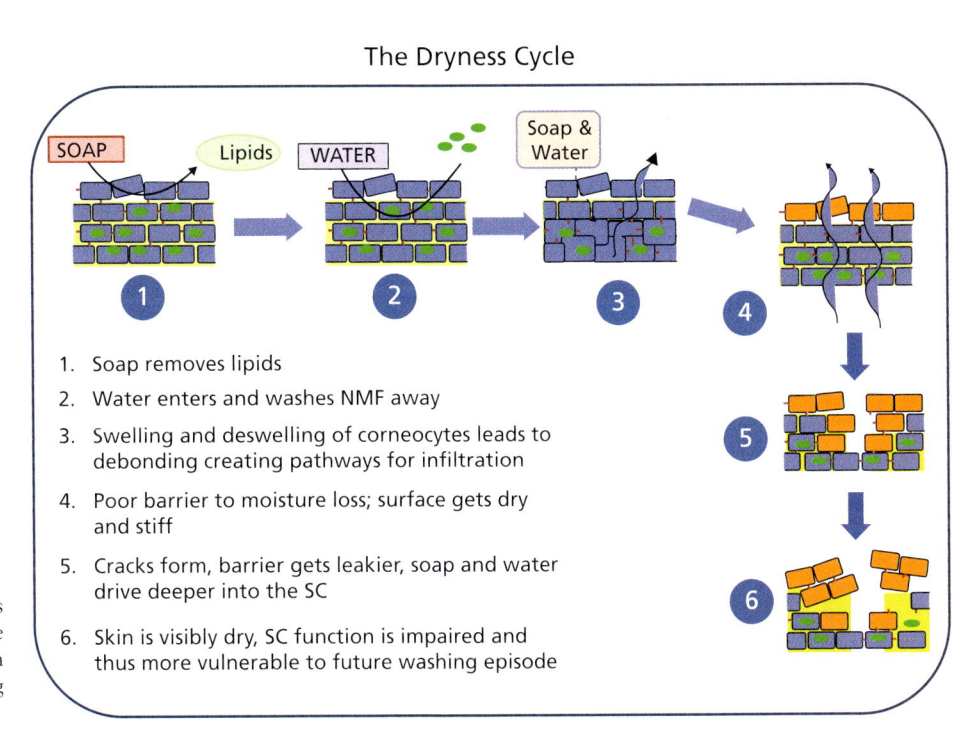

The Dryness Cycle

1. Soap removes lipids
2. Water enters and washes NMF away
3. Swelling and deswelling of corneocytes leads to debonding creating pathways for infiltration
4. Poor barrier to moisture loss; surface gets dry and stiff
5. Cracks form, barrier gets leakier, soap and water drive deeper into the SC
6. Skin is visibly dry, SC function is impaired and thus more vulnerable to future washing episode

Figure 9.8 Harsh cleansing leads to loss of lipids leaving skin more vulnerable to irritation, decreased barrier function and further damage to future washing episodes.

surrounding lipid matrix. The drying stress is often perceived as after-wash skin tightness usually lasting about 15 minutes while skin equilibrates. The detachment of corneocytes from the lipid matrix also creates micro pathways for infiltration of soap molecules into deeper layers causing progressive damage in sub-surface layers.

With loss of protective barrier lipids and Natural Moisturizing Factor to hold water in skin, the outermost cell layer becomes superficially dry, perhaps unperceivable at first but with two consequences. Dry corneocytes are stiff and inflexible making skin more vulnerable to cracking with fissures. The loss of barrier function increases skin vulnerability. The SC will compensate for the increased epidermal water loss by converting filaggrin to NMF, but as NMF gets depleted, this conversion needs to take place lower within the SC leaving the surface dry.

Desmosomes are sometimes called "molecular rivets" as they are proteins that connect corneocytes together. In the normal process of desquamation, the desmosomes are enzymatically degraded so that surface corneocytes are free to desquamate. However, loss of moisture at the surface impedes the process of desmolysis to leave surface cells connected together forming visible skin flakes. Initially seen as light powdery appearance, as dryness increase and skin is less able to hold moisture, the size of bound squames can increase to visible skin flakes.

With impaired barrier function, loss of NMF, and increased water loss, the SC is more vulnerable to subsequent washing events which continue to drive dryness deeper. While lotion application can help temporarily replace the moisture in the SC it cannot undo the soap damage, thus underscoring the need to reduce surfactant damage in the first place through mild cleansing.

Studies comparing mildness properties of soap and syndet cleansing bars

As we have shown, the effects of cleansers on skin are more than simply due to direct topical exposure. The potential for dryness is greatly impacted by weather, humidity, skin condition as well as intrinsic factors such as age and genetic skin type.

Controlled exposure trials

The first practical demonstration that syndet bars are fundamentally less damaging to skin than soap bars was a study published by Frosh and Kligman [1]. Using a new and simple method, the soap chamber test, they examined the skin irritation potential of all the cleansing bars they could purchase locally in Philadelphia at that time. One bar stood out as exceptionally mild compared with the rest of the marketplace (17 other bars tested) and this was a patented alkyl isethionate bar called Dove. Now that the Dove patent has expired a number of manufacturers sell similar isethionate syndet bars.

The difference in relative mildness of soap and isethionate/stearic acid syndet bars is easily demonstrated in the standard wash and rinse tests used by manufacturers of cleansing products. The forearm controlled application test (FCAT) and leg controlled application test (LCAT) are 5-day repeat washing tests. Skin condition is evaluated daily by a variety of techniques including visual dryness, superficial and deeper hydration measured instrumentally, TEWL to assess barrier performance, and erythema to assess irritation. As example of the comparison of soap to syndet cleansers in a FCAT, typical TEWL and dryness results are shown in Figure 9.9.

An increase in stratum corneum dryness has a negative effect on the mechanical properties of the corneum. Changes in stratum corneum elasticity/stiffness measured in a standard clinical test after washing with soap and syndet bars are shown in Figure 9.10. While soap washing increases skin stiffness markedly, the milder syndet bar maintains the original skin condition. Such effects are magnified further under low humidity and winter conditions and can lead to microcracks in the stratum corneum and increased water loss, plus increased vulnerability to penetration of external chemicals into skin.

Normal usage trials

Concern is sometimes expressed that industry standard tests are exaggerated and do not reflect real consumer experience. The evidence accumulated by manufacturers and published in peer-reviewed journals demonstrates that effects in standard

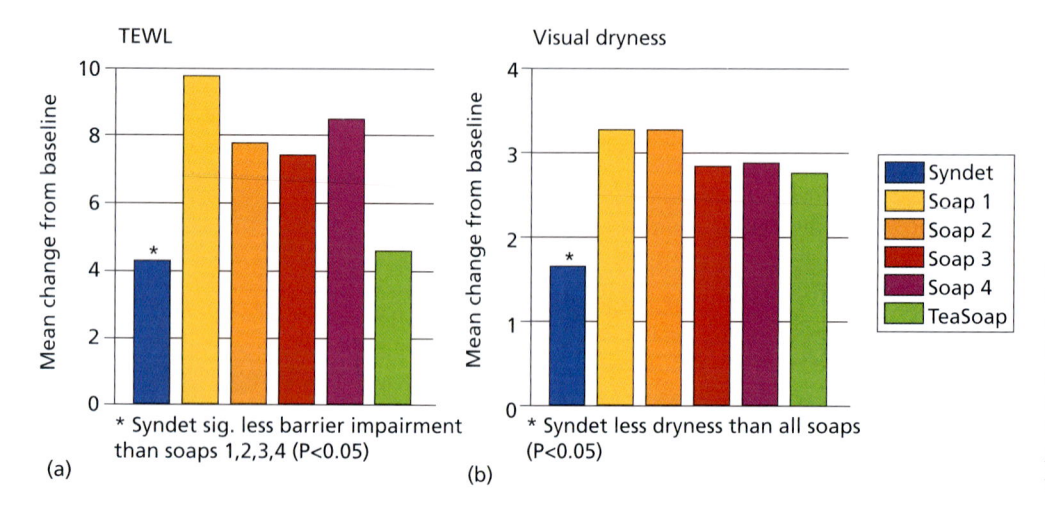

Figure 9.9 Skin changes after 5 days of twice daily washing with soaps and syndet using the forearm controlled application test (FCAT) method. (a) Transepidermal water loss rate and (b) Visual dryness are significantly lower for syndet bar as compared to regular soaps

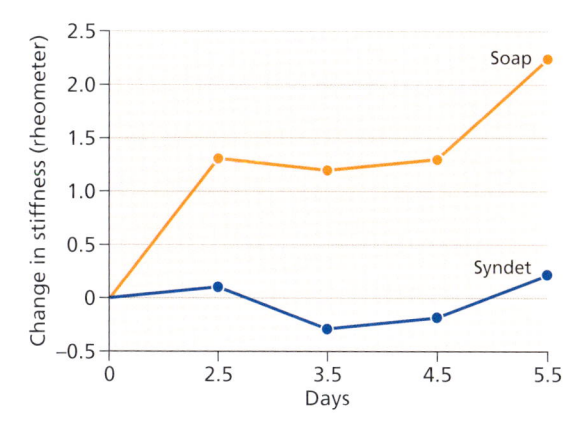

Figure 9.10 Changes in skin mechanical properties (stiffness) after 5 days of twice daily washing with soap and syndet using the FCAT method. Soap washing induced a progressive increase in stratum corneum stiffness as measured using a linear skin rheometer whereas the syndet bar did not induce stiffness.

tests are indeed predictive of what can be experienced in normal use under realistic but challenging environmental conditions. Figure 9.11 compares results of a controlled wash trial with a normal use study where women used soap or syndet for face washing for a week during the Canadian winter. They were not allowed to use a facial moisturizer during the study. Under the cold drying conditions of this study the soap users rapidly experienced intense drying and soreness whereas the syndet users were mostly able to tolerate the withdrawal of their normal after-wash moisturizer for a week. Despite differences in magnitude, the in-use trial was fully aligned with the controlled wash study indicating that controlled study results are very "real".

Benefits of mild cleansing for ashy skin

The mild cleansing effects discussed so far have focused on reducing the induction of dryness. However, there are also very real positive

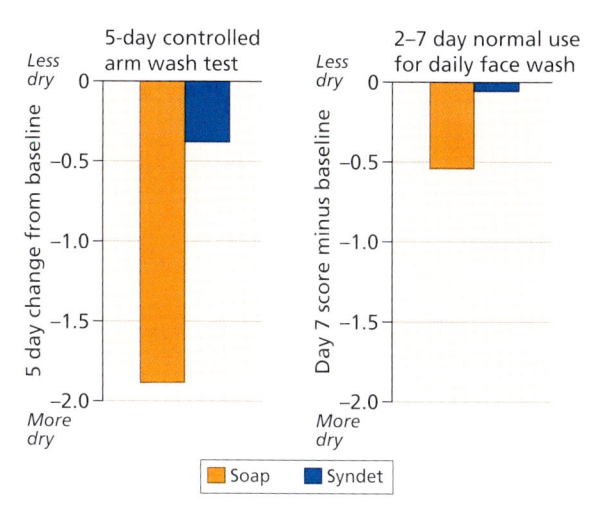

Figure 9.11 Skin dryness induced by soap and syndet bars in a 5-day controlled arm wash test compared to dryness induced by 2–7 days of normal use once daily for facial cleansing. Arm wash test carried out on the same subjects as the 7-day facial wash test. Most soap users were unable to continue soap use for a full week. Most syndet users were able to complete a full week of daily face washing – dryness scores are based on assessments made on day 7 for the whole panel.

benefits to mild cleansing. Ashy skin, sometimes referred to as grey skin, is a significant problem among darker skinned individuals. It is caused by refraction of light by a superficial layer of dryness leading to a dull cast. In a clinical trial of female subjects, Fitzpatrick Type IV–VI, with a moderate degree of visual skin ashiness, the subjects replaced their normal cleanser with the syndet bar provided and washed daily for 3 weeks. During this time, subjects refrained from using moisturizers on their arms or legs.

As shown in Figure 9.12, the severity of skin ashiness was significantly reduced on dorsal forearms and outer legs while visual dryness significantly improved on dorsal forearms and elbows. Subjects perceived significant improvement to moisturization,

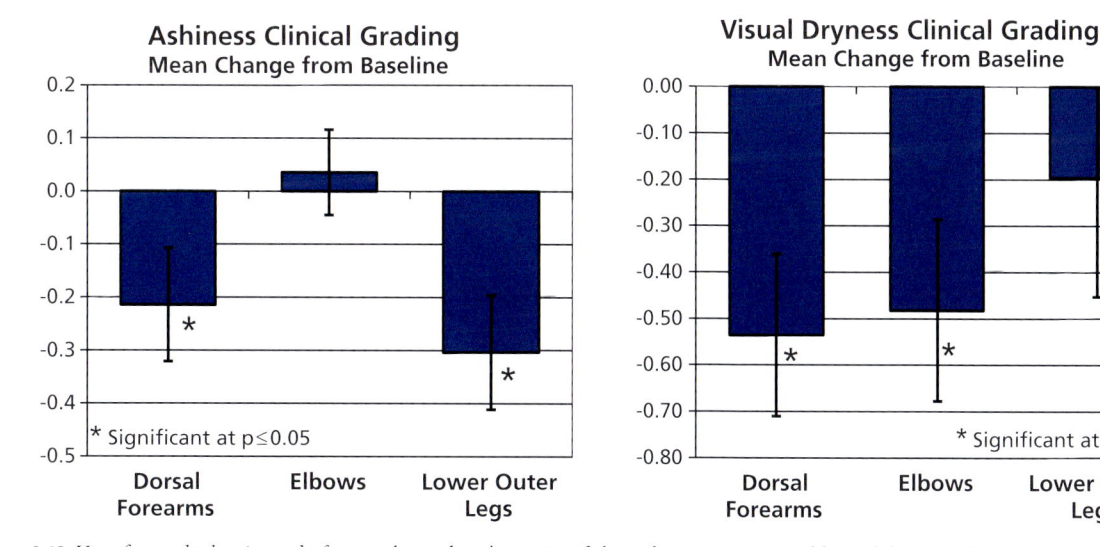

Figure 9.12 Use of a syndet bar instead of a soap bar reduced severity of skin ashiness on arms and legs while visual dryness significantly improved on forearms and elbows.

softness, and smoothness, as well as reduced itch, and dryness. These results demonstrate a mild, moisturizing syndet bar provides a positive skin condition benefit for ashy skin.

Benefits of mild cleansing for photodamaged skin

Facial photodamage is another area where mild cleansing can provide a positive skin benefit. In this clinical trial, 25 women, who were current soap users (non-syndet), with mild-to-moderate facial photodamage participated in a double-blind, split-face application face wash study. All subjects discontinued use of moisturizers 3 days prior to the study and were not permitted to use moisturizers or other skin care products for the duration of the study. Subjects washed their face using a split-face application with a syndet bar on one side, and a regular bar soap on the other twice daily for 4 weeks. As shown in Figure 9.13, the syndet bar showed significant improvement compared to the soap bar to dermatologist-assessed skin texture, brightness, clarity and tone within the first 2 weeks. Moreover, 3D texture of periorbital fine lines and wrinkles showed significant reduction with the syndet bar compared to the soap bar treated side. As expected, deeper wrinkles are not affected solely by use of cleanser and thus overall photodamage remained unchanged. Nevertheless, the superficial appearance of the photodamaged skin was shown to be significantly improved and these clinical effects were further confirmed in panellist self-assessments. Thus, across a range of parameters – dermatological, clinical, self-assessment, and objective instrumental measures, it is evident that the syndet bar improved skin appearance and barrier integrity compared to use of the harsh soap bar for daily cleansing in subjects with mild-to-moderate photodamage.

Practical implications of mild cleansing for patients with common skin disease

The studies described above [2-5] were based on a simple hypothesis that switching patients from their harsh soap bar cleanser to a milder syndet bar cleanser would minimize dryness and thus generally help improve skin condition. This same hypothesis extends directly to diseased skin conditions that suffer from a compromised skin barrier and are aggravated by dryness. In the following section we discuss clinical trials on a variety of patient populations to demonstrate the benefit of mild bar cleansing as part of the management program. The patient groups studied were atopic dermatitis, acne, and rosacea. The results show that patient symptoms were reduced and general skin quality improved.

Benefits of mild cleansing for adults and children with mild atopic dermatitis

A total of 50 patients with mild atopic dermatitis were enrolled for a 4-week double-blind study carried out under

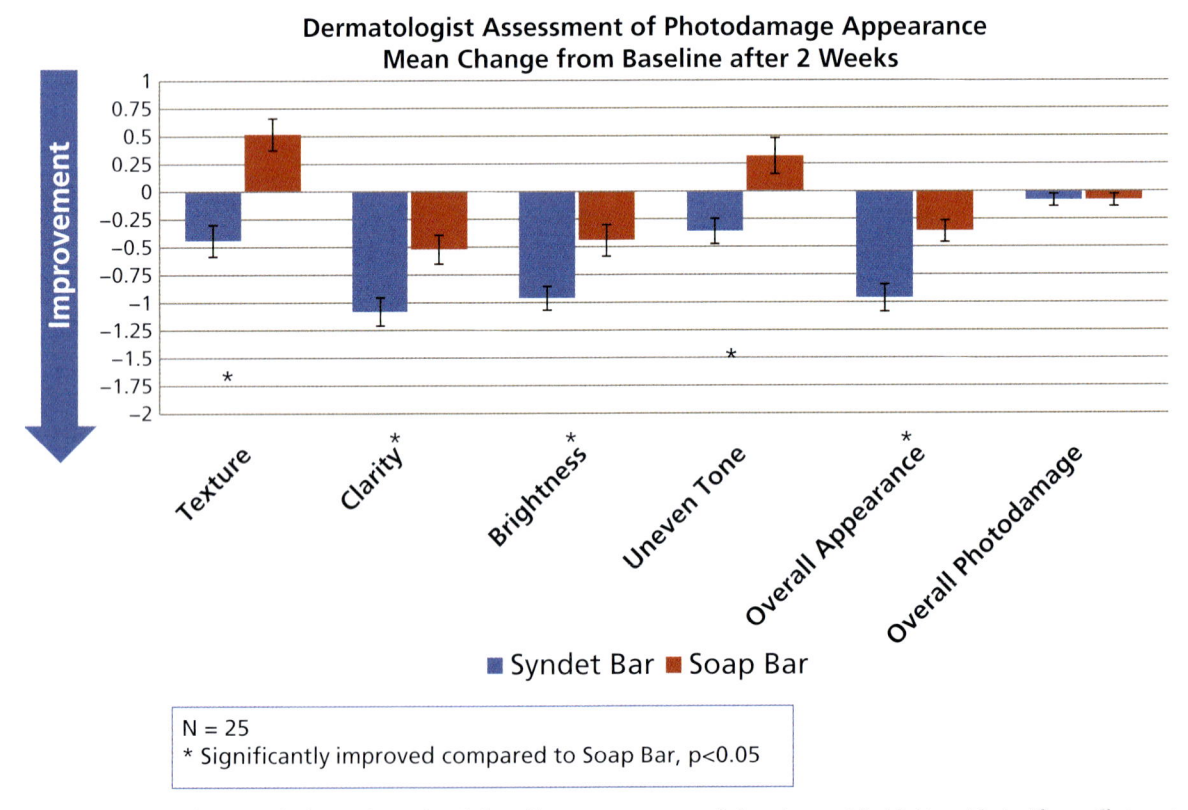

Figure 9.13 Use of a syndet bar instead of a soap bar reduced clinically assess appearance of photodamaged facial skin, with significant effects on texture, clarity brightness and tone.

the supervision of a certified dermatologist. One group of 25 patients (19 adults and 6 children > 15 years) used a marketed syndet cleansing bar instead of their normal cleansing bar for showering during the 4 weeks of the study. A second group of 25 patients (17 adults and 8 children) used a different syndet bar based on the same acyl isethionate cleansing system. Eczema severity was measured at baseline and 4 weeks using the eczema area severity index (EASI) clinical assessment system. Other evaluations at these times were dermatologist assessment of non-lesional skin, hydration by conductance meter, and patient self-assessment by questionnaire. Results indicated good compatibility with the syndet bar as a substitute for patient's usual bar cleanser for both adults and children. In addition, it was observed that the severity of eczematous lesions reduced with both bars, general skin condition was improved, and hydration was maintained. The main results are shown in Figure 9.14.

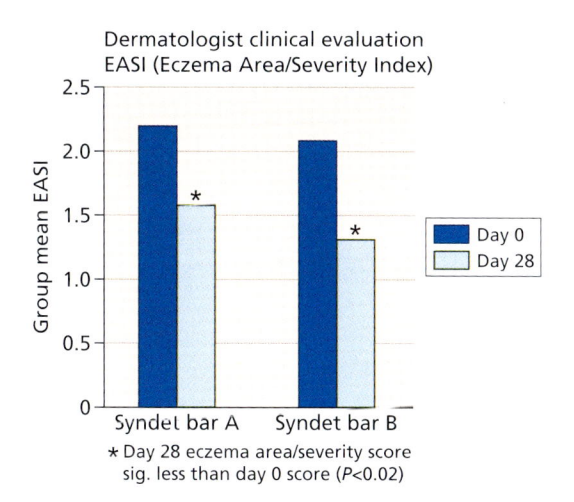

Benefits of mild cleansing for acne and rosacea patients

In one study, a group of 50 patients with moderate acne and using topical acne medications (benzamycin or benzamycin/differin) were split into two treatment cells (25 patients per cell) and instructed to use either a syndet bar or a soap bar for 4 weeks in place of their normal cleansing bar. Patient skin condition was assessed at baseline and after 4 weeks of use. Although the clinical differences between soap and syndet in this test were not statistically significant, there was a clear trend that patients using soap experienced worsening of measures relating to skin compatibility and irritation during the 4-week period of the study and little or no change in patients using the syndet bar (Figure 9.15).

A similar protocol was used in a study of rosacea patients. Seventy patients were enrolled and divided into two subgroups for a 4-week study period. Evaluations were performed at baseline and at 4 weeks. The results show a similar trend in favor of using the syndet bar (Figure 9.15).

The studies indicate a benefit for cleansing with a syndet bar as compared to a soap bar, for patients with disease compromised skin.

The future of cleansing bars

Bar soaps have been the most common product for skin cleansing for so long that most people never give them a second thought. Since the late 1990s there has been a slow but steady decline in bar sales in favor of liquid cleansing products in the developed markets, however globally, bars (both soap based and syndet) are continuing to grow and will remain an important format into the foreseeable future.

Like many market trends, the decline in developed markets is brought about by changes in consumer needs, habits, and attitudes. Cleansing liquids are becoming the product of choice for the shower, liquid soaps are increasingly used for hand cleansing, and quick foaming liquids, creams, and wipes have largely replaced soap bars for facial cleansing. Nevertheless, there is little doubt that low cost and universal access of cleansing bars will continue to make them a relevant format for hand, body and facial cleansing. New innovations will continue to bring new skin benefits to this well-established format.

This chapter describes the negative effects for skin associated with cleansing and provides evidence that there are real benefits for patients and consumers generally to use the mildest bar cleansers available. It has long been recognized that environmental factors facilitate the drying, irritating actions of surfactants and that people differ in their susceptibility to these effects. Only recently has it become evident that genetic variations are direct drivers of individual variations in susceptibility to develop dry and sensitive skin. It appears that loss-of-function mutations in the filaggrin gene

Dermatologist clinical evaluation EASI (Eczema Area/Severity Index)

(Bar chart: Syndet bar A — Day 0 ≈ 2.2, Day 28 ≈ 1.6*; Syndet bar B — Day 0 ≈ 2.1, Day 28 ≈ 1.3*)

*Day 28 eczema area/severity score sig. less than day 0 score ($P<0.02$)

Patient self assessment of change in skin condition from day 0 to day 28

Decreases from baseline			Increases from baseline		
Symptom	Change from day 0		Attribute	Change from day 0	
	Bar A	Bar B		Bar A	Bar B
Dryness	-1.5	-2.1	Complexion	0.2	1.3
Itching	-1.3	-2.8	Smoothness	0.7	2.7
Irritation	-1.1	-2.7	Softness	0.4	2.8
Tightness	-0.9	-1.3	Appearance	1.3	2.3
Tingling	-0.7	-1.4			

Red numbers - sig. diff from baseline at day 28 ($P<0.05$)

Figure 9.14 Changes in dermatologist and patient assessment of skin condition after 4 weeks' daily use of syndet cleansing bars by adult and child (7–15 years) patients with atopic dermatitis (AD). A total of 25 patients used bar A and 25 used bar B. The patients were patients with chronic AD stabilized using a variety of treatment regimens which they continued during the trial. The bars were similar in composition with the same acyl isethionate synthetic surfactant system and different ratios of emollients.

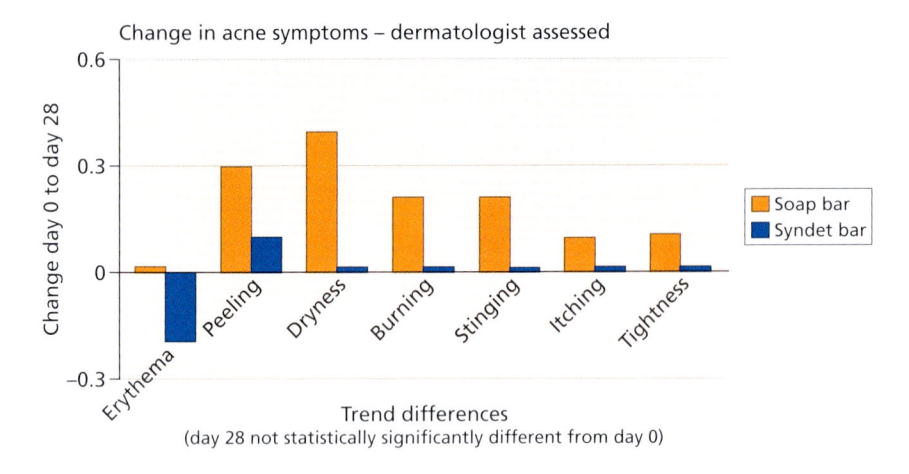

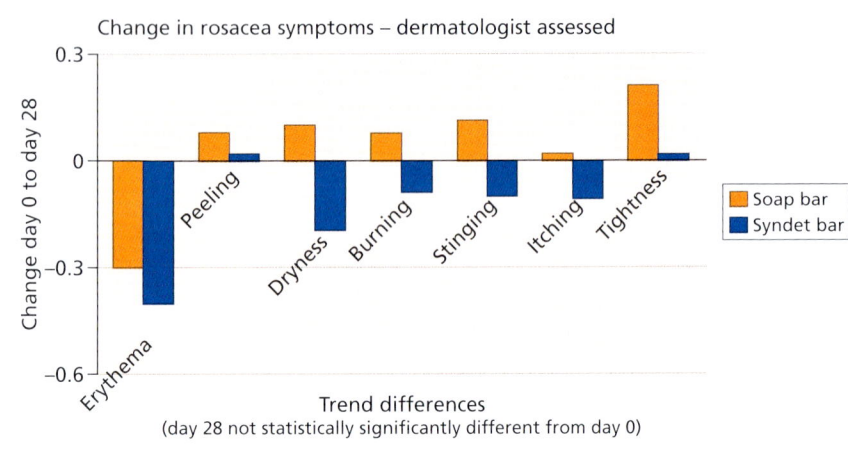

Figure 9.15 Dermatologist assessed changes in skin condition of patients with mild to moderate acne or mild to moderate rosacea after 4 weeks' use of soap or syndet bar for daily cleansing. In the acne study were 50 patients using topical benzamycin or benzamycin plus differin. In the rosacea study were 70 patients using topical metronidazole. The syndet bar was acyl isethionate synthetic surfactant and the soap bar was a standard 80/20 soap.

are relatively common in humans and are the cause of mild and severe forms of ichthyosis vulgaris and atopic dermatitis. The insight that filaggrin gene mutations and variations lead to a compromised barrier that makes skin vulnerable to dryness is changing how scientists and professionals think about dry skin and healthy skin functioning. Some people have a good barrier but others are much more susceptible to environmental challenges – including cleansing.

Gene profiling is not yet a routine diagnostic procedure but susceptibility to develop dry skin is a strong indication of a compromised barrier and the need for mild cleansing to prevent surfactant-induced exacerbation of a poor barrier. The future will see new and more precise diagnostic tests enabling dermatologists and healthcare professionals to more readily identify consumers and patients who have less than optimal stratum corneum functioning. In parallel, the need to identify mild products and good cleansing practice will come into sharper focus. It will be interesting to see if the future consumer product trend is a rebalancing from soap bars to milder syndet bars or if the trend will be a more direct move from bars to liquid cleansers. Most likely the market will develop in both directions – milder bars and more use of liquid cleansers.

Conclusions

Cleansing is a basic human need and cleansing bars are the universal way to satisfy this need. Liquid products may be gaining in popularity but it will be decades before bars become redundant, if ever.

Cleansing is a challenge to skin for everyone, but for patients with skin problems the choice of cleansing product is the difference between exacerbation and minimization of symptoms. There is ample evidence in the literature that syndet bars are milder than soap-based bars and better for patients with common dermatological conditions such as atopic dermatitis, eczema, acne, and rosacea. Not everyone needs to use a syndet bar, but it is fairly safe to say that all consumers and patients currently using harsh soap bars could experience a practical benefit by switching to a mild syndet bar.

References

1 Frosch PJ, Kligman AM. (1979) The soap chamber test: a new method for assessing the irritancy of soaps. *J Am Acad Dermatol* **1**, 35–41.
2 Current Stratum Corneum Research. (2004) Optimizing barrier function through fundamental skin care. *Dermatol Ther* 17(1), 1–68.

[A full issue of the journal (9 papers) dedicated to the biology of the stratum corneum barrier and the impact of cleansing and moisturizing products.]

3 Subramanyan K. (2004) Role of mild cleansing in the management of patient skin. *Dermatol Ther* **17**(1), 26–34.
4 Subramanyan K, Hawkins S, Johnson A (2005) Cosmetic benefits of mild cleansing syndet bars versus soap. Poster P1018 presented at American Academy of Dermatology Annual Meeting, Feb 18-22, 2005, New Orleans, LA.
5 Hawkins S, Feng L, Ananthapadmanabhan KP (2013) Reducing ashiness in skin of color – the impact of mild cleansing. Poster P1018 presented at American Academy of Dermatology Annual Meeting, Mar 22–24, 2012, Denver, CO.

Further reading

Ananthapadmanabhan KP, Lips A, Vincent C, Meyer F, Caso S, Johnson A, *et al.* (2003) pH-induced alterations in stratum corneum properties. *Int J Cosmet Sci* **25**, 103–112.

Ananthapadmanabhan KP, Subramanyan K, Rattinger GB. (2002) Moisturizing cleansers. In: LeydenJJ, RawlingsAV, eds. *Skin Moisturization*. New York: Marcel Decker, pp. 405–32.

Ananthapadmanabhan KP, Yu KK, Meyers CL, Aronson MP, (1996) Binding of surfactants to stratum corneum. *J Soc Cosmet Chem* **47**, 185-200

Ertel K, Keswick B, Bryant P. (1995) A forearm controlled application technique for estimating the relative mildness of personal cleansing products. *J Soc Cosmet Chem* **46**, 67–76.

Imokawa G. (1997) Surfactant mildness. In: RiegerMM, RheinLD, eds. *Surfactants in Cosmetics*. New York: Marcel Dekker, pp. 427–71.

Johnson AW. (2004) Overview. Fundamental skin care: protecting the barrier. *Dermatol Ther* **17**, 213–22.

Matts PJ. (2002) Understanding and measuring the optics that drive visual perception of skin appearance. In: MarksR, LevequeJL, VoegeliR, eds. *The Essential Stratum Corneum*. London: Martin Dunitz, p. 333.

Matts PJ, Goodyer E. (1998) A new instrument to measure the mechanical properties of human stratum corneum in vivo. *J Cosmet Sci* **49**, 321–33.

Meyers CL, Thorn-Lesson D, Subramanyan K. (2004) In vivo confocal fluorescence of skin surface: a novel approach to study effect of products on stratum corneum. *J Am Acad Dermatol* **50**, 130.

Misra M, Ananthapadmanabhan KP, Hoyberg K, *et al.* (1997) Correlation between surfactant-induced ultrastructural changes in epidermis and transepidermal water loss. *J Soc Cosmet Chem* **48**, 219–34.

Murahata RI, Aronson MP, Sharko PT, *et al.* (1997) Cleansing bars for face and body: in search of mildness. In: RiegerMM, RheinLD, eds. *Surfactants in Cosmetics*. New York: Marcel Dekker, pp. 427–71.

Nicholl G, Murahata R, Grove G, Barrows J, Sharko P. (1995) The relative sensitivity of two arm-wash methods for evaluating the mildness of personal washing products. *J Soc Cosmet Chem* **46**, 129–40.

Prottey C, Ferguson T. (19750) Factors which determine the skin irritation potential of soaps and detergents. *J Soc Cosmet* **26**, 29–46.

Rawlings AV, Harding CR. (2002) Moisturization and the skin barrier. *Dermatol Ther* **17**, 43–8.

Rawlings AW, Watkinson A, Rogers J, *et al.* (1994) Abnormalities in stratum corneum structure, lipid composition, and desmosome degradation in soap-induced winter zerosis. *J Soc Cosmet Chem* **45**, 203–20.

Strube D, Koontz S, Murahata R, *et al.* (1989) The flex wash test: a method for evaluating the mildness of personal washing products. *J Soc Cosmet Chem* **40**, 297–306.

Wihelm KP, Wolff HH, Maibach HI. (1994) Effects of surfactants on skin hydration. In: ElsnerP, BerardescaE, MaibachHI, eds. *Bioengineering of the Skin: Water and the Stratum Corneum*. Boca Raton, FL: CRC Press, pp. 257–74.

CHAPTER 10
Personal Cleansers: Body Washes

Keith Ertel and Heather Focht
Procter & Gamble Co, Cincinnati, OH, USA

> **BASIC CONCEPTS**
> - Dry skin on the body is a particular issue for most consumers. Leave-on lotion application is not always viewed as a convenient intervention, so relief is sought from alternative sources such as moisturizing personal cleansing products.
> - Body washes are a relatively new introduction into the armamentarium of personal cleansing products and their use is growing rapidly, particularly in developed countries.
> - Body washes present unique formulation challenges and benefit opportunities compared to traditional cleansing bar forms.
> - There are several distinct types of body washes. Of these, moisturizing body washes represent the greatest departure from traditional personal cleaners, having the potential to improve dry skin condition.
> - Moisturizing body washes vary widely in terms of their skin effects (i.e. their ability to mitigate dryness). A product must deposit an effective amount of benefit agent on the skin during the wash–rinse process. Understanding the basis for a product's designation as "moisturizing" is key.

Background

Cleansing to remove soils from the skin's surface is a basic human need that serves both a cosmetic and a health function. While cleansing needs for the face receive considerable attention and few question the logic of specialized facial cleansers, cleansing needs for the body are often given little thought, the assumption being that any personal cleanser will suffice. This view is somewhat surprising given that body skin accounts for more than 90% of the body's total surface area and, as we will show, consumers have diverse needs and expectations from a body cleanser.

Water alone cannot effectively remove all soils from the skin and surfactant-based materials have been the cleansing aids of choice throughout recorded history. Soap was among the first cleansing aids and some of the earliest references to soap preparation are found in Sumerian and Egyptian writings, although legend holds that the article we know as soap originated by chance at Mount Sapo in Ancient Rome when fat and wood ash from sacrifices were mixed with rainwater.

Regardless of its origin, soap was the cleansing aid of choice and remained largely unchanged for centuries. The next real step-change in personal cleanser technology occurred around the time of World War I, when the first non-soap surfactant was introduced. However, bars continued as the predominant form for body cleansing and it was not until the latter part of the 20th century that liquid personal cleansing products for the body (i.e. body washes) were introduced and began to gain a foothold in some regions.

Body washes are generally less messy in-use than bars (e.g. no soap mush), are more hygienic, and offer greater potential to deliver skin benefits, including dry skin improvement. However, body washes can be less convenient to transport and are generally more expensive on a per use basis than commodity cleansing bars. As a result, body wash adoption tends to reflect countries' economic development status.

Types of body wash

Body washes currently available in the market generally fall into three distinct categories. Regular body washes are products whose primary function is to provide skin cleansing. As such, they are typically based on a relatively simple chassis, although fragrance is sometimes used to define product character or to provide a higher order benefit (e.g. lavender scent may be used to produce a calming effect during use).

Moisturizing body washes are intended to provide a dry skin improvement in addition to performing the base skin cleansing function. However, there are different ways to define dry skin improvement for moisturizing body washes. In some cases a product's benefit is judged relative to another (drying) personal cleanser and "improvement" amounts to producing less dryness than the benchmark. In other cases a product's benefit is judged relative to an untreated control and "improvement" reflects the effect of the product relative to the condition of untreated skin.

Cosmetic Dermatology: Products and Procedures, Second Edition. Edited by Zoe Diana Draelos.
© 2016 John Wiley & Sons, Ltd. Published 2016 by John Wiley & Sons, Ltd.

Thus, moisturizing body washes can provide markedly different levels of dry skin improvement depending on the criterion used to judge their performance.

Finally, there are products that fall into a broad category best described as specialty body washes. These are extensions of regular and moisturizing body washes that contain ingredients intended to provide additional function or benefit. Examples include products that contain beads or other grit material (e.g. pulverized fruit seeds) to provide exfoliation and an enhanced dry skin benefit, and products that contain menthol or other sensates to provide a "cooling" or "tingling" sensation to the skin.

Major formula components of body washes

Water

Unlike their cleansing bar counterparts, body wash formulas contain a high percentage of water. This situation is a double-edged sword. On the one hand, eliminating the need to form materials into a bar that will hold its shape while maintaining good performance and wear characteristics removes a number of formulation constraints, and this introduces the possibility of incorporating relatively high levels of non-cleanser materials (e.g. benefit agents) into the formulation. On the other hand, the aqueous milieu present in liquid cleansers and body washes introduces issues not present in bars. For example, many benefit agents are lipophilic in nature and an improperly formulated liquid cleaner may exhibit phase separation or creaming, not unlike the separation of oil and water phases that occurs in some salad dressings. Chemical stability is also a consideration; the greater mobility afforded by a liquid environment increases the likelihood of molecular interactions, and water itself can participate in decomposition reactions (e.g. hydrolysis). An aqueous environment also increases the potential for microbial contamination. Thus, formulating a liquid cleanser or body wash presents a number of unique challenges, particularly if the product is intended to perform a function beyond simple cleansing such as delivering a benefit agent to the skin.

Surfactants

Surfactants are the workhorse ingredient in any personal cleansing product. Water is capable of removing some soils from the skin; however, sebum and many of the soils acquired on the skin through incidental contact or purposeful application (e.g. topical medicaments) are lipophilic in nature and are not effectively removed from the skin's surface by water alone. Surfactants, or surface-active agents, have a dual nature; part of a surfactant molecule's structure is lipophilic and part of it is hydrophilic. This structural duality allows surfactant molecules to localize at the interface between water and lipophilic soils and lower the interfacial tension to help remove the soil. Further, surfactants allow water to more effectively wet the skin's surface and to solubilize lipoilic soils after removal, which prevents the soils from redepositing on the skin during rinsing. Surfactants are also responsible for the formation of bubbles and lather, which most consumers view as necessary for effective cleansing.

As with cleansing bars, the surfactants used in liquid personal cleansers and body washes fall into two primary groups: soaps and non-soaps, also known as synthetic detergents or syndets. Soap is chemically the alkali salt of a fatty acid formed by reacting fatty acid with a strong base, a process known as saponification. The fatty acids used in soap manufacture are derived from animal (e.g. tallow) or plant sources (e.g. coconut or palm kernel oil). These sources differ in their distribution of fatty acid chain lengths, which determines properties such as skin compatibility and lather. Soap's properties are also affected by external factors such as water hardness; soaps are generally more irritating and lather and rinse more poorly in hard water. Some specialty body washes contain soaps derived from "natural" fatty acid sources such as coconut or soybean oil; these products will behave similarly to products containing soaps derived from traditional fatty acid sources.

Syndets, which are derived from petroleum, were developed to overcome shortcomings associated with soaps (e.g. the influence of water hardness on performance) and to expand the pool of available raw materials used in manufacture. Syndets vary widely in terms of their chemical structure, physicochemical properties, and performance characteristics, including skin compatibility. Syndets are not necessarily less irritating than soaps. Sodium lauryl sulfate is an example; many dermatologists view alkyl sulfates as model skin irritants. Most body washes are based on syndet surfactant systems, and because syndets have a wide range of performance characteristics, most body washes combine several surfactant types to achieve specific performance in the finished product. For example, alkyl sulfates, while having relatively poor skin compatibility, lather well. Combining an alkyl sulfate with an amphoteric surfactant such as cocamidopropyl betaine can improve both lather and skin compatibility. Thus, formulating a body wash with syndets involves choosing surfactants to optimize performance and aesthetics, balanced with cost considerations.

Skin benefit agents

Some body washes contain ingredients that are intended to provide skin benefits beyond simple cleansing. Dry skin, which is a pervasive dermatologic issue, is one of the most common benefit targets for body washes. Not surprisingly, moisturizing ingredients such as petrolatum, various oils, shea butter, or glycerin, which are found in leave-on moisturizers, are often used in moisturizing body washes. However, simply including a moisturizing ingredient in a rinse-off product is not sufficient; the product must deposit an effective amount of the material on skin during the cleansing and rinsing process. As noted earlier, standards for judging moisturizing efficacy differ. Clinical testing shows that moisturizing body washes vary widely in their ability to provide a dry skin benefit, and that some may actually worsen dryness and irritation.

In addition to moisturizing ingredients to improve dry skin, body washes might also contain particulates such as beads or pulverized fruit seeds to aid exfoliation. A particulate's size, surface morphology (i.e. smooth or rough), and in-use concentration will determine its ability to provide this benefit. Finally, body washes may contain ingredients that are intended to protect from or to reduce the effects of environmental insults. As with moisturizing ingredients, an efficacious amount of these materials must remain on skin after washing and rinsing.

Other ingredients

Body wash formulas contain additional ingredients that act as formulation and stability aids. The addition of polymers and salt alter a product's viscosity, which can modify performance characteristics or improve physical stability. Feel modifiers such as silicones are sometimes used to improve the in-use tactile properties of body washes that deposit lipophilic benefit agents on skin. Chelating agents such as ethylenediamenetetraacetic acid (EDTA) and antioxidants such as butylated hydroxytoluene (BHT) and are added to improve chemical stability, and buffering a body wash formula to a specific pH value can help inhibit microbial growth and improve the product's chemical and physical stability.

Color and fragrance are an important part of the in-use experience for many body washes. Colors are US Food, Drug, and Cosmetic Act (FD&C) approved dyes and are usually present in relatively low amounts, so the likelihood of experiencing an issue with a body wash product because of dye is low. Fragrances are also usually present in relatively low amounts, although the apparent concentration may seem higher as a result of "bloom" that results from lathering a body wash on a mesh cleansing puff, the recommended application procedure for many of these products. The incidence of issues with modern fragrances is low. Some body washes incorporate natural oils to impart fragrance but these products are not necessarily without potential issues because some of these natural materials can cause sensitization.

In-use performance considerations for body washes

Cleansing ability

The mechanical action associated with applying a personal cleanser to the body helps to loosen and remove some soils, but surfactants are the primary agents responsible for aiding soil removal, particularly lipophilic soils. However, surfactants and the cleansing products based on them differ in their abilities to remove sebum and lipophilic soils [1]. These cleansing performance differences are a greater consideration in body washes than in bars because of the relatively lower surfactant concentrations present in the former compared with the latter.

Because lipophilic soils present the greatest cleansing challenge, oil-based makeup materials are often used as model soils in tests intended to measure cleansing efficiency. These materials are poorly removed from the skin by water alone and their inherent color makes them easy to detect visually or instrumentally and measure on the skin's surface.

To test the cleaning efficiency of various methods of skin cleansing, we conducted a study comparing a moisturizing petrolatum-depositing body wash, a syndet detergent bar, and water for cleansing ability. A commercial oil-based makeup product served as a model soil and was applied to discrete treatment sites on the volar forearms of light-skinned females. The makeup was allowed to dry for 15 minutes and baseline colorimeter (L*) values were recorded at each site. Lather was generated from each cleansing product in a controlled manner and applied to a randomly assigned site for 10 seconds with gloved fingers. Sites were rinsed with warm water for 15 seconds, allowed to air dry for 30 minutes then chromameter measurements were repeated. Data were analyzed by a mixed-model procedure.

The results show that water has little effect on removing the model soil from the skin and while the makeup used in this study is perhaps an extreme challenge, it nonetheless exemplifies why personal cleansing products are needed for soil removal. Not surprisingly, both personal cleansing products removed a significantly greater amount of the model soil than did water ($P < 0.01$), but the petrolatum-depositing body wash showed significantly greater makeup removal (i.e. cleansing efficiency) than the syndet bar (mean ΔL^* values of 5.2 and 3.2, respectively; $P < 0.02$). Thus, this study shows that a petrolatum-depositing body wash can clean efficiently and demonstrates that consumers are not restricted to the traditional bar form for their skin cleansing needs.

Consumer understanding and need for moisturizing body washes

Patients with dry skin that accompanies a dermatologic condition often require a high level of skin moisturization and may be willing to tolerate poor moisturizer product aesthetics (e.g. skin feel) to obtain relief. A recent habits and practices study among a group of 558 adult females demonstrates that a consideration of consumers' varied moisturization needs and their desired product aesthetics must be made in order to create products that improve patient compliance. These participants answered questions that provided a range of information about their needs for body moisturization and their expectations for a moisturizing personal cleansing product (i.e. body wash).

Dry skin was a source of discomfort for a majority of participants; 62% said they were "very bothered" or "bothered" by discomfort due to dry skin, while 20% said they were "not bothered" by discomfort due to dry skin. Dry skin also drove these consumers to apply leave-on moisturizers; 68% said they "strongly agreed" or "agreed" that they needed to use a moisturizer every day because of their dry skin, while only 16% "disagreed" that their dry skin necessitated daily moisturizer application. With regard to moisturizing cleanser needs, 97% of the participants stated that they want more moisturization from their personal cleansing product. The needs fell into three groups that aligned with self-perceived body skin type. Women in one group (very dry skin, 32% of the population) want a body wash product that delivers a high level of moisturization and a substantial skin feel; women in a second group (dry skin, 35%

of the population) want a body wash product that delivers a moderate level of moisturization and a somewhat perceivable skin feel; and women in a third group (combination skin, 22% of the population) want a body wash that provides a low level of moisturization, rapid absorption of the moisturizing agent, and no residual skin feel.

This study is just one example of work conducted to understand female consumers' needs and expectations with regard to dry skin and moisturization. Traditionally, the needs and expectations of their male counterparts were at best little studied and poorly understood, or at worst assumed to be the same as those of females. To gain insights into male consumers' needs we conducted a habits and practices study among an adult panel representative of the US adult population comprising 303 males and 313 females. As in the study above, participants responded to a series of questions related to attitudes towards body skin condition, body skin care habits and practices, and attitudes towards various cosmetic interventions.

This consumer research showed a strong contrast between the sexes in terms of their usage of products to care for their body skin. Males were on the whole less likely to use a treatment on their body than were females. However, dry skin ranked high on the list of body skin care needs for both sexes. Moisturizer application was identified as the best treatment for dry skin, but males were less likely to apply moisturizer to their bodies than were females because of a perceived time constraint. Skin-feel parameters were also more important to males than females; males wanted to feel clean, not sticky or greasy. Surprisingly, the study results indicate that males are more likely to seek help from a dermatologist for their dry skin than females.

Moisturization from body washes

Dry skin on the body is a finding in many dermatologic conditions and the results presented in the previous section show that even in the absence of frank skin disease dry skin ranks as one of the most common body skin complaints for both sexes. Skin that is dry can itch, and flaking on "problem" areas such as legs, knees, and elbows is aesthetically unpleasing and can negatively impact self-confidence. Dry skin worsens with age, and low relative humidity, certain medications, and excessive hot water exposure are among the factors that can exacerbate dry skin. Personal cleansing products are also frequently cited as agents that cause or worsen dry skin via removal of essential skin lipids following excessive cleansing or cleansing with "harsh" surfactants.

Dry skin signals that there is an insufficient level of moisture in the stratum corneum. Dermatologists often recommend application of leave-on moisturizers to relieve symptoms and to provide an environment in which the skin can repair stratum corneum damage associated with dry skin. However, surveys show that a high percentage of dermatologists believe that their (female) patients do not moisturize as recommended, a lack of convenience being cited as the primary reason for the perceived non-compliance. This pattern is consistent with the results found in our consumer habits and practices research.

Coupling moisturization with an existing habit such as showering can improve compliance but, as noted earlier, there are different ways to define a moisturization or dry skin improvement benefit, and simply including a moisturizing ingredient in a body wash formula does not guarantee that it will deposit on skin or remain in a sufficient amount after rinsing to provide a benefit.

We conducted a leg wash clinical study using the industry standard method (leg controlled application test) comparing the dry skin improvement efficacy of a water control and three marketed moisturizing body wash products [2]. Treatment sites on the legs were washed in a controlled manner once daily for 7 days with the randomly assigned treatments. Expert visual scores and instrumental measurements collected at baseline and study end were used to assess the change in dry skin condition produced by the treatments. Expert scoring shows a range of skin effects from these moisturizing products (Figure 10.1). Two of the body washes delivered significant ($P < 0.05$) improvement in dry skin relative to the water control, while one of the products had little effect on visible dry skin. Skin capacitance measurements showed the former body washes improved stratum corneum hydration ($P < 0.05$), while the latter reduced stratum corneum hydration relative to the control ($P < 0.05$), i.e. it dried

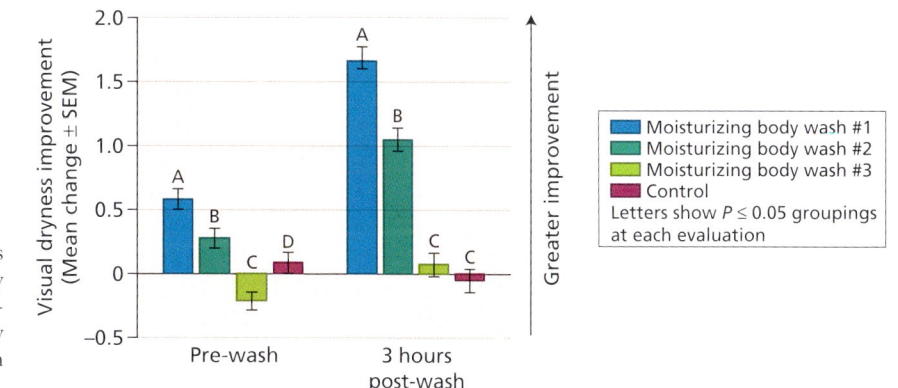

Figure 10.1 Expert dryness scores after 7 days of once-daily washing with marketed body wash products. The results show marked differences in the products' abilities to provide a dry skin improvement (i.e. a skin moisturization benefit).

the skin. Expert erythema scoring and transepidemal water loss (TEWL) showed a similar pattern; two of the body wash products improved skin condition relative to control, while the third significantly ($P < 0.05$) increased erythema and TEWL. This highlights the importance of understanding how products that are labeled as "moisturizing" perform clinically whenever possible. Simply recommending that a patient should use a moisturizing body wash may not produce an optimal benefit, and the wrong product recommendation could actually worsen skin condition.

The consumer research presented in the previous section also highlights the need for personal cleansing products that deliver different levels of moisturization and different use aesthetics. Many personal cleansers are available in versions that ostensibly are designed for different skin needs, but such products often involve relatively minor changes in formulation and performance. Body washes, because of the greater formulation flexibility they offer, provide an opportunity to develop product versions that offer different levels of performance to meet specific needs. For example, the habits and practices study conducted among females identified three primary consumer groups in terms of body skin moisturization and body wash performance needs. Body wash products were created that provide different levels of moisturization and dry skin improvement to meet the specific needs of these groups.

Who will benefit from using body washes?

The body wash is a relatively new-to-market personal cleanser form that will initially appeal to users with practical concerns or to users seeking experiential benefits such as better lather and in-use scent intensity, which are often greater than a bar can deliver. Where body washes really distinguish themselves from traditional bar forms, however, is in their ability to provide higher order skin benefits. As we have shown, some body washes can provide a marked skin moisturization benefit that can affect not only the quantity but also the morphology of dry skin flakes (Figure 10.2). A large segment of the population can benefit from using this type of personal cleansing product. However, the following are two examples of conditions that may derive a particular benefit from a moisturizing body wash.

Ashy skin

African-Americans and other dark-skinned individuals frequently suffer from ashy skin, a condition in which the skin's surface appears grayish or chalky as a result of excessive dryness. The condition is often exacerbated by soap bar use which is common among this population. Moisturizers or other oils can provide temporary relief but, as discussed earlier, convenience often limits willingness to use leave-on products. Petrolatum is an effective moisturizer but neat application to the skin is limited by both convenience and aesthetics. However, a

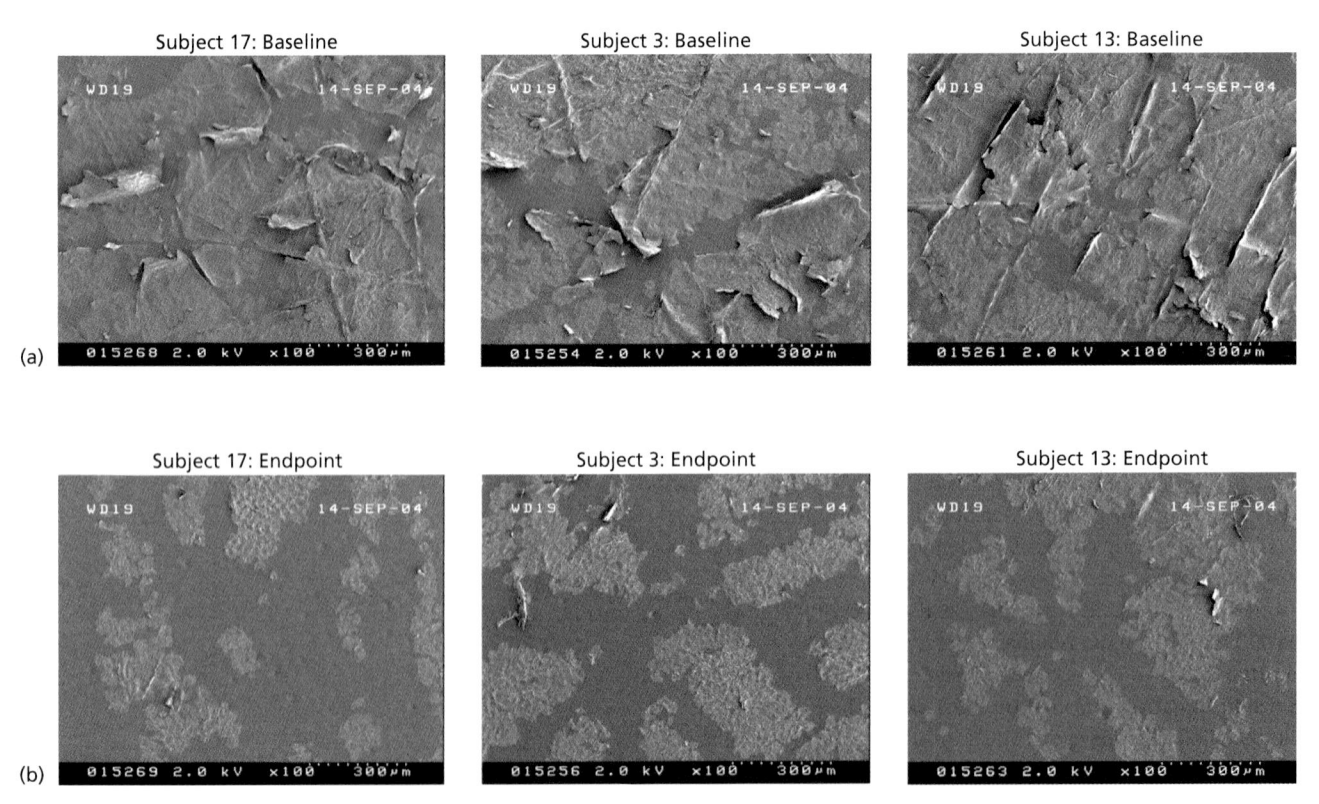

Figure 10.2 Scanning electron microscope (SEM) photomicrographs of skin flakes adhering to tape strips taken from subjects' legs before (a) and after (b) using a petrolatum-depositing body wash for 3 weeks. Baseline samples show numerous large, thick, dry skin flakes; endpoint samples show fewer and thinner flakes.

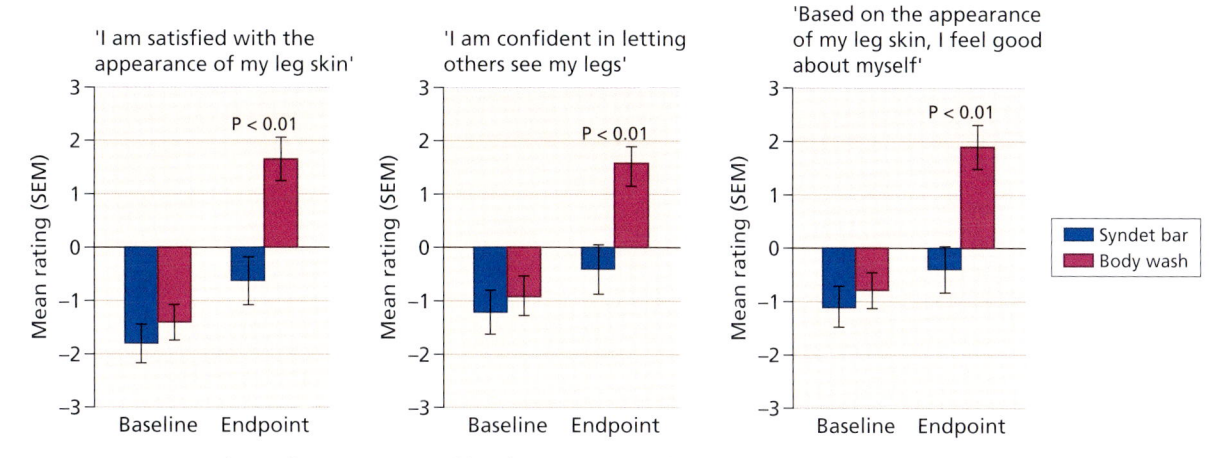

Figure 10.3 Responses to psychosocial questions answered by African-American subjects before and after using a syndet bar or petrolatum-depositing body wash for 4 weeks. Items were rated on a +3 (strongly agree) to –3 (strongly disagree) scale. Ratings were not significantly different at baseline ($P \geq 0.48$); endpoint ratings given by subjects assigned to use the body wash were significantly better than those given by subjects assigned to use the syndet bar ($P < 0.01$).

petrolatum-depositing body wash may circumvent these issues while still delivering a skin benefit.

To test this hypothesis, we conducted a study among a group of 83 African-American females who normally applied a leave-on moisturizer to relieve their ashy skin [3]. Subjects used a randomly assigned syndet bar or a moisturizing petrolatum-depositing body wash product for daily home showering for a 4-week period. Endpoint evaluations showed that the body wash produced significantly greater dermatologist-scored dry skin improvement and subject satisfaction for items such as ashy skin improvement and reducing itchy/tight feeling. Perhaps most importantly, subjects assigned to the petrolatum-depositing body wash noted marked improvement in their level of satisfaction with the appearance of their leg skin, their level of confidence in letting others see their legs, and in feeling good about themselves because of the appearance of their leg skin (Figure 10.3). These results indicate that proper personal cleanser choice can not only improve the physical symptoms of dry skin but also impact how users feel about themselves.

Atopic dermatitis

Atopic dermatitis is a chronically relapsing skin disorder that currently affects an estimated 10% of children and adults in the Western Hemisphere and whose incidence is growing worldwide. Symptoms include xerosis, skin hyperirritability, inflammation, and pruritus. Personal cleansing products are viewed as a triggering factor for atopic dermatitis and dermatologists frequently recommend that their patients avoid harsh cleansers. Therapy typically involves application of a prescription topical corticosteroid, using a mild cleanser for bathing or showering, and applying a moisturizer within 3 minutes of the bath or shower to seal in moisture [4]. The latter suggests that a moisturizing body wash may be ideally suited as a therapeutic adjunct in atopic dermatitis.

We conducted two studies among subjects undergoing treatment for mild to moderate active atopic dermatitis to examine the effect of using a moisturizing petrolatum-depositing body wash for cleansing. In both studies a moisturizing syndet bar, which is often recommended to patients undergoing therapy, was used as a control. In one study both cleansers were paired with 0.1% triamcinolone acetonide cream. Subjects applied the topical corticosteroid as directed and used their assigned personal cleanser for daily showering. After 4 weeks SCORAD for subjects who used the moisturizing body wash was significantly ($P < 0.01$) lower than for subject who used the bar. Subjects using the body wash also noted significantly ($P < 0.01$) greater improvement in skin dryness and itching.

The second study again involved subjects with mild to moderate active atopic dermatitis, but in this case subjects assigned to use the petrolatum-containing moisturizing body wash were prescribed a medium potency topical corticosteroid, while subjects assigned to use the moisturizing syndet bar were prescribed a standard high potency topical corticosteroid [5]. At study end the dermatologist investigator judged that subjects assigned to cleanse with the petrolatum-containing moisturizing body wash showed a significantly ($P < 0.01$) greater incidence of disease clearing than did subjects who used the syndet bar. The greater therapeutic response observed in the body wash group is important, but so is the fact that it was achieved using a lower potency topical corticosteroid, which can potentially reduce cost and the risk of steroid-related side effects. Subjects in the moisturizing body wash group also rated their skin condition better for a number of parameters related to their atopic condition. The results from both these studies indicate that therapeutic response in atopic dermatitis is influenced by personal cleanser choice and again highlight the importance of personal cleansing product choice when treating skin disease.

Conclusions

Body washes represent a new possibility in personal cleansing products, not only because of their ability to provide effective cleansing and deliver an improved in-use experience (e.g. lather amount, rinse feel, scent display) compared with bar cleanser forms, but also because they have a potential to improve skin condition by mitigating dry skin. Moisturizing body washes are in a position to meet a key consumer need for both men and women – dry skin improvement on the body. However, delivering a skin benefit from a rinse-off product is challenging and the product must leave an effective amount of benefit agent on the skin after washing and rinsing. Not surprisingly, moisturizing body washes vary widely in their ability to deliver a benefit and recommenders must understand these differences when evaluating moisturizing body wash products.

References

1 Bechor R, Zlotogorski A, Dikstein S. (1988) Effect of soaps and detergents on the pH and casual lipid levels of the skin surface. *J Appl Cosmetol* **6**, 123–8.
2 Ertel KD, Neumann PB, Hartwig PM, Rains GY, Keswick BH. (1999) Leg wash protocol to assess the skin mositurization potential of personal cleansing products. *Int J Cosmet Sci* **21**, 383–97.
3 Grimes PE. (2001) Double-blind study of a body wash containing petrolatum for relief of ashy, dry skin in African American women. *Cosmet Dermatol* **14**, 25–7.
4 Hanifin J, Chan SC. (1996) Diagnosis and treatment of atopic dermatitis. *Dermatol Ther* **1**, 9–18.
5 Draelos ZD, Ertel K, Hartwig P, Rains G. (2004) The effect of two skin cleansing systems on moderate xerotic eczema. *J Am Acad Dermatol* **50**, 883–8.

CHAPTER 11
Facial Cleansers and Cleansing Cloths

Thomas Barlage,[1] Susan Griffiths-Brophy,[1] and Erik J. Hasenoehrl[2]
[1]Procter & Gamble Company, Sharon Woods Technical Center, Cincinnati, OH, USA
[2]Procter & Gamble Company, Ivorydale Technical Center, Cincinnati, OH, USA

> **BASIC CONCEPTS**
> - History of facial cleansing.
> - How facial cleansers work.
> - Types of facial cleanser.
> - Selecting a facial cleanser.
> - Cleansing devices.

Do you think that choosing a cleanser to wash your face is a simple task? You may think so, but with the myriad of specialty cleanser product forms and devices that currently exist, the choice may prove daunting. Today, more than ever, facial cleansing plays an important role in the lives of many consumers. Cleansing is not only a means to remove dead skin, dirt, sebaceous oil, and cosmetics, but also a first step in the overall skin care routine, preparing skin for moisturizers and other treatments. Facial cleansing also plays an important role, well beyond skin care, in maintaining the psychological wellbeing of women by helping to provide a ritualistic sense of renewal and rejuvenation.

Dermatologists have a wide variety of cleansing technologies – ranging from water to a traditional bar of soap – at their disposal to meet the facial cleansing needs of different skin types and soil loads and can usually incorporate patient preference into selection as well. This chapter will (1) provide an overview of the many specialty facial cleanser technologies available; (2) recommend which technologies are best suited to each skin type and cleansing need; (3) provide an in-depth understanding of substrate-based facial cleansers; and, (4) give an overview of cleansing devices, which represent newest technology available for cleansing one's face.

A brief history of facial cleansing

The earliest form of facial cleansing existed well before *Homo sapiens* inhabited earth. Early facial cleansing consisted primarily of a quick splash or rinse of the face with cold water. In fact, this habit can still be observed in the animal kingdom today among many primates [1].

The first recorded use of facial cleansing utilizing more than water was among the ancient Egyptians in 10000 BC [2]. Egyptians were heavy users of makeups made from a base of metallic ores which contained natural dyes for color; this mixture was then painted onto the face. In this period, early Egyptians typically bathed and removed makeup in a river. Their cleansers consisted of animal fat mixed with lime and perfume, and were similar to some of the homemade natural soaps in use today. Facial cleansing and body cleansing were done with the same soap. During the Middle Ages, the crusaders brought back soap from the Far East to Europe which was used for bathing and facial cleansing. In the early 1900 s, bar soap was used to cleanse the face, and in the mid-1950 s, cold cream, an emulsified cleanser, was introduced.

In the past 20 years, specialty facial cleansers have become quite mainstream, a result of an explosion in cleansing technology which has led to a multitude of high-quality, relatively low-cost cleansers. More recently, cleansing devices have been introduced to the consumer. Over the years, technical developments in facial cleansing have focused on three primary areas: (1) better removal of exfoliated skin, dirt, soil, excess sebaceous oil, and makeup; (2) synthetic surfactants that induce less skin barrier damage and are thus less likely to dry skin; (3) incorporation of cleansing chemistry onto cleansing cloths; and (4) introduction of cleansing devices that assist the performance of facial cleansers.

Patients tend to take more care with cleaning and maintaining their face than the rest of their body. As such, consumer

Cosmetic Dermatology: Products and Procedures, Second Edition. Edited by Zoe Diana Draelos.
© 2016 John Wiley & Sons, Ltd. Published 2016 by John Wiley & Sons, Ltd.

product companies have developed many different technologies and cleansing forms that benefit different facial skin types, cleansing rituals, and soil loads. Since there is such a broad array of cleansing forms, specialty facial cleansers (including devices) have become a very fragmented category of products which utilize more different technologies than most other cleaning applications. Although a wide range of products is available, these products share four common goals: (1) to clean skin (removing surface dirt and all makeup); (2) to provide a basic level of exfoliation; (3) to remove potentially harmful micro-organisms (bacteria); and (4) to cause minimal damage to the epidermis and stratum corneum. Additionally, facial cleansers are required to remove a myriad of chemicals and biological materials, ranging from the latest waterproof makeup to excess skin oils and upper layers of stratum corneum (exfoliated skin).

How facial cleansers work

It is well-understood that the use of harsh surfactants and/or over-washing skin can result in over-removal or distortion of stratum corneum and intercellular lipids, which can lead to reduced skin barrier function [3].

While the wide array of facial cleanser technologies all provide basic levels of skin cleansing, they all clean skin slightly differently. The mechanisms by which cleansing is accomplished can be grouped into three main categories: (1) cleansing by chemistry; (2) cleansing by physical action; and (3) in many cases, cleansing by a combination of both chemistry and physical action.

Chemistry of cleansing

Two classes of chemicals are used in facial cleansers and are responsible for the cleaning effect: surfactants and solvents. Both of these types of chemicals interact with dirt, soil, and skin to remove unwanted material. Surfactants and solvents work via two different chemical mechanisms to effect removal of these materials. Understanding these mechanistic differences provides dermatologists with the insight needed to prescribe a cleansing regimen based on individual patient needs.

Surfactants

Surfactants or "**surf**ace **act**ing **ag**ents" are usually organic compounds that are amphiphilic, meaning they contain both hydrophilic groups and hydrophobic groups. The combination of both hydrophilic and hydrophobic groups uniquely makes surfactants soluble in both oil and water.

Surfactants work by reducing the interfacial tension (the energy that keeps water and oil separated) between oil and water by being adsorbed at the oil–water interface. Once adsorbed at the interface, cleaning surfactants assemble into a low-energy aggregate called a micelle. Surfactant needs to be present at high enough concentration to form a micelle, a level called the "critical micelle concentration" (CMC), which is also the minimum surfactant concentration required to clean sebaceous oil, cosmetics, etc. When micelles form in water, their tails form a core that encapsulates an oil droplet, and their (ionic/polar) heads form an outer shell that maintains contact with water. This process is called emulsification.

Surfactants clean skin by emulsifying oily components on the surface of skin with water. Once emulsified, the oil can be easily rinsed from skin during the post wash or rinse process. The stronger the surfactant, the more hydrophobic (oil-based) material removed, the greater the potential skin damage due to excessive removal of naturally occurring skin lipids, and the greater the ensuing compromise of optimal skin barrier function, therefore correct/careful formulation of these surfactants is required to ensure proper mildness. Recently marketed products, show that with careful formulation very strong surfactants such as sodium laurel sulfate (SLS) can be well tolerated by skin. All surfactant-based cleansers require water and generally include a rinsing step. They are best suited to removal of oily residue. Unfortunately, two problems have been associated with cleansing with surfactants (one real and one largely folk-lore). First, because of their powerful cleansing action, overuse may completely eliminate the protective lipid barrier on the surface of skin, resulting in irritation and dryness. Second, consumers for years have heard negative stories regarding the alkaline (pH around 9) nature of these products. Wrongly assuming that since skin pH is about 5, washing with these high pH surfactants can lead to an increase in skin pH. Recent data suggest that that the skins natural buffering capacity is more than adequate to eliminate any unwarranted impact of the pH of these products.

Classical surfactants used in facial cleansers are categorized into four primary groups: *cationic, anionic, amphoteric, and non-ionic*.

- **Cationic surfactants used alone** are generally poorly tolerated, and are now rarely used in skin care products without carful formulation into coaceravate systems.
- **Anionic surfactants**, such as linear alkyl sulfates, consist of molecules with a negatively charged "head" and a long hydrophobic "tail". Anionic surfactants are widely used because of their good lathering and detergent properties.
- **amphoteric (zwitterionic)** surfactants, such as the betaines and alkylamino acids, are well-tolerated and lather well, and are used in facial cleansers.
- **Non-ionic** surfactants, such as polyglucosides and sorbitan esters, consist of overall uncharged molecules. They are very mild (tolerated better than anionic, cationic surfactants on skin), but do not lather particularly well.

Some surfactants are harsh to the skin while others are very mild. Because of the wide variety of available surfactants, not all surfactant-based cleansers are the same. It is important for patients to use products that best fit their skin type. Today, most cleansers use synthetic surfactants.

Solvents

A solvent is a liquid that dissolves a solid or another liquid into a homogeneous solution. Solvent-based systems clean skin by dissolving natural sebaceous oil and external oils applied to skin via cosmetics and similar materials. Solvents work under the chemical premise that "like dissolves like". Solvents can be classified broadly into two categories: *polar* and *non-polar*. Typical non-polar solvents used in facial cleansing, such as mineral oil or petrolatum, are from the oil family, whereas typical polar solvents used in cleansing, such as isopropyl alcohol and ethanol, are from the alcohol family. Solvent-based cleansers are usually not used in conjunction with water; rather, they are applied and then "wiped" off with a tissue or cotton ball.

Solvent-based cleansers should be chosen carefully on the basis of cleansing need. Non-polar solvents work well for removing oil-based makeups and cosmetics but have little effect on water-based formulations. Similarly, alcohol-based systems work well on water-based makeups. It is also important to note that alcohol-based systems can dry skin, a benefit for younger consumers with acne-prone skin but a potential disadvantage for older consumers and those with dry skin. On the other hand, oil-based products can leave a greasy or oily residue, which is beneficial for consumers with dry skin, but undesirable for those with normal. However, recent studies have shown that a patient with oily skin can benefit from using an oil-based or emollient cleanser. By using an oil to cleanse the skin, dirt and excess oil are removed while leaving the skin conditioned. Hence, the skin is not totally void of the natural skin oils and the body does feel the need to generate excess oil. Choosing a solvent-based cleanser based on skin type is critical.

Physical cleaning

An alternative to chemical cleansing is physical cleaning of skin. Essentially physics, primarily in the form of friction, also plays an important role in cleansing. In facial cleansing, friction is generated primarily by the direct interaction of a washcloth, tissue, cotton ball, cleansing cloth, or mechanical device with the surface of skin. Friction works to help dislodge soils, as well as increase the interaction of chemical cleaning agents (surfactants and solvents) with soils. The role of friction will be covered in more detail in the section on substrate cleansers.

Types of facial cleanser

Seven primary and popular forms of facial cleansers exist (other rarely used forms exist but are not covered in this chapter). These cleansers can be categorized as follows: *lathering cleansers, emollient cleansers, milks, scrubs, toners, dry lathering cleansing cloths, and wet cleansing cloths*. Each form is described in detail below. A summary of cleansers, technologies, and uses is shown in Table 11.1.

Lathering cleansers

While lathering cleansers constitute one broad classification, they all have one unique characteristic that separates them from all other cleansing forms – they all generate lather when used in the cleansing process. Typically, these cleansers are formulated with a surfactant level greater than the CMC, such that excess surfactant can incorporate air and form lather. Additionally, these cleaners contain surfactants that have short hydrophobic chains; shorter chains enable faster and higher levels of lather.

Table 11.1 Cleanser technology and skin types.

Type of facial cleanser	Primary cleaning mechanism	Key characteristics	Primary recommended skin type
Liquid lathering cleansers	Emulsification	Forms lather when wet	Oily
Emollient cleansers	Emulsification	Non-lathering	Dry
Scrubs	Emulsification	Non-lathering, particulates provide exfoliation benefit	Dry, flakey
Milks	Dissolution	High conditioning, generally not used with water	Dry skin
Toners	Dissolution	Low viscosity liquid, pore tightening	Oily/young Acne prone
Dry cleansing cloths	Emulsification and physical removal	Provide multiple benefits: cleansing, conditioning, exfoliating, toning	All skin types
Wet cleansing cloths	Dissolution and physical removal	Provide multiple benefits: cleansing, conditioning, exfoliating, toning. Generally not used with water.	Dry skin
Cleansing device + cleanser	Mechanical dissolution and physical removal	Provide multiple benefits: cleansing, exfoliation, conditioning. Generally used with appropriate cleanser for skin type.	All skin types

Most lathering cleansers sold today utilize synthetic surfactants that have been especially designed to be mild to skin. These synthetic surfactants have little interaction with skin lipids and therefore produce substantially less skin damage than naturally derived surfactants. However, this quality also compromises to a small extent their capability to remove oil-soluble makeups. Many classes of surfactants are used in facial cleansers two common ones include sarcosinates and betaines [4]. Even formulations with newer surfactants tend to exhibit some skin barrier damage in clinical studies. Thus, lathering cleansers are generally warranted for patients with normal to oily skin or those who are removing a high cosmetic load (makeup, lipstick, or other cosmetic load). Interestingly, there is a strong consumer bias towards lathering cleansers since high levels of lather provide a very strong signal to consumers that the cleanser is working.

Lathering cleansers clean through the chemical process of emulsification. In other words, the cleanser emulsifies dirt and oils, by suspending or emulsifying materials, thus permitting them to be removed from skin during the rinse process. Many formulators of lathering cleanser products have tried to incorporate skin conditioning technologies that enable deposition of skin conditioners onto skin. Unfortunately, these technologies have generally been less successful at providing skin benefit ingredients than other cleansing forms.

Emollient (oil-based) cleansers

Emollient cleansers are a milder alternative to lather cleansers. Although they clean via emulsification, they do not form lather in the presence of water. Surprisingly, however they do form a structure that suspends dirt and makeup within formulation. Typically, these cleansers provide a very high level of soil removal without drying the skin to the same degree as lathering cleansers. Emollient cleansers generally consist of a special formulation of lathering surfactants in which either lathering is suppressed by an oil (e.g., mineral oil) or the surfactant forms a complex with another charged molecule to inhibit the formation of the air-water interface necessary to provide lather.

Clinically, emollient cleansers are generally less harsh on skin than lathering cleansers. However, consumers sometimes complain that emollient cleansers leave a residual film on skin that does not satisfy some cleansing expectations. Typically, these cleansers are best suited to those patients with high cleansing needs who also suffer from dry skin or patients with very oily skin.

Scrubs

Facial scrubs can be either lathering of emollient-based. They generally contain small particles of natural or polymeric ingredients. Scrubs are intended to provide a deep cleansing experience including a higher level of skin exfoliation due to abrasion with the particles. A non-exhaustive list of natural scrub particles includes seeds of many fruits (e.g., peach, apple, apricot), nut shells (e.g., almond, walnut), grains (e.g., oats, wheat), and sandalwood. Synthetic scrub particles include polyethylene or polypropylene beads. Because of their abrasive nature, patients with sensitive skin may not want to use these as their daily use cleanser. For those with sensitive skin, it is recommended that scrub cleansers be used only once or twice a week in normal cleansing routines, due to the abrasive nature of a facial scrub.

Cleansing milks

Milks are a form of cleansers that are generally not used in conjunction with water. Because they are not used in conjunction with a water rinse, cleansing milks are ideal for depositing beneficial agents, such as humectants, petrolatum, vitamins, and desquamatory ingredients, onto the skin. These cleansers are a good choice for cleaning dry or other diseased skin. One drawback is that the residual ingredients left on skin can make skin feel as though cleansing is incomplete. Milks work by dissolving, as opposed to emulsifying, oils and dirt. Typically they are applied like a lotion and then wiped off with a tissue, cotton ball, or towel.

Toners

Toners are a class of facial cleansers formulated to clean skin and minimize the appearance of pores. This class of cleanser utilizes solvency as the primary mode of cleaning. Toners are usually applied with a physical substrate, such as cotton balls, tissues, or wash cloths; however, some newer toners can be sprayed on and wiped off. In most cases, toners are used in the absence of water. Toner formulations generally utilize alcohol as the solvent of choice and some level of humectants. Toners usually exist in three strengths: (1) mild (0–10% alcohol, refresher); (2) medium (10–20% alcohol; tonic); and (3) strong (20–60% alcohol, astringent). More recently, some companies have developed two-phase toners, which consist of a solvent and an immiscible oil formulated to provide astringent benefits while minimizing the dry skin feeling. Typical uses of toners are makeup removal and pore cleaning associated with acne care. Toners are popular with teenagers and young adults because of the perceived acne benefits and pore tightening associated with this technology.

Substrate cleansers

Introduced in the early 2000s, cleansing cloths are disposable substrates that are pretreated with low levels of mild detergents. Cleaning is driven by both physics (friction from the interaction between cloth and skin) and chemistry (either emulsification or dissolution). This combined action often results in cleaner skin and offers several key advantages for product formulation. Conditioning ingredients can be incorporated into or placed on the substrate which can help to maintain surfactant mildness while providing the patient with additional skin benefits [5]. Additionally, the cloths themselves can be designed to meet the needs of different skin types.

Substrates used in cleansing cloths generally consist of natural fibers, such as cotton; synthetic fibers, such as rayon, polyester terphalate (PET) or polypropylene; or a blend of one or more of these fibers. Depending upon the fibers used and the nonwoven manufacturing process, the substrate texture can be tailored to meet differing expectations from very soft to rough, meaning that different exfoliation levels can be delivered to the consumer. Technologies used on cleansing cloths include the printing of a polymer on the cloth itself, which further improves exfoliation and cleansing capabilities.

Cleansing cloths utilize multiple cleansing mechanisms and can be formulated with as little as 25% of the surfactant used in liquid cleansers [6]. This lower surfactant level can translate to less skin damage. Another key trait of substrate cleansing cloths is that dirt, makeup and oil are picked up by and contained within the cloth. The visible dirt and oils on the cloth provide a subtle clue to patients that the cleansing step is complete, reducing over cleansing, another contributor to skin damage. Two popular forms of substrate-based cleansers exist today: (1) dry, or water activated cleansing cloths; and (2) wet cleansing cloths.

Dry lathering cleansing cloths

Dry cleansing cloths are disposable cloths that have lathering surfactants dried onto the cloths during the manufacturing process. They are purchased dry and are used after activated with water. These cloths generate a generous lather, similar to a liquid lathering cleanser, due to the cloth structure incorporating air as the cloth is rubbed together with water during use. The combination of rich lather and enhanced tactile feel of the cloth provides an enhanced cleansing experience to the consumer.

Many of these products contain and deposit on to stratum corneum moisturizing ingredients like petrolatum and glycerin. This enables dry cleansing cloths to deliver multiple skin care benefits in one product: (1) high level of cleansing; (2) high level of exfoliation; (3) minimal reduction in skin barrier function; (4) rich lather; (5) and, in the case of at least one product, significant moisturization [7]. This combination of benefits can eliminate the need for other specialty cleansing products such as toners and exfoliators.

One unique advantage of dry cleansing cloth technology, which enables multiple benefits, is that different ingredients can be placed in different "zones" on a cloth. This enables formulators to use ingredients that are not compatible in a liquid cleanser. Olay Daily Facials is one example in which the cleansing surfactant, skin conditioner, and fragrance are applied separately and to different zones of a cloth. This permits the product to deposit conditioning ingredients directly onto skin during washing. Studies have shown that separate addition of petrolatum onto a cleansing cloth provided hydration and transepidermal waterloss (TEWL) benefits and resulted in a smoother skin surface, a more compact SC, and well-defined lipid bilayers at the surface of the SC [8].

Wet cleansing cloths

Wet cleansing cloths are shipped pre-moistened and designed to cleanse without water or rinsing. They originated from disposable wipe technology for use with babies. However, these cleansing cloths have recently become quite popular for water-less cleansing and makeup removal. Wet cloths are non-lathering and since they are not rinsed with water they have the ability to incorporate and deposit small amounts of beneficial ingredients such a humectants and lipids onto the skin. Similar to dry cloths, differences in formulation and substrate choices enable wet cloths to suit varying skin types.

Wet cleansing cloths are often marketed as makeup removers and can be used either for full face cleansing or as a first step to remove makeup prior to traditional cleansing. As this product is not designed to be rinsed, there is generally a trade-off between efficacy and skin feel. Wet cloths formulated to remove difficult makeup require additional cleansing agents which can impact skin feel. Conversely, wet cloths that feel very refreshing may not have the level of surfactants needed to remove all makeup.

While wet cloths do not provide the typical cleansing experience, due to the fact that some patients do not like the cleansing agents left on the skin (when used without rinsing), wet cleansing cloths continue to be popular from a convenience standpoint. Patients can use wet cleansing cloths while on-the-go or when a sink or shower is not available.

Cleansing devices

Cleansing devices were recently introduced to patients and are motor-powered implements with a very soft brush head. The facial cleanser is applied to the brush head and generates later when pressed gently against the skin's surface. Cleansing devices clean the skin better than cleanser alone across any dirt substrate [9]. It has been demonstrated that surfactant-based cleansers work more efficiently with a device than an emulsion cleanser alone. Cleansing devices have the ability to clean the more difficult areas of the face, including the area at the base of the nose. However, harsh cleansers and facial scrubs containing large-sized exfoliant particles should not be used with cleansing devices. This could potentially cause the skin to become void of natural oils. Thus, it is very important to be selective in choosing the appropriate cleanser to use with a cleansing device.

Guide to selecting facial cleansers

Recommending a facial cleansing regimen can be a daunting task given the multitude of cleansing forms available. To choose the most appropriate cleanser, physicians should consider skin type, skin problems, and any skin allergies.

The following section provides a short reference guide and tools to help in selection of cleansers based on patient skin type, cleansing need, and preference. The selection guide is broken into three parts or strategies: (1) selection based on skin type; (2) selection based on cleansing form; and, (3) selection based on skin problems.

Selection based on skin type

The first step in selecting a facial cleanser is to assess the patient's skin type and to categorize it as dry, oily or normal. Once skin type has been determined, assess the skin for any problems, such as acne, excessive flakiness, and dryness. Table 11.1 systematically lists the main facial cleansers covered in this chapter, and highlights the key characteristics of each cleanser and the best cleanser for each skin type.

Selection based on cleanser form/cleansing ritual

The second strategy for selecting facial cleansers is to first assess a patient's cleansing ritual preference. Figure 11.1 depicts one of the main cleansing ritual preferences: no substrate/substrate and lathering/non-lathering. To use this approach most effectively, first, identify the quadrant of Figure 11.1 that best describes the patient's ritual preference, and then use Table 11.1 to select a facial cleanser that best matches the patient's skin type. This may be the best approach to selecting a cleanser when compliance with skin care is critical.

Selection based on skin problems

In many cases, cleanser selection may be somewhat subjective. The charts in the figures which follow provide a hierarchy of the primary benefits associated with facial cleansers ranked by cleanser type. The benefits described in this section are cleaning excess sebaceous oil, cleaning dirt and makeup loads, exfoliation, and mildness to skin. Considering these benefits when prescribing a cleansing routine may prove useful in providing a cleanser that fully meets patient expectation and needs.

Cleaning excess sebaceous oil

Removal of excess sebaceous oil is a significant concern of teens and young adults. Cleansing of sebaceous oil is best accomplished with either lathering products that emulsify the oils or toners that are specifically formulated to solubilize sebaceous oil. These products and can also give users a sense of control over oily skin by providing pore tightening benefits (Figure 11.2).

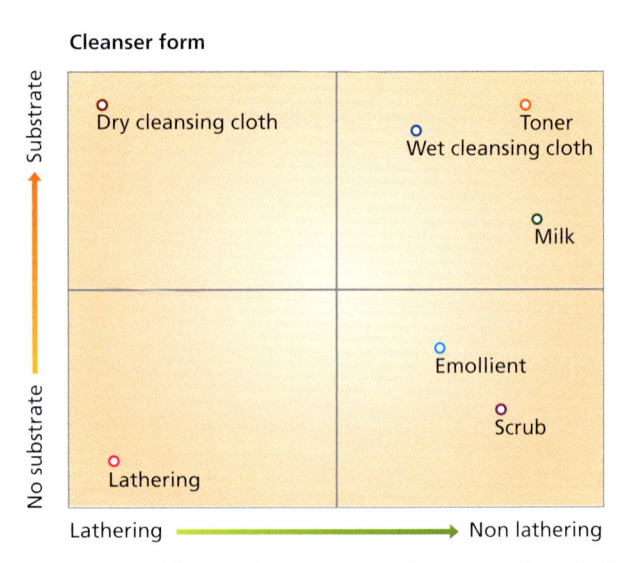

Figure 11.1 One of the main cleansing ritual preferences: no substrate/substrate and lathering/non-lathering.

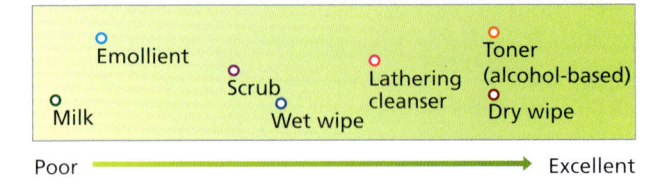

Figure 11.2 Products for the removal of excess sebaceous oil.

Cleaning dirt and makeup

One of the primary benefits of a facial cleanser is removal of high makeup loads and dirt. By a wide margin, dirt and makeup removal is best performed by substrate cleansers. The high cleansing capability of these cleansers is due to their capability to provide both physical and chemical cleaning, in addition to the substrates' ability to trap and hold dirt and oil within their fibers (Figure 11.3).

Exfoliation: removing dry dead skin cells

When high exfoliation is required, because of aging or for other reasons, products that provide physical cleansing are an appropriate choice because they also provide the highest level of exfoliation. Exfoliation is due to physical abrasion, which removes the top layers of skin. As a side note, most cleansers provide low to insignificant levels of exfoliation; thus, if exfoliation is the main skin need, a substrate-based cleanser or facial scrub is highly recommended (Figure 11.4).

Cleanser mildness

For much of facial cleansing history, cleanser mildness was a significant concern. Now, with new surfactant and cleansing technologies, most specialty facial cleansers (with the exception

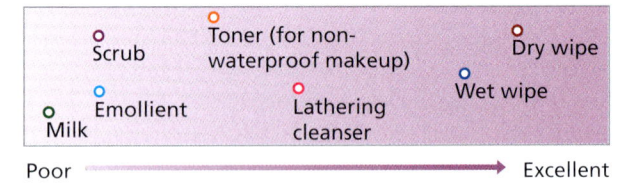

Figure 11.3 Products for the removal of dirt and makeup.

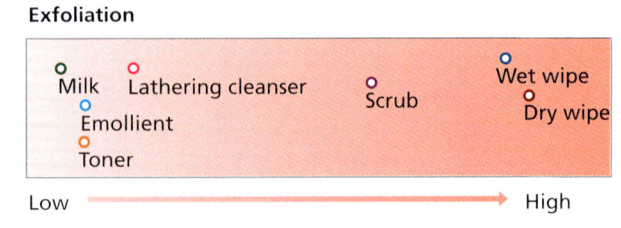

Figure 11.4 Products for the removal of dry, dead skin cells.

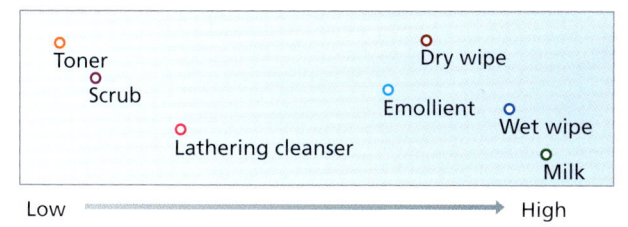

Figure 11.5 Products for patients for whom dry skin is a key complaint.

of toners) provide close to neutral or better mildness. This chart ranks cleansing forms for skin for patients for whom dry skin is a key complaint (Figure 11.5).

Summary

Many different facial cleansing forms exist today. All can be categorized on the basis of three factors: (1) the type of chemistry used, either surfactant or solvent-based; (2) whether or not the cleansing form creates lather; and (3) whether or not the cleansing form incorporates physical cleansing as well as chemical cleansing. All of these facial cleansing forms provide the basic level of cleansing required to maintain healthy skin; however, different skin types benefit from different cleansing forms, and patient preference drives usage and compliance.

The future of the facial cleansing category is bright. Significant innovation is expected to continue for the foreseeable future, particularly in substrate cleanser applications and formulations for removing the new and more durable makeups and mascaras that are entering the market. Technical development will continue to focus on low damage to skin and improved delivery of specially directed skin ingredients during the cleansing process.

References

1 Bolles RC. (1960) Grooming behavior in the rat. *J Comp Physiol Psychol* **53**(3), 306–310.
2 Nicholson PT, Shaw I. (2000) *Ancient Egyptian Materials and Technology*. Cambridge: Cambridge University Press.
3 Ananthapadmanabhan KP, Moore DJ, Subramanyan K, Misra M, Meyer F. (2004) Cleansing without compromise: the impact of cleansers on the skin barrier and the technology of mild cleansing. *Dermatol Ther* **17**(1), 16–25.
4 Paye M, Barel AO, Maibach HI. *Handbook of Cosmetic Science and Technology*, 2nd edn. London: Informa Health Care.
5 Kinderdine S, *et al.* (2004) *The evolution of facial cleansing: Substrate cleansers provide mildness benefits of leading soap and syndet*. P&G Beauty. Science poster presentation, 62nd Annual Meeting of the American Academy of Dermatology, February 6–11, 2004.
6 Unpublished data. P & G Beauty, Cincinnati, Ohio. *Comparison of surfactant level in Olay Foaming Face Wash, and Olay Daily Facials*.
7 McAtee D, *et al.* US patent 6280757 8-28-2001.
8 Coffindaffer T, *et al. Assessment of leading facial skin cleansers by microscopic evaluation of the stratum corneum*. P&G Beauty Science poster presentation. 62nd Annual Meeting of the American Academy of Dermatology, February 6–11, 2004.
9 Czetty, B, *et al. Powered devices for facial cleansing: Should they occupy space in the facial cleansing device toolbox?* Presented at the SCC Annual Scientific Meeting, December 2010.

CHAPTER 12
Hand Cleansers and Sanitizers

Duane Charbonneau
Procter and Gamble Company, Health Sciences Institute, Mason, OH, USA

BASIC CONCEPTS
- Hands are common sources for microbial contamination and microbial pathogen transfer.
- Cleansers and sanitizer products reduce transient microbes on the skin surface with the goal of reducing the spread of infectious disease.
- Hand cleansing products include liquid soaps with and without antimicrobial agents, alcohol-based hand sanitizers, and non-alcohol-based sanitizers.
- Hands with damaged skin harbor more transient microorganisms than healthy hands.
- Hand hygiene technologies have been demonstrated to reduce the spread of nosocomial infections.

Introduction

Hand cleansers and hand sanitizers were developed to reduce transient microbes on the skin to help limit the spread of infectious disease. This class of products includes liquid soaps, antimicrobial liquid soaps, alcohol-based hand sanitizers, and non-alcohol-based hand sanitizers.

Growing concern exists about the spread of infectious disease. Despite historical expectations that such disease would wane in the United States over the course of the 20th century, between 1980 and 1992, the death rate due to infectious diseases increased 58% from 41 to 65 deaths per 100 000 population [1]. In the United States, about 1 in 6 people contract a foodborne illness each year [2], resulting in an estimated 52 million cases annually. A growing number of outbreaks have been associated with Campylobacter or *Escherichia coli* O157:H7 through consumption of contaminated meats and produce in the home. Half of all cases of norovirus, the most common cause of food-borne illness in the US, occur in long-term care facilities [3]. Rotavirus, another viral cause of gastroenteritis, spreads by the fecal–oral route among children cared for in group settings [4]. More recently, the cross-species transfer of infectious viral agents to humans, which initiated the 2002–2003 outbreak of severe acute respiratory syndrome (SARS), the 2004 outbreak of H5N1-linked avian influenza [5], and the 2009 US outbreak H1N1-linked porcine influenza [6], have elevated concerns about the potential for human pandemics.

Healthcare associated infections have gained attention as the leading cause of death in US healthcare settings [7] and the fourth leading cause of death overall in Canada [8]. Pathogens once largely confined to healthcare facilities, such as methicillin-resistant *Staphylococcus aureus* (MRSA) and *Clostridium difficile* (*C. difficile*), have now moved into the community. Multi-drug resistant *Acinetobacter baummanii* has entered nursing homes and long-term care facilities through discharge of hospital patients into these settings [9]. The emergence of these antibiotic resistant organisms limits the therapeutic arsenal available to combat infection; moreover, it has become economically less desirable for pharmaceutical companies to develop and register novel antibiotics, further limiting potential new therapeutics.

Because of these concerns, reducing the burden of infectious disease must emphasize strategies to limit transmission. Good hygiene is a cornerstone of preventive measures, for the spread of infectious agents. Because hand contact plays such a crucial role in the transmission of infectious agents, effective hand hygiene products are a vital component of preventive regimens. This chapter reviews the formulation, mode of action and efficacy of hand cleansers and sanitizers, discusses regulatory and safety issues related to the use of antimicrobial ingredients, and proposes future directions for improving these products and technologies.

Hand microbiota

The skin is an ecosystem coinhabited by symbiotic and commensal microbes collectively termed the skin microbiome [10]. Most skin bacteria fall into four dominant phyla – Actinobacteria, Firmicutes, Bacteriodetes, and Proteobacteria – but a great deal of diversity exists at the species level [11]. Compared to the oral

---

Cosmetic Dermatology: Products and Procedures, Second Edition. Edited by Zoe Diana Draelos.
© 2016 John Wiley & Sons, Ltd. Published 2016 by John Wiley & Sons, Ltd.

or gut microbiota, the skin microbiota shows the greatest variability over time [12]. Although a core set of taxa inhabits skin surfaces, considerable intra-individual and interindividual variability in skin microbiome composition exists, reflecting both host and environmental influences. Diversity is greater between individuals: only 13% of bacterial phylotypes on the surface of the palms are shared between unrelated people [13]. Members of the same household share more of their skin microbiota, particularly on the palms, than people from different households [14]. The diversity of microbial populations within households arise from various internal and external sources, but surfaces with high contact bear the signature of the occupants' skin microbiome [15].

Microbes that inhabit the hand are generally divided into two categories: the transient and the resident microbiota (Figure 12.1). The transient microbiota are microbes that inadvertently become attached to the hands by touching contaminated materials and surfaces, such as raw food items during food preparation, body fluids in healthcare or group care settings, or fomites in the daily environment. Microbiota on the dominant and non-dominant hands of the same individual are quite significantly different [13], most likely because the dominant hand comes into contact with different types of surfaces than the non-dominant hand. Furthermore, the transfer of transient microbiota from hands to mouth or to other parts of the body, either in a single person or between individuals, is well documented in the literature. The classic example is the work of Gwaltney and others in the 1970 s [16,17], which demonstrated the importance of hand-to-hand transmission of the common cold virus.

The resident hand microbiota comprise the community of microbes that consistently inhabit the hand and routinely are not washed off with non-medicated soaps. A summary of bacteria reportedly isolated as resident flora is presented in Table 12.1. Handwashing alters overall community composition in a temporary, limited fashion, either because washing fails to remove

Table 12.1 Constituents of the resident microbiota of the hand.

Organism
Acinetobacter baumannii
Acinetobacter johnsonii
Acinetobacter lwoffii
Corynebacterium spp.
Enterobacter agglomerans
Enterobacter cloacae
Klebsiella pneumoniae
Propionibacterium acnes
Pseudomonas aeruginosa
Staphylococcus aureus
Staphylococcus epidermidis
Staphylococcus warneri
Streptococcus mitis
Streptococcus pyogenes

most taxa on the skin surface (resident taxa) or because depleted communities rapidly reestablish themselves [13]. In a University population, taxa such as Staphylococcaceae, Streptococcaceae, and Lactobacillaceae were relatively more abundant on hands that have been recently washed, whereas Proprionibacteria, Neisseriales, Burkholderiales, and Pasteurellaceae taxa became more abundant with longer times after handwashing [13]. Frequent exposure to certain transient microbes may lead to them becoming established as constituents of the resident microbiota. For example, nurses who perform similar tasks within a hospital share similarities in their resident microbiota but exhibit differences from those assigned to other tasks [18–21]. Furthermore, the resident hand microbiota of homemakers include microbes that are identical to those environmental isolates identified within the home [22].

The functional role of the skin microbiota in health and disease is incompletely understood, but it is speculated that the resident skin microbes are as essential to the health of the skin as the gut microorganisms are to overall health of the individual [23]. *Staphylococcus epidermidis*, a commensal bacterium, maintains health by modulating the host immune response (reviewed in [24]). However, the organism is also the most common cause of hospital-acquired infection, for example, when virulent forms create biofilms on in-dwelling medical devices such as catheters and heart valves [25]. *Proprionibacterium acnes*, a commensal skin bacterium, causes acne, an inflammatory disorder of the pilosebaceous unit that occurs when this structure matures during puberty. In addition, it is estimated that approximately 32% of the population carries the common pathogen, *Staphylococcus aureus* (*S. aureus*), as a member of the resident skin microbiota [23]. As many as 90% of patients with atopic dermatitis are colonized with *S. aureus* on lesional and non-lesional skin [26] and colonization rates are highest on acute lesions [27]. Treatment of

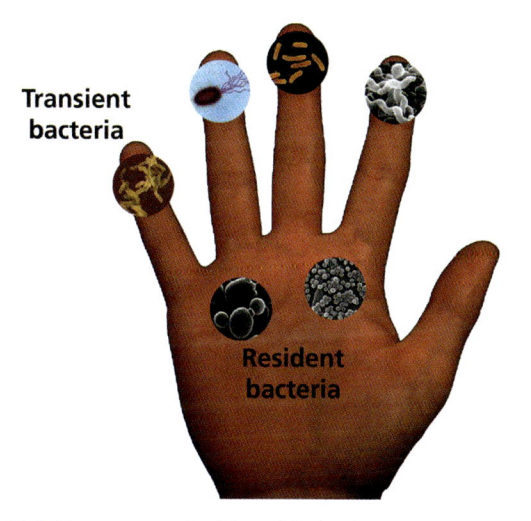

Figure 12.1 The common microbiota of the hand.

patients with atopic dermatitis leads to a more diversified skin microbiota [28,29].

Hand hygiene guidelines

The critical role of hand hygiene as means of infection control dates back to the mid-1800s, when the groundbreaking work of Professor Ignaz Semmelweis demonstrated a reduction in puerperal sepsis after initiating a mandatory handwashing policy for medical personnel [30]. By 1980, the role of hand transmission of bacterial and viral pathogens was well-documented [16,31]. Today, handwashing with soap and water, or hand antisepsis using antimicrobial washes or hand sanitizers, is the cornerstone of many infection control programs.

Guidelines for handwashing and hand antisepsis in healthcare settings were published by the Association for Professionals in Infection Control (APIC) in 1988 and updated in 1995 [32]. In 2002, the Centers for Disease Control and Prevention (CDC) published guidelines for hand hygiene in healthcare settings in collaboration with the HICPAC/SHEA/APIC/IDSA hand hygiene task force [33]. This guideline recommends using alcohol-based hand rubs routinely for hand antisepsis unless hands are visibly dirty, contaminated, or if exposure to spores is suspected; in such cases, washing with soap (non-antimicrobial or antimicrobial) and water is recommended.

In 2009, the World Health Organization (WHO) published Guidelines for Hand Hygiene in Healthcare as part of their "Clean Care Is Safer Care" Initiative [34]. The guidelines are intended to apply to all healthcare settings, whether care is delivered continually (as in healthcare institutions), or occasionally (e.g. home care by birth attendants). WHO recommended the adoption of alcohol-based hand rubs to rapidly and effectively inactivate a wide array of potentially harmful microorganisms on hands. Consistent with the earlier CDC guidelines, this body recommends the routine use of alcohol-based hand rubs unless hands are visibly soiled or contaminated. Posters and brochures depicting optimal methods for using hand rubs or washing with soap and water (and the situations in which they apply) are available online [35].

The US Food and Drug Administration (FDA) Food Code, most recently updated in 2013, contains specific hand hygiene guidance for retail and food service workers that describes when, where, and how to wash and sanitize hands [36]. The Food Code calls for proper handwashing with soap and water to control the transmission of enteric bacteria, enteric non-lipophilic viruses, and protozoan oocysts that may be encountered in settings where food is prepared. Alcohol-based hand sanitizers are not effective enough against these particular microbes. Furthermore, fatty or proteinaceous soils encountered during food preparation may interfere with alcohol efficacy [37]. Consequently, hand sanitizers that meet specific criteria described in section 2–301.16 of the Food Code may be used in retail and food service settings only after proper handwashing is used to remove soil.

Hand Hygiene Techniques and Compliance

When done properly, handwashing is considered to be the gold standard for removing transient pathogenic bacteria from the hands. The CDC has published a description of handwashing technique for healthcare settings in both text and pictorial poster format [38]. The CDC also promulgates general handwashing advice aimed at homes, schools and businesses as part of a "Handwashing: Clean Hands Save Lives" initiative [39]. The handwashing protocol for healthcare providers provides explicit descriptions for each step, including activating the faucet, the modes of scrubbing all aspects or the dorsal and palmar surfaces and fingers, drying the hands, and shutting off the faucet. It specifies that the full procedure should have a 60 second duration from start to finish. The description aimed at consumers is consistent with this healthcare protocol, but uses much simpler instructions, being most explicit about lathering and scrubbing for 20 seconds (see Table 12.2 for comparison).

Table 12.2 Comparison of hand hygiene instructions for healthcare workers and consumers.

Hand hygiene in healthcare settings[a]	Hand hygiene consumer guidelines[b]
Wet hands with water	Wet your hands with clean, running water (warm or cold), turn off the tap, and apply soap.
Apply enough soap to cover all hand surfaces	Lather your hands by rubbing them together with the soap. Be sure to lather the backs of your hands, between your fingers, and under your nails.
Rub hands palm to palm	Scrub your hands for at least 20 seconds. Need a timer? Hum the "Happy Birthday" song from beginning to end twice.
Right palm over left dorsum with interlaced fingers and vice versa	Rinse your hands well under clean, running water.
Palm to palm with fingers interlaced	Dry your hands using a clean towel or air dry them.
Backs of fingers to opposing palms with fingers interlocked	
Rotational rubbing of left thumb clasped in right palm **and vice versa**	
Rotational rubbing, backwards and forwards with clasped fingers of **right hand in left palm and vice versa**	
Rinse hands with water	
Dry hands thoroughly with a single-use towel	
Use towel to **turn off faucet**	
Your hands are now safe.	

[a] Centers for Disease Control/World Health Organization. Hand Hygiene in Health Care Settings. Hand Hygiene Basics 2012. www.cdc.gov/handhygiene/Basics.html.
[b] Centers for Disease Control and Prevention. Hand Washing: Clean Hands Save Lives. When and How to Wash Your Hands. 2013. www.cdc.gov/handwashing/when-how-handwashing.html.

The basic elements of proper handwashing are as follows:
- Wet your hands with clean, running water and apply soap.
- Lather well by rubbing the hands together, making sure to lather the back of the hands, the palms, between the fingers and under the nails.
- Scrub for at least 20 seconds.
- Rinse well.
- Dry your hands with a clean or disposable towel or air-dry them.

Although healthcare professionals recognize the importance of handwashing, observational studies indicate that compliance is poor. A CDC review of available studies found that the baseline level of compliance with hand hygiene guidelines among healthcare workers averaged 40% (range 5% to 81%) [33]. Handwashing compliance also tends to fall to lower levels at night [40], and fewer than 50% of hospital healthcare workers washed their hands after toileting [41].

A similar deficiency exists in the community. An observational study of food service workers found that 30% were compliant with standard guidelines [42]. Studies in public restrooms on a university campus indicated that 61% of the women and 37% of the men observed washed their hands with soap in the absence of a visual prompt; 97% of the women and 35% of the men washed their hands in the presence of a sign prompting handwashing [43]. When college students were evaluated in four restroom settings (presence of soap and water; soap and water and visual prompts; soap and water and hand sanitizers; or soap and water, hand sanitizers, and visual prompts), 72.9% of students either washed or just rinsed their hands, 58.3% practiced hand hygiene (using either soap or hand sanitizer), and 26.1% washed their hands for the adequate length of time [44].

The duration of handwashing averages about 8 to 9 seconds in both healthcare and community settings [45,46]. These conditions are not ideal, as evidenced by studies showing mean cell densities on the hands of homemakers to be 5.72 CFU before washing and a 5.69 CFU after handwashing [47]. Compliance with handwashing guidelines at a teaching hospital was shown to be inversely proportional to education levels, so understanding the guidelines is not the issue [48].

In certain situations where handwashing compliance is low, hand sanitizers, especially those with a persistent benefit, may be considered to promote hand hygiene if appropriate to the setting in question. However, merely providing the product is insufficient. University students typically do not use hand sanitizers when they are installed in restrooms without any reinforcement of their use [44,49]. However, prospective trials have shown that when hand sanitizers were provided in elementary school classrooms along with appropriate education about their use, or when sanitizers were used in the classroom as an adjunct to handwashing, intervention groups had significantly lower absenteeism due to illness [50–52]. Formulation choices must be appropriate to the target pathogens of concern. For example, alcohol-based hand sanitizers may exhibit limited effectiveness against norovirus unless alcohol concentrations are high enough or the formula is supplemented with other actives [53,54]. It bears repeating that substituting alcohol-based hand sanitizers for soap and water cleansing is inappropriate in food service settings; however, regimens that combine handwashing with the subsequent application of high efficacy hand sanitizers can be very effective in reducing hand contamination in food handling situations [55].

Antimicrobial handwash and hand sanitizer formulations

Antimicrobial handwashes are primarily water-based formulations composed of mixtures of surfactants, antimicrobial actives, perfumes, and, in some cases, emollients. Because frequent use of surfactants can be drying to the skin, emollients and other agents to improve skin feel are incorporated to improve the consumer experience with the hope of raising compliance.

In the US, antimicrobial actives for handwash and handrub products are regulated under the Food and Drug Administration's 1994 Tentative Final Monograph (TFM) for over-the-counter (OTC) antiseptic drug products [56]. The ingredients are classified into three categories:
I. Category 1 – Ingredients determined to be safe and effective;
II. Category 2 – Ingredients determined to be neither safe nor effective;
III. Category 3 – Ingredients for which there is insufficient evidence; however, the FDA is not objecting to marketing or sale of these products.

Only active ingredients in categories I and III can be lawfully marketed in products within the US. Antimicrobial actives used in handwashes include chlorhexidine gluconate, chloroxylenol, hexachlorophene, iodine and iodophors, quaternary ammonium compounds, and triclosan. Antimicrobial soaps vary in the nature of the active ingredient as well as their overall formulation. Each antiseptic agent has a distinct range of activity against various bacteria and viruses (reviewed in [33,34]). Apart from iodophors (at concentrations higher than used in antimicrobial washes or handrubs), neither alcohol or any of the agents listed above is reliably efficacious against spore-forming bacteria, such as against *Clostridium* spp. or *Bacillus* spp. [57]. Glove use and strict adherence to recommended handwashing protocols are critical if there is reason to suspect contamination with such microbes.

Hand sanitizers can be categorized into three main classes:
1. Alcohol-based: containing ≥ 62% alcohol.
2. Alcohol-based, supplemented: containing ≥ 62% alcohol plus antimicrobial agent.
3. Non-alcohol based: the main ingredient is water, with added surfactant and antimicrobial agent.

Previously in the US, the FDA's 1994 TFM classified ethanol 60–95% as a Category I agent (i.e., generally safe and effective for use in antiseptic handwash or healthcare worker handwash products) [56]. Although the TFM placed isopropanol 70–91.3% in category III (i.e., insufficient data to classify as effective), 60% isopropanol has subsequently been adopted in Europe as the reference standard against which alcohol-based hand-rub products are benchmarked [58].

Hand sanitizer product forms include liquids, gels and foams. Germicidal efficacy is based on the fact that they are leave-on products that rapidly kill microbes. Hand sanitizers based solely on alcohol as the antiseptic deliver an immediate benefit but provide no residual activity. Supplementation of the alcohol-based formula with chlorhexidine, quaternary ammonium compounds, or triclosan can provide more persistent activity, delaying the reestablishment of transient microbiota. Other combinations have also proved efficacious. For example, a synergistic combination of a humectant (octoxyglycerine) and preservatives has resulted in prolonged activity of an alcohol-based handrub against transient pathogens without raising the concentration of antimicrobial active [59]. An experimental alcohol-based surgical hand disinfectant containing a synergistic combination of farnesol and benzethonium chloride demonstrated both immediate and persistent activity against resident hand flora of volunteers [60].

In its 2009 guidelines, the WHO recommended two alcohol-based handrub formulations for hand hygiene in healthcare settings, taking into account cost and efficacy for resource-poor countries. The first has final concentrations of ethanol 80% v/v, glycerol 1.45% v/v, and hydrogen peroxide (H_2O_2) 0.125% v/v; the second has final concentrations of isopropyl alcohol 75% v/v, glycerol 1.45% v/v, and hydrogen peroxide 0.125% v/v. However, these formulations did not meet the most stringent European efficacy requirements for surgical hand disinfection (the prEN 12791 standard). Proposed modifications (raising alcohol content, reducing glycerol, modifying rub times) raise efficacy to the required standards [61–63].

The formulation of non-alcohol-based hand sanitizers or antimicrobial handwashes must take into consideration the bioavailability of the antimicrobial active. Certain surfactants may complex with or otherwise inactivate the antiseptic, which results in products with the same antimicrobial active having different levels of antimicrobial efficacy [64].

The final variable to be considered in formulating antimicrobial handwashes and hand rubs is pH. The relatively acidic pH of the skin plays a role in the innate antimicrobial hostility of the hand surface. The normal pH of the hands is approximately 4–5, but alkaline soaps often raise the skin pH. In one report, pH increased between 0.6 to 1.8 units after handwashing with plain soap and then gradually declined to baseline levels over a period of 45 min to 2 h [65]. A low pH matrix has been used in newer handwash formulations with triclosan.

Efficacy of antimicrobial handwashes and hand sanitizers

Historically, three approaches have traditionally been used to demonstrate the efficacy of antimicrobial hand soaps and hand sanitizers:

1. *In vitro* assays to assess potency and the spectrum and duration of activity.
2. *In vivo* models to assess germicidal activity against an artificial inoculate.
3. Clinical studies to demonstrate efficacy in reducing the burden of hand microbiota, limiting the transfer from one person to another, and reduction in infectious disease.

In 2013, the FDA issued a proposed rule to update the conditions for establishing that OTC antimicrobial products are generally recognized as safe and effective (GRASE) [66]. The proposal would to require manufacturers of antimicrobial hand or body washes to demonstrate that the products are more effective than plain soap and water in preventing illness and the spread of infection. Currently, the regulations rely on *in vivo* models of germicidal activity to determine efficacy. The proposed rule, which does not include over the counter antiseptic hand sanitizers or antiseptics used by healthcare professionals, is available for comment for 180 days, with a concurrent one-year period for companies to submit new data and information, followed by a 60-day rebuttal period [66].

In vitro assays for potency and spectrum of activity

Standard *in vitro* assays evaluate the minimum inhibitory concentration (MIC) for germicidal activity or assess the time to kill target organisms, using indicator bacteria or viruses of interest. The research community has debated the relevance of such assays for decades, as they describe the potency and spectrum of activity of a formulation or antiseptic under very specific laboratory conditions.

Other *in vitro* assays model the removal of transient flora from the hands by employing artificial substrates such as pig skin. The substrate is inoculated in a controlled fashion and microbial reductions following treatment with the antimicrobial formulation are assessed [60]. Efficacy is determined relative to either an untreated control or to a placebo lacking the active ingredient. Such models have been employed to establish a residual antimicrobial benefit such as that afforded by low pH hand sanitizers with triclosan. Formulations containing chlorhexidine were historically used as the gold standard for residual antimicrobial efficacy.

In vivo models with artificial inoculate to mimic transient flora

In Europe and the United States, regulatory bodies require that specific *in vivo* test protocols be used to demonstrate efficacy [34,67]. In both regions, these protocols involve artificially contaminating subjects' hands with large inoculums of indicator bacteria, treating the hands with the test formulation, neutralizing the active ingredient, and enumerating the remaining viable bacteria on the skin.

In Europe, the most widely accepted protocols are EN 1499 for hygienic antimicrobial hand washes and EN 1500 for hygienic leave-on hand sanitizers [67]. In both standard protocols, 12 to 15 subjects first wash their hands with a plain soap and water; inoculation is achieved by having the subjects immerse their hands half-way to metacarpals in a 24-hour broth culture of a non-pathogenic strain of *E. coli*; after drying, bacterial recovery is achieved by kneading the fingertips and palms separately into 10 mL of Trypticase Soy Broth with neutralizers. The hands are disinfected, contaminated again, and the antimicrobial treatments are applied for 30 to 60 seconds, with or without a rinsing step, depending on product type (rinse-off or leave-on). Bacterial recovery is performed as described above, and the extracted bacteria are enumerated using traditional microbiological plating techniques. The European standard protocols require that efficacy be determined relative to internal standards. With EN 1499, rinse-off antimicrobial hand soaps must provide a superior log reduction relative to a 60-second wash with plain soap (sapo kalinus). With EN 1500, leave-on products such as hand sanitizers must deliver a benefit no less than that observed with a 60-second application of 2-propanol (60% w/v).

In the United States, methods for determining efficacy are described in FDA's 1994 TFM for OTC Antiseptic Drug Products (although, as noted earlier, a proposed rule to amend the 1994 TFM has recently been promulgated) [56]. Currently, the standard method used to evaluate antimicrobial handwash and hand sanitizer formulations is the American Society of Testing and Materials (ASTM) protocol, E 1174. In this test, subjects refrain from utilizing any antimicrobial products for 1 week prior to the start of the study ("washout period"). At study initiation, the subjects perform a cleansing wash to remove transient bacteria. Then, in order to establish a baseline level of artificial contamination, the subjects' hands are treated with 4.5–5.0 mL of a 24-hour broth culture of either a non-pathogenic strain of *E. coli* or *Serratia marcescens*. Bacteria are recovered by separately placing each hand into a glove containing 75 mL of sampling solution containing neutralizers. The hand is massaged for 1 minute and bacteria are enumerated using traditional microbiological plating techniques. Following baseline treatment, another cleansing wash is performed and hands are re-inoculated. The test formulation is then applied according to the manufacturer's instructions for the product type in question (rinse-off antimicrobial soap or leave-on hand sanitizer). Following treatment, bacterial recovery is again achieved using the glove method, as described above. The cycle of cleansing wash, inoculation, treatment, and enumeration is performed 10 times. No internal standard is used. Efficacy is determined by the magnitude of the log reduction from baseline. Wash 1 must deliver a minimum 2-log reduction and Wash 10, a minimum 3-log reduction from baseline, respectively.

Table 12.3 Comparison of US and European standard methods for assessing presurgical hand antisepsis.

Parameter	US method	prEN 12791
Product application	Hands and lower forearm	Hands only
Number of applications	11 applications over 5 days	Single application
Sampling times	0, 3, 6 hours post-application	0, 3 hour post-application
Sample method	Glove juice	Fingertip sampling
Success criteria	Absolute bacterial reduction	Non-inferiority to reference standard

Besides the above-described standards for hygienic handwashes, a more stringent European standard, prEN 12791, applies to scrubs for presurgical antisepsis. Differences between this European Standard and the US standard are shown in Table 12.3.

The standard methods have been the subject of considerable critique [68]. Both European and US standard protocols employ treatment times and product volumes far outside the norm. A further critique of the US ASTM E1174 protocol is that bacteria are sampled from areas such as the back of the hand that are usually not involved in transmission. The relevance of the inoculum has also been challenged, as in the natural setting, transient bacteria would rarely be present without being incorporated into a soil matrix. Consequently, some investigators employ methodologies that incorporate the use of a soil matrix, such as chicken or hamburger, in lieu of simple inoculum with marker microbial organisms; these methods also focus on contamination of the palms of the hands [37,55,69]. In the presence of a greasy soil matrix such as chicken, the alcohol-based hand sanitizers lack appreciable efficacy, whereas hand sanitizers supplemented with more potent antimicrobial actives such as triclosan or benzalkonium chloride demonstrate a higher level of effectiveness (Figure 12.2).

Besides these standardized methodologies, a commonly used research tool is referred to as the fingerpad method [70]. With this approach, subjects who have previously refrained from using antimicrobial products have their fingerpads contaminated with either bacteria or viruses. The fingerpads are then treated with test product and the residual microbes are enumerated. With this protocol, the residual activity of a hand sanitizer was assessed by first treating the fingerpads with the sanitizer and then challenging with a bacterial or viral inoculate 3 hours later. Enumeration demonstrated that the hand sanitizer was protective for up to 3 hours post-application [71]. Another test model assesses the transfer of microbes to surfaces by applying fingerpads to agar or to hard surfaces such as metal disks [72].

Hence, several models besides the regulatory standards are useful for research purposes. The standard protocols are helpful for determining efficacy under defined conditions. Using

Untreated   **Triclosan-based**   **Alcohol-based**

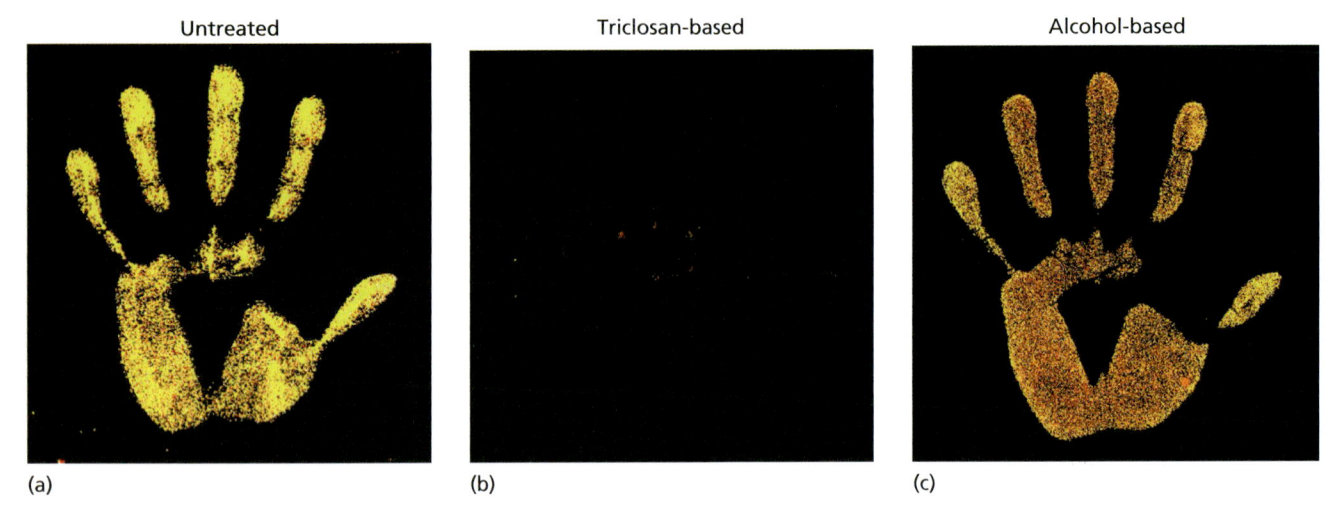

(a)   (b)   (c)

Figure 12.2 Effects of different hand sanitizer formulations on greasy soil.

large inocula allows small differences to be discerned; small changes potentially could have a public health impact. Although European and US standard protocols often yield similar conclusions regarding efficacy, this is not necessarily the case for all formulations [73,74]. A stringent assessment of the efficacy of a formulation could compare results with both testing methodologies.

In vivo models with artificial inoculate to mimic resident flora

Other models have been developed to assess the effects of antimicrobial cleansers on resident microbiota. A commonly used method is the Cade test, which measures the impact of several washes over a period of 5 days [25]. Like the ASTM E1174 test, the test begins with a washout period. This is followed by a 5-day baseline period, during which samples are collected over 2 days to control for day-to-day variations. Following the baseline assessment, subjects use the product multiple times daily over 2 days, during which hand microbiota are sampled. Efficacy is determined by comparing reductions from baseline during the treatment phase.

Clinical studies to demonstrate efficacy in reducing the burden of hand microbiota

Although prospective, randomized trials are generally considered the most rigorous approach to assess outcomes, some investigators argue that controlled clinical testing on human hands, with a well-designed protocol that simulates use conditions, is the most practical means to assess antimicrobial efficacy [68].

A few examples illustrate this approach. One study examined the ability of five, 30-second handwashes with a non-antiseptic lotion soap to remove a range of nosocomial pathogens applied to fingertips at 10^8 CFU [75]. A reduction of 10 to 15 CFU was observed after the first handwash but no further reductions occurred thereafter. Wiping hands with an antiseptic sponge (70% isopropyl alcohol or 10% povidone-iodine) removed the remaining contamination.

Another study examined the impact of three product types on existing hand microbiota using varying wash time durations in a healthcare setting [76]. Six hand hygiene interventions were implemented, in random order, immediately after patient care by 43 healthcare workers (26 nurses, nine nurse assistants, and eight physicians). The interventions were: handwashing with non-antiseptic soap for either 10 or 30 seconds; and handwashing with povidone iodine- or chlorhexidine-based soap for either 10, 30 or 60 s; and use of a commercially available alcohol-based handrub [76]. Log reductions in total bacterial counts were assessed by pressing the fingertips of the dominant hand onto agar both before and after the intervention in question. Relative efficacies (based on $\log_{10}$-transformed bacterial count reductions) were: alcohol-based handrub > antiseptic soap (60 s) > antiseptic soap (30 s) > antiseptic soap (10 s) > non-antiseptic soap (30 s) > non-antiseptic soap (10 s).

Alcohol-based hand sanitizers and soap and water washing were compared with for germicidal activity against rhinovirus [77]. Alcohol-based hand sanitizers were significantly more effective than handwashing with soap and water at reducing rhinovirus levels on artificially inoculated hands. Adding organic acids to the sanitizer formulation provided residual virucidal activity that persisted for at least 4 h.

Following the 2009 outbreak of H1N1 influenza (swine flu), the efficacy of soap and water and alcohol-based hand-rub preparations against live H1N1 influenza virus on the hands of human volunteers was evaluated [78]. Twenty vaccinated, antibody-positive healthcare workers had their hands contaminated with 1 mL of a 10^7 tissue culture infectious dose of live human influenza A virus (H1N1; A/New Caledonia/20/99). Five hand hygiene protocols were assessed: no hand hygiene (control); handwashing with soap and water; and the application of 1 of

3 alcohol-based hand rubs (61.5% ethanol gel, 70% ethanol plus 0.5% chlorhexidine solution, or 70% isopropanol plus 0.5% chlorhexidine solution). H1N1 concentrations were assessed before and after each intervention by viral culture and real-time reverse-transcriptase polymerase chain reaction (PCR). In the absence of hand hygiene, minimal reductions in H1N1 were observed after 60 minutes, whereas all four hand hygiene protocols eliminated viral contamination based on both culture results and PCR results.

Effects on the microbial burden of the hands have also been studied under real-world conditions. For example, two hand hygiene regimes (2% chlorhexidine gluconate-containing antiseptic wash and a waterless handrub containing 61% ethanol with emollients) were compared in a four-week, prospective randomized trial of among 50 full-time staff members (physicians, nurses, housekeepers, respiratory therapists) of a medical and a surgical intensive care unit at a large academic healthcare center [79]. Samples were obtained at baseline, on day 1, and at the end of 2 and 4 weeks. No significant differences in numbers of colony-forming units were observed between the two intervention groups at any time point.

In 2002, studies comparing the relative efficacy of plain soaps, antimicrobial soaps, and alcohol-based antiseptics for reducing counts of viable bacteria on hands (based on log10 reductions achieved in either existing hand microbiota or artificially contaminated hands) were summarized by the CDC [33]. In 2009, WHO published an updated review with particular reference to antisepsis in the healthcare setting. They concluded that antiseptic washes were generally more efficacious than plain soap and that alcohol-based rubs were generally more efficacious than antiseptic detergents in these settings [34]. On this basis, the use of alcohol-based hand sanitizers was recommended unless hands are visibly soiled.

A 2011 meta-analysis of 25 studies in which the efficacy of antimicrobial and non-antimicrobial handwashes were compared found that, in general, antimicrobial soap consistently produced statistically significantly greater reductions in the burden of microbiota relative to plain soap and water, provided group sizes were sufficient to detect a difference ($n > 20$). This was true regardless of the active ingredient evaluated (chlorhexidine gluconate, iodophor, triclosan, or povidone-iodine). The magnitude of the difference was small when existing hand contamination was examined (approximately 0.5-log CFU reduction difference); larger differences were observed when artificial inoculation with Gram-positive or Gram-negative bacteria was employed.

The efficacy of antimicrobial hand washes and hand sanitizers will vary depending on the antimicrobial spectrum of the active ingredients and bioavailability, the potency of the formulations employed, the specific microbial contaminants present, the type of setting (healthcare, schools, long-term care, food service), and levels of compliance with recommended practice. Product choices and hygiene regimens must be determined with these considerations in mind.

Effectiveness of antimicrobial hand washes and hand sanitizers in institutional and community settings

Impact on nosocomial infections

The causal connection between hand contamination and disease transmission has long been established [30,80], but because so many uncontrolled variables also play a role, substantiating the impact of hand hygiene practices on infection rates is challenging. A 2004 review of 1120 articles on the subject found "a lack of rigorous evidence linking specific hand hygiene interventions with the prevention of healthcare-acquired infections". Nevertheless, studies do exist that substantiate significant reductions in healthcare associated infections following hand hygiene interventions. For example, after an outbreak of methicillin-resistant *Staphylococcus aureus* (MRSA) in a neonatal intensive care unit that had persisted for 7 months, aggressive infection control measures failed to slow transmission until the hand and bath washes were changed to a preparation containing 0.3% triclosan [81]. This change halted the outbreak so effectively that at the time of publication, the unit had remained infection-free for 3½ years.

Another study compared the effectiveness of implementing two standardized hand hygiene programs in separate periods on reducing nosocomial infections among very low birth-weight infants in a neonatal intensive care unit [82]. In the first period, handwashing with plain fluid detergent was performed; in the second, a hand hygiene program employing an antimicrobial soap (4% chlorhexidine gluconate) along with alcohol-based hand rubs was instituted. The incidence of nosocomial infection after 72 hours of life fell from 18.8% on infants in the first period to 6.25% of infants in the second period. The rate of central venous catheter colonization also was significantly lower in the second period (5.8%) than in the first (16.6%).

Encouraging results have emerged in other healthcare settings. In 2005, the medical intensive care unit of a major US metropolitan hospital discontinued bathing patients daily with soap and water and substituted skin cleansing with no-rinse, 2% chlorhexidine gluconate-impregnated cloths. Daily bathing with the antimicrobial cloths resulted in a large, statistically significant decrease in the rate of central venous catheter associated bloodstream infections (from 5.31 to 0.69 cases per 1000 catheterization-days; $P = 0.006$).

The infection control benefits of alcohol-based hand sanitizers also have been substantiated. An observational survey in an inner-city, tertiary-care medical center, performed between 1998 and 2003, assessed the impact on the spread of infection with antibiotic resistant pathogens of providing wall-mounted dispensers of an alcohol-based handrub (62.5% ethyl alcohol with 0.3% triclosan) for staff hand hygiene in all inpatient and outpatient clinic rooms. [83]. All nosocomial infections with isolates of methicillin-resistant *Staphylococcus aureus* (MRSA), vancomycin-resistant *Enterococcus* (VRE), and *Clostridium difficile*-associated diarrhea were recorded occurring in the full

6-year time frame, and the handrub was made available after the first 3 years had elapsed. From the first to the second three-year period, a 21% decrease in new, nosocomially acquired MRSA (from 90 to 71 isolates per year; $P = .01$) and a 41% decrease in VRE (from 41 to 24 isolates per year; $P < .001$) were observed. The incidence of new infections with *C. difficile* was unchanged.

The use of alcohol-based handrubs is not optimal for all pathogens. Alcohol is ineffective against norovirus, *C. difficile*, and spore forming bacteria. After an outbreak of norovirus illnesses in long-term care facilities in New England, the state health departments determined that facilities in which staff were equally or more likely to use alcohol-based hand sanitizers than soap and water for routine hand hygiene had higher odds of a norovirus outbreak (adjusted odds ratio, 6.06; 95% confidence interval: 1.44–33.99) [84].

Studies have found alcohol to be relatively ineffective against Norwalk virus regardless of concentration in both suspension assays and in the ASTM standard finger pad assay [53]. Antiseptic handrubs containing 10% povidone-iodine (equivalent to 1% available iodine) were more efficacious against feline calicivirus (a surrogate for norovirus) than either alcohol-based products or triclosan-containing antimicrobial soaps, and sanitizers containing 99.5% ethanol are more virucidal against this microbe than formulations containing 62% ethanol, 70% isopropanol or 91% isopropanol [54]. An investigative, modified ethanol-based hand sanitizer (supplemented with a synergistic blend of polyquaternium polymer and an organic acid known to be active against non-enveloped enteric viruses) was significantly more efficacious in *in vitro* assays against human norovirus, human rotovirus, and poliovirus than a benchmark hand sanitizer product [85].

In summary, clinical evidence exists that hand hygiene regimens employing antimicrobial washes and hand sanitizers can substantially reduce healthcare acquired infections. However, the clinical experience also illustrates the ongoing challenge of optimizing hand hygiene regimens for various pathogens and institutional settings.

Effectiveness of hand hygiene in the community setting

Community-based clinical trials of hand hygiene regimes are complex and expensive to execute, and such interventions have been limited in scope. A 2008 meta-analysis of 30 community studies performed between 1960 and 2007 concluded that improvements in hand hygiene resulted in average reductions in gastrointestinal illness of 31% (95% confidence intervals [CI] = 19%, 42%) and average reductions in respiratory illness of 21% (95% CI = 5%, 34%). The review concluded that the most beneficial intervention for reducing such illnesses was hand-hygiene education coupled with use of non-antibacterial soap; it failed to find evidence of an added benefit with antibacterial handwashes [86].

Since then, prospective trials have documented the infection control benefits of alcohol-based hand sanitizers in the school setting. An 8-week prospective, randomized, controlled trial among third to fifth grade students at a single elementary school evaluated the use of an alcohol-based hand sanitizer for hand hygiene together with quaternary ammonium wipes for daily classroom surface disinfection, while control classrooms followed usual hand-washing and cleaning practices [87]. The adjusted absenteeism rate for gastrointestinal illness was significantly lower in the intervention group, but no difference was observed in the adjusted absenteeism rate for respiratory illness. In this study, norovirus was the only virus detected and was found less frequently on surfaces in intervention classrooms compared with control classrooms (9% vs. 29%).

A similar outcome was observed in a more extensive study conducted in two primary schools over a 17-week period that began before and lasted throughout the time frame of seasonal gastroenteritis [52]. The intervention consisted of consistent, teacher-monitored hand hygiene with an alcohol-based sanitizer in one of the two schools. The average number of gastroenteritis episodes was 0.31 in the intervention group and 0.53 in the control group ($P < 0.001$).

Hand hygiene in the home has been shown to be important in limiting community acquired MRSA. A study of risk factors for household transmission of community-associated MRSA found that household contacts of infected children who helped bathe the child or who shared skin balms or ointments with the child were more likely to be colonized, whereas household contacts who reported using antibacterial versus non-antibacterial soap for handwashing were less likely to be colonized with an isolate clonally related to the infection isolate from the child [88].

The above examples provide evidence that community use of antibacterial hand sanitizers and handwashes has infection control benefits. As noted earlier, in late 2013, the FDA issued a proposed rule that would to require manufacturers of antimicrobial hand or body washes to demonstrate that the products are more effective than plain soap and water in preventing illness and the spread of infection [89]. Given the challenges and prohibitive expense of conducting such studies routinely, the feasibility of this proposal has yet to be determined. A consumer product industry-sponsored expert panel has proposed the alternative of a surrogate infection model; it employs a modified but realistic hand contamination procedure with *Shigella flexneri* as a test organism to assess the efficacy of consumer antibacterial handwash products but this method needs further assessment [90]. The process of commenting on the proposed rule, generation of new data by interested parties, review and comment, and eventual publication of a final monograph is expected to take 2–3 years.

Handwash and hand sanitizer safety

Irritation associated with handwashes and hand sanitizers

Historically, skin irritation secondary to handwashing has been observed in up to 25% of healthcare workers [91]. The irritation is attributed to repeated contact with detergents, exacerbated by occlusion from wearing gloves [92]. Repeated handwashing with soap and water removes the protective lipid layer, compromising skin integrity and leading to redness, scaling and dermatitis. Allergic contact dermatitis to product constituents is a theoretical risk but reports of such reactions are rare [93]. Skin damage also alters the skin microbiota of healthcare workers: relative to healthy hands, damaged hands presented higher frequencies of *Staphylococcus aureus* (16.7% vs. 10%); Gram-negative bacteria (20% versus 6.7%); and yeast (26.7% vs. 20%, respectively) [94]. Moreover, when hands are damaged, handwashing becomes less effective in reducing microbial contamination [95]. Prospective multicenter studies conducted through the winter and summer seasons revealed that disinfection with an alcohol-based hand sanitizer is better tolerated than classic handwashing with mild soap and water [96], and its use improves compliance with hand hygiene guidelines in healthcare settings [92,97].

Recently, toxicological investigations of possible endocrine disruptor activity of triclosan have been performed in cell culture and in laboratory animals and reported in the literature [98–102].

Safety concerns specific to alcohol-based hand sanitizers

Several safety issues specific to alcohol-based products should be considered. In the occupational setting, precaution must be taken against excessive contact with alcohol, which could dilapidate the skin. In institutional settings, the flammability of these alcohol-based formulations should be considered so that dispensers are not located where the potential for ignition exists. In community settings, there have been reports of intentional ingestion by people with alcoholism [103] and accidental intoxication in children [104]. As previously discussed, conventional alcohol-based hand sanitizers have limited efficacy against norovirus or *C. difficile* and are not a substitute for handwashing in food service settings.

Development of microbial resistance to antimicrobial agents

A major question within the scientific community is whether widespread use of antimicrobial hand hygiene products, particularly by consumers, may lead to the development of resistance to the antimicrobial ingredients [38]. Most investigations of this question have focused on triclosan, which has been utilized as an antibacterial agent in consumer products for 30 years. Chronic, sub-lethal exposure of laboratory strains of *E. coli* to triclosan produced some clones with reduced susceptibility, but these were nevertheless inhibited by triclosan concentrations relevant to consumer use [105]. A comparative analysis of 256 clinical isolates of *P. aeruginosa* and *S. aureus* over a 10-year period found no difference in triclosan sensitivity between antibiotic sensitive and resistant strains [106]. A similar conclusion was drawn when comparing clinical isolates of methicillin-resistant or sensitive strains of *S. aureus* [107]. Furthermore,

continuous exposure of a triclosan-sensitive *S. aureus* strain to sub-inhibitory triclosan concentrations for one month did not decrease susceptibility either to triclosan or to other antibiotics. In addition, exposing mixed microbial communities derived from natural environments to triclosan for 6 months resulted in no change in sensitivity to triclosan or to antibiotics [108].

Investigations of this question have moved beyond the laboratory to community settings. A 2003 study, performed in three geographical areas in USA and UK, evaluated antibiotic and antibacterial cross-agent resistance in environmental and clinical samples from the homes of antibacterial product users ($n = 30$) and non-users ($n = 30$) [109]. Selected antibiotic-resistant and antibiotic-susceptible isolates were tested against four common antibacterial agents (triclosan, para-chloro-meta-xylenol, pine oil and quaternary ammonium compounds). No evidence of antibiotic and antibacterial agent cross-resistance was observed from homes of antibacterial product users and non-users. There was a higher increased prevalence of potential pathogens in non-user homes.

In 2005, a 12-month study of 224 households evaluated the impact of household use of antibacterial products and carriage of antimicrobial resistant bacteria on the hands [110]. Antibacterial product use did not lead to a significant increase in antimicrobial drug resistance after 1 year, nor did it have an effect on bacterial susceptibility to triclosan.

A 2011 study investigated antimicrobial and antibiotic susceptibilities of staphylococcal skin isolates from community users of antibacterial wash products compared to isolates from non-users [111]. The study compared three groups of 70 users: those that frequently used wash products containing triclosan; those that frequently used products containing triclocarban; and a control group that used no antibacterial wash products. The study found no evidence that the use of antibacterial wash products facilitated antibiotic resistance and antibiotic/antibacterial cross-resistance. No statistically significant difference in antibiotic resistance in Staphylococcus isolates was found between regular antibacterial wash product users and non-users. None of the isolates were resistant to vancomycin, and the rate of methicillin resistant *S. aureus* (MRSA) detected was appreciably less than that reported in the literature. The study found a definitive lack of antibiotic/antibacterial cross-resistance.

In summary, laboratory and epidemiologic research provides no evidence that use of triclosan in consumer products contributes to the societal burden of antibiotic resistance or decreases susceptibility to antimicrobials agents employed in hygienic antiseptic products.

Long-term effects on the skin microbiota

With the advent of the human microbiome project, there is growing interest in understanding the mutuality between human physiology and the microbiota that inhabit the human body. Although these complex relationships are still the subject of active research, regulatory bodies are considering requiring long-term safety studies in an effort to understand the impact of antimicrobial agents on the skin microbiome.

Future directions

Future epidemiological studies may better dimension the role of hand hygiene products and regimens in preventing infections in hospitals and long-term care institutions, as well as in the school, the workplace and the home. Developing improved products with a broad spectrum of activity and improved skin compatibility could be beneficial. Educational efforts on the best hand hygiene practices for health and safety can be developed for different audiences and settings using the variety of modern media channels that are now available. Ongoing research to extend our understanding of the skin microbiome and the broader implications of hand hygiene practices on the microbial ecology of the skin are needed.

References

1. Pinner RW, Teutsch S M, Simonsen L, et al. (1996) Trends in infectious diseases mortality in the United States. *Jama* **275**, 189–93.
2. Centers for Disease Control and Prevention Estimates of Foodborne Illness in the United States. (2011) www.cdc.gov/foodborneburden/2011-foodborne-estimates.html Accessed 28 May 2015.
3. Centers for Disease Control and Prevention Norovirus. Trends and outbreaks. (2013) www.cdc.gov/norovirus/trends-outbreaks.html Accessed 28 May 2015.
4. Centers for Disease Control and Prevention. Rotavirus. (2013) www.cdc.gov/rotavirus/index.html Accessed 28 May 2015.
5. Abbott A, Pearson H. (2004) Fear of human pandemic grows as bird flu sweeps through Asia. *Nature* **427**, 472–3.
6. Zimmer SM, Burke DS. (2009) Historical perspective – Emergence of influenza A (H1N1) viruses. *N Engl J Med* **361**, 279–85.
7. Klevens RM, Edwards JR, Richards CL, Jr., et al. (2007) Estimating healthcare-associated infections and deaths in U.S. hospitals, 2002. *Public Health Rep* **122**, 160–6.
8. Baker GR, Norton PG, Flintoft V, et al. (2004) The Canadian Adverse Events Study: the incidence of adverse events among hospital patients in Canada. *Cmaj* **170**, 1678–86.
9. Sengstock DM, Thyagarajan R, Apalara J, et al. (2010) Multidrug-resistant Acinetobacter baumannii, an emerging pathogen among older adults in community hospitals and nursing homes. *Clin Infect Dis* **50**, 1611–6.
10. Grice EA, Segre JA. (2011) The skin microbiome. *Nat Rev Microbiol* **9**, 244–53.
11. Grice EA, Kong HH, Renaud G, et al. (2008) A diversity profile of the human skin microbiota. *Genome Res* **18**, 1043–50.
12. Costello EK, Lauber CL, Hamady M, et al. (2009) Bacterial community variation in human body habitats across space and time. *Science* **326**, 1694–7.
13. Fierer N, Hamady M, Lauber CL, et al. (2008) The influence of sex, handedness, and washing on the diversity of hand surface bacteria. *Proc Natl Acad Sci USA* **105**, 17994–9.
14. Song SJ, Lauber C, Costello EK, et al. (2013) Cohabiting family members share microbiota with one another and with their dogs. *Elife* **2**, e00458.
15. Dunn RR, Fierer N, Henley JB, et al. (2013) Home life, factors structuring the bacterial diversity found within and between homes. *PLoS One* **8**, e64133.
16. Gwaltney JM, Jr., Moskalski PB, Hendley JO. (1978) Hand-to-hand transmission of rhinovirus colds. *Ann Intern Med* **88**, 463–7.
17. Hendley JO, Wenzel RP, Gwaltney JM, Jr. (1973) Transmission of rhinovirus colds by self-inoculation. *N Engl J Med* **288**, 1361–4.
18. Aiello AE, Cimiotti J, Della-Latta P, et al. (2003) A comparison of the bacteria found on the hands of 'homemakers' and neonatal intensive care unit nurses. *J Hosp Infect* **54**, 310–5.
19. McBride ME, Montes LF, Fahlberg WJ, et al. (1972) Microbial flora of nurses' hands. I. Quantitative differences in bacterial population between nurses and other occupational groups. *Int J Dermatol* **11**, 49–53.
20. McBride ME, Montes LF, Fahlberg WJ, et al. (1974) Microbial flora of nurses' hands. II. Qualitative differences in occupational groups. *Int J Dermatol* **13**, 197–204.
21. McBride ME, Montes LF, Fahlberg WJ, et al. (1975) Microbial flora of nurses' hands. III. The relationship between staphylococcal skin populations and persistence of carriage. *Int J Dermatol* **14**, 129–35.
22. Pancholi P, Healy M, Bittner T, et al. (2005) Molecular characterization of hand flora and environmental isolates in a community setting. *J Clin Microbiol* **43**, 5202–7.
23. Cogen AL, Nizet V, Gallo RL. (2008) Skin microbiota, a source of disease or defence? *Br J Dermatol* **158**, 442–55.
24. Christensen GJ, Bruggemann H. (2013) Bacterial skin commensals and their role as host guardians. *Benef Microbes* 1–15.
25. Uckay I, Pittet D, Vaudaux P, et al. (2009) Foreign body infections due to Staphylococcus epidermidis. *Ann Med* **41**, 109–19.
26. Hanifin JM, Rogge JL. (1977) Staphylococcal infections in patients with atopic dermatitis. *Arch Dermatol* **113**, 1383–6.
27. Park HY, Kim CR, Huh IS, et al. (2013) *Staphylococcus aureus* colonization in acute and chronic skin lesions of patients with atopic dermatitis. *Ann Dermatol* **25**, 410–6.
28. Bourrain M, Ribet V, Calvez A, et al. (2013) Balance between beneficial microflora and Staphylococcus aureus colonisation, *in vivo* evaluation in patients with atopic dermatitis during hydrotherapy. *Eur J Dermatol* **23**, 786–94.
29. Kong HH, Oh J, Deming C, et al. (2012) Temporal shifts in the skin microbiome associated with disease flares and treatment in children with atopic dermatitis. *Genome Res* **22**, 850–9.
30. Best M, Neuhauser D. (2004) Ignaz Semmelweis and the birth of infection control. *Qual Saf Healthcare* **13**, 233–4.
31. Hendley JO, Gwaltney JM, Jr. (1988) Mechanisms of transmission of rhinovirus infections. *Epidemiol Rev* **10**, 243–58.
32. Larson EL. (1995) APIC guideline for handwashing and hand antisepsis in healthcare settings. *Am J Infect Control* **23**, 251–69.
33. Centers for Disease Control and Prevention. (2002) Guideline for Hand Hygiene in Healthcare Settings: Recommendations of the Healthcare Infection Control Practices Advisory Committee and the HICPAC/SHEA/APIC/IDSA Hand Hygiene Task Force. *MMWR* **51** (No. RR-16). www.cdc.gov/handhygiene/Guidelines.html Accessed 28 May 2015.
34. WHO Guidelines on Hand Hygiene in Healthcare. (2009) First Global Patient Safety Challenge Clean Care Is Safer Care. Geneva: World Health Organization.
35. World Health Organization. (2014) *Clean Care is Safer Care. Five moments for hand hygiene.* Tools for 5 Moments. How to

handrub:how to handwash. www.who.int/gpsc/tools/Five_moments/en/ Accessed 28 May 2015.
36 U.S. Food and Drug Administration. (2013) *Food Code 2013.* www.fda.gov/Food/GuidanceRegulation/RetailFoodProtection/FoodCode/ucm374275.htm Accessed 28 May 2015.
37 Charbonneau DL, Ponte JM, Kochanowski BA. (2000) A method of assessing the efficacy of hand sanitizers, use of real soil encountered in the food service industry. *J Food Prot* **63**, 495–501.
38 Centers for Disease Control. (2012) *Hand Hygiene in Healthcare Settings.* Hand Hygiene Basics, 2012. www.cdc.gov/handhygiene/Basics.html Accessed 28 May 2015.
39 Centers for Disease Control and Prevention. (2013) *Handwashing, Clean Hands Save Lives. When and How to Wash Your Hands.* www.cdc.gov/handwashing/when-how-handwashing.html Accessed 28 May 2015.
40 Sahay S, Panja S, Ray S, et al. (2010) Diurnal variation in hand hygiene compliance in a tertiary level multidisciplinary intensive care unit. *Am J Infect Control* 2010; **38**, 535–9.
41 van der Vegt DS, Voss A. (2008) *Hand hygiene after toilet visits.* 18th European Congress of Clinical Microbiology and Infectious Disease [Abstract P1103].
42 Green LR, Selman CA, Radke V, et al. (2006) Food worker handwashing practices: an observation study. *J Food Prot* **69**, 2417–23.
43 Johnson HD, Sholcosky D, Gabello K, et al. (2003) Sex differences in public restroom handwashing behavior associated with visual behavior prompts. *Percept Mot Skills* **97**, 805–10.
44 Anderson JL, Warren CA, Perez E, et al. (2008) Gender and ethnic differences in hand hygiene practices among college students. *Am J Infect Control* **36**, 361–8.
45 Garbutt C, Simmons G, Patrick D, et al. (2007) The public hand hygiene practices of New Zealanders: a national survey. *NZ Med J* **120**, U2810.
46 Quraishi ZA, McGuckin M, Blais FX. (1984) Duration of handwashing in intensive care units: a descriptive study. *Am J Infect Control* **12**, 83–7.
47 Larson EL, Gomez-Duarte C, Lee LV, et al. (2003) Microbial flora of hands of homemakers. *Am J Infect Control* **31**, 72–9.
48 Duggan JM, Hensley S, Khuder S, et al. (2008) Inverse correlation between level of professional education and rate of handwashing compliance in a teaching hospital. *Infect Control Hosp Epidemiol* **29**, 534–8.
49 Burusnukul P, Broz CC. (2013) Drivers and motivators in consumer handwashing behavior. *Nutr Food Sci* **43**, 596–604.
50 Guinan M, McGuckin M, Ali Y. (2002) The effect of a comprehensive handwashing program on absenteeism in elementary schools. *Am J Infect Control* **30**, 217–20.
51 Azor-Martinez E, Cobos-Carrascosa E, Gimenez-Sanchez F, et al. (2014) Effectiveness of a multifactorial handwashing program to reduce school absenteeism due to acute gastroenteritis. *Pediatr Infect Dis J* **33**, e34–9.
52 Prazuck T, Compte-Nguyen G, Pelat C, et al. (2010) Reducing gastroenteritis occurrences and their consequences in elementary schools with alcohol-based hand sanitizers. *Pediatr Infect Dis J* **29**, 994–8.
53 Liu P, Yuen Y, Hsiao HM, et al. (2010) Effectiveness of liquid soap and hand sanitizer against Norwalk virus on contaminated hands. *Appl Environ Microbiol* **76**, 394–9.
54 Lages SL, Ramakrishnan MA, Goyal SM. (2008) In-vivo efficacy of hand sanitisers against feline calicivirus: a surrogate for norovirus. *J Hosp Infect* 2008; **68**, 159–63.
55 Edmonds SL, McCormack RR, Zhou SS, et al. (2012) Hand hygiene regimens for the reduction of risk in food service environments. *J Food Prot* **75**, 1303–9.
56 Food and Drug Administration. (1994) Tentative final monograph for healthcare antiseptic drug products; proposed rule. *Federal Register* **59**, 31441–52. www.federalregister.gov/articles/1994/06/17/94–14503/topical-antimicrobial-drug-products-for-over-the-counter-human-use-tentative-final-monograph.
57 Russell AD. (1991) Chemical sporicidal and sporostatic agents. In: BlockSS, ed. *Chemical Sporicidal and Sporostatic Agents*, 4th edn. Philadelphia, PA: Lea & Febiger, **1991**, 365–76.
58 European Committee for Standardization. (1997) *Chemical disinfectants and antiseptics – hygienic handrub – test method and requirements* (phase2/step2) [European standard EN 1500]. Brussels, Belgium, Central Secretariat.
59 Gaonkar TA, Geraldo I, Caraos L, et al. (2005) An alcohol hand rub containing a synergistic combination of an emollient and preservatives, prolonged activity against transient pathogens. *J Hosp Infect* **59**, 12–8.
60 Shintre MS, Gaonkar TA, Modak SM. (2007) Evaluation of an alcohol-based surgical hand disinfectant containing a synergistic combination of farnesol and benzethonium chloride for immediate and persistent activity against resident hand flora of volunteers and with a novel *in vitro* pig skin model. *Infect Control Hosp Epidemiol* **28**, 191–7.
61 Kampf G, Ostermeyer C. (2011) World Health Organization-recommended hand-rub formulations do not meet European efficacy requirements for surgical hand disinfection in five minutes. *J Hosp Infect* **78**, 123–7.
62 Suchomel M, Kundi M, Pittet D, et al. (2013) Modified World Health Organization hand rub formulations comply with European efficacy requirements for preoperative surgical hand preparations. *Infect Control Hosp Epidemiol* **34**, 245–50.
63 Suchomel M, Kundi M, Pittet D, et al. (2012) Testing of the World Health Organization recommended formulations in their application as hygienic hand rubs and proposals for increased efficacy. *Am J Infect Control* **40**, 328–31.
64 Fuls JL, Fischer G. (2004) Antimicrobial efficacy of activated triclosan in surfactant-based formulation versus *Pseudomonas putida*. *Am J Infect Control* **32**, E22.
65 Gunathilake HM, Sirimanna GM, Schurer NY. (2007) The pH of commercially available rinse-off products in Sri Lanka and their effect on skin pH. *Ceylon Med J* **52**, 125–9.
66 Food and Drug Administration. (2013) Safety and effectiveness of consumer antiseptics: Topical antimicrobial drug products for over-the-counter human use; proposed amedment of the Tentative Final Monograph; reopening of adminstrative record. *Fedral Register* **78**, 76444–78.
67 Rotter ML. (2004) European norms in hand hygiene. *J Hosp Infect* **56** Suppl 2, S6–9.
68 Rotter M, Sattar S, Dharan S, et al. (2009) Methods to evaluate the microbicidal activities of hand-rub and hand-wash agents. *J Hosp Infect* **73**, 191–9.

69 Hansen TB, Knochel S. (2003) Image analysis method for evaluation of specific and non-specific hand contamination. *J Appl Microbiol* **94**, 483–94.

70 Sattar SA, Ansari SA. (2002) The fingerpad protocol to assess hygienic hand antiseptics against viruses. *J Virol Methods* **103**, 171–81.

71 Zukowski C, Boyer A, Andrews S, et al. (2007) *Immediate and persistent antibacterial and antiviral efficacy of a novel hand sanitizer.* Presented at: 47th Interscience Conference on Antimicrobial Agents and Chemotherapy; Chicago, IL, September 17–20, 2007.

72 Mbithi JN, Springthorpe VS, Boulet JR, et al. (1992) Survival of hepatitis A virus on human hands and its transfer on contact with animate and inanimate surfaces. *J Clin Microbiol* **30**, 757–63.

73 Kampf G, Ostermeyer C, Heeg P, et al. (2006) Evaluation of two methods of determining the efficacies of two alcohol-based hand rubs for surgical hand antisepsis. *Appl Environ Microbiol* **72**, 3856–61.

74 Heeg P, Ostermeyer C, Kampf G. (2008) Comparative review of the test design Tentative Final Monograph (TFM) and EN 12791 for surgical hand disinfectants. *J Hosp Infect* **70** Suppl 1, 22–6.

75 Bottone EJ, Cheng M, Hymes S. (2004) Ineffectiveness of handwashing with lotion soap to remove nosocomial bacterial pathogens persisting on fingertips, a major link in their intrahospital spread. *Infect Control Hosp Epidemiol* **25**, 262–4.

76 Lucet JC, Rigaud MP, Mentre F, et al. (2002) Hand contamination before and after different hand hygiene techniques: a randomized clinical trial. *J Hosp Infect* **50**, 276–80.

77 Turner RB, Fuls JL, Rodgers ND. (2010) Effectiveness of hand sanitizers with and without organic acids for removal of rhinovirus from hands. *Antimicrob Agents Chemother* **54**, 1363–4.

78 Grayson ML, Melvani S, Druce J, et al. (2009) Efficacy of soap and water and alcohol-based hand-rub preparations against live H1N1 influenza virus on the hands of human volunteers. *Clin Infect Dis* **48**, 285–91.

79 Larson EL, Aiello AE, Bastyr J, et al. (2001) Assessment of two hand hygiene regimens for intensive care unit personnel. *Crit Care Med* **29**, 944–51.

80 Larson E. (1988) A causal link between handwashing and risk of infection? Examination of the evidence. *Infect Control Hosp Epidemiol* **9**, 28–36.

81 Zafar AB, Butler RC, Reese DJ, et al. (1995) Use of 0.3% triclosan (Bacti-Stat) to eradicate an outbreak of methicillin-resistant *Staphylococcus aureus* in a neonatal nursery. *Am J Infect Control* **23**, 200–8.

82 Capretti MG, Sandri F, Tridapalli E, et al. (2008) Impact of a standardized hand hygiene program on the incidence of nosocomial infection in very low birth weight infants. *Am J Infect Control* **36**, 430–5.

83 Gordin FM, Schultz ME, Huber RA, et al. (2005) Reduction in nosocomial transmission of drug-resistant bacteria after introduction of an alcohol-based handrub. *Infect Control Hosp Epidemiol* **26**, 650–3.

84 Blaney DD, Daly ER, Kirkland KB, et al. (2011) Use of alcohol-based hand sanitizers as a risk factor for norovirus outbreaks in long-term care facilities in northern New England, December 2006 to March 2007. *Am J Infect Control* **39**, 296–301.

85 Macinga DR, Sattar SA, Jaykus LA, et al. (2008) Improved inactivation of nonenveloped enteric viruses and their surrogates by a novel alcohol-based hand sanitizer. *Appl Environ Microbiol* **24**, 5047–52.

86 Aiello AE, Coulborn RM, Perez V, et al. (2008) Effect of hand hygiene on infectious disease risk in the community setting: a meta-analysis. *Am J Public Health* **98**, 1372–81.

87 Thomas JA, Sandora TJ, Shih MC, et al. (2009) Reducing absenteeism from gastrointestinal and respiratory illness in elementary school students: A randomized, controlled trial of an infection-control intervention. *Pediatrics* **121**, 1555–62.

88 Nerby JM, Gorwitz R, Lesher L, et al. (2011) Risk factors for household transmission of community-associated methicillin-resistant *Staphylococcus aureus*. *Pediatr Infect Dis J* **30**, 927–32.

89 Kuehn BM. (2014) FDA pushes makers of antimicrobial soap to prove safety and effectiveness. *Jama* **311**, 234.

90 Boyce JM, Dupont HL, Massaro J, et al. (2012) An expert panel report of a proposed scientific model demonstrating the effectiveness of antibacterial handwash products. *Am J Infect Control* **40**, 742–9.

91 Larson E, Friedman C, Cohran J, et al. (1997) Prevalence and correlates of skin damage on the hands of nurses. *Heart Lung* **26**, 404–12.

92 Kampf G, Loffler H. (2010) Hand disinfection in hospitals – benefits and risks. *J Dtsch Dermatol Ges* **8**, 978–83.

93 Berthelot C, Zirwas MJ. (2006) Allergic contact dermatitis to chloroxylenol. *Dermatitis* **17**, 156–9.

94 Rocha LA, Ferreira de Almeida EBL, Gontijo Filho PP. (2009) Changes in hands microbiota associated with skin damage because of hand hygiene procedures on the healthcare workers. *Am J Infect Control* **37**, 155–9.

95 de Almeida e Borges LF, Silva BL, Gontijo Filho PP. (2007) Handwashing: changes in the skin flora. *Am J Infect Control* **35**, 417–20.

96 Chamorey E, Marcy PY, Dandine M, et al. (2011) A prospective multicenter study evaluating skin tolerance to standard hand hygiene techniques. *Am J Infect Control* **39**, 6–13.

97 Kampf G, Loffler H, Gastmeier P. (2009) Hand hygiene for the prevention of nosocomial infections. *Dtsch Arztebl Int* **106**, 649–55.

98 Kumar V, Balomajumder C, Roy P. (2008) Disruption of LH-induced testosterone biosynthesis in testicular Leydig cells by triclosan, probable mechanism of action. *Toxicology* **250**, 124–31.

99 Kumar V, Chakraborty A, Kural MR, et al. (2009) Alteration of testicular steroidogenesis and histopathology of reproductive system in male rats treated with triclosan. *Reprod Toxicol* **27**, 177–85.

100 Gee RH, Charles A, Taylor N, et al. (2008) Oestrogenic and androgenic activity of triclosan in breast cancer cells. *J Appl Toxicol* **28**, 78–91.

101 Stoker TE, Gibson EK, Zorrilla LM. (2010) Triclosan exposure modulates estrogen-dependent responses in the female wistar rat. *Toxicol Sci* **117**, 45–53.

102 Zorrilla LM, Gibson EK, Jeffay SC, et al. (2009) The effects of triclosan on puberty and thyroid hormones in male Wistar rats. *Toxicol Sci* **107**, 56–64.

103 Emadi A, Coberly L. (2007) Intoxication of a hospitalized patient with an isopropanol-based hand sanitizer. *N Engl J Med* **356**, 530–1.

104 Anon. (2012) Alcohol-based hand sanitizers, severe intoxication in children. *Prescrire Int* **21**, 184.
105 Levy CW, Roujeinikova A, Sedelnikova S, *et al.* (1999) Molecular basis of triclosan activity. *Nature* 398, 383–4.
106 Lambert RJ. (2004) Comparative analysis of antibiotic and antimicrobial biocide susceptibility data in clinical isolates of methicillin-sensitive *Staphylococcus aureus*, methicillin-resistant *Staphylococcus aureus* and *Pseudomonas aeruginosa* between 1989 and 2000. *J Appl Microbiol* **97**, 699–711.
107 Suller MT, Russell AD. (2000) Triclosan and antibiotic resistance in *Staphylococcus aureus*. *J Antimicrob Chemother* **46**, 11–8.
108 McBain AJ, Bartolo RG, Catrenich CE, *et al.* (2003) Exposure of sink drain microcosms to triclosan, population dynamics and antimicrobial susceptibility. *Appl Environ Microbiol* **69**, 5433–42.
109 Cole EC, Addison RM, Rubino JR, *et al.* (2003) Investigation of antibiotic and antibacterial agent cross-resistance in target bacteria from homes of antibacterial product users and nonusers. *J Appl Microbiol* **95**, 664–76.
110 Aiello AE, Marshall B, Levy SB, *et al.* (2005) Antibacterial cleaning products and drug resistance. *Emerg Infect Dis* **11**, 1565–70.
111 Cole EC, Addison RM, Dulaney PD, *et al.* (2011) Investigation of antibiotic and antibacterial susceptibility and resistance in staphylococcus from the skin of users and non-users of antibacterial wash products in home environments. *Internat J Microbiol Res* **3**, 90–96.

CHAPTER 13
Shampoos for Normal Scalp Hygiene and Dandruff

James R. Schwartz,[1] Eric S. Johnson,[1] and Thomas L. Dawson, Jr.[2]
[1]Procter & Gamble Beauty Science, Cincinnati, OH, USA
[2]Agency for Science, Technology and Research (A*STAR), Institute for Medical Biology, Singapore

BASIC CONCEPTS
- Frequent scalp cleansing is important to prevent formation of unhealthy scalp.
- Three classes of shampoos can be delineated: (1) cosmetic shampoos and two types of therapeutic products; (2) standard and (3) cosmetically optimized therapeutics.
- Both therapeutic scalp care shampoos are effective for normal scalp to prevent unhealthy conditions and for dandruff/seborrheic dermatitis scalp to treat the condition and subsequently prevent its reoccurrence.
- All therapeutic shampoos are not equally efficacious, even though they may contain the same active.
- Cosmetically optimized therapeutic shampoos are desirable as they increase compliance long-term, due to having no aesthetic trade-offs and their affordability.
- All shampoos, including cosmetics, must be mild to the skin while being effective cleansers to minimize irritation that could initiate scalp problems.

Definition

Effective scalp care includes both treatment of conditions such as dandruff and seborrheic dermatitis as well as prevention of these conditions among susceptible individuals. This chapter covers product choice, explanation of benefits and mechanism and how best to maximize benefits via patient compliance and usage regimens.

Introduction

The scalp is a unique environment of the skin combining a high level of sebaceous lipid production with a physical covering of hair. The hair beneficially physically protects the scalp from UV light, increases the skin surface temperature and traps moisture vapor; but it can also detrimentally inhibit the cleansing efficiency of the scalp surface by shampoos. These conditions favor the colonization of *Malassezia* yeasts. Such colonization is normal as these are commensal scalp species and essentially everybody is culture-positive for such organisms. Under certain conditions, theses yeasts can become pathogenic, initiating skin reactions including inflammation and hyper-proliferation [1] leading to symptoms [2] of itch and flakes (see Figure 13.1), respectively. The mechanism by which *Malassezia* yeasts exert their pathogenicity, while likely not completely understood, is at least partially delineated. Lipases are secreted by the yeast into the surrounding medium to liberate fatty acids from the triglycerides of the sebaceous lipids that are constantly and copiously produced in the hair follicles and excreted onto the scalp surface. *Malassezia* selectively consume long chain saturated fatty acids to live, the unsaturated fatty acids left behind can then diffuse into the upper layers of the skin and be the initiators of inflammation. Cutaneous inflammation leads to hyper-proliferation in the epidermis resulting in immature stratum corneum cells with incompletely degraded adhesive function resulting in removal as macroscopic visible clumps/flakes.

The resultant condition is called either dandruff or seborrheic dermatitis (D/SD), depending on the severity of flaking and the presence of outward manifestations of inflammation (such as redness). The occurrence of the scalp condition places special requirements on effective scalp care and cleansing; in general, the lower the frequency of scalp cleansing, the greater the chances that scalp conditions such as D/SD will occur [3]. Since the sebaceous lipids are one of the key factors required for formation of D/SD, infrequent removal leads to the build-up of the pro-inflammatory by-products of *Malassezia* metabolism.

Cosmetic Dermatology: Products and Procedures, Second Edition. Edited by Zoe Diana Draelos.
© 2016 John Wiley & Sons, Ltd. Published 2016 by John Wiley & Sons, Ltd.

Normal Scalp	Dandruff	Seborrheic Dermatitis
A	B Loosely adherent white or gray flakes often occurring in patches.	C Larger, yellow greasy scales with underlying erythema.

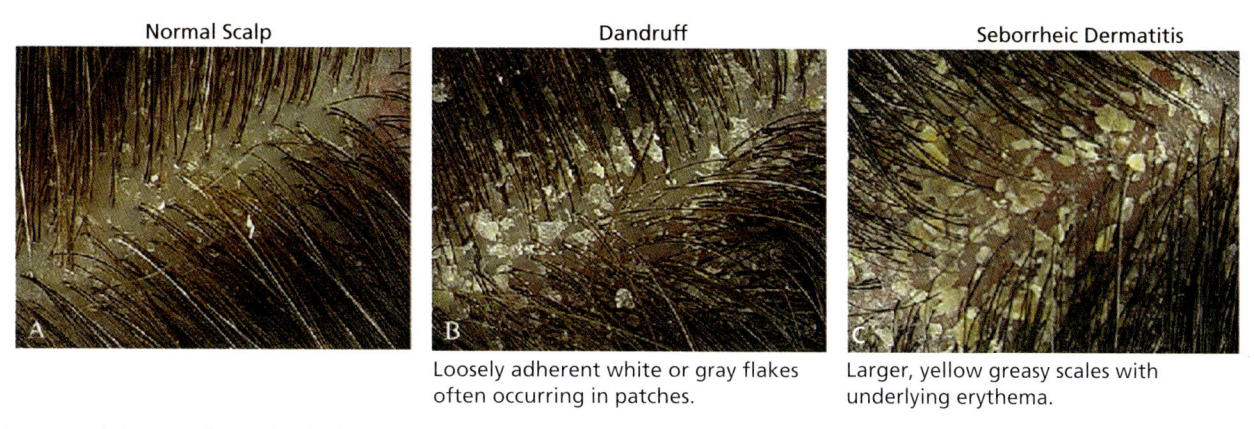

Figure 13.1 (A) Image of normal scalp skin. (B) Dandruff scalp image showing adherent white flakes. (C) Seborrheic dermatitis with more evidence of sebum yellowing on flakes and underlying erythema.

Product and formulation technology overview

Three categories of shampoos can be delineated (Figure 13.2). Cosmetic shampoos are primarily designed to cleanse the hair, but of course the scalp skin is cleansed simultaneously. Modern versions of these shampoos also condition the hair by depositing certain ingredients on the hair to improve cosmetic benefits such as ease of combing, shine maintenance and other attributes important to *all* consumers. Therapeutic scalp care shampoos (often termed "anti-dandruff") contain active ingredients to control the D/SD conditions, most often by reducing the *Malassezia* population on the scalp. Classical therapeutic products tend to focus on the drug active without full consideration of product in-use aesthetics. Cosmetically optimized therapeutic products also contain a drug active to achieve therapeutic benefits, but without the common aesthetic trade-offs (odor, hair conditioning) of therapeutic products. Cosmetically optimized therapeutic shampoos do not necessarily compromise on the magnitude of the therapeutic benefit. Recommendations involving the best products to use must take into consideration patient's needs for a pleasant use experience and delivery of cosmetic hair benefits. This is because compromises on these attributes significantly reduce patient compliance. No matter how therapeutically effective a product is, benefits will be minimized if usage frequency is compromised. This is a critically important situation in the case of D/SD since the condition is chronic and prophylaxis is the most effective long-term strategy.

The primary component (see Table 13.1) of all shampoos is the surfactant system which helps to remove sebaceous lipids, keratin debris, particulates from the environment, and residues from styling products. The surfactants are responsible for the lathering action of a product, the volume and quality of lather are perceived as important signals of cleansing action. Most of the surfactants tend to be negatively charged (anionic), though some contain both positive and negative charges in the same molecule (amphoteric) and others are uncharged (non-ionic); these latter types are considered co-surfactants and function to optimize the lather quality and amount and cleaning ability of the primary anionic surfactant.

The surfactant system is optimized to achieve two opposing objectives – cleaning effectively while minimizing irritation of the skin. All surfactants have the potential to irritate the skin to various degrees. The goal of the formulator is to achieve effective cleaning and lathering while minimizing the irritation potential of the product by using the right surfactants. The addition of co-surfactants can synergistically decrease irritation potential without harming cleaning. Some anti-dandruff actives also can minimize the irritation potential of surfactants

[Venn diagram: Cosmetic shampoos / Therapeutic shampoos, overlap = Cosmetically-optimized therapeutics]

- Mild to skin and hair for everyday
- Conditions hair while cleaning
- Pleasant fragrance and appearance
- Cost effective
- Does not harm scalp

- Can be harsh due to excessive cleaning
- Little or no hair conditioning
- Often very "medicinal" esthetics
- Can be prohibitively expensive

- Provides anti-dandruff technology

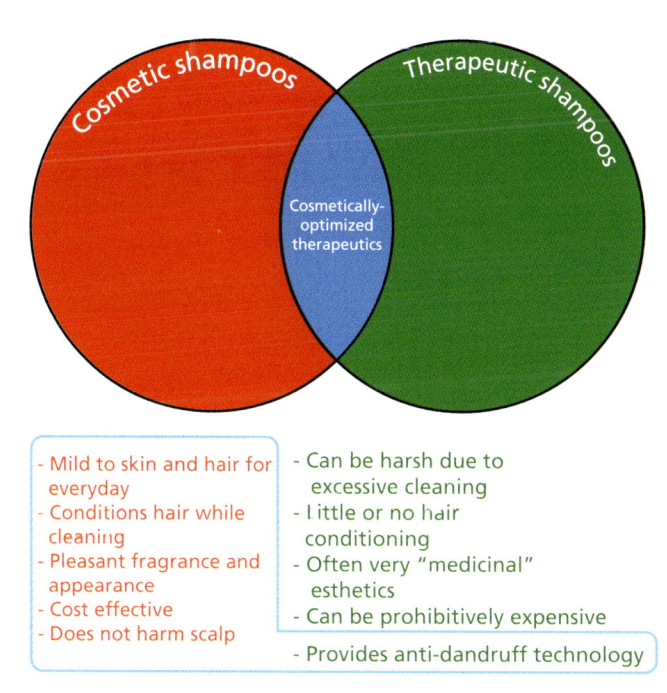

Figure 13.2 Representation of the shampoo segments, differentiating cosmetic from therapeutic shampoos and their key attributes. The category of cosmetically optimized therapeutics achieves therapeutic benefits without diminishing esthetic attributes.

Table 13.1 Summary of common formulation components of various shampoo types.

Function(s)		Material class(es)	Common examples	Cosmetic shampoo	cosmetically-optimized therapeutic	Standard therapeutic shampoo
Lather/cleaning		Primary surfactants	Sodium lauryl sulfate, ammonium lauryl sulfate, sodium laureth sulfate, ammonium laureth sulfate	Yes	Yes	Yes
	Optimization	Co-surfactants	Cocamidopropyl betaine, cocamide MEA	Yes	Yes	Yes
Hair conditioning agents	Shine, manageability	Silicones	Dimethicone, dimethiconol, amodimethicone	Yes	Yes	
	De-tangling, anti-static	Cationic polymers	Polyquaternium-10, cationic guar derivatives	Yes	Yes	
	Hydration	Humectants	Glycerin, urea	Some	Some	
	Hair health		Panthenol and derivatives	Some	Some	
Deposition aids	Benefit delivery	Cationic polymers	Polyquaternium-10, cationic guar derivatives	Yes	Yes	
Preservatives		Biocides	Isothiazalinone derivatives, parabens	Yes	Yes	Yes
Fragrance				Yes	Yes	Yes
Thickeners	Viscosity	Salts	Sodium chloride	Yes	Yes	Yes
		Particles	Glycol distearate	Some	Some	Some
Anti-dandruff components	Scalp care	Anti-fungals	Zinc pyrithione (ZPT), selenium sulfide, ketoconazole (see Table 13.2)		Yes	Yes
		Potentiators	Zinc carbonate		Some	

(see below); this is especially important for treatment of the D/SD condition which can be exacerbated by an irritating surfactant system.

In addition to surfactants for cleaning, shampoos contain a wide range of other materials to care for the hair and scalp, deliver cosmetic benefits, enhance the usage experience and to maintain the physical integrity of the product itself (preservatives, viscosity adjusters, pH control, etc.) Hair conditioning agents result in shiny, manageable hair and include such materials as silicones, cationic (positively charged) polymers that enhance deposition and retention of benefit agents to the hair fiber to provide conditioning and reduce static electricity, humectants to maintain hydration and materials that penetrate the hair shaft to maintain a healthy-looking appearance.

The cationic polymers mentioned as conditioning aids also are a critical component of the delivery system of many shampoos. While shampoos are first and foremost designed to clean, the delivery of additional hair and scalp benefits requires selected materials to be left behind after rinsing. The combination of oppositely charged surfactants and polymers results in an electrostatic association complex called coacervate which forms upon product dilution (lathering and rinsing). The coacervate is an aqueous gel that aids in the delivery of hair and scalp benefit agents to their respective surfaces.

The manipulation of surfactant and cationic polymer types and levels affects deposition efficiency, and together with the type and level of hair benefit agent(s), affects how much conditioning is delivered to the hair. This is the basis for a wide offering of shampoo versions, to meet the diverse hair and scalp needs of users to deliver cosmetic benefits and a pleasant in-use experience, especially in terms of how much hair conditioning is needed and desired. Standard therapeutic shampoos tend to be deficient in hair conditioning benefits. They also do not tend to have a range of versions to meet the esthetic needs of the user. Together these two factors limit compliance with classical therapeutic products.

Therapeutic scalp care shampoos will additionally contain active materials for resolving dandruff/seborrheic dermatitis (D/SD) and preventing its re-occurrence. Since the commensal scalp fungus *Malassezia* clearly plays a role in the etiology of the condition [1], the primary function of most scalp care active

Table 13.2 Overview of scalp care active materials.

Common actives	Primary mechanism	Typical amount used	Appearance	Odor	Usage
Most potent anti-fungal activity					
Zinc pyrithione (ZPT)	Anti-fungal	0.5–2%	White powder	Neutral	Wide. Positive impact on esthetics and hair care benefits.
Ketoconazole	Anti-fungal	1–2%	White powder	Neutral	Limited. Is expensive and requires regulatory approval.
Selenium sulfide	Anti-fungal	1–2%	Red powder	Sulfur-like	Limited. Color and odor affect esthetics.
Moderately potent anti-fungal activity					
Climbazole	Anti-fungal	0.5–2%	White powder	Neutral	Limited. Not accepted globally by regulatory bodies
Octopirox	Anti-fungal	0.5–2%	White powder	Neutral	Limited. Not accepted globally by regulatory bodies
Sulfur		1%	Yellow powder	Sulfur	Limited. Color and odor affect esthetics.
Least potent anti-fungal activity					
Salicylic acid	Keratolytic agent	1.8–3.0%	White powder	Neutral	Limited. Low anti-fungal potency.
Coal tar	Regulator of keratinization	0.5–1.0%	Black viscous liquid	Off-odor	Limited. Color and odor affect esthetics.

materials is anti-fungal; the most common are summarized in Table 13.2, grouped by their intrinsic anti-*Malassezia* potency. Some of the materials are accepted by global regulatory status agencies, while others are limited to use in only some geographical regions.

The most commonly used scalp active is zinc pyrithione (ZPT), a material developed as part of a program to identify biocides based on the naturally occurring antibiotic aspergillic acid [4]. Screening of over one thousand prospective anti-dandruff materials in the late 1950s led to the selection of ZPT; novel formulation work then led to commercialization of shampoos with ZPT in the early 1960s [5]. Since that time, the efficacy, ease of formulation, cost and compatibility with shampoo esthetic attributes has resulted in very broad use and acceptance of ZPT. The magnitude of therapeutic benefit delivered by ZPT-containing shampoos is formulation dependent (see below).

Other effective actives such as ketoconazole and selenium sulfide are used fairly broadly, but tend to be more limited to the classical therapeutic class of shampoos due either to cost, regulatory or esthetic limitations. Such products are generally used when especially difficult cases of D/SD occur. If such products are needed, subsequently switching to cosmetically optimized therapeutic shampoos should be advised for long-term prophylactic usage. Materials such as climbazole and octopirox have been used regionally, but have been limited by the lack of acceptance in some geographies such as the US by the FDA. Although the FDA does accept the safety and efficacy of salicylic acid, coal tar and sulfur, either low potency or poor esthetics have limited their broad utilization.

Unique attributes of scalp care products

The complexity of the shampoo delivery vehicle briefly described above, in combination with the unique attributes of the active material, results in seemingly similar products delivering different magnitudes of efficacy even though they contain the same level of the same active material. The pharmacological delivery factors are just as important in realizing efficacy as is the selection of active material. The case is well-illustrated for shampoos based on ZPT, in which both the physical form of the material as well as the shampoo composition affect resultant activity [1] by three factors (Table 13.3).

Retention of active on scalp

Regardless of the specific active material used in shampoos, activity is substantially dependent upon how much material is retained on the scalp surface after rinsing. As described above, this is a complex formulation technology task since cleaning is occurring simultaneously and, in the case of a shampoo, is the primary product benefit. Coacervate technology is used as a delivery system for ZPT (in addition to hair benefit agents) to control how much of a material like ZPT is retained on the scalp

Table 13.3 Formulation factors affecting the realization of full efficacy.

1. Retention of active material on scalp after rinsing.
2. Physical bio-availability: Spatial coverage of active on scalp surface and in infundibula.
3. Chemical bio-availability: Prevalence of bio-active species of active material.

after rinsing. The efficiency of this deposition can vary dramatically between commercial products and will directly affect the magnitude of efficacy [6]. The achievement of effective active delivery is a complex balancing of parameters to maximize delivery while not compromising the esthetic properties of the product. This is because the coacervate that efficiently deposits on the scalp also deposits on the hair and can compromise the perception of hair cleanliness if not optimized correctly. Successful formulation of cosmetically optimized therapeutic shampoos containing ZPT demands control over the coacervate formation upon dilution and rinsing. This is done by careful balancing of cationic polymer type and level and surfactant system optimizing to control the amount, texture and subsequent size of the coacervate gel phase formed. By controlling these factors the coacervate that deposits on the hair will provide ideal conditioning properties while also entraining ZPT on the scalp in a spatially optimized form (see below).

Spatial distribution of deposited active

While the amount of material remaining on the scalp surface is critically important, the physical distribution is just as important as it affects the bio-availability to *Malassezia* of what has been deposited. For a particulate material like ZPT, activity is derived from molecular dissolution into the surrounding medium, sebaceous lipids returning to and covering the scalp surface after shampooing (Figure 13.3 A). Thus the effective anti-fungal activity zone surrounding a given particle is limited by the contradictory rates of dissolution of ZPT and replenishment of new sebaceous liquid. Thus, to maximize activity, particles must be evenly spread out on relevant surfaces as their zones of activity are spatially limited.

There are two factors and two physical domains relevant to this spatial distribution. The two factors involved are the active particle morphology and the coacervate entrainment. There are two types of ZPT in use today, standard ZPT has a sub-micron size and a nondescript morphological shape. Optimized ZPT is used by one manufacturer where the morphology is platelet (see Figure 13.4) and the particle size has been optimized to 2.5 microns. Both of these parameters are designed to maximize the efficiency of scalp surface coverage to achieve uniform benefits throughout the micro-environment of the scalp. By use of platelet morphology particles, the spatial coverage is more efficient than use of a three-dimensionally symmetric particle. Particle size of the platelet also is important to achieve uniformity of coverage. Ideally, smaller particles are better, but they suffer from a trade-off that they are more difficult to retain through the rinsing step. Thus, practically, it has been observed [1] that an optimum particle size is 2.5 microns, which represents the average size of the optimized ZPT material. While the active material morphology plays a role in efficiency of spatial

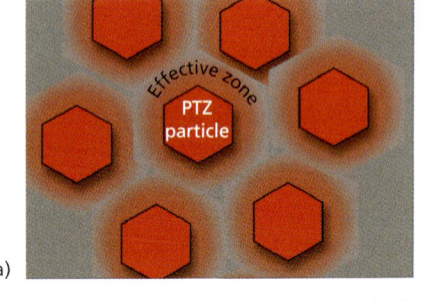

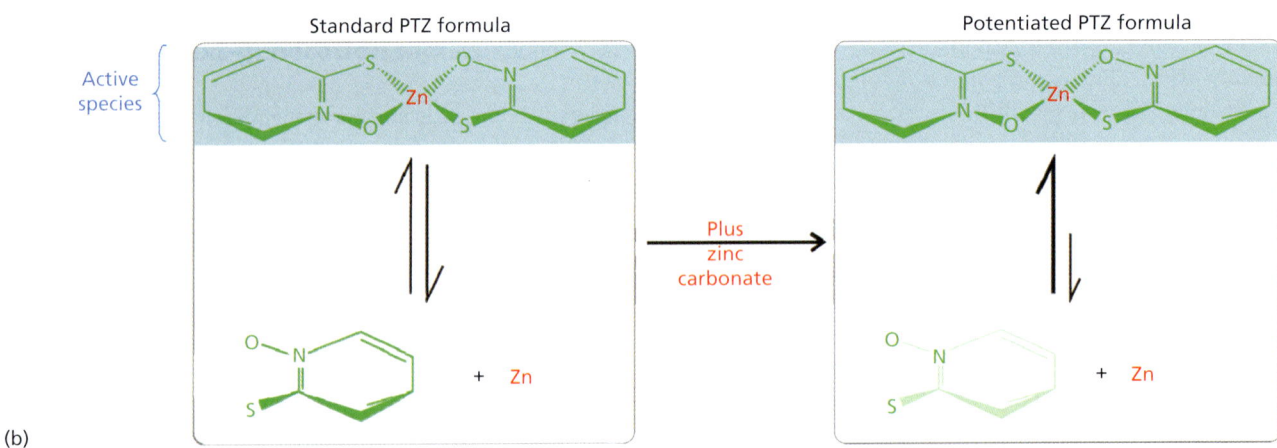

Figure 13.3 (a) Conceptual representation of the zone of inhibition of fungal growth surrounding ZPT particles and the importance of spatial distribution of particles to achieve uniformity of coverage. (b) ZPT can dissociate into component pyrithione (PT) and zinc (Zn) which reduces the presence of the intact bioactive species. The addition of zinc carbonate alters this equilibrium to maintain ZPT in its bioactive intact form.

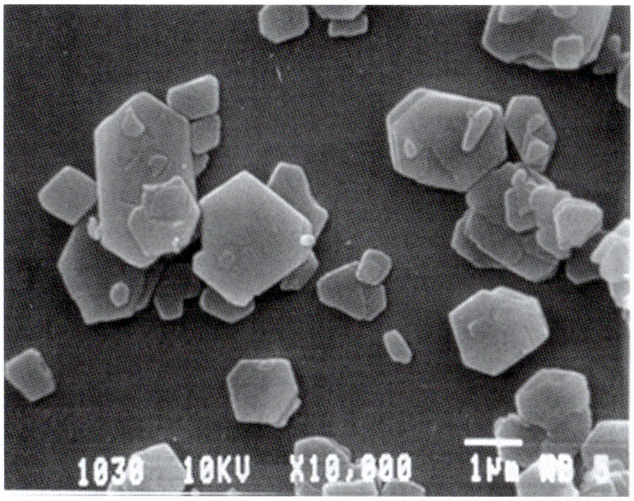

Figure 13.4 Electron micrograph of a unique form of ZPT, optimized for size and morphology to maximize the efficiency of surface coverage.

distribution of the active, the nature of the coacervate does as well. The particles are deposited on the scalp surface associated with the aqueous gel coacervate. The optimum coacervate for this purpose is one that forms into small dispersed gel particles entraining ZPT that facilitate even active distribution by easily flowing and not overly agglomerating the ZPT particles on the scalp surface. Use of a coacervate that forms large dispersed gel phases and is also thick or overly agglomerated in texture, while potentially increasing amount of ZPT deposited, inhibits its spatial distribution, thereby negating any benefits from increasing the amount deposited.

In addition to these two factors affecting spatial distribution, there are two domains in which the spatial distribution is considered relevant. The classical focus has been on the scalp surface, but it is now realized that *Malassezia* reside in the upper hair follicles (infundibula) and that effective D/SD treatment requires delivery of active materials to these relatively inaccessible spaces [7]. Specialized techniques such as confocal microscopy allow the quantification of both amount and spatial distribution of ZPT in the infundibulum, demonstrating the superior anti-dandruff efficacy that results from increasing ZPT bio-availability in the infundibulum [8].

Chemical bio-availability

The third factor affecting delivered efficacy is optimization of chemical bio-availability [9]. Chemically, ZPT is considered a coordination complex between inorganic zinc ion (Zn) and the pyrithione (PT) organic moiety. In such a material, the bonds are weak and an equilibrium exists between the intact species and the separate components (Figure 13.3B). Neither of the separated components (Zn and PT) are effective anti-fungals, thus to the extent this dissociation occurs, ZPT chemical bio-availability and resultant efficacy is reduced. By adding a common ion to the system (in the form of zinc carbonate), the equilibrium is shifted (exploiting LeChâtelier's Principle) to the intact and more effective ZPT; this unique potentiated ZPT formula thus maximizes bio-availability of the deposited material.

Another important aspect in product selection is that the cleaning activity of the shampoo not result in irritation of the scalp. For D/SD sufferers this would interfere with the natural cutaneous repair processes that occurs upon *Malassezia* population reduction. In addition to appropriate selection of the surfactant system as described above, some anti-fungal actives such as ZPT have been shown [10] to reduce the irritation potential of the surfactants as well.

Advantages and disadvantages of the use of therapeutic shampoos

The use of therapeutic shampoos for effective treatment of D/SD as well maintenance of normal scalp hygiene is very convenient since this is part of the normal habit and practice already. By choice of a cosmetically optimized therapeutic product, the therapeutic benefit can be achieved without any cosmetic benefit trade-offs that could result in reduced patient compliance. This product category also tends to be more affordable than standard therapeutic products, which also increases long-term (prophylactic) usage. Importantly, the cosmetic benefits can be delivered without reducing efficacy, i.e., classical therapeutic products are not necessarily any more effective than cosmetically-optimized therapeutic products. No diminution of benefit (i.e., tachyphylaxis) occurs upon long-term use of ZPT-based products; this is based on both designed clinical studies [11] as well as anecdotal evidence associated with over 50 years of usage history. The only disadvantage of using such scalp care products occurs when a strict therapeutic product is chosen. The expense and esthetic negatives that normally accompany such products limit patient compliance leading to frequent, frustrating condition re-occurrence; these products should be limited to the most recalcitrant of cases.

Table 13.4 Summary of advantages and disadvantages of using scalp care shampoos.

Advantages
- Convenient form for treatment and prevention of dandruff/seborrheic dermatitis
- For cosmetically optimized therapeutics, compliance is increased
  - Affordability
  - No esthetic trade-offs
- For ZPT-based products, over 50 years of safe utilization
- For ZPT-based products, no tachyphylactic responses

Disadvantages
- For straight therapeutic products, compliance is reduced
  - Can be very expensive
  - Can have substantial esthetic trade-offs

Effective use of products (see Table 13.5)

D/SD is a chronic condition characterized by frequent re-occurrence resulting in frustration on the part of the patient [12]. Initial treatment of the condition appears to be managed fairly effectively by either independent use of therapeutic anti-fungal shampoos or by combination with topical corticosteroid usage. However, preventative treatment is required for long-term management of the condition. Since the *Malassezia* easily recolonize, using a cosmetically optimized therapeutic product for each shampoo experience is the optimum method for preventing reoccurrence.

If cosmetic shampoo usage is alternated with therapeutic products, efficacy is decreased [13]: not only does the cosmetic shampoo have no active to deliver to the scalp, it washes off some of the deposited active material from the prior exposure to the active-containing shampoo. The desire to switch between a cosmetic shampoo and therapeutic product is motivated by either the real or perceived esthetic trade-offs in use of a therapeutic product. It has been shown [14] that therapeutic products do not provide all of the desired esthetic benefits and that this will drive patients to choose cosmetically optimized therapeutic shampoos for treating scalp conditions. Even with cosmetically optimized therapeutic products, there is often a *perception* that these products are not equivalent to cosmetic shampoos; while this may have been true in the past, modern technologies can deliver efficacious therapeutic and cosmetic benefits without the traditional trade-offs of standard therapeutic treatments.

A wide range of D/SD shampoo treatments are available [15] with widely ranging costs. By recommending a therapeutic product that has been cosmetically optimized and one that is affordable for on-going usage, the patient is best advised to use this product as their normal product to prevent reoccurrence.

Even by selection of an effective therapeutic product, how it is used can make a difference to the magnitude of benefit achieved. The length of time the lather is exposed to the scalp is generally not important as it is the material that is retained on the scalp after rinsing that provides the benefit. Using coacervate-based deposition technologies, it is the dilution that occurs during rinsing that triggers the deposition. Repeating the lathering and rinsing process twice will more thoroughly remove the sebaceous lipid and allow more active to be deposited.

D/SD symptoms occur year-around and should be treated all year. There is a mis-perception that it is a seasonal condition, primarily occurring in cold, dry seasons. This has been shown [13] not to be true. Winter months with less humid air combined with the tendency to wear darker clothing make the patient more able to detect the flaking symptoms under these conditions, but they occur throughout the year. Higher frequency of shampooing may occur in summer months resulting in a slight decrease in severity of symptoms.

Another critical usage factor involves whether a rinse-off conditioner is used after the shampoo [13]. Rinse-off conditioners that do not contain anti-dandruff actives remove a portion of the deposited active from the prior therapeutic shampoo exposure thereby reducing efficacy. If the patient desires use of a rinse-off conditioner, one containing anti-dandruff active should be recommended so that loss of retained active does not occur once the entire hair care regimen is practiced.

Benefits of use of scalp care shampoos

Resolution of D/SD is the primary motivation for initiation of use of therapeutic shampoos. The choice of shampoo should be motivated by, in order: efficacy, cosmetic hair benefits and cost. Assessing the relative efficacy of a product usually involves double-blind placebo-controlled clinical studies using medical experts to assess the severity of flaking and erythema; recent work has also extended measurement capability to molecular indicators of scalp condition as well [16]. A review of the comparative efficacy of products [3] supports that the most effective products are those that contain an effective anti-fungal, the most potent of which are ZPT, selenium sulfide and ketoconazole. Further rank-ordering within this group is somewhat difficult due to conflicting studies and the role that the specific formulation then plays. However, it is clear that cosmetically optimized therapeutics can be as effective as standard therapeutics; the marketing strategy used to position these products is not necessarily a good predictor of the true technical efficacy.

The use of certain scalp care shampoos also demonstrate the ability to deliver anti-irritancy effects [17]. There appears to be a wide range in activities depending on the specific active used. ZPT and especially the potentiated ZPT formula appear to be most effective at reducing irritation. Irritation and inflammation are early steps in the etiology of D/SD as well as many other scalp conditions. Thus, use of the zinc-based therapeutic products may well have general scalp health benefits beyond D/SD mitigation [18].

The scalp health benefits associated with use of anti-dandruff shampoos may extend to hair benefits as well. A number of studies have demonstrated (for example [19]) that use of these products can reduce the rate at which hair is lost. The mechanism for this benefit is not known, but may be speculated to originate in the reduction of inflammation referred to above as follicular inflammation may impede re-growth of lost hairs. A

Table 13.5 Summary of usage habits to maximize the therapeutic benefit.

1. Use the therapeutic shampoo for every shampooing to prevent a relapse
2. Use a therapeutic product that is cosmetically optimized and affordable
3. Shampoo as frequently as possible
4. Lather exposure time is not important but repeating the entire process can be beneficial
5. Product should be utilized all year
6. If a rinse-off conditioner is needed, use one that contains anti-dandruff active

further benefit of the scalp inflammation being reduced by these products is less itch and subsequent scratching which reduces hair damage and improves the quality and appearance of hair.

Summary

Normal scalp hygiene requires frequent and effective cleaning of the scalp. Cosmetic shampoos do this effectively while providing conditioning benefits for the hair. For many individuals, this frequent cleaning is sufficient to prevent adverse scalp effects. However, many still suffer from the symptoms of D/SD. For this group, therapeutic products are required that contain antidandruff actives that control the scalp *Malassezia* population. A subset of this class is cosmetically optimized therapeutics in which the product delivers the therapeutic benefits without loss of the typical cosmetic shampoo esthetics. This leads to much higher compliance, leading to effective long term care of the chronic condition. Other factors relevant for selecting the most useful product are that the active and shampoo composition be optimized to maximize the physical and chemical bio-availability of the active; this is especially true for ZPT-based treatments. Once the best shampoo is chosen, effective habits are required to realize the full benefit: frequent use without switching to cosmetic shampoos, use all year around and the use of a rinse-off conditioner that also contains anti dandruff active.

References

1 Schwartz J. (2007) Treatment of seborrheic dermatitis of the scalp. *J Cosm Dermatol* **6**, 18–22.
2 Elewski B. (2005) Clinical diagnosis of common scalp disorders. *J Invest Dermatol Symp Proc* 2005;**10**:190–3.
3 Schwartz J, Cardin C, Dawson Jr. T. (2005) Dandruff and seborrheic dermatitis. In: Barran R, Maibach H, eds. *Textbook of Cosmetic Dermatology*, 3rd edn. New York: Taylor & Francis, pp. 259–72.
4 Shaw E, Bernstein J, Losee K, Lott W. (1950) Analogs of aspergillic acid. IV. Substituted 2-bromopyridine-N-oxides and their conversion to cyclic thiohydroxamic acids. *J Am Chem Soc* **72**, 4362–4.
5 Snyder F. (1969) Development of a therapeutic shampoo. *Cutis* 5, 835–8.
6 Bailey P, Arrowsmith C, Darling K, Dexter J, Eklund J, Lane A, *et al.* (2003) A double-blind randomized vehicle-controlled clinical trial investigating the effect of ZnPTO dose on the scalp vs. antidandruff efficacy and antimicotic activity. *Internat J Cosm Sci* **25**, 183–8.
7 Schwartz J, Shah R, Krigbaum H, Sacha J, Vogt A, Blume-Peytavi U. (2011) New insights on dandruff/seborrhoeic dermatitis: the role of the scalp follicular infundibulum in effective treatment strategies. *Br J Derm* **165** Suppl 2, 18–23.
8 Schwartz J, Bacon R, Shah R, Mizoguchi H, Tosti A. (2013) Therapeutic efficacy of anti-dandruff shampoos: A randomized clinical trial comparing products based on potentiated zinc pyrithione and zinc pyrithione/climbazole. *Internat J Cosm Sci* **35**, 381–7.
9 Schwartz J. (2005) Product pharmacology and medical actives in achieving therapeutic benefits. *J Invest Dermatol Symp Proc* **10**, 198–200.
10 Warren R, Schwartz J, Sanders L, Juneja P. (2003) Attenuation of surfactant-induced interleukin 1α expression by zinc pyrithione. *Exog Dermatol* **2**, 23–7.
11 Schwartz J, Rocchetta H, Asawanonda P, Luo F, Thomas J. (2009) Does tachyphylaxis occur in long-term management of scalp seborrheic dermatitis with pyrithione zinc-based treatments? *Internat J Dermatol* **48**, 79–85.
12 Chen S, Yeung J, Chren M. (2002) Scalpdex. A quality-of-life instrument for scalp dermatitis. *Arch Dermatol* **138**, 803–7.
13 Schwartz J. (2004) A practical guide for the treatment of dandruff and seborrheic dermatitis. *J Am Acad Dermatol* **50**, p. 71.
14 Draelos Z, Kenneally D, Hodges L, Billhimer W, Copas M, Margraf C. (2005) A comparison of hair quality and cosmetic acceptance following the use of two anti-dandruff shampoos. *J Invest Dermatol Symp Proc* **10**, 201–4.
15 Schwartz R, Janusz C, Janniger C. (2006) Seborrheic dermatitis: An overview. *Am Fam Phys* **74**, 125–30.
16 Schwartz J, Messenger A, Tosti A, Todd G, Hordinsky M, Hay R, *et al.* (2013) A comprehensive pathophysiology of dandruff and seborrheic dermatitis – towards a more precise definition of scalp health. *Acta Derm Venereol* **93**, 131–7.
17 Margraf C, Schwartz J, Kerr K. (2005) Potentiated antidandruff/ seborrheic dermatitis formula based on pyrithione zinc delivers irritation mitigation benefits. *J Am Acad Dermatol* **52**(3), p. 56.
18 Schwartz J, Marsh R, Draelos Z. (2005) Zinc and skin health: Overview of physiology and pharmacology. *Dermatol Surg* **31**, 837–47.
19 Berger R, Fu J, Smiles K, Turner C, Schnell B, Werchowski K, *et al.* (2003) The effects of minoxidil, 1% pyrithione zinc and a combination of both on hair density: a randomized controlled trial. *Br J Dermatol* **149**, 354–62.

SECTION 2 Moisturizers

CHAPTER 14
Facial Moisturizers

Yohini Appa
Johnson & Johnson, New Brunswick, NJ, USA

> **BASIC CONCEPTS**
> - Facial moisturizers can be used to improve skin texture, treat dry skin, and provide sun protection.
> - Occlusives, humectants, emollients, and sunscreens are important ingredient categories in facial moisturizers.
> - The efficacy of a facial moisturizer can be measured via transepidermal water loss and corneometry.
> - Facial moisturizers can be an important adjunct in the treatment of facial dermatoses, such as atopic dermatitis and eczema.

Introduction

The face is the most conspicuous representation of age and health. While the eyes are considered the windows to the soul, the face is its billboard. No other body part demonstrates personal past history as convincingly as the face. Wrinkles form on the face well before the rest of the body and serve as an indicator of age and lifestyle. The relative color and luminosity of the facial skin represents overall health and emotional state. Facial skin can be dull to vibrant representing poor to excellent physical health. The face mirrors acute changes in well-being. For example, persons experiencing cardiac distress appear "ashen" while anger or embarrassment may be expressed as a reddened face. Thus, the face represents the current physical state of the individual. Moisturizers can enhance the appearance of the face and are thus important cosmeceuticals.

The face is rarely covered and constantly subjected to the elements. It is one of the most light-exposed areas of skin on the body, the other areas being the shoulders, upper chest, and forearms; as a result it receives high amounts of UV radiation. The incidence of cutaneous melanoma as measured by relative tumor density is highest on the face in subjects over the age of 50 years, a statistic that is interpreted as directly correlating to the amount of long term UV exposure [1]. This means that facial photoprotection is of great importance, thus the incorporation of efficacious UVA and UVB protection in daily facial moisturizers is worthwhile.

Facial skin is physiologically unique. It possesses numerous sweat glands and a relatively thin dermis. It is densely populated with sebaceous glands, possessing 400–900 glands per square centimeter [2]. The face is a major point of contact for sensory input, the facial skin possesses high innervation and is therefore more sensitive than skin elsewhere on the body [3]. The skin covering the face also has to allow for the subtleties of facial expressions and phonoation. Of all the areas on the body, the skin on the face has the highest level of hydration. When the ratio of transepidermal water loss (TEWL) to skin surface hydration was calculated in order to determine the most consistently hydrated area of the body, the forehead and cheek showed the lowest ratios (Figure 14.1).

Dry facial skin

Dry skin is a term used to describe the condition that arises when the normal functioning of the skin is compromised. More specifically, it is a manifestation of the consequences that arise from a loss of water from the outermost layer of the dermis: the stratus corneum (SC). The SC is formed when keratinocytes, cuboidal cells in the lower half of the epidermis, migrate from the basal layer to the most superficial layer, producing large amounts of the water-insoluble protein keratin along the way. The keratinization and migration process results in flattened, keratin-filled keratinocytes, referred to as corneocytes, which create an overlapping barrier with a "brick and mortar" appearance that is nearly waterproof. The gaps between the corneocytes, or "bricks," are filled with intercellular lipids, or "mortar" that is produced by keratohyaline granules. The SC layer is also referred to as the "dead layer" because by this point the cells have stopped synthesizing proteins and are unresponsive to cellular signaling. Cells in the SC are eventually sloughed off and replaced by more cells coming up through the epidermis,

---

Cosmetic Dermatology: Products and Procedures, Second Edition. Edited by Zoe Diana Draelos.
© 2016 John Wiley & Sons, Ltd. Published 2016 by John Wiley & Sons, Ltd.

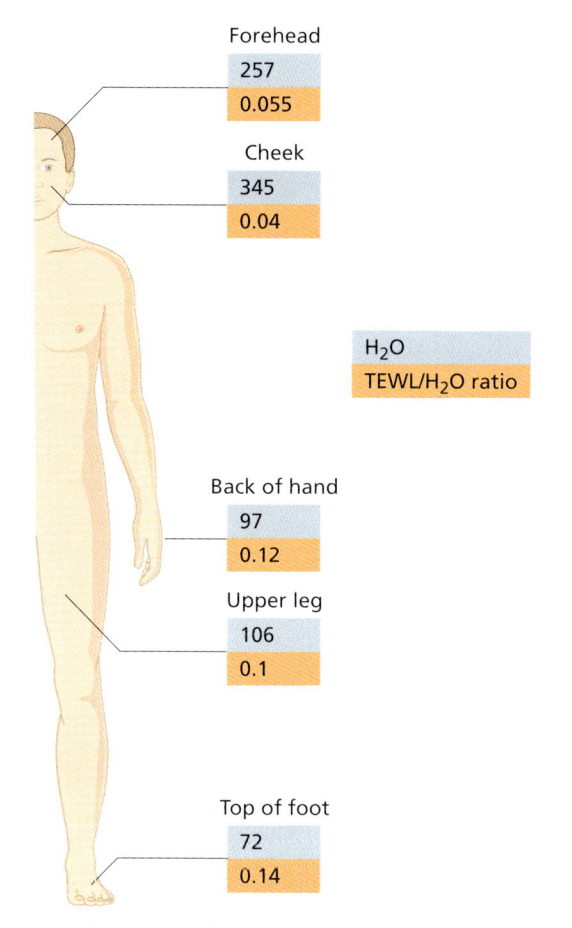

Figure 14.1 Skin surface hydration and transepidermal water loss (TEWL) and SciCon ratio.

- Forehead: 257 / 0.055
- Cheek: 345 / 0.04
- Back of hand: 97 / 0.12
- Upper leg: 106 / 0.1
- Top of foot: 72 / 0.14

H$_2$O / TEWL/H$_2$O ratio

thereby maintaining a continuous barrier. It normally takes 26–42 days for the epidermis to cycle completely [4].

The process of skin cell differentiation and maturation is a delicate balance that is easily disrupted. If the water content of the SC drops below 20% for an extended period of time, the enzymes involved in desquamation will be unable to function and the process of orderly epidermis cycling will be compromised. This especially apparent in dry facial skin.

There are many functions that the epidermal barrier performs:
1. Maintains a 20–35% water content;
2. Limits TEWL;
3. Preserve water homeostasis in the epidermis;
4. Sustains optimal lipid synthesis; and
5. Allows for orderly desquamation of SC cells.

A shift away from equilibrium in one of these five functions can result in a compromise of the barrier and the basic consequence is what we refer to as "dry skin." More specifically, when TEWL is increased to the point that the water content in the SC is reduced to below 10%, the clinical signs of xerosis will appear [5].

The orderly desquamation of the SC is a complex process which if disturbed can lead to a self-renewing cycle of dry skin. The corneocytes that make up the SC are highly interconnected and able to withstand a large amount of mechanical stress. When new cells are formed, enzymatic digestion of the proteins anchoring the old cells is required for removal. The level of humidity in the SC is a critical factor modulating the activity of these desquamatory enzymes, specifically stratum corneum chymotryptic enzyme (SCCE). When this process breaks down, desquamation becomes irregular and dead SC cells slough off in large clumps; representing the "flaking" seen in so many dry facial skin conditions [6].

The sebum-rich skin of the face can appear moisturized but possess a low water content. Sensory symptoms can include but are not limited to: dryness, discomfort, pain, itching, stinging, or tingling sensations. Tactile signs are rough, uneven, and sand-like feeling skin. Visible signs, which can be macroscopic or microscopic, are redness, dull surface, dry white patches, flaky appearance, and cracks and fissures. There are many causes for these signs and symptoms. In all, the presence of dry skin represents disorder in the complex system that continually renews the facial skin.

Facial moisturization

The physiologic goal of facial moisturization is to restore the elasticity and flexibility of the SC, thereby restoring its barrier function. Additionally, the reintroduction of humidity to the SC allows for proper functioning of desquamation enzymes and restores the natural skin renewal cycle. Kligman and Leyden [7] defined a moisturizer as "a topically applied substance or product that overcomes the signs and symptoms of dry skin." The esthetic goal of moisturization is achieving soft, supple, glowing, healthy looking skin, as subjectively evaluated by the end-user. Regular use of facial moisturizers mitigate and prevent signs of aging, especially when formulated with broad-spectrum sun protection for daytime use.

Because the face is one of the most sensitive areas of the body, a facial moisturizer must meet esthetic goals in addition to fulfilling a broad set of performance attributes. Consumers expect a facial moisturizer to reduce dryness, improve dull appearance, smooth and soften the skin, and increase suppleness [8]. Furthermore, these expectations must be achieved by a moisturizer with a minimal presence and pleasant sensory qualities.

A properly formulated moisturizer can supplement the function of the endogenous epidermal lipids and restore the epidermal barrier function. This allows the skin to continue its natural process of renewal and desquamation at a normal rate. The substances utilized by all moisturizers to achieve this desired effect fall into a handful of basic categories (Table 14.1). Humectants, such as glycerin, attract and hold moisture, facilitating hydration. Emollients, typically lipids or oils, enhance the flexibility and smoothness of the skin and provide a secondary soothing effect to the skin and mucous membranes. Occlusives create a hydrophobic barrier to reduce water loss from the skin. Emulsifiers work to bring together immiscible substances; they

Table 14.1 Function of common moisturizer ingredients. This listing represents the common ingredients found in a moisturizer formulation identifying the role of each of the substances in the ingredient disclosure.

	Humectant	Emollient	Occlusive	Emulsifier	Preservative
Dimethicone		X	X		
Trisiloxane		X			
Glycerin	X	X			
Glyceryl stearate				X	
PEG 100 stearate				X	
Potassium cetyl phosphate				X	
Behenyl alcohol			X		
Caprylyl methicone		X			
Hydrogenated palm glycerides		X			
Hexanediol	X	X			
Caprylyl glycol	X	X			
Cetearyl glucoside			X		
Cetearyl alcohol			X		
Methylparaben					X
Propylparaben					X
Methylisothiazolinone					X

are a critical element in the oil and water mixtures employed in moisturizer formulas. Preservatives prevent the premature breakdown of components and inhibit microbiologic growth. Fragrances not only add to the esthetic value but can also mask the odor of formulation ingredients.

These components make up the basic formulation of any moisturizer, and the choices available to achieve the preferred outcome are vast. The formulation of an acceptable and effective moisturizer for the face, one that will enable the natural processes of skin desquamation to occur and maintain healthy barrier function while meeting high esthetic standards, is as much an art as it is a science.

Facial moisturizer formulation

Facial moisturizers are typically oil-in-water emulsions. The water improves skin feel and offers an acceptable, universally tolerated base for the active ingredients. The water or oil solubility of components is inconsequential because both are present. Emulsions allow for a wide range of properties, such as slow to fast absorption rates depending on the final viscosity of the formulation. The fine-tuning of these properties is important for achieving the high esthetic expectations of a facial moisturizer. For example, a daily-use formula with high emollient content may feel heavy in a cream but be acceptable in liquid form. Conversely, overnight creams with antiaging additives may be thick in order to remain on the face during sleep and to slow the absorption of active components. Therefore, by utilizing a range of water to oil ratios, and varying humectant and emollient mixtures, the desired effects can be formulated within the acceptable esthetic parameters for a facial moisturizer.

Moisturizer ingredients and function

Humectants

The overall hydration level of the SC affects its mechanical properties. If the water level in the SC drops below 10%, its flexibility can be compromised and it becomes susceptible to damage from mechanical stress [9]. Humectants are key substances to maintain skin hydration. Natural humectants, such as hyaluronic acid, are found in the dermis, but external humectants can be externally applied in moisturizers. Humectants draw water from the viable epidermis and dermis, but can draw water from the environment if the ambient humidity is over 80%.

Humectants are water-soluble organic compounds that can sequester large numbers of water molecules. Glycerin, sorbitol, urea, and sodium lactate are all examples of externally applied humectants. Glycerin, also referred to as glycerol, is one of the most widely utilized compounds in cosmetic formulations because of its effects on multiple targets and its universal applications. Its chemical structure brings together the stability of three carbon atoms with three water-seeking oxygen atoms in an anisotropic molecule that is perfectly designed for use in skin and hair moisturizers. Glycerin also allows for the construction of different product physical forms that cover the spectrum from sticks to microemulsions to free-flowing creams that maintain stability over time.

The degree of purity to which glycerin can be manufactured not only ensures consistency and facilitates microbiologic stability, but also guarantees the minimization of allergic reactions by contaminants. The pure form of glycerin has been tested on thousands of patients and millions more have used it with extremely few reports of ill effects. Glycerin is generally classified as a humectant; however, this characteristic is not the sole reason for its ability to achieve skin moisturization, in fact, it performs a number of different functions that are not directly related to its water-holding properties.

Glycerin can restore the suppleness of skin without increasing its water content, a trait that is exploited by its use in the cryopreservation of skin, tissue, and red blood cells, where water would freeze and damage them. Glycerin enhances the cohesiveness of the intercellular lipids when delivered from high glycerin therapeutic formulations, thereby retaining their presence and function. Furthermore, glycerin has been identified as a contributor to the process of desquamation, a critical component of the dermal renewal cycle, through its ability to enhance desmosome digestion.

In addition to its direct, humectant effects on skin moisturization, endogenously produced glycerin has exhibited effects at the molecular level in knockout mouse model studies, confirming its role in maintaining SC hydration and barrier maintenance. A recent study showed that glycerin content was three times lower, SC hydration was reduced, and barrier function was impaired in mice deficient in the water/glycerin transporter protein, aquaporin-3 (AQP3) despite normal SC structure, protein–lipid composition and ion–osmolyte content. Glycerin, but not other small poly glycols, restored normal SC moisturization and TEWL values when applied to the AQP3-deficient mice, confirming that glycerin was physiologically necessary in the modulation of SC hydration and barrier maintenance [10].

Glycerin remains the gold standard for moisturization. The fact that it acts on so many different parameters with a nearly non-existent side-effect profile makes it a prime candidate for facial moisturizer formulations. It is also an excellent example of how moisturizer components, especially those used on the face, should be considered for their ability to enhance and protect the skin. Glycerin raises the bar for moisturizers in that it is capable of enhancing, or even rescuing, the intrinsic processes that are in place to maintain the orderly maturation of keratinocytes and the barrier function of the skin.

Occlusives

Humectants are only partially effective in moisturizing the skin. In order to maintain epidermal water content and preserve the barrier function of the SC, occlusive agents are employed in a role meant to complement the water-attracting nature of humectants. Occlusive agents inhibit evaporative water loss by forming a hydrophobic barrier over the SC and its interstitial areas. Occlusion is successful in the treatment of dry skin because the movement of water from the lower dermis to the outer dermis is a guaranteed source of physiologically available water. Moreover, these occlusive agents have an emollient effect, as is the case with behenyl alcohol.

Petrolatum and lanolin are two historically popular occlusives that are slowly being replaced by more sophisticated alternatives. Petrolatum is a highly effective occlusive, but it suffers from an unfavorable esthetic. Lanolin is not recommended for use in facial formulations because of its odor and potential allergenicity [11]. Newly constructed silicone derivatives have been employed in moisturizers for their occlusive properties, and they further enhance the esthetic quality of the formulation by imparting a "dry" touch. This technologic advancement is also an example of how the esthetic parameter of a facial moisturizer can have a major effect on compliance and willingness to apply.

Emollients

Emollients are agents, usually lipids and oils, designed to soften and smooth the skin. Lipids are non-polar molecules and as such they repel polarized water molecules, thereby limiting the passage of water to the environment. The most prevalent lipids in the SC, especially within the extracellular membranes, are ceramides. They comprise about 40% of the lipid content of the SC, the remainder of which is 25% cholesterol, 10–15% free fatty acids, and smaller quantities of triglycerides, stearyl esters, and cholesterol sulfate. These lipids are synthesized throughout the epidermis, packaged in lamellar granules, and eventually differentiate into multilamellar sheets that form the ceramide-rich SC water barrier [12].

The purpose of an emollient is to replace the absent natural skin lipids in the space between the corneocytes in the SC. Additional benefits include the smoothing of roughened skin thereby changing the skin's appearance, and providing occlusion to attenuate TEWL and enhance moisturization. Of the three components of skin moisturizers listed in the CTFA Cosmetic Ingredients Directory, emollients outnumber occlusives 2 to 1 and the humectants 10 to 1. This is an indication not only of the number of available compounds that can perform this function, but also the variety of lipids that can be utilized [13].

Fragrance

Fragrance is a component of facial moisturizers that is often dismissed as an unnecessary potential irritant, but this idea is becoming increasingly antiquated as the science supporting its proper use and evaluation is improved. Vigorous protocols have been developed that comprehensively and conclusively assess the tolerance of formulations on human subjects. Fragrances are screened separately first and then together in both normal and sensitive populations, and utilized at the minimum concentration required to mask the smell of certain components, if necessary. Fragrance improves the overall esthetic qualities of the moisturizer, which is an important component of any moisturizer formulation, especially one that is applied to the face.

Preservatives

Preservatives are also subject to the same rigorous testing protocols as fragrances. The preservative must be strong enough to completely inhibit bacterial growth, but must not be sensitizing or irritating. Preservatives are an important component in facial moisturizers to prevent the lipids in the formulation from becoming rancid. All facial moisturizers have some type of preservative, because there is really no such thing as a preservative-free formulation.

Photoprotection and facial moisturizers

Sunscreens could be considered to be the most globally effective ingredient added to a facial moisturizer. Because the incidence and mortality rates of skin cancer have been steadily rising in the USA, the use of sunscreen as a daily protectant has become more important to consumers. There are both immediate and long-term benefits from photoprotection. The immediate benefit is the prevention of a painful sunburn while long photoprotection results in reduced photodamage manifesting as wrinkling, inflammation, and dryness.

A key immediate event that leads to chronic photoaging is the production of proteases in response to UV irradiation at doses well below those that cause skin reddening. Matrix metalloproteinases (MMPs), for example, are zinc-dependent endopeptidases expressed in many different cell types and are critical for normal biologic processes. They may also be involved in desquamation processes, and overexpression would lead to early sloughing and increase in TEWL. With a proper sunscreen regimen, production of MMPs is minimized and their participation in chronic photoaging can be avoided. The addition of sunscreens to facial moisturizers also contributes to the prevention of reactive oxygen species (ROS) production, Langerhans cell depletion, and sensitivity to UV radiation, as is observed in polymorphous light eruption.

Facial moisturizer testing

The formulation of a moisturizer centers on the primary goal of delivering the perception of moisture to the skin. This includes not only adding moisture to the skin, but also the improvement of the barrier function and reinstating natural skin reparative processes. The testing of the efficacy of a moisturizer is based on barrier function assessment.

There are many ways to assess the barrier function of the skin based on SC integrity. Measurement of the TEWL is one method. A damaged SC allows water to evaporate resulting in high TEWL readings. These measurements are taken with an evaporimeter, which measures the amount of water vapor leaving the skin. The amount of water in the skin can also be measured via skin conductance. This technique, known as corneometry, measures the amount of low level electricity conducted by the skin. Because water is the conductor of electricity in the skin, the amount of current conducted is directly related to the water content. Thus, the efficacy of a moisturizer can be measured by its effect on water vapor loss and skin conductance.

Another method for evaluating skin dryness is D-squames. D-squames are circular, adhesive discs placed on the skin surface with firm pressure and then pulled away. The removed skin is observed and parameters such as the amount of skin removed, size of flakes, and coloration can be recorded. Differences between dry skin and normal moisturized skin are clearly evident upon examination of the disc, and further characterization can be carried out to differentiate levels of dryness and qualitative differences in desquamation.

The barrier function of the skin can be assessed following application of an irritant to the skin surface. The introduction of an irritant can cause erythema and scaling in the compromised SC. A frequent irritant used for the assessment of barrier function is sodium lauryl sulfate (SLS). The amount of erythema and TEWL is measured following scrubbing of the skin with SLS. Skin with a better barrier following use of an efficacious moisturizer will experience less damage than skin that possesses a compromised barrier.

Finally, after testing the efficacy of the formulation in a controlled, laboratory setting, its efficacy must be evaluated on a group of consumers. Consumer testing is usually carried out in a blind study involving 200–300 subjects, from geographically disparate locales in order to normalize any differences in skin types or backgrounds. This testing will introduce parameters that are evaluated subjectively by the population of subjects such as skin feel, perception of texture, ease of application, and scent, among other things, that define its esthetic qualities. The functional qualities of the moisturizer, such as "immediate comfort" and "long-lasting effect" will also be evaluated by the consumer group and incorporated into the overall assessment.

Use of facial moisturizers in common inflammatory dermatoses

The face presents a set of unique challenges regarding the treatment of skin disorders. What may be acceptable for treatment regimens elsewhere on the body, such as a strong occlusive such as petrolatum or a humectant such as urea, will be esthetically challenging to the user and stand in the way of compliance. While it is easy to think of esthetics as secondary to efficacy of treatment, it should be considered of primary importance where the face is concerned. This concept cannot be overstressed because the sensitivity of the facial skin to the sensory and olfactory qualities of moisturizers is much higher than the rest of the body.

It is generally believed that facial atopic dermatitis and various other facial skin diseases are associated with disturbances of skin barrier function as evidenced by an increase in TEWL, a decrease in water-binding properties, and a reduction in skin surface lipids. When chronic, inflammatory skin diseases manifest on the face, there is the challenge of reducing the lesion as quickly as possible to prevent it from worsening and further compromising the integrity of the skin involved. Because of the high sensitivity of the facial skin, what may start as a small lesion can quickly be exacerbated through physical intervention and quickly worsened. These problems can be addressed through the continual use of appropriate moisturizers, which have been shown to improve skin hydration, reduce susceptibility to irritation, and restore the integrity of the SC. Some moisturizers also supply the compromised SC with lipids that further accelerate barrier recovery. Moisturizers can serve as an important first-line therapeutic option for patients with atopic dermatitis and other chronic skin diseases [14].

Historically, moisturizers have been shown to have a steroid-sparing effect in patients with atopic dermatitis and eczema. Many of the elements in moisturizers, from lipids to emollients, have been shown to significantly improve the condition of the skin when used by patients with various dermatoses [15]. Glycerin has been implicated in the molecular mechanism controlling keratinocyte maturation, an important aspect of normal desquamation and barrier maintenance. Furthermore, its role in maintenance of hydration for the proper functioning of proteases, especially filaggrin, is critical to the successful treatment of eczemas [16,17].

Recently, a comprehensive clinical study provided evidence that moisturizers not only enhance the efficacy of topical corticosteroids in patients with atopic dermatitis, but may also prevent the recurrence of disease [15]. In general, the maintenance of the SC along with rapid repair of disruptions to the barrier that would otherwise become larger and increase inflammation and discomfort as well seem to be central tenets in the approach to treating potential dermatoses on the face with moisturization. Therefore, facial moisturizers may represent a valuable first-line treatment option for many dermatologic diseases and confer a number of important therapeutic benefits that go beyond the surface of the facial skin and have a critical role in the molecular mechanisms that maintain healthy skin.

Conclusions

Facial moisturizers fulfill an important need by providing skin comfort and alleviating dryness. Efficacious formulations contain ingredients that work directly to bring moisture to the skin, but also indirectly, as is the case with glycerin, induce the transport and retention of water molecules at the subcellular level. The goal of facial moisturizers is to enhance, or restart, the processes intrinsic to the skin's natural ability to maintain its barrier function through the multiple pathways utilizing proteases, lipids, cell differentiation and, eventually, desquamation, all while maintaining an esthetically pleasant presence.

References

1 Elwood JM, Gallagher RP. (1998) Body site distribution of cutaneous malignant melanoma in relationship to patterns of sun exposure. *Int J Cancer* **78**, 276–80.
2 Montagna W. (1959) *Advances in Biology of Skin*. Oxford, New York: Symposium Publications Division, Pergamon Press.
3 Montagna W, Kligman AM, Carlisle KS. (1992) *Atlas of Normal Human Skin*. New York: Springer-Verlag.
4 Baumann L. (2002) *Cosmetic Dermatology: Principles and Practice*. New York: McGraw-Hill.
5 Draelos ZK. (2000) *Atlas of Cosmetic Dermatology*. New York: Churchill Livingstone.
6 Watkinson A, Harding C, Moore A, Coan P. (2001) Water modulation of stratum corneum chymotryptic enzyme activity and desquamation. *Arch Dermatol Res* **293**, 470–6.
7 Kligman AM, Leyden JJ. (1982) *Safety and Efficacy of Topical Drugs and Cosmetics*. New York: Grune & Stratton.
8 Barton S. (2002) Formualtion of skin moisturization. In: Leyden JJ, Rawlings AV, eds. *Skin Moisturization*. New York: Marcel Dekker, pp. 547–84.
9 Rawlings AV, Canestrari DA, Dobkowski B. (2004) Moisturizer technology versus clinical performance. *Dermatol Ther* **17** (Suppl 1), 49–56.
10 Hara M, Verkman AS. (2003) Glycerin replacement corrects defective skin hydration, elasticity, and barrier function in aquaporin-3-deficient mice. *Proc Natl Acad Sci U S A* **100**, 7360–5.
11 Draelos ZK. (1995) *Cosmetics in Dermatology*, 2nd edn. New York: Churchill Livingstone.
12 Downing S, Stewart ME. (2000) Epidermal composition. In: Loden M, Maibach HI, eds. *Dry Skin and Moisturizers: Chemistry and Function*. Boca Raton: CRC Press, 2000: pp. 13–26.
13 Draelos ZK, Thaman LA. (2006) *Cosmetic Formulation of Skin Care Products.* New York: Taylor & Francis.
14 Lebwohl M. (1995) *Atlas of the Skin and Systemic Disease*. New York: Churchill Livingstone.
15 Ghali FE. (2005) Improved clinical outcomes with moisturization in dermatologic disease. *Cutis* **76** (Suppl), 13–8.
16 Hanifin JM. (2008) Filaggrin mutations and allergic contact sensitization. *J Invest Dermatol* **128**, 1362–4.
17 Presland RB, Coulombe PA, Eckert RL, *et al.* (2004) Barrier function in transgenic mice overexpressing K16, involucrin, and filaggrin in the suprabasal epidermis. *J Invest Dermatol* **123**, 603–6.

Further reading

Bikowski J. (2001) The use of therapeutic moisturizers in various dermatologic disorders. *Cutis* 68 (Suppl), 3–11.
Burgess CM. (2005) *Cosmetic Dermatology*. Berlin: Springer.
Crowther JM, Sieg A, Blenkiron P, *et al.* (2008) Measuring the effects of topical moisturizers on changes in stratum corneum thickness, water gradients and hydration *in vivo*. *Br J Dermatol* 159, 567–77.
Del Rosso JQ. (2005) The role of the vehicle in combination acne therapy. *Cutis* 76 (Suppl), 15–8.
Fisher GJ, Datta SC, Talwar HS, *et al.* (1996) Molecular basis of sun-induced premature skin ageing and retinoid antagonism. *Nature* 379, 335–9.
Fisher GJ, Varani J, Voorhees JJ. (2008) Looking older: fibroblast collapse and therapeutic implications. *Arch Dermatol* 144, 666–72.
Fisher GJ, Voorhees JJ. (1996) Molecular mechanisms of retinoid actions in skin. *FASEB J* 10, 1002–13.

Fisher GJ, Wang ZQ, Datta SC, *et al.* (1997) Pathophysiology of premature skin aging induced by ultraviolet light. *N Engl J Med* 337, 1419–28.

Fluhr J. (2005) *Bioengineering of the Skin: Water and Stratum Corneum*, 2nd edn. Boca Raton: CRC Press.

Friedmann PS. (1986) The skin as a permeability barrier. In: Thody AJ, Friedmann PS, eds. *Scientific Basis of Dermatology*. Edinburgh, London: Churchill Livingstone, pp. 26–35.

Held E, Jorgensen LL. (1999) The combined use of moisturizers and occlusive gloves: an experimental study. *Am J Contact Dermatol* 10, 146–52.

Jungermann E, Norman O, Sonntag V. (1991) *Glycerin: A Key Cosmetic Ingredient. Vol. 11, Cosmetic Science and Technology Series*. New York: Marcel Dekker.

Kafi R, Kwak HS, Schumacher WE, *et al.* (2007) Improvement of naturally aged skin with vitamin A (retinol). *Arch Dermatol* 143, 606–12.

Loden M, Maibach HI. (1999) *Dry Skin and Moisturizers: Chemistry and Function*. Boca Raton: CRC Press.

Orth DS. (1993) *Handbook of Cosmetic Microbiology*. New York: Marcel Dekker.

Page-McCaw A, Ewald AJ, Werb Z. (2007) Matrix metalloproteinases and the regulation of tissue remodeling. *Nat Rev Mol Cell Biol* 8, 221–33.

Rattan SI. (2006) Theories of biological aging: genes, proteins, and free radicals. *Free Radic Res* 40, 1230–8.

Streicher JJ, Culverhouse WC Jr, Dulberg MS, *et al.* (2004) Modeling the anatomical distribution of sunlights. *Photochem Photobiol* 79, 40–7.

Verdier-Sevrain S, Bonte F. (2007) Skin hydration: a review on its molecular mechanisms. *J Cosmet Dermatol* 6, 75–82.

CHAPTER 15
Hand and Foot Moisturizers

Teresa M. Weber,[1] Andrea M. Schoelermann,[2] Ute Breitenbach,[2] Ulrich Scherdin,[2] and Alexandra Kowcz[1]

[1] Beiersdorf Inc, Wilton, CT, USA
[2] Beiersdorf AG, Hamburg, Germany

> **BASIC CONCEPTS**
> - Xerosis of the hands and feet is common, caused by a paucity of sebaceous glands.
> - Moisturization of the hands and feet can prevent eczematous disease and aid in disease eradication.
> - Effective moisturizers provide occlusive lipophilic substances that act as protectants and barrier replenishers, as well as hydrophilic agents that function as humectants to bind and hold water.
> - Recent recognition of the role of aquaporins, special moisture regulating channels, in skin cells has provided the opportunity for a new moisturization technology, focusing on substances that stimulate and operate through aquaporins.

Introduction

The hands and feet are prone to dryness and impaired barrier function because of their unique functional roles, predisposing the skin to heightened irritant sensitivity and the development of dermatoses. Protective and regenerative moisturizing skin care is the foundation for averting and treating dry skin associated skin diseases and disorders.

Effective moisturizers provide occlusive lipophilic substances that act as protectants and barrier replenishers, as well as hydrophilic agents that function as humectants to bind and hold water. The importance of urea as a physiologic humectant and natural moisturizing factor is discussed. Application of moisturizers containing urea is shown to increase its concentration and exert ultrastructural changes in the stratum corneum, hydrate severely compromised skin, and support and enhance barrier function. In addition, the role of aquaporins and the underlying mechanisms of moisture homeostasis of the skin are discussed vis-à-vis new opportunities to create better actives and product formulations which can help regulate moisturization from within the skin.

Moisturization needs of the hand and foot

Skin of the hands and feet is different from other body sites. In particular, skin on the palms and soles is thicker, and has a high density of eccrine sweat glands; however, it lacks apocrine glands. These sites are highly innervated and involved in most of the daily activities of life. Repetitive use of the hands and feet accompanied by pressure and friction can promote the formation of areas of thickened keratinized skin or calluses, which can crack and fissure. Site-specific requirements for hygienic care and diseases common to these sites have been described [1]. In addition, the hands and feet have special skincare needs for efficacious moisturization as well as unique requirements for formulations that are compatible with their special sensory and functional roles and needs.

Hand skin is particularly susceptible to xerosis and dermatitis. Constant use of the hands, frequent washing, and environmental, chemical, and irritant exposure can provoke these problems. Further, because the hands are especially prone to injury and exposure to irritants and pathogens, specific skin protectant formulations can be highly beneficial to prevent irritation or occupational dermatoses such as hand eczema [2].

While the feet may be less likely to suffer from deleterious occupational exposures, environmental factors can have an impact on the moisture status of the foot skin. Cold, dry weather in winter, bare feet in summer, and the confinement of shoes can compromise the hydration state. Occlusive shoes and socks can also trap moisture and render the foot susceptible to microbial infections, especially from fungus, damaging the barrier function and dehydrating the skin. In addition, certain metabolic diseases can impact circulation and innervation of the extremities, which in turn affects skin hydration. In particular, reduced circulation and eccrine sweat gland activity in diabetics cause severe xerosis which can spiral into other severe foot problems.

Cosmetic Dermatology: Products and Procedures, Second Edition. Edited by Zoe Diana Draelos.
© 2016 John Wiley & Sons, Ltd. Published 2016 by John Wiley & Sons, Ltd.

Protective and regenerative moisturizing skin care is the foundation for treating all dry skin associated skin diseases and disorders. While the underlying cause of dry skin in any specific skin disorder needs to be addressed, frequently the symptomatic control of severe xerosis by appropriate moisturizers may reduce the need for more potent treatments, such as prolonged use of topical steroids and immune modulators, which can have detrimental side effects.

Moisturizing creams containing urea have been reported to improve the physical and chemical nature of the skin surface, with the manifest benefits of smoothing, softening, and making dry skin more pliable [2]. Traditional moisturizing emulsions have utilized non-physiologic emollients, humectants, and skin protectants to rehydrate the skin and reduce moisture loss. The identification and understanding of the structure and function of the stratum corneum barrier lipids and the role of water binding physiologic substances, collectively referred to as natural moisturizing factors (NMF), led to the development of formulations enriched in these actives. Recent recognition of the role of aquaporins, special moisture regulating channels, in skin cells has provided the opportunity for a new moisturization technology focusing on substances that stimulate and operate through aquaporins.

Moisturizing formulations and technologies

For thousands of years, oils, animal and vegetable fats, waxes and butters have been used to moisturize the skin. Recognized for their emollient or skin smoothing and softening properties, these substances were used to help restore dry skin to a more normal skin condition. The first significant advancement from these simple moisturizers occurred over a hundred years ago when emulsifiers were developed to create the first stable water-in-oil emulsion [3].

A simple emulsion can be defined as a heterogeneous system that contains very small droplets of an immiscible (or slightly miscible) liquid dispersed in another type of liquid. These emulsions consist of a hydrophilic (water loving) and a lipophilic (oil loving) portion, either of which can make up the external or internal phases of the emulsion system. The external phase generally comprises the majority of the emulsion while the smaller internal phase consists of the dispersed droplets. Most commonly used moisturizer formulations are either oil-in-water (O/W) emulsion systems, where aqueous components predominate, or water-in-oil (W/O), where the majority of ingredients are non-aqueous.

Emulsifiers are necessary components of emulsion systems as water-soluble and oil-soluble ingredients are not miscible. Emulsifiers are surface active agents that reduce the interfacial tension between the two incompatible phases to create stable emulsion systems. The properties of the chosen emulsifiers determine the final emulsion type.

Major progress in recent decades has enabled the formulation of increasingly complex emulsions (e.g. water-in-oil-in-water emulsions, multilamellar emulsions), which combine and stabilize many incompatible ingredients for moisturizing products with unique delivery characteristics that are both highly effective and aesthetically pleasing [4,5]. However, it is beyond the scope of this chapter to discuss the multitude of emulsion technologies which have been developed since the advent of the simple W/O system [6].

Occlusive materials and humectants are two major classes of moisturizing ingredients in many current moisturizers (Table 15.1). Occlusive materials coat the stratum corneum to inhibit transepidermal water loss (TEWL). Additionally, cholesterol, ceramides, and some essential and non-essential free fatty acids present in oils can help to replenish the natural lamellar barrier lipids that surround the squames in the stratum corneum, fortifying the barrier function of the skin. Some common examples of occlusive materials are petrolatum, olive oil, mineral oil, soybean oil, lanolin, beeswax, and jojoba oil. Petrolatum, lanolin, and mineral oil are considered occlusive materials, yet they also serve as emollients on the skin [7,8].

Humectants are materials that are capable of absorbing high amounts of water from the atmosphere and from the epidermis, drawing water into the stratum corneum for a smoother skin feel and look. Examples of well-known humectants include glycerin (or glycerol), sorbitol, urea, sodium hyaluronate, and propylene glycol. Glycerin is a widely used humectant with strong water binding capacity and holding ability, making it ideal for dry skin moisturizing formulations. Because of its importance in moisturizing products, it has been extensively reviewed elsewhere [9,10].

A number of commercially available hand and foot moisturizers incorporate combinations of both humectants and occlusive materials to deliver the optimal skin benefits (Table 15.2).

Natural moisturizing factors

The NMF are a collection of hygroscopic substances in the skin that act synergistically to confer effective water binding properties. The NMF has been reported to be composed of approximately 40% amino acids, 12% pyrrolidone carboxylic acid, 12% lactates, 7% urea, 18% minerals, and sugars, organic acids, citrates, and peptides [11]. These substances, derived largely from the breakdown products of the insoluble protein filaggrin, have an important role in maintaining moisture in the non-viable layers of the epidermis. Discovery of loss-of-function mutations in the filaggrin gene in many individuals with xerotic skin disorders including atopic dermatitis and psoriasis, and associated diminished levels of the NMF have confirmed the critical importance of filaggrin processing and these humectant substances in maintaining skin hydration and plasticity [12]. Due to the moisture gradient that exists from the well-hydrated dermis to the relatively moisture-deprived stratum corneum,

Table 15.1 Key classes of commonly used moisturizing ingredients.

Key classes	Moisturizing ingredients	Function in skin
Occlusives	Petrolatum Waxes Lanolin Mineral oil Cholesterol Ceramides Triglycerides and free fatty acids Sunflower oil Soybean oil Jojoba oil Olive oil Evening primrose oil Borage oil	Moisturization by occlusion of the stratum corneum and/or replenishment of lamellar barrier lipids
Humectants	Glycerin/glycerol Sorbitol Sodium hyaluronate Propylene glycol Amino acids* Lactate* Pyrrolidone carboxylic acid* Urea* Salts*	Draws water from the formulation base, atmosphere, and from the underlying epidermis to increase skin hydration *Natural moisturizing factor components – absorb large amounts of water even in relatively low humidities. Provide aqueous environment for key enzymatic functions in the skin

Table 15.2 Examples of commercially available hand and foot creams.

		Functions and claims	
Key ingredients		Hand cream	Foot cream
I	Glycolic acid, mineral oil, petrolatum	Exfoliation and moisturization by "occlusives" to both smooth and soften skin	Exfoliation and moisturization by "occlusives" to both smooth and soften skin
I	Glycerin, shea butter, almond oil, olive oil	Moisturization of hands and softening of cuticles	Moisturizes, soothes, and protects dry, cracked, and callused heels
III	Caprylic/capric triglycerides, glycerin, sunflower oil, olive oil, almond oil	Moisturization of hands, nails, and cuticles	Soothes and heals severely dry, cracked heels
IV	Beeswax, sweet almond oil	Moisturizes and softens dry skin	Prevents and heals cracked heels, calluses, corns, blisters
V	Lanolin, allantoin, glycerin, sunscreens: avobenzone, octinoxate	Moisturizes skin and helps treat the signs of aging	
VI	Glycerin, petrolatum, dimethicone, mineral oil	Helps form a protective moisture barrier; heals and protects dry hands with 24-hour moisturization	
VII	Urea, sodium lactate, glycerin	Gently exfoliates and moisturizes; relieves dry skin associated with hand eczema	Intensively moisturizes, smoothes and heals dry, cracked feet
VIII	Prescription urea (25%, 30%, 40%, or 50%), mineral oil, petrolatum	Healing and debriding of hyperkeratotic skin and nails	Healing and debriding of hyperkeratotic skin and nails

the cutaneous moisturization state is highly influenced by the occlusive barrier lipids in the stratum corneum and the humectant properties of the NMF [13]. Both are critical to retain moisture and resist TEWL and the dehydrating effects of the environment. Therefore, qualitative or quantitative changes in either the barrier lipids or the NMF components can alter skin hydration.

Urea is a major constituent of the water-soluble fraction of the stratum corneum [14]. Because of the high water binding capacity of urea, the water content in the skin depends on its concentration. In dry skin and in keratinization disorders, a deficit of urea is often found in the stratum corneum, confirming its importance in skin moisture balance. The concentration of urea has been reported to be reduced by approximately 50% in clinically dry skin compared to healthy skin [15,16]. The stratum corneum of unaffected psoriatic skin reveals no deficit in urea content, but levels in psoriatic lesions are reduced by 40% [17]. However, in patients with atopic dermatitis there is a deficit of about 70% in unaffected skin and about 85% in involved skin [18]. Urea has been demonstrated to be an effective moisturizer for a range of dry skin conditions [19], especially xerosis of the elderly [20,21]. Lodén has recently compiled a summary of clinical data on the treatment of diseased skin with urea-containing formulations [22]. Besides improvements in skin hydration, urea may be enhancing the levels of linoleic acid and ceramides [23], providing an additional skin benefit.

Urea is very soluble in water, but practically insoluble in lipids and lipid solvents. By its hydrogen-bond breaking effect, urea may expose water binding sites on keratin allowing the transport of water molecules into the stratum corneum, thereby leading to a plasticizing effect [24]. In addition, urea has proteolytic and keratolytic effects in concentrations above 10% [22]. These activities are exploited in prescription formulations of 12–50%, which are often employed for debriding purposes in keratinization disorders.

Lactic acid and salts of lactic acid, other efficacious components of NMF, have also been used to treat dry skin conditions [11]. Like urea, the principal moisturizing effect is brought about by their humectancy. However, additional benefits of barrier support and restoration may be attributed to these NMF as an increase in ceramide synthesis in keratinocytes treated with lactic acid has been reported [25].

Ultrastructural effects

Differential changes in skin hydration state and ultrastructure after the application of various moisturizing products can be observed using scanning electron microscopy (SEM) of frozen sections from skin biopsies [26]. Figure 15.1 depicts the epidermis of skin treated with a commercial lotion with 10% urea, sodium lactate, and glycerin (right), and treated with a vehicle lotion without urea, sodium lactate, and glycerin (left). From the SEM images it could be concluded that the product penetrated the entire stratum corneum, resulting in a more compact stratum corneum layer, with a 20–40% reduction in corneocyte thickness. When compared with an untreated control (not shown), the vehicle treatment did not have an influence on the stratum corneum thickness. The compaction of the stratum corneum by the urea product suggests an improved barrier function which has been confirmed in other clinical studies demonstrating a reduction in TEWL [23].

Clinical demonstrations of product efficacy of sodium lactate and urea formulations

Hand care
Several clinical studies were conducted to evaluate the ability of a fragrance-free, O/W emulsion containing 5% urea and 2.5% sodium lactate to fortify the skin of healthy subjects, and to moisturize, protect, and treat others with compromised hand skin.

Improvements in urea content
Thirty-one volunteers with healthy skin were enrolled in this study. Subjects refrained from the use of topical treatments for a period of 1 week and then applied the test product twice

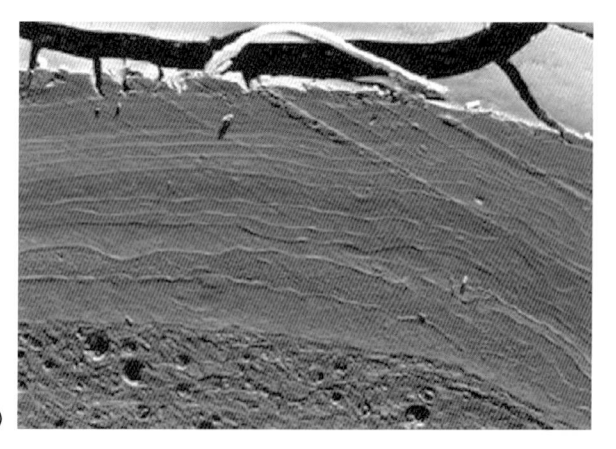

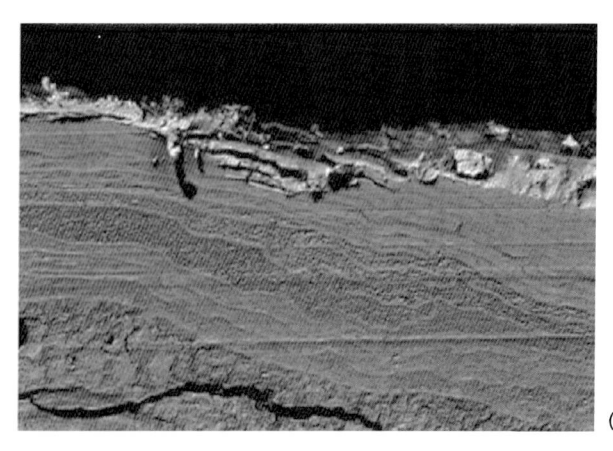

Figure 15.1 Freeze–fracture scanning electron micrographs of the stratum corneum of skin treated with a vehicle lotion (a) or the vehicle lotion containing 10% urea and sodium lactate (b).

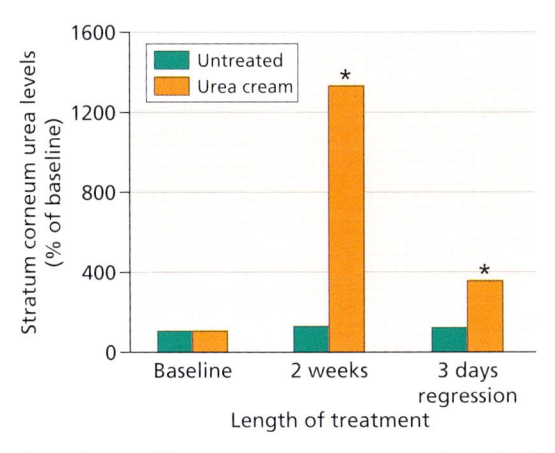

*Significant difference relative to untreated, p < 0.05

Figure 15.2 Stratum corneum urea content before application, after 2 weeks of daily use, and 3 days after discontinuing application of an oil-in-water emulsion containing 5% urea and 2.5% sodium lactate.

daily for 2 weeks. Urea content of the skin, moisturization state, and skin roughness were assessed at baseline, after 2 weeks of treatment, and 3 days after the last application. A significant increase ($p < 0.05$) in the urea content of the skin compared with untreated skin was observed (Figure 15.2) as well as significant improvements in skin hydration levels and roughness (data not shown). Franz cell porcine skin penetration studies confirmed the penetration and distribution of urea throughout the skin compartments 24 hours after application of a 5% urea body cream formulation: 54% in the stratum corneum, 7% in the viable epidermis, 22% in the dermis, and 17% in the receptor phase.

Improvement in eczema and xerosis

In a second 4-week controlled usage study, 23 subjects with hand eczema and 14 subjects with hand dermatitis/xerosis were enrolled. The subjects applied the test cream at least twice per day (morning and evening), and as often as needed. Clinical evaluations were made at baseline, and after 2 and 4 weeks of hand cream use for cracking/fissuring and dryness/scaling (0–8 scale), and erythema, edema, burning, stinging, and itching (0–3 scale). Subjects with eczema were also evaluated using an Investigator's Global Assessment for Eczema (0–5 scale). Digital photographs were taken at each of the clinical visits.

Significant improvements ($p < 0.05$) in clinical grading scores at week 4 relative to baseline were observed for dryness/scaling and cracking/fissuring, and the Investigators Global Assessment for Eczema (Table 15.3). Average irritation scores were also significantly reduced and negligible by week 4 for itching, stinging, and burning (data not shown).

Digital photographs captured the dry, compromised hand skin condition at the baseline visit, and demonstrated improvements that reflected the clinical assessments. Figure 15.3 shows the typical improvements observed in subjects at week 4 (right), compared with baseline (left).

Table 15.3 Mean clinical grading scores at baseline and after 4 weeks of daily use of a 5% urea and sodium lactate oil-in-water emulsion.

	Cracking/fissuring	Dryness/scaling	Eczema severity
Baseline	4.78	6.61	3.04
Week 4	2.91*	3.59*	1.66*

*Significant difference relative to baseline, $p \leq 0.05$.

In conclusion, appropriate hand care can both treat and prevent common dermatoses such as hand eczema.

Foot care

Patients with diabetes mellitus can exhibit a number of cutaneous manifestations as a result of changes in metabolic status and/or circulatory and neural degeneration [27]. Management of dry skin in these individuals is important to preserve barrier integrity which can help prevent bacterial and fungal infections. In particular, the heel skin can be very dry and scaly, prone to forming cracks and fissures which can lead to wounds that have difficulty healing.

A 6-week controlled usage study of a cream containing 10% urea, 5% sodium lactate, and glycerin as a daily treatment for the feet was conducted in 31 type I and II diabetic patients. This patient population was chosen because of their highly compromised foot skin condition. The subjects' heels were evaluated for roughness, scaling and cracking, and subjective irritation was also documented. Color photographs of the heels, taken before and after 6 weeks of treatment, documented the marked improvement in heel skin condition (Figure 15.4). In addition, significant reduction of roughness, scaling, and cracking was observed. In spite of the severely compromised skin condition at baseline, only one patient reported a mild irritation on the application site which did not interfere with his completing the study according to the protocol.

A second multicenter study of 604 patients with dry or severely dry, chapped feet and generalized xerosis (258, 42.7%), diabetes (179, 29.6%) or atopic dermatitis (113, 18.7%) was conducted in Germany and Austria. The patients applied a foot cream containing 10% urea, 5% sodium lactate, and glycerin at least twice daily for 2 weeks. While 319 patients used specific foot treatment products to care for their feet at the baseline visit, only 20 used other topical products in addition to the foot cream during the study period. The foot skin was clinically graded for xerosis, scaling, and cracking at baseline and after 2 weeks of treatment on a 5-point scale (none, slight, moderate, severe, or very severe). Table 15.4 documents the improvement in skin condition after 2 weeks of foot cream usage, showing significant and marked decreases in the percentage of patients with severe or very severe symptoms, and overall noticeable improvements in 95% of the patients. In this large patient population, the investigating dermatologists judged the tolerability to be very good or good in 96.7% of the patients, recommending continued product use.

144 HYGIENE PRODUCTS Moisturizers

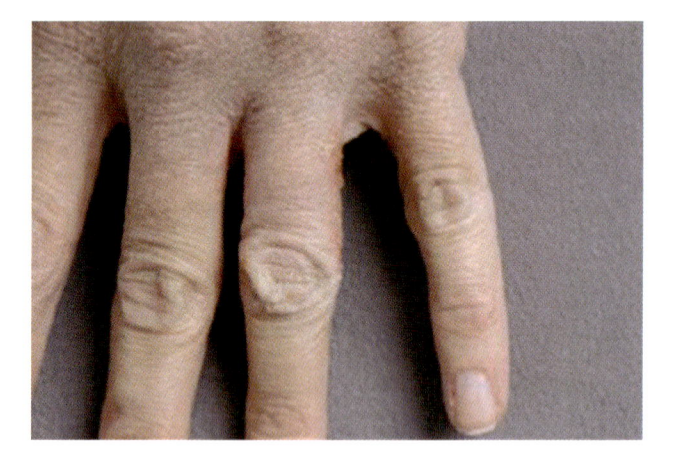

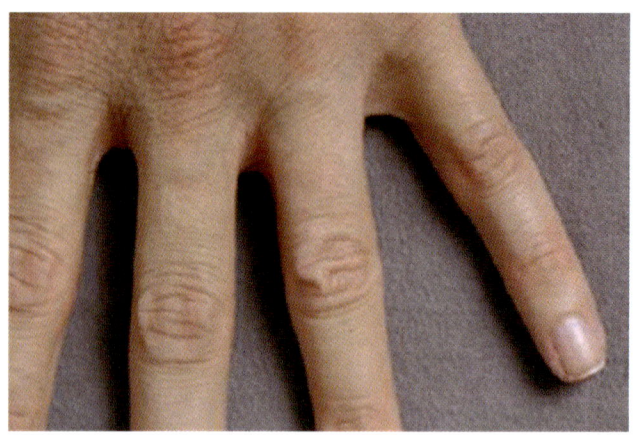

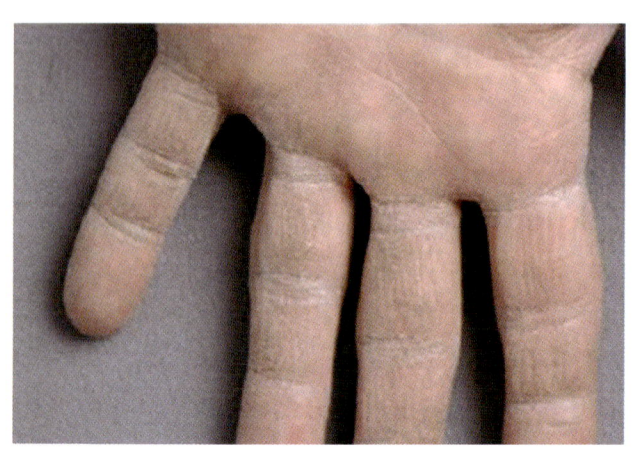

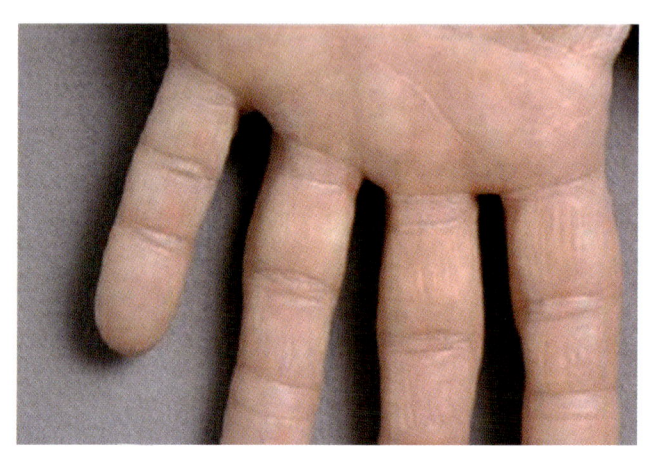

Figure 15.3 Improvement in hand eczema (top) and xerosis (bottom) after 4 weeks of daily usage (right) of a hand cream containing 5% urea and sodium lactate.

These data and many other published studies [19–23] support the therapeutic value and excellent safety profile of urea when administered topically to treat various dry skin conditions.

The future: Next-generation moisturizers

Water homeostasis of the epidermis is important for the appearance and physical properties of skin, as well as for the water balance of the body. Skin moisture balance depends on multiple factors including external humidity, uptake of water into the epidermis, skin barrier quality, and endogenous water binding substances. Biosynthesis and degradation of skin components is also influenced by water balance, impacting the moisturization state of the epidermal layers. In recent times, aquaporins (AQP), important hydration-regulating elements in the lower epidermis, have been described [28].

The first indications of the critical importance of AQP in regulating tissue hydration came from investigations of other organ systems, in particular the kidney [29]. Since their initial discovery, AQP genes have been cloned and, to date, 13 different genes (AQP1–13) have been identified [30]. The first proof for their relevance in skin came from Ma et al. [31] who produced knockout mice lacking AQP3, which exhibited reduced stratum corneum hydration. Studies confirmed the importance of these findings in dry human skin. Subjects whose epidermal barriers were damaged by a week-long tenside-based treatment that resulted in dry, compromised skin, showed a significant decrease in the number of AQP3 pores ($p = 0.04$). The pores were quantified by analysis of Western blots, and a 43% reduction in the dry skin samples was observed.

Further, in other skin conditions associated with skin dryness, a reduction in AQP3 has also been observed. Specifically, an age-related decline in AQP3 levels, as well as decreases associated with chronic sun exposure were reported [32].

Water and the moisturizing substances glycerol and urea have been found to be transported through the AQP in skin, providing moisture from within to the epidermis [33]. Expanding knowledge on the activity and regulation of AQP3 has led to the pursuit of a new class of actives that can modulate the expression of these water channels [34].

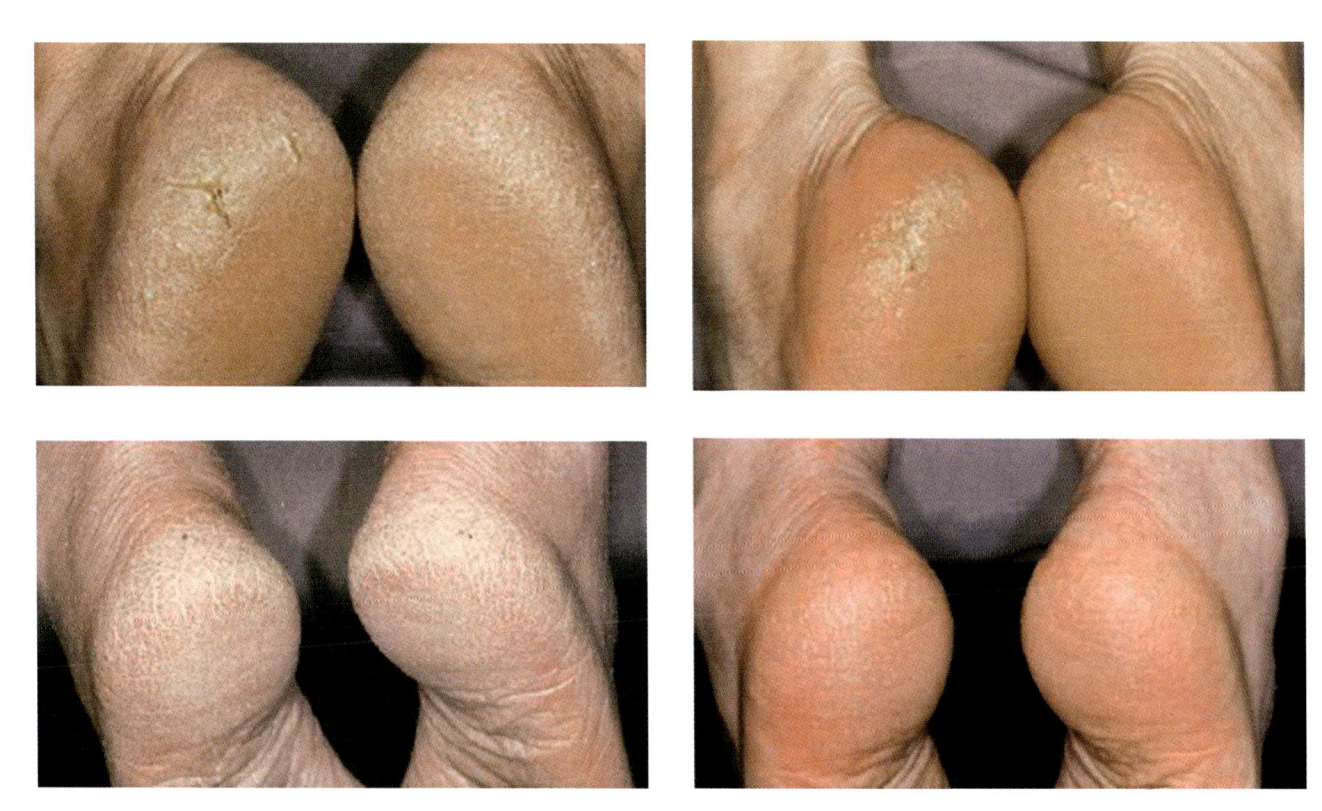

Figure 15.4 Improvement in diabetic foot skin after 6 weeks of daily usage of a foot cream containing 10% urea and 5% sodium lactate. Pretreatment photos (left) of two different subjects (top and bottom) and their corresponding week 6 photos (right).

Table 15.4 Clinical grading scores before and after 2 weeks of treatment. Percentage of patients with none or slight and severe or very severe symptoms (100% = 604 patients).

		None or slight (%)	Severe or very severe (%)
Xerosis	Baseline	5	67
	Week 2	69	6
Scaling	Baseline	22	44
	Week 2	79	6
Cracking	Baseline	26	32
	Week 2	66	8

Enhanced glycerol derivatives

In *vitro* studies on human keratinocytes demonstrated a significant increase in AQP3 levels by a specific enhanced glycerol derivative (EGD), glyceryl glucoside, designed and synthesized to confer specific structural and osmotic properties. Figure 15.5 depicts the enhanced AQP3 levels of EGD treated keratinocytes after 48 hours of incubation.

Additional *in vitro* and *in vivo* studies measuring AQP3 mRNA levels in human keratinocytes and skin confirmed these findings [35]. In contrast to glycerol treatment, EGD increased mRNA expression relative to the control. Further, to assess the efficacy of this new active, in vivo placebo-controlled studies were conducted. Figure 15.6 demonstrates the results of a study of 23 subjects, whose epidermal barriers were damaged by a tenside-based treatment, resulting in dry, compromised skin. The restoration of the epidermal barrier was assessed weekly by measuring TEWL on treated skin sites. The applied topical test lotions included a vehicle preparation, vehicle plus 6.5% glycerol, and the vehicle with 6.5% glycerol and 5% EGD.

After damaging the skin's barrier for 1 week, vehicle treatment was ineffective at restoring the barrier to baseline levels, exhibiting greater moisture loss levels in the skin. Treatment with the glycerol-containing vehicle showed a reduction of the TEWL compared with the vehicle. However, a superior and significant barrier restoration and fortification is observed with the glycerol–EGD containing formulation compared with both vehicle and vehicle with glycerol.

The moisturization and barrier-strengthening benefits of moisturizing formulations containing glyceryl-glucoside, urea and other components of the NMF were also investigated [36] Vehicle-controlled studies confirmed the additive benefits of these agents, underscoring the efficacy of addressing the deficiencies of xerotic skin conditions with topical formulations crafted with key ingredients that address the multiple factors in xerosis. Transported through the AQP3 channel, urea was

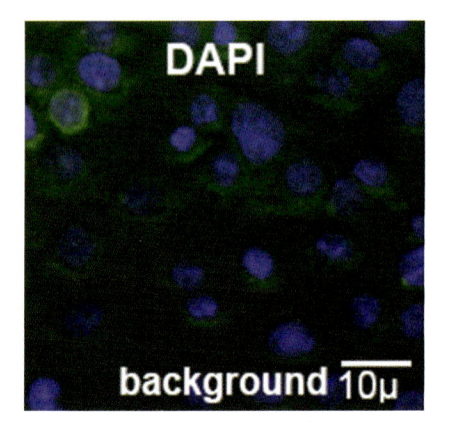

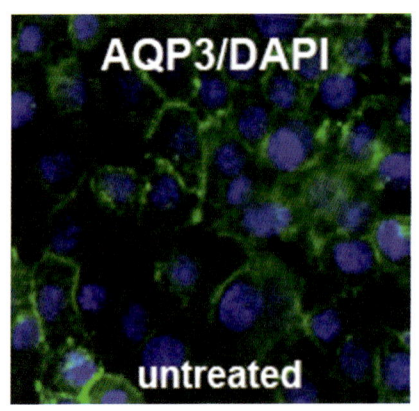

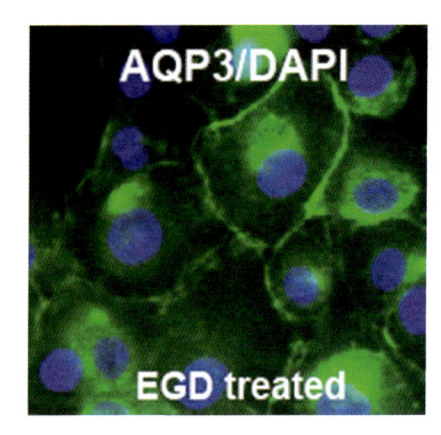

Figure 15.5 Immunohistochemical localization of the AQP3 protein in keratinocyte monolayers stained with a rabbit antihuman AQP3 antibody. Background control (left), untreated control (center), treatment with 3% enhanced glycerol derivative for 48 hours (right).

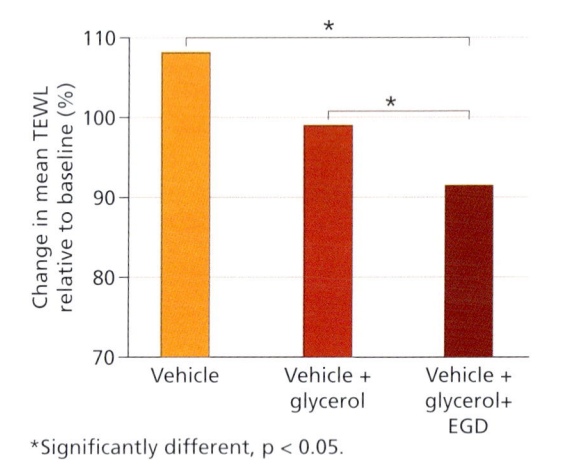

Figure 15.6 *In vivo* study of 23 volunteers with dry skin. Transepidermal water loss (TEWL) measurement after the following treatments: vehicle; vehicle with 6.5% glycerol; and vehicle with 6.5% glycerol and 5% enhanced glycerol derivative (EGD).

recently shown to upregulate expression of markers of keratinocyte differentiation, filaggrin, and lipid biosynthetic enzymes, responsible in part for the production of the lamellar lipids that constitute the barrier function, confirming a more complex regulatory function of this "tried and true" moisturizer that transcends its effect as a humectant [37].

Conclusions

Moisturizing substances have been used for thousands of years to improve the condition of compromised skin. The advent of stable emulsions and subsequent advancements in emulsion technologies provided improved elegance and efficacy for moisturizing products. More than 100 years of process refinements, discovery of new ingredients, and the growing understanding of NMF and biologic mechanisms that regulate the skin's moisture balance have contributed toward products with greatly enhanced stability, aesthetics, and efficacy. Elucidation of the multiple effects of urea, and the recent discovery and understanding of the function of AQP channels to regulate water balance and moisturization from within the skin provides a new appreciation of the complex mechanisms underlying moisture homeostasis of the skin. This knowledge provides new opportunities to create even better actives and multidimensional product formulations that address the multiple causes of xerotic skin conditions.

References

1. Draelos ZD. (2006) Cutaneous formulation issues. In: Draelos Z, Thamen L, eds. *Cosmetic Formulation of Skin Care Products*. New York: Taylor & Francis, pp. 3–34.
2. Zhai H, Maibach HI. (1998) Moisturizers in preventing irritant contact dermatitis: an overview. *Contact Dermatitis* **38**, 241–4.
3. Lifschütz I. (1906) Verfahren zur Herstellung stark wasseraufnahmefähiger Salbengrundlagen. Patent DE 167849.
4. Fluhr JW, Darlenski R, Surber C. (2008) Glycerol and the skin: holistic approach to its origin and functions. *Br J Dermatol* **159**, 23–34.
5. Epstein H. (2006) Skin care products. In: Paye M, Barel A, Maibach H, eds. *Handbook of Cosmetic Science and Technology*, 2nd edn. Boca Raton: CRC Press, pp. 427–39.
6. Schneider G, Gohla S, Kaden W, *et al.* (1993) Skin cosmetics. In: *Uhlmann's Encyclopedia of Industrial Chemistry*. Weinheim: VCH Verlagsgesellschaft, pp. 219–43.
7. Rajka G. (1995) Atopic dermatitis. In: Baran R, Maibach H, eds. *Cosmetic Dermatology*. London: Martin Dunitz, pp. 253–8.
8. Draelos ZD. (2005) Dry skin. In: DraelosZD, ed. *Cosmeceuticals*. Philadelphia: Elsevier Saunders, pp. 167–8.
9. Zocchi G. (2006) Skin feel agents. In: Paye M, Barrel A, Maibach H, eds. *Handbook of Cosmetic Science and Technology*, 2nd edn. Boca Raton: CRC Press, pp. 247–64.

10 Sagiv A, Dikstein S, Ingber A. (2001) The efficiency of humectants as skin moisturizers in the presence of oil. *Skin Res Technol* **7**, 32–8.

11 Harding CR, Rawlings AV. (2006) Effects of natural moisturizing factor and lactic acid isomers on skin function. In: Maibach HI, Lodén M, eds. *Dry Skin and Moisturizers: Chemistry and Function*, 2nd edn. Boca Raton: CRC Press LLC, pp. 187–209.

12 Fowler J. (2012) Understanding the role of natural moisturizing factor in skin hydration. *Practical Dermatol* **9**, 36–40.

13 Rawlings AV, Harding CR. (2004) Moisturization and skin barrier function. *Dermatol Ther* **17**, 43–8.

14 Swanbeck G. (1992) Urea in the treatment of dry skin. *Acta Derm Venereol* **177**, 7–8.

15 Mueller KH, Pflugshaupt C. (1979) Urea in dermatology I. *Zbl Haut* **142**, 157–68.

16 Mueller KH, Pflugshaupt C. (1982) Urea in dermatology II. *Zbl Haut* **167**, 85–90.

17 Proksch E. (1994) Harnstoff in der Dermatologie. *Dtsch Med Wochenschr* **119**, 1126–30.

18 Wellner K, Wohlrab W. (1993) Quantitative evaluation of urea in stratum corneum of human skin. *Arch Dermatol Res* **285**, 239–40.

19 Schölermann A, Filbry A, Rippke F. (2002) 10% urea: an effective moisturizer in various dry skin conditions. *Ann Dermatol Venereol* **129**, 1S422, P0259.

20 Schoelermann A, Banke-Bochita J, Bohnsack K, *et al.* (1998) Efficacy and safety of Eucerin® 10% urea lotion in the treatment of symptoms of aged skin. *J Dermatol Treat* **9**, 175–9.

21 Norman RA. (2003) Xerosis and pruritus in the elderly: recognition and management. *Dermatol Ther* **16**, 254–9.

22 Lodén M. (2006) Clinical evidence for the use of urea. In: Lodén M, Maibach HI, eds. *Dry Skin and Moisturizers. Chemistry and Function*, 2nd edn. Boca Raton: Taylor & Francis, pp. 211–25.

23 Pigatto PD, Bigardi AS, Cannistraci C, Picardo M. (1996) 10% urea cream (Eucerin) for atopic dermatitis: a clinical and laboratory evaluation. *J Dermatolog Treat* **7**, 171–6.

24 McCallion R, Wan Po AL. (1993) Dry and photo-aged skin: manifestations and management. *J Clin Pharm Ther* **18**, 15–32.

25 Rawlings AV, Davies A, Carlomusto M, *et al.* (1995) Effect of lactic acid isomers on keratinocyte ceramide synthesis, stratum corneum lipid levels and stratum corneum barrier function. *Arch Dermatol Res* **288**, 383–90.

26 Richter T, Peuckert C, Sattler M, *et al.* (2004) Dead but highly dynamic: the stratum corneum is divided into three hydration zones. *Skin Pharmacol Physiol* **17**, 246–57.

27 Nikkels-Tassoudji N, Henry F, Letawe C, *et al.* (1996) Mechanical properties of the diabetic waxy skin. *Dermatology* **192**, 19–22.

28 Hara-Chikuma M, Verkman AS. (2008) Roles of aquaporin-3 in the epidermis. *J Invest Dermatol* **128**, 2145–51.

29 Agre P. (2006) Aquaporin water channels: from atomic structure to clinical medicine. *Nanomed Nanotechnol Biol Med* **2**, 266–7.

30 Verkman AS. (2008) Mammalian aquaporins: diverse physiological roles and potential clinical significance. *J Exp Med* **10**, 1–18.

31 Ma T, Hara M, Sougrat R, *et al.* (2002) Impaired stratum corneum hydration in mice lacking epidermal water channel aquaporin-3. *J Biol Chem* **27**, 17147–53.

32 Dumas M, Sadick NS, Noblesse E, *et al.* (2007) Hydrating skin by stimulating biosynthesis of aquaporins. *J Drugs Dermatol* **6** (Suppl), 20–4.

33 Hara M, Verkman AS. (2003) Glycerol replacement corrects defective skin hydration, elasticity, and barrier function in aquaporin-3-deficient mice. *Proc Natl Acad Sci USA* **100**, 7360–5.

34 Draelos Z. (2012) Aquaporins; An introduction to a key factor in the mechanism of skin hydration. *J Clin Aesthet Derm* **5**(7), 53–56.

35 Schrader A, Siefken W, Kueper T, Breitenbach U, *et al.* (2012) Effects of glyceryl glucoside on AQP3 expression, barrier function and hydration of human skin. *Skin Pharm. Skin Physiol* **25**, 192–199.

36 Weber TM, Kausch M, Rippke F, Schoerlermann AM, Filbry A (2012) Treatment of xerosis with a topical formulation containing glyceryl glucoside, natural moisturizing factors, and ceramide. *J Clin Aesthet Dermatol* **5**, 29–39.

37 Grether-Beck S, Felsner I, Brenden H, *et al.* (2012) Urea uptake enhances barrier function and antimicrobial defense in humans by regulating epidermal gene expression. *J Invest Derm* **132**(6), 1561–72.

CHAPTER 16
Sunless Tanning Products

Angelike Galdi, Peter Foltis, and Christian Oresajo

L'Oréal Research, Clark, NJ, USA

> **BASIC CONCEPTS**
> - Tanned skin is considered attractive among fair-skinned individuals.
> - Self-tanning preparations containing dihydroxyacetone (DHA) induce a temporary safe staining of the skin simulating sun-induced tanning.
> - Self-tanners are formulated into sprays, lotions, creams, gels, mousses, and cosmetic wipes.
> - The tanning effect of DHA begins in the deeper part of the stratum corneum before expanding over the entire stratum corneum and stratum granulosum resulting in the production of brown melanoidins.
> - DHA products do not confer photoprotection unless sunscreen filters are added to the formulation.

Introduction

Social norms for tanning in the USA have dramatically changed in recent times. The presence of a tanned body at one time conveyed the social status of an outdoor laborer. Now, having a tan, especially during the winter months, indicates affluence.

More information has become available regarding the deleterious effects of UV exposure. [1–3]. The public is beginning to understand the dangers, thereby modifying their lifestyle choices towards safer practices. However, the change has been slow because sun exposure behavior is in part influenced by psychologic and societal factors [4–6]. Self-tanning preparations are becoming an increasingly important option for those desiring the tanned look but not exposing themselves to undue harm.

Sunless tanning products

Definition

Self-tanning products, or sunless tanners, are preparations that when applied topically impart a temporary coloration to the skin mimicking skin color of naturally sun-tanned skin. Depending on the formulation and the active ingredients, the onset of color formation can be anything from immediate to several hours and can last up to 1 week.

Self-tanning formulations were introduced in the 1960s. Consumers' acceptability soon waned because of unattractive results such as orange hands, streaking, and poor coloration. Because of these drawbacks, consumers today still associate sunless tanning with these undesirable results. However, improved formulations have appeared on the market. Refinements in the dihydroxyacetone (DHA) manufacturing process has aided in the creation of formulations that produce a more natural-looking color and better longevity.

Active ingredients

The most widely used and most efficacious active ingredient in self-tanners is DHA. It is the only ingredient that is currently recognized as a self-tanning agent by the US Food and Drug Administration (FDA) [7]. DHA-based sunless tanners have been recommended by the Skin Cancer Foundation, the American Academy of Dermatology Association, and the American Medical Association [8–10]. DHA is a triose and is the simplest of all ketoses (Figure 16.1).

Mechanism of action of DHA

Ketones and aldehydes react with primary amines to form Schiff bases [11]. This is similar to the Maillard reaction, also known as non-enzymatic browning, and involves, more specifically, the reaction between carbohydrates and primary amines [12].

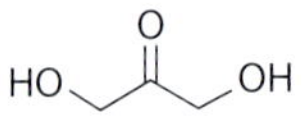

Figure 16.1 Chemical structure of dihydroxyacetone (DHA).

Cosmetic Dermatology: Products and Procedures, Second Edition. Edited by Zoe Diana Draelos.
© 2016 John Wiley & Sons, Ltd. Published 2016 by John Wiley & Sons, Ltd.

DHA is able to penetrate into the epidermis because of its size. Pyruvic acid is formed from DHA and either can react with sterically unhindered terminal amino groups in the amino acids of epidermal proteins. The epsilon amino group of lysine and the guanido group of arginine are particularly susceptible to nucleophilic attack by the reactive carbonyl oxygen. Epidermal proteins contain high concentrations of both of these amino acids. Based on photoacoustic depth profilometry, the tanning effect of DHA begins in the deeper part of the stratum corneum layer (15–22 μm) before expanding over the entire stratum corneum and stratum granulosum [13,14]. Subsequent steps of the reaction mechanism are not fully understood. The resultant products are brown in color and are collectively referred to as melanoidins.

Alternate actives

As previously stated, US federal regulations recognize only DHA as a sunless tanning agent [7]. Alternative technologies exist, however, with the capability to impart an artificial tan to the skin.

Reducing sugars other than DHA can act as Maillard reaction intermediates and therefore have the potential for use as sunless tanning agents [15]. Reducing sugars, in basic solution, form some aldehyde or ketone. This allows the sugar to act as a reducing agent in the Maillard reaction of non-enzymatic browning. Reducing sugars include glucose, fructose, glyceraldehyde, lactose, arabinose, and maltose.

Unfortunately, a large amount of heat energy is required to trigger the glycation reaction between glucose, the most commonly known reducing sugar, and free amines. Such properties render many reducing sugars useless for sunless tanning products. An exception is the keto-tetrose, erythulose. Although this reducing sugar produces a more gradual tan than DHA, it has been utilized as a self-tanning enhancer for years.

As corporations continue to aggressively pursue new sunless tanning technologies, reducing sugars may provide the next generation of self-tanning actives.

Formulation challenges

The content of DHA in self-tanning products depends on the desired browning intensity on the skin and is normally used in the range 4–8%. Depending on the type of formulation and skin type, a tan appears on the skin about 2–3 hours after use. During product storage, the pH of a DHA-containing formulation will drift over time to about 3–4. At this pH, DHA is particularly stable. In order to ensure end product stability, certain key factors must be considered.

pH and buffers

The pH of DHA-containing formulation drops during storage. The resulting pH lies in the range of 3–4. In the past, buffering was recommended to keep the pH at a level of 4–6. However, investigations have since shown that the storage stability of DHA could be increased when formulations are kept at a pH of 3–4 and buffering at a higher pH enhances the degradation of DHA [16]. The pH of a formulation may be adjusted to approximately 3–4 by using a small amount of citric acid or using acetate buffers as they do not affect DHA stability [17].

Processing and storage of DHA

Storage and heating of DHA above 40 °C should be avoided as it causes rapid degradation. During manufacturing processes that require heating (as in the case of emulsions), DHA should not be added until the formulation has been cooled down to below 40 °C. Additionally, finished products containing DHA should be sold in opaque, or other UV-protective packaging, as well as resealable packaging, to limit exposure to air.

Nitrogen-containing compounds

Amines and other nitrogen-containing compounds should be avoided in DHA-containing formulations. This includes collagen, urea derivatives, amino acids, and proteins. The reactivity of DHA towards these compounds can lead to its degradation, therefore resulting in the loss in efficacy and acceptability of resulting color. However, some commercial formulations combine DHA with nitrogen-containing containing compounds (e.g. amino acids). This combination provides a perceptual advantage to customers as provides within tanning 1 hour as a result of the accelerated reaction between DHA and amino acids. This tan is not substantive, however, and most of it is easily washed off [17].

Sunscreens

A tan achieved with DHA alone does not offer sun protection comparable to that of sunscreens. However, it is possible to combine DHA with sunscreens to achieve a product with sun protection. Inorganic sunscreens such as titanium dioxide, zinc oxide, and nitrogen-containing sunscreens should be avoided as they induce rapid degradation of DHA.

As a final stability check, periodic determination of DHA dosage is recommended to ensure end product and long-term stability and efficacy. A simple high performance liquid chromatography (HPLC) method exists using an amine column with acetonitrile/water (75 : 25) as a mobile phase. Detection is at 270 nm.

Delivery vehicles

Creams and lotions

Self-tanning creams and lotions tend to be the most widely used of all of the self-tanning vehicles. Our studies have confirmed that although conventional, creams and lotions are preferred by consumers because of their ease of use and reduced likelihood of having streaky color results. This is most likely because of the extended play time (e.g. rub-in time) offered by cream and lotion vehicles.

In selecting the appropriate ingredients for formulation, the use of non-ionic emulsifiers is recommended over ionic emulsifiers because of improved stability of the DHA [16]. Additionally, xanthan gum and polyquaternium-10 may be used for thickening emulsions.

Emollients have an important role in many self-tanning formulations as they impart hydration to the skin, play time during application, and a smooth and silky after feel. Types of emollients include oils, waxes, fatty alcohols, silicone materials, and certain esters.

Emulsions with DHA are particularly susceptible to microbial attack. Parabens, phenoxyethanol, and mixtures thereof are recommended [16].

Gels and gelees

Thickening formulations containing DHA, particularly to produce a clear gel, is relatively difficult because many of the conventional thickeners are not compatible with DHA. Studies have found that hydroxyethylcellulose, methylcellulose, and silica are good choices, whereas carbomers, PVM/MA decadiene crosspolymer, and magnesium aluminum silicate are not acceptable as they cause rapid degradation of DHA [16].

Silicones such as dimethicone and cyclomethicones have increased in popularity over recent years, particularly for producing water-in-silicone emulsions (typically classified as gelees). Gelees are similar in appearance to gels; however, they tend to offer improved play time and skin feel over gels as they contain high levels of the silicone emollients.

Regulatory considerations

The US FDA considers sunless tanning actives as color additives as they impart color to the skin. According to 21CFR70, color additives are defined as: "A dye, pigment, or other substance…that, when added or applied to a food, drug or cosmetic or to the human body or any part thereof, is capable (alone or through reaction with another substance) of imparting a color thereto" [18].

The actives permitted in the sunless tanning products in the USA are limited to those approved for use as such. The following color additives appear in the Code of Federal Regulations in Tables 16.1 and 16.2.

Labeling requirements are also specified under current FDA guidelines. All sunless tanning products that do not contain sun protection factor (SPF) protection must be labeled with the following warning statement (US Code of Federal Regulations): "Warning – This product does not contain a sunscreen and does not protect against sunburn. Repeated exposure of unprotected skin while tanning may increase the risk of skin aging, skin cancer and other harmful effects to the skin even if you do not burn" [18].

Table 16.1 Color additives exempt from certification per 21CFR73 2003 (US Code of Federal Regulations).

Aluminum powder	Copper powder	Luminescent zinc
Annatto	Dihydroxyacetone	Manganese violet
β-Carotene	Disodium EDTA copper	Mica
Bismuth citrate	Ferric ammonium ferrocyanide	Potassium sodium copper
Bismuth oxychloride	Ferric ferrocyanide	Pyrophyllite
Bronze powder	Guaiazulene	Silver
Caramel	Guanine	Sulfide
Carmine	Henna	Titanium dioxide
Chromium oxide greens	Iron oxides	Ultramarines
Chlorophyllin	Lead acetate	Zinc oxide

Table 16.2 Color additives per 21CFR73 2003 (US Code of Federal Regulations).

Citrus Red No. 2	D&C Red No. 17	D&C Yellow No. 10
D&C Blue No. 4	D&C Red No. 21	D&C Yellow No. 11
D&C Blue No. 6	D&C Red No. 22	Ext. D&C Violet No. 2
D&C Blue No. 9	D&C Red No. 27	Ext. D&C Yellow No. 7
D&C Brown No. 1	D&C Red No. 28	FD&C Blue No. 1
D&C Green No. 5	D&C Red No. 30	FD&C Blue No. 2
D&C Green No. 6	D&C Red No. 31	FD&C Red No. 3
D&C Green No. 8	D&C Red No. 33	FD&C Red No. 4
D&C Orange No. 4	D&C Red No. 34	FD&C Red No. 40
D&C Orange No. 5	D&C Red No. 36	FD&C Yellow No. 5
D&C Orange No. 10	D&C Red No. 39	FD&C Yellow No. 6
D&C Orange No. 11	D&C Violet No. 2	Orange B
D&C Red No. 6	D&C Yellow No. 7	Phthalocyaninato2-Copper
D&C Red No. 7	D&C Yellow No. 8	

Product attributes

Coloration

The onset of coloration starts at approximately 2–3 hours and will continue to darken for 24–72 hours after a single application, depending on formulation and skin type. Because DHA forms covalent bonds with epidermal proteins, the tan will not sweat off or wash away with soap or water. The color gradually fades over 3–10 days, in conjunction with stratum corneum exfoliation. Any product or process that increases the rate of cell turnover or removes portions of the stratum corneum will decrease the longevity of the color. Thus, preparations containing alpha- and beta-hydroxyacids and retinoids, as well as microdermabrasion creams and the process of shaving, decrease the longevity of coloration from self-tanning products.

Evaluation

Various spectrophotometric methods can be used to evaluate the coloration parameters of self-tanners such as onset of color and longevity of color. The most popular is the L*a*b* standard from Commission Internationale d'Eclairage (CIE). The three coordinates of CIELAB represent the lightness of the color (L* = 0 yields black and L* = 100 indicates diffuse white), its position between red/magenta and green (a*, negative values indicate green while positive values indicate magenta), and its position between yellow and blue (b*, negative values indicate blue and positive values indicate yellow). The total color difference between any two colors in $L^*a^*b^*$ can be approximated by treating each color as a point in a three-dimensional space (with three components: L^*, a^*, b^*) and taking the Euclidean distance between them (ΔE). ΔE is calculated as the square root of the sum of the squares of ΔL*, Δa* and Δb* [19]. It is generally recognized that 1.5 ΔE units is the minimal difference detectable to the eye. Comparisons to baseline readings can yield onset of tanning (usually readings at 30 minutes, 60 minutes, etc.) and longevity of tanning (readings at 48 hours, 72 hours, etc.).

Moisturization

The recent trend in cosmetic products is to be multifunctional. Moisturizing formulations are increasing in popularity in keeping with this trend. Formulations with 8–24 hour hydration claims are not uncommon. Current self-tanners are formulated into sprays, lotions, creams, gels, mousses, and cosmetic wipes. In general, there are no obstacles to obtaining satisfactory levels of hydration, although there are some compromises that may have to be made. Alcohol is often incorporated to achieve quick drying formulations. The trade-off is sacrificing some level of hydration. This can be offset with humectants such as glycerin or sodium hyaluronate.

Trends in sunless tanning

Daily use moisturizers/glow

Face and body moisturizers with low levels of DHA have grown in popularity over the past 5 years. Although not new to the market, the concept of using a daily moisturizer that imparts gradual color was particularly well-received by the faint in heart who were afraid of making mistakes and/or turning orange with the use of traditional sunless tanners. Typically formulated with 1–3% DHA, glow moisturizers are easy to apply and, depending on the formulation and user's skin tone, may impart a darker shade to the skin after 1–3 applications.

No-rub mists

No-rub sunless tanning mists have been sought out as the less expensive alternatives to the airbrushing trend. These multiangle applicator systems allow for simple, even, and often hands-free application. The formulation base systems are typically hydroalcoholic or aqueous solutions, therefore allowing for quick-drying properties.

Sunless tanning spray booths

A growing trend is the professional whole body application in aerosolized form. The suitably clad consumer is sprayed with a uniform fine mist. The consumer is instructed to close their eyes or wear suitable eye protection, hold their breath or wear nose plugs to avoid inhalation, and wear a shower cap to protect the hair. While the cost is generally higher for this application compared to self-application of a consumer product, the results tend to be more uniform and controlled.

Sunless tanning products with UV protection

The tan imparted by sunless tanners is not adequate to protect against UVB and UVA damage. Sunless tanners must therefore carry the required FDA warning statement [19]. Sunless tanning products that do contain sunscreen are growing in popularity because of their multifunctional properties. If sunless tanners do carry an SPF claim, the product labeling and testing must comply with the FDA Sunscreen Monograph published in 2011.

Conclusions

With an increasing awareness of the harmful acute and chronic effects of UV damage, sunless tanning use remains a popular alternative to tan seekers. Modern day formulations are efficacious, well-tolerated, easy-to-use, and provide natural looking results. A probable increase in patient compliance of safe sun practices can therefore be anticipated.

References

1. Jemal A, Siegel R, Ward E, *et al.* (2006) Cancer statistics, 2006. *CA Cancer J Clin* **56**, 106–30.
2. American Cancer Society. (2006) *Cancer Facts and Figures 2006: American Cancer Society.*
3. Elwood JM (1993). Recent developments in melanoma epidemiology, 1993. *Melanoma Res* **3**, 149–56.
4. Garvin T, Wilson K. (1999) The use of storytelling for understanding women's desires to tan: lessons from the field. *Professional Geographer* Vol. 51, **2**, 297–306.
5. Cokkinides V, Weinstock M, Glanz K, Albano J, Ward E, Thun M. (2006) Trends in sunburns, sun protection practices, and attitudes toward sun exposure protection and tanning among US adolescents, 1998–2004. *Pediatrics* **118**, 853–64.
6. Cokkinides V, Weinstock MA, O'Connell MC, Thun MJ. (2002) Use of indoor tanning sunlamps by US youth, ages 11–18 years, and by their parents or guardian caregivers: prevalence and correlates. *Pediatrics* **109**, 1124–30.
7. United States Code of Federal Regulations 21CFR 73.2150, 2002.
8. www.skincancer.org
9. www.aad.org
10. www.ama-assn.org
11. Morrison RT, Boyd RN. (1973) *Organic Chemistry*. Boston, MA: Allyn and Bacon.

12 Lloyd RV, Fong AJ, Sayre RM. (2001) In Vivo formation of Maillard reaction free radicals in mouse skin. *J Invest Dermatol* **117**, 740–2.
13 Puccetti G, Tranchant JF, Leblanc RM. (1999) The stability and penetration of epidermal applications visualized by photoacoustic depth profilometry. Sixth Conference International Society of Skin Imaging, Skin Research and Technology, Berlin, Germany.
14 Puccetti G, Leblanc R. (2000) A sunscreen-tanning compromise: 3D visualization of the actions of titanium dioxide particles and dihydroxyacetone on human epiderm. *Photochem Photobiol* **71**, 426–30.
15 Shaath N. (2005) *Sunscreens Regulation and Commercial Development*. Boca Raton, FL: Taylor & Francis Group.
16 Chaudhuri R. Dihydroxyacetone: Chemistry and Applications in Self-Tanning Products. White Paper; 7.
17 Kurz T. (1994) Formulating effective self-tanners with DHA. *Cosmet Toiletries* **109**, 55–60.
18 United States Code of Federal Regulations. 21CFR740.19, 2003.
19 Minolta. (1993) Precise Color Communication, Color Control from Feeling to Instrumentation. Minolta Camera Co. Ltd.

CHAPTER 17
Sunscreens

Dominique Moyal,[1] Angelike Galdi,[2] and Christian Oresajo[2]
[1]La Roche-Posay Laboratoire Dermatologique, Asnières sur Seine, France
[2]L'Oréal Research and Innovation, Clark, NJ, USA

> **BASIC CONCEPTS**
> - Photoprotection is required for both UVB and UVA radiation.
> - Organic and inorganic filters are used in sunscreens.
> - Sunscreen filters must be carefully combined to achieve esthetically pleasant products with photo-stability and well-balanced UVB-UVA photoprotection, as defined by UVAPF being at least one-third of the SPF value.
> - International acceptance of the same UV filters would benefit the consumers.
> - There is a need for harmonization of testing methods and labeling to afford the same information of efficacy to the consumers.

Introduction

Human skin exposure to UVR from sunlight can cause many adverse effects. These involve both UVB (290–320 nm) and UVA (320–400 nm). UVB rays are mainly responsible for the most severe damage being acute such as sunburn, and long-term skin cancer included. They directly impact DNA and proteins [1]. Unlike UVB, UVA rays are not directly absorbed by biologic targets [2] but can still dramatically impair cell and tissue functions:

- UVAs penetrate deeper into the skin than UVB. They particularly affect connective tissue inducing the production of detrimental reactive oxygen species (ROS) which in turn damage DNA, cells, vessels, and tissues [3–8].
- UVAs are potent inducers of immunosuppression [9,10] and their contribution to the development of malignant melanoma and squamous tumors is a growing concern [11,12].
- Photosensitivity reactions and photodermatoses are primarily mediated by UVAs [13].

It is important to note that under all weather conditions, the UVA irradiance is at least 17 times higher than the UVB irradiance.

For all these reasons, sunscreens must evidently contain both UVA and UVB filters to protect skin from these two associated harmful rays.

Regulatory status of sunscreens

With increased knowledge about UV-induced skin damage and particularly the effects of UVA, public educational programs have been developed, emphasizing on the proper use of sun-screening products. Many new UV filters have been made available in the last decade with improved efficacy and safety, of a slow process in some countries for regulatory reasons. In the US as example, some UVA and UVB filters are still not approved for use, albeit marketed elsewhere since many years without any safety issue for consumers. The availability of efficient sunscreen products depends not only upon the regulatory status of the UV filters but on the ability to inform the consumer about product efficacy with appropriate labels based on sun protection factor (SPF) and UVA protection level.

Sunscreen products can be classified in two main categories according to their purpose:

1. *Primary sunscreens.* Products directly intending to protect skin from the effects of the sun, such as beach sunscreens and products used for outdoor activities.
2. *Secondary sunscreens.* Products that have a primary use other than skin protection, such as daily moisturizing creams, anti-wrinkle/antiaging creams, whitening skin products and make-up products. In these products, sun protection is necessary to optimize the claimed effect. For this category of products, sun

---

Cosmetic Dermatology: Products and Procedures, Second Edition. Edited by Zoe Diana Draelos.
© 2016 John Wiley & Sons, Ltd. Published 2016 by John Wiley & Sons, Ltd.

protection is an additional claim, i.e. not their main objective, despite becoming essential for daily exposed areas.

Sunscreen classification

Sunscreen products can also be classified in terms of regulatory status. Sunscreen products enter legally in the cosmetic category in the European Union (EU), non-EU Europe countries (e.g. Russia), most African and Middle-Eastern countries, India, Latin America, and Japan. They are classified as "special" cosmetic products in China (special cosmetics), Korea and Ethiopia (functional cosmetics), South Africa (under SABS standard), Australia (under standards) [14], and Taïwan (medicated cosmetics). As all products claiming a SPF, they belong to the over-the-counter (OTC) drugs in the USA [15]. In Canada, they can be either OTC drugs or natural health products (NHP), where in such a case the sunscreening agents should only be "natural" ingredients: titanium dioxide, zinc oxide.

Approved UV filters

In the EU, 27 UV filters are listed in Annex VII of the Cosmetics Directive. Zinc oxide both under non-nano and nano forms should be added in 2015. In the USA, 16 filters are included in the sunscreen monograph (Table 17.1). There are two main regulatory methods to market OTC products: monograph or a New Drug Application (NDA). The latter is necessary to obtain the approval of a formula containing a new UV filter, a new concentration for an approved active ingredient, or a new mixture of approved actives.

A Time and Extent Application (TEA) is a new procedure established by the FDA in 2002, for an active ingredient already approved abroad. It allows the FDA to accept commercial data obtained on external markets in place of use of an authorized drug on the US market. However, toxicologic data file required for a TEA is very similar to that for an NDA.

The following 8 UV filters are currently eligible for evaluation through a TEA procedure.

1 Isoamyl p-methoxycinnamate (amiloxate) 10% max.
2 Methyl benzylidene camphor (enzacamene) 4% max.
3 Octyl triazone 5% max.
4 Methylene bis-benzotriazolyl tetramethylbutylphenol (bisoctrizole) 10% max.
5 Bis-ethylhexyloxyphenol methoxyphenol triazine (Bemotrizinol) 10% max.
6 Diethylhexyl butamido triazone (Iscotrizinol) 3% max.
7 Terephthalylidene dicamphor sulfonic acid (Ecamsule) 10% max.
8 Drometrizole trisiloxane 15% max.

Unfortunately the TEA process is not working because FDA has not approved a sunscreen ingredient through this process since it began. Many stakeholders in USA consider that FDA has failed consumers as the UV filters available abroad offer enhanced protection and that the lack of reliable process is a disincentive to innovation.

In Australia, 26 UV filters are accepted by the Therapeutic Goods Administration (TGA) and in Japan 31 UV filters are allowed.

When comparing the approved UV filters in EU and the USA, only 11 filters appear in common. Terephtalilydene dicamphor sulfonic acid (TDSA) is available in the USA under NDA for four formulas only.

Because of the importance of being well-protected against UVA radiation, there are many new UVA filters or broad UVB/UVA filters, which have been developed and approved in EU, Australia, and Japan. It is obvious that the number of these filters is highly limited in the USA (Table 17.2). In addition, the

Table 17.1 Sunscreens approved in the USA.

Sunscreen approved in the USA	Maximum concentration (%)
p-Aminobenzoic acid (PABA)	15
Avobenzone	3
Cinoxate	3
Dioxybenzone	3
Ensulizole (phenylbenzimidazole sulfonic acid)	4
Homosalate	15
Meradimate (menthyl anthranilate)	5
Octinoxate (octyl methoxycinnamate)	7.5
Octisalate (octyl salicylate)	5
Octocrylene	10
Octyl dimethyl PABA	8
Oxybenzone (Benzophenone-3)	6
Salisobenzone	10
Titanium dioxide	25
Trolamine salicylate	12
Zinc oxide	25

Table 17.2 Regulatory approval status for the main UVB/UVA and UVA filters.

Benzophenone-3 (Oxybenzone)	EU, Japan, Australia, Canada, USA
BMDM (avobenzone)	EU[1], Japan[1], Australia[1], Canada[2], USA[2]
TDSA (Ecamsule, Mexoryl ®SX)	EU, Japan, Australia, Canada, USA (NDA)
DTS (Mexoryl ®XL)	EU, Japan, Australia, Canada
DPDT (Neo-Heliopan ®AP)	EU, Australia
DHHB (Uvinul ®A+)	EU, Japan, Australia[3]
MBBT (Tinosorb ®M)	EU, Japan, Australia
BEMT (Tinosorb ®S)	EU[4], Japan[2], Australia[4]
Titanium dioxide	EU, Japan, Australia, Canada, USA
Zinc oxide	Japan, Australia, Canada, USA

[1] Max at 5%.
[2] Max at 3%.
[3] Only in primary sunscreens.
[4] Max at 10%.

use of avobenzone in the USA has some limitations. Combinations with some other UV filters, such as titanium dioxide and enzulizole, are not permitted and the maximum level according to the sunscreen monograph is restricted to 3% whereas up to 5% is approved by regulation in EU, Australia, Korea and 10% in Japan.

Mutual recognition of UV filters safety by the authorities of these countries would have positive repercussions on the international situation which can benefit consumers.

Development of sunscreens

- A proper sunscreen product must fulfil the following critical requirements:
- Provide efficient protection against UVB and UVA radiation;
- Being stable to heat and to UVR (photo-stable);
- Being user-friendly to encourage frequent application and provide reliable protection; and
- Cost-effective.

In order to protect against both UVB and UVA, the sunscreen product must contain a combination of active ingredients within a complex vehicle matrix.

Active ingredients can be either organic or inorganic UV filters. According to their chemical nature and their physical properties, they can act by absorbing, reflecting, or diffusing UVRs.

Organic UV filters

How do organic filters work?

Organic filters are active ingredients that absorb UVR energy to a various extent within a specific range of wavelengths according to their chemical structure [16], which, absorbing energy, is called a chromophore. The latter consists of electrons engaged into multiple bond sequences between atoms, generally conjugated double bonds. An absorbed UV photon contains energy enough to cause electron transfer to a higher energy orbit in the molecule [16]. The filter that was in a low-energy state (ground state) is converted into a higher excited energy state. From an excited state, different processes can occur:

- The filter molecule can simply deactivate from its excited state and resume its ground state while releasing the absorbed energy as unnoticeable heat.
- Structural transformation or degradation may occur and the filter losses its absorption capacity. The filter is then said to be photo-unstable.
- The excited molecule can interact with its surroundings, other ingredients of the formula, ambient oxygen, and thus lead to the production of undesirable reactive species. The filter is said to be photoreactive.

The behavior of the filter under UV exposure is a critical point that needs to be investigated when new sunscreen products are being developed.

Inorganic UV filters

Pigment grade powders of metal oxides such as titanium dioxide or zinc oxide have been used for many years in combination with organic filters to enhance protection level in the longer UVA range. Unlike organic filters, they act by reflecting and diffusing UVR. However, as a result of the large particle sizes, these powders also diffuse light from the visible range of the sun spectrum therefore tending to leave a white appearance on the skin. To overcome this drawback, which affects cosmetic acceptance, nano-sized powders of both titanium dioxide and zinc oxide have been made available. Decrease in particle size to nano form leads to changes in the protective properties of titanium dioxide: the smaller particles shift the protection range from the longer UVA toward the UVB.

Zinc oxide has better absorption in the long UVA than titanium dioxide, but it is not very efficient both in the UVB and UVA range when used alone.

Because of possible photocatalytic activity, inorganic particles are frequently coated with dimethicone or silica for maintenance of their efficacy. Nano-sized titanium dioxide (<100 nm), when combined with organic UV filters, allows high SPF products to be developed with a lower dependence on organic UV filters hence a lower concentration of these showing more a synergetic than an additive effect.

Steps toward more efficient sunscreens

As far as UVB protection is concerned, a large choice of filters has been available since long. They are photo-stable, at the exception of the most common, ethylhexyl methoxy cinnamate (EHMC). The choice of UVA filters depends on the countries and is limited in the USA, as previously mentioned. Inorganic pigments offer a poor level of protection against UVA when used alone. Benzophenones are photo-stable but are primarily UVB filters with some absorption in the short UVA range (peak at 328 nm).

Butyl methoxy dibenzoyl methane (BMDM or avobenzone) has a high potency in the UVA1 range peaking at 358 nm; however, it undergoes significant degradation under UV exposure leading to a decrease in its UVA protection efficacy. Research on the photochemistry of filters has led to identifying some potent photo-stabilizers (e.g. octocrylene) of avobenzone and developing new UVA filters that show photo-stable. Since 2005, diethylamino hydroxybenzoyl hexyl benzoate (DHHB) was approved in all countries, excepted in the USA and Canada. This UVA1 filter has UV-spectral properties similar to BMDM but DHHB is photo-stable.

In order to provide full protection in the entire UVA range, it is necessary to have efficient absorption in the short UVA range. TDSA or Mexoryl SX™ (Chimex, Le Thillay, France), with a peak at 345 nm at the boundary between short and long UVA wavelengths, was first approved in EU in 1993. This was followed by the approval of the broad UVB/UVA filter drometrizole trisiloxane (DTS or Mexoryl XL) with two peaks (at 303 and 344 nm) in 1998. Since 2000, another short UVA filter, disodium phenyl dibenzimidazole tetrasulfonate [DPDT] or Neo-Heliopan AP® (Symrise, Holzminden, Germany, peak at 334 nm) and broadband UVB/UVA filters (MBBT, Tinosorb M and BEMT, Tinosorb S) have been approved in EU. All these filters are photo-stable.

Formulation of sun protection products

The efficacy of the formulations depends upon a wide variety of factors.

First, the formulator must consider the chemical structure and the concentration of filtering agents to design a specific absorption profile and to reach a given high level of protection. As far as broad and well-balanced UVB/UVA protection is concerned, there is a specific issue in formulating UVA photo-stable filtering systems.

UV filters are either hydrophilic or lipophilic and, when combined, a synergetic effect can be observed. This property is used to obtain higher efficacy against UVB and UVA radiation and to limit the concentration of filters.

Different approaches can be used to improve the solubility and the photo-stability of the UV filters.

Combinations of highly efficient and photo-stable filters provide an optimally balanced protection against both UVA and UVB [17]. Studies [18–20] have shown that the protection against UV-induced skin damage provided by sunscreen products with same SPF but different UVA protection factor is markedly different, emphasizing the importance of high UVA protection in preventing cell damage.

Only well balanced sunscreen products characterized by a UVAPF/SPF protection factor ratio at least 1/3, containing photo-stable sunscreens with absorption over the entire UV spectrum of sun radiation have been shown maintaining intact essential biologic functions.

The combined needs of products with high sun protection factor (SPF), of a well-balanced UVB-UVA spectrum, photo-stable, respecting stringent regulations, with pleasant sensory results is increasingly important. To increase efficacy, improving the compliance of consumers is a key factor, implying to develop products with a good spreadability and aesthetically appealing, of a pleasant skin feeling and transparency on the skin. A suitable solubility and a homogeneous distribution of UV filters in both the product and onto skin are essential for maximizing efficacy.

Different strategies based on non-absorbing material can be used to correct the spreading and boost the efficiency of the product. Film-forming polymers are very often used to obtain more evenly spread product and to enhance SPF.

Criteria and methods for evaluating the efficacy of sunscreen products

The methods for assessing the efficacy of sunscreen products must take into account the photo-instability of products to avoid an overestimation of protection. *In vivo* SPF and *in vivo* UVAPF (Persistent Pigment Darkening) test methods take photo-degradation into account. Appropriate UV doses are used to induce erythema on human skin for SPF determination or pigmentation for UVAPF determination.

When *in vitro* methods are used, they should also take into account this issue to provide relevant evaluation.

Determination of the sun protection factor (SPF)

In 2010, the International standardization organisation (ISO) working group 7 in charge of the sun protection methods within the technical committee TC 217 Cosmetics products published the first ISO standard on the determination of the sun protection factor SPF [22]. This ISO standard (ISO 24444) is based upon the international test method for SPF determination 2006 [23]. This ISO standard has been adopted by the EU and South Africa in 2010, by Australia, Mercosur, Japan, Mexico in 2012 and Canada in 2013 (Table 17.3). In 2011, the US Food and Drug Agency (FDA) published a final monograph [15] including an *in vivo* SPF test method which is based on the International SPF test method 2006 and similar to the ISO

Table 17.3 ISO Standards adoption/recognition.

	Europe	Australia 2012	South Africa 2013	USA 2011	Canada 2013	Mercosur 2012	Mexico 2012
In vivo SPF	ISO 24444	ISO 24444	ISO 24444	FDA 2011	FDA 2011 ISO 24444	Interna2006 FDA 1999 or updates (ISO 24444; FDA 2011)	FDA 2011 ISO 24444
In vivo UVA	ISO 24442	No	ISO 24442 JCIA 1995	No	ISO 24442	JCIA 1995 or Updates (ISO 24442)	ISO 24442
In vitro UVA	ISO 24443	ISO24443	ISO24443	FDA 2011	ISO 24443 Colipa 2011 FDA 2011	Colipa 2009 or all updates (Colipa 2011, ISO 24443)	Colipa 2011, ISO 24443, FDA 2011

24444. However, there is no recognition of ISO 24444 by FDA USA and no recognition of the FDA method by some countries. This situation implies retesting for the same products when marketed in these countries and finally raises ethical and cost issues.

SPF labeling

In some countries like EU, Australia, South Africa, Mexico the SPF values used for the labeling are submitted to restrictions. Minimum SPF varies from 2 to 6 and harmonization on the SPF cap has made progress, SPF50+ being the most frequently adopted cap (Table 17.4).

Table 17.4 Efficacy criteria and labeling

	EU2006	USA [a] 2011	Australia TGA 2012	Australia [b] NICNAS 2013	South Africa [c] 2013	Canada [d] 2013
Type of sunscreen	Primary	All with SPF	Primary and secondary with SPF > 15	Secondary with SPF ≤ 15 and make-up	All with SPF	Primary
SPF min	6	2	4	4	6	2
SPF max	50+ (at least 60)	Not decided	50+ (at least 60)	Make-up 50+ (at least 60) secondary sunscreens max 15	50+ (at least 60)	50+ (above 50)
Restricted SPF numbers	6,10,15,20,25, 30,50, 50+	No	4,6,8,10,15,20,25,30, 40,50,50+	Make-up 4,6,8,10,15,20,25,30, 40,50,50+ Other secondary: 4,6,8,10,15	6,10,15,20,25, 30,40, 50,50+	No
UVA criteria	Ratio SPF/UVAPF ≤ 3 + λc ≥ 370 nm	λc ≥ 370 nm	Ratio SPF/UVAPF ≤ 3 + λc ≥ 370 nm	Ratio SPF/UVAPF ≤ 3 + λc ≥ 370 nm	Ratio SPF/UVAPF ≤ 3 + λc ≥ 370 nm	λc ≥ 370 nm and/or Ratio SPF/UVAPF ≤ 3
UVA labeling	UVA logo	Broad spectrum if at least SPF 15 and λc ≥ 370 nm	Broad spectrum	Broad spectrum	UVA logo	Broad spectrum if λc ≥ 370 nm if SPF ≥ 15 and λc ≥ 370 nm, decreases the risk of skin cancer and early skin aging if SPF/UVAPF ≤ 3 UVA logo

	Mercosur 2012	Mexico 2012
Type of sunscreen	Primary	Primary
SPF min	6	6
SPF max	99	50+
Restricted numbers	No	6,10,15,20,25,30,50, 50+
UVA criteria	Ratio SPF/UVAPF ≤ 3 + λC ≥ 370 nm	Ratio SPF/UVAPF ≤ 3 + λC ≥ 370 nm
UVA labeling	ND	UVA logo

[a] Broadspectrum property not mandatory.
Sunscreens that are not broad spectrum or that lack an SPF of at least 15 must now carry a warning: "Skin Cancer/Skin Aging Alert: Spending time in the sun increases your risk of skin cancer and early skin aging. This product has been shown only to help prevent sunburn, not skin cancer or early skin aging."
Sunscreens that are broadspectrum can carry the following sentence: "if used as directed with other sun protection measures, decreases the risk of skin cancer and early skin aging caused by the sun."
[b] UVA criteria not mandatory for make-up products below SPF30 (mandatory for all primary and other secondary sunscreens).
[c] UVA criteria not mandatory only if UVA protection is claimed.
[d] UVA criteria not mandatory only if UVA protection is claimed (broadspectrum or UVA logo).
If broadspectrum and SPF ≥ 15, the following statement may be made: "decreases the risk of skin cancer and early skin aging caused by the sun".
If not broadspectrum or with a SPF < 15, the following warning is required: "**Skin Cancer/Skin Aging Alert:** Spending time in the sun increases your risk of skin. Cancer and early skin aging. This product has been shown only to help prevent sunburn **not** skin cancer or early skin aging".
Note 1: New Zealand adopted the Australian Standards 2012 (AS/NZS 2604:2012) for sunscreen products evaluation and classification but it is not mandatory.
Note 2: UVAPF determination for ratio SPF/UVAPF can be done using either *in vivo* UVA or *in vitro* UVA methods depending on the local regulations, λc can only be measured using *in vitro* methods.

Table 17.5 Main differences between the ISO 24443:2012 and the FDA 2011 methods, and influence of the test conditions on the critical wavelength results.

Parameters	FDA 2011	ISO 24443:2012	Differences in results
Plates	PMMA 2 to 7 µm	PMMA 5 µm	Between 2 and 5 µm: + 2 nm; 5 µm to be used for harmonization
Product amount	0.75 mg/cm^2	1.3 mg/cm^2	No significant difference due to product amount
Irradiation dose	4 MEDs (8 J/cm^2)	1.2 J/cm^2 x UVAPF0	Difference due to the UV dose : 1 nm
Number of plates	At least 3	At least 4	No difference if 3 or 4 plates

Determination of UVA protection level

The EU issued a recommendation on 22 September 2006 [24] to use a persistent pigment darkening (PPD) method similar to the JCIA method [25] or any *in vitro* method able to provide equivalent and reliable results. In addition, the critical wavelength which is an evaluation of the width of the absorbance of the sunscreen product must be at least 370 nm. The EU Commission also recommends that the methods used should take into account photo-degradation.

Japan (JCIA) was first to publish in January 1996 an official *in vivo* method to assess UVA protection level, adopting the PPD method for assessment of the UVA efficacy of sunscreen products [25]. Korea and China adopted this method in 2001 and 2007, respectively. Finally, the *in vivo* UVA method has been standardized by ISO TC217 and published in 2011 under the reference ISO 24442 [26], now adopted or accepted in many countries (Table 17.3).

In 2007, the European Cosmetic industry (Colipa now Cosmetics Europe) published a guideline on the determination of UVA protection factor using an *in vitro* method. This method has been developed to provide UVA protection factors which are correlated with *in vivo* UVA protection factors, i.e. an alternative to the *in vivo* method [27]. This method was revised in 2011 [28, 29] and then published as ISO standard (ISO 24443) in 2012 [30]. This method allows determining both the UVA protection factor and the critical wavelength value.

In 2011, the US FDA published a final rule including a method to determine the critical wavelength [15]. This method is however not harmonized with the ISO 24443 standard and can lead to different results. A summary of the main differences between the two methods is provided in Table 17.5.

To obtain the critical wavelength value, the absorbance of the thin film of the sunscreen is integrated (starting from 290 nm) sequentially across the UV wavelength spectrum until the integration reaches 90% of the total absorbance of the sunscreen in the UV region (290–400 nm).

UVA protection criteria

Combining both the measure of the level of UVA protection and the critical wavelength method to measure the broadness of UVA absorbance has been first proposed for assessing UVA protection of sunscreen products by the EU Commission [24] and further adopted by other regulations such as Australia, Mercosur, Mexico and Canada (Table 17.4). The UVA protection factor (UVAPF) value must be at least 1/3 that of the SPF.

The critical wavelength value must be at least 370 nm to qualify the product as "broadspectrum" in the USA and Canada (see Table 17.4). The critical wavelength determination (λ_c) addresses the broadness of the protection rather than the specific protection in the UVA. Products with widely different UVA protection factors may have identical critical wavelengths and studies have shown that for products of a critical wavelength >370 nm, the higher the UVA protection level the better the protection against damages induced by UVA rays [31].

Conclusions

Over the past 20 years, an increasing number of publications have reported the damaging effects of UVA rays which induce molecular, cellular and clinical damage. This lead to photoaging, immune system depression, altered gene expression, oncogenes and tumor suppressor gene modulation partly responsible for skin cancer development.

In parallel to this increased knowledge, a significant progress in sunscreen technology has been achieved, with a variety of UVA filters being developed. Formulators combined them with UVB filters to reach high photo-stable protection with a minimal concentration of active ingredients. However, some restrictions (USA) ground in the availability of the potent UVA filters making the UVA protection level limited. A need for harmonization of testing methods and labeling, to afford the same information of efficacy to the consumers, appears crucial.

It is important that a minimal proportionality between UVA and UVB protection be ensured to avoid high UVB protection with low UVA protection. Accordingly, a UVAPF / SPF ratio of at least one-third has been adopted by many countries.

References

1 Urbach F. (2001) The negative effect of solar radiation: a clinical overview. In: Giacomoni PU, ed. *Sun Protection in Man, ESP Comprehensive Series in Photosciences*, Vol. 3. Amsterdam: Elsevier Sciences, pp. 41–67.

2 Peak MJ, Peak JG. Molecular photobiology of UVA. (1986) In: UrbachF, GangeRW, eds. *The Biological Effects of UVA Radiation*. New York: Praeger Publishers, pp. 42–52.

3 Lavker RM, Kaidbey K. (1997) The spectral dependence for UVA-induced cumulative damage in human Skin. *J Invest Dermatol* **108**, 17–21.

4 Lavker R, Gerberick G, Veres D, Irwin C, Kaidbey K. Cumulative effects from repeated exposures to suberythemal doses of UVB and UVA in human skin. *J Am Acad Dermatol* 1995; **32**, 53–62.

5 Lowe NJ, Meyers DP, Wieder JM, Luftman D, Bourget T, Lehman MD, et al. (1995) Low doses of repetitive ultraviolet A induce morphologic changes in human skin. *J Invest Dermatol* **105**, 739–43.

6 Séité S, Moyal D, Richard S, de Rigal J, Lévêque JL, Hourseau C, et al. (1997) Effects of repeated suberythemal doses of UVA in human skin. *Eur J Dermatol* **7**, 204–9.

7 Séité S, Moyal D, Richard S, de Rigal J, Lévêque JL, Hourseau C, et al. (1998) Mexoryl SX: a broadspectrum absorption UVA filter protects human skin from the effects of repeated suberythemal doses of UVA. *J Photochem Photobiol B Biol* **44**, 69–76.

8 Moyal D, Fourtanier A. (2004) Acute and chronic effects of UV on skin. In: Rigel DS, Weiss RA, Lim HW, Dover JS, eds. *Photoaging*. New York: Marcel Dekker, pp. 15–32.

9 Moyal D, Fourtanier A. Effects of UVA radiation on an established immune response in humans and sunscreen efficacy. *Exp Dermatol* 2002; **11** (Suppl 1), 28–32.

10 Kuchel J, Barnetson R, Halliday G. (2002) Ultraviolet A augments solar-simulated ultraviolet radiation-induced local suppression of recall responses in humans. *J Invest Dermatol* 2002; **118**, 1032–7.

11 Garland CF, Garland FC, Gorham EC. (2003) Epidemiologic evidence for different roles of ultraviolet A and B radiation in melanoma mortality rates. Ann Epidemiol (AEP) pp. 13395–404.

12 Agar NS, Halliday GM, Barnetson RS, et al. (2004) The basal layer in human squamous tumors harbors more UVA than UVB fingerprint mutations: a role for UVA in human skin carcinogenesis. *Proc Natl Acad Sci USA* 2004; **101**, 4954–9.

13 Moyal D, Binct O. (1997) Polymorphous light eruption (PLE): its reproduction and prevention by sunscreens. In: LoweNJ, ShaatN, PathakM, eds. *Sunscreens: Development and Evaluation and Regulatory Aspects*, 2nd edn. New York: Marcel Dekker, pp. 611–7.

14 *TGA Australian regulatory guidelines for sunscreens* (Nov 2012).

15 Department of Health and Human Services, Food and Drug Administration (USA). (1999) Sunscreen drug products for over-the-counter human use. *Fed Register* **43**, 24666–93.

16 Health Canada's Health Products and Food Branch (2013) *Sunscreen Monograph*, 7 July 2013.

17 Kimbrough DR. (1997) The photochemistry of sunscreens. *J Chem Ed* **74**, 51–3.

18 Marrot L, Belaidi J, Lejeune F, Meunier J, Asselineau D, Bernerd F. (2004) Photo-stability of sunscreen products influences the efficiency of protection with regard to UV-induced genotoxic or photoaging-related endpoints. *Br J Dermatol* **151**, 1234–44.

19 Fourtanier A, Bernerd F, Bouillon C, Marrot L, Moyal D, Seité S. (2006) Protection of skin biological targets by different types of sunscreens. *Photodermatol Photoimmunol Photomed* **22**, 22–32.

20 Moyal D, Fourtanier A. (2001) Broad spectrum sunscreens provide better protection from the suppression of the elicitation phase of delayed-type hypersensitivity response in humans. *J Invest Dermatol* **117**, 1186–92.

21 Damian DL, Halliday GM, Barnetson RSC. (1997) Broad spectrum sunscreens provide greater protection against ultraviolet-radiation-induced suppression of contact hypersensitivity to a recall antigen in humans. *J Invest Dermatol* **109**, 146–51.

22 ISO 24444 (2010) *Cosmetics – Sun protection test methods – In vivo determination of the sun protection factor (SPF)*.

23 Colipa, JCIA, CTFA SA, CTFA. (2006) *International Sun Protection Factor (SPF) Test Method*.

24 24 European Commission Recommendation on the efficacy of sunscreen products and the claims made relating thereto. OJL 265/39, (26.9.2006).

25 Japan Cosmetic Industry Association (JCIA). (1995) *Japan Cosmetic Industry Association measurement standard for UVA protection efficacy*. 15 November 1995.

26 ISO 24442 (2011) *Cosmetics – Sun protection test methods – in vivo determination of sunscreen UVA protection*.

27 Matts P, Alard V, Brown MW, Ferrero L, Gers-Barlag H, Issachar N, Moyal D. (2010) The COLIPA in vitro UVA method: a standard and reproducible measure of sunscreen UVA protection. *Internatl J Cosm Sci* **32**, 35–46.

28 Colipa. (2011) Method for *in vitro* determination of UVA protection. *COLIPA Guidelines*.

29 Moyal D, Alard V, Bertin C, Boyer F, Brown MW, Kolbe L, Matts P, Pissavini M. (2013) The revised COLIPA *in vitro* UVA method. *Int J Cosm Sci* **35**, 35–40.

30 ISO 24443 (2012) UVA *in vitro* Cosmetics – Sun protection test methods – Determination of sunscreen UVA photoprotection *in vitro*.

31 Fourtanier A, Moyal D, Seité S. (2012) UVA filters in sun-protection products: regulatory and biological aspects. *Photochem Photobiol Sci* **11**(1), 81–89.

SECTION 3 Personal Care Products

CHAPTER 18
Antiperspirants and Deodorants

Eric S. Abrutyn
TPC2 Advisors Inc., Boquete, Chiriqui, Republic of Panama

> **BASIC CONCEPTS**
> - Antiperspirants are US Food and Drug Administration (FDA) regulated drugs to be used in the underarm axilla vault only.
> - Antiperspirants are primarily complexes of aluminum (e.g. aluminum chlorohydrate) and aluminum zirconium (e.g. aluminum tetrachlorohydrex-GLY).
> - Deodorants, not to be confused with antiperspirants, are cosmetics and do not typically contain any aluminum-type salt complexes.
> - Antiperspirants are associated with few dermatologic issues; slightly irritating under certain conditions, but not scientifically associated with breast cancer or Alzheimer disease.

Introduction

This chapter deals with the technologies for wetness and odor protection of the human axilla, how they are applied, and potential adverse effects of use of these products on a regular basis. Antiperspirants and deodorants have been used for centuries, evolving from simple fragrances that masked offensive odors to today's complex ingredients based on aluminum and zirconium chemistries that act to slow or diminish sweat production. Odors (scents) and sweating have a biologic significance. Body scents are primeval and most likely evolved genetically to attract the opposite sex. Sweating is regulated by the sympathetic nervous system and is an important body temperature regulator, especially in warm weather climates or during heavy exercise, and functions to remove waste and toxic by-products of the body. The axilla area of the body represents a small contribution to sweating to control body temperature and removal of biologic by-products, so the controlling of sweat from this area has fewer health risks than other areas of the body. There is little scientific evidence that supports the idea that the use of antiperspirants, based on aluminum or aluminum–zirconium chemistry causes appreciable lasting adverse effects other than possible temporary and reversible irritation.

Physiology

Sweat glands and how they work

Sweat by itself is odorless and only establishes a characteristic odor when exposed to moisture (humidity) in the presence of bacterial flora on the skin surface, breaking down the sweat's composition and resulting in unpleasant odors. The use of antimicrobial agents is a good defense in preventing odor development from bacteria and yeast present on the skin. Another defense is the reduction of excretion from the eccrine gland to minimize the appearance of uncomfortable or unsightly wetness production.

According to *Gray's Anatomy* [1], most people have several million sweat glands distributed over their bodies, to include the underarm axilla and thus providing plenty of opportunity for underarm odors to develop. Skin has two types of sweat gland: eccrine glands and apocrine glands (Figures 18.1 and 18.2). Eccrine glands open directly on to the surface of the skin and exude sweat in the underarm, subsequently contributing to odor formation. These glands are located in the middle layer of the skin called the dermis, which is also made up of nerve endings, hair follicles, and blood vessels. Sweat is produced in a long coil embedded within the dermis where the long part is a duct that connects the gland to the opening (pore) on the skin's surface. When body temperature rises, the autonomic nervous system stimulates these glands to secrete fluid on to the surface of skin, where it then cools the body as it evaporates. The composition of the eccrine gland secretion is about 55–60% fluid, mostly water with various salts (primarily: sodium chloride, potassium chloride) and various electrolytic components (ammonia, calcium, copper, lactic acid, potassium, and phosphorus). The warmth and limited air flow is conducive to allowing for rapid decomposition of organic matter made up of primarily low molecular weight volatile fatty acids (Figure 18.3). These fatty acids and the steroidal compounds produce the recognizable body odors.

Cosmetic Dermatology: Products and Procedures, Second Edition. Edited by Zoe Diana Draelos.
© 2016 John Wiley & Sons, Ltd. Published 2016 by John Wiley & Sons, Ltd.

18. Antiperspirants and Deodorants   161

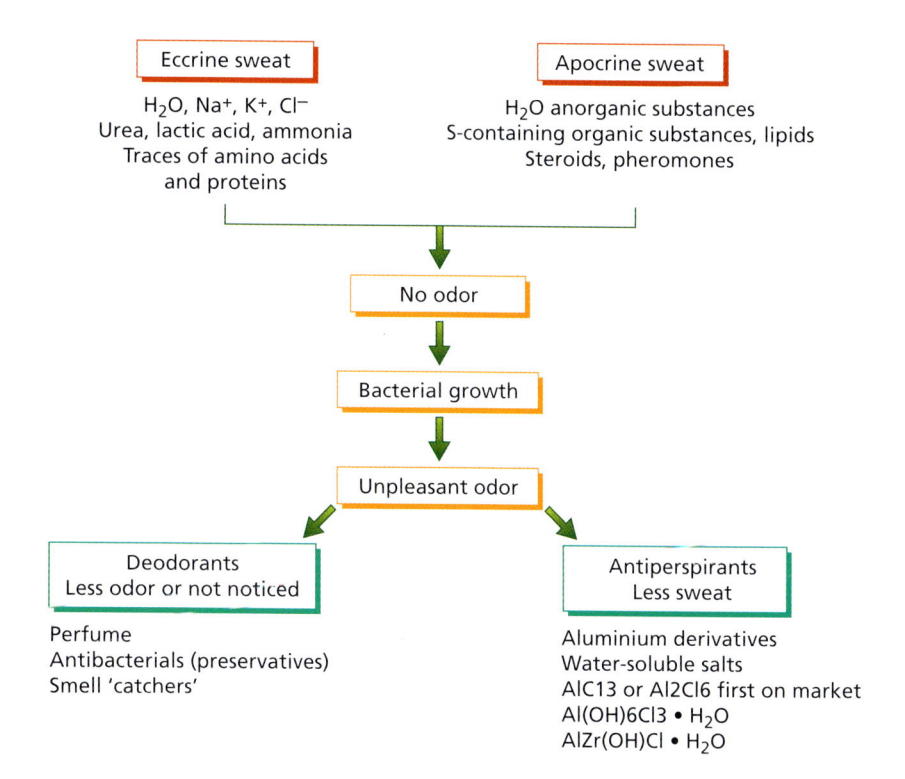

Eccrine sweat
H_2O, Na^+, K^+, Cl^-
Urea, lactic acid, ammonia
Traces of amino acids
and proteins

Apocrine sweat
H_2O anorganic substances
S-containing organic substances, lipids
Steroids, pheromones

→ No odor
→ Bacterial growth
→ Unpleasant odor

Deodorants
Less odor or not noticed
Perfume
Antibacterials (preservatives)
Smell 'catchers'

Antiperspirants
Less sweat
Aluminium derivatives
Water-soluble salts
AlC13 or Al2Cl6 first on market
$Al(OH)6Cl3 \cdot H_2O$
$AlZr(OH)Cl \cdot H_2O$

Figure 18.1 Underarm sweat gland mechanism.

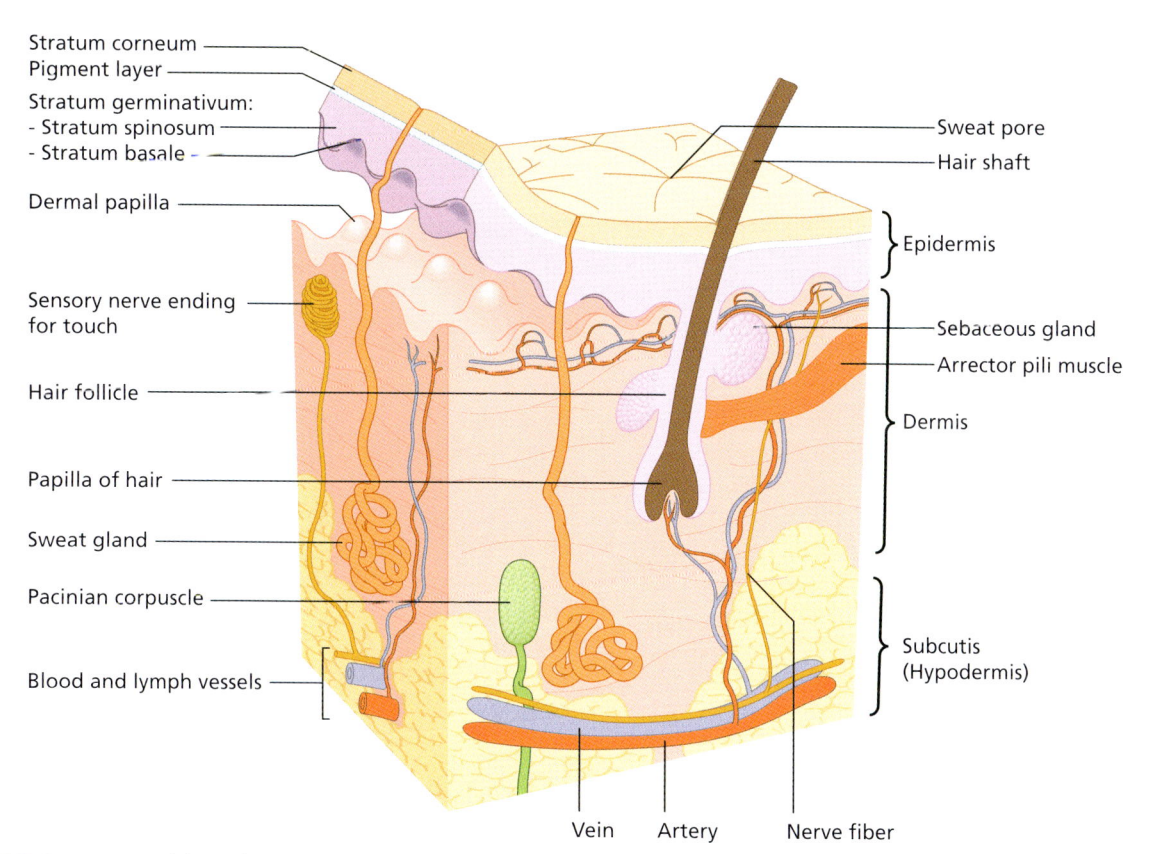

Figure 18.2 Cross-section of skin and sweat glands.

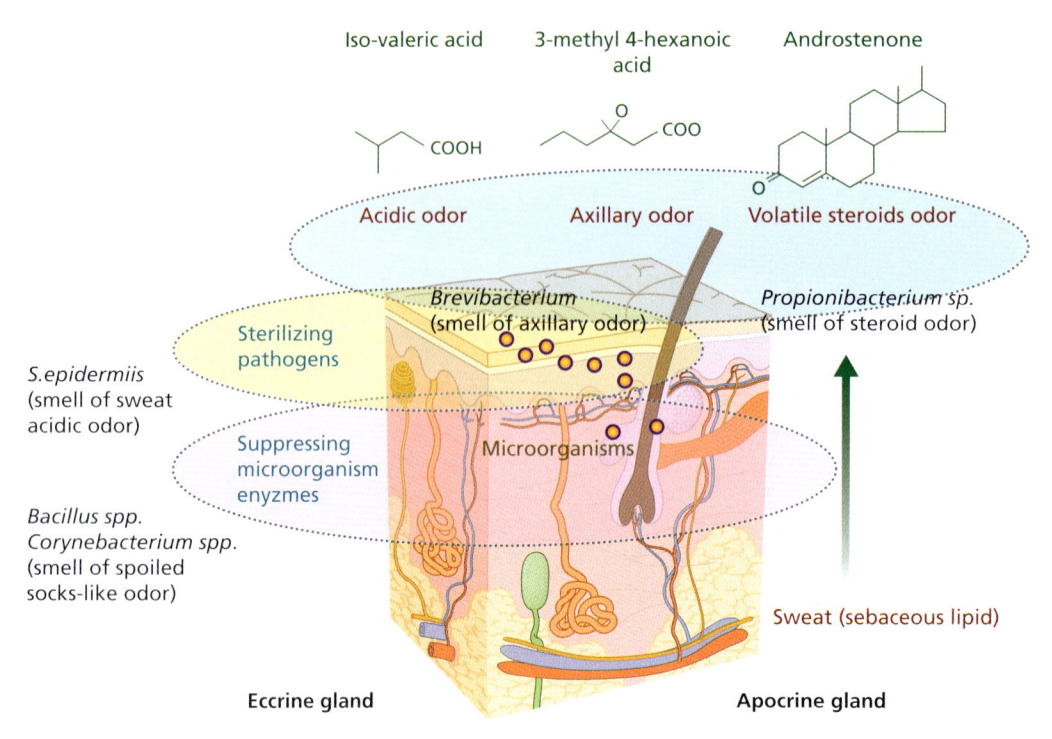

Figure 18.3 Sweat metabolism cycle.

The apocrine glands are triggered by emotions. These glands are dormant until puberty, at which time they start to secrete. Apocrine glands secrete a fatty substance. When under emotional stress, the wall of the tubule glands contract to push the fatty exudates to the surface of skin where bacterial flora begin breaking it down.

In a regulatory monograph [2] the FDA, through the Food Drug and Cosmetic Act, defines antiperspirants as an over-the-counter (OTC) drug when applied topically to reduce production of underarm sweat (perspiration). They are considered drugs because they can affect the function of the body by reducing the amount of sweat that reaches the skin surface. In the USA, OTC drugs are subjected to monograph rules, which define standards and requirements, premarket approval process, acceptable actives, and allowable formulation percentages of actives. Other countries' regulations vary in content and scope. Some countries consider antiperspirants as cosmetics and not affecting the biologic physiology of the body; as such they are not held to the same strict standards as in the USA. As an example, Canada (2008) ruled that antiperspirants were no longer be considered a drug; their use only needs to comply with cosmetic regulations.

Wetness and odor control and testing

The consumer typically confuses what antiperspirants and deodorants do, mostly caused by a misunderstanding of marketing claims and product positioning. For the most part, antiperspirants are based on aluminum-based cationic salt chloride complexes (as well as complexes with zirconium acid salts) and are referred to as "actives" on the back label of consumer antiperspirant products.

There are numerous types of antiperspirant actives listed in the FDA monograph as well as in the US Pharmacopia (USP) [3]. Antiperspirant actives are responsible for blocking sweat expulsion through the formation of temporary plugs within the sweat duct, thus stopping or slowing down the flow of sweat to the surface of the eccrine gland.

A theory of wetness control that has been accepted over the years is that the hydrated aluminum or aluminum–zirconium cationic salt chloride is transported to the eccrine gland, interacting with the protein contained within the gland. In this basic protein environment, the antiperspirant active is reduced, producing a gelatinous proteinaceous plug. By plugging the gland, sweat is prohibited from transporting to the surface, causing osmotic pressure. Eventually, this plug is pushed out of the eccrine gland and the gland is allowed to operate again in a normal fashion. This can take 14–21 days for all the eccrine gland to begin firing; known as a wash-out period.

Without going into detail, one can describe how antiperspirants are tested for their Wetness Inhibiting Performance ("WIP"™) effectiveness. The FDA prescribes a methodology for testing the effectiveness of an antiperspirant by having participants tested in a controlled environment – 30–40% relative humidity at approximately 100°C. Sweat is continuously collected during 20-minute intervals and reported as the production or percentage change in production over the average of two 20-minute collection periods. To be accepted as a participant

---

Trademarked 2008 and property of Eric Abrutyn, TPC2 Advisors Ltd., Inc., Republic of Panama Corporation.

one must exceed production of 100 mg collected sweat per 20-minute period and should not exceed more than 600 mg difference between the highest and lowest sweat production within the test population. The results of testing need to meet a minimum of 20% sweat reduction in 50% of the test population in order to be considered an antiperspirant.

Deodorants cover odor through a variety of mechanisms, which include the neutralization or counteracting of odoriferous axilla odor through the retardation of the odor development, or the reduction in perception of odor through masking of the odor. Masking is basically accomplished via use of fragrances and other volatile components. Neutralization is the chemical reaction to modify low molecular weight fatty acids that are excreted from the apocrine gland. One type of neutralization agent is antimicrobials that disrupt cell barrier viability causing the bacterial microbes to perish (triclosan is one popular example). Deodorants are designed to minimize underarm axilla odor, not to reduce or eliminate perspiration. So, deodorants are best for those people who do not have a problem with sweating yet want to feel fresh and odor free. It is important to note that deodorants have no antiperspirant physiologic activity, but antiperspirants can function both as antiperspirants and deodorants; thus, consumers needing odor and wetness control will require the use of antiperspirants to achieve their needs.

Chemistry and formulation of antiperspirants

It is important to have some understanding of the chemistry of antiperspirants to gain a better appreciation of their physiologic action in the axilla mantle. Antiperspirants are divided into two categories of functional aluminum-based and zirconium-based actives (typically: aluminum chlorohydrate, aluminum zirconium tetrachlorohydrex-GLY, aluminum zirconium trichlorohydrex-GLY, or aluminum chloride) plus an inactive formula matrix for consumer acceptable esthetics.

The basic building block of antiperspirant actives is based on aluminum chemistry in which elemental aluminum is reduced in an acidic medium to produce what is traditionally known as aluminum chlorohydrate (ACH) with an atomic ratio of 2 : 1 aluminum to chloride. These inorganic cationic polymer salts are classified as octahedral complexes of a basic aluminum hydroxide, stabilized with an anionic chloride to maintain their water solubility. Within the monograph boundaries [2], the atomic ratio of aluminum to chloride can range from 2 : 1 to 1 : 1 within three different segmentations (aluminum chlorohydrate, aluminum sesquichlorohydrate, and aluminum dichlorohydrate).

Antiperspirant actives can also be complexed with hydrated acidic zirconium cationic salts of chloride to make what is traditionally known as aluminum zirconium chlorohydrate (ZAG or AZG). Like ACHs, AZGs can have various ratios of atomic aluminum to zirconium of 2 : 1 to 10 : 1 and atomic total metals to chloride of 0.9 : 1 to 2.0 : 1. These AZG complexes can be buffered with glycine (an amino acid) to stabilize the complex and mitigate the acidic harshness which could result when applied to underarm axilla.

There is a growing interest in aluminum-free odor and wetness controlling products. One product that has emerged is based on a natural stone "crystal." "Crystal" products are made from a mineral known as potassium alum, also known as potassium aluminum sulfate and contain aluminum. Unlike aluminum salts used in antiperspirants, alum does not prohibit sweating; it only helps control the growth of bacteria that can cause an underarm odor.

Delivery systems

The formulation matrix delivery system is the key to effectiveness of antiperspirant active performance and acceptable consumer application. The most common delivery systems are roll-ons (either aqueous or cyclosiloxane suspensions), aerosol (hydrocarbon propellant suspensions), extrudable clear gels (water-in-cyclosiloxane emulsions), extrudable opaque soft solids (anhydrous cyclosiloxane suspension pastes), or sticks (anhydrous cyclomethicone suspension solids) (Figure 18.4). Within each form there are typical inactive ingredients that support a stable formula with consumer-acceptable esthetics so as not to interfere with the WIP™ delivery of the antiperspirant active.

Although this chapter does not focus on details of formulation development, this subject can be researched in more detail in the literature [4,5]. In general, aqueous-based hydrous formulas (mostly based on roll-on and clear gel delivery systems) will have some type of emulsifier or stabilizing agent. In the case of aqueous roll-ons, they tend to be polyethylene glycol (PEG) or polypropylene glycol (PPG) ethoxylated alcohols (INCI e.g.: PEG-2, PEG-20) and for clear gel emulsions they are based on PEG and PPG alkoxylated functional siloxanes (INCI e.g.: PEG/PPG-18/18 dimethicone copolymer). Anhydrous-based formulas (typically: solid sticks, some types of roll-ons, extrudable creams) include cyclosiloxane (preferably cyclopentasiloxane) for transient solvent delivery of the active and its eventual evaporation to leave no residue on the skin, solidification agent (INCI e.g.: stearyl alcohol, hydrogenated castor oil, and miscellaneous fatty acid ester wax), and dispersing agent (INCI e.g.: PPG-14 butyl ether). Most antiperspirant formulas include other ingredients for cosmetic purposes, such as fragrance, antioxidants (BHT – butylated hydroxytoluene), chelating agents (disodium EDTA – disodium edetate), soft feel powders (talc, corn starch, and corn starch modified), and emollients and/or moisturizers (petrolatum, mineral oil, fatty acid esters, non-volatile hydrocarbons). These ingredients have been used in the industry for well over 25 years with accepted safety profiles; reviewed by Cosmetic Ingredient Review (www.cir-safety.org/) and other governmental or medical agencies.

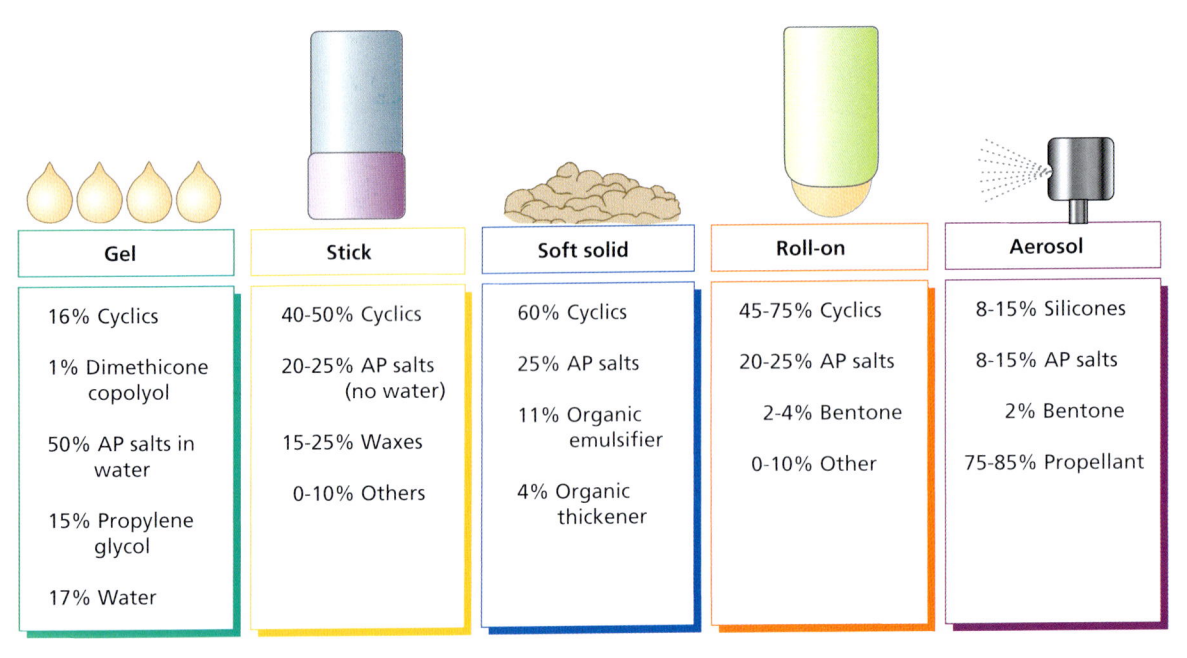

Gel	Stick	Soft solid	Roll-on	Aerosol
16% Cyclics	40-50% Cyclics	60% Cyclics	45-75% Cyclics	8-15% Silicones
1% Dimethicone copolyol	20-25% AP salts (no water)	25% AP salts	20-25% AP salts	8-15% AP salts
50% AP salts in water	15-25% Waxes	11% Organic emulsifier	2-4% Bentone	2% Bentone
15% Propylene glycol	0-10% Others	4% Organic thickener	0-10% Other	75-85% Propellant
17% Water				

Figure 18.4 Antiperspirant formula matrix delivery systems.

Dermatologic concerns

Each manufacturer of antiperspirants keeps a thorough record of adverse effects as reported by the consumer. For the most part, there is a low incident of adverse effects when the product is use as prescribed. Issues tend to revolve around skin irritation and sensitization. These adverse effects are reversible with cessation of use. Irritation can be brought about for a number of reasons, but most often by application on broken skin (e.g. from shaving) or sensitivity to the fragrance or one of the metallic components of the antiperspirant active. Switching brands or fragrance types is one remedy to alleviate adverse effects. In some cases a person is so sensitive to an antiperspirant active that he or she can no longer use a product containing an aluminum-based antiperspirant.

Health concerns regarding antiperspirants have been discussed in the literature over the last 40–50 years and mostly relate to breast cancer or Alzheimer disease. According to the Alzheimer's Association (www.alz.org/index.asp), the linkage of aluminum and Alzheimer disease is most likely linked to a single study in the 1960s where an abnormally high concentration of aluminum was observed in the brains of some Alzheimer patients. However, "After several decades of research," reports the Alzheimer's Association, "scientists have been unable to replicate the original 1960s study." In fact, there is still no scientific correlation on the cause and effect relationship for contracting Alzheimer disease. The research community is generally convinced that aluminum is not a key risk factor in developing Alzheimer disease. Public health bodies sharing this conviction include the World Health Organization, the US National Institutes of Health, the US Environmental Protection Agency, and Health Canada.

According to the National Cancer Institute (NCI) and the American Cancer Society, rumors connecting antiperspirant use and breast cancer are largely unsubstantiated by scientific research. The rumors suggest that antiperspirants prevent a person from sweating out toxins and that this helps the spread of cancer-causing toxins via the lymph nodes. The NCI discusses two studies that address the breast cancer rumor. A 2002 study of over 800 patients at the Fred Hutchinson Cancer Research Institute found no link between breast cancer and the use of antiperspirant and/or deodorant [6]; and a study of 437 cancer patients, published in 2003 in the *European Journal of Cancer Prevention*, found no correlation between earlier diagnosis of breast cancer and antiperspirant and/or deodorant use [7]. The NCI's analysis of the second study was that it "Does not demonstrate a conclusive link between these underarm hygiene habits and breast cancer. Additional research is needed to investigate this relationship and other factors that may be involved."

Through the evaluation of these and other independent studies, it can be concluded that there is no existing scientific or medical evidence linking the use of underarm products to the development of breast cancer. The FDA (Food & Drug Administration), the Mayo Clinic, the American Cancer Society, and the Personal Care Products Council (formerly Cosmetic, Toiletry, and Fragrance Association) have come to a similar conclusion.

Sweating is necessary to control body temperature, especially during times of exercise and warm or hot surroundings. In a small portion of the population the sympathetic nervous system can go awry, affecting the complex biologic mechanism of perspiration, resulting in either excessive perspiration (hyperhidrosis) or little or no perspiration (anhidrosis). Currently, there are no known cures for hyperhidrosis but there are a number of treatment options: injectable treatment such as botulinum toxin type A (Botox), topical agents such as prescribed antiperspirants, oral medications, and surgery.

Based on information from the International Hyperhidrosis Society, over 87% of people with hyperhidrosis say that OTC antiperspirants do not provide sufficient relief. Thus, it is important for the medical community to understand the other options available to treat excessive sweating. Botox, a drug that has been approved for use as an injectable treatment in the axilla area, works to interrupt the chemical messages (anticholinergic) released by nerve endings to signal the start of sweat production. It is important to understand how to administer Botox in a manner that will not cause medical issues; thus only a trained practitioner should administer treatment. Unfortunately, Botox is not a permanent solution, and patients require repeat injections every 6–8 months to maintain benefits.

There are other options for treating excessive sweating, but none have been demonstrated to be either safe or effective for use by consumers. Most systemic medications, in particular anticholinergics, reduce sweating but the dose required to control sweating can cause significant adverse effects (e.g. dizziness), thus limiting the medications' effectiveness. Iontophoresis is a simple and well-tolerated method for the treatment of hyperhidrosis without long-term adverse effects; however, long-term maintenance treatment is required to keep patient's symptom free. Psychotherapy has been beneficial in a small number of cases.

Strengths and weakness of antiperspirants

Based on all the information known about antiperspirants one would surmise there are few weaknesses regarding their use. Basically, they serve the purpose of reducing the discomfort and potential observation of underarm wetness, and can lead to reduced underarm offensive odors. Except in the case of hyperhidrosis, antiperspirants serve to provide cosmetic esthetics and social acceptance. It is important to note that, even if used twice a day, antiperspirants do not completely stop axilla sweating, but provide a significant reduction in the amount of sweating produced in the axilla. With almost 70 years of use for antiperspirant actives, there is almost no association with adverse effects when properly used in the underarm area. So, the risk–benefit is minimal and is balanced by the ability to maintain a more comfortable and socially appealing state.

Conclusions

Because they are regulated in the USA and other countries as drugs, it is foreseen that introduction of new antiperspirant actives will be restricted. To introduce new antiperspirant actives, one would have to go through an extensive New Drug Application process, requiring costly studies on safety and effectiveness. Aside from the introduction of new antiperspirant drugs, dermatologists need to continue monitoring the introduction of unregulated new ingredients that would be included in existing or new formula matrices. For over 5500 years, every major civilization has left a record of its efforts to mask body odors. The early Egyptians recommended following a scented bath with an underarm application of perfumed oils (special citrus and cinnamon preparations).

References

1 *Gray's Anatomy: The Anatomical Basis of Clinical Practice*, 39th edn. (2004) CV Mosby.
2 USA Department of Health and Human Services: Food and Drug Administration. (2003) Antiperspirant Drug Products for Over-the-Counter Human Use, Final Rule. 68 CFR, Part 110. www.fda.gov/cder/otcmonographs/Antiperspirant/antiperspirant_FR_20030609.pdf
3 USP 27/NF 22 (2004) United States Pharmacopeial Convention, Rockville, MD, pp. 83–91; 93–106.
4 Abrutyn E. (1998) *Antiperspirant and Deodorants: Fundamental Understanding*. IFSCC Monograph Series No. 6. Weymouth, Dorset, UK: Micelle Press.
5 Abrutyn E. (2000) Antiperspirant and deodorants. In: ReigerMM, ed. *Harry's Cosmetology*, 8th edn. New York: Chemical Publishing Company, Inc.
6 http://jncicancerspectrum.oxfordjournals.org/cgi/reprint/jnci; 94/20/1578.pdf (Vol. 94, No. 20, Pg 1578, October 16, 2002).
7 McGrath KG. (2003) An earlier age of breast cancer diagnosis related to more frequent use of antiperspirants/deodorants and underarm shaving. *Eur J Cancer Prev* **12**, 479–85.

CHAPTER 19
Blade Shaving

Kevin Cowley,[1] Kristina Vanoosthuyze,[1] Gillian McFeat, and Keith Ertel[2]

[1]Gillette Innovation Centre, Reading, UK
[2]Procter & Gamble Co., Cincinnati, OH, USA

> **BASIC CONCEPTS**
> - Hair removal practices have their roots in antiquity. While modern global attitudes towards hair removal vary, consumers around the world use blade shaving as a method to effect hair removal.
> - Modern blades and razors are the product of extensive research and technologically advanced manufacturing procedures; these combine to provide the user with an optimum shaving experience.
> - Effective blade shaving involves three steps: preparation, including skin cleansing and hair hydrating; hair removal, including the use of an appropriate shaving preparation; and post-shave skin care, including moisturizer application.

Introduction

Like many personal care practices, the roots of shaving lie in the prehistoric past. Hair removal for our cave dwelling ancestors was probably more about function than esthetics; hair could provide an additional handle for an adversary to grab during battle, it collected dirt and food, and it provided a home to insects and parasites. Flint blades possibly dating as far back as 30 000 BC are some of the earliest examples of shaving implements. Archaeological evidence shows that materials such as horn, clamshell, or shark teeth were used to remove hair by scraping. Pulling or singeing the hair, while somewhat more painful, were also methods used to effect hair removal.

Attitudes towards hair became more varied in ancient times. The Egyptian aristocracy shaved not only their faces, but also their bodies. The ancient Greeks viewed a beard as a sign of virility but Alexander the Great, who is said to have been obsessed with shaving, made the practice popular among Greek males. Greek women also shaved; a body free from hair was viewed as the ideal of beauty in Greek society. Shaving was viewed as a sign of degeneracy in early Roman society, but an influx of clean-shaven foreigners gradually changed this attitude. For affluent Romans, shaving was performed by a skilled servant or at a barbershop, which was popularized in ancient Rome as a place of grooming and socializing. Shaving implements at this time were generally made from metals such as copper, gold, or iron.

The barbershop took on an expanded role in the Middle Ages. In these shops barbers provided grooming services and routinely performed other duties such as bloodletting and minor surgical and dental procedures. Shaving injuries were common and the striped pole that is today associated with barbershops has its origin in these times, its red and white stripes symbolizing blood and the bandages that were used to cover the wound, respectively.

The Industrial Revolution heralded a number of advancements in shaving technology. The straight razor was first introduced in Sheffield, England and became popular worldwide as a tool for facial shaving. While an improvement over earlier shaving implements, the straight razor dulled easily, required regular sharpening or stropping and a high skill level, and shaving injuries were still a problem, which earned it the nickname of "cutthroat razor". Many credit Jean Jacques Perret with inventing the safety razor in 1762. His device, which he apparently did not patent, consisted of a guard that enclosed all but a small portion of the blade. Variations on the design followed from other inventors, many using comb-like structures to limit blade contact with the skin. The Kampfe Brothers filed a patent in 1880 for a razor, marketed as the Star Safety Razor that used a "hoe" design in which the handle was mounted perpendicular to the blade housing. The blade, essentially a shortened straight razor, was held in place by metal clips. While generally successful, the blade in the Star Safety Razor still required stropping before each use.

In 1904 King C. Gillette introduced the real breakthrough that brought shaving to the masses. Unlike its predecessors, the Gillette Safety Razor used an inexpensive disposable blade that was replaced by the user when it became dull. The new razor quickly gained popularity due a variety of promotional efforts, including a blades and razors marketing model pioneered by Gillette.

Cosmetic Dermatology: Products and Procedures, Second Edition. Edited by Zoe Diana Draelos.
© 2016 John Wiley & Sons, Ltd. Published 2016 by John Wiley & Sons, Ltd.

Shaving was not only promoted to males. The practice of shaving among females was prompted by the May 1915 issue of Harper's Bazaar Magazine that featured a picture of a female model wearing a sleeveless evening gown and sporting hairless axillae. The Wilkinson Sword Company built on the idea by running a series of advertisements targeting women in the 1920s to promote the idea that underarm hair was not only unhygienic, it was also unfeminine. Sales of razor blades doubled over the next few years.

Razor developments during the next several decades were primarily limited to improvements in single blade technology, including the switch from carbon steel to stainless steel blade material in the 1960s introduced by Wilkinson Sword. This prevented corrosion thus increasing blade life. The next major change occurred in 1971 with the introduction of the Trac II, the first multi-blade razor. Innovation has continued along this track and today consumers can choose from a variety of razor models having multiple blades contained in a disposable cartridge, with specialized designs available to meet the shaving needs of both sexes. The relatively simple appearance of these devices belies their sophistication; they are the product of years of development and technically advanced manufacturing processes.

Of course, not all shaving is done with a blade. Electric razors remove hair without drawing a blade across the skin. There are two basic types of electric razors, both relying on a scissor action to cut hairs using either an oscillatory or circular motion. When the razor is pressed against skin the hairs are forced up into holes in the foil and held in place while the blade moves against the foil to cut the trapped hairs. Colonel Jacob Schick patented the first electric razor in 1928. Electric razors were for many decades confined to use on dry skin, but some modern battery-powered razors are designed for use in wet environments, including the shower.

Hair biology basics

Much of the hair targeted for removal by shaving or other means is terminal hair (i.e. hair that is generally longer, thicker, and more darkly pigmented than vellus hair). In prepubescent males and females this hair is found primarily on the head and eyebrow regions, but with the onset of puberty terminal hair begins to appear on areas of the body with androgen-sensitive skin, including the face, axillae, and pubic region. Further, vellus hairs on some parts of the body, such as the beard area, may convert to terminal hairs under hormonal influence.

The pilosebaceous unit

A pilosebaceous unit comprises the hair follicle, the hair shaft, the sebaceous gland, and the arrector pili muscle. The hair follicle is the unit responsible for hair production. Hair growth is cyclical, and depending on the stage of hair growth, the follicle extends to a depth as shallow as the upper dermis to as deep as the subcutaneous tissue during the active growth phase.

The hair shaft is the product of matrix cells in the hair bulb, a structure located at the base of the follicle. The hair shaft is made up primarily of keratins and binding material with a small amount of water. A terminal hair shaft comprises three concentric layers. Outermost is the cuticle, a layer of cells that on the external hair are flattened and overlapping. The cuticle serves a protective function for external hair, regulates the water content of the hair fiber, and is responsible for much of the shine that is associated with healthy hair. The cortex lies inside the cuticle and is composed of longitudinal keratin strands and melanin. This layer represents the majority of the hair shaft and is responsible for many of its structural qualities, e.g. elasticity and curl. The medulla is the innermost layer found in some terminal hairshafts, made up of large loosely connected cells which contain keratin. Large intra- and intercellular air spaces in the medulla to some extent determine the sheen and colour tones of the hair.

Each hair follicle is associated with a sebaceous gland. This gland lies in the dermis and produces sebum, a lipophilic material composed of wax monoesters, triglycerides, free fatty acids, and squalene. Sebum empties into the follicle lumen and provides a natural conditioner for the forming and already extruded hair. The arrector pili muscle is a microscopic band of smooth muscle tissue that connects the follicle to the dermis. In certain body sites, when stimulated the arrector pili muscle contracts and causes the external hair to stand more erect, resulting in the appearance of goose bumps.

Hair growth cycle

Hair growth is not a continuous process but occurs over a cycle that is conveniently divided into three stages; at any given time hairs on a given body site are at various points in this cycle. The dermal papilla orchestrates the hair growth cycle. Anagen is the phase of hair follicle re-growth and hair generation. During this stage the hair follicle grows downward into the dermis and epidermal cells that surround the dermal papilla undergo rapid division. As new cells form they push the older cells upward. The number of hairs in anagen varies according to body site. At any given time approximately 80% of scalp hairs are in anagen. This is lower for beard and moustache hairs (around 70%) and only 20–30% for the legs and axillae. The length of the anagen phase also varies; on the scalp anagen typically lasts from 3–6 years, in the beard area this is closer to 1 year and in the moustache area anagen lasts from 4–14 weeks. Anagen is typically 16 weeks for the legs and axillae. The time in anagen determines the length of the hair produced [1].

Anagen is followed by catagen, a transitional phase in the hair growth cycle that sets the stage for production of a new follicle. In catagen the existing follicle goes through controlled involution, with apoptosis of the majority of follicular keratinocytes and some follicular melanocytes. The bulb and suprabulbar regions are lost and the follicle moves upward, being no deeper than the upper dermis at phase end. The dermal papilla becomes more compact and moves upward to rest beneath the hair follicle bulge. On the scalp catagen lasts from 14–21 days.

Telogen is a phase of follicular quiescence that follows catagen. The final cells synthesized during the previous cycle are dumped at the end of the hair shaft to form a "club" that holds the now non-living hair in place. These hairs are lost by physical action (e.g. combing) or are pushed out by the new hair that grows during the next anagen phase. The percentage of follicles in telogen also varies by body site (e.g. 5–15% of scalp follicles are normally in telogen, whereas 30% of follicles on the beard area are normally in telogen and 70–80% of leg and axillae hairs). Telogen typically lasts for 2–3 months, although this is slightly longer for leg hairs [1].

Properties of hair – impact on shaving

The beard area of an adult male contains between 6000 and 25000 hair fibers and beard growth rate has been reported in the literature to be 0.27 mm per 24 hours, although this can vary between individuals [2]. There are two types of hair fiber found in the beard area. Fine, non-pigmented vellus hairs are distributed amongst the coarser terminal hairs. While the literature abounds in publications on the properties of scalp hair, studies of beard hair are relatively scarce. Tolgyesi et al. [3] published the findings of a comparative study of beard and scalp terminal hair with respect to morphological, physical and chemical characteristics. Scalp fibers were reported to have half the number of cuticle layers compared to beard hairs from the same subject (10–13 in facial hair, 5–7 in scalp hair). Scalp fibers also had smaller cross-sectional areas (approximately half the area) and were less variable in shape than beard hairs, which exhibited asymmetrical, oblong and trilobal shapes. These differences can be seen in (Figure 19.1). Thozur et al. [4] further showed considerable variations in beard hair follicle shape and diameter within and between individuals. A number of factors contribute to this variation including anatomical location, ethnicity, age and environmental factors.

The structural properties of the hair impact shaving. The force required to cut a hair increases with increasing fiber cross-sectional area [5]. Thus, it requires more force to cut a larger fiber. Indeed, it requires almost three times the force to cut a beard hair compared to a scalp or leg hair. An important property of hair is that the force required to cut it can be greatly reduced by hydrating the hair. Hydration causes the hair to become significantly softer and much easier to cut so that it offers less resistance than dry hair to the blade and minimizes any discomfort.

The human hair follicle and the surrounding skin are richly innervated. In particular the terminal hairs of the human skin are supplied with several types of nerve endings most of which are sensory in nature. It is hypothesized that discomfort associated with shaving (during shaving or post-shave) is a result of localized skin displacement and/or the rotation and extension of the beard fiber in its follicle. The current neurological literature clearly demonstrates that such local cutaneous distortions bring about the release of various chemical communicators (histamine, prostaglandins, bradykinins, etc.) that will heighten the sensitivity of the response of pain-mediating nerve endings for a period of time [6]. The contribution to shaving comfort and irritation remains to be elucidated.

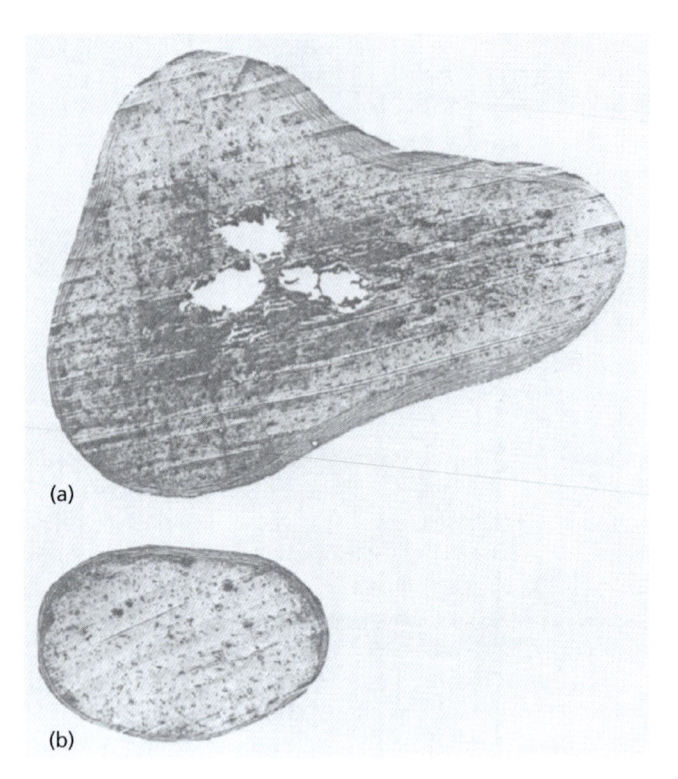

Figure 19.1 Optical micrographs of hair cross-sections taken from the beard (a) and scalp (b) area of the same subject. Beard fibers have a greater cross-sectional area and more cuticle layers than scalp hair [3]. Magnification 915×.

Shaving can also cause irritation due to physical damage. There is evidence to suggest that shaving irritation involves the removal of irregular elevations of the skin by the razor blade particularly around follicular openings [7,8]. The topography of the skin is highly variable and combined with the presence of hairs this creates a very irregular terrain over which an incredibly sharp blade traverses (Figure 19.2). This can result in irritation, generally

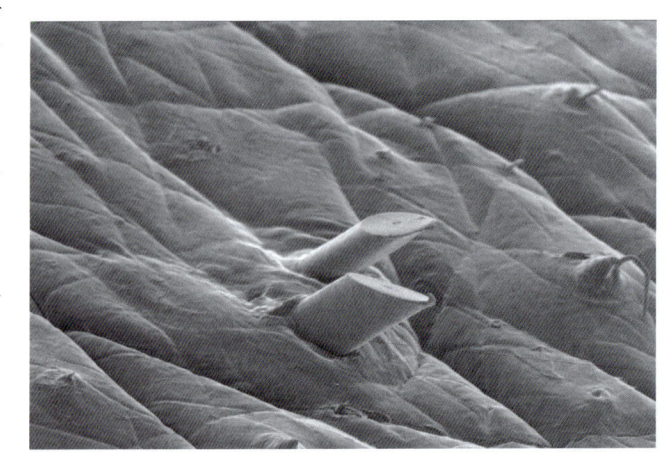

Figure 19.2 A scanning electron micrograph of a replica of an area of cheek on a male face. The topography of the skin is highly variable and combined with the presence of hairs this creates a very irregular terrain over which an incredibly sharp blade traverses.

characterized in this context by the presence of attributes such as nicks/cuts, redness, razor burn, sting or dryness. Indeed, shaving-related skin irritation is one of the most frequently noted male cosmetic complaints in Europe and the US [9]. In order to achieve a close and comfortable shave with minimal irritation it is essential to use a good quality, sharp blade and adopt a shave care regimen designed to remove as much hair as possible while inflicting minimal damage to the underlying skin.

Shaving and the razor explored

Since the invention of the safety razor, consumer product industries have invested a considerable amount of time, money and expertise in improving the design of the razor and blade in order to provide a closer, more comfortable and safer shave.

To date, few reports have been available in the literature detailing the shaving process and the mechanisms involved. The following section aims to provide an overview of the razor and the complex mechanisms by which the blade cuts the beard hair and interacts with the underlying skin.

Evolution of the system razor

With a system razor only the cartridge containing the blades is replaced, unlike a disposable razor which is thrown away in its entirety when blunt.

In the first double edge razor systems, the consumer had to position and tension a single blade within the handle. As a result, there was variability and inconsistency in how the blade interacted with the skin. In contrast, the advanced shaving systems of today are precisely assembled during manufacture.

Figure 19.3 shows a cross-section of a double edge razor with the key parameters of the cartridge geometry indicated. The shaving angle is the angle between the center plane of the blade and a plane tangent to the guard. The blade exposure is the amount by which the tip of the blade projects beyond the plane tangent to the cap and guard. Altering any of these parameters has both good and bad effects. For example, an increase in blade exposure brings the blades into closer contact with the underlying skin and hair, increasing the closeness of a shave at the expense of more nicks and cuts, and discomfort. A reduction in the shaving angle improves comfort but reduces cutting efficiency. Consequently, all aspects of the double edge blade system were compromises and the user was able to adjust the razor to suit their individual preferences [10]. Modern systems have reduced the need to compromise and achieved the previously unattainable: improving closeness, safety and comfort simultaneously. The improvement in closeness is attributed to, and exploits the mobility of the hairs within the follicle. Observation of the movement of hairs during shaving has shown that they are not cut through immediately upon contact with the blade; rather, they are carried along by the embedded blade tip, and effectively extended out of the follicle. This extension is primarily due to the distortion of the soft tissue between the hair root and the skin surface layers. Due to the visco-elastic nature of the tissue, once severed, the hair rapidly retracts back into the follicle. If a second blade follows closely behind the first, it can engage the hair in the elevated state, cutting it further down the hair shaft, before it has time to fully withdraw into the follicle [10]. By having multiple blades, this process can be exploited to give a measurable improvement in closeness. It is therefore possible to use a lower blade exposure to achieve closeness while minimizing skin contact and thus the potential for nicks, cuts and discomfort.

Simply adding more blades to razors is not a new idea (the first US patent for a five-blade razor was filed in 1929, US1920711) and from the above it is clear that on its own this will not deliver a great shave. In addition to precisely controlling the razor geometry, it is essential that the underlying skin is carefully managed to ensure a safe and comfortable shave. Adding more blades improves closeness by virtue of hair extension and probability of cutting, but can also create drag and discomfort. The pressure exerted on the skin by the additional blades can cause the skin to bulge between the inter blade span. By spacing the blades closer together, both the drag and skin bulge are reduced and a more uniform stress is placed on the skin leading to a safer, more comfortable shave (Figure 19.4). Of note, the act of cutting hairs during a shave can cause the blades to deflect and can take the blade span away from its optimal value. Recent innovations include the introduction of a blade stabilizer that supports each blade in a multiple-blade cartridge and helps to maintain the optimal distance between blades during shaving (Figure 19.5).

Manipulating these parameters can greatly alter the characteristics of a shave; consequently cartridge geometry and blade spacing are carefully controlled and set during manufacturing using specifications determined through extensive research. This ensures that the user receives a targeted and consistent shave with the optimum blade–skin contact.

Cutting edge technology

A further critical component of the shaving process, and central to an optimal shave, is the razor blade edge. The narrower the blade edge the more easily it can cut through a hair, leading to a more comfortable shave compared with less fine blade edges. Depending on the razor blade, the radius of the sharpened tip

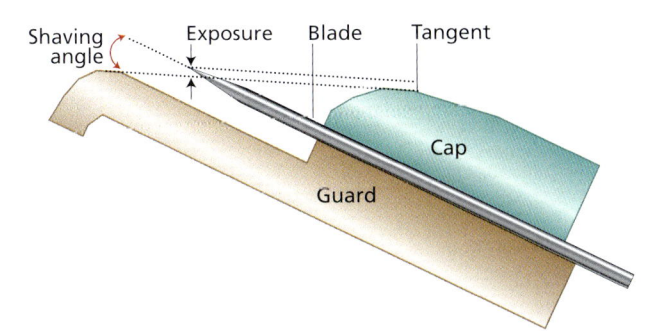

Figure 19.3 Cross-section of a double-edge razor showing exposure geometry.

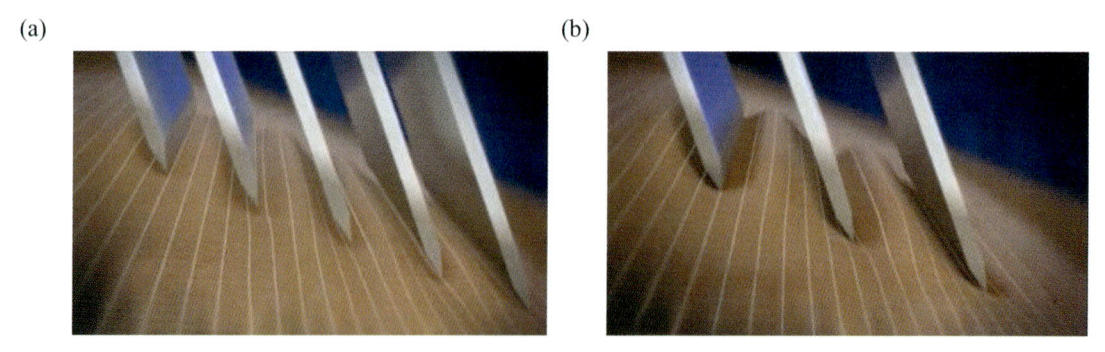

Figure 19.4 Model of multiple blade razors and skin management: five blade razors with lower inter-blade distance (a) distribute the shaving force more evenly onto the skin than fewer blades with a larger inter-blade span (b), thus reducing the height of the skin bulges between the blades for a more comfortable shave.

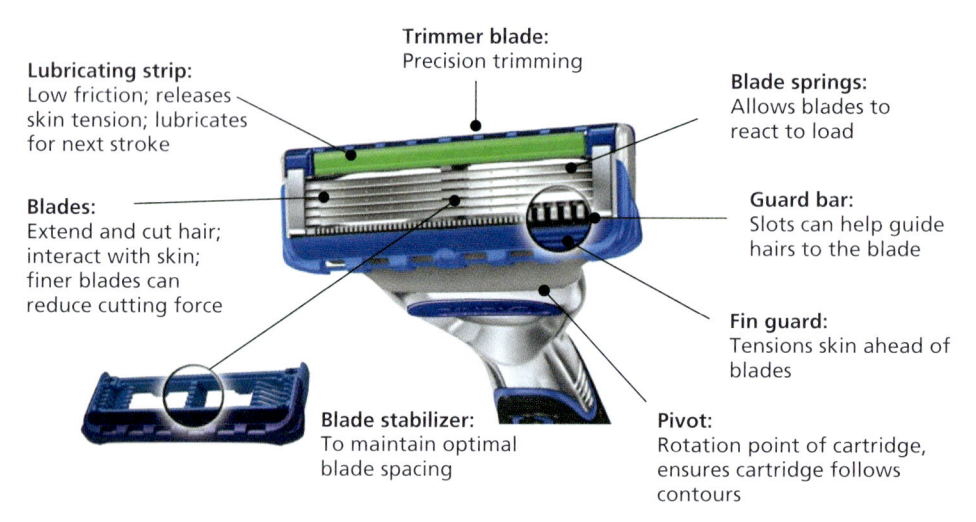

Figure 19.5 The key components of a razor and their functions.

in advanced systems can be around 25 nm [11], ~2500 times less than the radius of an average beard hair [3]. However, if the blade is too narrow it can collapse under the cutting force. Thus, the industry strives to produce the finest blade edge possible while retaining blade edge strength. This is typically achieved by treating a stainless steel substrate with thin film coatings such as diamond-like carbon to enhance edge strength or platinum–chromium to enhance corrosion resistance. The blades are further coated in a telomer-like material to create a low friction cutting surface. This greatly reduces the force required to cut hair, minimizing hair "pulling" and leading to lower localized stresses in the skin (Figure 19.6) [12].

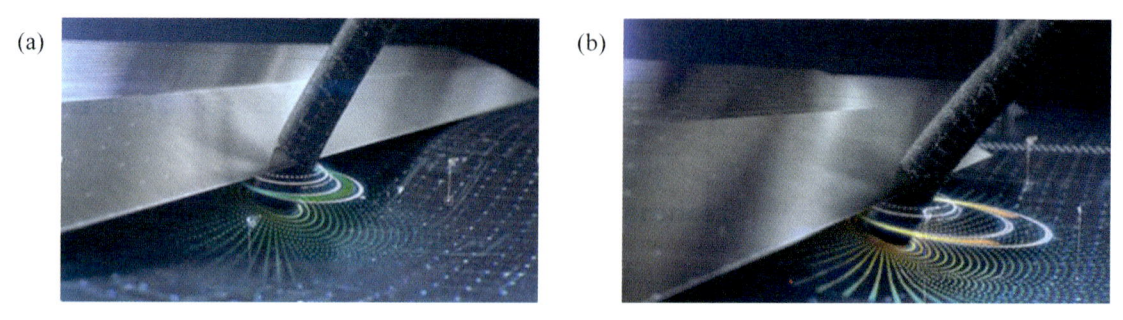

Figure 19.6 Illustration showing computer modeling of the stress in skin caused by hair cutting force. Finer blades (a) cut with less force versus thicker blades (b). This results in reduced stress in the surrounding skin [12].

Additional key components of a modern razor are shown in (Figure 19.5). First introduced in 1985, lubricating strips are now found on most disposable and permanent system cartridges. The strips distribute water soluble lubricant following each shaving stroke, resulting in a significant reduction in drag of the cartridge over the skin and allowing additional strokes to be taken comfortably even after most of the shaving preparation has been shaved off. The strips also allow the skin to release freely from the tension created by the skin guard. The guard on modern razors is typically comprised of rigid plastic or soft, flexible microfins which precede the blades. These microfins gently stretch the skin ahead of the first blade, thus presenting a smoother surface to be shaved and causing beard hairs to spring upward so they can be cut more efficiently [8]. Some advanced razors have micro slots in the guard bar designed to guide hairs to the blade prior to being cut. Additional features include pivoting heads that allow the cartridge to follow the contours of the face and also trimmer blades at the back of the cartridge that allow the user to easily shave tricky places like sideburns and under the nose or create accurate lines around facial hair. The introduction of oscillating wet shaving systems increases razor glide compared with non-oscillating systems for improved comfort.

Such advances in blade edge and razor technology, coupled with an understanding of the needs of the consumer, have significantly enhanced the quality, closeness, safety and comfort of the shave. This is most evident when combined with a shave care regimen designed to maximize hair removal and minimize skin damage.

The shaving process

Drawing a sharpened implement across the skin's surface has the potential to cause damage, and blade shaving in the absence of water or a shave preparation can result in the immediate appearance of uplifting skin cells and perturbation of stratum corneum barrier function, with an increase in dryness observed several days subsequent to the initial damage [13]. Body site will likely influence the response to this insult since the number of stratum corneum cell layers varies over the body surface, averaging 10 layers on the cheek or neck and 18 layers on the leg [14]. The potential for damage is compounded by non-uniform skin surface topography and the presence of hair (Figure 19.2), which when dry is relatively tough.

A few simple steps can help prepare the skin and hair for an optimum shaving experience. First, the skin should be thoroughly cleansed. Cleansing removes surface soils that can interfere with the shaving process and also helps hydrate the hair [15]. The latter is especially important; shaving during or after showering or bathing is ideal but, short of this, the area to be shaved should be washed with a cleanser and warm water. In some situations applying a warm, wet towel or cloth to the skin for a few minutes before shaving may also help. Hair is mostly keratin, and keratin has a high affinity for water. Hydrating softens the hair to make it more pliable and easier to cut; the force required to cut a hair decreases dramatically as hydration increases (Figure 19.7). Short-term hydration will also improve

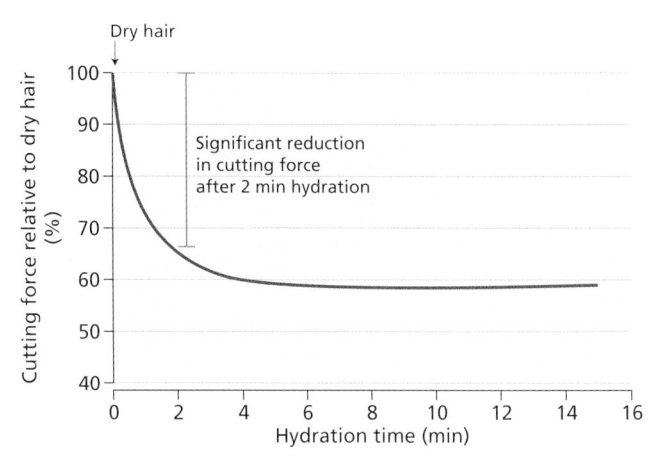

Figure 19.7 Effect of hydration time on force required to cut (beard) hair. The most significant reduction occurs over the first 2 minutes.

the skin's elasticity [16], making it better able to deform and recover as the blade is drawn over its surface. However, more is not necessarily better; prolonged soaking can macerate skin and cause the surface to become uneven, making effective hair removal more difficult and increasing the risk of damaging the skin. Excessive soaking can also deplete the stratum corneum of substances such as natural moisturizing factor (NMF) that help it hold onto water [17], which can exacerbate any dryness induced by the shaving process.

A preparation such as a shaving gel or cream can also improve the shaving experience. A preparation serves several functions. The physical act of rubbing preparation onto the skin can remove oils and dead skin cells from the surface and aid in the release of trapped hairs, with the potential to improve the efficiency of the cutting process [11]. Shaving preparation formulas typically contain a high percentage of water, which provides an additional hydration source for the hair and skin. Finally, shaving preparations are usually based on surfactants and contain other ingredients such as oils or polymers. For reasons already noted hydrating hair and skin is important for the shaving process, but hydration increases the coefficient of friction for an object sliding across the skin's surface [18]. The surfactants, oils, and polymers in shave gels can reduce friction to improve razor glide, provide a cushion between the blade and skin, and improve cutting efficiency.

Equipment and technique are also important for an optimum shaving experience. The razor should be in good condition with a sharp blade. A dull blade will not cut the hair cleanly and will pull the hair, increasing discomfort and the likelihood of nicks and cuts. Shaving in the direction of hair growth with a light pressure is preferred to reduce pulling, at least for the first few strokes. These preliminary strokes can be followed up with strokes against the grain if additional hair removal is needed. On the face, feeling the beard with the hand can help identify hair growing patterns and guide stroke direction. Skin on some areas of the body, such as the underarms, has a naturally uneven

Table 19.1 Summary of some differences between males and females related to hair characteristics and blade shaving behaviors and attitudes.

	Male	Female
Onset of shaving behavior	Most males begin shaving between the ages of 14 and 15	Most females begin shaving between the ages of 11 and 13
Body areas shaved	Most male shaving occurs on the face and neck areas. The average male shaves an area of ~300 cm^2	Female shaving is focused on the leg and underarm areas. The average female shaves an area of ~2700 cm^2
Relative hair density	Higher hair density. On average the male face has 500 hair follicles per cm^2 [7]	Lower hair density. On average the leg and axillae have 60–65 hair follicles per cm^2 [7]
Hair growth pattern	Hair on the face tends to grow in multiple directions	Hair on the legs tends to grow in the same direction; hair in the underarm area typically grows in multiple directions
Location where shaving occurs	Males tend to shave at the bathroom sink	Females tend to shave in the shower or bath
Attitudes towards shaving	Males tend to view shaving as a skill	Females tend to view shaving as a chore

or very pliable surface. Pulling the skin taut on these areas during shaving can improve the efficiency of the hair removal process and reduce nicking or cutting. In all cases the razor should be rinsed often to keep the blade surface clean.

Following the shave, skin should be thoroughly rinsed with water to remove all traces of shaving preparation, since these products are generally surfactant-based and leaving surfactant in contact with the skin can induce or exacerbate irritation. Rinsing with cool water can have a soothing effect on the skin. Applying a moisturizer can also have a soothing effect and will hydrate the skin to help prevent dryness. Moisturizers can also speed the barrier repair process and thus help to mitigate any stratum corneum damage that might result from shaving [15].

The benefits of a good regimen apply generally to the blade shaving needs for both sexes. However, there are differences between males and females in terms of hair characteristics and blade shaving behaviors and attitudes. As a result, razors for females are often designed to accommodate body specific needs. Some of these differences are summarized in Table 19.1.

Challenges within male blade shaving

Some situations may require extra care during the shaving process. For the growing number of men with self-perceived sensitive skin, the need or desire to shave on a regular basis can be challenging. In a survey of more than 1800 dermatologists, over 90% of responders agreed that the selection of shaving products was important for men with sensitive skin [19]. Individuals, including those prone to sensitive skin, should adopt an appropriate regimen that includes thoroughly hydrating the hair before shaving, liberally applying a shaving preparation and shaving with an advanced multiple-blade razor.

Pseudofolliculitis barbae (PFB) is a condition distinct from sensitive skin that affects individuals with very tightly curled hair, and is particularly prevalent among those who are of African descent. In PFB hairs may grow parallel to, rather than out from, the skin's surface and in some cases the tip of the hair curves back and grows into the surface of the skin, causing inflammation. This presents clinically as papules in the beard area with occasional pustules or hypertrophic scarring, all of which usually develop in response to shaving, and may be exacerbated by subsequent shaving. Recommendations to reduce PFB frequently include avoidance of shaving and if this is not possible, shaving with a single-bladed razor at least every 3 days [20,21]. However, there is a lack of clinical evidence to support such recommendations and thus there is a need for randomized, blinded clinical trials comparing the use of multi- and single-edged razors, different shaving techniques and shaving frequencies to determine the optimal shaving recommendations for patients with PFB [22]. Emerging clinical data suggest that PFB is not exacerbated by daily shaving with a multiple-blade razor as part of a shaving regimen that includes pre-shave hair hydration and post-shave moisturization steps [23].

Summary

Fundamental understanding of blade shaving has evolved dramatically in recent years leading to the development of sophisticated products that more effectively address the hair removal and skin care needs of men and women. Extensive research and technologically advanced manufacturing procedures are paving the way for future innovations with a deeper understanding of skin and hair.

References

1 Richards R, Meharg, G. (1991) *Cosmetic and Medical Electrolysis and Temporary Hair Removal: A Practice Manual and Reference Guide.* Medric Ltd, ISBN 0969474601.
2 Saitoh M, Uzuka M and Sakamoto M. (1969) Rates of hair growth. *Adv Biol Skin* **9**, 183–201.
3 Tolgyesi E, Coble DW, Fang FS, Kairinen EO. (1983) A comparative study of beard and scalp hair. *J Soc Cosmet Chem* **34**, 361–82.
4 Thozhur SM, Crocombe AD, Smith AP, Cowley K, Mullier M. (2007) Cutting characteristics of beard hair. *J Mater Sci* **42**, 8725–37.

5. Deem D, Rieger MM. (1976) Observations on the cutting of beard hair. *J Soc Cosmet Chem* **27**, 579–92.
6. Michael-Titus A, Revest P, Shortland P, Britton R. (2007) *The Nervous System: Basic Science and Clinical Conditions*. Oxford: Elsevier Health Sciences.
7. Bhaktaviziam C, Mescon H, Matoltsy AG. (1963) Shaving. I. Study of skin and shavings. *Arch Dermatol* **88**, 874–9.
8. Hollander J, Casselman EJ. (1937) Factors involved in satisfactory shaving. *JAMA* **109**, 95.
9. Elsner P. (2012) Overview and trends in make grooming. *Br J Dermatol* **166**(S1), 2–5.
10. Terry, J. (1991) Materials and design in Gillette razors. *Mat Design* **12**, 277–81.
11. Cowley K, Vanoosthuyze K. (2012) Insights into shaving and its impact on skin. *Br J Dermatol* **166**(S1), 6–12.
12. Zupkosky PJ, Vanoosthuyze K. (2013) *Dermatological assessment of the skin tolerance of a daily shave with a 5-blade razor for men with sensitive skin*. Poster presented at: 71st Annual Meeting of the American Academy of Dermatologists; 1–5 Mar 2013; Miami Beach, FL.
13. Marti VPJ, Lee RS, Moore AE, Paterson SE, Watkinson A, Rawlings AV. (2003) Effect of shaving on axillary stratum corneum. *Int J Cosmet Sci* **25**, 193–8.
14. Ya-Xian Z, Suetake T, Tagami H. (1999) Number of cell layers of the stratum corneum in normal skin – relationship to the anatomical location on the body, age, sex and physical parameters. *Arch Dermatol Res* **291**, 555–9.
15. Draelos D. (2012) Male skin and ingredients relevant to male skin care. *Br J Dermatol* **166**(S1), 13–16.
16. Auriol F, Vaillant L, Machet L, Diridollou S, Lorette G. (1993) Effects of short-term hydration on skin extensibility. *Acta Derm Venereol [Stockh]* **73**, 344–7.
17. Visscher MO, Tolia GT; Wickett RR, Hoath SB. (2003) Effect of soaking and natural moisturizing factor on stratum corneum water-handling properties. *J Cosmet Sci* **54**, 289–300.
18. Highley DR, Coomey M, DenBeste M, Wolfram LJ. (1977) Frictional properties of skin. *J Invest Dermatol* **69**, 303–5.
19. Vanoosthuyze K, Zupkosky PJ, Buckley K. (2013) Survey of practicing dermatologists on the prevalence of sensitive skin in men. *Int J Cosmet Sci* **35**(4), 388–93.
20. Alexis AF, Barbosa VH. (2013) *Skin of Color: A Practical Guide to Dermatologic Diagnosis and Treatment*. New York, NY: Springer, p. 128.
21. Quarles FN, Brody H, Johnson BA, *et al.* (2007) Pseudofolliculitis barbae. *Dermatol Ther* **20**, 133–6.
22. Coley MK, Alexis AF. (2009) Dermatologic conditions in men of African ancestry. *Expert Rev Dermatol* **4**(6), 595.
23. Daniels A, Gustafson CJ, Zupkosky PJ, *et al.* (2013) Shave frequency and regimen variation effects on the management of pseudofolliculitis barbae. *J Drugs Dermatol* **12**, 410–18.

PART III

Adornment

SECTION 1 Colored Facial Cosmetics

CHAPTER 20
Facial Foundation

Sylvie Guichard and Véronique Roulier

L'Oréal Research, Chevilly-Larue, France

> **BASIC CONCEPTS**
> - Facial foundation places a pigment over the skin surface to camouflage underlying defects in color and contour.
> - Facial foundations must be developed to match all ethnicities and facial needs.
> - New optic technologies have allowed modern facial foundations to create a flawless facial appearance more effectively.
> - Facial foundations impact skin health because they are worn daily for an extended period.

Introduction

Complexion makeup is anything but a trifling subject. The practice is deeply rooted in human history. It has evolved along with civilizations, fashions, scientific knowledge, and technologies to meet the various expectations depending on mood, nature, culture, and skin color. A prime stage to beautifying the face, complexion makeup creates the "canvas" on which coloring materials are placed. Women consider it as a tool to even skin color, modify skin color, or contribute to smoothing out the skin surface. To fulfill these different objectives, substances extracted from nature took on various forms over time until formulation experts developed a complex category of cosmetics including emulsions, poured compacts, and both compact and loose powders. These developments have improved the field of skin care providing radiance, wear, and sensory effects.

It remains a challenge to adequately satisfy the varying makeup requirements of women from different ethnic origins, who do not apply products in the same way and do not share the same diverse canons of beauty. It is therefore necessary to gain a thorough understanding of the world's skin colors.

Finally, as a product intended to be in intimate contact with the skin, facial foundations must meet the most strenuous demands of quality and safety. This has motivated evaluation teams to develop methods for assessing product performance.

Complexion makeup – an ancient practice

Modifying one's self-appearance by adding color and ornament to the skin of the face and body skin is hardly a recent trend [1-3]. From Paleolithic times, man has decorated himself with body paint and tattoos for various ritual activities. In the Niaux Cavern (Ariège, France), the cave of Cougnac (Lot, France), and the Magdalenian Galleries of le Mas d'Azil (Ariège), the past ages have left evidence of these practices. Along with the flint tools in the Magdalenian Galleries at le Mas d'Azil ochre nodules were found that look like "sticks of makeup" as well as grinding instruments, jars, spatulas, and needle-like "rods" 8–11 cm long, tapered at one end and spatula-shaped on the other end, suitable for applying body paint.

From the earliest of ancient civilizations, there are cosmetic recipes containing a variety of ingredients which are often closer to magic than to rational chemistry, aimed particularly at modifying the complexion. Usually used exclusively by high dignitaries, cosmetics were intended to whiten the complexion.

Ancient Mesopotamia (2500 BC)
The queen and the princes of Ur used cosmetics consisting of a mixture of mineral pigments based on Talak (from which the word "talc" is derived). Nowadays such cosmetics are still commonly used in some parts of the Middle East.

Ancient Egypt (3rd millennium BC)
The priests used plaster to cover their faces. It was also desirable for women to exhibit very white skin without blemishes, as these were indications of a privileged life of leisure. The complexion was whitened with mixtures of plaster, calcium carbonate, tin oxide, ground pearls, and lead carbonate (ceruse) mixed with animal grease, waxes, and natural resins. Evidence of the complexity of the ancient recipes has been determined

---

Cosmetic Dermatology: Products and Procedures, Second Edition. Edited by Zoe Diana Draelos.
© 2016 John Wiley & Sons, Ltd. Published 2016 by John Wiley & Sons, Ltd.

by chemical analyses carried out jointly by the Centre National de la Recherche Scientifique, L'Oréal's Recherche department, the Research Laboratory of the Museums of France, and the European Synchrotron Radiation Facility on the content of cosmetic flasks found in archeologic excavations [4]. The earliest cosmetic formulary is attributed to Cleopatra – *"Cleopatrae gyneciarum libri."*

Ancient Greece

In Ancient Greece, the white, matte complexion symbolizing purity was obtained through generous application of plaster, chalk, kaolin (*gypsos*), and ceruse (*psimythion*), but Plato was already denouncing the harmfulness of these cosmetics.

Ancient Rome

Ancient Rome raised the use of makeup to the level of an art form. In addition to cosmetics that enhance the beauty of face and body, cosmetics were applied to improve appearance and hide flaws, notably those caused by the aging process.

Women of the upper classes "coated" their face with complex mixtures with recipes reported in Ovid's *Cosmetics* or in Pliny the Elder's *Natural History*. For instance, hulled barley, powdered stag antlers, narcissus bulbs, spelt, gum, and honey were the components of a mixture to make the face shiny. Dried crocodile excrement, ceruse, vegetal extracts, as well as lanolin or suint (also known as *oesype*) were used to whiten the complexion.

Recently, an analysis was made of an ointment can, christened *Londinium*, discovered in London when excavating a temple dated at the middle of the 2nd century AD. It contained glucose-based polymers, starch, and tin oxide. The white appearance of the cream reflects a certain level of technological refinement [5].

From the Middle Ages to the 19th century

In Europe, from the Middle Ages up to the middle of the 20th century, good breeding and good manners were associated with a white complexion. In the Middle Ages, makeup was based on water, roses, and flour, which did not prevent ceruse from making a strong comeback in the Renaissance. It was then subsequently mixed with arsenic and mercury sublimates to give the complexion a fine silver hue.

Toxic effects of these cosmetics, however, was beginning to worry the authorities. In 1779, following the onset of a number of serious cases, the manufacture of "foundation bases" was placed under the control of the Société Royale de Médicine, which had just been set up in 1778. The toxic components were then removed. This measure seems to have made them disappear from the market, but it was not until 1915 that the use of ceruse was officially prohibited.

In 1873, Ludwig Leichner, a singer at the Berlin Opera, sought a way to preserve his skin tone by creating his own foundation base from natural pigments. In 1883, Alexandre Napoléon Bourjois devised the first dry or pastel foundation. Bourjois was about to launch his first dry blush, Pastel Joue.

With the birth of the cosmetics industry, products were widely distributed. Modern manufacturing techniques with production on an industrial scale coupled with the beginning of mass consumer use started at the beginning of the 20th century.

20th century: the industrial era and diversification

In the 20th century, fashionable powders for the complexion became more sophisticated [6,7]. Market choice extended with the launch of new brands such as Gemey, Caron, and Elizabeth Arden.

The 1930s saw the development of trademarks such as Helena Rubinstein and Max Factor created by professional movie and Hollywood makeup artists. The products were suited to the requirements of the movie studios. Extremely opaque, tinted with gaudy colors, they were compact and difficult to apply. After the success of Max Factor's Pancake and Panstick cosmetics, use of the word "makeup" became widespread. Initiated by Chanel in 1936, the fashion in Europe and the USA began to switch from white to a tanned complexion.

Even though women were more inclined to wear cosmetics, makeup was still not part of everyday life. Pancake makeup, a mixture of stearate, lanolin, and dry powders, was not easy to apply. Technical advances gradually made products more practical. The box of loose powder was equipped with a sieve in 1937 (Caron). In 1940, Lancôme launched Discoteint, a creamy version of its compact. Coty micronized its powder (Air Spun) in 1948. Yet, it was not until the 1950s that a real boom occurred in the number of products on the market. Compact makeup was made available in creamy form; foundation became a fluid cream (Gemey, Teint Clair Fluide, 1954). It was the start of a great diversification of formulations: fluids, dry or creamy compacts, sticks, and powders. Makeup became multifaceted, with more sophisticated effects, including moisturizing, protection from damaging environmental factors, and other skincare properties in addition to providing color.

Since then, complexion makeup has followed the continuous changes in regulations and advances in biologic knowledge, especially in the area of skin physiology. Over the last decades, it has benefitted from technologic progress in the field of raw materials, as well as from enhanced understanding and gains in optics and physical chemistry. Finally, makeup was enriched with the diversity of cultures from all over the world prompted by globalization. The beginning of the 21st century opens a new era of visual effects, sensory factors, and multiculturalism.

Formulation diversity

Women expect foundations to effect a veritable transformation that hides surface imperfections, blemishes, discolorations, and wrinkles, while enhancing a dull complexion and making shiny skin more satiny. Whereas making up the eyes and the lips is generally done playfully, the complexion receives more attention. It

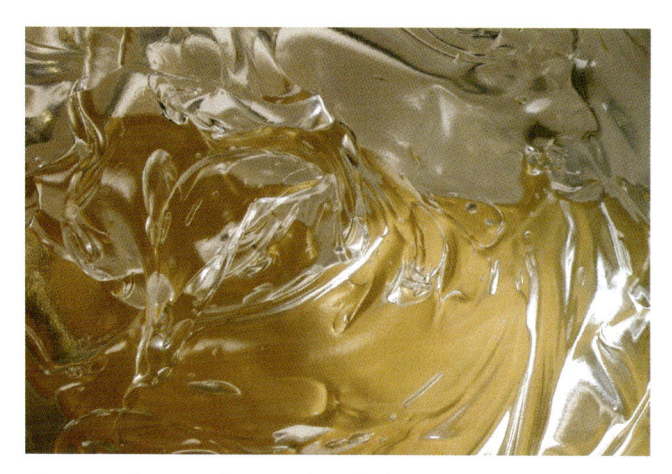

Figure 20.1 Diversity of textures: from fluid emulsion to paste dispersion.

is in this area that women display their greatest expertise and are the most demanding. Women have high expectations for their foundation including:
- Guaranteed evenness and concealment of flaws;
- Hiding of wrinkles and pores;
- Good adherence to the skin;
- Matting of lustrous skin;
- Excellent wear all day long;
- Unaltered color over time;
- Pleasant, easy application; and
- Appropriate for sensitive skin.

Variety of formulations

In order to satisfy diverse demands, a large number of products types and forms have been developed (Figure 20.1):
- Fluid foundations;
- Compact, easy-to-carry foundations with adjustable effects; and
- Powders to be used alone or in combination with a fluid foundation.

Fluid foundations: emulsions

Fluid foundations include both oil-in-water (O/W) and water-in-oil (W/O) emulsions. Until the 1990s, most foundations were O/W emulsions. Generally intended for mixed to oily skin, they are characterized by:
- Very rapid drying, which can complicate even application;
- Poor coverage;
- Reduced wear;
- Appropriate for mixed to oily skin with their external aqueous continuous phase, which makes them feel fresh on the skin.

In the 1990s, the first W/O formulations revolutionized the foundation market. The external oil continuous phase gives textures with longer drying times more suitable for perfect product application. The progressive coating of pigments has improved their dispersion in the oil phase and helped to stabilize the emulsion.

Throughout the years, the oil phase has been diversified mainly as a result of introducing silicone oils, first in conventional then in volatile forms. Silicone oils have dramatically changed the cosmetic attributes of facial foundation. Foundation no longer has to be spread evenly over the face. Its slickness makes it slide on the skin evenly with a single stroke without caking. The use of volatile oils, siliconated or carbonated, gave rise to the design of long-lasting foundations. As the volatile phase evaporates, the tinted film concentrates on the skin. Adhering during drying on the skin surface, the tinted film withstands friction and does not stain clothes.

Thus, the "non-transfer" facial foundation was born.

In the 21st century, combining volatile oils with different volatilities will lead to novel cosmetic attributes; the oily phase gradually evaporates accompanying finger strokes during application. Today, 90% of the foundations on the market are water/silicone/oil emulsions. Over the past few years, the chemistry of the emulsifying agents have also expanded as new functionalized emulsifiers become available. Either endowed with moisturizing effects or able to enhance optical properties, they contribute to the comfort and the performance of facial foundations.

Over the past few years, with the push toward a more natural-looking result and a nude, no-makeup look, formulae have become lighter, making them more transparent. Formulae with a smaller amount of opaque powders, which increase coverage and mask blemishes, remain just as effective due to the addition of transparent fillers that produce a blurring effect.

To go with such a trend, formulators designed entirely fluid products by working with high concentrations of alcohol in invert emulsions. By combining oils with various volatilities within a completely anhydrous galenical structure, formulators were then able to produce evanescent textures that leave a veil of color on the skin In 2012/2013, the market witnessed the creation of veritable foundation "essences", products pushed to the extreme limit of fluidity. This precise combination of different oils, being natural or synthetic, volatile or long lasting, produces a thin veil of color.

Compact foundations

Compact foundations are made up of waxes and oils in which powders and pigment phases are dispersed under heat, but compact foundations can be greasy, heavy, and streaky. The more recent use of esters and siliconated oils has made it possible to lighten the texture and improve application qualities. Volatile oils also help the facial foundation film remain unaltered for a longer time and provide long-lasting coverage. Compact foundations display the advantage of being adjustable with a sponge, which is ideal for concealing localized defects. Packaging the foundation in compact cases makes it practical for touching up during the day.

Waterpacts are a special compact type that contain water. They consist of W/O or O/W emulsions rich in waxes that are poured into the compact under heat. The water content makes it necessary to use waterproof packaging. These solid emulsions are difficult to manufacture and preserve, but they have the huge advantage of making the compact fresh as well as practical in use.

Compacts can also be packaged as sticks for more precise and localized strokes, such as around the eyes.

Powders

Compact powders are distinct from loose powders as they represent the "portable to go" version of loose powders. They are composed of fillers and pigments. A binder containing 10% oils and grease ensures the compact powder particle cohesion, while also providing comfort and ease of application. To make a high-quality powder a suitable milling procedure must be used in order to disperse the pigments finely and evenly throughout the powder phase.

Loose powders

A loose powder is characterized by weak particle cohesion. It does not contain binder or may contain just enough to provide a degree of cohesion that controls the final product volatility. Loose powders are generally applied with a puff, but manufacturers are developing tricks for easy application by using more finely tuned application brushes. Unlike with a puff, the powder does not scatter.

Compact powders

There are different kinds of compact powders:

- Finishing powders provide sheer coverage and are used for touch-up during the day. They are usually applied with a sponge over a foundation to mask facial shine. The fillers used in these powders tend to be organic, because they are more transparent. They also have the advantage of absorbing sebum while still leaving a natural look. The formulation challenge is to find a good balance between texture quality and the ease in placing the proper amount of powder on the applicator.
- Powder foundations are compact or loose powders whose covering power is equivalent to that of a foundation (i.e. better than a finishing powder). They can be used instead of foundation, for instance by women who dislike fluid textures. The loose powder version known as mineral makeup is currently enjoying considerable success.
- Two-way cakes, which are available in compact form, can be used either wet or dry. This kind of powder is popular with Japanese women. Using it dry gives the same kind of makeup as a powder foundation, while using it wet gives more even coverage. This dual usage requires the vast majority of the fillers to be hydrophobic. Treated fillers, coated with silicone oils that cannot be wetted, are mostly used. In this way, the compact remains unaltered after contact with water and does not cake. These two-way cakes are formulated to provide fuller coverage than powder foundations. They give a very matte appearance that will not wear off in hot, humid conditions such as in the Asiatic climate.

The main drawback of all powders is a certain discomfort relative to foundation, mainly because of the absence of any moisturizing effect (Table 20.1).

Table 20.1 Products categories overview.

Skin type target	Formulations characteristics	Name of category	Main objectives
All types of skin but adapted to Asian routine	Uncolored formulations To be applied under foundation	Foundation base	Application: Lasting effect – spreadability Moisturizing effect – matt finish
All types of skin	Weakly colored	Tinted creams BB creams	Skincare attributes Skincare and make-up performances
All types of skin	Weakly colored but pearly	Bronzers Highlighters	Healthy "glow" effect, suntan color
All types of skin	Greens, purples, blues, apricot	Complexion correctors	Correction of discoloration (red spots by green tints) Complexion freshener (apricot – blue)
All types of skin	Low to full coverage	Fluid foundations	Wear – matt finish Antiaging – radiance
Normal to oily skin	Low to full coverage	Compacted powders, such as two-way cakes (adapted to Asian routine)	Matt finish – complexion evenness
Normal to dry skin	Medium to full coverage	Compact foundation	Evenness – adjustability of the result. Comfort – mobility
Normal to oily skin	Weak to medium coverage	Waterpacts (poured emulsions)	Same properties as compacts, plus freshness and hydrosoluble actives
Eye contour	Medium to full coverage	Concealers	Hides dark circles under the eyes
All types of skin	Transparent to opaque (mineral makeup)	Loose powders	Matt finish and adhesion – evenness

Color creation

At the core of foundation formulations there is a combination of colored powders that must be:

- As finely dispersed as possible with optimal stability; and
- Able to create a natural-looking tinted film once smeared over the skin.

To achieve this end, the formulator has available various colorants that comply with the different cosmetics legislations (positive lists) and are thus certified to be harmless, chemically pure, and microbiologically clean. These are inorganic pigments such as metallic oxides – yellow, red, and black iron oxides – to which colored and uncolored pearls can be added to give a lustrous effect. To brighten foundations (especially the darkest ones) blue pigment can be substituted for black (Figure 20.2).

For improved pigment dispersion and formula stability, the process of pigment coating has gradually become the standard. In water/silicone emulsions, a silicone coating is most frequently used. Coating with an amino acid aims at developing products for sensitive skin.

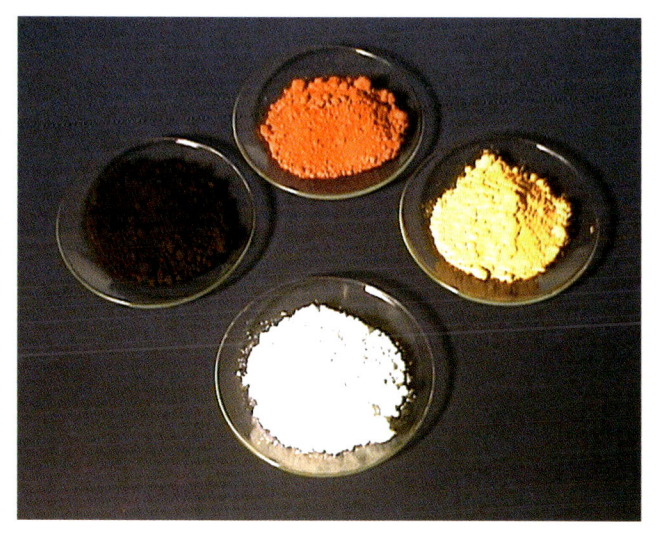

Figure 20.2 The four iron oxides used in foundations.

Pigments and coverage

The amount of titanium oxide pigment in the product is an indication of its ability to cover skin flaws (i.e. the level of coverage provided). A foundation is characterized by theoretical coverage on a scale from 7 (natural effect) to 50 (corrective makeup). However, this ignores the optical properties of the product, which may also be able to mask skin defects through a soft focus effect [8]. It also does not take into account the influence of texture, which will determine how transparent or opaque the colored deposit is according to the ability of the product to spread evenly as a thin layer over the skin.

Importance of fillers

Fillers are all the non-pigment powders introduced in the product to provide:

- Covering power;
- The ability to absorb sebum and sweat so as to make the skin velvety and fix the color to the skin;
- Fineness and smoothness, which enhances cosmetic qualities of the textures; and
- Spreadability, which makes application easier.

Both form and chemical nature govern the final qualities of fillers (Figure 20.3a–c). Talc is an example of a spreadable, lamellar powder that is widely used for its extreme softness and absorbing power. Kaolin, starches, and calcium carbonate used to be widely employed but they have now been superseded by:

- Different varieties of silica, sometimes porous forms;
- Polymers such as nylon and polymethylmethacrylate (PMMA); and
- Mica platelets that can also be coated.

Not only are these powders essential to the basic properties of a product, but they also contribute to its optical properties. Transparent or opaque, lustrous, matte, or soft focus, they help to achieve the desired finish on the skin.

While fillers remain a necessary ingredient in powders, smaller amounts are introduced in foundations. Formulators favour optically transparent particles rather than white, opaque fillers.

When applied, the product is lighter and more transparent, and does not create a caked or mask-like look.

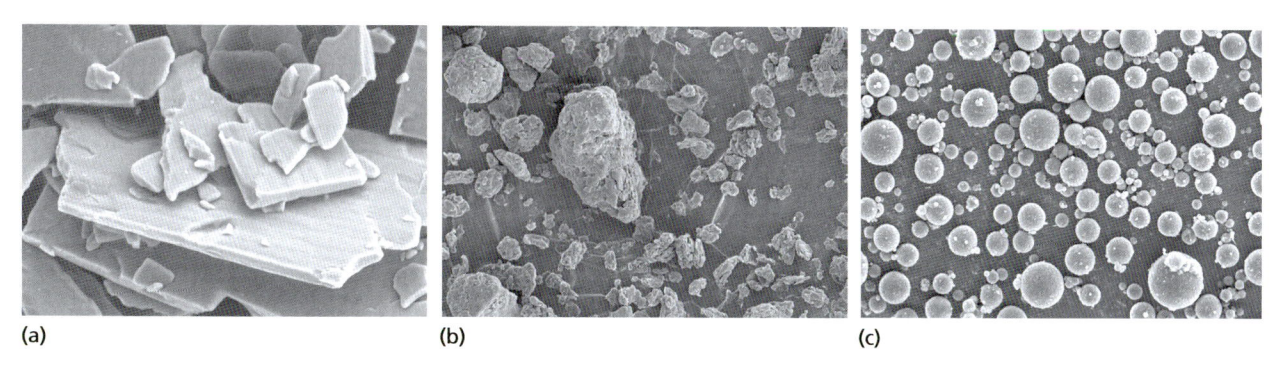

(a) (b) (c)

Figure 20.3 Shape variety of fillers (a–c).

When color and skincare combine

Progress in formulation technologies has allowed scientists to stabilize pigments in skincare formulae designed to provide short- and long-term results, such as protection, anti-ageing treatment, and long-lasting moisture.

Reconciling comfortable texture and the masking properties of desaturated color had been the goal of products designed towards the user's skincare routine: such products were very successful in South Korea, then called BB creams (blemish balm cream).

European versions were just as successful by combining effective skincare with a healthy glow/radiance (BB) or corrective (CC) color.

From 2010, these products opened a new category of hybrid formulations conceived to provide coverage (through blurring or color) while being effective through their active ingredients. These simple, multi-use products combining skincare and make-up cosmetics are very popular among women, making the frontier between both categories increasingly fuzzier.

Facial foundation application

Most women usually apply their facial foundation first when applying cosmetics. They may choose to modify their complexion color or make it more glowing and even without changing the color. Whatever effect is desired, makeup is used to recreate an ideal of color and finish peculiar to each individual according to ethnic and cultural practices. It must also be adapted to suit the woman's routine: application of a single product, use over a base or under a powder, stroked on by finger or by sponge.

There is a great diversity in the use of complexion makeup. The formulator must address several issues. Being familiar with the various skin color characteristics is a primary requisite for recreating the shades that closely match the ethnic origin of the user. For any given product, this is a necessary prerequisite for creating a range of shades that will likely satisfy the women throughout the world, whether Caucasian, Hispanic, African, or Asian.

A large study carried out on a widely representative panel demonstrated significant differences in the colorimetric characteristics of skin color of six ethnic groups living in nine different countries [9,10]. The recorded measurements enabled the definition of a wide color space showing the various color spectra typical of each ethnic group's skin color mesh and overlap (Figure 20.4).

Further studies showed that the variety of makeup routines reflected the ethnic origin and cultural heritage which determines whether a woman feels positive toward her natural skin color. For many women, skin color is a major factor in their cultural identity. Complexion makeup is the easiest way to achieve even skin color by erasing surface color variations or correcting color unevenness. Some women wish to appear more deeply "tanned" than their natural color. This behavior is commonly found in Caucasian and Hispanic women. Japanese women, however, desire their makeup to give them a lighter complexion (Figure 20.5) [10].

The formulator works within this defined scope to develop shades matching natural skin colors. To meet women's expectations, it is necessary to analyze how women self-perceive their complexion. By identifying skin colors within a definite color range and precisely identifying the makeup habits of women over the world, it is now possible to formulate a variety of shades that match up with the wishes of all women.

Emphasis on quality, safety and confirmed performance

Complexion makeup creates an intimate relationship between the skin and a complex formulation that is left on for hours. Before being marketed, every product has to undergo a battery of tests to confirm its safety and performance. There are several steps in this process.

Design stage

The formulator must ensure high quality ingredients are used by defining specifications and analytical controls and carrying out screening for the non-toxicity of the ingredients with *in vitro* tests on reconstructed skin models. Each raw material used must be cleared for safety and have a proper toxicologic dossier.

Formulation stage

It is necessary to:
- Evaluate stability by subjecting products to thermal cycles to accelerate aging.
- Confirm the level of microbiologic preservation of the formulas using challenge tests. The selected method of preservation and the nature of the preservatives depend on the technology involved (powder emulsion, anhydrous compact). The risk of microbiologic contamination increases with the water content. It also depends on the packaging; a pump bottle provides better protection than a jar.
- Check it is harmless through using alternate methods: *in vitro* testing and including tests run on reconstructed skin model, e.g. (EpiSkin®, L'Oréal Episkin SNC, Lyon, France); clinical tests (simple patch test [SPT] and repeated patch test [RPT]); and, finally, user tests under dermatologic controls, carried out on the product's targeted skin types, particularly on sensitive skins and using wide ranging, representative panels. Use testing under ophthalmologic controls is carried out systematically on products intended to mask under-eye rings.

Performance stage

The performance of the product must be studied to ensure that it complies with consumer wishes and to obtain an unbiased

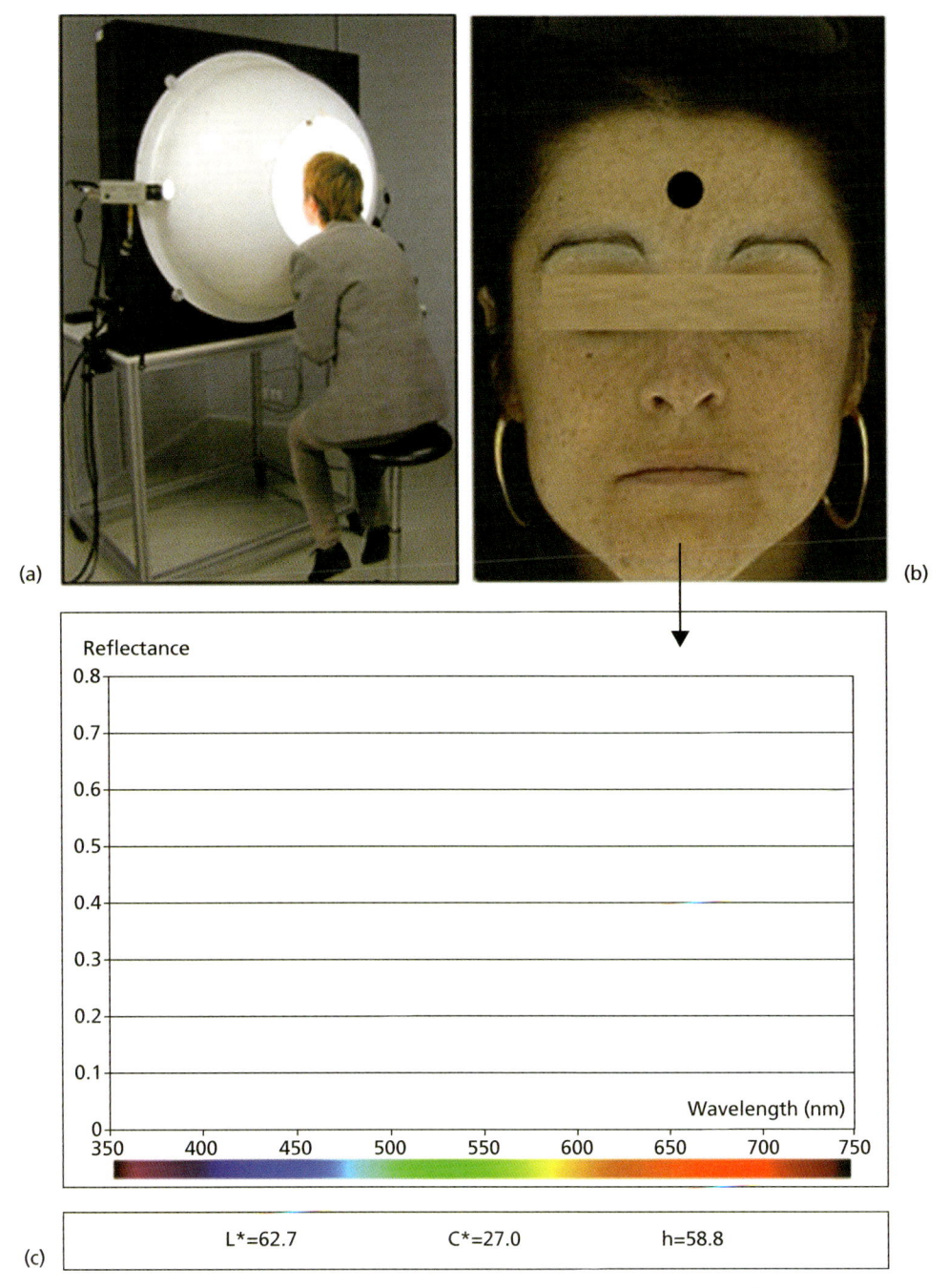

Figure 20.4 (a) The color of the forehead was measured using a spectroradiometer inside a Chromasphere™. (b) The volunteer placed her face into the Chromasphere. A standardized camera was used to acquire pictures of the face. (c) A spectroradiometer measured the reflectance of forehead in the visible field 400–700 nm every 4 nm. The recorded spectrum was expressed in the CIE 1976 standard colorimetric space L*C*h D65/10 ° where each color is described through three coordinates that reflect perception by human eye. h, Hue angle (angular coordinate); C*, chroma (radius coordinate); L*, lightness (z axis).

opinion on advertising claims and consumer complaints. Sensorial analysis tests provide qualitative and quantitative assessments of a product's features by a trained panel of experts, as well as by untutored panels performing the tests under the formula's normal user conditions.

Additionally, a complexion product can be tested with the conventional methods used for skincare cosmetics:

- Measurement of moisturizing effects using SkinChip® (L'Oréal, Chevilly-Larue, France) or Corneometer® (Courage & Khazaka, Köln, Germany).
- Effects on skin firmness with using the Dermal Torque Meter® (Dia-Stron Ltd, Andover, UK).
- Image analysis on skin imprints or, even better, projection of light fringes involving no contact with skin (i.e. skin in real

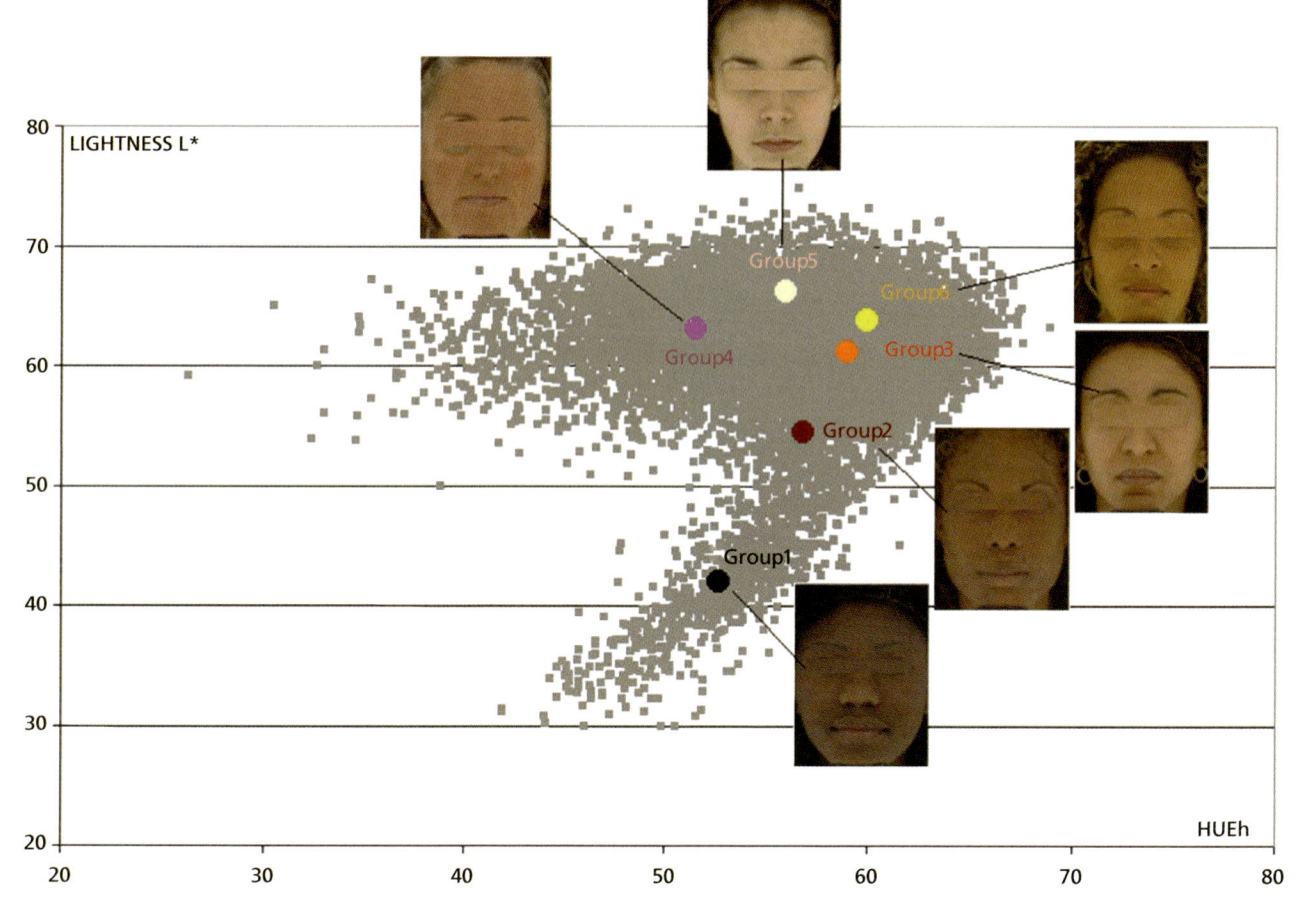

Figure 20.5 The worldwide skin color space depicted in (h, L*) and split in six groups of skin tones that reflect the color diversity.

conditions with makeup as applied) to assess antiwrinkle performance.

Also specific tests:
- Color appraisal using the Chromasphère® (L'Oréal, Chevilly-Larue, France): the difference in the color of the skin before and after applying makeup quantifies the improvement in color evenness and change in color effect. Moreover, it makes it possible to monitor both. As a result, the manufacturer can claim that its makeup effects last a given number of hours.
- Evaluation of the matt finish with a suitable device (Samba® [Bossa Nova Technologies, Venice, CA, USA]).

Conclusions and prospects

Beauty is diverse. Textures, tones, matte or lustrous results, play time, and sensoriality must all come together to give a woman a simple means to recreate her ideal complexion. Complexion makeup products today benefit from knowledge of physical chemistry, resulting in better understanding of the relationships between chemical composition, texture, and application behavior. Facial foundations benefit from technologic advances in optics, which has generated formulations that are sheer, glowing, matte, able to provide soft focus concealment of flaws, while simultaneously giving shades that mirror the natural hues of the skin.

Complexion makeup products have been expanded to deliver multisensory effects and address ethnic diversity issues. From simple emulsions applied by finger, facial foundations have evolved into mousses, creamy compacts, and soft powders that can be applied by brush or sponge, and layered. Facial foundations contribute to beauty of the face respecting the women's own skin, but also addressing their culture and ethnic diversity [11,12]. New forms, new optical effects, and new application methods will permit users to attain their ideal complexion irrespective of origin or own canons of beauty.

References

1 Claude C. (2006) Histoire du maquillage du teint: une vision croisée des cultures, des modes et des évolutions technologiques. Thèse pour l'obtention du Diplôme d'Etat de Docteur en Pharmacie Faculté Paris V.

2 Gröning K. (1997) *La Peinture du Corps*. Arthaud Editions.
3 Gründ F. (2003) *Le Corps et le Sacré*. Editions du Chêne Hachette Livre.
4 Walter P, Martinetto P, Tsoucaris G, Breniaux P, Lefebvre MA, Richard G, *et al.* (1999) Making make-up in ancient Egypt. *Nature* **397**, 483–4.
5 Evershed RP, Berstan R, Grew F, Copley MS, Charmant AJH, Barham E, *et al.* (2004) Formulation of a Roman cosmetic. *Nature* **432**, 35–6.
6 Chanine N, Deprund MC, De La Forest F, *et al.* (1996) *100 Ans de Beauté*. Atlas Editions.
7 Pawin H, Verschoore M. (2001) *Maquillage du Teint du Visage*. Paris: Encyclopédie Médicale Chirurgicale, Cosmétologie Dermatologie Esthétique Editions Scientifiques et Médicales Elsevier.
8 Takayoshi I, Miyoji O. (2002) Appealing the technical function of the optical characteristic foundation from the view point of marketing. *Fragrance J* **30**, 59–63.
9 Caisey L, Grangeat F, Lemasson A, Talabot J, Voirin A. (2004) Skin color and make-up strategies of women from different ethnic groups. *Int J Cosmet Sci* **28**, 427–37.
10 Baras D, Caisey L. Skin, lips and lashes of different skins of color: typology and make-up strategies. In AP Kelly and SC Taylor, *Dermatology for Skin of Color*. McGraw-Hill, Berkshire, UK, pp. 541–9.
11 Mulhern R, Fieldman G, Hussey T, Lévêque JL, Pineau P. (2003) Do cosmetics enhance female Caucasian facial attractiveness? *Int J Cosmet Sci* **25**, 199–205.
12 Korichi R, Pelle-de-Queral D, Gazano G, Aubert A. (2008) Why women use make-up: implication of psychological traits in make-up functions. *J Cosmet Sci* **59**, 127–37.

CHAPTER 21
Camouflage Techniques

Anne Bouloc
Vichy Laboratoires, Cosmétique Active International, Asnières, France

> **BASIC CONCEPTS**
> - Camouflage makeup is used to cover facial defects of contour and color.
> - Camouflage makeup must be artistically applied to achieve an optimal result.
> - Camouflage techniques can improve quality of life.
> - Camouflage therapists can train patients in the proper application techniques for cosmetics.

Introduction

Camouflage techniques can be helpful in patients who do not achieve complete or immediately attractive results from dermatologic therapy. Because appearance is one of the pivotal factors influencing social interactions, facial blemishes and disfigurements are a psychosocial burden in affected patients leading to low self-esteem and poor body image. Camouflage makeup can normalize the appearance of skin and improve quality of life. Training in camouflage techniques is essential because the application is different from regular foundations. This chapter discusses the use of camouflage cosmetics.

Definitions

Camouflage cosmetics were introduced more than 50 years ago to improve the appearance of World War II pilots who had sustained burns. The products provided an opaque cover over the damaged skin areas. Modern high quality camouflage products provide an excellent coverage, but with a more natural appearance (Figure 21.1).

There are several brands of camouflage makeup on the market. They aim to conceal skin discoloration and scars and to impart a natural, normal appearance. Camouflage products differ from makeup products purchased over the counter. They contain up to 25% more pigment, as well as fillers endowed with optical properties. Camouflage makeups are waterproof and designed to cover and mask a problem, but must be mixed to match the patient's skin tone. The goals of camouflage cosmetics are to provide [1]:

1. *Color:* Camouflage makeup must match all skin tones as it should blend into the color of the area on the face it is intended to cover evenly.
2. *Opacity:* Camouflage makeup must conceal all types of skin discoloration, yielding as natural and normal an appearance as possible.
3. *Waterproof:* Camouflage makeup must be rain and sweat-resistant, remaining unaltered with athletics (e.g. swimming).
4. *Holding power:* Camouflage makeup must adhere to skin without sliding off.
5. *Longer wear:* Camouflage makeup must provide the assurance of long wear with easy reapplication, if necessary.
6. *Ease of application:* Camouflage makeup must be easy to apply. Too many steps and color applications may create patient confusion.

There are several different types of camouflage cosmetics:

1. *Full concealment:* A method referring to complete coverage of the damaged skin and extending beyond the boundaries of the injured area. High coverage foundation creams or cover creams should be used for full concealment.
2. *Pigment blending:* A method that involves selection of a cover cream that matches the color of patient's foundation.
3. *Subtle coverage:* A light application of foundation cream that conceals only moderately.

Contouring is used to minimize areas of hypertrophy or atrophy present in facial scars, using highlighting or shading to create the illusion of smoothness.

Camouflage makeup application procedures

It is important to remember that camouflage makeup is most effective when applied over skin with color abnormalities or discoloration. The size of the defect is immaterial, because it is as easy to cover a large blemish as a smaller one. However, the

---

Cosmetic Dermatology: Products and Procedures, Second Edition. Edited by Zoe Diana Draelos.
© 2016 John Wiley & Sons, Ltd. Published 2016 by John Wiley & Sons, Ltd.

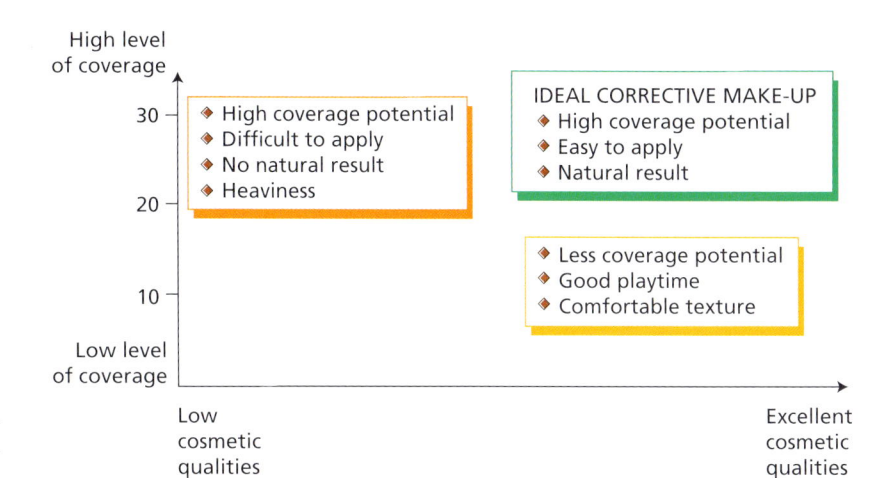

Figure 21.1 Ideal corrective makeup: a compromise between coverage and cosmetic qualities. After Sylvie Guichard, L'Oréal Research.

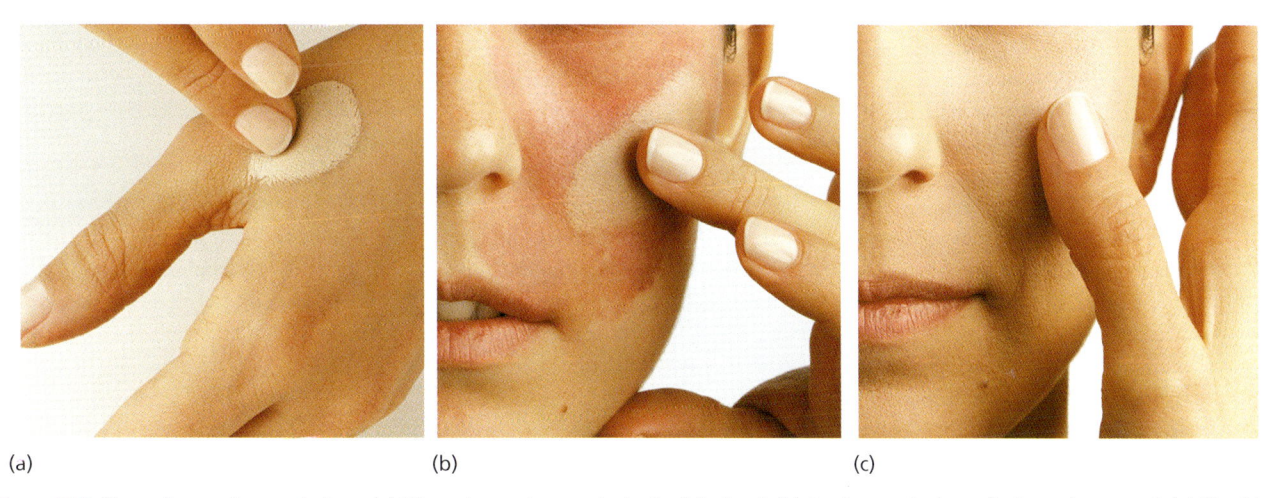

Figure 21.2 Camouflage makeup technique. (a) Warm the product on the back of the hand. (b) Apply over the imperfection to be covered. (c) Blend in round the edges.

camouflage of texture abnormalities is more challenging. Rough scars are more difficult to conceal than smooth scars because unevenness is exaggerated after camouflaging [2].

This section of the chapter presents the steps necessary to complete a camouflage makeup application procedure for a given patient. First, patients should be asked about prior experience in attempting to camouflage their lesions with or without medical makeup. If they have no experience, the necessary steps should be discussed in detail. Second, the patient's skin should be cleansed with a product selected according to patient's skin type. For an optimal camouflage result, the skin should be well exfoliated and moisturized. If using a camouflage product without sun protection factor (SPF) protection, a sunscreen-containing moisturizer should be selected otherwise a bland moisturizer can be used.

Third, the camouflage product must be selected to match the patient's skin. The camouflage therapist should identify the underlying tones that contribute to skin color: haemoglobin produces red, keratin produces yellow, and melanin produces brown [3]. Thinner skin possesses more red tones while thicker skin appears more yellow. For this reason, it is almost impossible to mimic natural skin color with only one shade.

Fourth, the camouflage therapist must understand color. There are three color coordinates: hue, value, and intensity.

1. *Hue* is the coordinate for the pure spectrum colors commonly referred to as "color name" – red, orange, yellow, blue, green, violet – which appear in the hue circle or rainbow. Each different hue is a different reflected wavelength of light. White light splitting up through a prism has seven hues: red, orange, yellow, green, blue, indigo, and violet.
2. *Value* is defined as the relative lightness or darkness of a color. Adding white to a hue produces a high value color, often called a tint. Adding black to a hue produces a low value color, often called a shade.

3. *Intensity*, also called chroma or saturation, refers to the brightness of a color. A color is at full intensity when not mixed with black or white – a pure hue. The intensity of a color can be altered, making it duller or more neutral by adding gray to the color.

Matching a color from one manufacturer to another one is a very difficult procedure because of the variety of shades that can be produced by combining various colors and the tints of the color that can be made by varying the amount of white. Judgment of color should always be made on the skin and never in the container because what seems to be the same shade may appear quite different on the skin.

The use of neutralizers in camouflaging is somewhat controversial. Some experts think it is possible to neutralize undesirable skin discoloration [2]. For example, green undertoner neutralizes a red complexion and lavender undertoner negates a yellow complexion. Other authors think that makeup undertoners do nothing but create a third color [4]. They consider that when two colors are mixed, the result is a third color. Mixing opposite colors on the color wheel (e.g. green and red or yellow and purple) will result in an unattractive gray–brownish color that must be concealed with a color that matches the skin, which adds an extra step and thickness to the makeup.

For contouring, several products have to be applied. Hypertrophic scars appear lighter than surrounding skin, and have to be camouflaged applying a darker product than to surrounding skin. Atrophic scars, however, appear darker than surrounding skin, and have to be corrected using lighter product.

Once the shades have been selected, the camouflage therapist may apply them to the back of the hand as a painter uses a palette to warm and soften the product (Figure 21.2a). Camouflage products are either applied with a sponge in a patting motion or with the fingertips (Figure 21.2b). The patting motion applies the product to the surface of the skin and does not clog pores, which allows the skin to retain its natural characteristics. Distinct borders are eliminated by blending the edges (Figure 21.2c).

A camouflage product often is not used over the entire face like a regular facial foundation, but the surrounding skin must be matched as closely as possible. Patients have to be reminded that skin color on the hands does not really correspond to skin color of the face. The application is generally followed up with an application of powder which sets and waterproofs the camouflage product. The setting powder used should be translucent so that the camouflage product does not change color. For patients with very dry skin, it is not necessary to use a powder as the oils are quickly absorbed into the skin.

Many patients may prefer using only one shade even when the color match is not perfect. Men may not wish to mix colors. It might be of interest to show the patient the coverage with one shade and the coverage using more than one shade while demonstrating that color blending is relatively easy and worthwhile.

For men, common skin flaws must be reproduced in order to prevent a "mask-like" appearance [5]. Beard stubble can be recreated by using different sponges and a brown or black pigment that mimics surface irregularities. Other colored powdered blushes can be used on the cheeks to simulate the natural glow of youth and around the eyes and mouth to attract the attention on other parts of the face [6]. Pictures should be taken before and after the application to document the cosmetic results.

Finally, the cosmetics must be removed each evening prior to bed. Removing camouflage makeup is more difficult than regular makeup. Alcohol or acetone-based removers are too irritating for sensitive skin, thus it is better to use water-soluble cream-type makeup remover. The remover is applied generously to emulsify the makeup followed by wiping with cotton pads. The face is then rinsed with tepid water and patted dry [7].

Other camouflage therapies

A few other options than camouflage makeup therapies have been suggested. Dihydroxyacetone, the main ingredient in self-tanning creams, has been proposed for camouflaging in patients with vitiligo [8]. It may be a cheap, safe, and effective alternative especially for the hands and the feet as cover creams are waterproof but not rubproof.

Medical tatooing under local anesthesia has also been tried to create the appearance of hair in hairless areas [9]. The pigment used is made of ferrous oxide, glycerol, and alcohol. A test on a small area should be performed to evaluate the outcome. The needle should be introduced into the dermis similarly to the natural hair pattern of the patient.

Medical indications for camouflage makeup

There are various medical indications for camouflage makeup. The lesion requiring camouflage can be permanent or temporary. The best results are obtained with macules, but papules, nodules, or scars can also be camouflaged. Macular lesions for camouflaging include pigmentary disorders such as vitiligo (Figure 21.3), chloasma (Figure 21.4), lentigenes, postinflammatory hypopigmentation or hyperpigmentation (Figure 23.5); hypervascular disorders such as telangiectasia (Figure 21.6) and angioma (Figure 23.7); and tattoos. Papulonodular lesions for camouflaging include discoid lupus, acne (Figure 21.8), dermatosis papulosa nigra, and facial scars.

After a graft for oncologic surgery, or for other postsurgical scars, there may be variation in pigmentation and/or relief and corrective cosmetics may be of interest. Depending on the skin's ability to heal, camouflage therapy can be applied 7–10 days after most surgical procedures. However, the premature use of makeup following epidermal damage may cause a secondary infection or tattooing effect.

There may be transient injuries or lesions of the skin that can be camouflaged with makeup. An injury may produce hematoma and oedema that should be concealed for occupational

21. Camouflage Techniques 189

Figure 21.3 Perioribital hyperpigmentation: (a) before and (b) after camouflage.

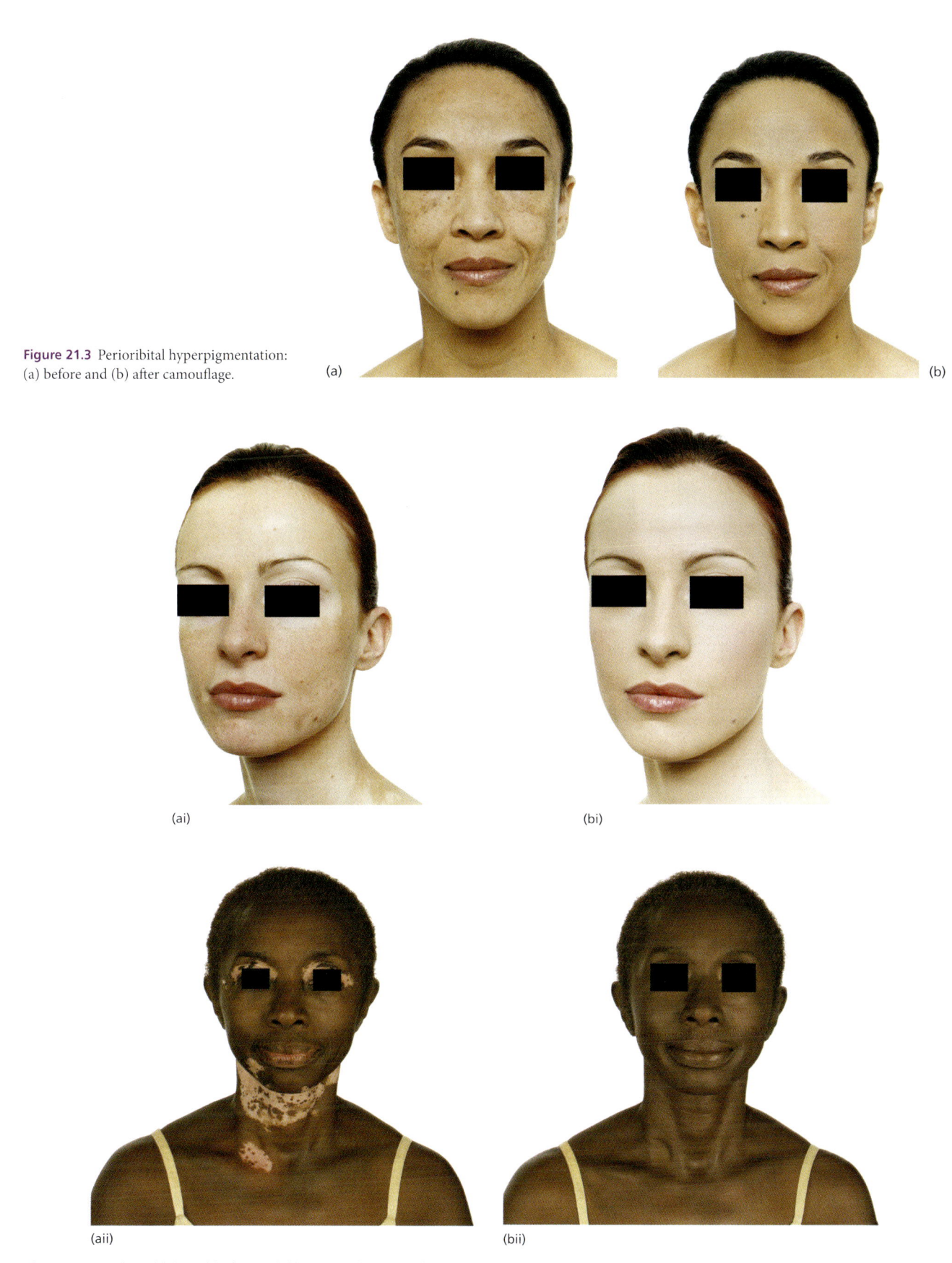

Figure 21.4 Vitiligo: (a) (i & ii) before and (b) (i & ii) after camouflage.

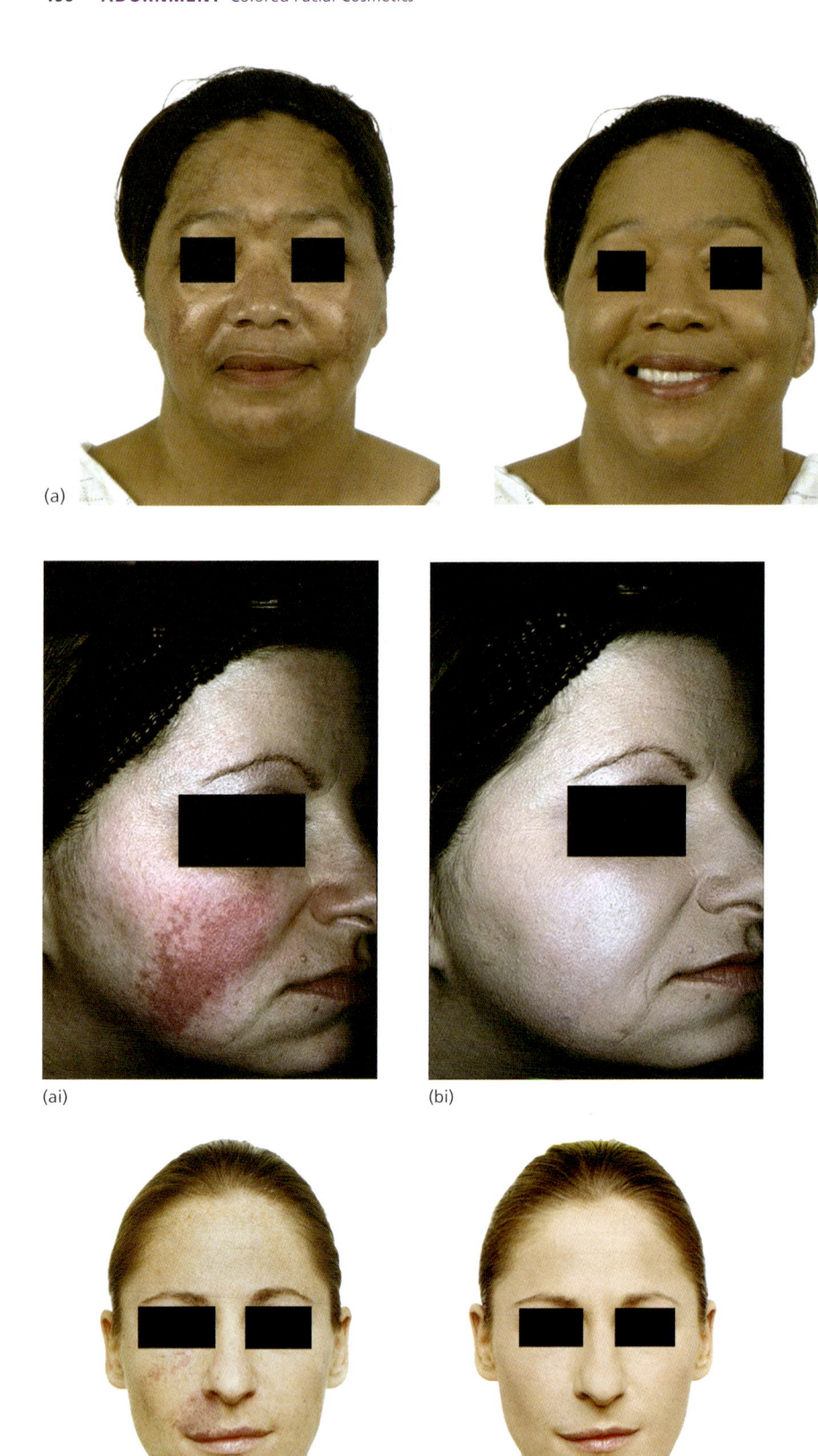

190 ADORNMENT Colored Facial Cosmetics

Figure 21.5 Melasma: (a) before and (b) after camouflage.

Figure 21.6 Vascular malformation: (a) (i & ii) before and (b) (i & ii) after camouflage.

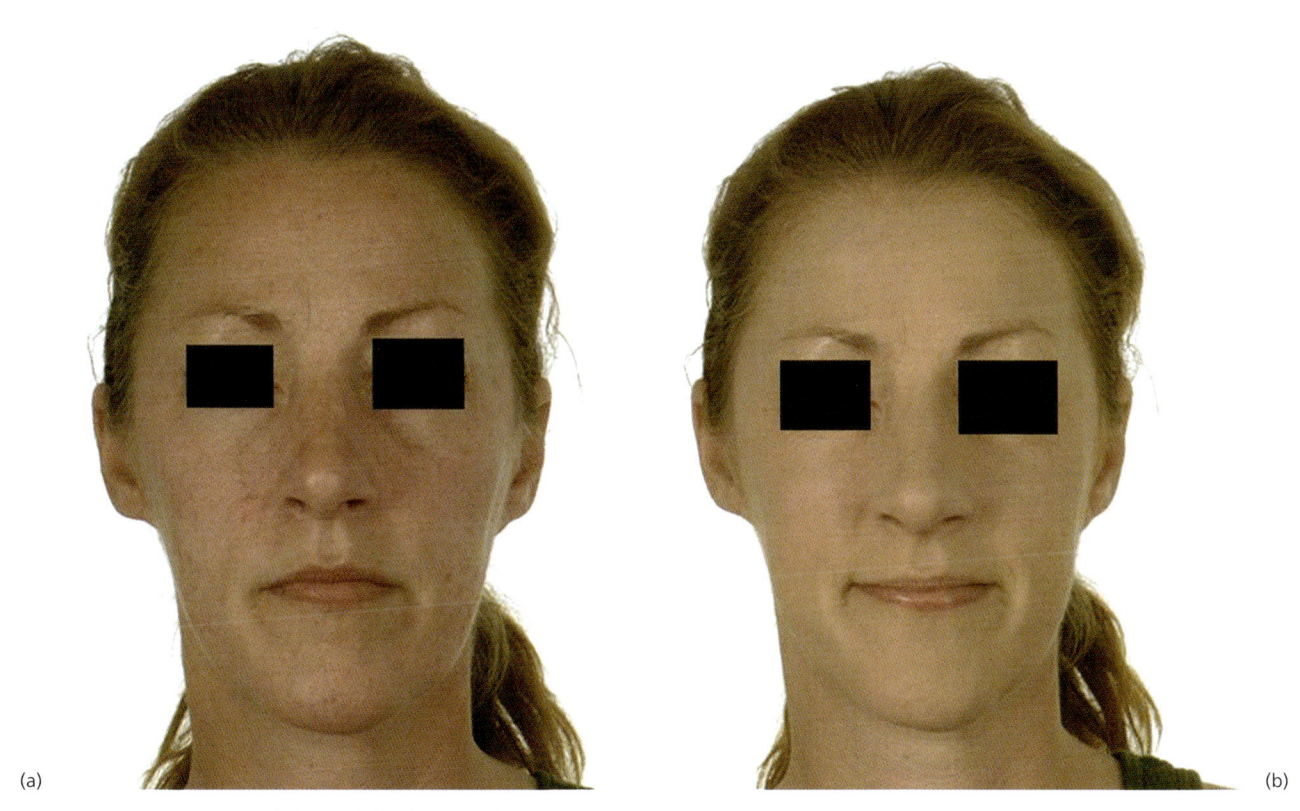

Figure 21.7 Telangiectasia: (a) before and (b) after camouflage.

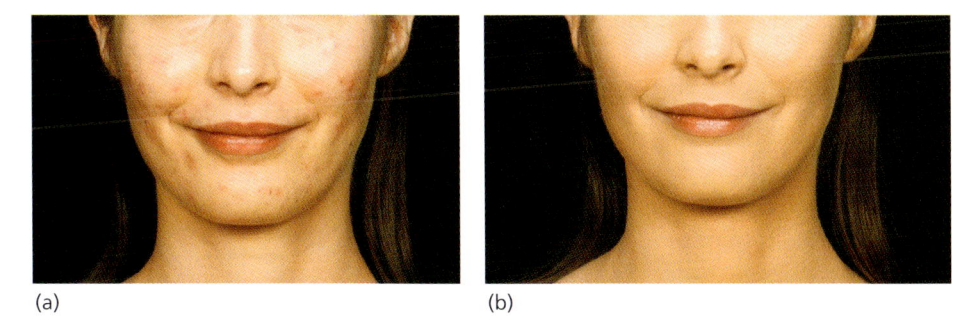

Figure 21.8 Acne: (a) before and (b) after camouflage.

reason or social event. Corrective makeup can also be used after medical procedures such as laser resurfacing, peels, and microdermabrasion to camouflage erythema. After filler injections, redness may also appear. Laser hair removal will induce temporary redness, but following some lasers the skin may become purpuric. Camouflage makeup optimizes the patient's postprocedure appearance. Indeed, if the patient knows he or she will be red, he or she will require an appointment at the end of the day or of the week. With corrective makeup, patients are able to go straight back to work. Similarly, after filler or botulinum toxin injections, hematomas may appear which can be camouflaged with corrective makeup.

Beginning a camouflage clinic

It is important to offer patients camouflaging makeup knowledge [6]. In general, the dermatologist will delegate this activity to a staff member. Many physicians find that a camouflage therapist can bring an added value to the practice by enhancing patient recovery.

The room for teaching camouflaging techniques should contain a table with a mirror and fluorescent bulbs to provide adequate light. A chair should be placed in the room tall enough to allow the camouflage therapist to stand. Several camouflage products should be available in various shades to match the different skin colors.

The camouflage therapist

In the USA, camouflage therapists are state-licensed and medically trained skincare professionals, with both clinical knowledge and therapeutic skill [5]. They do not treat patients but educate them by providing information on the best way to go about applying camouflage makeup. In other countries of the world such a degree does not exist. Camouflage therapists should obtain appropriate training and education. They should be trained to select and apply cosmetics beyond the application of standard cosmetics. Their training should include the study of facial anatomy, highlighting and contouring techniques, and prosthetic makeup techniques similar to those used in the stage and motion picture industry.

The camouflage therapist should be a good communicator to teach patients how to apply various products, which the patient can easily reproduce without assistance. Camouflage therapists should be genuinely interested in the patient's well-being. Therefore, they should be mature enough to work with people who have a severely damaged appearance.

The camouflage therapist must record the patient's history and identify needs based on the patient's perception of the problems. Because of the clinical knowledge and personal qualities required, a trained nurse would be an ideal camouflage therapist [7,10].

The camouflage therapist can design a cosmetic treatment plan. During the interview four issues should be addressed [5]:
1. The ability of the patient to follow simple instructions.
2. The patient's social activities and job environment.
3. The patient's prior makeup experience.
4. The financial status of the patient.

Camouflage makeup and quality of life

Psychosocial aspects of skin disease has important implications for optimal management of patients. The presence of abnormal visible skin lesions may result in significant psychologic impairment. Health-related quality of life (QOL) is a measurement method to describe physical, social, and psychological well-being and to assess the burden of disease on daily living. Several general measures have been developed [11]. Surprisingly, women who used facial foundation reported a poorer QOL than those who did not. This was interpreted to mean that more severely impacted patients are more likely to hide the disorder using camouflage cosmetics, albeit inadequately. Yet, wearing makeup may improve appearance and looking better translates into feeling better. Those who feel better show signs of higher self-esteem.

Many studies have been performed in order to demonstrate the effects of corrective makeup on patients' QOL [12,13,14] and remove misconceptions that the use of cosmetics can be tedious and difficult for ordinary people. A wide range of facial blemishes and disfigurements such as pigmentary disorders, vascular disorders, scars, acne, rosacea, lupus, lichen sclerosus, and keratosis pilaris have been included in these studies. QOL questionnaires were completed before the first application and after applying corrective makeup. Results show that corrective cosmetics are well-tolerated and patients report high satisfaction rates. There is an immediate improvement in skin appearance and no significant adverse effects. Corrective cosmetics rapidly improve QOL, which persists with continued use. There was no difference in QOL according to the type of facial disfigurement or the size of the affected area. Not only were patients improved with pigmentary or vascular disorders, but also with scars.

Camouflage therapy can help patients cope with skin disorders that affect appearance. The cosmetics can be used long-term without difficulty. Camouflage therapy is of great help to patients who cannot be medically improved.

Conclusions

Camouflage techniques help affected patients cope with the psychologic implications of facial blemishes or disfigurements. Covering visible signs of the disease minimizes stigmatization. Today's high quality camouflage products provide excellent good coverage with a natural appearance. Many physicians find that a camouflage therapist can bring an added value to the practice by enhancing patient recovery.

References

1. Westmore MG. (2001) Camouflage and make-up preparations. *Dermatol Clin* **19**, 406–12.
2. Draelos ZK. (1993) Cosmetic camouflaging techniques. *Cutis* **52**, 362–4.
3. LeRoy L. (2000) Camouflage therapy. *Dermatol Nurs* **12**, 415–6.
4. Westmore MG. (1991) Make-up as an adjunct and aid to the practice of dermatology. *Dermatol Clin* **9**, 81–8.
5. Rayner VL. (1995) Camouflage therapy. *Dermatol Clin* **13**, 467–72.
6. Deshayes P. (2008) Le maquillage médical pour une meilleure qualité de vie des patients. *Ann Dermatol Venereol* **135**, S208–10.
7. Rayner VL. (2000) Cosmetic rehabilitation. *Dermatol Nurs* **12**, 267–71.
8. Rajatanavin N, Suwanachote S, Kulkllakarn S. (2008) Dihydroxyacetone: a safe camouflaging option in vitiligo. *Int J Dermatol* **47**, 402–6.
9. Tsur H, Kapkan HY. (1993) Camouflaging hairless areas on the male face by artistic tattoo. *Dermatol Nurs* **5**, 118–20.
10. McConochie L, Pearson E. (2006) Development of a nurse-led skin camouflage clinic. *Nurs Stand* **20**, 74–8.
11. Balkrishnan R, McMichael AJ, Hu JY, *et al.* (2006) Correlates of health-related quality of life in women with severe facial blemishes. *Int J Dermatol* **45**, 111–5.
12. Boehncke WH, Ochsendorf F, Paeslack I, Kaufmann R, Zollner TM. (2002) Decorative cosmetics improve the quality of life in patients with disfiguring diseases. *Eur J Dermatol* **12**, 577–80.
13. Holme SA, Beattie PE, Fleming CJ. (2002) Cosmetic camouflage advice improves quality of life. *Br J Dermatol* **147**, 946–9.
14. Balkrishnan R, McMichael AJ, Hu JY, *et al.* (2005) Corrective cosmetics are effective for women with facial pigmentary disorders. *Cutis* **75**, 181–7.

CHAPTER 22
Lips and Lipsticks

Catherine Heusèle, Hervé Cantin, and Frédéric Bonté
LVMH Recherche, Saint Jean de Braye, France

> **BASIC CONCEPTS**
> - The lips possess a complex anatomy consisting of mucosa and skin.
> - Lipsticks are designed to enhance the appearance of the lips.
> - Lipstick is an anhydrous paste of oils and waxes in which pigments are dispensed along with other coloring agents.

Introduction

Lip makeup is an essential element in seduction and women frequently use lipsticks to make their faces more attractive. The lips are muscular membranous folds surrounding the anterior part of the mouth. This tissue is both mucosa and skin and has a complex anatomy. Labial tissue has a dense population of sensory receptors, is very sensitive to environmental stress, can present pigmentation defects, and is modified during aging. Lipstick formulations are most widely used to enhance the beauty of lips and to add a touch of glamour to women's makeup. The lipstick that we know today is a makeup product composed of anhydrous pastes such as oils and waxes in which are dispersed pigments and other coloring agents designed to accentuate the complexion of the lips. This chapter draws together our knowledge of the biology of this special tissue, and gives detailed information on the formulation elements of lipsticks.

Lip anatomy

The lips are muscular membranous folds surrounding the anterior part of the mouth. The area of contact between the two lips is called the stomium and forms the labial aperture. The external surfaces of the lips are covered by skin, with its hair follicles, sebaceous glands, and sweat glands; the inner surface is covered by the labial mucosa, a non-stratified, non-keratinized epithelium bearing salivary glands. The transitional zone between these two epithelia is the red vermilion border of the lips (Figure 22.1). It has neither hair follicles nor salivary glands, but sebaceous glands are present in about 50% of adults [1]. The red area is also keratinized, with rete ridges more marked than in the neighboring cutaneous zone.

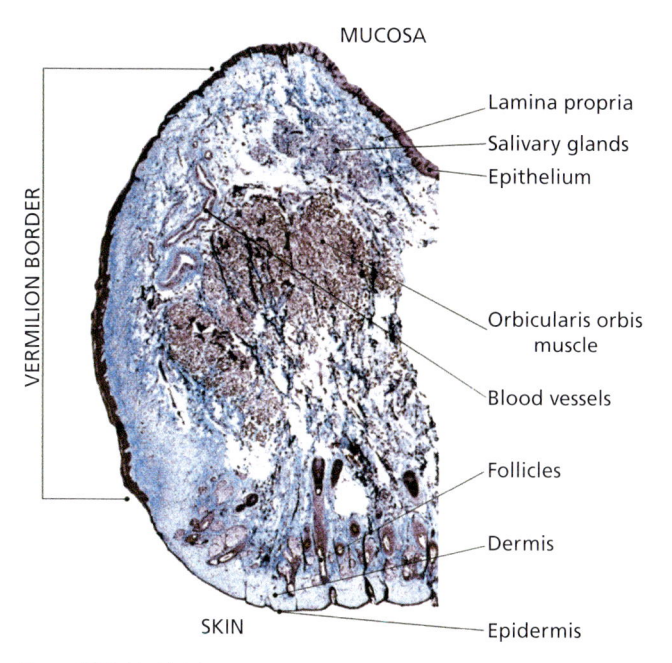

Figure 22.1 Lip histology.

Several studies have identified an intermediate area between the vermilion zone and the mucosa that does not contain a cutaneous annex; it is covered by a stratified epithelium that lacks a stratum granulosum but does have a thick parakeratin surface layer. This intermediate zone increases with age [2–4].

The deeper region of this soft tissue forming the lips is made up of a layer of striated muscle, the orbicularis orbis muscle, and loose connective tissue. The muscle makes a hooked curve towards the exterior at the edge of the vermilion area which gives the lips their shape.

Cosmetic Dermatology: Products and Procedures, Second Edition. Edited by Zoe Diana Draelos.
© 2016 John Wiley & Sons, Ltd. Published 2016 by John Wiley & Sons, Ltd.

Immediately above the transition between the skin and the vermilion zone is the Cupidon arch, a mucocutaneous ridge, also called a white roll, or the white skin roll. Its physical appearance and lighter color seem to be essentially caused by the configuration of the underlying muscle [5]. This region is rich in fine, unpigmented, "vellous" hairs that may influence the appearance of this zone.

The lips have great tactile sensitivity. Labial tissue has a dense population of sensory receptors, including Meissner corpuscles, Merkel cells, and free nerve endings. The sensitivity of the lips is somewhere between that of the tongue and the fingertips [6].

Labial epidermis

The epidermis of the vermilion region is twice as thick (180 µm) as the adjacent skin [4,7,8]. It still has the markers of cutaneous epidermis differentiation, even though it has fewer keratinized layers than the skin [9]. Barrett et al. [4] found that the distribution of cytokeratins (CK) differed from that of the intermediate zone, with a loss of the skin cytokeratins CK1 and CK10 and the presence of the mucosal cytokeratins CK4, CK13, and CK19. CK5 and CK14 were still present in the basal layer and occasionally in the suprabasal layer. CK8, CK18, and CK20 were found only in Merkel cells. Involucrin was present in all the zones, but its restricted distribution in the stratum granulosum of the skin extended to the stratum spinosum and the parabasal keratinocytes of the lip zone and the mucosa. Loricrin, profilaggrin, and filaggrin were found in the stratum granulosum of the orthokeratinized zones but not after the junction between the vermilion zone and the intermediate zone.

The corneocytes in the mucosa are flat, smooth cells. In contrast, most of the corneocytes on the surface of the vermilion border are seen to have microvilli on all their internal surfaces when examined under the high power microscope [10]. These projections are rarely seen on the corneocytes of the adjacent skin [11]. The cell turnover of the epidermis of the vermilion border seems to be more rapid than that of the adjacent skin cells. The vermilion border also appears to lose water three times as fast as the cheeks and to have only one-third the conductance. Thus, the lips function as a barrier but their capacity to retain water is much poorer than that of facial skin [1].

Hikima et al. [11] showed that the surface of the lips, like the surface of the skin, has cathepsin D-like activity and chymotrypsin-like activity. These enzymes are involved in the hydrolysis of corneodesmosomes, and hence in the release of corneocytes from the skin surface.

Like the skin, the vermilion border epithelium contains melanocytes and there is melanin in the cytoplasm of basal cells [4]. However, as the melanin pigmentation is light and associated with reduced keratinization, the color of the hemoglobin is seen more clearly. There are also Langerhans cells in this zone [8]. Cruchley et al. [12] used immunodetection of CD1a to show that there were more Langerhans cells per unit area of the lips than in abdominal skin.

Sallette et al. [13] recently showed that there is more neuropeptide-type neurotransmitter in the epidermis of the lips than in the eyelids, which seems to indicate that the lips are better innervated.

Lip dermis and lamina propria

The epithelium of the vermilion border lies on a layer of connective tissue, which ensures the continuity of the cutaneous dermis and the lamina propria. This tissue is composed of collagen fibers and a network of elastic fibers.

There is a thin layer of fatty tissue between the muscle and the dermis in the cutaneous part of the lips with many attachments between the muscle and the skin [14]. The deep part of the lamina propria of the mucosa lies above the hypodermis of the subcutaneous zone. The invaginations at the junction between the epithelium and the connective tissue of the vermilion border are higher than those of the skin [15]. These papillae contain blood capillaries. The capillary loops in the vermilion border are higher than those of the skin, which accentuates the red color of the lips because of the hemoglobin in them [16].

The lymph drainage of the red border is not uniform; it flows towards the cutaneous system on the external side of the lips and towards the mucosal system on the inner side [17].

Lip topology

The description of lip topology first interested legal medicine because each individual has a different organization, much like fingerprints. The study of lip prints is called cheiloscopy. The development of kiss-proof lipsticks led legal medicine to develop protocols for revealing latent prints at a crime scene [18]. Lip prints can be classified in several ways and their distributions in populations have been quantified [19–22].

Sensitivity of lips to the environment

As the lips have little cornified tissue or melanin they are very sensitive to chemical, physical, or microbial damage. Their prolonged exposure to sunlight, particularly for fair-skinned people, may lead to the appearance of actinic cheilitis and even spinocellular carcinoma [23]. Pogoda and Preston-Martin [24] suggested that frequent applications of sunscreen can have a positive protective effect. Smoking has also been found to be a major risk factor for lip cancers.

Aging of the lips

The esthetic consequences of aging of the superficial lip tissues (sagging, distension, and ptosis) are aggravated by changes in the shape of the bone and dental infrastructure and the aging of the underlying muscles and adipose tissue. The orientation of the labial aperture changes with a drooping of the lateral commissures: from a concave curve in newborns and children to a horizontal line in adults, and then to an inverted curve in the elderly. In profile, the lips, particularly the lower lip, recede with age. The upper lip becomes lower and enlarged [3,22]. Tissues become less extensible and elastic because of repeated mechanical stresses and the weakening of the orbicularis orbis muscle with age [3,25].

The vermilion border becomes larger, longer, and thicker at the corners of the mouth [2]. While wrinkles develop in the skin around the lips with age, the outline of the lips themselves becomes sunken [22]. The depth and organization of the lips varies greatly from one person to another and some young people have deep furrows. Both the spatial resolution and the tactile sensitivity of the lips decrease with age [3,6,25,26]. There may also be histologic signs of solar elastosis. The superficial microcirculatory network (both papillary and mucosal) may become smaller and less dense (reticular and mucosal), together with an apparent thinning of the lips in older people who have lost their teeth [15].

Cosmetic surgery can be used to "refresh" and to fill the tissue to rejuvenate the lips. This might involve reducing the upper lip or recovering the shape of a young lip by a series of interventions to reinforce the shape and projection of the lips and restructure the Cupid's bow, better define the lip outline, and lift the corners of the mouth. This surgery is accompanied by a rejuvenation of the perioral region, including removal of peribuccal wrinkles, peeling, laser resurfacing, and dermabrasion [27–30].

Lip plumpness and cheilitis

Cheilitis can be caused by a cold or dry environment, repeated pressure on the lips – as it can develop in players of wind instruments – or by defective dental work. It can also occur in people taking oral retinoids, or from a lack of dietary vitamin B_{12} (riboflavin), B_6 (pyridoxine), nicotinic acid, folic acid, or iron [31].

Hikima *et al.* [11] reported that the corneocytes at the edges of dried out lips become flattened and their surface area increased. This suggests that the turnover of these cells is slowed in dried out lips. The degree of visible dryness is also correlated with a reduction in cathepsin D, one of the enzymes involved in desquamation, but the chymotrypsin-like activity remains unchanged.

The upper lip seems to dry out less than the lower lip as it is less exposed. While the hydration measured by the capacitance does not seem to change with age, the loss of water via the lips decreases [25]. Clinically assessed drying out increases with age [22].

Defects of lip pigmentation

Pigmentation defects, particularly ephelides and lentigos, may also occur. The lips of some populations, like those from Thailand, may become dark because of the accumulation of melanin in the basal layer of the epidermis without any increase in the number of melanocytes [32]. This disorder may be congenital, caused by smoking, or an allergic reaction to a topical compound. Smoking can also increase pigmentation of the buccal mucosa in darker-skinned people (Africans, Asians, Indians) [33].

Lipsticks

Lipstick, a symbol of feminine beauty and sensuality and a method of attracting attention, has a very long history. The red color and bloom (lively, plump) of the lips was first accentuated in the ancient world. Today, a woman uses lipstick to highlight her individuality, character, and seductive capacity and to underline her smile [34]. It is everything but an empty gesture; it reflects the image that the woman has of herself and what she wants to project in society.

In the 18th century, people distinguished between the red coloring used for the lips and the rouge used for the cheeks. Many rather toxic substances have been used in the past. The red coloring material used can be of animal, vegetable, or mineral origin. It could be obtained from the cochineal beetle imported from Mexico, the purple dye extracted from molluscs, red sandalwood from Brazil, or the orcanette root. The minerals most frequently used were lead oxide (minium), mercuric sulfate (cinnabar), and antimony.

The popularity of lipstick exploded in the 20th century with the use of lip makeup based on a colored paste made from grapes and sold in little jars. These were deep colors. The mouth became much fuller with the arrival and spread of talking movies in the 1930s. The first "indelible" or "kiss-proof" lipstick was the lipstick Rouge Baiser sold by the French chemist Paul Baudecroux in 1927. Red, pouting lips became all the rage in the 1950s, while in the 1990s lip gloss or brilliant was produced as a paste rather than a stick.

Lipstick formulation

The lipstick that we know today is a makeup product composed of anhydrous pastes in which are dispersed pigments and other coloring agents designed to accentuate the complexion of the lips. It is formed into a stick by pouring the hot material into a mold. A classic lipstick formula is:
- Wax (about 15%) which is solid at room temperature. It provides hardness and creaminess when applied;
- Waxy paste (20%) helps lubricate the lipstick after application;
- Oil (30%) for dispersing the pigments;
- Texturing agents (about 10%) to improve the texture;
- Coloring agents, pigments, and/or pearls (20%) to give color;
- Preserving agents and antioxidants (1%) to stabilize the formulation;
- Perfume (1%);
- Active ingredients including UV filters to improve long-term benefit.

Waxes

The wax may be of vegetable, animal, or synthetic origin. They are solid at room temperature and must be melted for use. They create a crystalline network within the formulation that gives the lipstick its shape. The wax is chosen to give the stick a suitable hardness so that it does not break during application. They also give the lipstick a rather matte appearance (Table 22.1).

Lipsticks are currently made using specific fractions of wax that provide specific fusion points. These refined fractions are whiter and more odorless than the original waxes, which were a complex mixture of natural lipids.

Table 22.1 Waxes.

Origin	Wax	Properties	Source	Appearance
Animal	Beeswax	Composed of fatty acids and alcohols Thickener	Bees	Relatively solid, give a lustrous appearance
Plant	Carnuba wax	Harder than bees wax Very slightly acid, but brittle Often used mixed with bees wax	From the leaves of the carnuba palm (Brazil)	Relatively hard, and give a lustrous appearance
	Candelilla wax	Very hard wax	From the candelilla plant	Matte appearance
Mineral	Paraffin Ozokerite	Non-stick Non-polar White, fairly transparent and odorless	Paraffin is obtained from oil refining	More malleable

Table 22.2 Waxy pastes.

Origin	Name	Properties	Source	Appearance
Synthetic	Polybutene	Adherence Brilliance Extremely hydrophobic	Synthesis from ethylene	Very viscous transparent, viscous liquid
Synthetic	Methyl hydrogenated rosinate			

Waxy pastes

They are called pastes because they are semi-solid forms of wax at room temperature (Table 22.2). They contribute to the cosmetic function of the lipstick by helping to keep the color on the lips. They can do this because they are sticky and because their fusion point is close to the temperature of the lips, thus enabling the stick to melt during application.

Oils

These hydrophobic liquids are solvents for the coloring agents that allow them to diffuse so as to develop their color. The oils provide comfort, lubrication during application, and contribute greatly to the cosmetic effect. They may also provide brilliance and subtlety (Table 22.3). Castor oil has been used for many years but is now less often utilized. It has excellent pigment-dispersing properties because of its polarity; its main inconvenience is its unpleasant taste and odor (caused by oxidation). It is gradually being replaced by stable, odorless, fatty acid esters.

Table 22.3 Oils.

Name	Properties	Source	Appearance
Di isostearylmalate	Emollient Not oxidized Colorless Odorless	Synthetic	Colorless liquid
Trimethylolpropane triisostearate	Emollient Comfort	Synthetic	Colorless, viscous liquid
Polyglyceryl-2 triisostearate	Emollient Comfort Dispersant	Synthetic	Transparent pale yellow liquid

Texturing agents

These components can be very different; they provide moisturizing, brightness, and subtlety. For example, polyamide powders bring softness, silica beads provide subtlety and a matte finish, titanium dioxide flakes give a soft-focus effect, while bismuth oxychloride gives a satin, shimmering effect.

Pigments

Pigments are synthetic substances or of mineral origin. They are fine powders when dry and are used because they are very opaque and have great coloring properties (Table 22.4).

The solid powders are suspended and dispersed in oil. The covering property of a lipstick depends on its pigment content; these pigments can hide the underlying lip color. International regulations strictly limit the use of pigments. Only a restricted number can be used on the face because of the risk of ingestion. The pearly

Table 22.4 Pigments and coloring agents.

Component	Origin
Titanium (IV) oxide – mica	Mineral
Ferrous oxide (II)	Mineral
Ferric oxide (III)	Mineral
DC Red 33	Organic
DC Red 27	Organic
DC Red 21	Organic
DC Red 7	Organic
DC Red 6	Organic
DC Red 28	Organic
DC Red 30	Organic

and metallic effects are obtained with composite materials, often multilayered. These are interference pigments because they create long wavelength interference patterns in natural light. Holographic effects may be obtained by liquid crystals (cholesterol derivatives) or multilayer plastic slabs (terephthalates).

Antioxidants and preserving agents

The most frequently used antioxidants are the β-carotenes (provitamins A), ascorbic acid, and tocopherol, which are all powerful, natural antioxidants. The preserving agents are used to control bacterial proliferation. There are few preserving agents (phenoxyethanol mainly) in anhydrous products such as lipsticks.

Perfume

Perfume provides the desired smell to the lipstick. It is generally used as an oil-based concentrate that is miscible with the other oils in the formulation.

Active ingredients

These are used to provide their specific properties to the finished product and often permit claims of antiaging or moisturizing. They must be included at the considered concentration to be effective. Vitamin A, as β-carotene, vitamin E (tocopherol), and vitamin C are classically used in lipstick. Sunscreen can be used to protect the lips against UV rays for an antiaging quality.

Lip glosses and brilliances

A lip brilliance is a makeup product that generally has low covering qualities but reflects light and gives the lips a shiny appearance. A brilliant lipstick has a gloss effect. So, by extension, the term lip gloss includes lip brilliants.

Lip glosses nourish the lips and give them a light, wonderfully supple appearance and a long-lasting sparkle. Their crystalline effect is brought about by their ultra-brilliant, transparent base. They may be used over a lipstick to give a new sparkle to the lipstick color, or simply provide the lips with a very pure, superfine color. Its formulation differs from that of lipstick only in the quantity and nature of the components classically used in lipsticks.

Lip glosses are frequently sold in small flasks and are applied with a special applicator. They are not applied directly to the lips, so they do not need to have a solid structure like a lipstick. The wax content is lower and the content of waxy paste higher.

Conclusions

Lipsticks and lip glosses are essential to a women's makeup, and have a key role in the affirmation of her personality and well-being. These skin surface products – thanks to their simple formula that contains a limited number of constituents – are usually well accepted and adverse reactions are very rare.

Pink, purple, even blue, the colors follow the fashion trends, and, most of the time, they are coordinated with clothes and nail polishes. The shapes and textures that women appreciate remain quite classic. Indeed, if raw materials are constantly evolving, cosmetic regulations worldwide lay down some new restrictions to the manufacturers of the beauty sector. Nevertheless, these regulatory evolutions still allow the creation of ever more innovative and qualitative products.

References

1 Kobayashi H, Tagami H. (2005) Functional properties of the surface of the vermilion border of the lips are distinct from those of the facial skin. *Br J Dermatol* **150**, 563–7.
2 Binnie WH, Lehner T. (1970) Histology of the muco-cutaneous junction at the corner of the human mouth. *Arch Oral Biol* **15**, 777–86.
3 Fogel ML, Stranc MF. (1984) Lip function: a study of normal lip parameters. *Br J Plast Surg* **37**, 542–9.
4 Barrett AW, Morgan M, Nwaeze G, *et al.* (2005) The differentiation profile of the epithelium of the human lip. *Arch Oral Biol* **50**, 431–8.
5 Mulliken JM, Pensler JM, Kozakewich HPW. (1993) The anatomy of vermilion bow in normal and cleft lip. *Plast Reconstr Surg* **92**, 395–404.
6 Stevens JC, Choo KK. (1996) Spatial acuity of the body surface over the life span. *Somatosens Mot Res* **13**, 153–66.
7 Lafranchi HE, de Rey BM. (1978) Comparative morphometric analysis of vermilion border epithelium and lip epidermis. *Acta Anat* **101**, 187–91.
8 Heilman E. (1987) Histology of the mucocutaneous junctions and the oral cavity. *Clin Dermatol* **5**, 10–6.
9 Kuffer R. (1982) Pathologie de la muqueuse buccale et des lèvres. *Encyclopédie Médicochirurgicale (Paris), Dermatologie*, **12830** A10.
10 Muto H, Yoshioka I. (1980) Relation between superficial fine structure and function of lips. *Acta Dermatol Kyoto Engl Ed* **75**, 11–20.
11 Hikima R, Igarashi S, Ikeda N, *et al.* (2004) Development of lip treatment on the basis of desquamation mechanism. *IFSCC Magazine* **7**, 3–10.
12 Cruchley AT, Williams DM, Farthing PM, *et al.* (1994) Langerhans cell density in normal human oral mucosa and skin: relationship to age, smoking and alcohol consumption. *J Oral Pathol Med* **23**, 55–9.
13 Sallette J, Al Sayed N, Laboureau J, Adem C, Soussaline F, Breton L. (2006) Neuropeptide Y may be involved in human lip keratinocytes modulation. *J Invest Dermatol* **126**, suppl 3, s13.
14 Choquet P, Sick H, Constantinesco A. (1999) *Ex vivo* high resolution MR imaging of the human lip with a dedicated low field system. *Eur J Dermatol* **9**, 452–4.
15 Wolfram-Gabel R, Sick H. (2000) Microvascularisation of lips in ageing edentulous subjects. *Surg Radiol Anat* **22**, 283–7.
16 Iwai I, Yamashita T, Ochiai N, *et al.* (2003) Can daily-use lipstick make lips more fresh and healthy? A new lipstick containg α-glucosyl hesperidin can remove the dull-color from lips. 22nd IFSCC Conference, pp. 162–77.
17 Ricbourg B. (2002) Vascularisation des lèvres. *Ann Chir Plast Esthet* **47**, 346–56.
18 Ball J. (2002) The current status of lip prints and their use for identification. *J Forensic Odontostomatol* **20**, 43–6.
19 Sivapathasundharam B, Prakash PA, Sivakumar G. (2001) Lip prints (cheiloscopy). *Indian J Dent Res* **12**, 234–7.
20 Hirth L, Göttsche H, Goedde HW. (1975) Lips print: variability and genetics. *Humangenetik* **30**, 47–62.

21. Hirth L, Goedde HW. (1977). Variability and formal genetics of labial grooves. *Anthrop Anz* **36**, 51–7.
22. Lévêque JL, Goubanova E. (2004) Influence of age on the lips and perioral skin. *Dermatology* **208**, 307–14.
23. Calvalcante ASR, Anbinder AL, Carvalho YR. (2008) Actinic cheilitis: clinical and histological features. *J Oral Maxillofac Surg* **66**, 498–503.
24. Pogoda JM, Preston-Martin S. (1996) Solar radiation, lip protection, and lip cancer risk in Los Angeles County women (California, United States). *Cancer Causes Control* **7**, 458–63.
25. Caisey L, Gubanova E, Camus C, Lapatina N, Smetnik V, Lévêque JL. (2008) Influence of age and hormone replacement therapy on the functional properties of the lips. *Skin Res Technol* **14**, 220–5.
26. Wohlert AB. (1996) Tactile perception of spatial stimuli on the lip surface by young and older adults. *J Speech Hearing Res* **39**, 1191–8.
27. Simon E, Stricker M, Duroure F. (2002) Le vieillissement labial: composantes et principes thérapeutiques. [The lip ageing.] *Ann Chir Plasti Esthét* **47**, 556–60.
28. Aiache AE. (1997) Rejuvenation of the perioral area. *Dermatol Clin* **15**, 665–72.
29. Guerrissi JO. (2000) Surgical treatment of the senile upper lip. *Plast Reconstr Surg* **92**, 938–40.
30. Ali MJ, Ende K, Maas CS. (2007) Perioral rejuvenation and lip augmentation. *Facial Plast Surg Clin North Am* **15**, 491–500.
31. Zugerman C. (1986) The lips: anatomy and differential diagnosis. *Cutis* **38**, 116–20.
32. Kunachak S, Kunachakr S, Kunachark S, Leelaudomlipi P, Wongwaisatawan S. (2001) An effective treatment of dark lip by frequency-doubled Q-switched Nd:YAG laser. *Dermatol Surg* **27**, 37–40.
33. Sarswathi TR, Kumar SN, Kavitha KM. (2003) Oral melanin pigmentation in smoked and smokeless tobacco users in India: clinicopathological study. *Indian J Dent Res* **14**, 101–6.
34. Dong JK, Jin TH, Cho HW, *et al.* (1999) The esthetics of the smile: a review of some recent studies. *Int J Prosthodont* **12**, 9–19.

CHAPTER 23
Eye Cosmetics*

Sarah A. Vickery, Robyn Kolas, and Fatima Dicko
Procter & Gamble Cosmetics, Hunt Valley, MD, USA

> **BASIC CONCEPTS**
> - Mascara is intended to darken, thicken, and lengthen the lashes to make them more noticeable. Careful selection of mascara film materials and new applicator technologies are enhancing women's ability to quickly and effectively accentuate these characteristics.
> - Other eyelash products, beyond mascara, such as lash perms and lash tints are becoming more prevalent and are beginning to gain mainstream acceptance. These new products are changing the way women think about eyelash beauty.
> - Eyebrows are groomed or shaped via the removal or trimming of hairs. Eyebrows can be accentuated, or sparse growth can be filled in via the addition of eyebrow cosmetics.
> - Eyeshadow is color applied to the upper eyelids that is used to add depth and dimension to the eyes, thus drawing attention to the eye look or eye color.
> - Eyeliner is used to outline the eyelids, serving to define the eyes and to make the eye look more bold or to give the illusion of a different eye shape.
> - New eye cosmetic products are being introduced that feature enhanced long wear, new applicator surfaces, novel color effects, sustainable natural materials, improved application, and even lash growth.

Definition

This chapter will give a broad introduction to eye cosmetics. Mascara, eyeshadows, eyeliners and eyebrow cosmetics will be presented along with the physiology of eyelashes and future trends in the category.

Eye cosmetic history

Cosmetics have been used to decorate the eyes for thousands of years. In ancient Egypt materials like charcoal and Kohl were mixed with animal fat to create ointment for darkening the lashes and eyelids. They used eye cosmetics for the same reasons that we do now: in youth to attract by accentuating and drawing attention to the eyes, and in age to preserve beauty as it starts to fade [1,2].

Moving forward to more modern times, in the eighteenth and nineteenth centuries, men would condition their hair and mustaches with a touch-up product for graying hair called Mascaro. This was also used in stage makeup as both an eyelash and brow cosmetic. In the nineteenth century women darkened their lashes with lamp black, which they could collect simply by holding up a plate to catch the soot above a lamp or candle flame. They also used cake mascara (soap, wax and pigment wetted with a moistened brush) to darken their lashes or they could plump their lashes with petroleum jelly. Since then a wide variety of innovations have changed both the way we decorate eyes and the penetration of these products into daily use by the majority of women [3].

The first half of the twentieth century saw a range of new product forms emerge including liner pencils, melted wax dripped onto lashes, eyelash curlers, eyebrow pencils, lash dye, cream mascara (toothpaste style tube with brush), false lashes, liquid drops, and even turpentine based waterproof mascara. As the century progressed, more and more women were using eye cosmetics, driven in part by the makeup of the popular actresses in the Hollywood movies and also because of new distribution systems, such as Maybelline's mail order mascara, and availability at local stores. By the late 1930s the majority of women applied cosmetics around their eyes [4].

In 1957, Helena Rubenstein launched the first modern day mascara – a tube of mascara cream with the applicator stored inside the tube. No longer was the mascara applicator separate from the mascara formulation. This efficient and more sanitary design took off quickly, and by the 1960s, this became the standard form of mascara. Once this new product form was established, the applicator quickly changed from a simple grooved aluminum rod to the ubiquitous twisted wire brush applicator that is the predominant applicator today.

By the 1970s, waterproof mascaras were more appealing than the past turpentine-based versions due to the availability of purified petroleum-based volatile solvents. Fibers were

---

* Original chapter by Sarah A. Vickery, Peter Wyatt and John Gilley
Cosmetic Dermatology: Products and Procedures, Second Edition. Edited by Zoe Diana Draelos.
© 2016 John Wiley & Sons, Ltd. Published 2016 by John Wiley & Sons, Ltd.

introduced into mascaras for a "lengthening" benefit. Eyeshadows, due partly to the growth of iridescent pigments in the 1960s, were available in a broad range of matte and sparkling colors. By the 1980s and into the 1990s the rapidly improving performance of polymers resulted in more durable eye cosmetics that would glide on with ease and maintain their effect for hours [5].

Eyelash physiology

Eyelashes are terminal hairs growing from follicles around the eye. Like all hair, the eyelash is a mixture of dead cells that have been keratinized, binding material, melanin granules, and small amounts of water. Keratin makes up ~95% of the total lash composition, providing lash insolubility and chemical resistance. The outer surface is comprised of a series of overlapping transparent scales called cuticle cells that protect the inside, called the cortex. The cortex contributes to the eyelash's shape, mechanical properties, and color. Eyelashes vary by ethnicity, and as a result, can have an elliptical or circular cross section with an average diameter of 60–120 microns, tapering to a fine, barely pigmented tip [6–8]. Figure 23.1 is a series of scanning electron micrographs that show the shape, cross section, and surface morphology of an eyelash.

While hair over the body is likely there for thermal insulation and proximity sensation, eyelashes protect the eye from debris and signal the eyelid to reflexively close when something is too close to the eye. Chemically, eyelashes are the same as scalp hair, and structurally, the eyelash is very close to curly hair [9]. Eyelashes have a substantially shorter, slower growth phase than scalp hair, hence their shorter length [6–7], and they typically last for about 3 months before falling out [9]. An active follicle, during the anagen (growth) cycle will typically produce a lash at approximately 0.12–0.14 mm/day, about half the growth rate of scalp hair. Roughly three quarters of the eyelash follicles are in the telogen (resting) phase at any point in time [6–7].

The direction that the eyelash protrudes from the eyelid is based on the follicle's position in the skin. The curvature of the lash is derived from the plane curved, "comma-shape" of the follicle, which is about 2 mm long. As the lash forms inside the follicle, and the protein strands are bonded together, the lash shape that is formed corresponds to the shape of the follicle they are formed within [8–9]. Eyelashes are arranged around the eye in a narrow band 1–2 mm wide, growing in imperfect rows of five to six in the upper and three to four in the lower eyelid [10]. Lashes are longer (8–12 mm) and more numerous (90–200) on the upper eyelid, while lower eyelid lashes number 75–80 and are typically 6–8 mm long [8]. For a single person, lash length varies dramatically, and although lash cycle duration is similar, longer lashes grow faster and for longer than shorter lashes [9].

There are a number of ailments to which the eyelashes are prone, the most common of which are listed in Table 23.1.

Table 23.1 Common eyelash ailments.

Ailment	Description
Madarosis, or hypotrichosis	Thinning, or loss, of eyelid and eyebrow hairs. Can be caused by aging, physical trauma, burns, x-ray therapy, overuse of glued false lashes, and trichotillomania (impulse to pull out one's hairs, including eyelashes).
Stye	A stye can be caused, among other things, from a bacterial infection of the eyelash follicle's sebaceous glands, leading to an inflammation of skin tissue around the eyelash follicle.
Poliosis	Lashes losing their pigmentation with age, caused by less melanin granules being present in the lashes. Gray lashes are pigmented, just with less pigment than those of a younger person. Completely un-pigmented lashes would be white.
Trichiasis	This is the abnormal growth of lashes directed towards the eyeball, causing irritation and possibly leading to infection.
Ectropion	Weakening in the muscles that hold the eyelids firmly against the eyeball, causing the eyelid (usually the lower eyelid) to turn outward, giving the eye a red-rimmed appearance. This is usually associated with aging, but can also be attributed to scarring around the eyelid, or nerve damage.
Entropion	Weakening in the muscles that hold the eyelids firmly against the eyeball, causing the eyelid (usually the lower eyelid) to turn inward. This can result in severe discomfort and possible cornea damage as the eyelashes rub on the eyes, and requires medical intervention.

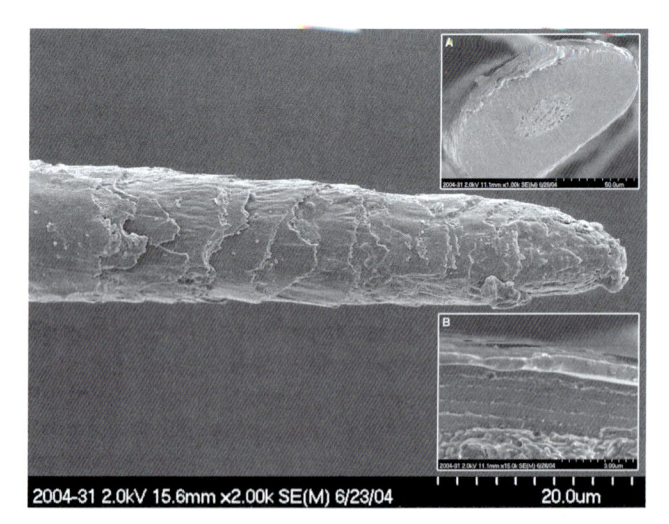

Figure 23.1 Eyelash SEM images. The eyelash tapers to a fine tip. The cross section may be circular or elliptical (A), and the surface is composed of overlapping cuticle cells (B).

Mascara

Over 70% of women who wear cosmetics wear mascara. In fact, mascara is a product that women tend to be absolutely passionate about. When asked which cosmetic they would choose if they could only choose one, over fifty percent of women would choose mascara. Mascara is intended to darken, thicken, and lengthen the lashes to make them more noticeable. Through careful selection of materials, mascara films can be produced to accentuate these characteristics. Mascara formulations can be roughly divided into two different types, water-resistant and waterproof.

Mascara composition

Water-resistant mascaras typically deliver a combination of waxes, polymers, and pigments in a water-based emulsion to the lashes. The water helps contribute to the enhanced lash attributes by absorbing into the lash, bloating its diameter by as much as 30% and in many cases forcing the lashes to curl. The waxes are emulsified into the water creating a thick, creamy texture that glides onto the lashes in a thick film that resists fading, abrasion, and flaking throughout the day, but is still easily removed with warm water and soap. Polymers are often included to bind the mascara to itself as well as to the lashes. Advances in polymer technology over the last twenty years have led to very substantive films that last throughout the day, even though they are delivered to the lash in an aqueous medium [11].

Consumers who desire the longest lasting mascara will select the anhydrous waterproof formulations that contain little to no water and deliver very durable, but difficult to remove films. Waterproof mascaras usually use hydrocarbon solvents and anhydrous raw materials. They provide a long wearing film on the lashes which is very resistant to water, smudging and smearing. Its anhydrous nature makes it more difficult to both apply and remove; however, it may have more eye irritation potential [11].

A list of common water-resistant and waterproof mascara ingredients and their functions can be found in Table 23.2.

Additional ingredients can be added to a formulation to enhance particular eyelash characteristics. A common method for producing lengthening mascara is to include fibers in the formulation so that, when applied, the fibers will extend beyond the natural ends of the eyelashes. Similarly, large light-weight hollow particles may be incorporated into the mascara film to create a thicker film for bolder lashes. Synthetic or natural polymers with novel properties can also be incorporated to induce a curling effect on the lashes.

Other forms of mascara are available such as clear mascaras, waterproofing topcoats, pearlescent topcoats, and lash primers. Recently, many double-sided mascara products have been introduced which include a basecoat formula and a topcoat formula that deliver different benefits, such as adding volume, extending wear and also providing appearance and decoration benefits. This breadth of cosmetic options gives consumers many choices to groom and decorate their lashes.

Mascara applicator technology

Consumers will typically judge a better mascara applicator as one that creates precise groups of lashes that are uniformly spaced apart [12]. However, different consumers apply their mascara for different end looks – some aspiring for only a few (spiky) clumps of lashes, others working towards well separated lashes. The twisted wire brush has been the mainstay mascara applicator for 50 years. As seen in Figure 23.2, it is simply a metal wire bent back upon itself into two parallel wires. Bristles, typically made of nylon, are inserted between the bent wire and it is twisted around to form a helical arrangement of

Table 23.2 Water-resistant and waterproof mascara ingredients and function.

Class	Material type	Examples	Function
Water-resistant solvent	Carrier fluid	Water, propylene glycol	Deliver mascara ingredients to lashes in liquid vehicle
Waterproof solvent	Carrier fluid	Isododecane, cyclomethicone, petroleum distillates	Deliver mascara ingredients to lashes in liquid vehicle
Film former	Polymers/binder	Cellulosic polymers, acrylates copolymer/xanthan or acacia gum	The main constituent of the mascara film and serves to bind the other ingredients together in the wet and dried film
Structurant	Waxes/clays	Beeswax, carnauba wax/bentonite clay	Provides body and structure to the mascara film during application and wear
Surfactant or emulsifier	Anionic/non-ionic, etc.	Sodium laureth sulfate/TEA soap, polysorbates	In a formulation with two immiscible substances, an emulsifier stabilizes the two dissimilar parts of the formulation, preventing separation
Colorant	Pigments	Iron oxides, mica, ultramarines	Provides color to the mascara film
Care or attribute	Hair treatment/lengthening, etc.	Panthenol, keratin/Nylon or silk fiber	An ingredient included for a specific effect in the mascara film
Preservatives	Anti-microbial/pH adjuster/chelator	Parabens, potassium sorbate/citric acid/EDTA	Prevents contamination of harmful micro-organisms such as bacteria, mold and fungus

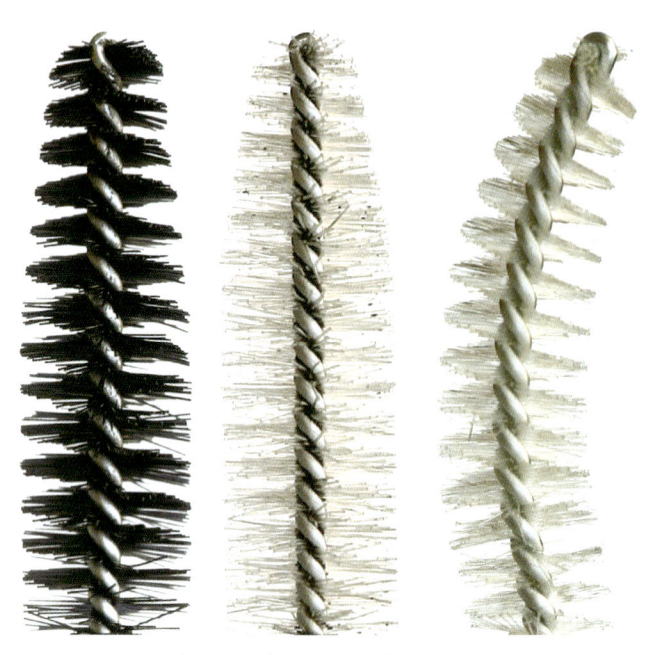

Figure 23.2 Twisted wire brush mascara applicators.

bristles. The bristles are very effective at depositing mascara onto lashes, but the inconsistent spacing between bristles on the brush can lead to excessively large clumps of lashes, uneven lash separation, and the need for compensatory grooming of the lashes.

The skill of the consumer plays a large part in achieving her desired look in a timely manner, and the twisted wire applicator has seen many adjustments over the years to make mascara application easier and quicker for consumers to achieve their desired lash appearance. Innovations include tapering the end of the applicator, curving the brush, hollow bristles, changing the diameter or length of the applicator, and even cutting shapes out from the applicator's profile to create channels within the collection of bristles. Despite the wide variety of twisted wire applicator innovations, the bristles all converge around a central shaft and the spacing between adjacent bristles is highly variable. This limits the consistency of both lash clump size and gaps between clumps of lashes.

In the last eight years, technology advancements have enabled a whole new category of molded mascara applicators to emerge. The precisely engineered surfaces of a molded applicator, shown in Figure 23.3, give control over the placement, number, and physical properties of bristles or other grooming surfaces. The result is consistent gaps between bristles, enabling the bristles to penetrate deeper into the lashes for increased mascara transfer and more efficient and regular separation of lashes. In addition, the varieties of colors, shapes, and textures that can be created are almost limitless and offer new opportunities to delight consumers. A few examples of these are shown in Figure 23.4. These molded applicators now have the ability to be molded in various shapes and sizes to form configurations that fit the shape of the eye [13].

Other eyelash treatments

The ability to change the appearance of eyelashes extends beyond mascara. For example, false eyelashes or eyelash extensions are designed to add thickness, fullness and length to natural eyelashes. False eyelashes significantly change the way the entire eye

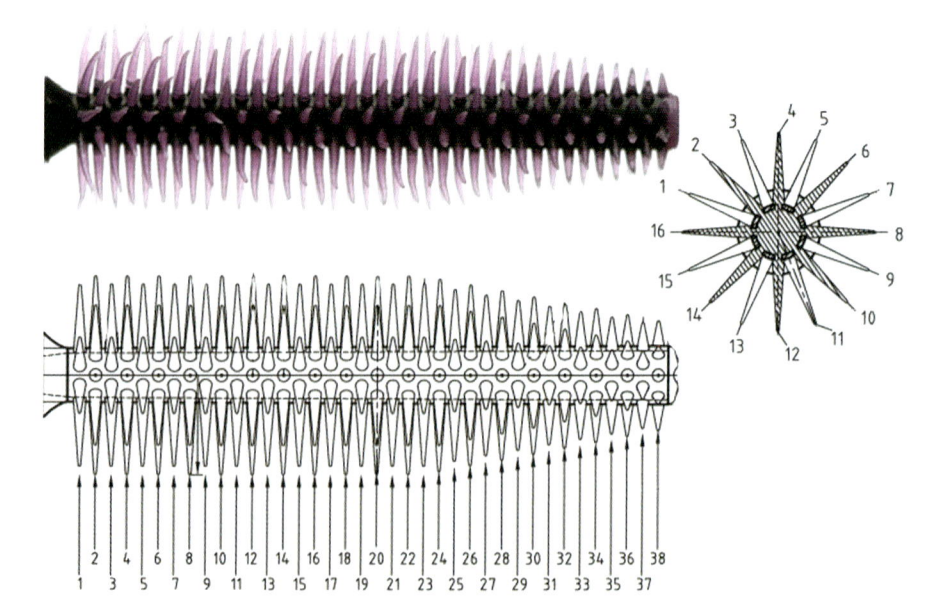

Figure 23.3 Molded mascara applicator with precisely engineered parallel bristles.

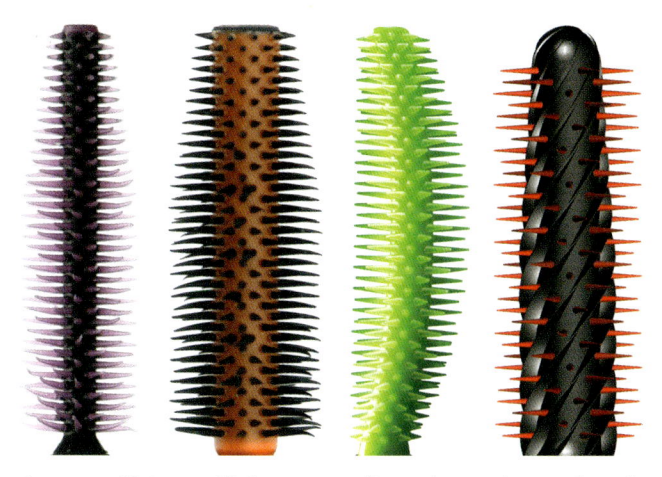

Figure 23.4 Various molded mascara applicator designs showing the wide range of possibilities that are possible with this versatile applicator type.

looks. False eyelashes can come in two different types: temporary and semi-permanent. The temporary eyelashes are applied with glue designed specifically for the purpose. One can use a variety of different types and colors of glues to adhere false eyelashes to natural lashes. False eyelashes may be applied as entire strips or as individual groups of lashes. They are adhered to the eyelid with a non-permanent adhesive. This allows easy application and removal at the end of the day.

Lash tinting involves application of a semi-permanent dye for color that lasts about a month. This is a two part product, just like permanent coloring for scalp hair. An oxidative cream is mixed with an oxidizing agent and then applied onto the lashes and left for 15 to 20 minutes. The dye forms while it is penetrating into the lashes. Currently there are no color additives approved by FDA for permanent dyeing or tinting of eyelashes and eyebrows [14].

Lash perming is done by rolling the lashes of the top eyelid around a thin cotton tube. The lashes are then coated with a high pH gel that penetrates into the lashes and breaks disulfide bonds holding together keratin protein strands in the cortex. After about 15 minutes, a second neutralizing coat is applied to the lashes to neutralize the high pH and reform bonds between protein strands to hold the lash in its new shape after the cotton cylinder is removed. While the FDA has approved these chemicals for use on scalp hair, it has not yet approved them for use around the eyes [14].

Eyelash extensions are synthetic fibers that are bonded to individual lashes, usually with a cyanoacrylate adhesive. Typically, 30–80 lashes per eyelid will have eyelash extensions applied, and they typically last one to two months, after which they must be touched up due to the natural growth cycle of lashes.

Eyelash transplants involve relocating scalp follicles to the eyelids. Small incisions are made in the top and bottom eyelids into which are placed the transplanted follicles. Manual curling and trimming is necessary because the scalp follicles will continue to grow hair for years in a relatively straight direction.

Blepharopigmentation, or eyelid tattooing, involves application of pigmentation into skin at the edges of the eyelid to simulate either eyeliner or the appearance of lashes. This is permanent but can be reversed with laser surgery.

Over the past ten years a number of products have launched with claims that suggest physiological stimulation of lash growth for darker, thicker, longer, and curlier lashes. Many of these make use of prostaglandin analogues that are similar to drugs used for treating glaucoma, but are known to have the above (beneficial) side effects [15]. The only FDA-approved treatment to stimulate the growth of eyelashes is Bimatoprost ophthalmic solution 0.03% (marketed under the brand name Latisse). Bimatoprost lengthens lashes by increasing the percentage of eyelash follicles in the anagen growth phase. It also stimulates melanogenesis, causing the lashes to appear darker and also increasing the size of the dermal papilla, which affects lash thickness and fullness [16]. Other products may contain one or many of a variety of peptides, vitamins, natural extracts or conditioning agents delivered as a serum, mascara primer or in mascara form. These products claim to either nourish eyelash follicles to improve growth or the lashes themselves to reduce breakage or eyelash fallout, however there is little to no independent clinical data to support these claims.

Eyebrows

Eyebrows are the strips of short hairs growing from the ridge above a person's eye socket. Throughout history, cultures have focused on eyebrow grooming as a way to frame the features of the face. Trends in desirable eyebrow thickness and shape in Western culture have changed during the twentieth century, from the very thin, tweezed brows of the 1920s and 1930s to the ungroomed, natural brow of the 1980s. The current trend is toward a thicker but well-shaped eyebrow "customized" for each person's face, and eyebrow grooming specialists and salons have become prevalent [17].

Eyebrow shaping is accomplished by trimming and by removing unwanted hairs from the brow area using tweezers, wax, or via a technique called threading. Threading originates from Middle Eastern and Asian cultures and involves twisting a thread around the unwanted hairs and then pulling to remove them from the follicle.

Consumers that wish to accentuate their eyebrows, or fill in sparse or uneven growth, may use a variety of brow cosmetics. Brow powders and pencils are available in neutral shades and are generally selected in a shade that matches or is slightly lighter than the person's natural brow color. Gels are available in both colored and uncolored versions, are applied with a mascara-type applicator or spoolie (a stand-alone twisted wire brush) and usually contain polymers meant to hold brows in a particular style much like hair gel for scalp hair.

Treatments for eyebrows are similar to those available for eyelashes/eyelids and include dyeing, tattooing and artificial brows or eyebrow "wigs" [18]. As with eyelashes, many serums are available which claim to aid or enhance brow growth.

Eyeshadow

Eyeshadow is color applied to the upper eyelids. It is used to add depth and dimension to the eyes, thus drawing attention to the eye look or eye color. The predominant form is powder, both pressed and loose, but eyeshadow is also available in other forms, such as creams, sticks, and liquids. In recent years, "baked" eyeshadows have become widely available. These are prepared in slurry or liquid form, rather than by pressing into compacts. The solvent is evaporated from the slurry, leaving only the pigments – this gives denser and truer pigmentation and improves application and wear due to the lack of binder present. Eyeshadows are very similar to blushes and pressed powder in terms of their key ingredients (see Chapter 20). They normally are comprised of pigments and pearls, and fillers bound together with a volatile or non-volatile binder. They may also contain other powder particles such as boron nitride or polytetrafluoroethylene to improve slip and pay-off on application. An eyeshadow primer, typically composed of a volatile solvent base, silicones and film formers, may be applied prior to eyeshadow application in order to extend wear and reduce creasing on oily eyelids.

Eyeliners

Eyeliner is used to outline the upper and lower eyelids. This serves to define the eyes against the backdrop of the face. Eyeliner can also be used to make the eye look more bold or to give the illusion of a different eye shape. They are typically available in liquid form and wood or mechanical pencils. Wood pencils excel at creating a softer, more natural look. Mechanical pencils tend to be a bit bolder, and the gel forms are great for gliding easily across the eyelid. Liquid liners can create a distinctively defined eye and provide longer wear, but are difficult to apply correctly. Most eye pencils are comprised of colorants dispersed in a waxy matrix for ease of application and to help the color adhere to the skin. Liquid liners, though not as popular as the pencil form, contain colorants that are dispersed in volatile solvents so they can be applied with a brush or pen-like applicator.

Product application

Eyeshadow application techniques vary according to the look you are trying to achieve, but generally, an appealing look can be achieved using three complimentary shades in light, medium and dark. The lightest shade highlights the area below the eyebrow, the medium shade is applied to the creased area, and the darkest shade is reserved for the area immediately above the upper eyelashes. Matte, silky shadows tend to blend nicely and are often preferred for mature eye skin over iridescent or sparkly shades which can highlight fine lines or puffiness. Eyeshadow can be applied with a dry applicator for a more natural look, or with a wet applicator for a more intense, dramatic look.

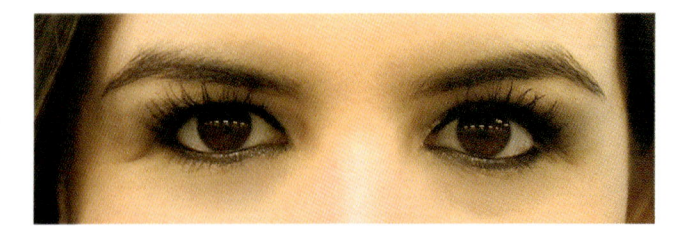

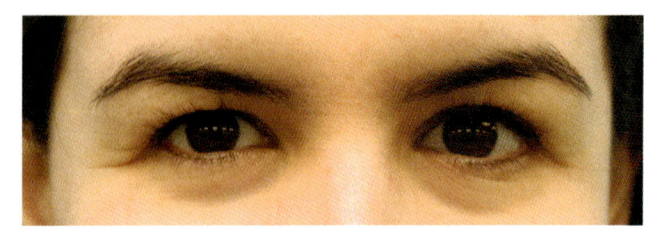

Figure 23.5 The impact of eye cosmetics on eye beauty.

Generally, eyeliner is applied to the outer two thirds of the lower lid below the lashes and to the entire upper lid above the lashes in a thin line. An angled brush can be used to gently soften the look. Although dark liners draw a lot of attention to the eyes, softer shades of brown, especially in the day time, can be used to avoid looking too harsh.

Curling the lashes with an eyelash curler prior to mascara application will make the eyes seem more wide open and bright. Usually, mascara is applied generously to upper lashes and to a lesser extent to the lower lashes. Color choice of mascaras can change the look obtained. For instance, on light-haired individuals brown mascara can be used for a softer, more natural look. Black or brown-black is best for deeper skin tones or for a more dramatic look.

Figure 23.5 shows the effect of applying eye cosmetics.

Safety and regulatory considerations for eye area cosmetics

Most countries or regions regulate cosmetics to a varying degree of complexity, largely due to safety considerations. Since cosmetics touch and interact directly with the human body, the various regulations are in place to ensure that consumers are not exposed to materials that may be harmful. This does of course stem from various safety incidents that have occurred with personal care products. For instance, consumers can have allergic reactions to lash dyes, which were becoming a popular product in the 1930s. In one case, an allergic reaction to a lash dye led to one consumer becoming blind [4]. Ultimately this was one of many causes in the United States that led to FDA oversight of cosmetics, and in particular it led to a positive list of colorants that could be used for eye area cosmetics [19]. In later years other regulatory bodies, such as the European Commission, adopted similar restrictions to the FDA's on colorants for use in the eye area [20].

One notable regulatory discussion in the area of eye cosmetics in recent years is the use of Carbon Black (also referred to as D&C Black No 2). Carbon Black is a fine-particle pigment produced from the partial combustion of hydrocarbon gas or oil and is a desirable cosmetic ingredient, particularly in eye cosmetics, because it can deliver much darker blacks than iron oxides. There has been considerable debate about the potential carcinogenicity of Carbon Black. In 2004, the FDA concluded research into the safety of the use of Carbon Black in cosmetics and ruled that the pigment is safe for use, but is subject to batch certification for purity due to the potential presence of PAH contaminants which are a byproduct of the production process [21].

Due to intimate contact with the human body, all cosmetics should be adequately preserved from microbiological insults. This is especially true for eye cosmetics where contact with a contaminated product could lead to an eye area infection and the possibility of more serious complications.

The future of eye cosmetics

For a mature category like eye cosmetics, it is surprising how much potential still exists for product innovation. New products are being introduced that feature enhanced long wear, new applicator surfaces, novel color effects, sustainable natural materials, improved application, and even lash growth.

Long wear

In the past, there have been two primary classes of mascara: water resistant and waterproof. Water-resistant mascara can be removed with warm water and soap, whereas waterproof mascara is usually removed with a makeup remover product. Both types are applied and removed during the same day. This does not allow for a consumer to enjoy the beauty benefits of mascara all of the time.

Although many consumers desire a semi-permanent mascara benefit, current options are longer wearing waterproof mascaras or semi-permanent lash stain products that are only designed to eliminate reapplication during the day while also being easily removable by the user using soap and water or a makeup remover product. These technologies do not last through showering and sleeping and are therefore not appropriate for wear beyond one day. Furthermore, the beauty look of existing semi-permanent lash stain products provides darkness, but not the level of thickening consumers desire from a mascara; moreover, they typically degrade quickly after the first day of wear [22].

To address the strong consumer need of semi-permanent mascara, new longer lasting formula technologies have been developed to be abrasion resistant, flexible and insoluble in soap and water so that the initial beauty look is maintained for multiple days. These technologies achieve extended wear benefits through various formula design elements. One example is the choice of polymers. Polymers must be screened for film flexibility, abrasion resistance and water and surfactant resistance. Another design element is balancing the ratio of polymer to other nonvolatiles in the formula such that there is sufficient polymer to form a continuous phase. Studies have shown that a continuous film modifies many film properties including gloss, film flexibility and abrasion resistance. As the pigment volume concentration increases, film flexibility decreases and abrasion resistance remains the same or improves. The more this pigment volume concentration is increased, the more the film will become brittle and abrasion resistance will decrease rapidly. Scanning electron microscopy can be used to compare the morphologies of mascara films applied to false lashes as shown in Figure 23.6.

Pushing the applicator envelope

In addition to new benefits from advancements in molded applicator technology, the mascara application experience is being

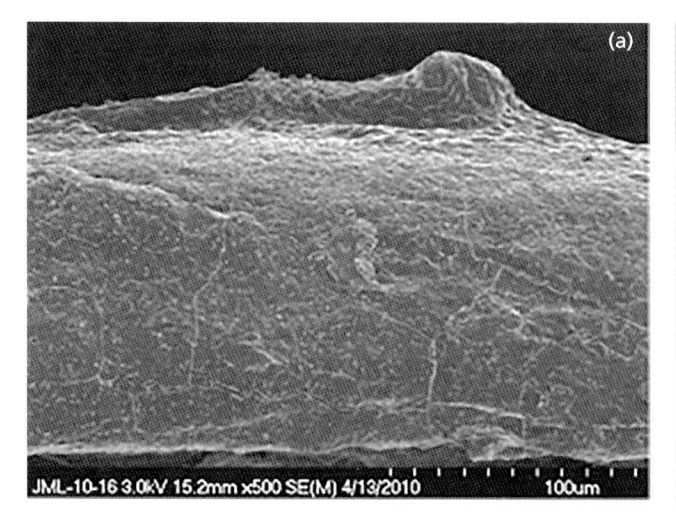

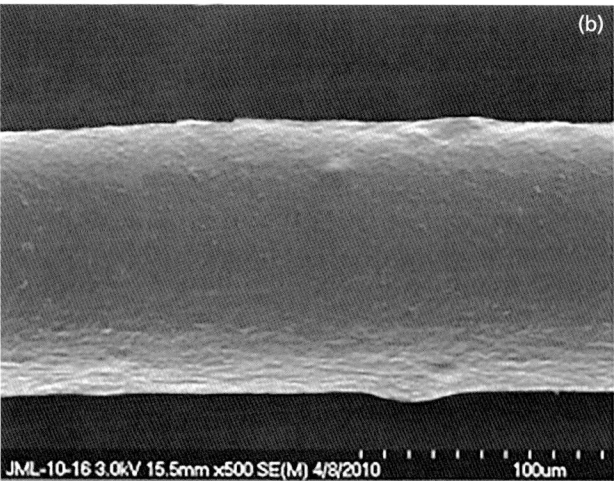

Figure 23.6 SEM images of mascara film morphology. Rough mascara film of a long wearing waterproof mascara that lasts a day (a), and microscopically smooth continuous mascara film of a semi-permanent mascara that lasts multiple days (b).

improved with automated applicators that use vibrating or rotating brushes to take away some of the skill necessary to achieve beautiful lashes. These applicators can be held up against the lashes while they work for the consumer by exposing more of the applicator surface to the lashes, encouraging more deposition of mascara and more grooming of the lashes. Other innovative eye makeup tools are being developed to make the application of makeup easy. These tools are not only meant for applying mascara, but also for curling and perming the eyelashes. They include heated mascara brushes, bristle-free tips, expandable brushes, precision tips, corkscrew bristles and disposable mascara wands.

Lash conditioners and growers

As consumers have become more sensitive to the impact that beauty products have on the health and condition of their skin and hair, cosmetic companies have started to adopt healthy hair actives commonly used for scalp hair into products intended to improve or repair eyelashes. As mentioned previously, products are also coming onto the market that claim to actually stimulate and enhance lash growth. While there are regulatory considerations that make these products controversial, if approved for consumer use, they may negate the need of some women to use mascara to achieve beautiful lashes.

References

1. Kunzig R. (1999) Style of the Nile. *Discover* September, p. 80.
2. Ahuja A. (1999) Chemistry and eye makeup – science. *Times*, September 22.
3. Geibel V. (1991) Mascara. *Vogue* August.
4. Riordan T. (2004) *Inventing Beauty: A History of the Innovations that have Made us Beautiful*. New York: Broadway Books, pp. 1–31.
5. Balaji Narasimhan R. (2001) Pearl luster pigments. *Paintindia* **51**, 67–72.
6. Elder MJ. (1997) Anatomy and physiology of eyelash follicles: relevance to lash ablation procedures. *Ophthal Plast Reconstr Surg* **13**, 21–5.
7. Na J, Kwon O, Kim B et al. (2006) Ethnic characteristics of eyelashes: a comparative analysis in Asian and Caucasian females. *Br J Dermatol* **155**, 1170–6.
8. Liotet S, Riera M, Nguyen H. (1977) Les cils: Physiologie, structure, pathologie. *Arch Opht* **37**, 697–708.
9. Thibaut E, De Becker E, Caisey L, et al. (2010) Human eyelash characterization. *Br J Dermatol* **162**: 304–310.
10. Montagna W, Ford DM. (1969) Histology and cytochemistry of human skin. 3. The eyelid. *Arch Dermatol* **100**, 328–35.
11. Cunningham J. (1996) Color cosmetics. In: Williams D. F, Schmitt WH, eds. *Chemistry and Technology of the Cosmetics and Toiletries Industry*. New York: Blackie Academic & Professional.
12. Sheffler RJ. (1998) The revolution in mascara evolution. *Happi* April, pp. 48–52.
13. Wall Street Journal Online (2013) *Makeup to Women: Apply Yourself. Finally, Cosmetics That Promise to Be Faster and More Precise; Shoppers Toss the Mirror and Buy.* http://online.wsj.com/news/articles/SB10001424127887323419104578372311872888312 (accessed 4 June 2015).
14. US Food and Drug Administration. (2013) *Eye cosmetic safety*. www.fda.gov/Cosmetics/ProductandIngredientSafety/ProductInformation/ucm137241.htm (accessed 4 June 2015).
15. Wolf R, Matz H, Zalish M, Pollack A, Orion E. (2003) Prostaglandin analogs for hair growth: great expectations. *Dermatology* **9**, 7.
16. Cohen JL. (2010) Enhancing the growth of natural eyelashes: the mechanism of bimatoprost-induced eyelash growth. *Dermatol Surg* **36**(9), 1361–71.
17. Sherrow V. (2006) *Encyclopedia of Hair: A Cultural History*. Westport (CT): Greenwood Press; Eyebrows; pp. 118–20.
18. O'Donoghue MN. (2000) Eye cosmetics. *Dermatol Clin* [Internet] 2000 Oct [cited 2014 Jan 27]; **18**(4), 633–9. Available from ScienceDirect: www.sciencedirect.com/science/article/pii/S073386350570214X
19. US Federal Regulations. FDA. 21C.F.R. Part 700, Subchapter G.
20. EC Directive 76/768/EC, OJ L 262, p. 169 of 27.9.1976.
21. Color additives subject to certification; D&C Black No. 2. Final rule. Fed Regist. 2004 Jul 28; **69**(144), 44927–30.
22. Dempsey JH, Fabula AM, Rabe TE, et al. (2012) Development of a semi-permanent mascara technology. *Int J Cosmetic Sci* **34**, 29–35.

SECTION 2 Nail Cosmetics

CHAPTER 24
Nail Physiology and Grooming

Anna Hare[1] and Phoebe Rich[2]
[1]Emory School of Medicine., Atlanta, GA, USA
[2]Oregon Health & Science University, Portland, OR, USA

> **BASIC CONCEPTS**
> - Knowledge of nail unit anatomy and physiology and an understanding of nail plate growth and physical properties are important prerequisites for understanding nail cosmetics.
> - Disruption and excessive manipulation of certain nail structures, such as the hyponychium and eponychium/cuticle, should be discouraged during nail cosmetic procedures and nail salon services.
> - In addition to beautifying natural nails, nail cosmetics are beneficial in camouflaging unsightly medical and infectious nail problems, especially during the lengthy treatment period.
> - Some nail cosmetics provide a protective coating for fragile, weak, and brittle nails.
> - Proper nail grooming is crucial for maintaining nail health.
> - Although most nail cosmetics are used safely, it is important to be aware of potential complications associated with nail cosmetic materials and application processes.

Introduction: Nail physiology

Nail unit anatomy
Understanding nail unit anatomy and pathophysiology is essential to maximizing the benefits of nail cosmetics without inducing pathology via cosmetic materials and procedures. The nail unit is composed of the nail matrix, proximal and lateral nail folds, the hyponychium, and the nail bed (Figure 24.1).

Table 24.1 lists common nail signs and definitions relevant to nail cosmetics.

Nail matrix
The nail matrix is comprised of germinative epithelium from which the nail plate is derived (Figure 24.2). The majority of the matrix lies under the proximal nail fold. The distal portion of the nail matrix creates the white lunula, visible through the proximal nail plate on some digits. It is hypothesized that the white color of the lunula can be attributed to both incomplete nail plate keratinization and loose connective tissue in the underlying dermis. The proximal nail matrix generates the dorsal (superficial) nail plate, while the distal nail matrix generates the ventral (inferior) nail plate. This concept is crucial to understanding nail pathology. Preserving and protecting the matrix during nail cosmetic processes is essential for proper nail plate formation. Significant damage to the nail matrix can result in permanent nail plate dystrophy.

The nail plate is derived from the nail matrix and composed of closely packed, keratinized epithelial cells called onychocytes. Cells in the matrix become progressively flattened and broadened and lose their nuclei as they mature into the nail plate. The nail plate is curved in both the longitudinal and transverse planes, allowing adhesion to the nail bed and ensheathment by the proximal and lateral nail folds. Longitudinal ridging may be present on both the dorsal and ventral surface of the nail plate. Mildly increased longitudinal ridging on the dorsal nail plate is considered a normal part of aging. Ridging on the ventral surface of the nail plate is caused by the structure of the underlying nail bed and vertically oriented blood vessels. The composition and properties of the nail plate are further discussed below.

Nail folds
The nail folds surround and protect the nail unit by sealing out environmental irritants and microorganisms through tight attachment of the cuticle to the nail plate. This barrier formed by the cuticle, or eponychium, is essential to prevent-

---

Cosmetic Dermatology: Products and Procedures, Second Edition. Edited by Zoe Diana Draelos.
© 2016 John Wiley & Sons, Ltd. Published 2016 by John Wiley & Sons, Ltd.

208 **ADORNMENT** Nail Cosmetics

Table 24.1 Common nail signs associated with or helped by nail cosmetics.

Nail sign	Definition	Association
Onycholysis	Separation of the nail plate from the nail bed	Vigorous cleaning of hyponychium exacerbates. Polish hides
Onychorrhexis	Increased longitudinal ridging	Associated with aging, distal notching. Polish may help
Onychoschizia	Lamellar splitting of the free end of the nail plate	
Paronychia	Inflammation of the nail fold	
Dyschromia yellow	Staining of the surface of the nail plate yellow from the dye in nail polish	
Green/black discoloration	*Pseudomonas* is a bacterium that generates a green–black pigment that discolors the nail plate	
Nail bed changes as in psoriasis, onychomycosis		

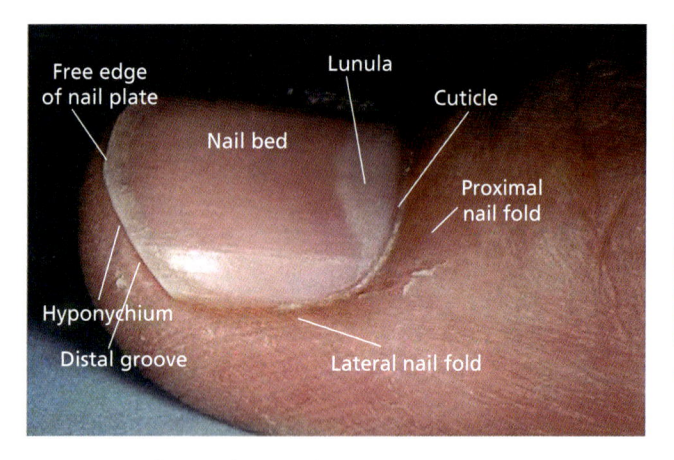

Figure 24.1 Nail unit with lines indicating important structures.

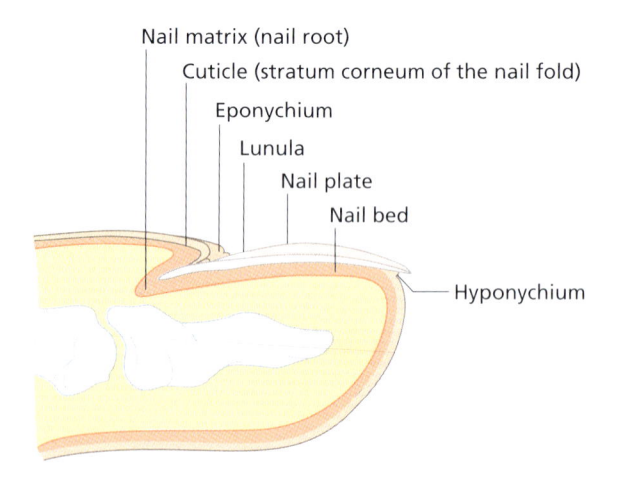

Figure 24.2 Diagram of the nail unit.

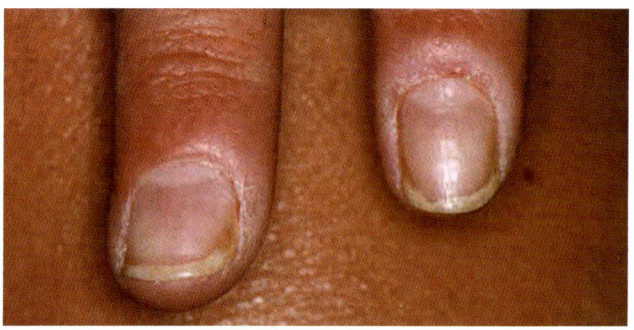

Figure 24.3 Paronychia.

ing invasion of irritants, moisture, bacteria, and yeasts under the nail fold. Disruption of this barrier, as often occurs in cosmetic nail procedures when the cuticle is cut or pushed back, can result in infection or inflammation of the nail fold, termed paronychia (Figure 24.3). Chronic paronychia may disrupt the underlying nail matrix and subsequently lead to nail plate dystrophy.

Hyponychium

The hyponychium is the cutaneous margin underlying the free edge of the nail plate. It is contiguous with the volar aspect of the fingertip. The nail bed ends at the hyponychium. The hyponychium functions like the cuticle, acting as an adherent seal to protect the nail unit. Overmanipulating of the hyponychium during nail grooming can result in onycholysis, or separation of the nail plate from the nail bed. This space created between the nail plate and bed retains moisture, creating an ideal environment for potential pathogens, such as yeast, bacteria, or fungi.

Nail bed

The nail bed is thin, 2–5 cell layer thick epithelium that underlies the nail plate. It extends from the lunula to the hyponychium. The nail bed is composed of longitudinal, parallel rete ridges with a rich vascular supply. This vascularity is responsible for the pink coloration of the bed as well as longitudinal ridges on the

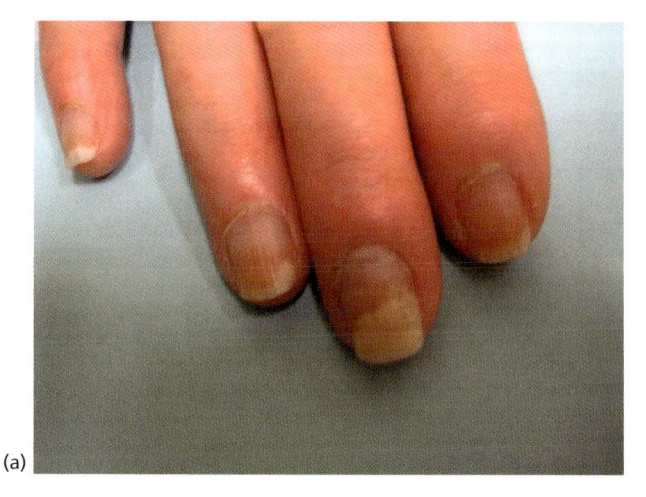

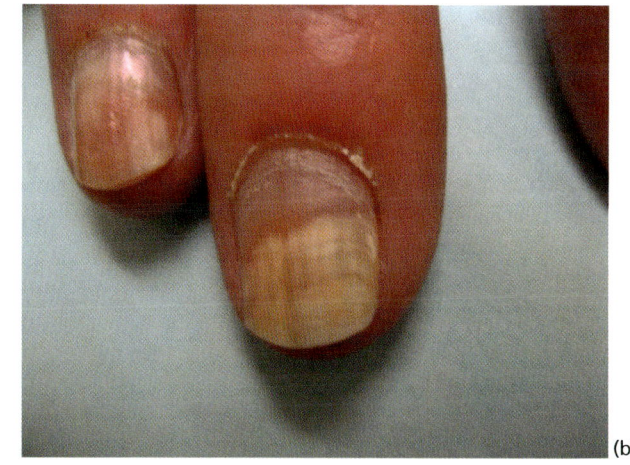

Figure 24.4 (a & b) Onycholysis.

ventral surface of the nail plate. In chronic onycholysis, when the nail plate is separated from the nail bed for an extended duration, the nail bed epithelium may become keratinized, form a granular layer, and lead to permanent onycholysis (Figure 24.4).

Other structures
The distal phalanx lies immediately beneath the nail unit. The extensor tendon runs over the distal interphalangeal joint and attaches to the distal phalanx 12 mm proximal to the proximal nail fold. Given that there is little space between the nail unit and distal phalanx, minor injury to the nail unit may extend to the periosteum and lead to infection.

Nail growth
Normal nail growth has been cited to vary from less than 1.8 mm to more than 4.5 mm per month. Average fingernail growth is 0.1 mm per day, or 3 mm per month. This information is useful when determining the duration of nail pathology. For example, if splinter hemorrhages are located 6 mm from the proximal nail fold, it can be estimated that they occurred from injury approximately 2 months prior. Based on this growth rate, fingernails grow out completely in 6 months. Toenails grow at one-third to half of the rate of fingernails and take 12–18 months to grow out completely.

Several factors affect the rate of nail growth. Age affects nail growth rate, with nail growth peaking at 10–14 years and declining after 20 years. Nail growth is proportional to finger length, with fastest growth of the third fingernail and slowest growth of the fifth fingernail, and faster nail growth has been noted in the dominant hand. Nails grow slower at night and during the winter. Other factors causing slower nail plate growth include lactation, immobilization, paralysis, poor nutrition, yellow nail syndrome, antimitotic drugs, and acute infection. Pregnancy, psoriasis, and nail biting are other factors linked to faster nail growth. Table 24.2 summarizes factors influencing nail growth.

Physical properties of nails

Nail composition
The nail plate is composed mainly of keratin, which is embedded in a matrix of non-keratin proteins. There is wide variation in reported percentage of inorganic elements found in the nail plate. Several elements, including sulfur, calcium, iron, aluminum, copper, silver, gold, titanium, phosphorus, zinc, and sodium, are constituents of the nail plate. Of these elements, sulfur, contained in the cysteine bonds that cross-link nail plate keratin, has the greatest contribution to nail structure and comprises approximately 5% of the nail plate. Some studies attribute brittle nails to decreased cysteine levels. Cytokeratin 16 and 17 are present in normal nails but diminished in brittle nails [10].

There is a popular misconception that calcium content is responsible for nail hardness. However, calcium comprises less than 1% of the nail plate by weight [1], and no current evidence supports association between calcium deficit and brittle nails or shows increased nail strength with calcium supplementation. In fact, in kwashiorkor, a condition of nutritional deficiency caused by insufficient protein intake, nails are thin and soft and with increased nail plate calcium.

Water content of the normal nail plate is reported to range between 10% and 30%. The most commonly accepted value is 18% water content in normal nails and 16% in brittle nails. However, a study aimed at confirming this demonstrated no statistically significant difference between normal and brittle nails [2]. In addition, this study showed lower water content than previously thought, with a mean water content of 11.90% in normal nails and 12.48% in brittle nails. Some limitations in this study were noted, including analysis of only the distal nail plate (clippings) and variable time between sample collection and analysis, allowing interval water loss.

Lipids, including squalene and cholesterol, are also constituents of the nail plate and comprise 5% of the nail plate by weight. These lipids are thought to diffuse from the nail bed to the nail

Table 24.2 Nail cosmetic products: ingredients and uses.

Product	Ingredients	Application procedures	Benefits of use	Potential complications
Nail polish	Film former: nitrocellulose Thermoplastic resin: (toluene sulfonamide formaldehyde resin) Plasticizer: dibutyl pthalate Solvents and pigments	Polish is applied in several coats with a small brush and allowed to dry by evaporation	Provides an attractive glossy smooth decorative surface and camouflages nail defects Protects nail from dehydration and irritants	Yellow staining of nail plate. Potential for allergy to toluene sulfonamide formaldehyde resin and other ingredients
Nail hardener	May contain formaldehyde in a nail polish base, also may have fibers that reinforce the nail	Application similar to nail polish which is applied in several coats	Forms several layers of protection on the nail plate	Potential allergy to formaldehyde and possible brittleness
Acrylic nail extensions DO GEL AND S	Acrylic monomer, polymer, polymerized to form a hard shell attached to the nail plate or to a plastic tip glued to the nail	Monomer (liquid) and polymer (powder) mixed to form a paste and polymerized with a catalyst to a harden the product	Cover unsightly nail defects, may help manage onychotillomania and habit tic disorder	Possible allergy to acrylates, inflexibility of artificial nail may cause injury to nail unit
Cuticle remover	Contains potassium hydroxide or sodium hydroxide plus humectants	Applied to cuticle for 5–10 minutes to soften cuticle adhered to nail plate	Gently removes dead skin attached to the nail plate without mechanical trauma	Over removal of cuticle and result in the potential for paronychia and secondary bacteria and *Candida* infections. Can soften the nail plate
Nail polish remover	Acetone, butyl acetate, ethyl acetate, may also contain moisturizer such as lanolin or synthetic oils	Wiped across nail plate with cotton or tissue to remove nail polish	Removes polish smoothly without removing layers of nail plate	May dehydrate the nail plate and periungual tissue

plate. The water binding capacity of brittle nails is less than that of normal nails which may be due to an abnormality in lipid content, keratin, or keratin-associated proteins or lipid content [9,10].

Nail flexibility

Most references to nail strength and hardness actually refer to nail flexibility. A flexible nail will bend and conform to physical force, whereas a hard nail is brittle and breaks more easily. Nail flexibility is aided by plasticizers, which are liquids that make solids more flexible. Examples of nail plasticizers are water and lipids. Flexibility is decreased by solvents, such as nail polish removers, which remove both water and lipids, and detergents, which remove lipids.

Nail brittleness is caused by loss of flexibility. Brittle nails are a common complaint and are found in 20% of the general population and more commonly in females (Figure 24.5). Brittleness encompasses several nail features including onychoschizia, which is lamellar peeling of distal nail plate (Figure 24.6); splitting and notching, sometimes associated with ridges; and fragility of the distal nail plate, including lamellar splitting of the free end of the nail plate. Several attempts have been made to define brittleness with objective measurements, including Knoop hardness, which evaluates indentation at a fixed weight; modulus of elasticity, which describes the relationship between force/area and deformation produced; tensile strength; and a brittleness grading system.

Although there are systemic and cutaneous conditions that may cause brittle nails, exogenous causes are more common. These include mechanical trauma, exposure to solvents and extraction of plasticizers, and repeated hydration and drying of nails.

Nail thickness

Thickness of the nail plate is determined primarily by matrix length and rate of growth. Measurements of distal plate thickness demonstrate greatest thickness in the thumbnail, followed by the second, third, fourth, and fifth fingernails. Thickness also is influenced by sex, with males having an average nail plate thickness of 0.6 mm, compared to 0.5 mm in females.

Nail grooming principles

Nail care

Several principles of nail care should be observed during nail grooming to maintain normal nail structure.

Manicures and pedicures are the processes of grooming the fingernails and toenails respectively at home or in a nail salon (Figure 24.7). The procedure involves soaking the nails to soften prior to trimming and shaping the nail plate. Excess cuticle is removed from the nail plate using a chemical cuticle remover and often a metal implement. The nails are then finished with a

Figure 24.5 (a–c) Brittle nails.

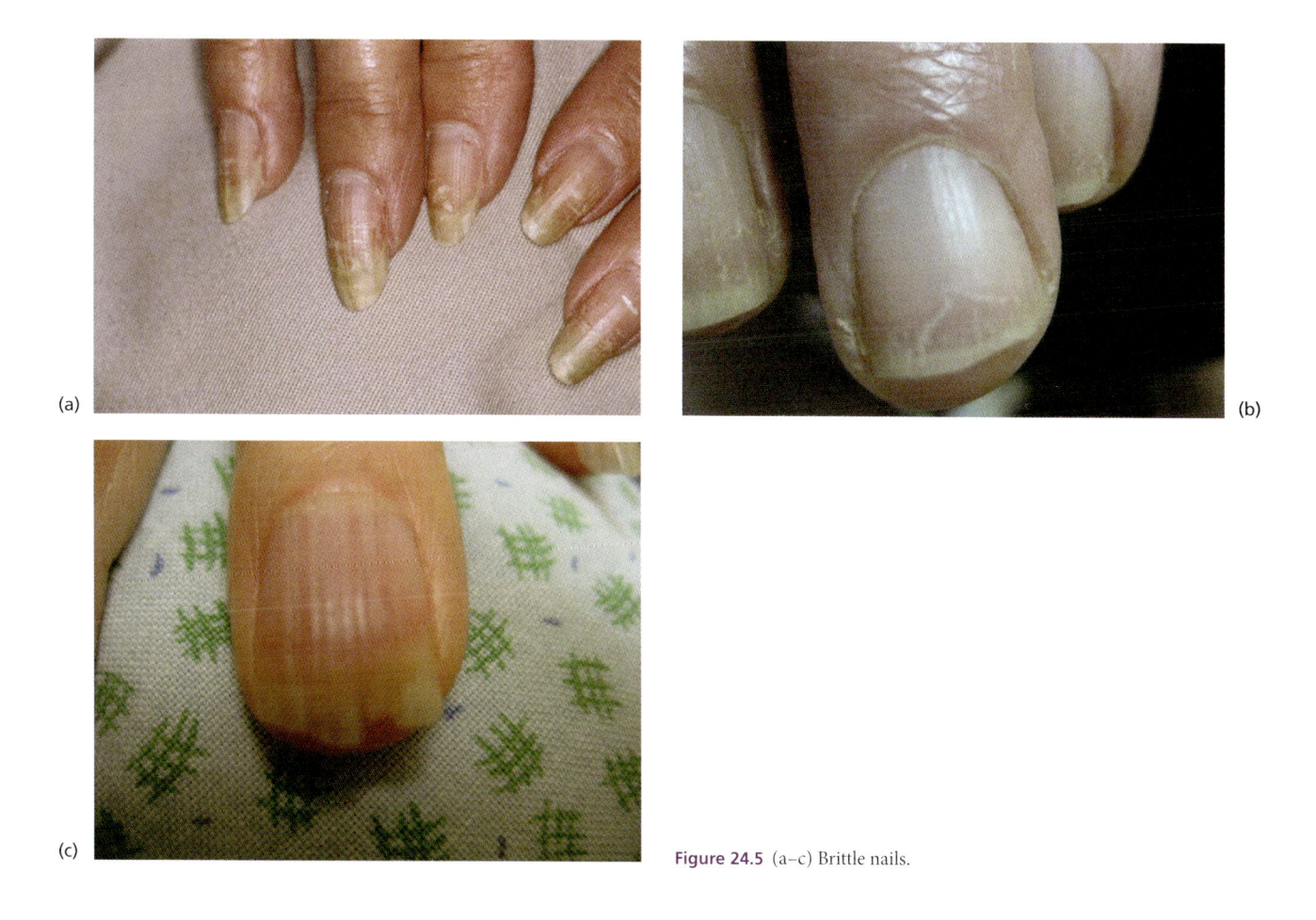

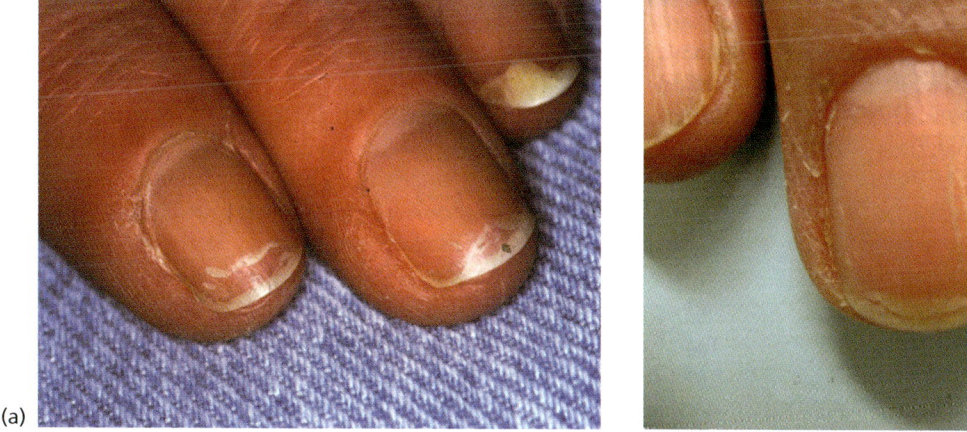

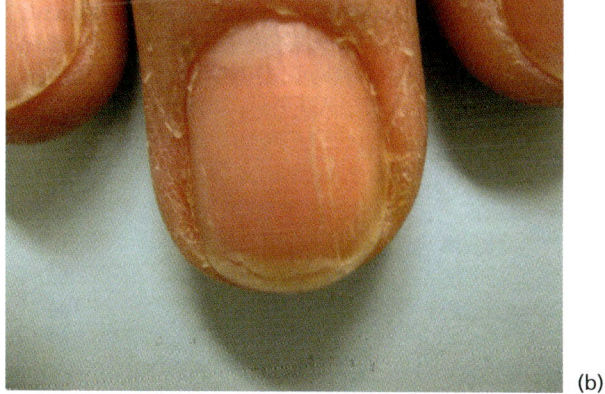

Figure 24.6 Onychoschizia, distal lamallar peeling of the nail plate.

shiny, smooth coat of nail enamel, commonly called nail polish, sandwiched between a base coat and top coat, or the nails may be buffed to a soft luster.

Other procedures such as acrylic, gel or silk wrap enhancements may be added to the basic manicure to extend nail length, improve shape, hide damaged nails, or increase durability of nail colors. These nail extension procedures involve applying product to the natural nail or to a plastic tip glued to the nail. The material are applied and shaped before curing or polymerizing to form a hard surface.

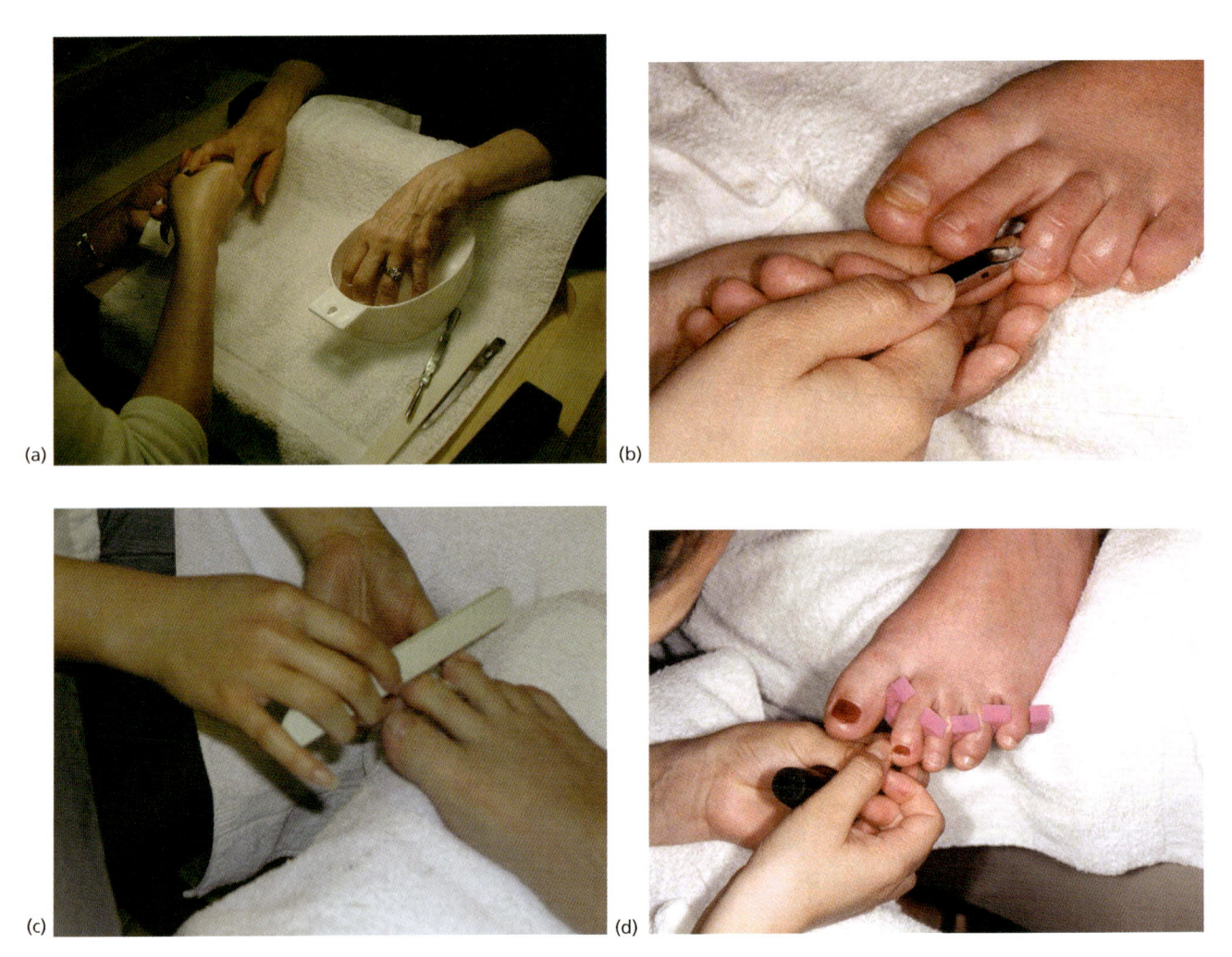

Figure 24.7 (a) Manicure; (b–d) Pedicure.

Nail trimming

Most nail experts advocate shaping nails with an emery board rather than clipping or cutting nails. Filing should be carried out with the file exactly perpendicular to the nail surface to avoid inducing onycholysis. Proper filing of the free edge of nail plate reduces sharp edges that may catch and cause nail plate tearing. If nails must be clipped or cut, this should be performed after they have been hydrated which maximizes nail flexibility and prevents breakage during trimming. Nails should also be kept as short as possible. Long nails, especially those that are brittle, may act as a lever and create onycholysis.

Nail buffing and filing

The dorsal nail plate surface is often filed to remove shine from the natural nail plate at nail salons prior to application of nail products or artificial nails. Care must be taken to avoid excessive filing, especially with electric drills. The nail plate is approximately 100 cell layers thick. If filing must be done, only 5% of the nail plate thickness, or approximately five cell layers, should be removed which is just enough to remove the shine of the dorsal nail plate in order to facilitate adherence of the product to the nail plate. Limited buffing to reduce nail ridging is acceptable, but excessive buffing thins the nail plate and should be avoided.

Nail painting

Classic nail polish contains ingredients allow it to be painted on smoothly, harden, and adhere to the nail (Table 24.2). This polish typically lasts 2–7 days without chipping or cracking. Gel polish became popular for its increased durability over time, lasting around 2 weeks. Application typically requires smoothing the nail via filing, which can weaken the nail plate, though application of a thick coating, which is dried using UV or LED light, may have a mitigating effect by protecting the nail. Removal is often performed in a nail salon, and requires either filing the false nail coat off, which can damage the native nail if filing extends below the gel coat, or considerable soaking in acetone followed by scraping, which contributes to drying of the nail. Shellac, a recent development often called a hybrid of the two, can be painted on in coats with time to harden under UV light between coats. Removal requires 10–15 minutes of soaking in acetone before scraping off.

Recent concern has arisen over potential increased risk of skin cancer due to exposure of the hands to UV light used to cure these nail coatings. However, research examining this risk has noted that the risk is very small and can be minimized further with the use of white cotton gloves with the fingertips cut off, and application of water resistant sunscreen to the dorsal hands prior to salon services involving UV light [3,4].

Care for brittle nails

Brittle nails should be treated by avoiding nail trauma and increasing flexibility by maintaining nail hydration. Nails should be kept short to prevent lifting of the nail plate, disruption of the hyponychium, and onycholysis. In addition, nails should be trimmed after they have been hydrated and are the most flexible. Avoiding solvents and frequent cycling between hydration and desiccation of nails also helps maintain flexibility. Humectants hydrate the nail plate and increase flexibility and reduce brittleness. However, frequent use of hand moisturizers is not necessarily recommended. In one study of 102 participants, nail brittleness was positively associated with frequency of professional manicures, use of nail polish remover, family history of brittle nails, and higher frequency of hand moisturizer use [2]. There is also controversy over avoidance of nail cosmetics in the management of brittle nails. The use of nail polish remover, an organic solvent, results in drying of the nails and can increase brittleness [5]. Filing nails thins the nail plate and increases nail desiccation [5]. However application of nail polish can be protective. Coating the nail with a protective layer of nail enamel can prevent dehydration by sealing the moisture in the nail plate and preventing rapid evaporation [5], as well as protecting the nail plate from some environmental irritants. Biotin has also been advocated for brittle nails, but results are inconclusive. One open label study by Scher *et al.* showed that 2.5 mg biotin daily for 6 to 15 months improved brittle nails and onychoschizia in all subjects [10]. The recommended dose of biotin for brittle nails is 2.5–5 mg/day, which is 100–200 times the recommended daily allowance. Given that biotin has relatively few side effects, most experts recommend its use, in addition to the above grooming recommendations.

Adverse effects from nail grooming

Nail cosmetics are safely used by millions of people worldwide. In addition to enhancing the appearance of normal nails, cosmetics are useful for improving the appearance of unsightly nail dystrophy caused by medical disease, such as psoriasis (Figure 24.8), onychomycosis (Figure 24.9), or trauma. Although nail cosmetics rarely cause problems, it is important to be aware of possible adverse effects related to procedures or to materials used in nail cosmetics, and to guide or patients toward safe use of nail cosmetics and nail salon services. (Figure 24.10).

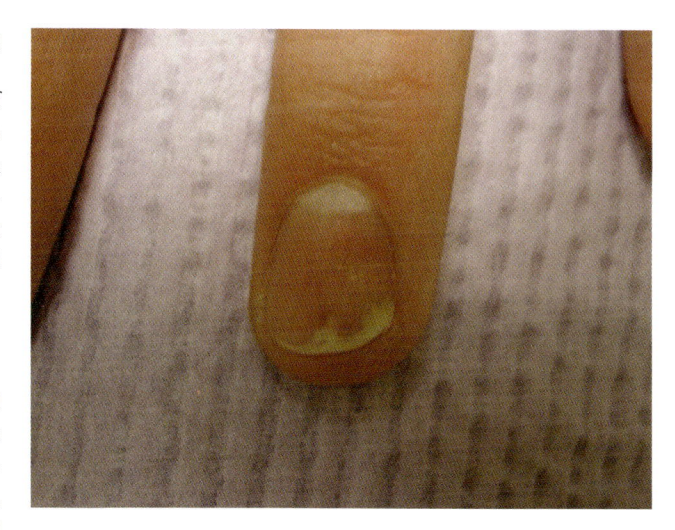

Figure 24.8 Psoriasis: salmon patch oil drop discoloration.

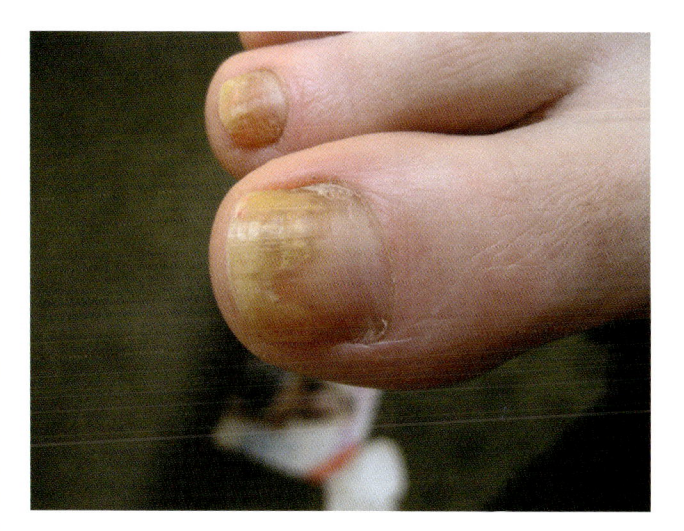

Figure 24.9 Onychomycosis.

Allergic reactions to nail cosmetic ingredients

Allergic contact dermatitis from nail cosmetics not common and occurs it occurs on periungual skin, as well as the eyelids, face, and neck, caused by touching these areas with freshly polished fingernails (Figure 24.11). The most common allergen in nail polish is tosylamide-formaldehyde resin (TSFR) with sensitization occurring in up to 3% of the population. TSFR, a product that increases adhesion, gloss, and flow of nail polish, is found in most brands of nail polish available in concentrations ranging from around .1 to 25% in dried polish(6). Some "hypoallergenic" labeled products have replaced TSFR with ester resins, though these products may still contain other allergens and testing of these products has found TSFR present in a few [7]. Formaldehyde, another allergenic ingredient used for nail hardening, is often used in conjunction with and correlated with TSFR concentration [6]. Gel nail polish, popular for

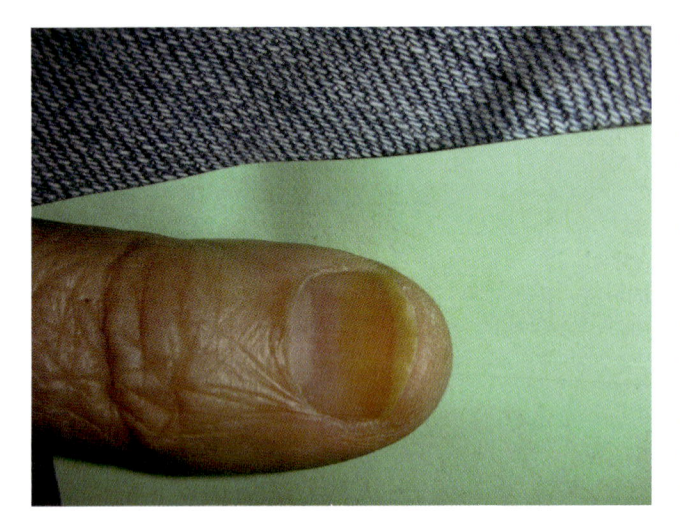

Figure 24.10 Yellow staining from nail polish.

its increased durability, often contains methyl acrylate, which can also result in sensitization and cause contact dermatitis. Other potential allergens are cyanoacrylate nail glue, formaldehyde in nail hardeners, and ethylmethacrylate in sculptured nails.

Irritant reactions

Common nail products that cause irritant reactions to periungual skin include acetone or acetate nail polish removers and cuticle removers with sodium hydroxide. Reactions are manifested as an irritant dermatitis of the periungual skin and as brittle nails, including onychoschizia. Prolonged use of nail polish can induce development of keratin granulations on the nail plate. This commonly is seen when fresh coats of nail enamel are applied on top of old enamel for and left in place for an extended period of time. These granulations cause superficial friability of the nail plate (Figure 24.12).

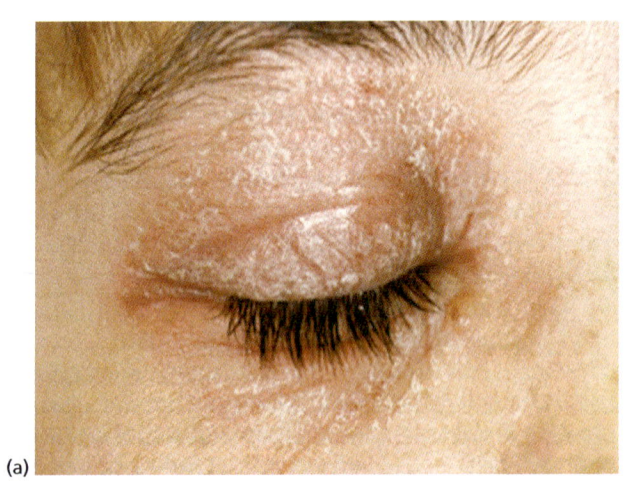

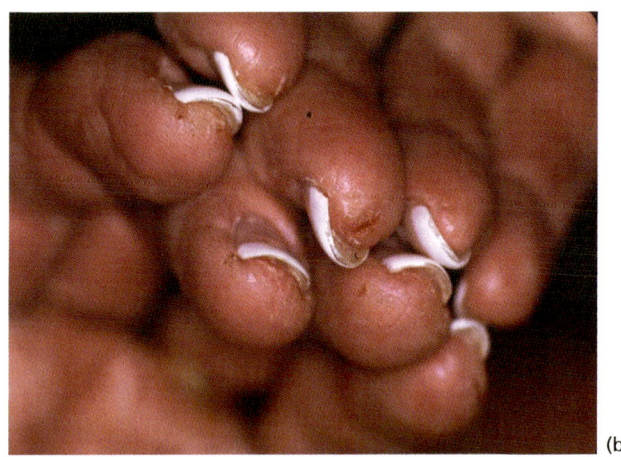

Figure 24.11 Allergic contact dermatitis from nail cosmetics. (a) On the eyelid. (b) On periungal skin caused by acrylates.

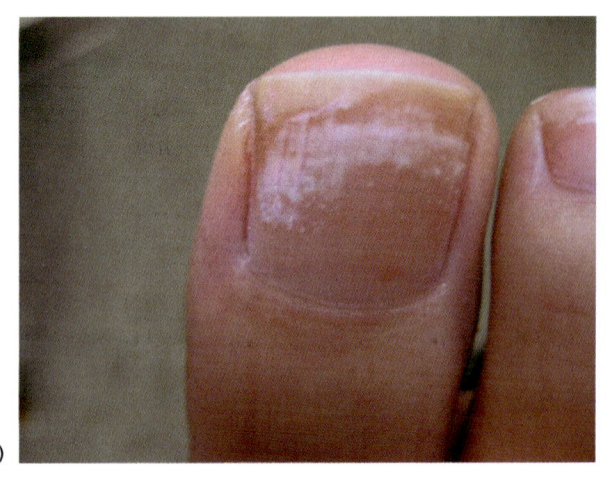

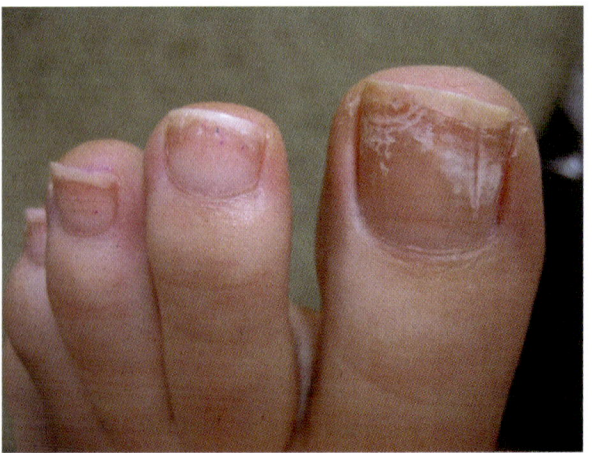

Figure 24.12 (a & b) Keratin granulations.

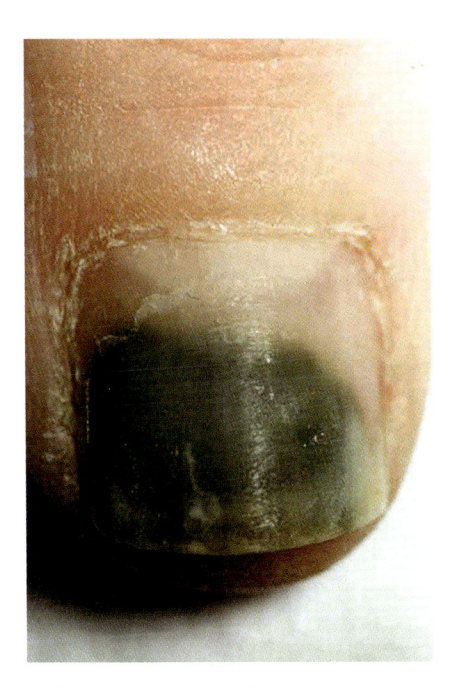

Figure 24.13 Infection caused by *Pseudomonas*.

Table 24.3 Information for patients for safe nail cosmetic use.

- Be sure that the salon sterilizes instruments, preferably with an autoclave. Some salons offer instruments for clients to purchase
- Stinging, burning, or itching following a nail salon treatment may be signs of an allergic reaction to a cosmetic ingredient. Remove the product and seek medical evaluation by a dermatologist
- If using artificial nail extensions, keep them short. Long nails can cause mechanical damage to the nail bed. Remove extensions at the first sign of onycholysis and avoid enhancements until the nail is reattached
- Do not allow nail technician to cut or clip cuticles. Cuticles serve an important protective function and should not be cut. They may be pushed back gently with a soft towel after soaking the nails or bathing

Source: Rich, 2001 [8]. Reproduced with permission of John Wiley & Sons.

Nail cosmetic procedures

Several nail problems, including paronychia, onycholysis, and thinning of the nail plate, may be mechanically induced by cosmetic procedures. Paronychia, or inflammation of the proximal nail fold, is often caused by cutting or pushing back the cuticle, leading to separation of the proximal nail fold and cuticle from the nail plate. Sharp manicure instruments used to clean under the nail plate may induce onycholysis and create an environment for secondary bacterial and fungal infection. Onycholysis may be exacerbated by long artificial nails because of increased mechanical leverage. Nail drills or excessive filing and buffing of the surface of the nail plate may lead to thinning of the nail plate and weak, fragile nails. Breaks in the integrity of the nail unit allow access of microorganisms such as *Candida* and *Pseudomonas* (Figure 24.13) and result in exacerbation of paronychia and onycholysis. Some basic principles for safe use of nail cosmetics are outlined in Table 24.3.

Conclusions

Nail cosmetics is a multibillion dollar industry which continues to grow. Thorough knowledge of nail anatomy and physiology is essential for the safe use and development of nail cosmetics.

References

1. Reid IR. (2000) Calcium supplements and nail quality. *New England J Med* **14**, 343(24), 1817.
2. Stern DK, Diamantis S, Smith E, *et al.* (2007) Water content and other aspects of brittle versus normal fingernails. *Journal of the American Acad Dermatol* **57**(1), 31–6.
3. Diffey BL. (2012) The risk of squamous cell carcinoma in women from exposure to UVA lamps used in cosmetic nail treatment. *Br J Dermatol* **167**(5), 1175–8.
4. Markova A, Weinstock MA. (2013) Risk of skin cancer associated with the use of UV nail lamp. *J Invest Dermatol* **133**(4), 1097–9.
5. Murdan S, Hinsu D, Guimier M. (2008) A few aspects of transonychial water loss (TOWL): inter-individual, and intra individual inter-finger, inter-hand and inter-day variabilities, and the influence of nail plate hydration, filing and varnish. *Eur J Pharmaceut Biopharmaceut: official journal of Arbeitsgemeinschaft fur Pharmazeutische Verfahrenstechnik eV.* **70**(2), 684–9.
6. Sainio EL, Engstrom K, Henriks-Eckerman ML, Kanerva L. (1997) Allergenic ingredients in nail polishes. *Contact Derm* **37**(4), 155–62.
7. Hausen BM. (1995) A simple method of determining TS-F-R in nail polish. *Contact Derm* **32**(3), 188–90.
8. Rich P. (2001) Nail cosmetics and camouflaging techniques. *Dermatol Ther* **14**(3), 228–36.
9. Forslind B. (1970) Biophysical studies of the normal nail. *Acta Derm Venereol* **50**, 161–8.
10. Sasaki M, Kugbata M, Akamatsu H. (2008) Biochemical analysis of keratin in the brittle nail. *J Invest Dermatol* **128**, 591.
11. Hochman LG, Scher RK, Meyerson MS. (1993) Brittle nails: response to daily biotin supplementation. *Cutis* **51**(4), 303–305.

Further reading

Baran R, Dawber RPR, de Berker DAR, Haneke E, Tosti A. (2001) *Diseases of the Nails and their Management*, 3rd edn. Malden, MA: Blackwell Science.

Chang RM, Hare AQ, Rich P. (2007) Treating cosmetically induced nail problems. *Dermatol Ther* **20**, 54–9.

DeGroot, AC, Weyland JW. (1994) Nail cosmetics. In: *Unwanted Effects of Cosmetics and Drugs used in Dermatology*, 3rd edn. New York, Oxford: Elsevier, 524–9.

Draelos Z. (2000) Nail cosmetic issues. *Dermatol Clin* **18**, 675–83.

Iorizzo M, Piraccini B, Tosti, A. (2007) Nail cosmetics in nail disorders. *J Cosmet Dermatol* **6**, 53–6.

Paus R, Peker S, Sundberg JP. (2008) Biology of hair and nails. In: BologniaJL, JorizzoJL, RapiniRP, eds. *Dermatology*, 2nd edn. Elsevier, pp. 965–86.

Rich P. (2008) Nail surgery. In: Bolognia JL, Jorizzo JL, Rapini RP, eds. *Dermatology*, 2nd edn. Elsevier, pp. 2259–68.

Schoon DD. (2005) *Nail Structure and Product Chemistry*, 2nd edn. Thompson Corporation.

Scher RK, Daniel CR. (2005) *Nails: Diagnosis, Therapy, Surgery*, 3rd edn. Elsevier.

CHAPTER 25
Colored Nail Cosmetics and Hardeners

Paul H. Bryson
OPI Products Inc, Los Angeles, CA, USA

> **BASIC CONCEPTS**
> - Nail lacquers contain resins that create a thin, resistant film over the nail plate.
> - Adding color to the nail plate surface is accomplished with a variety of nail lacquers including a basecoat, color coat, and topcoat.
> - Nail hardeners cross-link nail protein to increase strength, but overuse may contribute to brittle nails.
> - Nail lacquers are resistant to contamination and cannot spread nail infectious disease.

Introduction

The use of colored nail polish and nail hardeners has increased among consumers with the rise of the manicure industry. With nail salons found in almost every strip mall, painting nails is a very popular service for the customers of the professional manicurist. The use of nail cosmetics is well rooted in history. Ancient Chinese aristocrats colored their nails red or black with polishes made with egg white, bees wax, and gelatin. The Ancient Egyptians used henna to dye the nails a reddish brown color (J. Spear, editor of *Beauty Launchpad*, Creative Age Publications, Van Nuys, CA, personal communication). In the 19th and early 20th centuries, "nail polish" was a colored oil or powder, which was used to rub and buff the nail, literally polishing and coloring the nail simultaneously. Modern nail polish was created in the 1920s, based on early nitrocellulose-based car paint technology [1].

The term "nail polish" is somewhat of a misnomer for modern products, because no actual polishing is involved in its application. The product is composed of dissolved resins and dries to a hard, glossy coat, so the technically correct name is "nail lacquer." However, the terms "nail polish," "nail enamel," "nail varnish," "nail paint," and "nail lacquer" are used interchangeably. Several specialty products have developed from nail lacquer, including basecoats, topcoats, and hardeners. A newer technology involves pigmented UV-curable resins. This chapter discusses the current use of these modern formulations (Table 25.1).

Application techniques

These nail products are applied by painting the nail with a brush. In best manicuring practices, old nail lacquer is removed with a solvent followed by application of a basecoat, two coats of colored nail lacquer, and a topcoat allowing sufficient time for drying between coats. The basecoat increases the adhesion of the colored nail lacquer to the nail while the topcoat increases the chip-resistant characteristics of the colored nail lacquer. These products are applied on both natural and artificial nails. Nail hardener is only applied to natural nails, either as a basecoat or a stand alone product. UV-curing nail "lacquers" are hardened with a UV light after application; no evaporation is necessary. In all cases, best practice dictates that the products be kept off the skin. Failure to do so can result in eventual, irreversible sensitization and allergic contact dermatitis [2].

Proper nail cosmetic application dictates the maintenance of excellent hygiene in the nail salon. Unsanitary procedures may result in medical problems [3]. Nail technicians must use cleaned, disinfected, or disposable nail files and tools. Clipping or cutting the cuticles before applying nail lacquer can also lead to infection. Infections with staphylococcus [4] and herpetic whitlows [5] have been attributed to unsanitary manicures. Nail technicians should not perform services on diseased nails.

Lacquers, topcoats, and basecoats

Nail lacquers contain six primary ingredients: resins, solvents, plasticizers, colorants, thixotropic agents, and color stabilizers. By law, all ingredients must be disclosed on the product packaging, usually by means of the International Nomenclature for Cosmetic Ingredients (INCI) names. Understanding the chemistry nomenclature is important for isolating the causes of allergic contact dermatitis. Each of these ingredients is discussed in detail.

Cosmetic Dermatology: Products and Procedures, Second Edition. Edited by Zoe Diana Draelos.
© 2016 John Wiley & Sons, Ltd. Published 2016 by John Wiley & Sons, Ltd.

Table 25.1 Overview of product types.

Product class	Nail lacquer	Basecoat	Topcoat	Nail hardener	UV curable
Coating created by	Solvent evaporation	Solvent evaporation	Solvent evaporation	Mainly solvent evaporation; some polymerization of formalin may occur	Polymerization
Resin type or mix	Balanced	Biased toward adhesion	Biased towards glossiness, hardness	Balanced or biased towards adhesion	Balanced; resin formed by reacting directly on nail
Pigment	Yes	Little or none	Little or none	Usually none	Yes
Removal	Easily dissolves in solvent	Easily dissolves in solvent	Easily dissolves in solvent	Easily dissolves in solvent	Soften by acetone soak, then peel
Benefits	Attractive color; can be applied over natural nails or enhancements	Helps color coat last longer; protects natural nail from staining	Helps color coat last longer; some contain optical brighteners or UV protectants	Strengthens natural nail by cross-linking proteins; may be used as a basecoat	Attractive color; tough cured-in-place resin protects nail

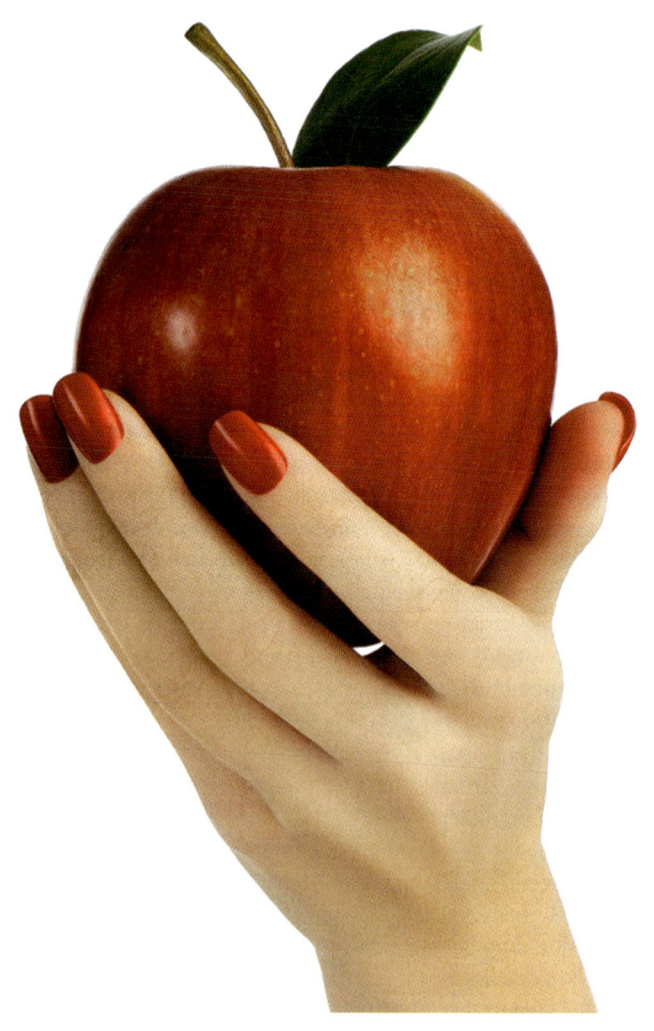

Figure 25.1 Lacquered nails. (Source: OPI Products, Inc., Los Angeles, CA. Reproduced with permission.)

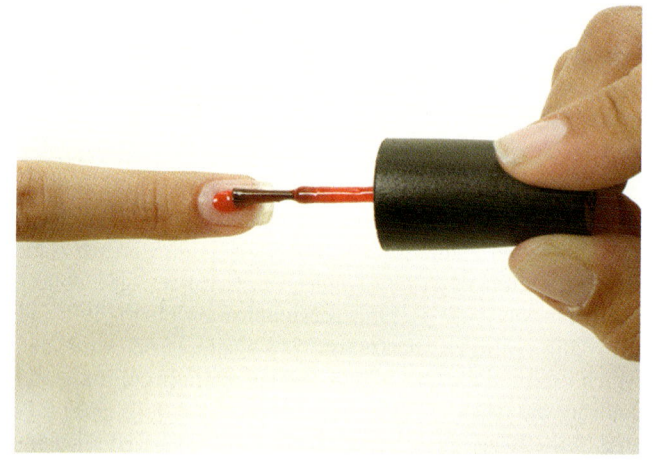

Figure 25.2 Painting a nail. (Source: OPI Products, Inc., Los Angeles, CA. Reproduced with permission.)

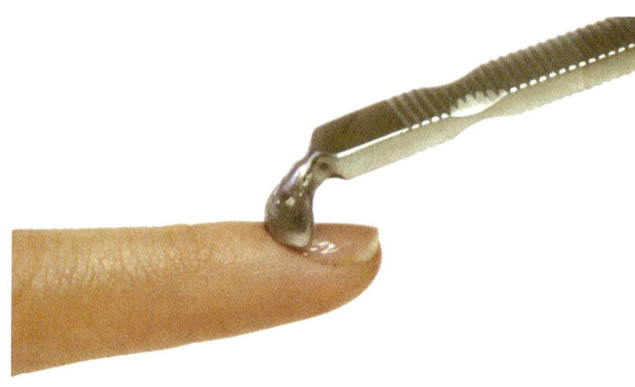

Figure 25.3 Be careful with the cuticle. (Source: OPI Products, Inc., Los Angeles, CA. Reproduced with permission.)

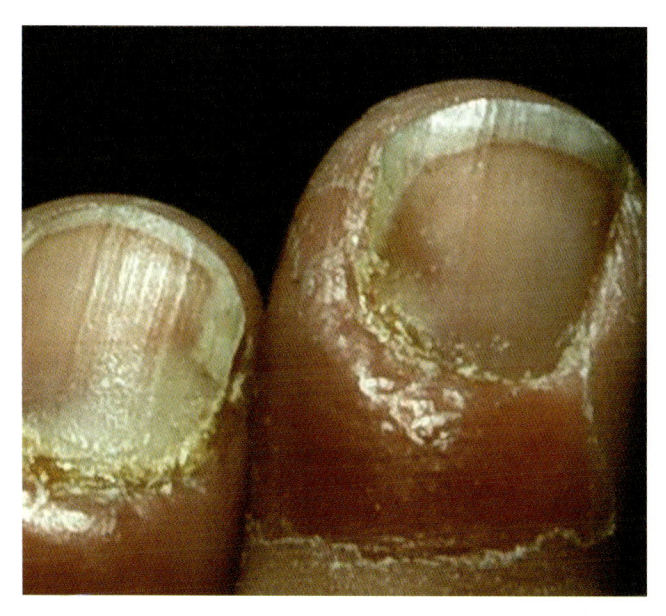

Figure 25.4 Infected nail. (Source: Nails Magazine. Reproduced with permission.).

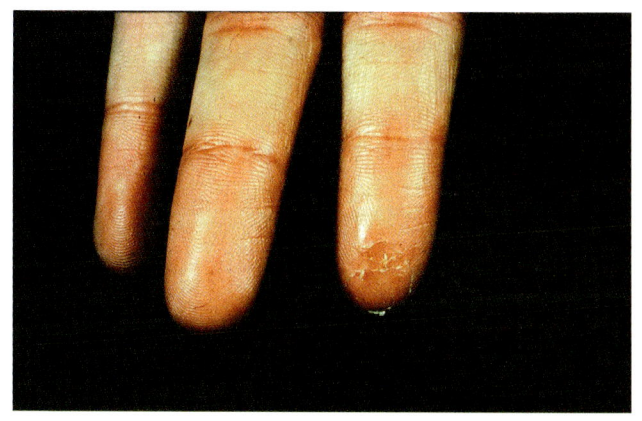

Figure 25.5 Dermatitis on the finger. (Source: Nails Magazine. Reproduced with permission.).

Resins

Resins hold the ingredients of the lacquer together while forming a strong film on the nail. Chemically, the resins are polymers – long-chain molecules – that are solid or gummy in their pure state. Two types of resins are used. Hard, glossy resins give the lacquered nail its desired appearance; these include nitrocellulose and the methacrylate polymers or co-polymers (usually labeled by their generic INCI name, "acrylates co-polymer"). Topcoat formulations have a higher percentage of these harder resins. Softer, more pliable resins, which enhance adhesion and flexibility, include tosylamide/epoxy resin, tosylamide/formaldehyde resin, and several polyester resins. Basecoats incorporate a higher proportion of pliable resins. Of all the resins, tosylamide/formaldehyde resin is the most commonly implicated in allergic reactions [6] affecting not only the fingers, but other parts of the body by transfer [7].

Solvents

Solvents are the carriers of the lacquer. They must dissolve the resin, suspend the pigments, and evaporate leaving a smooth film. The drying speed must be controlled to prevent bubbling and skinning; thus faster drying is not necessarily better. Optimum drying speed requires a careful blend of solvents. Ethyl acetate, n-butyl acetate, and isopropyl alcohol are common solvents; other acetates and alcohols are also occasionally employed. All solvents have a dehydrating and defatting action on the skin, but this usually occurs during the removal of the lacquer, not its application.

Formerly, toluene was a commonly used solvent, but the industry trend is to move away from it in response to expressed health concerns. Research indicates that toluene exposure for a nail technician and consumer is far below safe exposure limits [8]; however, consumer perceptions are negative for toluene, necessitating its replacement. A related chemical, xylene, has already virtually vanished from the industry. Ketones such as acetone or methyl ethyl ketone are not amenable to suspension of pigments and are therefore used at low levels, if at all, in lacquers, although these substances will dissolve the resins effectively and therefore are useful as lacquer removers.

A few water-based nail "lacquers" are now on the market. Because of their slow drying time and lesser durability, they are unlikely to replace solvent-based products in the foreseeable future. If they are ever perfected, they will completely take over the industry, because water is cheaper, non-flammable (which reduces shipping costs), and odorless.

Plasticizers

Plasticizers keep the resins flexible and less likely to chip. Camphor and dibutyl phthalate (DBP) have long been used for this purpose; however, the EU maintains its 2004 ban of DBP, despite authoritative findings regarding its safety in nail lacquer [9]. Because many manufacturers sell globally, DBP has largely been replaced by other plasticizers, including triphenyl phosphate, trimethyl pentanyl diisobutyrate, acetyl tributyl citrate, ethyl tosylamide, and sucrose benzoate.

Colorants

Colorants are selected from among various internationally accepted pigments. They are mostly used in the "lake" form, meaning that the organic colorants have been adsorbed or co-precipitated into inorganic, insoluble substrates such as the silicates, oxides, or sulfates of various metals. A shimmer effect is created by minerals such as mica, powdered aluminum, or polymer flakes. Guanine from fish scales is falling out of favor but is still occasionally used.

Following INCI convention, most colorant materials are labeled by their international "Color Index" (CI) numbers. This is a convenient way to identify colors, which have different national

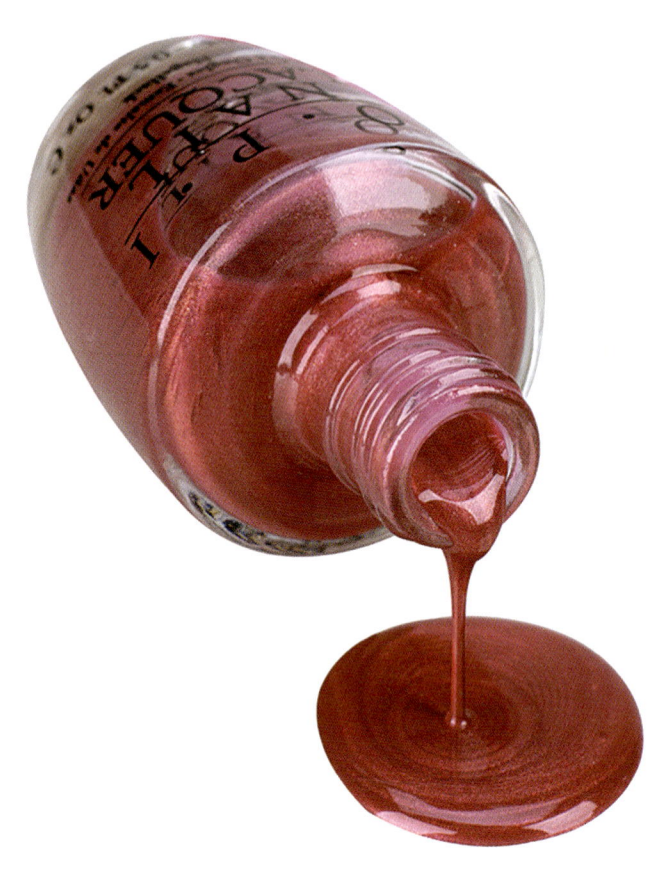

Figure 25.6 Nail lacquer. (Source: OPI Products, Inc., Los Angeles, CA. Reproduced with permission.)

Color stabilizers

Color stabilizers, such as benzophenone-1 and etocrylene, are added to prevent color shifting of the lacquer on exposure to UV light. These substances are better known as sunscreens, but their use in nail lacquer is to protect the color. Some specialty topcoats have a high level of UV protectants, for application over colored nail lacquer to prevent fading during tanning booth use.

Minor ingredients

Minor ingredients may include vitamins, minerals, vegetable oils, herbal extracts, or fibers such as nylon or silk. Some companies may include adhesion-enhancing agents in lacquers or basecoats, or other proprietary ingredients whose functions they elect not to disclose (Table 25.2).

Antifungal agents

Antifungal agents may be added to nail lacquer for therapeutic purposes. However, as of this writing, there is only one prescription US Food and Drug Administration (FDA) approved antifungal nail lacquer, a topical solution of 8% ciclopirox (Penlac®, Sanofi-Aventis, Bridgewater, NJ, USA). According to *FDA Consumer Magazine*, "There are no approved non-prescription products to treat fungal nail infections … fungal infections of the nails respond poorly to topical therapy … the agency ruled that any OTC product labeled, represented or promoted as a topical antifungal to treat fungal infections of the nail is a new drug and must be approved by FDA before marketing" [11]. Furthermore, the FDA's policy is to "prohibit claims that non-prescription topical antifungals effectively treat fungal infections of the scalp and fingernails" [12].

Preservatives

Preservatives are not present in nail lacquer. Regulatory authorities inquired if microbial cross-contamination could occur when the same nail lacquer bottle and brush are used on multiple clients. In response, a series of experiments was performed to investigate microbe survival in nail lacquer. The results indicate that nail lacquers do not support microbial growth in the laboratory or salon (OPI Products Inc., and Nail Manufacturers Council, unpublished data) [13]. The solvents are sufficiently hostile to microbes that no preservative is required. This does not apply to water-based products, because water is required for microbial growth. Although solvent-based water-free lacquer is hostile to microbes, it would be a mistake to assume that it has any curative value for nail fungus or other infections.

Nail hardeners

The oldest known method of fingernail hardening, is fire. On the early American frontier, the combat sport called "rough and tumble" or "gouging" allowed fingernails to be used as weapons, and expert "gougers" hardened their nails by heating them over candles [14]. The heat of the candle flame caused cross-linking of the nail proteins.

designations. Labeling colorants by their CI numbers is either legal or *de facto* accepted by most regulatory agencies around the world; even so, out of deference to local custom, colors are often declared binonially (e.g. CI 77891/Titanium Dioxide).

One difficulty with international designations is that some closely related colorant chemicals and their lakes are lumped under one CI number. An example is the ubiquitous CI 15850, which covers D&C Red #6, D&C Red #7, and all the various lakes of both. Normally, the manufacturer can provide more specific information if needed.

Colorants sometimes cause staining of the nail. Although uncommon, it is more often seen with colors at the red end of the spectrum. It can usually be prevented by using a basecoat between the lacquer and the natural nail [10]. Topcoats can also cause apparent yellowing, but this is usually the product rather than the natural nail – as can be easily seen by removing the product [10].

Thixotropic agents

Thixotropic agents provide flow control and keep the lacquer colorants dispersed. They are usually clay derivatives such as stearalkonium bentonite or stearalkonium hectorite. Most topcoats and basecoats are uncolored and do not require these additives. Silica is also sometimes used as a thickener.

Table 25.2 Common ingredients of nail lacquer and related products.

Ingredient category and examples	Function
Hard resins	
Nitrocellulose	Gloss
Acrylates co-polymer	Toughness
Soft resins	
Tosylamide/formaldehyde resin	Flexibility
Polyvinyl butyral	Adhesion
Solvents	
Ethyl acetate	Carrier for the resin and pigment
Butyl acetate	Removing lacquer
Isopropyl alcohol	Soaking and removing UV-cured colors
Acetone (removers only)	
Monomers and oligomers	
Polyurethane acrylate oligomer	Hardens to hold color on nail
Hydroxypropyl methacrylate	Only in UV-curable colors, not standard lacquer
Various other acrylates and methacrylates	
Photoinitiators	
Benzoyl isopropanol	Initiates the light cure reaction
Hydroxycyclohexyl phenyl ketone	Only in UV-curable colors, not standard lacquer
Colorants	
FDA/EU approved colorant	Esthetic
Mica	
Plasticizers	
Camphor	Keeps resin flexible to prevent chipping
Dibutyl phthalate (formerly)	
Thixotropic agents	
Stearalkonium hectorite	Controls flow
Stearalkonium bentonite	Suspends pigment until use
UV stabilizers	
Benzophenone-1	Prevents light-induced color fading
Etocrylene	
Hardeners	
Formalin	Hardens nail protein by cross-linking
Dimethyl urea	Only in hardener products
Hydrolyzed proteins	
Keratin	Thought to bond with formalin and nail protein
Wheat, oats, etc.	Usually used in hardeners

Modern nail hardeners contain a chemical cross-linking agent. Otherwise, their composition is similar to ordinary nail lacquer. As with lacquers, care must be taken to avoid skin contact during application to avoid allergic sensitization, particularly to the most common hardener, formalin (hydrated formaldehyde). Formalin cross-links proteins primarily by reacting with their nitrogen-containing side groups, forming methylene bridges [15]. Overuse causes too many cross-links, reducing the flexibility of the protein and causing brittleness, yellowing, and cracking of the nails. Manufacturers generally recommend avoiding overuse by cycling the products, alternating between the hardener and a non-hardening topcoat every week or two.

Other hardeners include dimethyl urea (DMU), which is does not cross-link as aggressively as formalin. It is also less allergenic [16]. Glyoxal, a relative of formaldehyde, is larger and less able

222 ADORNMENT Nail Cosmetics

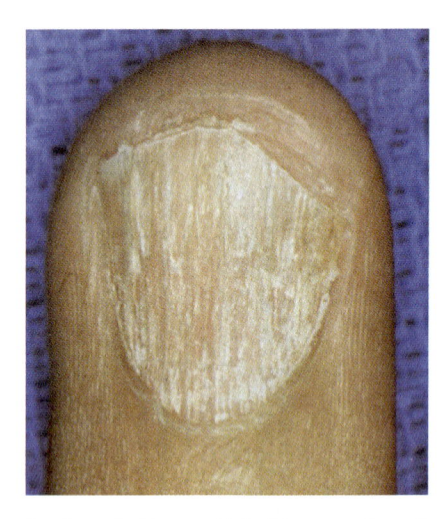

Figure 25.7 Brittle nail. (Source: Nails Magazine. Reproduced with permission.)

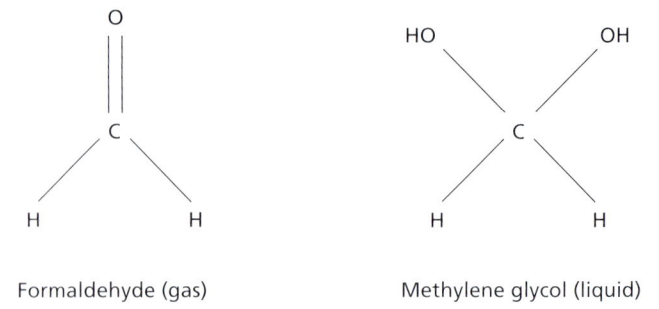

Figure 25.8 Formaldehyde versus methylene glycol. Reproduced by permission of OPI Products, Inc.

to penetrate the skin, also contributing to reduced allergenicity. Hydrolyzed proteins are common additives in hardeners and may chemically bond to the formalin. Many nail hardeners are simply clear lacquers with no cross-linking agents at all. These products rely on the strength of the resins to protect the nails. Until DMU or some other alternative proves itself, the most effective nail hardeners will likely continue to rely on formalin.

Formaldehyde issues

Formalin, formaldehyde, and tosylamide/formaldehyde resin warrant some additional discussion. True formaldehyde is a highly reactive gas. Obviously, it cannot be a part of nail products in that form. It is therefore combined with water to make a product traditionally called "formalin." Formalin contains water (~40%) and a reaction product of water and formaldehyde, properly known as methylene glycol (~60%). Published literature [17] on the hydration of formaldehyde reveals a chemical equilibrium constant for this reaction, which confirms the near complete conversion of formaldehyde to methylene glycol. This chemical equilibrium constant yields the presence of 0.0787% free formaldehyde in formalin. A nail hardener that is 1.5% formalin, therefore contains ~0.0007% or 7 parts per million of formaldehyde. This is not to dismiss "formaldehyde allergy", which causes significant suffering to some patients, but it would be more accurately known as methylene glycol or formalin allergy (Figure 25.8).

The near-complete conversion of formaldehyde to methylene glycol, which is far less volatile, undoubtedly explains why a California study showed that formaldehyde gas levels in nail salons were not above the normal background levels found in other settings such as offices [8]. This is significant because the only identified cancer risk associated with formaldehyde exposure results from inhalation in industrial settings [18], not cosmetic skin or nail exposure.

Tosylamide/formaldehyde resin is also a cause for controversy solely because of the word "formaldehyde" in its name. It is an inert macromolecule, created by reacting tosylamide and formaldehyde. However, the formaldehyde is consumed in the reaction, and any leftover formaldehyde is hydrated to methylene glycol by the water molecules generated in the reaction. Hence the formaldehyde content of the resin is essentially nil. However, allergies nevertheless occur; it has been speculated that trace formaldehyde is responsible but sensitization to tosylamide/formaldehyde resin can occur in the absence of formaldehyde sensitization [19,20], and tests indicate that side products of the synthesis reaction can be responsible for the resin allergies [21] (Figure 25.9).

A final concern occasionally raised regarding formaldehyde is its absence. Because formaldehyde-releasing agents have a long history as preservatives in other forms of cosmetics, it is sometimes mistakenly assumed that formaldehyde was added to nail lacquer for preservative purposes. As a result, publicity regarding "formaldehyde-free" products has inspired fears of microbial cross-contamination via nail lacquer brushes. As noted above, experiments have shown that solvent-based nail lacquer is hostile to microbes and needs neither formaldehyde nor any other preservative.

UV gel "lacquers" (aka UV gel polish)

UV-cured nail enhancements, UV curing lamps, and their safety aspects are discussed elsewhere (D.D. Schoon, Chapter 26); however, a relatively new class of UV-curing nail "lacquers" merits mention here. The same pigments are used as in standard nail lacquer but instead of a solvent/resin base (a true lacquer), curable methacrylate or acrylate oligomers and monomers are used, with little or no solvent. A photoinitiator causes polymerization of the monomers on exposure to UV light, leaving a polymer/pigment coat. Unlike the products to create nail enhancements, these curable colored products are not used to sculpt nails, but are designed to apply as a thin coat of color, resembling conventional lacquer. Hybrid systems also exist, which combine traditional lacquer technology with UV curable components.

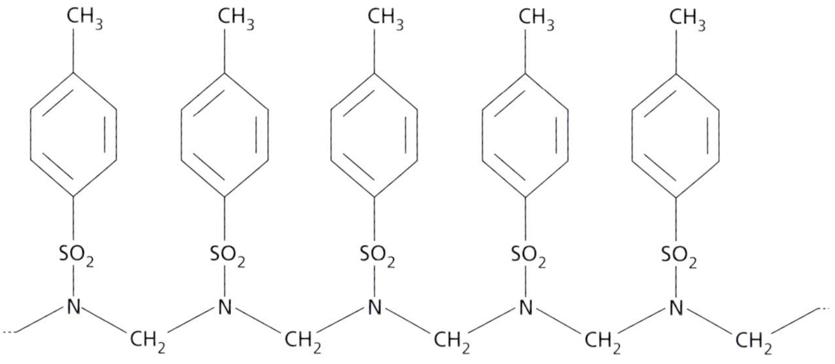

Figure 25.9 Tosylamide formaldehyde resin. Reproduced by permission of OPI Products, Inc.

Allergic sensitization may result from repeated skin exposure to uncured or incompletely cured monomers; the fully cured polymer is inert. Allergies to the photoinitiators and pigments are also possible. Good manicuring technique can mitigate these risks, but once an allergy is established it is irreversible. It is important to note, that due to oxygen inhibition of the curing reaction, a thin layer of uncured gel remains at the surface of the nail; properly trained nail technicians will remove this final layer to avoid sensitization.

The low-power UVA lights used to activate the photoinitiator are comparable to summer sunshine [10], so the use of UV cured nail products poses no hazard to healthy skin, despite misguided media reports to the contrary (Table 25.3). The curing lights use either conventional UV fluorescent bulbs with a typical peak wavelength (λ-max) of 365 nanometers (nm), or the much faster light-emitting diodes (LED) with λ-max of 395 nm or 405 nm. Since 405 nm is slightly outside the UVA range – the visible light range is understood to start at 400 nm – there is a widespread erroneous assumption that a 405 nm LED is "not UV" and therefore "safer". This is a misunderstanding; the λ-max is not the sole frequency emitted by a bulb or diode, only the most predominant frequency, and the output of a 405 nm LED definitely contains some UVA. Though this low UV exposure is quite safe, promoting the LED as a "non-UV" system is inaccurate.

Nail lacquer removers

In contrast to nail enhancements for nail elongation purposes, no polymerization takes place during the drying of nail lacquer; the resin is simply deposited on the nail as the solvent evaporates. Therefore, removing nail lacquer is easy: it can be redissolved and wiped off with a solvent-soaked cloth pad, tissue, or cotton ball (Figure 25.11). Any solvent that dissolves the resin, and is safe for skin exposure, can be successfully used. Although UV-curable nail colors are polymerized, they are far less cross-linked than enhancements, and can be removed with a short acetone soak.

Table 25.3 Common health effects of nail color ingredients

Ingredients	Health concerns
Resins	Possible allergies, particularly to tosylamide/formaldehyde resin
Solvents	Dehydration and defatting of skin and nails
	Irritant dermatitis
UV-curable acrylates/methacrylates	Allergy after repeated exposure to uncured monomer or oligomer
Photoinitiators	Possible allergies
	Possible photosensitization
Colorants	Occasional staining
	Occasional allergies
Plasticizers	Possible allergies
	Camphor exposure is contraindicated for some patients with fibromyalgia
Thixotropic agents	None known
UV stabilizers	Possible allergies
Hardeners (cross-linkers)	Formalin sensitization and allergies are common
	Overuse may cause brittleness or splitting of nail
	Not recommended for nails that are already brittle
Hydrolyzed proteins	Possible allergies
	May trigger gluten sensitivity via transfer to mouth

Acetone, chemically known as dimethyl ketone or 2-propanone, is the preferred solvent, because it is the least physiologically hazardous. Other removers are based on ethyl acetate or methyl ethyl ketone (MEK). Ethyl acetate has the advantage of not damaging acrylic nails, so it is used for removing lacquer from nail elongation enhancements. However, because of air quality regulations in California and Utah, ethyl acetate, MEK, and most other acetone alternatives are prohibited for nail lacquer

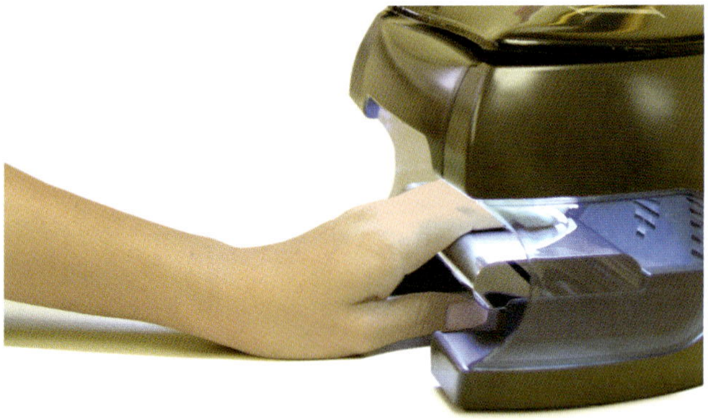

Figure 25.10 UV curing lamp. (Source: OPI Products, Inc., Los Angeles, CA. Reproduced with permission.)

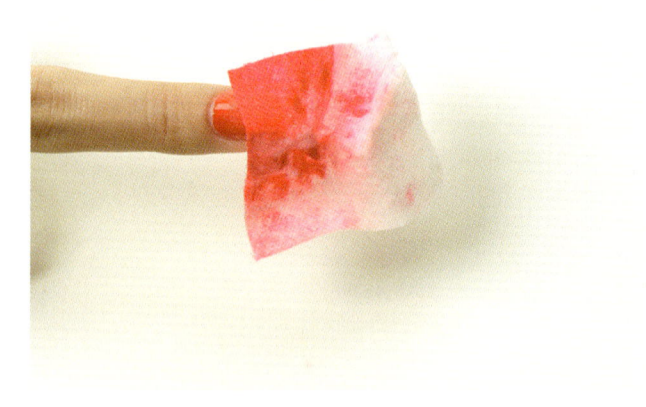

Figure 25.11 Polish remover in action. (Source: OPI Products, Inc., Los Angeles, CA. Reproduced with permission.)

removers, and other states and countries are considering similar actions. Acetone is exempt because its atmospheric breakdown produces less photochemical smog than almost any other solvent. One other "clean air" solvent, methyl acetate, is allowed in California, but has been avoided by most manufacturers because of toxicity concerns; those who use it add an embittering agent to deter accidental ingestion. Other hazardous solvents such as methanol and acetonitrile are seldom used, and are not California-compliant (Figure 25.11).

All solvents can have significant drying and defatting effects on the skin, leading to irritation. This can be mitigated by using a lacquer remover with added moisturizers, or by using lotion afterwards. Drying and cracking of the nail can also result; oiling the nail is the most common way to counteract this. Some removers contain fragrances or botanical additives, which may pose allergy risks.

Low-odor, non-volatile removers have been created based on methylated vegetable oils and/or various dibasic esters. As with water-based nail lacquer, however, the slow speed of nail polish removal with these products prevents them from finding general marketplace acceptance. These products are less damaging to the skin barrier.

Conclusions and future developments

Arguably the largest potential for future improvement lies in cleaner application techniques, not new products. As more cases of manicure-transmitted infection are publicized, customers and governments will demand that nail technicians practice proper sanitation and disinfection.

Most manufacturers are looking to develop "greener" products, whether in perception or reality. Toluene and DBP have been almost totally abandoned by the industry, and efforts continue to find a functional substitute for formalin. As for removers, most likely only acetone will survive the regulatory concerns. Water-based and the increasingly popular UV-cured products have the potential to reduce solvent emissions, but still have unresolved disadvantages compared to traditional lacquers. Research continues in the realm of nail polish, as adding nail color is a commonly practiced form of adornment.

References

1. Gorton A. (1993) History of nail care. *Nails*, February. Torrance, CA: Bobit Business Media.
2. Schultes SE. (ed.) (2007) *Miladay's Standard Nail Technology*, 5th edn. New York: Thomson Delmar Learning, pp. 129–32.
3. Baran R, Maibach HI. (2004) *Textbook of Cosmetic Dermatology*. New York: Taylor & Francis, p. 295.
4. Lee W. (2005) Bill targets nail salon outbreaks. *Los Angeles Times*, August 25, p. B-1.
5. Anon. (2002) Nightmare manicure: woman who says she got herpes from manicure is awarded $3.1 million *ABCNews.com*, May 29.
6. Linden C, Berg M, Färm G, Wrangsjö K. (1993) Nail varnish allergy with far reaching consequences. *Br J Dermatol* **128**, 57–62.
7. Frosh PJ, Menne T, Lepoittevin JP. (2006) *Contact Dermatitis*, 4th edn. Basel: Birkhäuser, p. 499.
8. McNary JE, Jackson EM. (2007) Inhalation exposure to formaldehyde and toluene in the same occupational and consumer setting. *Inhalat Toxicol* **19**, 573–6.
9. Dibutyl phthalate – Summary risk assessment (2003, with 2004 addendum), European Commission Joint Research Centre, Institute for Health and Consumer Protection, European Chemicals Bureau, Italy.
10. Schoon DD. (2005) *Nail Structure and Product Chemistry*, 2nd edn. New York: Thomson Delmar Learning.
11. Kurtzweil P. (1995) Fingernails: Looking good while playing safe. *FDA Consumer Magazine*, December.

12 US Food and Drug Administration (1993) *Answers*, September 3. Available from: www.fda.gov/bbs/topics/ANSWERS/ANS00529.html; retrieved 5 June 2015.

13 Nail Manufacturers Council (NMC) data, publication forthcoming.

14 Fischer DH. (1989) *Albion's Seed: Four British Folkways in America*. Oxford: Oxford University Press, p. 738.

15 Kiernan JA. (2000) Formaldehyde, formalin, paraformaldehyde and glutaraldehyde: What they are and what they do. *Microscopy Today* **00-1**, 8.

16 Schoon DD. (2005)*Formaldehyde vs. DMU; What's the Difference?* Vista, CA: Creative Nail Design. Available from: www.beautytech.com/articles/out.php?ID=354; retrieved August 25, 2008.

17 Winkelman JGM, Voorwinde OK, Ottens M, Beenackers AACM, Janssen LPBM. (2002) Kinetics and chemical equilibrium of the hydration of formaldehyde. *Chem Engineering Sci* **57**, 4067–76.

18 International Agency for Research on Cancer (IARC) – Summaries & Evaluations (Group 2A) (1995) Formaldehyde. 62, 217. Available at: www.inchem.org/documents/iarc/vol62/formal.html; retrieved 5 June 2015.

19 Fuchs T, Gutgesell C. (1996) Is contact allergy to toluene sulphonamide-formaldehyde resin common? *Br J Dermatol* **135**, 1013–14.

20 Final Report on Hazard Classification of Common Skin Sensitisers (January 2005), National Industrial Chemicals Notification and Assessment Scheme, Australian Government, Department of Health and Ageing, p. 106.

21 Hausen BM, Milbrodt M, Koenig WA. (1995) The allergens of nail polish. (I). Allergenic constituents of common nail polish and toluenesulfonamide-formaldehyde resin (TS-F-R), *Contact Dermatitis* **33**(3), 157–64.

CHAPTER 26
Cosmetic Prostheses as Artificial Nail Enhancements

Douglas Schoon

Schoon Scientific and Regulatory Consulting, Dana Point, CA, USA

> **BASIC CONCEPTS**
> - Artificial nail enhancements are commonly used to address malformed fingernails.
> - The major forms of artificial nail enhancements include nail wraps, liquid and powder, or UV gels.
> - Methacrylate monomer liquid systems remain the most widely used type of artificial nail enhancement.
> - Proper application of artificial nail enhancements can avoid infection and sensitization.

Introduction

The natural nail plate can not only be cosmetically elongated and enhanced to beautify the hands, but also to effectively address discolored, thin, and weak or malformed fingernails. When used properly, these cosmetic products and services provide great value and enhance self-esteem. Artificial nails not only add thickness and strength to the nail plate, they extend its length, typically 0.25–0.75 inches. A skilled nail technician can closely mimic the length and shape of the final product to create natural-looking artificial nails. Certain techniques utilizing custom blending of colored products allow the appearance of the nail bed to be extended beyond its natural boundary, which can dramatically lengthen the appearance of the fingers (Figure 26.1). Different types of artificial nail coatings are applied to provide a range benefits, as well as numerous decorative colors and designs, collectively known as "nail art."

A typical nail salon client wears artificial nail products to correct problems they are having with their own natural nails such as discoloration, splitting, breaking, unattractive or deformed nails (i.e. median canal dystrophy or splinter hemorrhages). There are several basic types from which to choose: nail wraps, liquid and powder, UV gels or UV gel polish/manicures. An overview of each type is given in Table 26.1.

Liquid and powder

Liquid and powder systems (aka acrylic nails) were the original artificial nail enhancements designed to extend the length of the natural nail plate. These systems were similar to certain dental products made from methacrylate monomers and polymers. Methacrylates are structurally different from acrylates, have different safety profiles, and should not be confused with one another. The literature frequently confuses methacrylates with acrylates and/or incorrectly suggests they are a single category (i.e. [meth] acrylate). The first structure shown in Figure 26.2 has a branching methyl group (–CH3) attached to the double bond of ethyl methacrylate. The branching changes both the size (10% larger) and shape of the methacrylate molecule, which reduces the potential for skin penetration. This helps explain why methacrylate monomers are less likely to cause adverse skin reactions than homologous acrylate monomers (i.e. ethyl acrylate and ethyl methacrylate). It is also one important reason why artificial nails containing acrylates are more likely to cause adverse skin reactions than those based solely on methacrylate monomers [1]. The polymer powders are polymerized to very high molecular weights and therefore unlikely to cause adverse skin reactions.

Methacrylate monomer liquid systems are among the most widely used type of artificial nail enhancement in the world. The "liquid" is actually a complex mixture of ethyl methacrylate (60–95%) and other di- or tri-functional methacrylate monomers (3–5%) that provide cross-linking and improved durability, inhibitors such as hydroquinone (HQ) or methyl ether hydroquinone (MEHQ) (100–200 p.p.m.), UV stabilizers, catalysts such as dimethyl tolyamine (0.75–1.25%), flexibilizing plasticizers and other additives. The "powder" component is made from poly methyl and/or ethyl methacrylate polymer beads (approximately 50 80 μm), coated with 1–2% benzoyl peroxide as the polymerization initiator, colorants, opacifiers such as titanium dioxide, and other additives.

Liquid and powder systems are applied by dipping a brush into the monomer liquid, wiping off the excess on the inside lip of a low volume container (3–5 mL) called a dappen dish. The

---

Cosmetic Dermatology: Products and Procedures, Second Edition. Edited by Zoe Diana Draelos.
© 2016 John Wiley & Sons, Ltd. Published 2016 by John Wiley & Sons, Ltd.

Table 26.1 The three main types of artificial nail enhancements.

Type	Chemistry	Also known as	Hardener
Nail wraps	Cyanoacrylate monomers	Fiberglass wraps, resin wraps, no-light gels, silk or paper wraps	Spray, drops, powder, or fabric treated with an tertiary aromatic amine
Liquid and powder	Methacrylate monomers and polymers	Acrylic, porcelain nails, solar nails	Polymer powder treated with benzoyl peroxide; monomer liquid contains tertiary aromatic amine
UV gels	Urethane acrylate or urethane methacrylate oligomers/monomer, expoxidized methacrylate or acrylates.	Gel nails UV gels Soak-off gels	Low-power UVA lamp to activate the photoinitiator and tertiary aromatic amine catalyst
UV gel polish/manicure	Urethane acrylate or urethane methacrylate oligomers/monomer, expoxidized methacrylate or acrylates. solvents,e.g. acetone, ethyl acetate.	Permanent polish UV polish	Low-power UVA lamp to activate the photoinitiator and tertiary aromatic amine catalyst

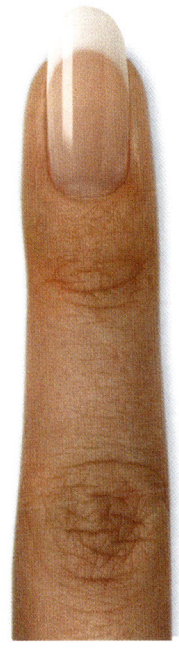

Figure 26.1 The use of custom-blended colored powders with methacrylate monomers to "illusion sculpt" and extend the apparent length of a short nail bed while also correcting a habitually splitting nail plate. (Source: Creative Nail Design, Inc., Vista, CA, USA. Reproduced with permission.)

Ethyl methacrylate
$C_6H_{10}O_2$
Molecular weight 114 Daltons

Ethyl acrylate
$C_5H_8O_2$
Molecular weight 100 Daltons

Figure 26.2 Chemical structure differences between methacrylates and acrylates.

excess monomer is removed by wiping the brush on the edge of the dappen dish. The tip of the brush is drawn through the polymer powder, also in a dappen dish, and a small bead or slurry forms at the end of the brush. Three to six beads are normally applied and smoothed into shape with the brush. Pink powders are applied over the nail bed and white powders are used to simulate the free edge of the nail plate. The slurry immediately begins to polymerize and hardens on the nail within 2–3 minutes. Over 95% of the polymerization occurs in the first 5–10 minutes, but complete polymerization can take 24–48 hours [2]. After hardening, the nail is then shaped either by hand filing or with an electric file to achieve the desired length and shape. The finished nail can be buffed to a high shine or nail color applied.

Length is added to the nail plate in one of two ways:

1. Adhering an ABS plastic nail tip to the nail plate with a cyanoacrylate adhesive, coating the tip with the liquid and powder slurry, and filing as described above. This technique is called "tip and overlay."
2. A non-stick (Mylar© or Teflon© coated paper) form is adhered underneath the free edge of the natural nail and used as a support and guide to which the liquid and powder slurry is applied, then shaped and filed. This technique is called "nail sculpting."

Proper preparation of the natural nail's surface is the key to ensuring good adhesion. Before the service begins, natural nails should be thoroughly scrubbed with a clean, disinfected, soft-bristled brush to remove contaminants from the service

228 ADORNMENT Nail Cosmetics

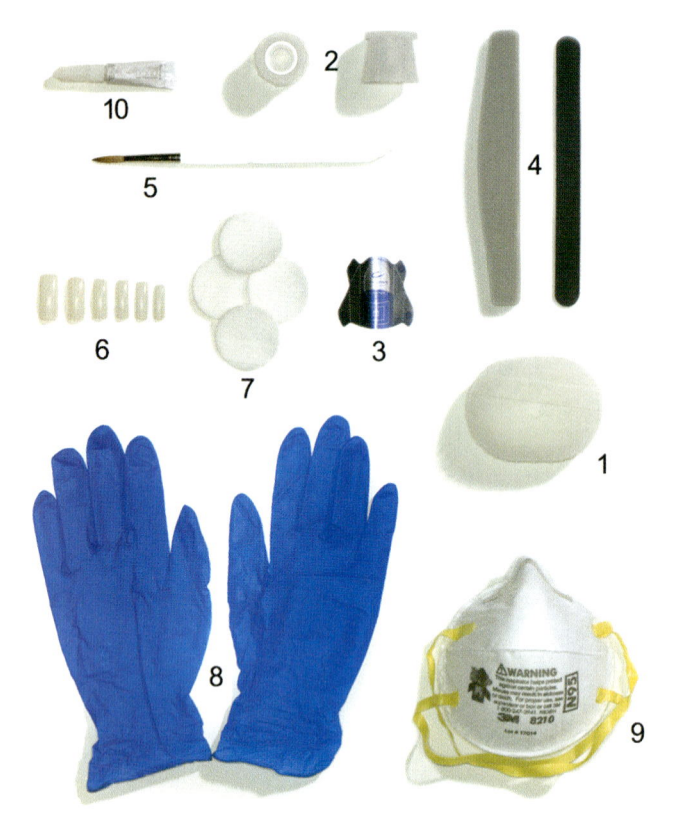

Figure 26.3 Equipment used to create liquid and powder artificial nails. 1, Nail scrub brush; 2, Dappen dishes containing liquid and powder; 3, Mylar nail form; 4, Abrasive files; 5, Nail enhancement application brush; 6, ABS preformed nail tips; 7, Plastic-backed cotton pad; 8, Nitrile gloves; 9, N-95 dust mask. (Source: Paul Rollins Photography, Inc. Geyserville, CA, USA.)

thereby covering the area of new growth. This process is called "rebalancing" and is essential to maintaining the durability and appearance of the artificial nail. Rebalancing is done primarily with services designed to be long lasing, e.g. liquid and powder nails and UV gels. Other types of nail coatings and some UV gels typically are removed completely and replaced.

UV gels

Products that cure under low intensity UVA lights, typically with major spectral outputs from 410–350 nm. These are used to create artificial nails called "UV gels or UV polish". UVB and UVC are not used to create UV gel nails [4]. Traditionally, UVA fluorescent style lamps were used in these units. Newer types of UV nail lamps utilize instead LED (light emitting diodes) technology to produce the UVA needed to polymerize UV curable nail coatings of any type. LED produce narrow band width emissions centered at either 405 or 395 nm, which allow faster and more efficient curing. Due to significant differences in curing times, artificial nail coatings are formulated to properly cure with a specific type of UV nail lamp, either LED or fluorescent-style (Figures 26.4 and 26.5).

of the nail plate as well as underneath the free edge (Figure 26.3). This removes surface oil and debris that can block adhesion. The nail is then lightly filed with a low grit abrasive file (180–240 grit) to increase surface area for better adhesion. Nail surface dehydrators containing drying agents such as isopropyl alcohol are applied to remove surface moisture and residual oils. Adhesion promoting "primers" may then applied to increase surface compatibility between the natural nail and artificial nail product. These adhesion promoters contain proprietary mixtures of hydroxylated monomers or oligomers, carboxylic acids, etc. In the past, methacrylic acid was frequently used but has fallen out of favor because of its potential as a skin and eye corrosive [3].

Rebalancing

As the natural nail grows, the artificial nail advances leaving a small space of uncoated nail plate. Every 2–3 weeks the nail technician will file the artificial nail down to one-third its thickness, reapply fresh product, and reshape the artificial nail,

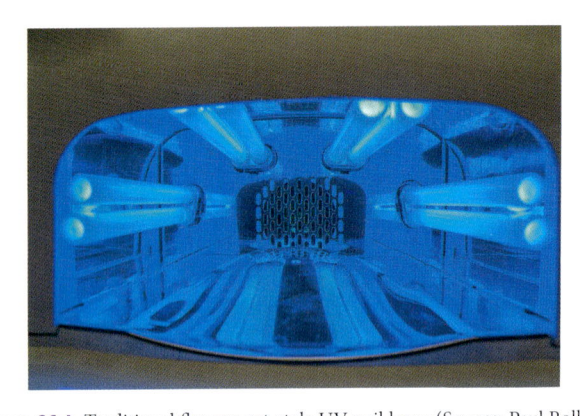

Figure 26.4 Traditional fluorescent-style UV nail lamp (Source: Paul Rollins Photography, Inc. Geyserville, CA, USA.)

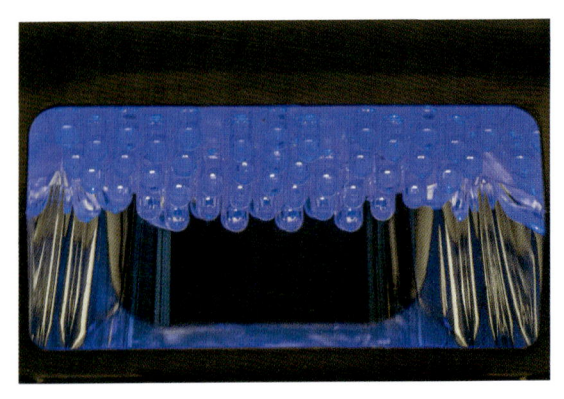

Figure 26.5 Newer LED-style UV nail lamp (Source: Paul Rollins Photography, Inc. Geyserville, CA, USA.)

Unlike liquid and powder systems, UV gels are not mixed with another substance to initiate the curing process. Historically, UV gels have been blends of polymerization photoinitiators (1–5%), urethane or epoxy acrylate oligomers, and durability improving, cross-linking monomers (approximately 75–95%), and catalysts such as dimethyl tolyamine (0.75–1.25%). Newer formulations using urethane methacrylate oligomers and monomers lower the potential for adverse skin reactions.

Rate of cure is a hindrance for UV-curable artificial nails. Slow cure rates allow atmospheric oxygen to prevent curing of the uppermost layers of UV gel products. This layer can also be observed with certain types of liquid monomers, e.g. lower odor or "odorless" products that utilize hydroxyethyl or hydroxypropyl methacrylate as the main reactive monomer. This residual sticky surface layer is called the "oxygen inhibition layer" [5]. Skin contact with this layer should be avoided since it contains unreacted monomers, of in the case of UV curing products, unreacted monomer or oligomers.

UV gels can be clear, tinted, or heavily colored. The natural nail is cleaned, filed, dehydrated, and coated with adhesion promoters. The UV gel is then applied to the nail, shaped, and finished in the same fashion as two-part liquid and powder systems and produces very similar looking results. In most cases, the same equipment used to create other types of artificial nails is used (Table 26.2). Most often UV gel curing achieved by placing the artificial nail under a UVA lamp for 2–3 minutes per applied layer or 10–30 seconds per layer for LED cured UV nail coatings. Because UVA does not efficiently penetrate more than a few millimeters into the UV gel, these products are applied and cured in several successive layers. UV gels are also applied over ABS nail tips or non-stick nail forms to lengthen the appearance of the natural nail.

Nail wraps

Methyl and ethyl cyanoacrylate monomer is used not only for adhering ABS nail tips to the natural nail, but also to create artificial nail coatings called "nail wraps." This technique is not widely used, but accounts for at least 1% of the worldwide market [6].

The natural nail is precleaned, shaped, and filed as described above, but the cyano functional group provides tremendous adhesion to the natural nail plate, eliminating the need for adhesion-promoting primers (Figure 26.6). Nail enhancements

Table 26.2 Specialized equipment used to create artificial nail enhancements.

Item	Description
Brush	Natural or synthetic hair brush for application, spreading, and shaping of monomer and oligomers products on the nail plate
Dappen dish	Small containers that hold liquid artificial nail monomer, oligomers, or polymer powders during the application process
Manual files	Wooden or plastic core boards coated with abrasive particles (e.g. silicon nitride, aluminium oxide or diamond) used to shape, shortening, smooth, thin, or buff both natural and artificial nails
Electric files	Handheld, variable speed, rotary motors that securely hold barrel-shaped abrasive bits and are used for the same purposes as manual files
Nippers	Small clippers sometimes used to remove old artificial nail product from the nail plate
Wood stick	A thin, pencil-shaped, plastic implement used to remove cuticle tissue from the nail plate
Buffers	Block shape, high grit abrasive buffers use for shape refining (180–240 grit) or buffing to a high shine (>1000 grit)
UV lamp	Electrical device that holds either 4 or 9 W UVA producing bulbs and is used to cure UV gel nail products
Cotton pads	Disposable pads or balls used to remove old nail polish and/or dusts after filing
Scrub brush	Soft bristle, disinfectable brushes used to clean natural and artificial nails
Nail forms	Mylar© or Teflon© coated paper used as a support and guide to extending artificial nails beyond the natural nail's free edge
Nail tips	Preformed ABS plastic tips adhered to the natural nail to support artificial nail products and create nail extensions beyond the nail's free edge
Wrap fabric	Loosely woven silk, linen, or fibreglass strips adhered to the natural nail plate with cyanoacrylate monomer to create nail wraps
Droppers	Used to transfer product from larger containers into dappen dishes or to apply nail wrap curing accelerators
Scissors	Slightly curved blades use for trimming or cutting natural nails and wrap fabrics
Disinfectant container	Containers designed to hold EPA registered disinfectants needed to properly disinfectant tools and implements
Remover bowl	Container that holds solvents (e.g. acetone) for artificial nail removal

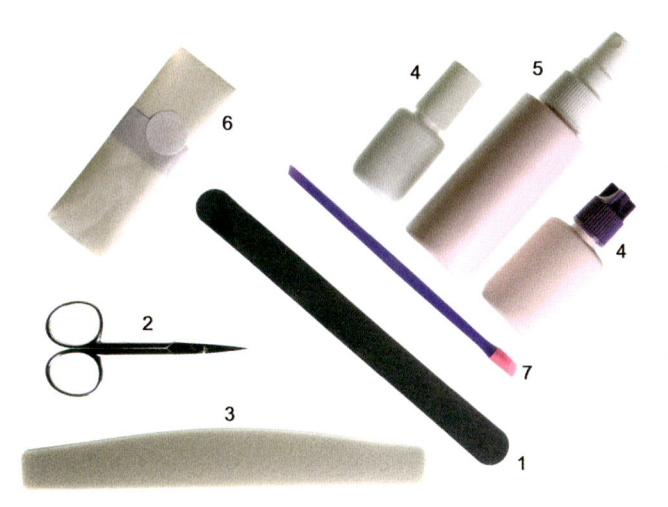

Figure 26.6 Materials needed to apply nail wraps. 1, Abrasive file for nail preparation and final shaping; 2, Scissors for cutting fabric; 3, Block buffer for high-shining; 4, Cyanoacrylates; 5, Spray-on catalyst; 6, Silk fabric; 7, Pusher to gently remove skin from the nail plate. (Source: Paul Rollins Photography, Inc. Geyserville, CA, USA.)

relying on cyanoacrylate monomers do not contain other cross-linking monomers and therefore are inherently weaker than cross-linking artificial nail enhancement systems. To improve durability and usefulness, a woven fabric (silk, linen, or fiberglass) is impregnated with cyanoacrylate monomer and adhered to the nail plate. Even so, these types of coatings are not strong enough to be sculpted on a non-stick nail form and cannot be extended beyond the free edge of the natural nail plate, unless the nail wrap is applied over an ABS nail tip, as previously described. Usually, cyanoacrylate monomers are very low viscosity, mobile liquids, but they are sometimes thickened with polymers (e.g. polymethyl methacrylate) and used without a reinforcing fabric. Such systems are referred to as "no-light gels."

Cyanoacrylate monomers are applied without the use of a brush, directly from the container's nozzle and will cure upon exposure to moisture in the nail plate, but the process can be greatly hastened by solvent mixtures containing a tertiary aromatic amine such as dimethyl tolylamine (0.5–1%), which is either sprayed on, applied with an dropper, or impregnated into the woven fabric. After curing (5–10 seconds), the nail wrap coating can be shaped and buffed to a high shine or nail color applied. This technique is also used to mend cracks or tears in the nail plate, by using the cyanoacrylate monomer to adhere a small piece of fabric over the broken or damaged area of the plate.

Artificial nail removal

Improper removal of artificial nails can lead to nail damage; however, they can be safely removed if the proper procedures are followed. Acetone (dimethyl ketone) is the preferred remover for artificial nail products, but ethyl acetate and methyl ethyl ketone (MEK) is also used. The artificial nails are placed in a small bowl and immersed in solvent. Nail wraps based on cyanoacrylates are the easiest to remove because they are not cross-linked polymers and have lower solvent resistance; usually requiring less than 10 minutes immersion for full removal. Liquid and powder products are cross-linked polymers structures that can take 30–40 minutes to swell and break apart for gentle, non-damaging removal from the nail plate. UV gels are also cross-linked polymer structures and these urethane acrylate or methacrylate based artificial nails have inherently greater solvent resistance so removal can take 45–60 minutes. The removal process is greatly accelerated by pre-filing to remove the bulk of the artificial nail coating. Care must be taken. Improper removal can cause significant damage to the nail plate. Prying or picking off the artificial nails can lead to onycholysis [7]. A common myth is that artificial nail should be regularly removed to allow nails to "breathe"; in reality they should only be removed when there is a need.

Gel manicure/polish

A new type of nail coatings called UV gel manicures (aka Gel Polish or Gel Lacquer) became popular in 2010 and their popularity continues. These nail coatings provide value to deformed or misshapen nails by coating them with a long-lasting colored coating capable of camouflaging visible nail defects, e.g. splint haemorrhages, nail bed bruising, etc. Gel polish is a unique type of artificial nail coating designed for removal and subsequent replacement on a two or three week schedule. These types of colored nail coatings are designed to duplicate the look of nail polish, but are polymerized by UV so the resultant films are far superior in scratch resistance and durability, which also makes them more difficult to remove.

Improper removal may cause small, roundish white spots, typically 2–5 mm, often with an irregular borders. These appear on the surface of the nail plate immediately following incorrect removal of the coating. These have been observed after incorrect removal of other types of nail coatings, as well, even traditional nail polishes. These areas of surface damage somewhat resemble white superficial onychomycosis (WS0), but are not caused by an infectious organisms; instead as result of damage to the nail surface. Over aggressive removal techniques used in the salon are a leading cause of this type of damage, but some wearer pick, peel or bite the coating from their own nail plate. Excessive filing of the nail plate before or after application of any nail coating is the cause of any nail plate thinning that may result.

When nail plates with these white spots are magnified (186–3830×) via scanning electron microscopy as in Figure 26.7, the observed modes of failure reveal that the damage is caused by prying and/or scraping residual coating from the plate. The damage shown in Image 1 is caused by upward prying, while Images 2 and 3 are from scrapping. Image 4 shows pieces of residual coatings remaining adhered to the plate after the removal process; usually a result of not enough contact time with the solvent remover to sufficiently soften nail coating before removal. This type of surface

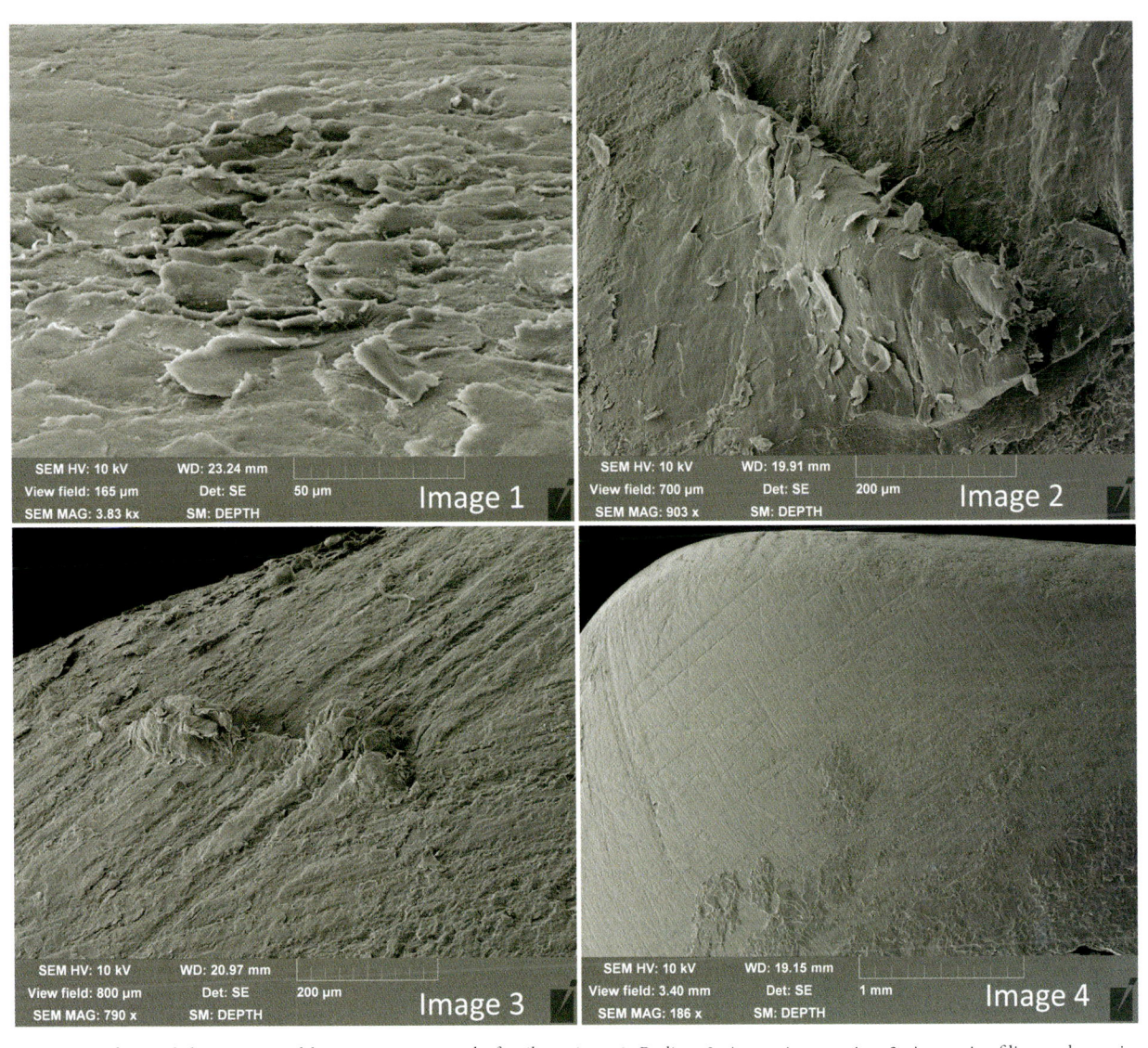

Figure 26.7 Surface nail damage caused by improper removal of nail coatings; 1. Peeling, 2. Aggressive scraping, 3. Aggressive filing and scraping, 4. Residual nail coating left on the nail plate when removal time is improperly shortened. (Source: Doug Schoon, Schoon Scientific, Dana Point, CA, USA.)

nail damage is completely avoidable if the appropriate amount to time is allowed for properly soften nail coatings before removal. Surface damage may occur more easily after nail plates are soaked for more than a minute in solvents such as acetone or water, since these may soften the nail's surface making it temporarily more susceptible to damage from any implements used to pry, push or force off residual nail coats. Those wearing nail coatings applied in a salon should be warned not to self-remove their nail coatings or avoid overly aggressive and damage removal methods.

Adverse reactions

Both nail technicians and those wearing artificial nails can develop adverse skin reactions if steps are not taken to avoid prolonged and/or repeated skin contact with artificial nail products. For example, the product should be applied to the nail plate in such a manner that skin contact is avoided (i.e. a tiny free margin left between the eponychium and artificial nail). Typically, reactions are a result of many months of overexposure to eponychium, hyponychium, or lateral side walls (Figure 26.8).

Reactions can appear as paronychia, itching of the nail bed and, in extreme cases, paresthesia and/or loss of the nail plate [8,9]. Onycholysis can be a result of allergic reactions, but the nail plate is resistant to penetration from external agents and this condition is more likely to be caused by overly heavy handed, aggressive filing techniques with coarse abrasives or overzealous manicuring of the hyponychium area [10]. Allergic contact dermatitis can affect the chin, cheeks, and eyelids as a result of touching the face with the hands [11]. Filings and dusts may contain small amounts of unreacted monomers and oligomers, because it can take more than 24 hours for the artificial nails to finish the curing process.

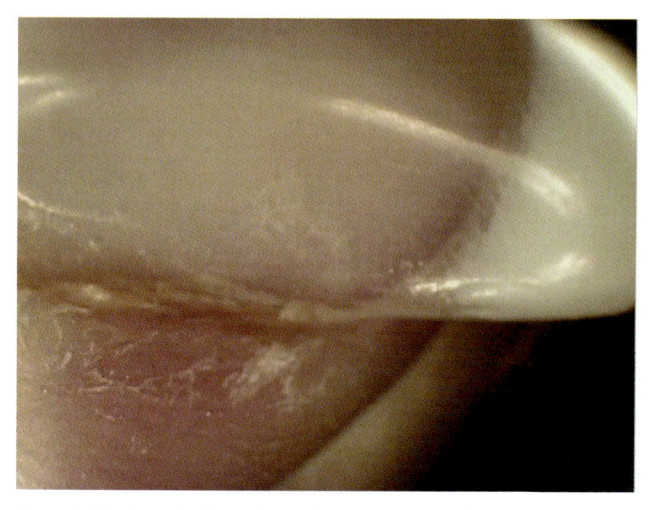

Figure 26.8 Example of an adverse skin reaction caused by repeated contact to the skin. (Source: Paul Rollins Photography, Inc. Geyserville, CA, USA.)

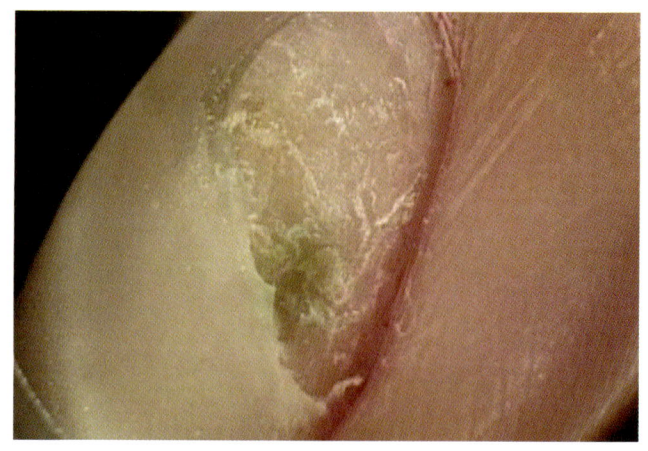

Figure 26.9 Example of a nail infection growing underneath an artificial nail. (Source: Paul Rollins Photography, Inc., Geyserville, CA, USA.)

Nail technicians should be instructed to wash their hands thoroughly before touching the face or eye area. They should be warned to avoid contact with the dusts and filings, especially the oxygen inhibition layer created on the surface of UV gels and odorless monomer liquid systems (see above), which can contain substantial amounts of unreacted ingredients. Gloves (nitrile) and/or plastic-backed cotton pads should be used to remove the oxygen inhibition layer as skin contact should be avoided. The UV bulbs in the curing lamps should be changed every 2–4 months (depending on usage) to ensure thorough cure and lessen the amount of unreacted ingredients, thereby lowering the potential for adverse skin reactions. For liquid and powder systems, it is common for technicians to use excessive amounts of liquid monomer, creating a wet consistency bead. Nail technicians should avoid applying beads of product with a wet mix ratio because this can lower the degree of curing and increase the risk of overexposure to unreacted ingredients. Nail technicians should be instructed to avoid all skin contact with uncured artificial nail products or dusts and not to touch them to client's skin prior to curing.

Nail damage and infection

Avoiding the use of heavy grit abrasives (<180 grit) or electric files directly on the nail plate will lessen the potential for damage and injury (e.g. onycholysis). Plate damage can occur when nail technicians aggressively file the natural nail, rather than use safer, smoother abrasive files (>180 grit). These gentler methods also increase the surface area for better adhesion, but without overly thinning or damaging the nail plate.

Methyl methacrylate (MMA) monomer is sometimes used illegally in artificial nail monomer liquids because of its low cost when compared to better alternatives (e.g. ethyl methacrylate [EMA]). MMA has very poor adhesion to the natural nail plate so technicians who use these liquid monomers frequently abrade away the uppermost layers of the natural nail plate to achieve significantly more adhesion by allowing for deposition into the more porous layers underneath. However, this poor technique can compromise the nail plate's strength and durability, so liquid monomer MMA containing products should be avoided [12]. The other artificial nail systems described in this chapter have improved adhesion and do not require technicians to heavily abrade the nail plate in order to achieve proper adhesion.

Infections can occur underneath the artificial nail to produce green or yellow stains (Figure 26.9). Several types of bacteria and dermatophytes can cause such infections (*Pseudomonas aeruginosa, Staphylococcus aureus, Trichophyton rubrum*). To avoid this, state regulations require nail technicians to properly clean and disinfect all implements in an Environmental Protection Agency (EPA) registered disinfectant to avoid transmission of pathogenic organisms, and to dispose of all single-use items. Clients should wash their hands, scrubbing under the nails with a clean and disinfected, soft-bristled brush before receiving any services.

Education

Almost every US state requires specialized nail training and education, typically 300–750 hours depending on the state, to obtain a professional license and some states have continuing education requirements. The textbooks teach a surprisingly wide range of topics including anatomy and physiology of the skin and nails, product chemistry, an overview of common nail related diseases and disorders, contamination and infection control and universal precautions, safe working practices, as well as manicuring, pedicuring, and the artificial nail techniques described in this chapter [13–15].

Multilingual information sources for proper use and other safety information can be found from a wide range of sources, including the EPA [16] and Nail Manufacturers Council [17].

UV nail lamp safety

An observation by MacFarlane and Alfonso [18] inaccurately reported UV nail lamps to be a source of "high-dose UV-A" light and incorrectly compared UV tanning beds with UV nail lamps claiming these may cause NMSC (non-melanoma skin cancer). The authors mistakenly assumed that UV bulb "wattage" is a measure of UV exposure to the skin, when wattage is actually a measure of energy usage, and were in error to rely solely on UV bulb wattage to estimate the actual amount of UV exposure to skin. They also made incorrect comparisons to UV tanning beds, when the skin is not tanned or burned by salon UV nail lamps when they are properly used to provide salon services. To address the concerns raised, three scientific studies have determined that UV nail lamps are safe as used in nail salons. Lighting Sciences [19] concluded that UV-B output is less than that which occurs in natural sunlight, approximately equal to spending an additional 17 to 26 seconds in sunlight each day and UVA exposure was found equivalent to an extra 1.5 to 2.7 minutes, depending on the type of nail lamp used. Massachusetts General Hospital and the Alpert Medical School at Brown University [20] confirm the safety of UV nail lamps stating that dermatologists and primary care physicians may reassure patients regarding the safety of these devices. Concerning the potential for developing skin cancer, UV nail lamps do not appear to significantly increase lifetime risks, and they point out that UV medical lamps used in therapeutic skin treatment are considered safe. When compared to these medical devices the authors stated, "...one would need over 250 years of weekly UV nail sessions to experience the same risk exposure." Markova and Weinstock [23] and Dowdy and Sayre [21] tested six major brands of UV nail lamps to the appropriate International testing standards [22] and determined they did not release excessive amounts of UV. Risk was determined to be low for developing NMSC (non-melanoma skin cancer) and found to be 11–46 times lower in risk than natural noonday sunlight.

The study authors also considered that dorsum of the hand is four times more UV resistant than the hands or cheeks, making it the most UV resistant part of the body, providing a further margin of safety [23] and that the natural nail plate has a natural UV resistance equal to that of a high SPF sunscreen [24]. They concluded that the UV nail lamps tested are safe as used in nail salons and are unlikely to increase risks of NMSC.

References

1. Baran R, Maibach HI. (2005) Cosmetics for abnormal and pathologic nails. *Textbook of Cosmetic Dermatology*, 3rd edn. Taylor & Francis, London/New York, pp. 304–5.
2. Schoon D. (1994) Differential scanning calorimeter determinations of residual monomer in ethyl methacrylate fingernail formulations and two addendums. Unpublished data submitted by the Nail Manufacturers Council to the Cosmetic Ingredient Review (CIR) Expert Panel.
3. Woolf A, Shaw J. (1998) Childhood injuries from artificial nails primer cosmetic products. *Arch Pediatr Adolesc Med* **152**, 41–6.
4. Newman M. (2001) Essential chemistry of artificial nails. *The Complete Nail Technician*. London: Thompson Learning, p. 41.
5. Schoon D. (2005) Liquid and powder product chemistry. *Nail Structure and Product Chemistry*, 2nd edn. New York: Thomson Delmar Learning, p. 138.
6. Kanerva S, Fellman J, Storrs F. (1966) Occupational allergic contact dermatitis caused by photo bonded sculptured nail and the review on (meth) acrylates in nail cosmetics. *Am J Contact Derm* **7**, 1–9.
7. Schoon D. (2005) Trauma and damage. *Nail Structure and Product Chemistry*, 2nd edn. New York: Thomson Delmar Learning, p. 52.
8. Fisher A, Baran R. (1991) Adverse reactions to acrylate sculptured nails with particular reference to prolonged paresthesia. *Am J Contact Derm* **2**, 38–42.
9. Fisher A. (1980) Permanent loss of fingernails from sensitization and reaction to acrylics in a preparation designed to make artificial nails. *J Dermatol Surg Oncol* **6**, 70–6.
10. Baran R, Dawber R, deBerker D, Haneke E, Tosti A. (2001) Cosmetics: the care and adornment of the nail. *Disease of the Nails and their Management*, 3rd edn. Oxford: Blackwell Science, p. 367.
11. Fitzgerald D, Enolish J. (1994) Widespread contact dermatitis from sculptured nails. *Contact Derm* **30**, 118.
12. Nail Manufactures Council (NMC). (2001) *Update for Nail Technicians: Methyl Methacrylate Monomer*. Scottsdale, AZ: Professional Beauty Association, www.probeauty.org/NMC
13. Jefford J, Swain A. (2002) *The Encyclopedia of Nails*. London: Thompson Learning.
14. Frangie C, Schoon D, et al. (2007) *Milady's Standard Nail Technology*, 5th edn. New York: Thomson Delmar Learning.
15. Schoon D. (2005) Trauma and damage. *Nail Structure and Product Chemistry*, 2nd edn. New York: Thomson Delmar Learning.
16. United States Environmental Protection Agency (2007) Protecting the Health of Nail Salon Workers, Office of Pollution Prevention and Toxics. EPA no. 774-F-07-001.
17. Nail Manufacturers Council (NMC). A series of safety related brochures for nail technicians. Scottsdale, AZ: Professional Beauty Association. www.probeauty.org/NMC.
18. MacFarlane D, Alfonso C. (2009) Occurrence of nonmelanoma skin cancers on the hands after UV nail light exposure. *Arch Dermatol* **145**(4), 447–9.
19. Lighting Sciences Inc., 7826 East Evans Road, Scottsdale, Arizona 85260 U.S.A. www.lightingsciences.com, (personal communication)
20. Markova A, Weinstock M. (2012) Risk of skin cancer associated with the use of UV nail lamp. *J Invest Dermatol* **133**, 929–35.
21. Dowdy JC, Sayre RM. (2013) Photobiological safety evaluation of UV nail lamps. *Photochem Photobiol* **89**, 961–7.
22. ANSI/IESNA RP-27.3-96, *Recommended Practices for Photobiological Safety for Lamps – Risk Group Classification & Labeling*.
23. Olson RL, Everett MA. (1966) Effect of anatomic location and time on ultraviolet erythema. *Arch Dermatol* **93**, 211–5.
24. Stern D, Creasey A, et al. (2011) UV-A and UV-B penetration of normal human cadaveric fingernail plate. *Arch Dermatol* **147** (No 4).

SECTION 3 Hair Cosmetics

CHAPTER 27
Hair Physiology and Grooming

Maria Hordinsky,[1] Ana Paula Avancini Caramori,[2] and Jeff C. Donovan[3]

[1] Department of Dermatology, University of Minnesota, Minneapolis, MN, USA
[2] Department of Dermatology, Complexo Hospitalar Santa Casa de Porto Alegre, Porto Alegre, Brazil
[3] Division of Dermatology, University of Toronto, Toronto, Canada

> **BASIC CONCEPTS**
> - The hair follicle is a complex structure that produces an equally complex structure, the hair fiber.
> - Human hair keratins consist of at least 19 acidic and basic proteins which are expressed in various compartments of the hair follicle.
> - The science behind modern shampoos and conditioners has led to the development of rationally designed products for normal, dry, or damaged hair.

Definitions

The use of hair cosmetics is ubiquitous among men and women of all ages. Virgin hair is the healthiest and strongest but basic grooming and cosmetic manipulation cause hair to lose its cuticular scale, elasticity, and strength. Brushing, combing, and shampooing inflict damage on the hair shaft, much of which can be reversed with the use of hair conditioners. In this chapter, the physiology of hair, grooming techniques including the science and use of shampoos and conditioners, are reviewed.

Physiology

Hair follicle
The hair follicle is a complex structure that demonstrates the ability to completely regenerate itself – hair grows, falls out and then regrows. Plucked hairs can regrow. Important cells for the development of hair follicles include stem cells in the bulge region and dermal papilla cells [1]. Hair follicle stem cells are described as being present just below the entrance of the sebaceous duct into the hair follicle. The hair follicle's complexity is further appreciated when examining the organization of follicles in the scalp and the complexity of its vascular complex and nerve innervation. Scalp hair follicles present in groups of one, two, three, or four follicular units (Figure 27.1).

The hair follicle is defined histologically as consisting of several layers (Figure 27.2). It is the interaction of these layers that produces the hair fiber. The internal root sheath consists of a cuticle which interdigitates with the cuticle of the hair fiber, followed by Huxley's layer, then Henle's layer. Henle's layer is the first to become keratinized, followed by the cuticle of the inner root sheath. The Huxley layer contains trichohyalin granules and serves as a substrate for citrulline-rich proteins in the hair follicle. The outer root sheath has specific keratin pairs, K5–K16, characteristic of basal keratinocytes and the K6–K16 pair characteristic of hyperproliferative keratinocytes, similar to what is seen in the epidermis. Keratin K19 has been located in the bulge region [2,3].

The complexity of the hair follicle is further demonstrated by the fact the follicle cycles from the actively growing phase (anagen), through a transition phase (catagen), and finally a loss phase (telogen). The signals associated with the transition from anagen, catagen to telogen are the subject of current research activities in this field.

Product of the hair follicle: the hair fiber
The hair follicle generates a complex fiber which may be straight, curly, or somewhere in between. The main constituents of hair fibers are sulfur-rich proteins, lipids, water, melanin, and trace elements. The cross-section of a hair shaft has three major components, from the outside to the inside: the cuticle, the cortex and the medulla [4].

Fibers can be characterized by color, shaft shape – straight, arched, or curly – as well as microscopic features. The cuticle can be defined by its shape – smooth, serrated, or damaged, and

---

Cosmetic Dermatology: Products and Procedures, Second Edition. Edited by Zoe Diana Draelos.
© 2016 John Wiley & Sons, Ltd. Published 2016 by John Wiley & Sons, Ltd.

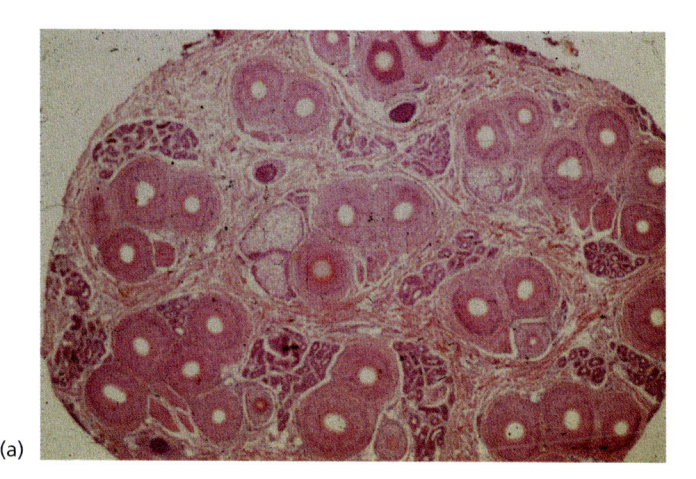

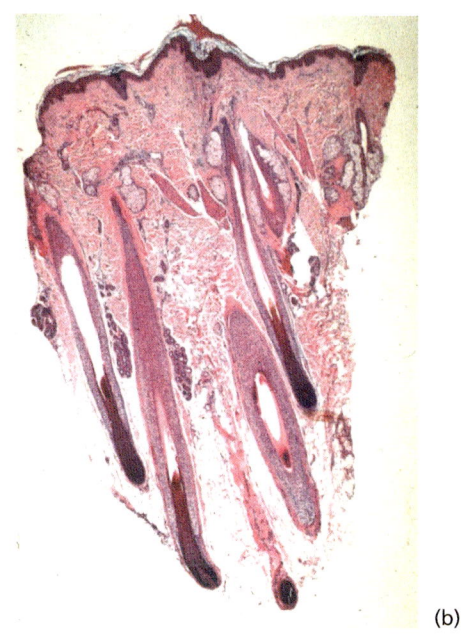

Figure 27.1 (a) Horizontal section of a 4 mm scalp biopsy specimen demonstrating follicular units containing 1, 2, 3, or 5 anagen follicles. (b) Vertical section of a 4-mm scalp punch biopsy specimen from a normal, healthy Caucasian female in her early twenties.

whether or not it is pigmented. The cortex can be described by its color and the medulla by its distribution in fibers. It can be absent, uniform, or randomly distributed. Lastly, fibers can be abnormal and present with structural hair abnormalities such as trichoschisis or trichorrhexis nodosa. Both of these structural abnormalities can commonly be seen in patients with hair fiber injury related to routine and daily cosmetic techniques including application of high heat, frequent perming as well as from weathering, the progressive degeneration from the root to the tip of the hair initially affecting the cuticle, then later the cortex [3].

The cuticle is also composed of keratin and consists of 6–8 layers of flattened overlapping cells resembling scales. The cuticle consists of two parts: endocuticle and exocuticle. The exocuticle lies closer to the external surface and comprises three parts: b-layer, a-layer, and epicuticle. The epicuticle is a hydrophobic lipid layer of 18-methyleicosanoic acid on the surface of the fiber, or the f-layer. The cuticle protects the underlying cortex and acts as a barrier and is considered to be responsible for the luster and the texture of hair. When damaged by frictional forces or chemicals and subsequent removal of the f-layer, the first hydrophobic defense, the hair fiber becomes much more fragile.

The cortex is the major component of the hair shaft. It lies below the cuticle and contributes to the mechanical properties of the hair fiber, including strength and elasticity. The cortex consists of elongated shaped cortical cells rich in keratin filaments as well as an amorphous matrix of sulfur proteins. Cysteine residues in adjacent keratin filaments form covalent disulfide bonds, which confer shape, stability, and resilience to the hair shaft. Other weaker bonds such as the van der Waals interactions, hydrogen bonds and coulombic interactions, known as salt links, have a minor role. These bonds can be easily broken just by wetting the hair. It is the presence of melanin in the cortex that gives hair color; otherwise, the fiber would not be pigmented [4].

The medulla appears as continuous, discontinuous, or absent under microscopic examination of human hair fibers. It is viewed as a framework of keratin supporting thin shells of amorphous material bonding air spaces of variable size [4]. Fibers with large medullas can be seen in samples obtained from porcupines or other animal species. Other than in gray hairs, human hairs show great variation in their medullas.

Human hair keratins

Human hair keratins are complex and, until recently, research suggested that the hair keratin family consisted of 15 members, nine type I acidic and six type II basic keratins, which exhibited a particularly complex expression pattern in the hair-forming compartment of the follicle (Figure 27.2). However, recent genome analyses in two laboratories has led to the complete elucidation of human type I and II keratin gene domains as well as a completion of their complementary DNA sequences revealing an additional small hair keratin subcluster consisting of genes *KRT40* and *KRT39*. The discovery of these novel genes brought the hair keratin family to a total of 17 members [3].

The human type II hair keratin subfamily consists of six individual members which are divided into two groups. Group A members hHb1, hHb3, and hHb6 are structurally related, while group C members hHb2, hHb4, and hHb5 are considered to be rather distinct. Both *in situ* hybridization and immunohistochemistry on anagen hair follicles have demonstrated that hHb5 and hHb2 are present in the early stages of hair differentiation in the

236 ADORNMENT Hair Cosmetics

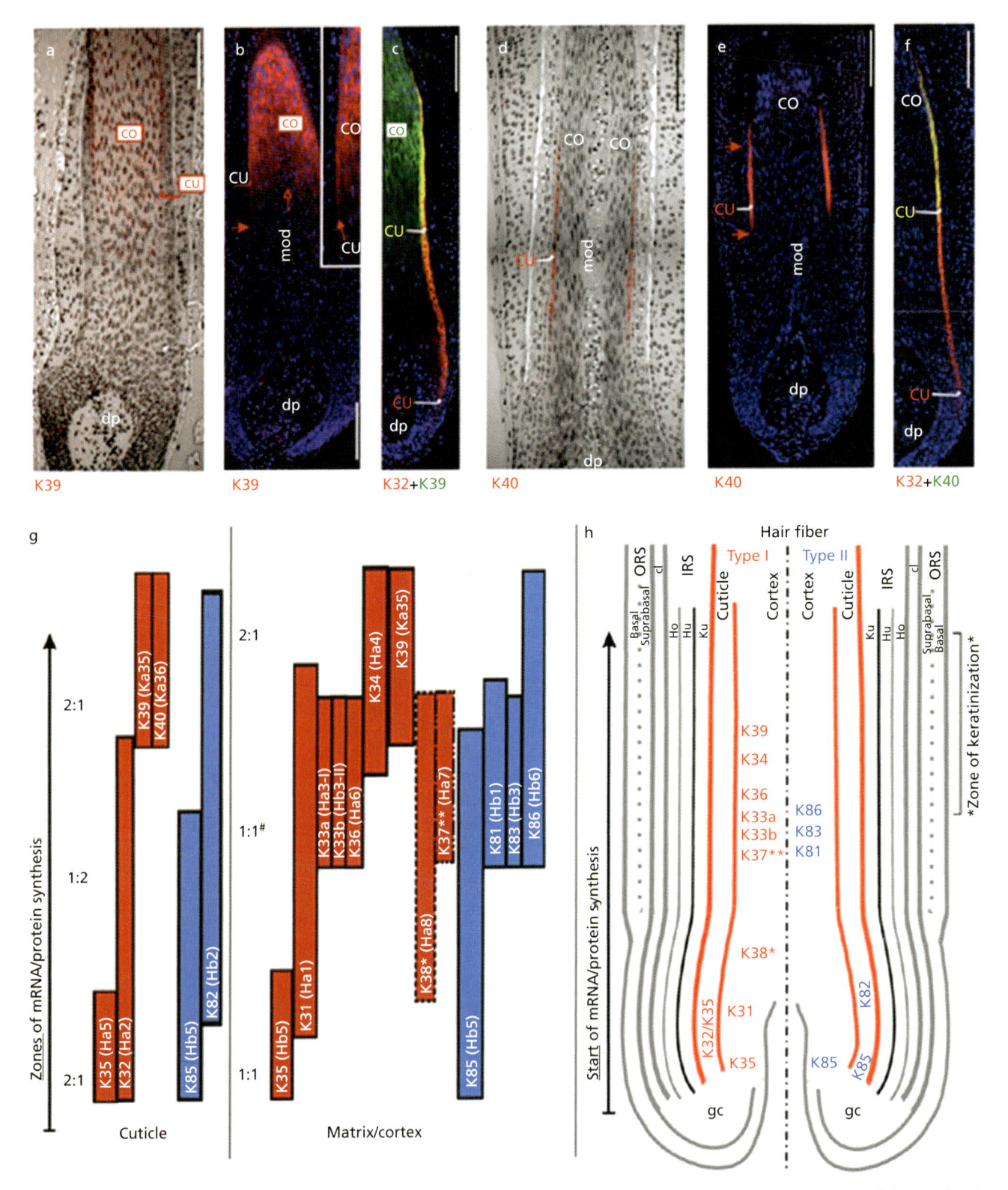

Figure 27.2 Schematic presentation of the complex pattern of hair keratin expression in the human hair follicle. (Source: Langbein, 2007 [2]. Reproduced with permission of Nature Publishing.)

matrix (hHb5) and cuticle (hHb5, hHb2), respectively. Cortical cells simultaneously express hHb1, hHb3, and hHb6 at an advanced stage of differentiation. In contrast, hHb4, has been undetectable in hair follicle extracts and sections, but has been identified as the most significant member of this subfamily in cytoskeletal extracts of dorsal tongue [3].

Grooming

Shampoos: formulations and diversity

Cleaning hair is viewed as a complex task because of the area that needs to be treated. The shampoo product has to also do two things – maintain scalp hygiene and beautify hair. A well-designed conditioning shampoo can provide shine to fibers and improve manageability, whereas a shampoo with high detergent properties can remove the outer cuticle and leave hair frizzy and dull.

Formulations

Shampoos contain molecules with both lipophilic and hydrophilic sites. The lipophilic sites bind to sebum and oil-soluble dirt and the hydrophilic sites bind to water, permitting removal of the sebum with water rinses. There are four basic categories of shampoo detergents: anionics, cationics, amphoterics, and non-ionics (Table 27.1). A typical shampoo will typically have two detergents. Anionic detergents have a negatively charged hydrophilic polar group and are quite good at removing sebum; however, they tend to leave hair rough, dull, and subject to static electricity. In contrast, ampotheric detergents contain both an anionic and a cationic group allowing them to work as cationic detergents at low pH and as anionic detergents at high pH. Ampotheric detergents are commonly found in baby shampoos and in shampoos designed for hair that is fine or chemically treated [5].

The number of shampoo formulations on the market can be overwhelming but when the chemistry behind those marketed for "normal hair" or "dry hair" is understood, recommending the best product becomes easier (Table 27.2). Shampoos for "normal" hair typically have lauryl sulfate as the main detergent and provide good cleaning of the scalp. These are best utilized by those who do not have chemically treated hair. Shampoos designed for "dry hair" primarily provide mild cleansing but also excellent conditioning. An addition to shampoo categories has been the introduction of conditioning shampoos which both clean and condition. The detergents in these types of shampoos tend to be amphoterics and anionics of the sulfosuccinate type. These work well for those with chemically damaged hair and those who prefer to shampoo frequently. For individuals with significant sebum production, oily hair shampoos containing lauryl sulfate or sulfosuccinate detergents can work well, but can be drying to the hair fiber.

Hydrolyzed animal protein or dimethicone are added to conditioning shampoos, also commonly called 2-in-1 shampoos. These chemicals create a thin film on the hair shaft to increase manageability and even shine. For individuals with tightly kinked hair, conditioning shampoos with both cleaning and conditioning characteristics that are a variant of the 2-in-1 shampoo can be beneficial. These shampoos can be formulated with wheat-germ oil, steartrimonium hydrolyzed animal protein, lanolin derivatives, or dimethicone and are designed for use either weekly or every 2 weeks.

Conditioners

Conditioners can be liquids, creams, pastes, or gels that function like sebum, making hair manageable and glossy appearing. Conditioners reduce static electricity between fibers following combing or brushing by depositing charged ions on the hair shaft and neutralizing the electrical charge. Another benefit from conditioners is improved hair shine which is related to hair shaft light reflection. Conditioners may also improve the quality of hair fibers by reapproximating the medulla and cortex in frayed fibers [5,6].

There are several hair conditioner product types including instant, deep, leave-in, and rinse. The instant conditioner aids with wet combing; the deep conditioner is applied for 20–30 minutes and works well for chemically damaged hair. A leave-in conditioner is typically applied to towel dried hair and facilitates combing. A rinse conditioner is one used following shampooing and also aids in disentangling hair fibers.

There are at least four conditioner categories, summarized in Table 27.3. The quaternary conditioners are cationic detergents. The film-forming conditioners function by coating fibers with a thin polymer layer. Protein-containing conditioners contain small proteins with a molecular weight of 1000–10 000 Da.

Table 27.1 Four categories of shampoo detergents.

1. Anionics.
    Lauryl sulfate
    Laureth sulfates
    Sarcosines
    Sulfosuccinates

2. Cationics.

3. Amphoterics.
    Betaines such as cocamidopropyl betaine
    Sultaines
    Imidazolinium derivatives

4. Non-ionics.

Table 27.2 Categories of shampoos are available for the following hair types.

Normal hair
Dry hair
Oily hair
Tightly kinked hair

Table 27.3 Categories of hair conditioners.

Category	Primary ingredient
Cationic detergent	Quaternary ammonium compounds
Film-former	Polymers
Protein-containing	Hydrolyzed proteins
Silicones	Dimethicone
	Cyclomethicone
	Amodimethicone

These penetrate the hair shaft and are thought to increase fiber strength temporarily. Silicone conditioners form a thin film on the hair shaft and, by doing so, reduce static electricity and friction. Dimethicone is the most common form of silicone used.

Conclusions

The hair follicle is recognized as being a complex structure consisting of at least 17 different keratins as well as lipids, water, melanin, and trace elements. The follicle produces an equally complicated structure, the hair fiber which may be straight, wavy, or curly. Hair is cited as a factor contributing to attractiveness and is frequently styled to convey cultural affiliations [4].

References

1 Cotsarelis G, Millar SE. (2001) Towards a molecular understanding of hair loss and its treatment. *Trends Mol Biol* 293–301.
2 Langbein L, Rogers MA, Praetzel-Wunder S, Böckler D, Schirmacher P, Schweizer J. (2007) Novel type I hair keratins K39 and K40 are the last to be expressed in differentiation of the hair: completion of the human hair keratin catalog. *J Invest Dermatol* **127**, 1532–5.
3 Langbein L, Rogers MA, Winter H, Praetzel S, Schweizer J. (2001) The catalog of human hair keratins. II. Expression of the six type II members in the hair follicle and the combined cataloging of human type I and type II keratins. *J Biol Chem* **34**, 35123–32.
4 Gray J. (2008) Human hair. In: McMichael A, Hordinsky M, eds. *Hair and Scalp Diseases*. New York: Informa Healthcare, pp. 1–17.
5 Draelos ZD. (2008) Nonmedicated grooming products and beauty treatments. In: McMichael A, Hordinsky M, eds. *Hair and Scalp Diseases*. New York: Informa Healthcare, pp. 59–72.
6 McMullen R, Jachowicz J. (2003) Optical properties of hair: effect of treatments on luster as quantified by image analysis. *J Cosmet Sci* **54**, 335–51.

CHAPTER 28
Hair Dyes

Rene C. Rust[1] and Harald Schlatter[2]

[1] GSK/Stiefel, Brentford, Middlesex, UK
[2] Procter & Gamble German Innovation Centre, Schwalbach am Taunus, Germany

> **BASIC CONCEPTS**
> - Hair dyes are a cosmetic product category that can be traced back thousands of years. Modern hair dyes have been developed since the late 19th century and are now available in a broad range of products delivering a variety of color results and usage conditions.
> - Hair dyes constitute a large product category – over 70% of women in the developed world color their hair at least once, and many do so regularly. Psychologic aspects of color transformation are a key decision driver for using hair color products; especially dyeing gray hair can contribute significantly to the confidence and self-perceived attractiveness of many people.
> - Within the category, permanent or oxidative hair dyes represent the largest market share with around 80% of all products. A combination of hydrogen peroxide and an alkalizing agent (typically ammonia) form the basis to lighten the natural hair color while at the same time depositing oxidatively coupled dyes inside the hair shaft.
> - Additional considerations for people using permanent hair dyes regularly include a high maintenance routine, and the need for special care and attention to the hair because of the associated changes to the hair structure.
> - Because of the complex chemistry of hair dyes, safety and regulatory criteria are important aspects of modern hair dyes. Special emphasis needs to be put on proper safety and use instructions, together with recent technology advances these enable to further minimize a potential allergy risk.

Introduction

Modern hair dyes offer a broad range of products and a variety of color results. They constitute a large category – over 70% of women in the developed world color their hair at least once, and many do so regularly. The number one reason for dyeing hair is to cover gray hair and look younger, but more women now use hair dyes as a means to change their appearance. Within the category, permanent or oxidative hair dyes represent the largest market share with around 80% of all products. A combination of hydrogen peroxide and an alkalizing agent (typically ammonia) form the basis to lighten the natural hair color while at the same time forming wash-resistant dyes inside the hair shaft. Due to the complex chemistry of hair dyes, safety and regulatory criteria are important aspects of modern hair colorants. Special emphasis needs to be made on proper safety and instructions for use – together with recent technology advances these enable potential allergy risk to be further minimized.

Definitions

Natural hair color manifests itself in a vast multitude of shades and tones – from the lightest blonde and warmest brunette to the most vibrant red and deepest black. Yet, for thousands of years humans have attempted to enhance or change their natural hair color, initially with the help of natural preparations such as kohl and henna [1], nowadays with modern products which offer a broad range of color results and gray coverage.

Hair dyes can be defined as products that alter the color appearance of hair temporarily or permanently, by removing some of the existing color and/or adding new color. They constitute a significant category in the cosmetics market – it is estimated that over 70% of women in the developed world have used hair color, and a large proportion of those do so regularly [2]. Consumers have the choice between home hair dye kits, and having their hair dyed professionally at a salon. While each woman may have a very individual reason for coloring her hair, covering gray can be considered a universal key motivator. Other desired performance aspects include enhancing the existing color, choosing a color different from the natural hair, or achieving a more striking appearance.

Product subtypes

- Temporary hair dyes.
- Semi-permanent hair dyes.
- Permanent (oxidative) hair dyes.
- Hair bleaching.

Cosmetic Dermatology: Products and Procedures, Second Edition. Edited by Zoe Diana Draelos.
© 2016 John Wiley & Sons, Ltd. Published 2016 by John Wiley & Sons, Ltd.

240 **ADORNMENT** Hair Cosmetics

Table 28.1 Overview of hair dye product types.

Hair dye product types	Dye technology	Level of lastingness
Temporary	Preformed FD&C and D&C dyes	Wash out (with one wash)
Semi-permanent	Preformed HC and disperse dyes	Wash out (with 6–8 washes)
Demi-permanent	Oxidative dyes, reduced peroxide concentration	Wash out (with up to 24 washes)
Permanent	Oxidative dyes	Permanent (grows out)
Bleaching	Oxidative bleaching, no dye deposition	Permanent (grows out)

D&C, dyes to be used in drugs and cosmetics; FD&C, dyes allowed to be used in food, drugs and cosmetics; HC, dyes to be used in hair colorants.

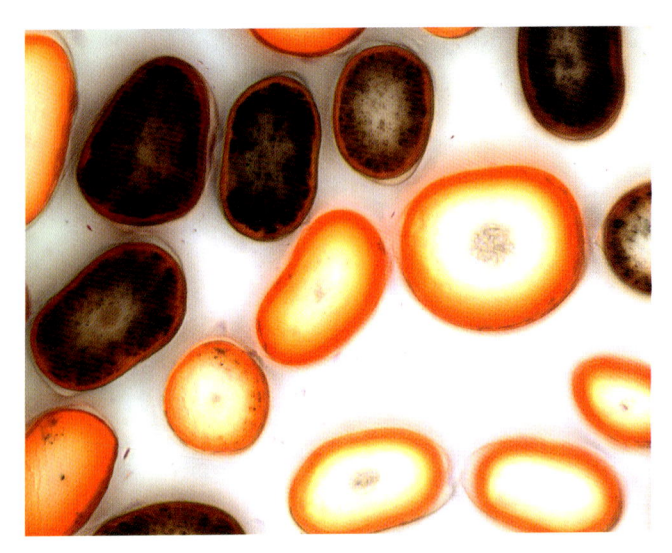

Figure 28.1 Hair cross-section showing color penetration after semi-permanent dyeing.

A wide range of products for changing the color of hair is available to consumers. Today's hair dyes can partially remove (lift) natural hair color, add (deposit) new artificial color, or indeed do both at the same time. They offer a variety of results, from a subtle color refresher to a significant change in the natural hair color, based on very different dye technologies. The classification of hair dyes is based on the permanency of the induced color change (Table 28.1). It should be noted that home and salon hair dyes are fundamentally based on the same technologies, while there are key differences in shade and application variety.

Temporary dyes

Temporary dyes or color rinses are usually formulated with high molecular weight acid or dispersed dyes, which have little affinity for hair and are quite soluble in the dye base. The dye is complexed with a cationic polymer to decrease solubility and increase affinity for hair, and the complex dispersed in the dye base by surfactants. The complex coats the outside of the hair shaft and excess can be rinsed off [3]. The binding forces between hair substrate and dyes are low, which determines their temporary effect, as they are easily washed out with the next use of shampoo.

Each product contains a mixture of generally two to five color ingredients to achieve the desired shade [4]. Typical product forms include shampoos and sprays. While color results are very limited (no lightening, no permanent gray coverage), temporary dyes represent a good option to test colors or refresh dyed hair.

Semi-permanent dyes

Semi-permanent hair dyes use a combination of preformed (direct) dyes to obtain results that last up to 6–8 shampoos. The dyes are generally characterized by their low molecular weight, allowing them to diffuse into the outer cuticle layers without binding firmly to the hair protein (Figure 28.1). Nitro-dyes are the most important group of dyes used in semi-permanent colorants [5]. These uncharged (non-ionic) dyes are barely influenced by negative charges on the surface of the hair. As a result, and because of their relatively small size, they are able to penetrate into the hair cuticle. Washing hair opens the cuticle, allowing the added color molecules to be washed out of the cuticle layer because of their solubility in water.

The products contain a mixture of preformed dyes and are usually left on the hair for approximately 20–30 minutes to achieve a meaningful color change. Color results are limited (no lightening, subtly blending away first grays).

Demi-permanent and permanent dyes

Demi-permanent and permanent hair dyes involve oxidative chemistry, requiring different product components to be mixed just before they are applied. Oxidative dyes are the most frequently used and commercially most relevant hair dyes. Within this category two differentiated product groups exist: permanent and demi-permanent dyes. The primary distinctions between those two groups are the type and level of alkalizing agent and the concentration of peroxide, which determine the efficacy of color change and formation in the hair and impact color longevity, gray coverage, and lightening performance.

Demi-permanent colors typically use 2% hydrogen peroxide (concentration on head) and low levels of alkalizer (usually monoethanolamine, not ammonia), leading to a less efficient dye penetration (ring dye effect; Figure 28.2). They wash out after up to 24 shampoo treatments. While they can be used to enhance and brighten natural color and blend or cover up gray hair up to 50%, they have little or no lightening potential.

Permanent colorants use up to 6% peroxide (concentration on head) and typically contain ammonia as alkalizer to bring the pH of the final product to 9.0–10.5. This allows complete penetration across the cortex (Figure 28.3). Permanent colorants are the most versatile and long-lasting hair dye products and are also available in the widest spectrum of shades. Permanent dyes can lighten hair significantly, change color in subtle

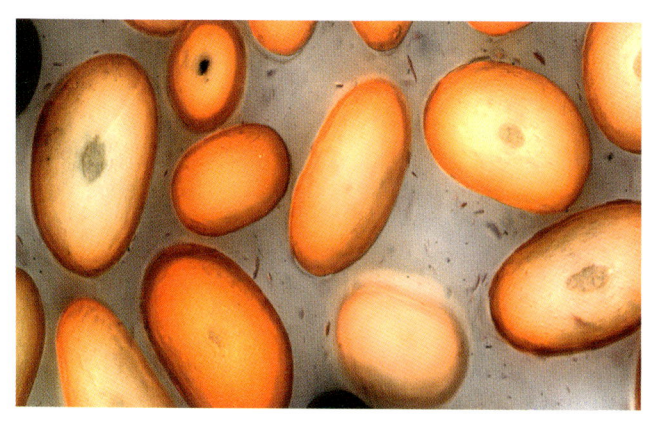

Figure 28.2 Hair cross-section showing color penetration after demi-permanent dyeing.

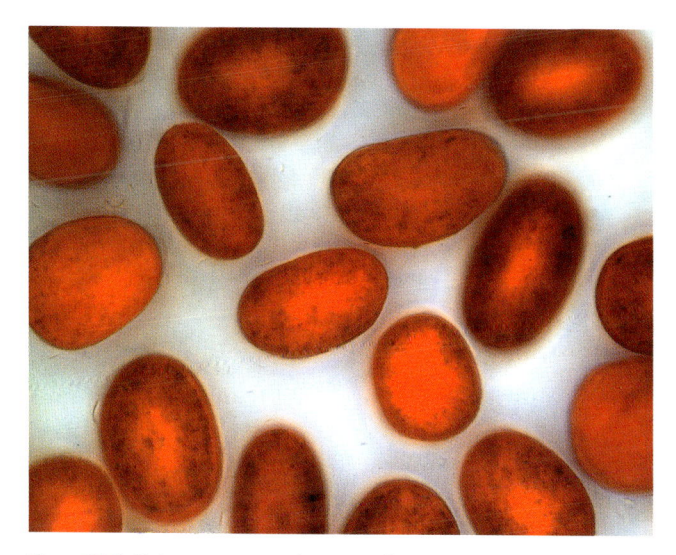

Figure 28.3 Hair cross-section showing color penetration after permanent dyeing.

or dramatic ways, and provide 100% gray coverage, even on resistant gray hair. Reapplication is required every 4–6 weeks to avoid a noticeable root line from re-growing, not colored hair.

Bleaches

Most hair bleaches are products that lighten hair without adding a new color. In addition to hydrogen peroxide and ammonia they contain persulfates to boost and accelerate the bleaching efficacy. Bleaching is the most efficient method of lightening natural and precolored hair. In the case of a partial bleaching, especially on very dark hair, the results can be an unwanted yellow to orange-colored shade due to residual melanin residues in the hair's cortex.

Bleaches can lift the natural hair color most significantly and are often used with special techniques to apply highlighting effects to hair. Just as with permanent dyes, regular reapplication is needed to prevent visible re-growth of the naturally darker hair.

Chemistry

Natural hair pigmentation

The natural coloration of hair is caused by the presence of melanin in the cortex of the hair shaft, which occurs in the form of minute pigment granules formed by melanocytes during the growth of the hair in the lower parts of the follicle. All natural hair color shades are created by just two types of melanin: the more common brownish black eumelanin, and the less common reddish yellow pheomelanin. The final color of hair is determined by the total amount of melanin it contains, by the size of the pigment granules, their distribution in the hair shaft, and by the ratio between the two melanin types [6]. Black hair contains eumelanin in high concentration, whereas blonde and red hair contains less pigment overall – and also higher ratios of pheomelanin.

Despite clear differences in molecular size and general properties, the two melanin types are biogenetically related and develop from a common metabolic pathway involving dopaquinone as a key intermediate [7]. The pigments are present as oval or spherical granules, generally in the range 0.2–0.8 μm in length, and constitute less than 3% of the total hair mass [4]. Production of the pigment particles is located in specialized cells, the melanocytes, deep within the hair follicle. Melanocytes are embedded in the dermal papilla of the hair bulb where they secrete tiny packages called melanosomes into the surrounding keratinocytes.

Natural hair color changes are often observed over the years from birth to old age. Many fair-haired children gradually become darker and by middle age have brown hair. Graying hair affects all to a greater or lesser extent as part of the aging process. It seems to appear earlier in dark- than in light-haired people, and is less common in people of African descent. Graying of the hair is usually a gradual process and irreversible.

The reason for going gray is not the production of a new "gray" pigment, but rather it is the cessation of production of the melanin pigment. Hence gray hair is simply the appearance of a pigmentless hair fiber. The gray to white appearance of non-pigmented hair fibers is due to scattering of light both at the surface and inside the keratin fiber. The increase in the total number of non-pigmented hair fibers on a person's head is the cause of the bulk appearance of the hair color going towards gray with increasing age. The precise molecular and cellular causes of hair depigmentation are still under discussion. Hereditary factors seem to be predominant, meaning that a change in gene expression leads to the exhaustion of the pigmentary potential of each individual hair follicle which leads to reduced melanogenic activity with increasing age. It is likely that the reduced activity is due to the loss of the pigment forming melanocytes from the bulb and the outer root sheath of the aging hair follicle. Another theory is that melanocytes become inactive with age, and may also turn into fully committed pigment cells at the wrong place within the hair follicle, where they are ineffective for providing color to hair [8]. Melanocyte activity is under cyclic control in line with the growth cycle of the hair follicle leading to an apoptosis-driven regression in the catagen and telogen phases.

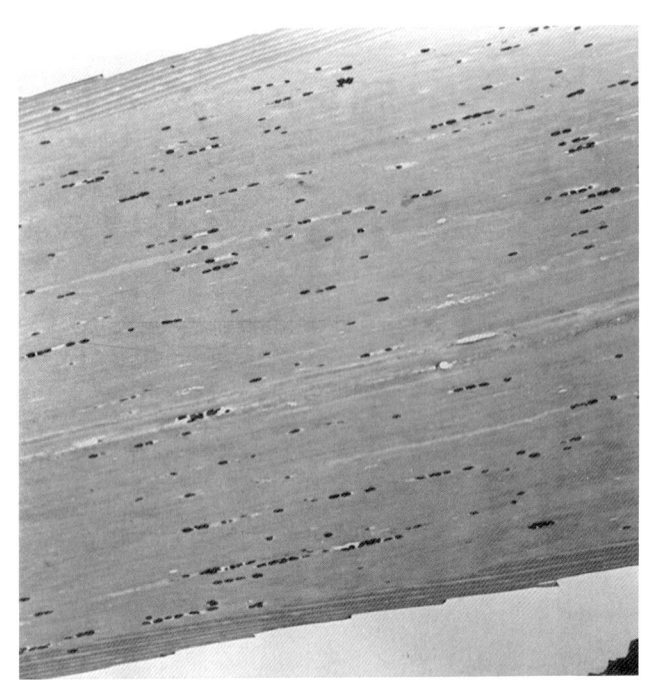

Figure 28.4 Longitudinal section of hair fiber showing melanin distribution across the cortex.

Theories on the mechanism behind the gradual depigmentation of the hair fiber include impaired DNA repair, anti-apoptotic signals, loss of telomerase, and antioxidant mechanisms [8]. A key role is currently attributed to oxidative stress in the lower hair follicle induced by excess levels H_2O_2 caused by intrinsic production of the melanogenesis pathway [8].

For products designed to change the natural color of hair it is important to consider that the melanin granules are distributed throughout the cortex of the hair shaft, showing the greatest concentration towards the outer edge (Figure 28.4). The cuticle layer of the hair shaft typically carries no natural pigments and is therefore transparent. It is therefore imperative for any effective hair dye product to penetrate past the cuticle layer into the cortex of the hair fiber.

Permanent hair dyes

There are two chemical processes that take place during the permanent dyeing process, both of which contribute to the final color. The first is the oxidation of the melanin pigments, lightening the underlying color. The second is the oxidation of the dye precursors to form the actual colored chromophores [10]. Important to note is that only the chromophores formed inside the hair are retained permanently, the remainder are washed away. Consequently another important design parameter for permanent colorants is that the rates of diffusion of dye precursor in to the fiber and the rate of oxidation of the primaries must be balanced [10].

Melanin bleaching

Permanent hair dyes and hair bleach products have the capability to lighten the natural color of hair by removing some of the existing pigment. Melanin is an impressively stable and resistant molecule, as a recent study demonstrated by giving evidence of melanin molecules being preserved in three fossil marine reptiles for nearly 200 million years [11]. Therefore, melanin bleaching requires a highly active technology that enables it to partly break down and dissolve the melanin granules in the hair shaft. During a complete bleaching procedure the melanin granules are dissolved completely, leaving behind what appears under the microscope as a tiny cavity in the cortex of the hair. The process can be described as oxidative degradation of the melanins, leading to a variety of smaller degradation products. The reaction is diffusion-controlled and therefore time dependent [4]. It has been reported that pheomelanins are more resistant to photobleaching, and probably also chemical bleaching, than eumelanins [12].

Oxidative dye formation

Permanent hair dyes are based on the oxidation by hydrogen peroxide of so-called dye precursors or primary intermediates which typically belong to the chemical groups of p-diamines and p-aminophenols, in the presence of various couplers (for examples see Figure 28.5). To start the process, the highly alkaline pH of the dye formulations swells the hair fiber and allows the small active molecules to penetrate into the cortex where the dye formation takes place in three main steps. The first step of the dye formation process is the oxidation of the primary intermediates to highly active imines. If no coupler is present, these imines will react with their unoxidized form to give polynuclear brown or black colored complexes. In the presence of couplers (sometimes called color modifiers) the imines then react preferentially with the coupler molecules at the most nucleophilic carbon atom on the structure. In step 3 this coupled reaction product is oxidized to form wash-resistant indo dyes (for an overview of the dye formation process see Figure 28.6).

Couplers do not themselves produce color but modify the color produced by the oxidation of the primary intermediates (Table 28.2). The final color is a function of the amounts and the properties of the individual primary intermediates and couplers in the composition. The choice of primary and coupler is large hence leading to the possibility to formulate a large range of colors. The size and solubility of the chromophores formed in the hair makes them particularly resistant to removal by washing, and means they undergo little fading [5].

Formulation

All permanent hair dyes are generally marketed as two component kits because of the different components working as oxidizer and alkalizer respectively. One component (tint) contains the dye precursors and an alkalizer (typically ammonia or monoethanolamine) in a surfactant base, and the other is

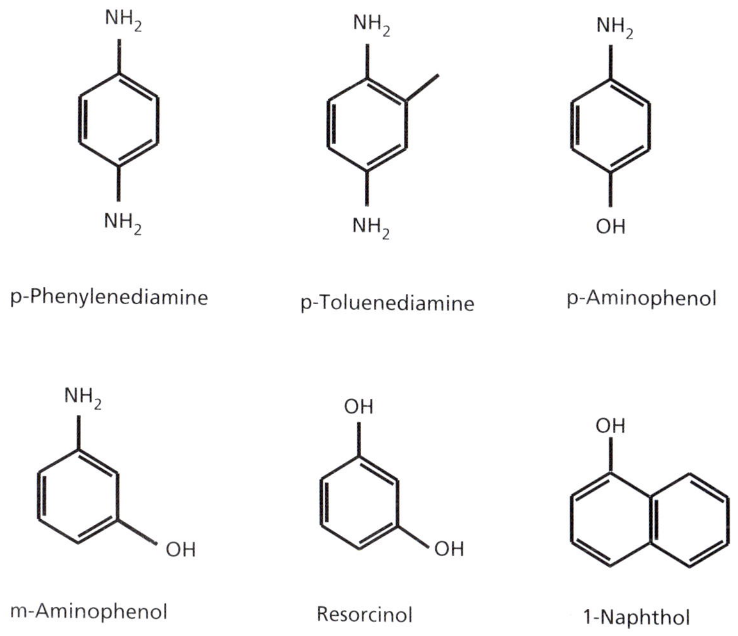

Figure 28.5 Some typical oxidative dye precursors (top) and couplers (bottom).

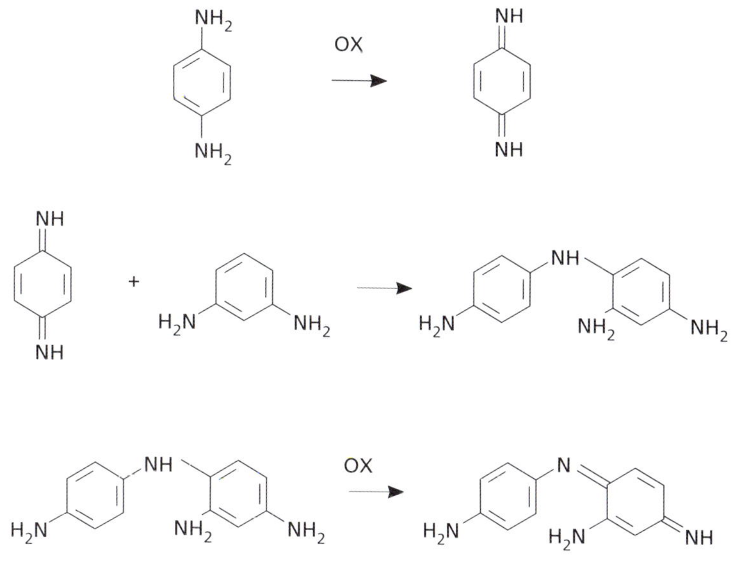

p-Phenylenediamine   p-Toluenediamine   p-Aminophenol

m-Aminophenol   Resorcinol   1-Naphthol

Figure 28.6 The three main steps in oxidative dye formation (here with p-phenylenediamine and m-phenylenediamine).

Table 28.2 Variety in color results given by different couplers in the presence of p-diamines and p-aminophenols.

Coupler	Color on hair with p-diamines	Color on hair with p-aminophenols
m-Phenylenediamine	Bluish brown–black	Reddish brown
1-Napthol	Blue–violet	Red
Resorcinol	Greenish brown	Light brown
3-Aminophenol	Warm brown/magenta	Red–brown
o-Aminophenol	Warm brown	Warm brown

a stabilized solution of hydrogen peroxide (developer). These two components are mixed immediately prior to use and then applied to the hair. The developer component is in liquid form, whereas the tint is usually either a cream or a liquid. Which product form to use is mainly a matter of individual preference, liquids might be easier to mix while creams might be applied with less dripping.

Table 28.3 summarizes common hair dye components and their functions, while also naming some specific examples as they would appear in the ingredients list of a marketed product.

Table 28.3 Overview of common hair dye ingredients.

Component	Function	Sample ingredients
Peroxide	Oxidant, bleaching	Hydrogen peroxide
Alkalizer	Swell hair, bleaching	Ammonia, monoethanolamine (MEA), aminomethylpropanol (AMP)
Dye precursors	Impart color	p-Aminophenol, 1-naphtol, p-phenylenediamine, 4-amino-2-hydroxytoluene
Solvent	Dye vehicle	Water, propylene glycol, ethanol, glycerin
Surfactant	Foaming, thickening	Sodium lauryl sulfate, ceteareth-25, cocoamide MEA, oleth-5
Buffer	Stabilizing	Disodium phosphate, citric acid
Fatty alcohols	Emollients	Glyceryl stearate, cetearyl alcohol
Quaternary compounds	Conditioning	Polyquaternium, cetrimonium chloride

Advantages and disadvantages

Coloring hair, if performed well with satisfactory results, can have a profoundly beneficial effect that can be life-transforming; however, there are some considerations to take into account when weighing up advantages and challenges of the use of hair colorant products.

Advantages

The key strength of hair dye products lies in their transformational potential. Changing one's hair color can have a dramatic physical effect but, more importantly, it can also have a strong beneficial impact on a psychological level. Patients may not only feel more attractive and younger looking, they also report increased confidence both in their private and work environments which can be very important for individuals and therefore should not be discounted or belittled [2]. In our appearance- and youth-obsessed society coloring gray hair is a simple yet powerful and impactful tool in the arsenal of appearance-enhancing and "anti-aging" procedures and products.

Another advantage of modern hair dyes is the variety of technologies and benefits that it offers. Virtually everyone can find a product that suits them and their personal requirements, and new innovative technologies continuously expand the range of offered visual effects, treatment experiences, and shades.

Challenges

Even though only a small fraction of the population is affected (see section on 'Safety and regulatory considerations' for more detail), most hair dyes, mainly permanent, oxidative hair colorants (with the exception of pure bleaching products) have the potential to cause allergic reactions. Recent technological advances, however, have led to the development of new hair dye technologies reducing the risk of developing allergy whilst delivering permanent hair color change. More details on the risk of allergies with hair dyes will be provided in the relevant section of this chapter.

All oxidative hair dyes, including demi-permanent, permanent, and bleaching products, contain ingredients such as hydrogen peroxide and ammonia, which may cause skin irritation. To minimize these risks, it is imperative that usage instructions are followed carefully, and that all products are kept well out of the reach of children.

It should also be mentioned that permanent hair dyes require a certain amount of upkeep and maintenance from the user. Visible root re-growth, especially if the natural hair color has been significantly changed, necessitates the regular reapplication of product to maintain high quality appearance benefits. This is one of the main reasons why a large group of consumers who color their hair choose to do so themselves, at home, rather than visiting a professional hairdresser every single time they feel the need to recolor.

Lastly, one drawback of hair dyes, again mainly relevant to oxidative products, lies in the fact that hydrogen peroxide at alkaline pH conditions can alter the hair structure, leading to undesirable sensorial attributes described by consumers as poor shine, poor feel, and reduced strength [13]. It should be noted that these problems mostly occur with frequent use, and with high levels of lift or bleaching or even wrong use of the products. Therefore, these effects on the hair structure can be reduced with the right application techniques. More details on these structural changes will be provided in the section "Impact of hair dyes on hair structure".

Product choice and application

The most important step in hair dyeing is the right choice of product, considering both the type of hair dye and the color shade. Individuals with no previous experience in using hair colorants who want to blend away some first grays, or who want a subtle enhancement of their natural color, are perhaps best advised to choose a semi-permanent colorant. If the person has a higher percentage of gray (up to 30%) and wants to stay close to their natural hair color, a demi-permanent product could be the best solution. Covering higher levels of gray and/or achieving significant changes in the natural hair color will require the application of a permanent hair dye product. Even within permanent hair color category there are now different technologies available that allow the creation of a broad range of visual effects and color quality from intense block colors to transparent shades that allow for a more subtle blending of the new hair color with the natural hair color.

Once the right type of hair dye has been identified, the key decision is to identify the right shade. The final color result is a combination of the existing hair color and the shade produced by the colorant – shade guides on the packaging are usually very helpful in exploring which result should be expected based on those two parameters. For home hair dyes a useful guideline is to stay within two shade differences of one's natural color, and – if in doubt – choose a lighter over a darker shade. To be sure about the outcome of the coloring process, which will also be affected by the condition of the hair and previous treatments, a strand test can be helpful. For this test a small strand of hair (0.25 inch) is cut from the darkest part of the hair, or area with the most gray hair, and covered with the product for the time recommended for the hair color. Checking after different time points enables the optimum processing time to accomplish the desired end result to be determined.

Another check that should always be completed before coloring hair is an allergy alert test. The test should be carried out 48 hours prior to product use and involves applying a small amount of the product to an area of the body skin (typically recommended is the inside of the elbow). If a rash or redness, burning, or itching occurs the patient may be allergic to certain product ingredients and must not use the tested product. If an individual has such a reaction following an allergy alert test, it is strongly advised to consult a dermatologist or physician.

Lastly, it is very important, especially for first time color users, to read the product usage directions carefully. Oxidative colorants require the mixing of several components before application and each product might be slightly different in terms of how it should be mixed and used. It is therefore imperative for a successful color result and experience to follow the recommended procedure step by step.

Impact of hair dyes on hair structure

Oxidative coloring and bleaching have been shown to cause several changes to the hair structure, especially with frequent use (Figure 28.7). Alkaline peroxide partially removes the outer hydrophobic surface barrier of hair, called the f-layer, made of 18-methyl eicosanoic acid. This layer functions a natural protection or conditioning system of hair and its destruction leads to significant changes in important hair properties such as feel and behavior when it is exposed to changes of the environment [14]. At the protein level, peroxide at alkaline pH conditions attacks certain amino acids which are part of the hair fiber structure, especially cystine, leading to oxidative degradation products. The resulting physicochemical changes of the hair surface are irreversible and can lead to hair that feels coarse, is more difficult to comb, lacks shine, and is weakened [11,13]. Importantly, hair that has been treated and thus changed by oxidative treatments is more prone to physical and environmental stress and subsequent damage [16] and therefore needs to be regularly treated with care and conditioning products.

Recent technology strategies to minimize fiber damage

While the above described hair fiber changes can be mainly attributed to hydrogen peroxide itself, it is also well known that hydrogen peroxide at high pH is likely to form reactive radical species which can be an additional source of fiber damage during hair coloration. The reaction is catalyzed by the presence of redox metal ions such as copper and iron which are prevalent in tap water. It has been reported that the addition of metal

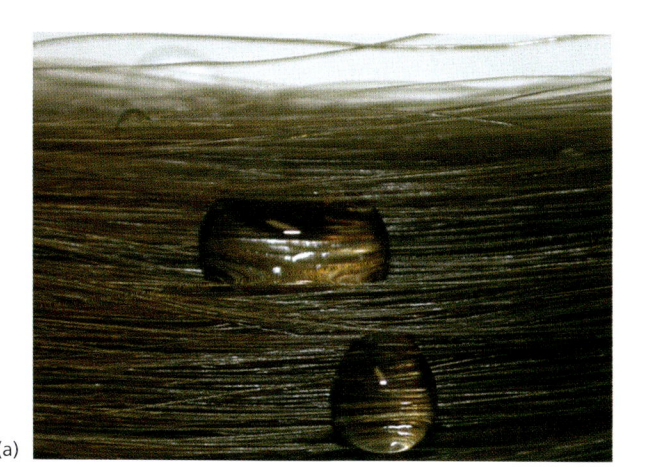

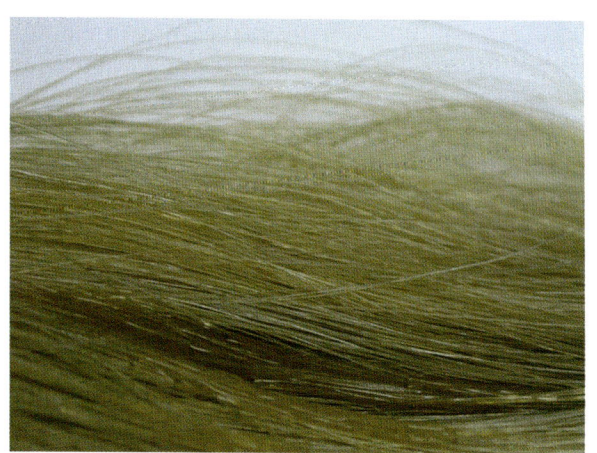

Figure 28.7 Change in surface hydrophobicity before (a) and after (b) bleaching.

chelating agents to oxidative colorants can reduce the surface damage caused in the presence of copper in tap water [17]. Key is to find a chelant that selectively binds to transition metal ions such as copper in the presence of high concentration of water hardness ions, especially calcium. N,N'-ethylenediamine disuccinic acid (EDDS) has been found to fulfill this requirement and has therefore since been introduced into hair color and hair care products [15].

Caring for colored hair

Based on the described changes to the hair surface structure, it is important that consumers take the right steps to care for their hair before, and especially after coloring. This will help in keeping good color results for as long as possible, and also in protecting the weakened hair structure from further damage from daily wear and tear.

The first step in treating colored hair correctly is to use the most appropriate application technique when re-coloring. Covering visible re-growth only requires the hair dye to be used on the hair sections affected – the hair roots. This will help to protect the bulk of the hair from unnecessary exposure and over-processing.

The basis for a suitable hair care routine after dyeing should be the use of a shampoo and conditioner specifically developed for colored hair. They contain ingredients that are tailored to the altered hydrophilic surface conditions of the hair and help to smoothen the cuticle surface, protecting it against mechanical damage. Secondly, sun exposure should be minimized because UV radiation not only contributes to hair damage but also has a direct impact on color fading by inducing degradation of the hair dye molecules in the hair shaft. Lastly, it should be pointed out that water exposure is a big contributor to color fading (also called wash fading). It can therefore be beneficial to adjust the wash frequency of freshly colored hair accordingly.

Safety and regulatory considerations

As part of cosmetics, hair dyes are thoroughly safety regulated by global regulatory authorities such as the US Food and Drug Administration (FDA) or EU Cosmetic Directive or Regulation (1223/2009 EC), and their scientific advisory board, the Scientific Committee on Consumer Safety (SCCS, formerly SCCP, SCCNFP) [18,19]. Hair dyes are one of the most thoroughly studied cosmetics and consumer products and there is an overwhelming amount of safety data on hair dyes [20]. Despite the extensive safety testing and close safety regulation regimen, two safety concerns are typically associated with hair dyes: skin allergy and allegations regarding a slightly increased cancer risk.

Allergy

Like other products such as certain foods or drugs, hair dyes can cause allergic reactions in a few individuals. Allergic reactions to hair dyes are well known but still relatively rare when compared to the daily global use of millions of hair colorants. In general allergic reactions to hair dyes are classified as delayed hypersensitivity or type IV reactions. Type IV reactions are normally localized to the area where the product is applied. Only in very rare exceptional cases more severe and spreading symptoms like facial edema can occur. Type IV reactions are triggered by a different immune-response mechanism than type I allergies, which are more typically reactions to food or drug ingredients and in severe cases may lead to life-threatening symptoms.

Key hair dye allergens

Key hair dye actives such as para-phenylenediamine (pPD), but also para-toluenediamine (pTD), are well known skin sensitizers. pPD is part of the standard patch test series in certain countries; pTD is part of the hairdresser patch test series [21]. This is particularly important as pPD and pTD are key dye precursors for the vast majority of oxidative permanent hair dyes and virtually present in all black, brownish and blond shades. Beside pPD and pTD, various other hair dye ingredients have been identified as allergens. In 2006 and 2013, EU's SCCS published a Memorandum on hair dye chemical sensitization [22]. The SCCS concludes that 13 hair dyes fulfil the criteria of extreme sensitizers, 23 of strong and 20 of moderate sensitizers. This assessment is based on the intrinsic allergy potential of hair dyes only. It does not consider use concentrations and actual consumer exposure to these hair dyes during hair coloring, and hence is of limited relevance for the actual allergy induction risk for the consumer. In fact, many hair dyes including some of those classified as strong or extreme sensitizers are commonly used because they are non-relevant allergens among consumers and clients, due to their low use concentrations.

A new risk assessment approach for the allergy induction of hair dyes has been jointly developed by academia and industry experts. This Quantitative Risk Assessment Approach (QRA) for hair dyes builds on the allergy potential, but introduces use concentration and actual consumer exposure to individual hair dyes during hair coloring to estimate the actual allergy induction risk for hair dye users. In fact, pPD was shown to be tolerated by most users while sensitive individuals may indeed develop an allergic reaction. Other hair dyes also being classified as strong allergens do not represent a significant allergy risk according to the QRA approach, which is confirmed by in market surveillance data [23].

Allergy prevalence of hair dye allergy

There are different ways to quantify the actual hair dye allergy frequency and prevalence:

1. Number of allergic reactions to hair colorants

Actual hair dye allergic reactions are relatively rare given the wide and frequent use of hair colorants. According to a study of hair dye manufacturers looking at the number of reported allergy cases after hair dye use in various different European countries, 0.2–4.3 hair dye allergic reactions are reported per one million sold product units (undesirable effects, UEfs, reasonably attributed to product use, causality assessment likely and very likely). UEfs vary between reporting countries and manufacturers, but overall show to be rather stable. Reporting rates of home use products are altogether higher than the reporting rates for salon uses [24].

2. Number of patients with newly diagnosed allergy for key hair dye ingredients like pPD

The allergy incidence against key hair dyes like pPD and pTD among patients undergoing patch testing have been monitored over several decades in different countries. Incidence rates vary between countries and are usually in the area of 5% in the US and the EU and slightly higher in Asian countries. The allergy incidence against pPD has been more or less stable over the past years [25]. While a few authors have concluded that pPD allergy incidence among patch-tested individuals has slightly increased over the years [26], most authors conclude that pPD allergy incidence is stable or even slightly decreasing [27–29].

3. Number of individuals in the general population being allergic to key hair dye ingredients like pPD

The actual pPD allergy prevalence in the general population was assumed to be significantly lower compared to the incidence among dermatological patients undergoing diagnostic patch testing routine. Using the methodology of clinical epidemiology (CE) and drug utilization research (DUR) a prevalence of 1% pPD allergy in the general population was estimated [30]. According to a recent study, the prevalence against the key hair dye allergen pPD in the general population was indeed confirmed to be slightly less than 1% [31].

It is important to note that pPD, as one of the most frequently cited key hair dye allergens, is also widely used elsewhere. While hair dyes are commonly regarded as one of the contributors to pPD allergy, several other key uses have been identified to substantially contribute to the overall pPD allergy rates. One key contributor being identified in the recent past is black henna tattooing. Such temporary henna tattoos are often added with pPD to darken them and make them longer lasting. Black henna tattoo inks have been found to have PPD concentrations as high as 15% to 30%, i.e. a use concentration one order of magnitude higher than the maximally allowed pPD use concentrations in hair dyes in the EU; moreover it was left on the skin and not rinsed after approximately 30 minutes like most permanent hair colorants [32].

Beside black henna tattoos, pPD is also widely used in black textile dyes, leather dyes, printing inks, photograph developer and the rubber industry. A study of the German "Informationsverbund Dermatologischer Kliniken, IVDK" could attribute only 22% of all pPD allergy cases to hair dyeing including clients, 23% to different occupational exposures including hairdressers and 12% to clothing and shoes. About 44% of the pPD allergy cases could not be linked to any specific exposure or product use. The majority of pPD allergy cases could not be attributed to hair colorant use, but resulted from sources other than hair dye exposure [33].

Are children at higher risk to develop hair dye allergic reactions?

Most permanent hair colorant products come with advice not to be used by children. In the EU, hair colorants are mandated to be labeled with a disclaimer that the products are not to be used by children less than 16 years old. A similar disclaimer is mandatory also in the US. This however is not related to a higher risk of younger individuals developing an allergic contact dermatitis. In fact, several studies have shown that age is irrelevant with regard to the allergy risk and that younger individuals are not at higher risk for developing an allergic contact dermatitis compared to adults [34,35]. The recommendations given by manufacturers and mandated by some regulators are more driven by the opinion that users of respective hair colorants are mature enough to understand the potential allergy risk and to follow the usage and safety instructions properly, including allergy risk mitigation measures.

Allergy Alert Test

In order to minimize the risk of an allergic reaction during use, which can be severe, most hair dye manufacturers recommend conducting an Allergy Alert Test (sometimes called pre-test or skin sensitivity test) with the colorant and shade of interest 48 hours before the actual hair coloration. Pending manufacturer's guidance, a small proportion of the colorant of interest should be applied at a small skin site either behind the ear or the lower arm 48 hours before the coloration. In case of any adverse reaction, consumers and clients are advised not to color and seek medical advice. While some dermatologists and also the European Commission's SCCS raised questions regarding the suitability of the Allergy Alert Test, e.g. with regard to false negatives or an allergy risk resulting from the exposure through the test, manufacturers claim that the Allergy Alert Test is an important allergy risk management measure and recommend the procedure. Similarly, some regulators in the US require the Allergy Alert Test or pre-test to be recommended in the product use instructions.

Permanent hair dyes with reduced allergy risk

While some direct, non-permanent colorants work without pPD and pTD, permanent hair colors offering the full color spectrum and long lasting color performance usually require pPD or pTD as key building block of mainly black, brown and most blond shades. For many years hair dye manufacturers have been investigating hair dyes with reduced allergy risk, as replacements for pPD and pTD. The key challenge in this quest was to find the right balance between optimal color performance (gray coverage, shade space) and reduced allergy risk.

A first invention was the pPD derivative hydroxyethyl-p-phenylenediamine, which can replace pPD and pTD and deliver some shade variability. While still classified as strong sensitizer, its allergy potential is reduced compared to pPD and pTD. Cross-reactions to existing pPD and pTD allergies however cannot be excluded [36]. It is used in few commercial products.

The latest innovation in this area is 2-methoxymethyl-p-phenylenediamine (ME-PPD) with further reduced allergy potential. It is classified as moderate sensitizer and offers full color performance and gray coverage. Pre-market data indicate a negligible allergy induction risk during use of ME-PPD [37]. Also cross-reactivity versus existing pPD-allergy is reduced and is in the range of approximately 30% [38]. Net, ME-PPD may be suitable for pPD-allergic individuals but only following thorough and close dermatological examination and consultation to exclude the individual cross-allergy and elicitation risk. ME-PPD was first introduced in commercial products in 2014.

Overall it is too early to conclude whether any of the above pPD and pTD alternatives with lower allergy induction potency will be able to successfully replace pPD or pTD. Future consumer acceptance and in-market allergy surveillance data will be needed to further verify suitability of either of the alternatives.

In summary, for the time being, hair dye allergy remains an issue for a small number of consumers and therefore the following safety measures can help to minimize the allergy risk [39]:

- Consumers should read and follow the usage instructions of hair colorants carefully. All hair dyes carry clear allergy warning labels, making users aware of the potential allergy risk.
- For permanent and most semi-permanent hair colorants, consumers are advised to conduct an Allergy Alert Test (product tolerance test) with the product and shade of interest 48 hours before hair coloring, by following the recommendations coming with each product. However, the absence of a reaction at the test site is no guarantee that a reaction will not occur during hair coloring. In case of a skin reaction at the test site, consumers should not color their hair and seek dermatologic advice. When consumers experience initial signs of an adverse reaction at the scalp during the hair coloring session, the hair dye should be rinsed off immediately.
- Consumers may develop an allergy to hair dyes over time also as a result of products other than hair dyes. Temporary black henna tattoos are one important contributor to pPD allergy in humans [40,41]. This emphasizes the importance of conducting an Allergy Alert Test.
- Professional hairdressers should follow occupational safety measures, such as wearing protective gloves during preparation, application, and rinsing of hair colorants [42].
- In the case of consumers who have a diagnosed allergy against a specific hair dye ingredient, hair dyes should not be applied before they have consulted with their dermatologist. Some hair dyes are known to cross-react (e.g. pPD and pTD).

Overall, it should be emphasized that the vast majority of consumers can safely use hair colorants and that following the use and safety instructions plus the above guidance, will help to minimize the allergy risk for the small number of individuals at risk of allergic reaction to hair dyes.

Cancer

Cancer concerns were raised early in the context of oxidative hair dyes, because of their chemical nature. Numerous epidemiologic studies into hair dye safety have been conducted since then, the vast majority concluding that there is no association of hair dye use and an increased cancer risk. Occasional, single epidemiologic studies reporting a slightly increased risk for certain cancer types such as bladder cancer have not been confirmed by multiple epidemiologic studies. Early in 2008, leading cancer experts of the International Agency of Cancer Research (IARC, a subsidiary of the WHO) reviewed all relevant studies and scientific papers published to date and concluded that there is no evidence that personal hair dye use is associated with any increased cancer risk ("not classifiable as to its carcinogenicity in humans" (Group 3)) [43]. The US Cosmetic Ingredient Review (CIR) panel came to the same conclusion.

Early in 2000 the EU Commission launched a big hair dye safety campaign in joint collaboration with leading hair dye manufacturers. More than 100 individual hair dyes have been re-assessed and validated, including updated safety studies provided by manufacturers. Many hair dyes not relevant or in use any more have been taken off the list of approved hair dyes. After almost 10 years' work, the SCCS concluded that for hair dyes marketed in the EU, no clear indications for an excess of cancer risk was demonstrated, which is in line with the judgement of the aforementioned IARC working group [44]. Net, initial or occasionally raised cancer concerns have been thoroughly reviewed by global leading expert panels and safety regulators and disproved to be relevant for today's modern hair colorants.

Conclusions

Modern hair dyes are an effective tool in altering the natural color of hair and to cover gray hair. Different product types offer a wide range of results, from subtly enhancing color to dramatic color changes and complete gray coverage. While the potentially huge beneficial effect on people's perceived attractiveness and self-esteem is undisputed, a thorough understanding of the different available technologies and their benefits and challenges is essential to advise consumers on the most suitable products to use.

Most relevant are permanent hair colors, allowing a full color variability, most efficient gray coverage and long durability. While the vast majority of consumers do tolerate today's permanent colorants, a small number of consumers and clients may show an allergic reaction, mainly to the key hair dye allergens pPD and pTD. Allergy risk management measures have been developed to reduce the risk of allergic reactions for both, hair dye consumers and hairdressers.

Most recently, hair dye alternatives to pPD and pTD with significantly reduced allergy risk have been developed and introduced in the market. The pre-market studies indicate a negligible allergy risk with these new technologies; however, future consumer acceptance and in-market surveillance will be needed to further confirm these data.

The main future challenge in hair coloring lies in preventing or even reversing hair graying via stimulating melanocyte activity at the molecular or even genetic level. The recently reported modulation of hair follicle melanocyte behavior with corticotropin-releasing hormone peptides could be a first step towards that direction [45].

Acknowledgment

The authors thank Frauke Neuser for her contributions to the first edit of this chapter.

References

1. Zviak C. (1986) *The Science of Hair Care*. New York: Marcel Dekker.
2. Gray J. (2005) *The World of Hair Colour*. London: Thomson.
3. Brown K. (2000) Hair coloring products. In: Schlossman M, ed. *The Chemistry and Manufacture of Cosmetics*, Vol. II Formulating. Carol Stream, IL: Allured Publishing, pp. 397–454.
4. Robbins CR. (2002) *Chemical and Physical Behavior of Human Hair*. New York: Springer.
5. Corbett JF. (1998) *Hair Colorants: Chemistry and Toxicology*. Cosmetic Science Monographs. Weymouth, UK: Micelle Press.
6. Schwan-Jonczyk A. (1999) *Hair Structure*. Darmstadt, Germany: Wella AG.
7. Prota G, Ortonne JP (1993) Hair melanins and hair color: Ultrastructural and biochemical aspects. *J Invest Dermatol* **101**, 82S–9S.
8. Wood, J. M. Decker H, Hartmann H, Chavan B, Rokos H, Spencer JD, Hasse S, Thornton MJ, Shalbaf M, Paus R, Schallreuter KU. (2009) Senile hair graying: H_2O_2-mediated oxidative stress affects human hair color by blunting methionine sulfoxide repair. *FASEB* **23**(7), 2065–75.
9. Nishimura EK, Granter SR, Fisher DE. (2005) Mechanisms of hair graying: incomplete melanocyte stem cell maintenance in the niche. *Science* **307**, 720–4.
10. Brown KC, Pohl S, Kezer AE, Cohen D. (1985) Oxidative dyeing of keratin fibers. *J Soc Cosmet Chem* **36**, 31–7.
11. Lindgren J, Sjoevall P, Carney RM, Uvdal P, Gren JA, Dyke G, Pagh B, Shawkey MD, Barnes KR, Polcyn MJ. (2014) Skin pigmentation provides evidence of convergent melanism in extinct marine reptiles. Nature doi: 10.1038/nature12899.
12. Wolfram LJ, Albrecht L. (1987) Chemical and photobleaching of brown and red hair. *J Soc Cosmet Chem* **38**, 179–91.
13. Jachowicz J. (1987) Hair damage and attempts to its repair. *J Soc Cosmet Chem* **38**, 236–86.
14. Lodge RA, Bhushan B. (2006) Wetting properties of human hair by means of dynamic contact angle measurement. *J Appl Polym Sci* **102**, 5255–65.
15. Wortmann FJ, Schwan-Jonczyk A. (2006) Investigating hair properties relevant for hair "handle". Part I: hair diameter, bending and frictional properties. *Int J Cosmet Sci* **28**, 61–8.
16. Takada K, Nakamura A, Matsua N, Inoue A, Someya K, Shimogaki H. (2003) Influence of oxidative and/or reductive treatment on human hair (I): Analysis of hair damage after oxidative and/or reductive treatment. *J Oleo Sci* **52**, 541–8.
17. Marsh JM, Flood J, Damaschko D, Ramji N. (2007) Hair coloring systems delivering color with reduced fiber damage. *J Cosmet Sci* **58**, 495–503.
18. European Union Cosmetics Regulation EC 1223/2009: http://eur-lex.europa.eu/LexUriServ/LexUriServ.do?uri=CONSLEG:2009R1223:20130711:en:PDF.
19. SCCP/1501/12 Notes of guidance for testing of cosmetic ingredients for their safety evaluation, 8th revision, adopted by the SCCS during the plenary meeting of December 1, 2012. http://ec.europa.eu/health/scientific_committees/consumer_safety/docs/sccs_s_006.pdf
20. Nohynek GJ, Fautz R, Benech-Kieffer F, Toutain H. (2004) Toxicity and human health risk of hair dyes. *Food Chem Toxicol* **4**, 517–43.
21. Diepgen TL, Coenraads PJ, Wilkinson M, Basketter DA, Lepoittevin JP. (2005) Para-phenylendiamine (PPD) 1% pet. is an important allergen in the standard series. *Contact Dermatitis* **53**, 185.
22. SCCS Memorandum on hair dye Chemical Sensitization (SCCS/1509/13), adopted at its 18th plenary meeting February 26 2013; http://ec.europa.eu/health/scientific_committees/consumer_safety/docs/sccs_s_007.pdf
23. Goebel C, Diepgen TL, Krasteva M, Schlatter H, Nicolas JF, Blömeke B, Coenraads PJ, Schnuch A, Taylor JS, Pungier J, Fautz R, Fuchs A, Schuh W, Gerberick GF, Kimber I. (2012) Quantitative risk assessment for skin sensitisation: consideration of a simplified approach for hair dye ingredients. *Regul Toxicol Pharmacol.* **64**(3), 459–65.
24. Krasteva M, Bons B, Tozer S, Rich K, Hoting E, Hollenberg D, Fuchs A, Fautz R. (2010) Contact allergy to hair colouring products. The cosmetovigilance experience of 4 companies (2003–2006). *Eur J Dermatol.* **20**(1), 85–95. doi: 10.1684/ejd.2010.0808.
25. Gerberick GF, Ryan CA. (2005) Hair dyes and skin allergy. In: Tobin DJ, ed. *Hair in Toxicology: An Important Biomonitor*. London: CRC Press, pp. 212–28.
26. McFadden JP, White IR, Frosch PJ, Sosted H, Johansen JD, Menne T. (2007) Allergy to hair dye. *Br Med J* **334**, 220.
27. Uter W, Lessmann H, Geier J, Schnuch A. (2003) Contact allergy to ingredients of hair cosmetics in female hairdressers and clients: an 8-year analysis of IVDK data. *Contact Dermatitis* **49**, 236–40.
28. DeLeo VA. (2006) p-Phenylenediamine. *Dermatitis* **17**, 53–5.
29. Wetter DA, Davis MDP, Yiannias JA, et al. (2005) Patch test results from the Mayo Clinic Contact Dermatitis Group, 1998–2000. *J Am Acad Dermatol* **53**, 416–21.
30. Thyssen JP, Menne T, Schnuch A, Uter W, White I, White JM, Johansen JD. (2009) Acceptable risk of contact allergy in the general population assessed by CE-DUR – A method to detect and categorize contact allergy epidemics based on patient data. *Regulat Toxicol Pharmacol* **54**, 183–7.
31. Diepgen T. (2013) Annual ACDS Meeting Abstracts, *Dermatitis* **24**(4), 1–15.
32. Gawkrodger DJ, English JS. (2006) How safe is patch testing to PPD? *Br J Dermatol* **154**(6), 1025–7.
33. Schnuch A, Lessmann H, Frosch PJ, Uter W. (2008) Para-phenylenediamine: the profile of an important allergen. Results of the IVDK. *Br J Dermatol.* **159**(2), 379–86.
34. Felter SP, Robinson MK, Basketter DA, Gerberick GF. (2002) A review of the scientific basis for uncertainty factors for use in the quantitative risk assessment for the induction of allergic contact dermatitis. *Contact Derm* **47**, 257–66.

35 Cassimos C, Kanakoudi-Tsakalidis F, Spyroglou K, Ladianos M, Tzaphi R. (1980) Skin sensitization to 2,4-dinitrochlorobenzene (DNCB) in the first months of life. *J Clin Lab Immunol* **3**, 111–13.

36 Frosch PJ, Kuegler K, Geier J. (2011) Patch testing with hydroxyethyl-p-phenylenediaminesulfate – cross-reactivity with p-phenylenediamine, *Contact Derm* **65**, 96–100.

37 Goebel C, Troutman J, Hennen J, Rothe H, Schlatter H, Gerberick GF, Bloemeke B. Introduction of a methoxymethyl side chain into p-phenelyenediamine attenuates its sensitizing potency and reduces the risk of allergy induction. *Tox Appl Pharm* **174**(2014), 480–7.

38 Blömeke B1, Pot LM, Coenraads PJ, et al. (2015) Cross-elicitation responses to 2-methoxymethyl-p-phenylenediamine under hair dye use conditions in p-phenylenediamine-allergic individuals. *Br J Dermatol* **172**, 976–80.

39 Schlatter H, Long T, Gray J. (2007) An overview of hair dye safety. *J Cosmet Dermatol* **6**, 32–6.

40 Onder M. (2003) Temporary holiday "tattoos" may cause lifelong allergic contact dermatitis when henna is mixed with PPD. *J Cosmet Dermatol* **2**, 126–28.

41 Nawaf AM, Joshi A, Nour-Eldin O. (2003) Acute allergic contact dermatitis due to para-phenylenediamine after temporary henna painting. *J Dermatol* **30**, 797–800.

42 Dickel H, Kuss O, Schmidt A, Diepgen TL. (2002) Impact of preventive strategies on trend of occupational skin disease in hairdressers: population based register study. *Br Med J* **324**, 1422–3.

43 Baan R, Straif K, Grosse Y, Secretan B, Ghissassi FE, Bouvard V, et al.(on behalf of International Agency for Research on Cancer, IARC). (2008) Carcinogenicity of some aromatic amines, organic dyes and related exposures. *Lancet Oncol* **9**, 322–3.

44 SCCS Opinion on reaction products of oxidative hair dye ingredients formed during hair dyeing processes (SCCS/1311/10), adopted during its plenary meeting of 21 September 2010; http://ec.europa.eu/health/scientific_committees/consumer_safety/docs/sccs_o_037.pdf.

45 Kauser S, Slominski A, Wei ET, Tobin DJ. (2006) Modulation of the human hair follicle pigmentary unit by corticotropin-releasing hormone and urocortin peptides. *FASEB J* **20**, 882–95.

CHAPTER 29
Permanent Hair Waving

Annette Schwan-Jonczyk[1], Gerhard Sendelbach[2], Andreas Flohr[3], and Rene C. Rust[4]

[1] Private Practice, Darmstadt, Germany
[2] Darmstadt, Germany
[3] Wella/Procter & Gamble Service GmbH, Darmstadt, Germany
[4] GSK/Stiefel, Brentford, Middlesex, UK

BASIC CONCEPTS

- Permanent hair waving is a chemical/mechanical treatment aimed at modifying hair protein to achieve and retain curly shapes.
- During the permanent waving process the hair is wound on rods, then first treated with a reduction agent– typically thioglycolate – followed by an oxidation step with hydrogen peroxide. The first reduction step chemically reduces the cystine inside the hair, breaking the sulfur–sulfur-bridge of the cystine molecule. The hair fiber is weakened and can now conform to its new shape. The oxidation step then chemically locks the new molecular confirmation of the hair proteins.
- The intensity as well as the durability of the treatment depends on a variety of parameters which can be chemical or mechanical in nature. As with all other hair transformations involving reactive chemistry, results vary with the texture and quality of the hair.
- Due to the chemical nature and the complexity of the application process, for personal safety and to avoid undesirable hair damage, permanent waving products are typically applied by a stylist in a salon. In salon applications permanent waving chemistry may also be mixed with conventional hair masks to create special effects.

Introduction

Since ancient cultures, curly hair has been regarded one of the most prominent signs of femininity and beauty. Women with straight hair purchased expensive wigs or spent hours for hair ondulation with water and heat for a temporary success. A ground-breaking invention was made by Carl Nessler in 1906 who offered, for the first time, irreversible hair shaping to clients by means of heat and borax.

Improvements followed during the 20th century by the creation of "cold waves," using sulfite or thioglycolate as actives, still the most popular waving agents in home and salon perms.

Hair physiology

Hairs are composed of cells packed in tight cell bundles that grow out from up to 3 mm skin depth. About 5 million hairs cover the human body and scalp classified as vellus hairs (5–10 μm in diameter) or terminal hairs (5–120 μm in diameter). The human head has 100,000– 50,000 fibers, which grow approximately 1 cm per month through rapid cell division in the living, lowest part of their hair follicle, known as the hair bulb. Each strand of hair is made up of three regions, the medulla, the cortex, and cuticle.

The innermost structure of the hair, the medulla, is not always present and is an open, spongiform region. The highly structural and organized cortex, or middle layer of the hair, is the primary source of mechanical strength and water uptake. The cortex contains melanin, which colors the fiber based on the number, distribution and types of melanin granules. It is currently under discussion if either the shape of the follicle determines the shape of the hair, or if the way the hair forms and hardens determines the shape of the hair follicle. There are ethnical differences in hair shape and structure, for example Asian hair typically has a round fiber diameter and is normally straight. Hair fibers with oval and irregularly shaped diameters are generally wavier or even curly. The hair surface contains flattened cells, known as the cuticle, which forms an imbricate structure resembling shingles on a roof. The hair surface is covered with a single molecular layer of lipid ("f-layer") which gives the hair surface hydrophobic properties. However, when the hair fiber swells, for example induced by chemical treatments, its complex structure changes and the cuticle layer is opened making the hair more porous. The cuticle provides protection and support for the inner spindle-shaped "cortical cells," which make up 80% of the hair mass. During hair growth, the interdigitated cells are organized into a three-dimensional network resembling a jigsaw puzzle. This construction contributes to cell cohesion and hair fiber strength (Figure 29.1).

Cosmetic Dermatology: Products and Procedures, Second Edition. Edited by Zoe Diana Draelos.
© 2016 John Wiley & Sons, Ltd. Published 2016 by John Wiley & Sons, Ltd.

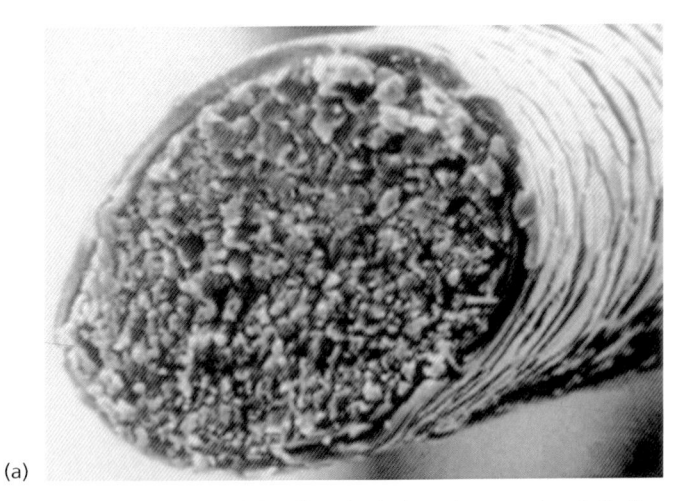

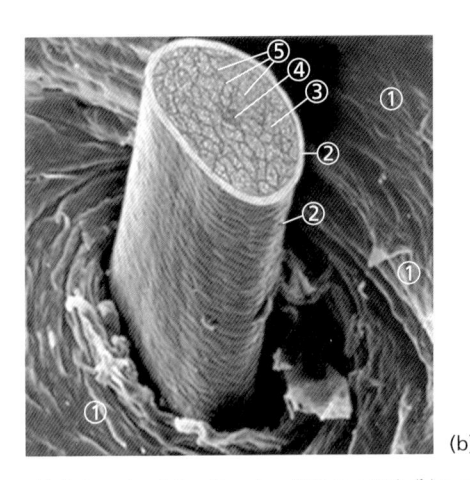

Figure 29.1 (a) The fracture plane of a hair fiber clearly shows the composite of a fibrillar core with flattened cuticle cell coating (SEM ×1420). (b) Just emerging hair: 1, scalp surface; 2, cuticle pattern of hair fiber surface; 3, interior of the hair with cortical cells; 4, medullary cells; 5, cell membrane.

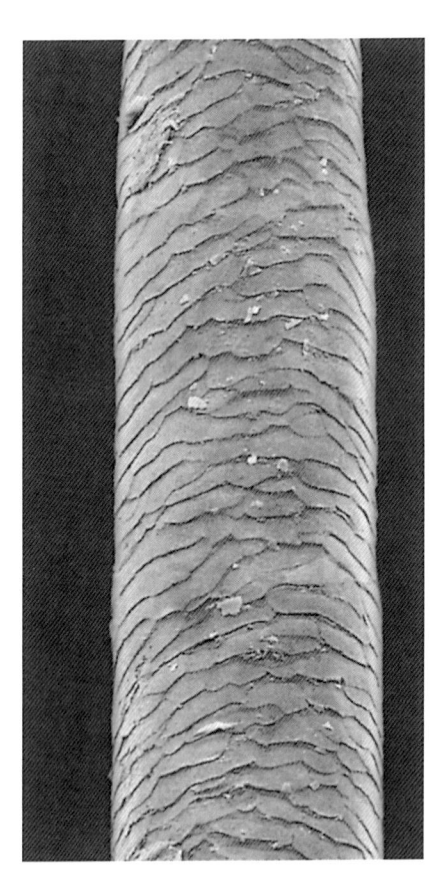

Figure 29.2 The intact cuticle pattern of the hair fiber near the scalp (SEM ×800).

While all hair fibers contain a cuticle, only thicker hair fibers with a diameter greater than 75 μm contain a central area of hollow cells, the medulla (Figure 29.2). For animals, the medulla also enhances thermal insulation.

The active growth period of scalp hair is known as the anagen phase and is limited to 3–6 years. Then the hair disconnects from the papilla, a period known as the catagen phase, and enters a 2-months resting phase, known as the telogen phase, and is subsequently lost through shedding. Hair shedding and renewal results in an average loss of up to 100–125 scalp hairs per day. With constant hair growth and no cutting, bulk hair may reach up to 1 m in length – depending on the genetically determined length of the hair growth cycle (for more hair growth details, the reader is referred to more detailed references [1,2]).

Permanent wave hair relevant properties

Hair geometry
Usually, scalp hair is visualized as a circular fiber but cross-sections of individual hairs reveal variation in hair shape. The typical appearance of a person's hair is determined by its special mixture of thick, thin, elliptical, kidney-shaped, and triangular cross-sectional shapes [3]. "Unmanageable" hair often comprises a high percentage of irregular hair shapes. Irregular hair geometry, small diameter, and large hair diameter all create permanent waving challenges. Hair thickness has a large influence on the shape and hold of permanent wave curls as well [4].

Hair and water interaction
Although hair is not soluble in water, its interaction with water is of particular importance for permanent waving [2,6]. The hair surface is naturally hydrophobic, and permanent waving lotions contain surfactants for enhanced wetting, the first step in the curling process. Under certain climatic conditions, hair adsorbs atmospheric water up to 30% of its own weight.

Although feeling dry at ambient temperature, hair still contains 15% water. Excess water can be bound by capillary forces.

The hair water content dictates its chemical reactivity as water widens the hydrogen-bond network of protein side chains and acts as the vehicle for all permanent waving ingredients. Proper water balance is important for a successful permanent waving. Moreover, as water functions as a plasticizer for hair, permed hair loses curls more rapidly after washing or exposing it to humid conditions, which can be measured in a curl retention test [7].

In presence of water, hair displays its amphoteric character. A hair is at the "isoionic point" when the positive and negative charges of hair proteins are at an equilibrium. The natural "intrinsic point of neutrality" of hair is pH 6, which is the point of greatest stability of the hair structure. This intrinsic point of neutrality must be restored after permanent waving to maintain the structural integrity of the hair.

Closely related to hair fiber water hydrophilicity is its thermal behavior. Dry hair can withstand temperatures during heat styling for a short time when it is dry; it is recommended not to exceed 200°C on virgin hair, and 180°C on chemically treated hair. In the wet state, however, hair can suffer structural damage at much lower temperatures, sometimes even below 100°C.

Hair aging

Hair fibers undergo longitudinal aging when exposed to external factors such as grooming or environmental influences [2,6,8]. The hair emerges at the scalp surface in a virgin state, but can suffer structural damage due to mechanical effects (e.g. friction during styling), temperature changes (e.g. heat styling), or UV-radiation. Free radicals can further induce structural damage at the surface and the cortex of the hair fiber via chemical oxidation.

The result of this range of insults is chemical and mechanical wear of the hair. Some of the chemical changes are cleavage of the hair's proteins, conversion of amino acids, oxidation of cystine to cysteic acid, and decomposition of histidine. As a consequence, stability and elasticity of the hair, especially at its ends, decreases, flexibility is reduced, and hair fibers get more rigid and brittle, a process termed "hair weathering". Unsightly split ends often occur and the hair tends to feel dry (Figure 29.3).

The structural differences between hair roots and hair ends require special attention in hair permanent waving because the ends of hair – due to their structural and chemical changes – react faster to the perming process and tend to break more easily.

Hair chemical structure

The protein content of a normal hair at ambient conditions is approximately 80 wt% [2,9]. Further components are approximately 5 wt% internal lipids; <1 wt% trace elements and metals; 14 wt% water. Of the 22 amino acid types found in hair, the most important is "L-cystine" (56-89-3), a sulfur-containing amino acid (Figure 29.5), which facilitates covalent cross-linking between two different protein chains. Up to the high amount of 9 mol% (750 µmol/g hair) [10] is typical for cornified tissues, such as hair, nail, hooves, horn, or cornea. Because of the

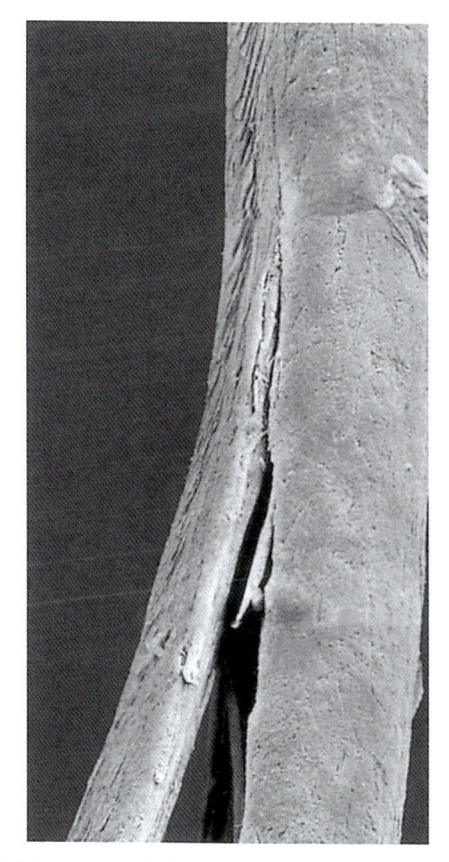

Figure 29.3 The worn cuticle-free split end of hair (SEM ×800).

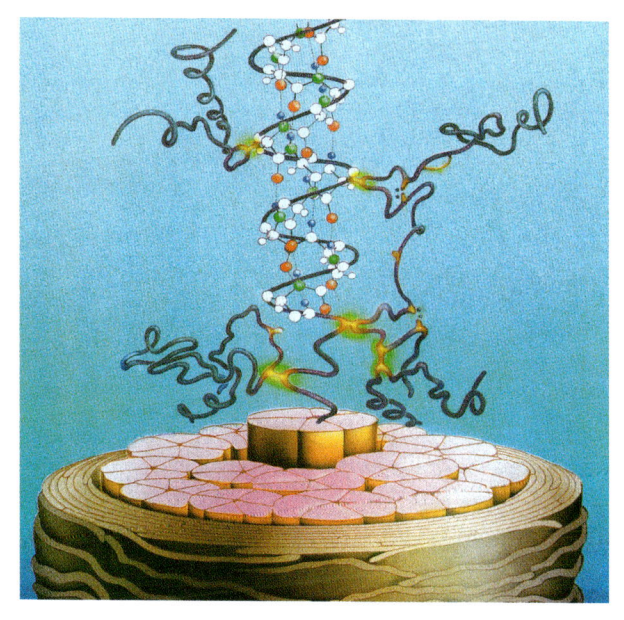

Figure 29.4 Coiled (alfa-helical) and amorphous molecules of hair proteins are cross-linked by disulfide bonds inside the cortical cells. Helical proteins are stabilized by hydrogen bonds.

covalent cross-links between amino acids of different proteins, hair demonstrates high mechanical strength and shear resistance, insolubility in water, but is also prone to swelling.

Figure 29.5 Chemical formula of the amino acid "cystine".

Two types of proteins constitute the hair content: low and high sulfurous proteins. It is their typical arrangement that differentiates hair proteins from proteins in the rest of the body:
- About 50% of the proteins are present in an unorganized, amorphous form, called matrix proteins, which feature frequent disulfide bridges.
- The rest of the proteins typically coil up to form a helical configuration in certain sections, to constitute micro fibrils, which are embedded in and anchored to the matrix proteins.

Figure 29.4 shows the network of hair proteins, with the "disulfide bonds" marked in yellow, which gives hair properties similar to a fiber-reinforced plastic [11] or the elastic rubber of a tire. This special architecture is the source of hair's elasticity.

Perming agents cleave disulfide bonds in these matrix proteins, causing the plasticization that is necessary for shaping hair.

However, an excess of a reducing agent is necessary to achieve this, as cross-linked sulfur proteins in the cuticle make the hair mantle hard to dissolve and penetrate.

Additional support of the chemical network is provided by the acid and basic amino acids in hair protein which make up more than 40% of the hair's substance. These form low energy bridges, salt linkages, and hydrogen bonds, which are also cleaved and reformed during the permanent waving process.

Chemophysical principles of hair waving

Because of hair's great elasticity and strong resilient forces, it quickly resumes its original straight shape after being re-shaped without structural changes. Therefore it has to be softened and subsequently re-hardened chemically to maintain a conformation change. Especially with permanent waving, it is important to select a reversible reaction to allow repeated treatments without hair destruction. The sulfur bridges of the amino acid cystine, linking the proteins, are best suited [6,12,13].

The conditions for permanent waving to be well tolerated are:
- Low temperature (20–50°C), convection or contact heat;
- Short process time (5–30 minutes); and
- Mildness to the skin

A permanent wave occurs with two solutions:
1. *Solution 1*: the "perming lotion" comprising a thiol-compound as reducing agent, designed to split about 20–40% of hair cystine bonds.
2. *Solution 2*: a "fixing lotion" usually comprising hydrogen peroxide as the oxidizing agent, designed to rebuild cystine bridges between proteins at new sites in the curled hair shape (Figure 29.6).

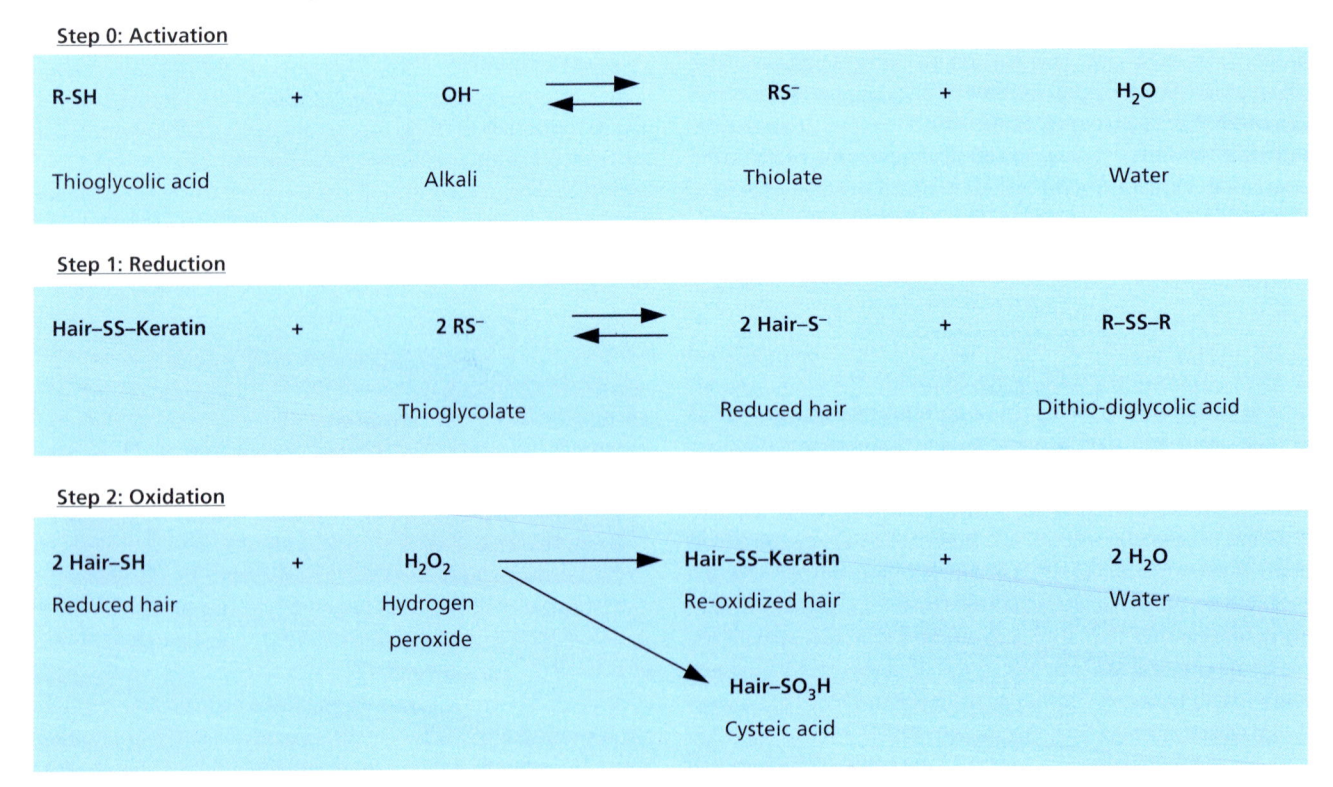

Step 0: Activation

R-SH	+	OH$^-$	⇌	RS$^-$	+	H$_2$O
Thioglycolic acid		Alkali		Thiolate		Water

Step 1: Reduction

Hair–SS–Keratin	+	2 RS$^-$	⇌	2 Hair–S$^-$	+	R–SS–R
		Thioglycolate		Reduced hair		Dithio-diglycolic acid

Step 2: Oxidation

2 Hair–SH	+	H$_2$O$_2$	→	Hair–SS–Keratin	+	2 H$_2$O
Reduced hair		Hydrogen peroxide		Re-oxidized hair		Water
			↘	Hair–SO$_3$H		
				Cysteic acid		

Figure 29.6 Chemical reaction formulas 0–2.

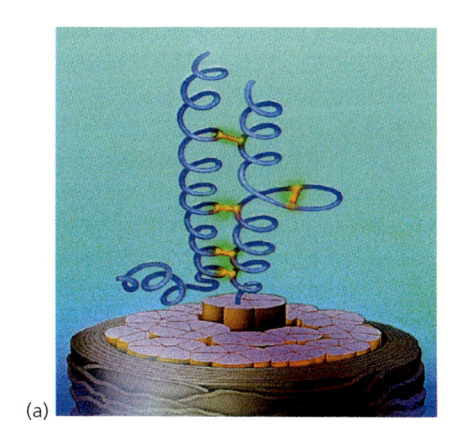

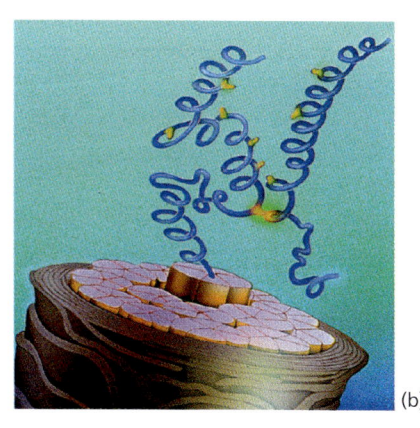

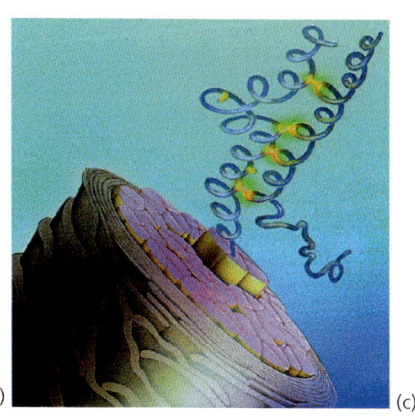

Figure 29.7 (a) Sulfur bridges between the proteins are closed. (b) Part of the sulfur bridges are being cleaved, proteins shift, take on the form. (c) Sulfur bridges are being rebuilt at a different site, neutralizer fixes the new shape.

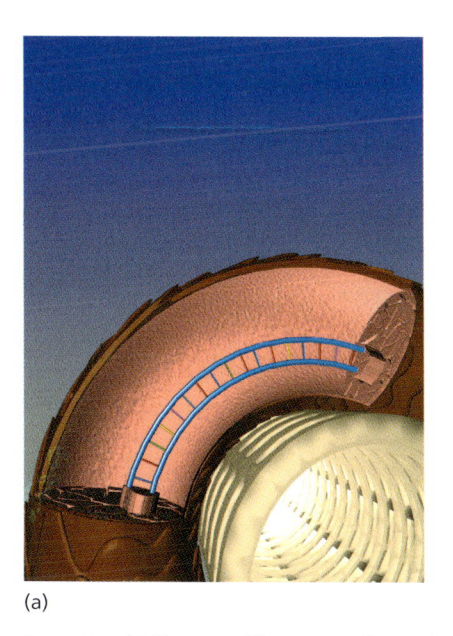

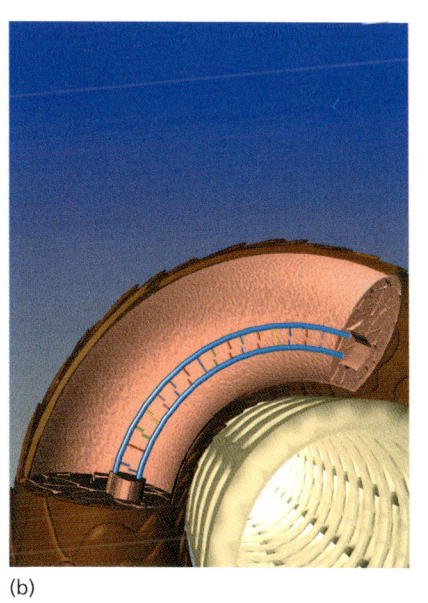

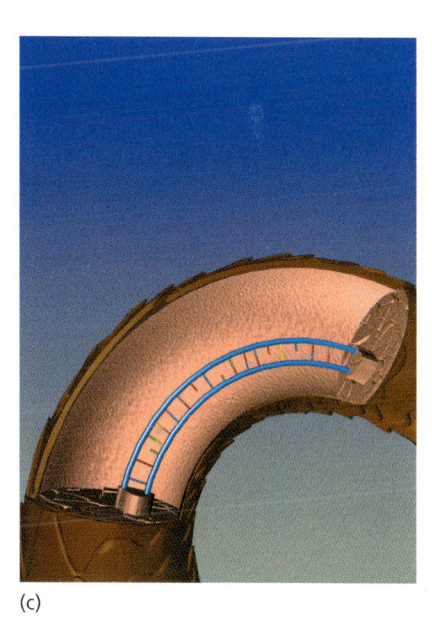

Figure 29.8 (a) Shampooed hair is wound on curlers while still moist. Bending strain is applied to the protein chains. (b) Perm-wave lotion 1 is applied to the hair and cleaves part of the sulfur bridges by the reducing (thioglycolic acid) and the alkalizing agent. Hair is softened, proteins creep and adjust to the shape of the curler. (c) Neutralizing process: an acid neutralizer (peroxide) rebuilds the sulfur bridges at different sites and the new shape is permanent.

It is crucial to keep in mind that permanent waving is a two-step procedure with the chemical reaction and physical effects running in parallel to achieve sufficient results (Figures 29.7 and 29.8) [14-16]: reduction of disulfide-bonds, softening of hair, lateral swelling and length contraction, stress development and protein flow, then re-oxidation of cystine bonds and de-swelling, and fixation of the new curly shape. Table 29.1 summarizes how hair reacts chemically and physically during each of the permanent waving steps.

Usually only 85% of the cleaved disulfide is reformed during neutralization. Some hair cystine oxidizes to give cysteic acid (Figure 29.6, formula 2), which renders hair more hydrophilic, incompletely cross-linked, and more vulnerable to subsequent treatments. Therefore, permed hair gradually loses its curl and relaxes to a straight hair conformation again (for additional details, the reader is referred to Robbins [2] and Wickett and Savaides [17]).

Perm products and types

Permanent waving products contain an elaborate mixture of ingredients to make the reactions controllable and appropriate for different hair types, such as normal hair (N-type), sensitive hair (S-type), coarse hair (F-type), and coloured/bleached hair (C- or G-type).

Typical formulations for a one-component perm lotion and a fixing lotion are shown in Table 29.2. Each ingredient is listed by

Table 29.1 The usual steps of perming.

Steps in practical permanent waving	Hair reacts chemically/physically
1. Ask and consult the client concerning the desired hairstyle (curly head or gentle waves)	–
2. Assess the hair quality regarding the hair thickness, hair and scalp health, split ends	–
3. Shampoo the hair with a mild shampoo to remove fat and residual cosmetics	Water swells hair by 15% in diameter, about 2% in length and softens it at the same time
4. Apply a conditioning pre-product, aqueous or oily	Hair surface, root to tip differences in hair structure are equalized, lowers chemical reactivity of hair tips
5. Divide hair into sections with comb to get flat and small hair tresses	–
6. Take/use endpapers, wrap them around the weathered hair tips, wind the hair tightly on curlers; up to 60 on one head of hair	Paper helps to align tip end hair fiber, protects and delays instant reaction. Moistened hair is usually wound on a rigid rod. Bending hair around the curler produces a slight tension on hair
7. Use gloves, protect clients face with cotton plugs	Protection for hands and face/neck skin against dripping solution
8. Apply the permanent waving lotion (about 75 mL), avoid dripping	Fluid penetrates into the hair, starts chemically reducing it from outside in, softens hair
9. Apply heat by means of a hairdryer, heat processor or use ambient temperature	Heat accelerates: (a) penetration; (b) the reduction step; (c) move-ability of hair proteins
10. Develop process time of permanent waving lotion with heat for 5–20 minutes	Reductive cleavage of the hair cystine-network proceeds, hair swells up to 50%, contracts approx. 2%, generates internal stress, which relaxes by creeping and flowing of the protein mass The hair substance is transferred from an elastic into a "plastic" state adopting the shape of the curler
11. Monitor curl development unwinding a test curler	Although wet, unwound test lock shows degree of wave/hair deformation (measurable by an electronic test curler), cystine side chains changed their position relative to each other
12. Rinse-off thoroughly the permanent waving lotion (with water, up to 3 minutes)	Chemicals are diluted, removed from hair, reaction stops, but physical swelling and shrinking onto the curler peaks by osmotic forces
13. Apply a neutralizing liquid or foam. Process the neutralizer for up to 10 minutes followed by rinsing and unwinding the hair	Re-oxidation of cysteine to cystine by hydrogen peroxide restores hair's protein network again, fixing new cystine cross-links at different positions. Residual cystine oxidizes to cysteic acid De-swelling and hardening occurs Unwinding the hair results in curl relaxation
14. Apply an acid conditioning product as after treatment	Restores hairs neutrality, also neutralizes residual perm molecules. The deformation process is now complete
15. Dry and style the hair by means of a brush or setting curlers and a hairdryer	Curl relaxation starts in wet hair, brushing, combing diminishes curl retention. Best: air drying

its International Nomenclature of Chemical Ingredients (INCI) name as it would be found on the packaging; each ingredient has its own distinct role in making the solution active, efficacious, pleasant to the hair, and odor free (for different formulations see [18,19]).

Role of permanent waving product ingredients

This section reviews the individual ingredients important in achieving a successful permanent waving solution [20].

Reducing agents

Reducing agents, most commonly ammonia or sodium salts of thioglycolic acid (TGA), have been used since the late 1950s to avoid skin and hair irritation while producing a lasting hair curl. Other alternatives are glycerol monothioglycolate (GMT), which is active at neutral pH levels. Cysteine [21] and cysteamine (2-mercaptoethylamine) are typically used for perming Asian hair. Thiolactic acid, with less reducing power, can be used as co-reducing agent. Many home permanent waves contain sulfites.

Alkalizing additives

Alkalizing additives, such as ammonia or monoethanol amine, are included in the formulation to achieve the appropriate pH at which the reducing agent as well as the hair disulfide is activated, normally pH 7–9.5 (Figure 29.6, step 0). Glycerol monothioglycolate, the active component of an "acidic wave" works best at pH 7; TGA requires a pH of 8.5–9. Hair damage is often related to products with higher pH levels.

Table 29.2 Ingredients in a typical perm solution 1 and neutralizer solution 2.

Ingredient	Content % w/w	Action
Ammonium thioglycolate 70%	14	Waving agent
Ammonium hydrogen carbonate	5	Buffer
Ammonia 25%	1	Alkalizing agent
1,2 Propylene glycol	2	Carrier
Styrene/PVP copolymer	0.1	Opacifier
Polyquaternium-6 [poly(dimethyl diallyl ammonium chloride)]	0.2	Conditioning agent
Perfume	0.4	Fragrance
Coceth-10 (alkyl polyglycol ether)	0.4	Solubilizing agent
Water	76.9	Basis
pH	8.2–8.5	
Neutralizer		
Hydrogen peroxide 50%	5	Oxidizing/fixing agent
Ammonium hydrogen phosphate	0.3	Stabilizing agent
Phosphoric acid	0.1	Stabilizing agent
EDTA	0.2	Complexing agent
Perfume, conditioning agent, surfactant, water		As in perm solution
pH	2.5–3.5	

Buffer salts

Buffer salts, such as ammonium (hydrogen) carbonate, affect the alkalinity. These ingredients buffer the working pH because with hair being a natural ion exchanger, its pH is typically reduced when it comes into contact with the perm solution.

Carriers

Carriers (e.g. urea, ethanol, or 2-propanol) enhance penetration of actives into hair and thus the effectiveness of the perm product.

Surfactants

Surfactants are included to ensure wet-ability of the originally hydrophobic hair surface. They also facilitate foaming of perm solutions or neutralizers so they can be better applied avoiding dripping. In permanent wave foams, the type and concentration of surfactants are especially critical for skin compatibility [13].

Conditioning ingredients

Conditioning ingredients such as polymers are often included in perm products to allow good manageability of the new shape and mask the somewhat harsh tactile properties of hair after permanent waving.

Complexing agents

Complexing agents in thioglycolate-based perm lotions prevent intensive red–violet colouring with iron contamination. Complexing agents are added to the neutralizing lotions to avoid decomposition and boosting of hydrogen peroxide.

Opacifiers

Opacifiers, such as styrene-vinyl-pyrrolidone-copolymers, and coloring agents (e.g. azulene) give a pleasant appearance to the product but also help with the application of the product.

Thickeners

Thickeners (e.g. cellulose derivatives or polyacrylate salts) are used to convert fluid preparations to gels which enhance accuracy during application as they prevent dripping from the hair and enable a more intensive perm treatment of the hair root area.

Solubilizing agents

Oily fragrances require a solubilizing agent for better integration into the product formulation.

Neutralizers

Neutralizer ingredients are in principle oxidizing agents, mostly hydrogen peroxide at concentrations of approximately 0.5–3% and acid at pH 2–4.5. Advantages of including neutralizers in perming products are:
- Low solution concentrations;
- Excellent environmental compatibility; and
- Physiological safety.

Moreover, at acid pH hydrogen peroxide has no bleaching power for the natural hair colour, but specifically re-oxidizes hair cysteine to cystine and truly neutralizes the alkaline hair. However, metal salts can catalyze the rapid decay of hydrogen peroxide, which contains as stabilizer inorganic phosphates, phenacetin, or 4-acetaminophenol.

As alternatives, bromate salts are used. The concentration is approximately 6–12 wt% at pH 6–8.5. Bromate-based neutralizers are preferentially used in Asia because they do not lighten dark hair. Less widely used are sodium perborate and percarbamid.

Different product types

The majority of commercial waving and neutralizing lotions are aqueous solutions, but a few are designed as gels, creams, or aerosol permanent waves [17,18].

Preparations chiefly differ in:
- Mixture of reducing agent;
- Concentration of reducing agent;
- pH-value;
- Form of application.

Alkaline perms

Alkaline perms are alkalinized with ammonia to a pH 9–9.5. Because of the frequent association of these formulations with skin irritations, these products were largely replaced by mildly alkaline preparations at pH 7.5–9.

Acidic and neutral permanent wave

Acidic and neutral permanent wave preparations mostly contain glycerol monothioglycolate (GMTG) as reducing agent. This allows easy control of the processing behavior, leaves hair with a pleasant feel, and the danger of over-waving is reduced. It is often retained in hair for a sustained period of time, imparts an unpleasant smell, and causes sensitization of hairdressers' hands even by touching hair that was processed weeks ago. Therefore, esters must not be used according to the technical directives for dangerous substances in hair salons [22].

Thermal waves

Thermal waves produce heat during the perming procedure. Hydrogen peroxide reacts with excess of thioglycolic acid to release heat. Such warming is meant to generate a pleasant feeling on the client's head and to render the addition of external heat unnecessary.

Sulfite perms

Perming lotions containing ammonium sulfite are used in home applications for permanent waving. At neutral pH 7 and without thiols, they work best on healthy, undamaged hair. However, stable "Bunte" salts are typically formed during their chemical reaction with hair which can lead to poor fixation, a rough hair feel and hair damage especially on tinted or fine hair.

An overview of product types is summarized in Lee et al. [23].

Regulatory aspects of permanent hair waving

Permanent waving formulations are regulated by different legislations in a variety of regions and countries [20]. For example, the *EC Cosmetics Directive*, Annex III, Part 1 [24], restricts the pH of permanent wave preparations with thioglycolic acid, its salts and esters to pH 7–9.5, and for the acid and salts, pH 6–9.5 for esters. The maximum concentration calculated as thioglycolic acid is 8 wt% ready for use in home applications and 11 wt% for professional use. A special warning label is required and hydrogen peroxide concentrations are limited to 12% [24].

In the USA, the Cosmetic Ingredient Review (CIR) expert panel considers 15.4 wt% maximum of thioglycolic acid as safe in permanent wave products. The CIR recommendations are respected by the manufacturers.

In Japan, permanent wave products are classified as quasi-drugs. Thioglycolic acid and its salts are permitted, as is cysteine, but concentration and pH are restricted by the regulatory bodies, whereas these don´t permit thioglycolic esters

Perming practice – how to achieve a perfect curl

The question of perming safety is not only a function of product composition, but also depends on the use conditions [6,25]. Therefore, each package of perms on the market contains a list of instructions for the hairdresser or consumer. Table 29.2 summarizes the recommended steps and how hair answers (i.e. reacts), chemically and physically.

Any deviations from this course of action will be specified in the instructions for use. The correct execution of each step should produce the desired result, a curl lasting up to 3 months, a well-preserved hair structure, and an easy styling of the hair assembly (Figure 29.9).

In salons where hairdressers use long-lasting perms, an appropriate permanent wave must be selected to achieve the best result. The hair thickness and quality must be assessed to determine if the hair is healthy or damaged. If the hair feels rough, is of a lighter colour, or possesses split ends, it may have a porous structure produced by previous weathering, bleaching, colouring, or permanent waving. This increased porosity allows the perming lotion to react faster. Damaged hair requires bigger curlers, a reduced perm strength, and shortened processing time.

Heat from a drying hood (45°C) accelerates the chemical reaction, but should not be used for people with sensitive scalp skin as it might increase the risk of skin irritations.

To ensure that the desired waving result has been achieved, a test curl should be performed. A test curl is loosely unwound from a curler after several minutes to determine the degree of curl achieved and whether to extend the processing time.

After thoroughly rinsing off the perming lotion, complete hair neutralization is strongly advised as the second fundamental step in perming. Three to ten minutes are recommended to obtain a lasting perm, to re-oxidize the hair, and to neutralize the alkalinity of the reducing step. Hair only gains its physical strength and integrity back after thorough neutralization.

Application of an acidic conditioning lotion as an after-treatment, removes residual peroxide, restores the hair internal pH to neutrality, helps to stabilize the hold of the curl, and makes it less prone to future damage.

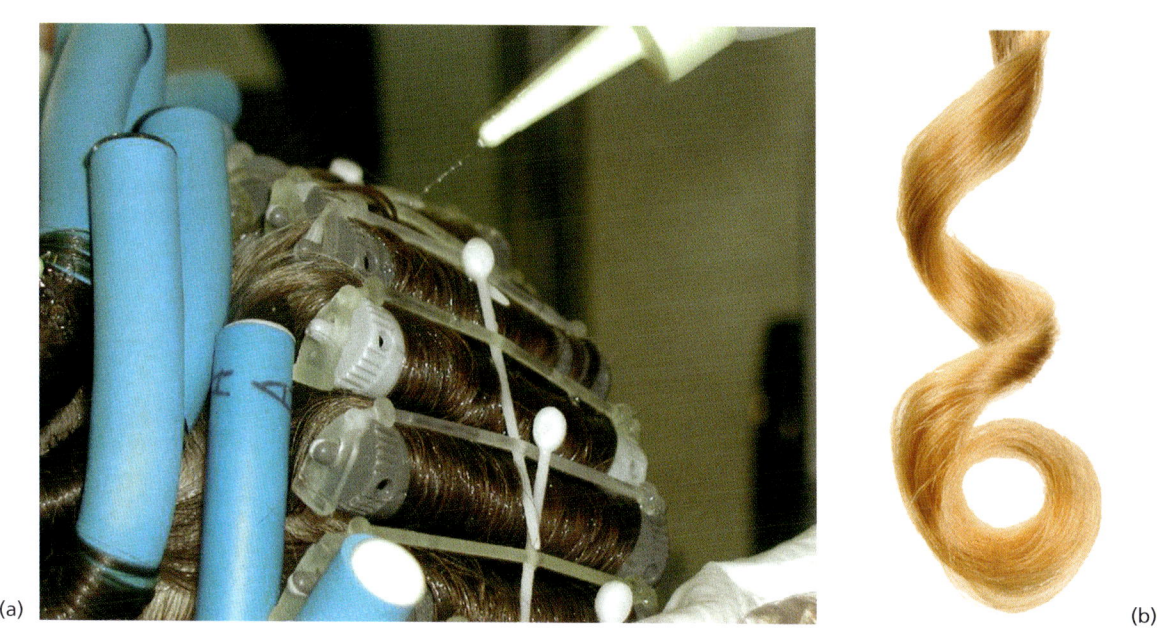

Figure 29.9 Hair, properly wound, fixed on rollers, and wetted by the perming lotion (a) delivers perfect locks (b).

Safety of and adverse reactions to perm products

Safety requirements from consumer expectations are adequately summarized by the EU Cosmetics Directive: "A cosmetic product put on the market within the Community must not cause damage to human health when applied under normal or reasonably foreseeable conditions of use" [24].

Therefore, as permanent wave preparations contain reactive chemicals, these have to pass a complete toxicological characterization. Essentially, the potential for:
- acute systemic toxicity;
- local compatibility and irritation;
- sensitizing potential, allergenicity;
- mutagenicity;
- tumorigenicity;
- teratogenicity; and
- percutaneous absorption.

Based on experience with the safety of waving products over many years and regularly updated statistics published by intoxication advisory centers, manufacturers today have a solid foundation of knowledge about perming formulations. Statistics of adverse reactions from cosmetic products sold between 1976 and 2004 revealed only 1.1 undesired effects per 1 million packages sold [26]. This confirms that cosmetic products are very safe (for more detailed information about toxicological test methods and safety assessment processes see references [20,27,28]).

However, even though a perm product has been approved as safe by legal authorities, occasional hair or skin damage can occur from incorrect use and application:

- consumers apply a home wave without reading/understanding instructions; or
- new hairdressers in salons are untrained and less skilful.

The first sign of a failure in permanent waving is a lack or excess of curliness. This is typically not only caused by the wrong choice of product, but also excessive development time, and temperature, and especially incomplete rinsing of the active substances and shampoo components may lead to undesired results. Surfactant residues, residual reducing and/or oxidizing agents left in the hair can encourage irreversible side reactions such as incomplete re-oxidation and cysteic acid formation.

Moreover, the stylist or the client may try to "repair" the unexpected result by repetition of the permanent waving process, which is not recommended as multiple treatments, as well as the combination of perming and bleaching or colouring in the same session lead to heavily damaged hair. Electron microscopy reveals residual softening; even severe damage and complete removal of the hair surface (Figures 29.10 and 29.11).

Other instrumental methods can further detect the degree of damage. These include hair tensile testing, elasticity, curl hold, swelling behavior, and static charging [2,20]. Chemical damage of hair may also be assessed by analyzing dissolved hair proteins [29,30] and hair lipids [30]. Residual presence of cystine and cysteic acid are signs of a weakened hair structure [30]. Table 29.3 lists examples for hair and skin symptoms indicating mistakes during a perm treatment [25,31–34]).

Although ammonium thioglycolate has been reported to have a low sensitization potential, occasionally sensitization, skin irritation, contact dermatitis [33,34], or seborrhea might occur [32]. If itching, burning, and redness occur, they are typically confined to the neck and scalp margins after prolonged con-

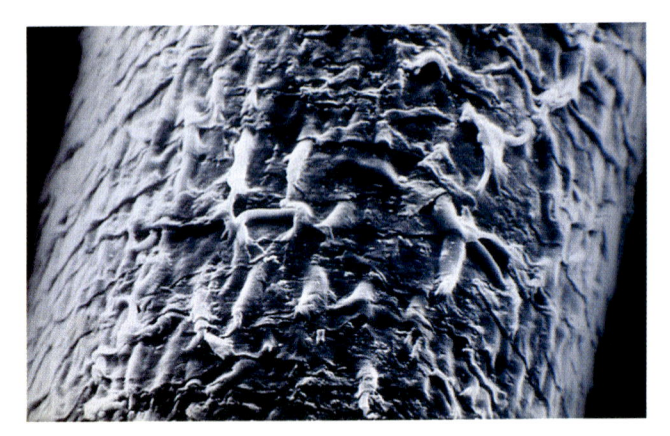

Figure 29.10 The curtain-like structure of a hair surface indicates heavy perming damage.

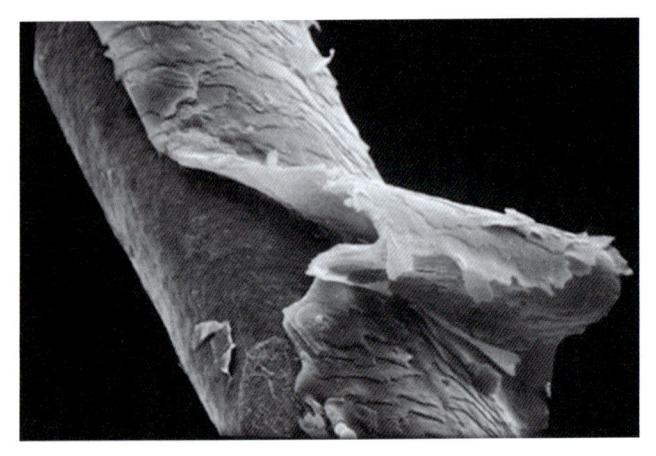

Figure 29.11 A bleach applied immediately after a perming treatment chips off the cuticle as a whole (SEM ×700).

tact with perm solution [31]; however, high levels of alkalinity and heat [33,34] may also precipitate irritation. Scalp skin damage seldom occurs. Scalp skin, which contains keratin proteins like hair, is less reactive to reduction by thioglycolate. This contributes to a lower swelling response of the skin than hair (22% vs. 38%) and the lower cystine content and hydrophobic nature of skin vs. more cystine and hydrophilicity in hair [35]. The skin is more susceptible to surfactants, however, causing the hairdresser's hands to be affected by an allergy to perms. High exposure to surfactants for example by frequently shampooing clients´ hair, can lead to the skin of the hairdressers hands to be softened and displaying a reduced barrier function. In this case, monothioglycolate esters found in acid waves may cause skin reactions [31].

Permanent hair waving is a sophisticated process that can achieve a powerful transformation of the appearance of a person with longer hair. Due to the complexity of the use of perming products, considerable experience and care is needed during and after the application process, to ensure a desirable outcome of the treatment as well the personal safety.

Table 29.3 Symptoms of hair/skin damage by perm products.

Symptom	How it happened
Hair loss (rarely)	Telogen hair effluvium Temporary contact allergic reaction
Hair breakage	False hair quality diagnosis
Near root	Perm choice too strong for fine or pre-damaged/ bleached hair Stress on root hair by tight winding or rubber band Winding against hair growth direction
In hair length	Hair growth with thinning diameters Winding on curlers with " fish hooks" Incomplete neutralization
Near tip ends	Forgot pre-treatment with equalizer Processing without wrap end paper protection Excess perm solution stored by hair tips
Hair modification (consumer complaints)	
Unwanted kinky curls	Permanent waving power of product too high Curler thickness too thin Processing time with heat too long
Limp hair/curls without springiness	Loose winding, impaired protein creep Time set incorrectly, application levels too low,
Wet hair feels plastified, spongy, extensible	Over-processed by extended application Loss of keratin elasticity Increased hydrophilicity Neutralization too short
Dry hair feels rough, brittle, poor combability, "matting", is dull, ready to break	Intermediate rinsing too short Increased hair surface friction by shrunken cuticle cells Loss of hair lipids and proteins
Highlighted natural colour or tint	Dissolution of natural pigment/tint Excess perm conditions
Skin damage	
Redness	Too much heat (heat rollers, hood defect)
Pustules	Skin swelling during extensive pre-wash
Irritant skin	Soaked cotton pads for face protection not removed

References

1 Jollès P, Zahn H, Höcker H, eds. (1997) *Formation and Structure of Human Hair*. Basel: Birkhäuser Verlag.
2 Robbins CR. (2012) *Chemical and Physical Behaviour of Human Hair*, 5th edn. Berlin, Heidelberg: Springer Verlag.
3 Schwan-Jonczyk A, Schmidt CU. (2007) Hair geometry changes during lifespan. Proceedings of the 15th International Hair Science Symposium, HAIRS 07, Banz.
4 Robbins CR. (1983) Load elongation of single hair fiber coils. *J Soc Cosmet Chem* **34**, 227–39.
5 Wolfram L, Dika E, Maibach HI Hair anthropology, or Swift JA. The transverse dimensions of human head hair. (2007) In: BerardescaE, LevequeJL, MaibachHI, eds. *Ethnic Skin and Hair*. New York: Informa Healthcare.

6. Schwan-Jonczyk A, Arlt T, Maresch G, Schonert D. (2003) *Curls, Curls, Curls*. Darmstadt: Wella AG (inhouse publication).
7. Franbourg A, et al. (2005) Evaluation of product efficacy. In: Bouillon C, Wilkinson J, eds. *The Science of Hair Care*. Boca Raton, FL: CRC Press, pp. 351–76.
8. Swift JA. (1997) *Fundamentals of Human Hair Science*. Weymouth UK: Micelle Press.
9. Franbourg A, Leroy F. (2005) Hair structure and physicochemical properties. In: Bouillon C, Wilkinson J, eds. *The Science of Hair Care*. Boca Raton, FL: CRC Press, pp. 351–76.
10. Marshall RC. (1986) Nail, claw, hoof and horn keratin. In: Bereiter-Hahn J, Matoltsy AG, Richards KS, eds. *Biology of the Integument II*. Berlin: Springer Verlag, pp. 722–38.
11. Zahn H. (1977) Wool as a biological composite structure. *Lenzinger Ber* **42**, 19–34.
12. Umprecht JG, Patel K, Bono KP. (1977) Effectiveness of reduction and oxidation in acid and alkaline permanent waving. *J Soc Cosmet Chem* **28**, 717–32.
13. Lang G, Schwan-Jonczyk A. (2004) Haarverformungsmittel (Hair waving preparations). In: Umbach W, ed. *Kosmetik und Hygiene*, 3rd edn. Weinheim: Wiley-VCH Verlag, pp. 264–78.
14. Schwan A, Zang R. (1993) *Method and apparatus for the shaping treatment of hair wound on to rollers, including human hair*. Wella AG EP0321939B1.
15. Borish ET. (1997) Hair waving. In: Johnson D, ed. *Hair and Hair Care, Cosmetic Science and Technology*, Vol. 17. Marcel Dekker, pp. 167–90.
16. Garcia ML, Nadgorny EM, Wolfram LJ. (1990) Letter to the Editor: Physicochemical changes in hair during permanent waving. *J Soc Cosmet Chem* **41**, 149–53.
17. Wickett R, Savaides A. (1993) Permanent waving of hair. In: Knowlton J, Pearce S, eds. *Handbook of Cosmetic Science and Technology*, 1st edn. Oxford: Elsevier Sciencc, pp. 511–34.
18. Shipp JJ. (1996) Hair care products. In: Williams DF, Schmitt WH, eds. *Chemistry and Technology of the Cosmetics and Toiletries Industry*, 2nd edn. Chapman & Hall.
19. Dallal JA. (2000) Permanent waving, hair straightening and depilatories. In: Rieger MM, ed. *Harry's Cosmeticology*, 8th edn. New York: Chemical Publishing, Chapter 32.
20. Clausen T, Schwan-Jonczyk A, Lang G, Clausen T, Liebscher KD, et al. (2006) Hair preparations. In: *Ullmann's Encyclopedia of Industrial Chemistry*, 7th edn, Vol. A 12, Weinheim: Wiley, pp. 571.
21. Shansky A. (2008) Antichaotropic salts for stabilizing cysteine in perm solutions. In: Koslowsky AC, Allured J, eds. *Hair Care: From Physiology to Formulation*. Carol Stream, IL: Allured, pp. 341–6.
22. Technische Regeln für Gefahrstoffe, Friseurhandwerk TRGS530 (2007) GMBL, Bundesministerium für Arbeit und Soziales.
23. Lee AE, Bozza JB, Huff S, Mettric R. (1988) Permanent waves: an overview. *Cosmet Toiletr* **103**, 37–56.
24. EU Council Directive of 27 July 1976 on the approximation of the laws of the Member States relating to cosmetic products (76/768/EEC).
25. Meisterburg M, Riehl U, et al. (2007) *Friseurwissen (0Hairdresser's knowledge)*. Schmidt W, ed. Troisdorf, Germany: Bildungsverlag EINS. Available at www.bildungsverlag1.de
26. IKW information. (2008) Undesireable effects of cosmetics. Available at www.ikw.org.
27. Draelos ZD. (2000) Safety and performance. In: Rieger MM, ed. *Harry's Cosmeticology*, 8th edn. New York: Chemical Publishing, Chapter 34.
28. Hourseau C, Cottin M, Baverel M, Meurice P, Riboulet-Delmas G. (2005) Hair product safety. In: Bouillon C, Wilkinson J, eds. *The Science of Hair Care*. Boca Raton, FL: CRC Press, pp. 351–76.
29. Han M, Chun J, Lee J, Chung C. (2008) Effects of perms on changes of protein and physicomorphological properties in human hair. *J Soc Cosmet Chem* **59**, 203–15.
30. Hilterhaus-Bong S, Zahn H. (1989) Protein and lipid chemical aspects of permanent waving treatments. *Int J Cosmet Sci* **11**, 164–74, 221–34.
31. Wilkinson JD, Shaw S. (2005) Adverse reactions to hair products. In: Boullion C, Wilkinson J, eds. *The Science of Hair Care*. Boca Raton, FL: CRC Press, p. 521.
32. Bergfeld WF. (1981) Side effects of hair products on the scalp and hair. In: Orfanos CE, Montagna W, Stüttgen G, eds. *Hair Research*. Berlin: Springer Verlag, pp. 507–12.
33. Ishihara M. (1981) Some skin problems due to hair preparations. In: Orfanos CE, Montagna W, Stüttgen G, eds. *Hair Research*. Berlin: Springer Verlag, pp. 536–42.
34. Orfanos CE, Sterry W, Leventer T. (1979) Hair and hair cosmetic treatments. In: Orfanos CE, ed. *Hair and Hair Diseases*. Stuttgart: G. Fischer Verlag, pp. 853–85.
35. Robbins CR, Fernee KM. (1983) Some observations on the swelling of human epidermal membrane. *J Soc Cosmet Chem* **34**, 21–34.

CHAPTER 30
Hair Straightening

Harold Bryant, Felicia Dixon, Angela Ellington, and Crystal Porter
L'Oréal Institute for Ethnic Hair and Skin Research, Chicago, IL, USA

> **BASIC CONCEPTS**
> - Hair is straightened to improve manageability and provide style versatility.
> - To straighten hair, an alteration of the cortex must occur.
> - To achieve temporary straightening – a lower energy process – hydrogen bonds and salt linkages are altered while permanent straightening is achieved through the modification of covalent bonds, which requires more energy.
> - Permanent hair straightening can be accomplished with ammonium thioglycolate, sulfites, and hydroxide.

Introduction

The desire for straight hair was once attributed to a "universal" vision of beauty and social status associated with straight hair; however, recent information links this style preference to improved manageability and style versatility. In order to achieve the straight look, it is necessary to transform the natural hair configuration, which has been linked to the shape of the follicle. Bernard et al. [1,2] found that the asymmetric protein expression in curved follicles was associated with the formation of curly hair. At this time, it is not possible to straighten hair by changing the shape of the follicle. However, it is possible to straighten hair based on its chemical composition. For mature hair, the composition is generally the same and consists of roughly 90% protein with smaller quantities of water, lipids, and minerals but does not vary by degree of curl, despite differences that exist in the early stages of hair production. To understand how hair can be transformed, it is important to know the different components of hair. Hair is made-up of three macro structures including the cuticle, cortex, and medulla, the latter being of little significance. The major morphologic part of the hair is the cortex, which is made up of highly organized α-helical proteins packed in a cystine-rich matrix. To straighten hair, an alteration of the cortex must occur.

There are three types of bonds in hair: hydrogen, electrostatic salt linkages, and covalent, each consecutively requiring more energy to break. Based on the bonds that can be affected, there are two categories of straightening: temporary and permanent. To achieve temporary straightening, a lower energy process is required involving alteration of hydrogen bonds and salt linkages while permanent straightening is achieved through the modification of covalent bonds, which requires more energy. Thermal appliances can be used to disrupt and rearrange the weaker hydrogen bonds and salt linkages required for temporary straightening. Depending on the approach, the results can last from a few days to several months. However, permanent straightening is obtained through a chemical process that alters the protein structure by cleaving and reforming covalent bonds, preventing the hair from returning to its natural curly state until it grows out from the scalp.

The following are usually considered when choosing the type of hair straightening process or treatment: degree of curl, degree of desired straightness, point of service, convenience, environmental conditions, and the desired frequency of straightening. All of these are important; however, the degree of curl in hair may be the most influential because it impacts other desired attributes. It is often subjectively described and ranges from various degrees of wavy to tightly curled. These descriptors are relative and can be confusing because they often overlap. Thus, the L'Oréal Curl Classification was recently developed to quantitatively describe the degree of curl in hair (Figure 30.1) [3]. This classification used hair from around the world and identified eight distinct curl types, where the degree of curl increases directly with number. People with curl types I–IV often have concerns about hair frizz and volume while higher curl types are more concerned about manageability. Thermal techniques can be used to achieve straight hair for all curl types but, typically, curl types V and above are difficult to straighten permanently without the use of hydroxide-based systems.

Cosmetic Dermatology: Products and Procedures, Second Edition. Edited by Zoe Diana Draelos.
© 2016 John Wiley & Sons, Ltd. Published 2016 by John Wiley & Sons, Ltd.

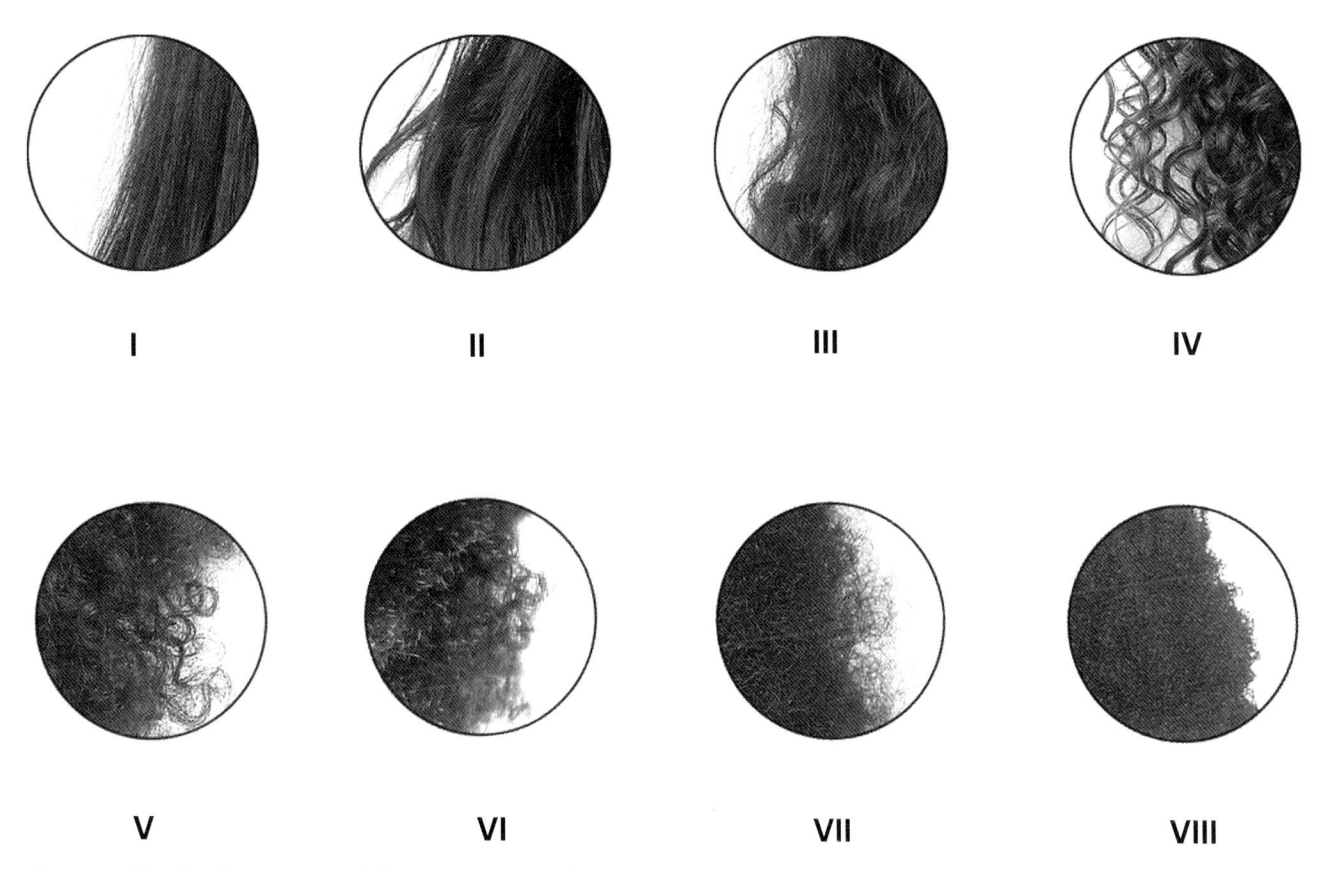

Figure 30.1 Hair classification types to differentiate the degree of curl in hair.

Hair straightening appliances and chemicals are centuries old; however, instrument designs and formulations have evolved to improve effectiveness while limiting the negative attributes. New materials are used for the heated surface of flat irons and product formulas have been modified and developed to protect hair and scalp and aid in the ease of application. In some markets, the combination of heat and chemicals is often used. This chapter briefly reviews the most common straightening practices, including a description of the procedures and perceived advantages and disadvantages.

Thermal processing

The use of thermal appliances dates back to the Egyptian period and is still considered to be a necessity to most women in today's world. In the Egyptian period, hot metal was used to straighten hair. A less aggressive method was popularized in the late 1800s with the invention of the blow-dryer; the handheld version for home use became available in the 1920s. This increased the ability for women with curl types I–IV to have a variety of temporary and permanent styles (hot waving).

Because curl types V–VIII were inherently more resistant to reconfiguration, there was a specific need to straighten these hair types. This was achieved with the popularization of the hot comb combined with pressing oil, attributed to Madame C.J. Walker in the early 1900s. The hot comb, still in use today, is a metal comb heated to temperatures reaching 450°F. Whether utilizing a hot comb, professional tongs heated in a Marcel oven, or one of the electronic devices such as a blow-dryer, curling iron, or flat iron, the process involves using heat and mechanical stress. These common thermal appliances represent an alternative way for people with naturally curly hair to achieve manageability and straight hair styles.

The combination of heat and mechanical stress, in the form of combing or brushing while blow-drying and smoothing with the other devices, straightens hair by rearranging hydrogen bonds. Once straightened, the new configuration of the hair is only temporary and will revert back to its natural state after exposure to moisture from any source such as environmental conditions and perspiration. Temperatures of thermal appliances typically range from 150–232°C (302–450°F). While thermal processing is considered temporary in terms of styling, it can have a permanent effect on hair. For example, the proteins in hair can start to denature at high temperatures. Protein denaturation is a process by which proteins are irreversibly altered by an external stimulus, and for hair can result in decreased fiber integrity. The denaturation temperature is 235–250°C (455–482°F) and 155–160°C

(311–320°F) for dry and wet hair, respectively [4–6]. The upper temperature limits for some of the appliances exceeds the denaturation temperature for wet and dry hair so care must be taken to avoid repeated applications and overheating.

Of all heat appliances currently available to straighten hair, the flat iron is rapidly becoming the most popular; therefore, it is the focus of technologic advancements. Important attributes of a good flat iron are the ability to provide even heat and maintain a consistent temperature. Recent improvements in temperature control promote thermal stability and coatings, including ceramic and titanium, provide durability and reduced friction. Reduced friction is critical to maintaining a smooth cuticle surface and reducing breakage during thermal processing. Other advances in materials include the incorporation of pure ceramic heating elements and minerals (tourmaline) that allow manufacturers to make claims about the positive effects of ions and far infrared radiation on the final state of the hair.

The product offerings associated with the use of thermal appliances typically contain hydrocarbon-based ingredients (e.g. petrolatum and mineral oil) and polymers (e.g. silicone-derived, cationic, and non-ionic) to condition, protect, and accommodate styling preferences. Because blow-drying typically starts in the wet state when hair is vulnerable to damage, conditioning polymers (e.g. polyquaternium 10) that improve wet combing by reducing frictional forces are typically used. Prior to heat application, products that contain ingredients such as sugars and silicones can be applied. Sugars help to increase thermal integrity while silicones protect the hair by acting as a thermal barrier. Silicones also can function as lightweight films whereas hydrocarbons are often used when a heavier coating is desired for style preferences.

Reducing agents

Reducing treatments are traditionally known to curl hair (hot and cold permanent waving); however, they can also be used to straighten hair. The chemistry involves a two-step process where the disulfide bonds in hair keratin are cleaved in the first (reducing) step followed by oxidization in the second step to form new disulfide bonds (Scheme 30.1). The difference between straightening and waving using reducing agents is the configuration of hair prior to oxidation and the form of the product during the reducing step. The reducing product for waving the hair is usually a liquid and the hair is curled using rollers before oxidizing. For straightening, the product is usually in the form of a thick cream so that the viscosity of the product can assist in holding hair fibers in a straightened configuration during manipulation. The most commonly used reducing agents in this process are ammonium thioglycolate (thiols) and sulfite.

Ammonium thioglycolate

Thioglycolate straighteners come in several product strengths. Treatment procedures and strength should be based on the hair attributes according to product recommendations. For curl types V–VIII, these products usually leave the hair with residual curl so the result can be disappointing if a straight style is desired. In addition, the hair can feel dry as a result of the treatment; thus, products that contain glycerin are used to provide moisture. Thioglycolate straighteners can be used on hair that has been previously colored or permed; however, it is not recommended for bleached or relaxed hair.

In addition to traditional thiol straighteners, a new technique is becoming popular that includes the incorporation of heat with thiol-based cream products. These treatments are used

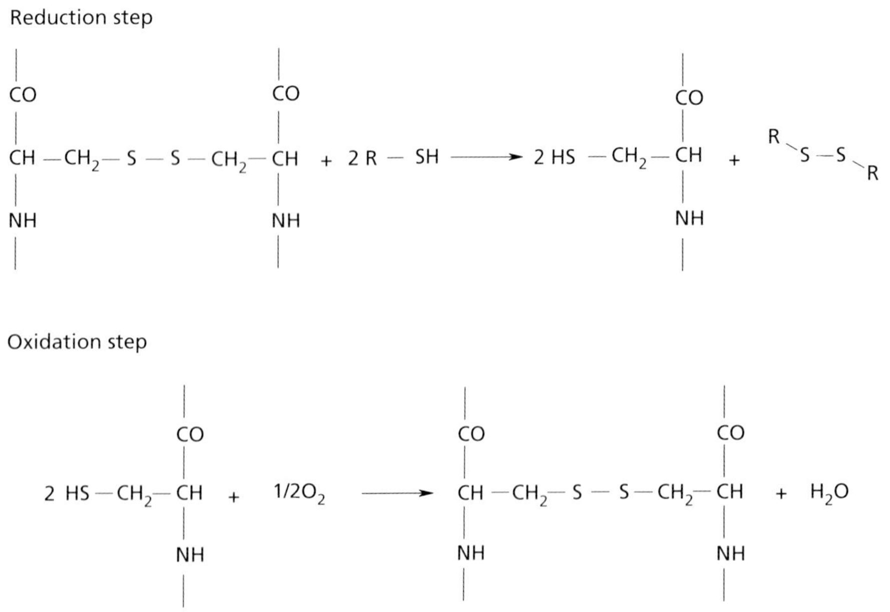

Scheme 30.1

Table 30.1 Common names for thiol-based straighteners that use heat.

Culture that introduced the technique	Popular thiol-based treatments
Japanese/Filipino	Hair rebonding
	Thermal reconditioning and restructuring
	Ion retexturizing
	Bio ionic system
	Japanese hair restructuring
	Straightening and reconditioning
	Japanese straightening perm
Brazilian	Chocolate, strawberry, kelp, milk, sugar, passion, mint, gold, orchid, French, gumbo, etc. treatment (or brushing)
	Brazilian keratin treatments (may contain up to 2% formaldehyde)

Note: To be comprehensive, it is cautiously noted that products containing or that are altered with formaldehyde (formol) at higher than approved levels (0.2% as an antimicrobial) are sometimes used to straighten hair. However, formaldehyde is classified as a probable human carcinogen by the Environmental Protection Agency and should not be used to straighten hair.

Even though sulfite straighteners have been around for decades, they are less common than hydroxide relaxers because they tend to result in less effective straightening of highly curled hair (types VI–VIII). However, they are believed to be less irritating to the scalp. The decrease in straightening efficacy may be related back to the reactivity of the disulfide bonds, which depends on the pH of the active solution. The maximum reactivity is reached at pH 4–6, but sulfites are not stable at such low pH conditions [8,9]. Because of this, commercial products generally range in pH from 6.5 to 7.5. At pH 7, only about 15% of the cystine residues can be reduced [10]. The first step of the reaction mechanism involves a reduction of the cystine via a nucleophilic reaction similar to thioglycolate, with the exception of the formation of Bunte salt (Scheme 30.2). To lock the hair into the desired conformation, a neutralizing solution is used which typically contains sodium carbonate or bicarbonate. The application procedure is similar to that of a thioglycolate straightener except no oxidant is used, resulting in poor or modest straightening.

to permanently straighten and/or reduce volume in curl types I–V. They are commonly used on Asian and Brazilian hair and go by several names that are listed in Table 30.1. Even though there are several names, they all use similar processes to achieve hair characteristics that consumers describe as straight, soft, and shiny. The main point of differentiation between this new treatment and the traditional straightening method is the application of heat prior to the oxidation step for the Asian and Brazilian treatments. Details about the specific procedure can be found in the appendix. This straightening technique is not recommended for natural hair that is higher than curl type V, particularly hair from people of African descent because it is inherently more fragile than other hair [7].

After a period of time, the processes described above will need to be repeated to the new hair growth because of its natural configuration. The treatment should only be performed on the new growth, referred to as a "touch-up," to minimize overlapping of treatments which may result in overprocessed hair. It is recommended that the time between treatments is maximized, with a minimum of 6 weeks, depending on the rate of hair growth.

Sulfite

Sulfites are an additional class of reducing agents that can be used for hot waving or straightening depending on the procedure.

Hydroxide straighteners

According to legend, Garrett A. Morgan was the first person to stumble upon a chemical to permanently straighten hair in the early 1900s [11]. While experimenting with substances to reduce the heat of friction during sewing, he wiped his hands on a cloth that was made of curly pony fur. Later, he found that the fur had been straightened. Following trials on different types of hair, including his own, he started selling the G.A. Morgan Hair Refining Cream. To this day, the identity of this substance is a mystery, but the first known composition for chemically straightening hair was formulated in household kitchens in the 1930s. This contained a chemical mixture of potato starch, lard, egg, and sodium or potassium hydroxide. Because of its corrosive nature, it was advised to protect or base the scalp with petrolatum before treatment. The use of this concoction led to the development of relaxers.

The first commercially available relaxer, based on sodium hydroxide (lye), was introduced in the 1950s by Johnson Products. Even though the relaxer formula included petrolatum, basing the scalp was still a requirement to minimize scalp irritation. The relaxer technology continued to improve in the early to mid 1960s with the invention of the no-base relaxer. This version incorporated higher percentages of petrolatum and mineral oil in the formula and decreased the amount of sodium hydroxide to make it less irritating, thus it claimed to eliminate the need to base the scalp.

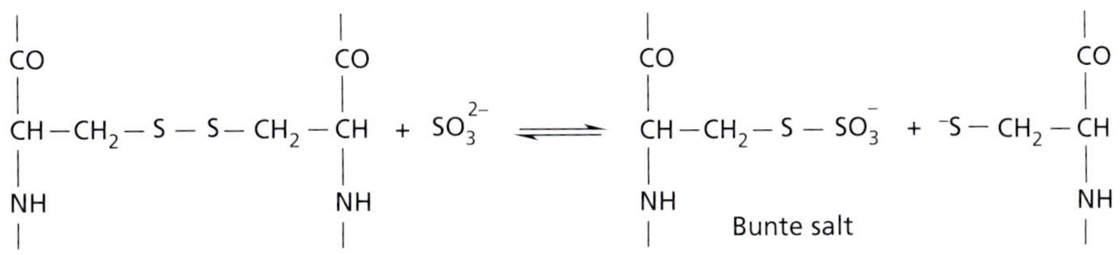

Scheme 30.2

$$\text{CH(CO)(NH)}-\text{CH}_2-\text{S}-\text{S}-\text{CH}_2-\text{CH(CO)(NH)} + \text{SO}_3^{2-} \rightleftharpoons \text{CH(CO)(NH)}-\text{CH}_2-\text{S}-\text{SO}_3^- + {}^-\text{S}-\text{CH}_2-\text{CH(CO)(NH)}$$

Bunte salt

In the late 1970s, the first no-lye relaxer was marketed that significantly reduced the amount of irritation during treatment [12]. The technology uses a two-part system where a calcium hydroxide cream is mixed with a guanidine carbonate liquid activator to produce guanidine hydroxide.

Several other relaxer versions were introduced over time that improved the product attributes, the cosmetic properties, and integrity of the hair. This was achieved through the addition of conditioning agents such as cationic polymers and by incorporating various alkali metal hydroxides in both product forms, mix or no-mix [13,14]. The most commonly used hydroxides are sodium, guanidine, lithium, and potassium (see Table 30.2 for definitions of key terms).

Chemistry of relaxing

Amino acid analysis of relaxed hair hydrolysates indicates lanthionine is the primary product of the reaction. The formation of lanthionine can occur via two pathways. The first is through a binuclear nucleophilic substitution reaction [10]. The second is beta-elimination that is initiated by abstraction of the hydrogen beta to the disulfide (Scheme 30.3) [15]. This results in the formation of dehydroalanine, cysteinate ion, and sulfur. Dehydroalanine is a highly reactive intermediate that continues to react with cysteine and lysine moieties in hair to form lanthionine and lysinoalanine, respectively. It can also react with ammonia to form beta-aminoalanine. The new thioether bonds (lanthionine) are stable in the presence of reducing agents, such as thioglycolate or sulfite, compared to cystine. This is evidenced by the decrease in solubility of hair protein and the inability to permanently curl relaxed hair.

While lanthionization is popularly believed to be the cause of permanent straightening of curly hair, Wong et al. [16] believe that it is not the critical step in hair straightening. They propose that the permanent straightening depends on supercontraction of the fiber. They report that fiber supercontraction is what "locks" the fiber into the straight configuration and the formation of lanthionine is a by-product rather than a requirement.

Table 30.2 Vocabulary list of select terms related to straightening curly hair.

Relaxer	Hydroxide technology used to permanently straighten curly hair. It is sometimes mistakenly referred to as a "perm"
Lye relaxer	Technology that commonly utilizes sodium hydroxide as the active ingredient
No-lye relaxer	Non-sodium hydroxide-based system that includes but is not limited to guanidine and lithium hydroxides. Some of these products require mixing prior to use; those that do not are sometimes referred to as no-lye no-mix
No-base relaxer	A relaxer that may not require basing the scalp with a petrolatum product prior to relaxer application
Texturizer	A lower concentration version of relaxer used to permanently reduce or loosen curl in hair
Perm	Thiol-based products used to permanently curl hair according to a sequential reduction–oxidation process

Application

The relaxer process involves a chemical reaction in addition to mechanical manipulation, which involves the action of smoothing the hair into the desired configuration during application. This can be accomplished with the back of a comb, an application brush, or the fingers. However, the most recommended tool is a comb. Applicator brushes can increase the chance of scalp irritation and the use of fingers is not suggested because of the caustic nature of the relaxer ingredients. The initial relaxer is applied to the full length of the fiber. Subsequent treatments are only applied to new growth, which typically occurs within 6–8 weeks. The exact period of time should be determined based on the amount of new hair growth, which varies with the individual. For example, hair growth rates can range from approximately 4 mm/month to 18 mm/month [17].

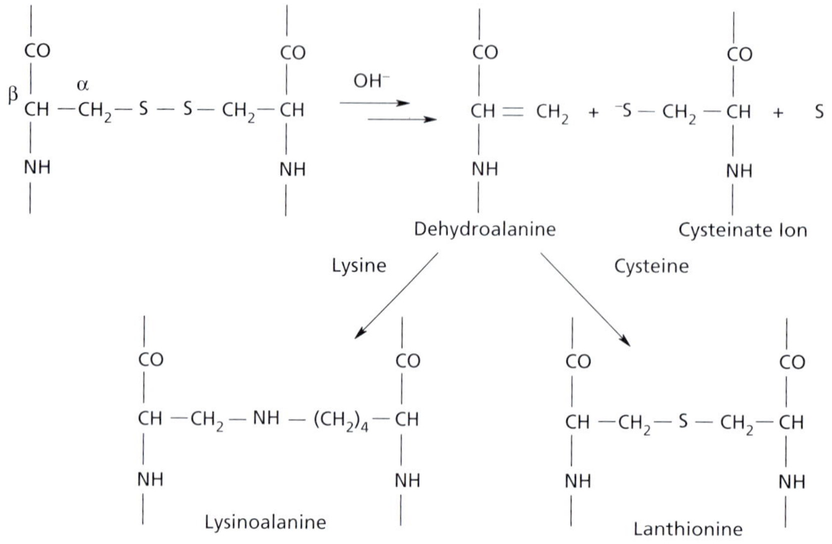

Scheme 30.3

Several key factors are used to determine the relaxer type, such as hair diameter, degree of curl, porosity, and type of prior chemical treatments. To help maintain the integrity of hair, it is important to follow the directions on the package carefully. Overprocessing and improper neutralization are problems that are commonly associated with relaxer misuse. Similar to thermal processing, repeat application on the same section of hair and treating the hair longer than the recommended time can result in overprocessing and may result in hair breakage. Determination of proper application time can be achieved by performing the recommended strand test. To insure proper removal of the relaxer, hair should be rinsed thoroughly followed by the application of a neutralizing shampoo, sometimes referred to as chelating or decalcifying. These shampoos are acidic with a pH typically ranging from 4.5 to 5.5. The neutralizing step is an important part of the relaxer process because it helps return the hair to a neutral pH. This is necessary because, at high pH, hair swells up to 70–80% during relaxing making the hair susceptible to damage [18].

Effect of relaxers on hair

In 2006, Yang and Barbosa [19] performed a national study to obtain consumer perceptions of relaxers. From this study, consumer responses on the effects from relaxer use were grouped into three categories including scalp irritation, hair quality, and relaxer efficiency. Users of lye technology reported a higher incidence of scalp irritation while no-lye users experienced more hair quality issues. The same study showed that consumers were more likely to take action for hair quality issues and more often seek advice from a stylist as opposed to consulting a dermatologist or physician. In a separate study, it was noted that those who frequently obtain services at a salon, more than 50% of them were unaware of the specific relaxer type being used [20].

All hydroxide-based relaxers follow the same chemistry and are designed to straighten hair but to varying degrees. Due to the high pH, relaxers cause swelling of the fiber, cuticle abrasion, loss of the hydrophobic lipid layer, an increase in porosity, a loss in tensile strength, and an increase in plasticity.[1] All of these affects weaken the hair compared with its natural state. The swelling and de-swelling of the hair during the process may in part, be responsible for loss in fiber strength as it can result in cracks proposed to be related to the change in osmotic pressure also associated with permanent waving [18]. In addition to cracks, cuticle swelling may cause cuticle erosion. Figure 30.2 shows the progression of the cuticle surface during the relaxer

---

[1] Plasticity: a material property whereby it undergoes irreversible deformation when a high enough force is applied.

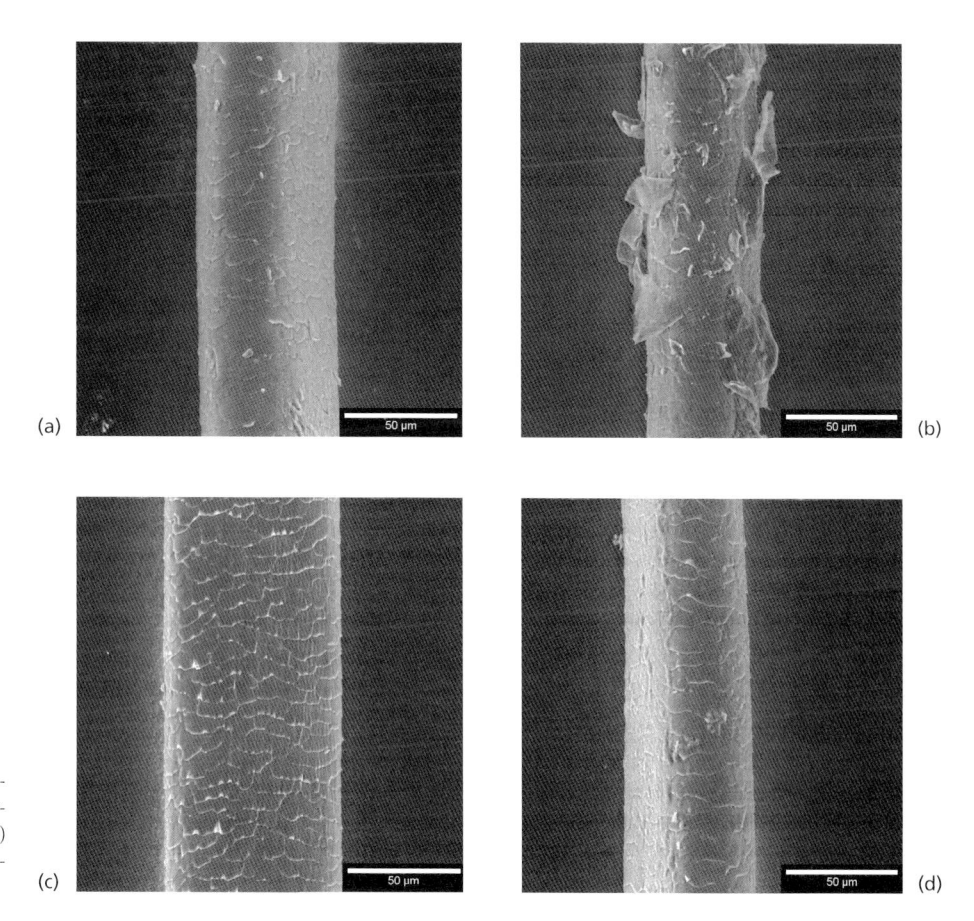

Figure 30.2 Scanning electron micrograph images of hair fibers under different treatment conditions, (a) virgin; (b) after relaxer rinse only; (c) after neutralization; (d) after conditioning.

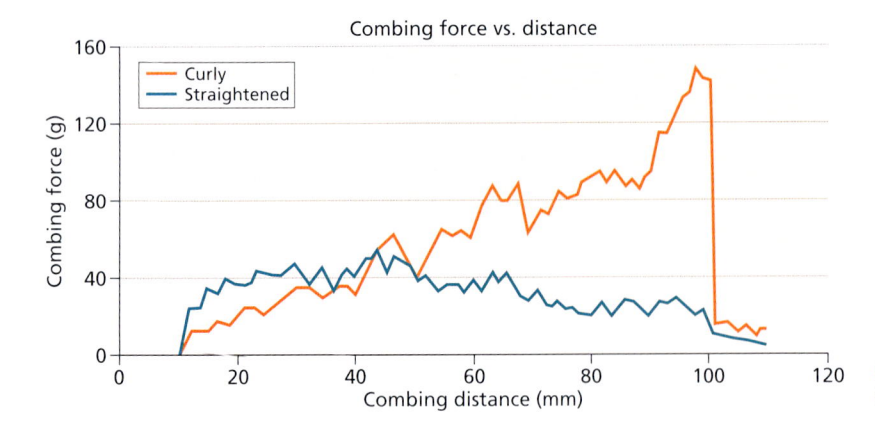

Figure 30.3 Combing profiles of curly and straightened hair.

process. After the relaxer has been rinsed from the hair before neutralizing, the image shows the presence of cuticle scales that have been abstracted from the hair fiber but still remain on the hair. After neutralizing, the loose cuticle scales are removed. The images representing neutralized and conditioned fiber surfaces show that while relaxers erode cuticle layers from the hair, some amount of the protective layer is still present.

In addition to the cuticle, the cortex, which is mainly responsible for the hair's strength, is also affected during relaxing. The original protein linkages in hair are altered, and when this occurs the hair becomes more fragile. The decrease in break stress and increase in break extension indicates that the hair becomes weaker and is more prone to deformation after relaxing. Even though hair quality is compromised, the straightened configuration of hair increases combability as shown in Figure 30.3. This in turn helps to decrease breakage that is known to be associated with combing curly hair and mitigates further decreases in mechanical properties [21].

It is important to follow relaxer services with post-relaxer treatments such as conditioners to further enhance manageability and improve the quality of hair. A good conditioner should exhibit the following qualities: improved wet and dry combing, flyaway reduction, and surface protection of the hair. These qualities can be achieved by adding conditioning agents that will reduce the frictional force during combing. Key ingredients commonly used are conditioning agents such as polyquaternium-6, behentrimonium chloride, and hexadimethrine chloride. In addition, ceramides and panthenol are linked to increasing the cuticle integrity and relative strength of hair [22].

Although sodium hydroxide (lye) and guanidine (no-lye) relaxers straighten the hair via the same chemical pathway, some important differences exist between the two technologies. It is well established through published and unpublished studies that the guanidine systems are milder to the scalp causing less incidence of irritation [23]. In addition, unpublished laboratory studies indicate that guanidine systems create more lanthionine (7.4% vs 5.2% lanthionine) in the same time than the sodium hydroxide systems. The majority of sodium hydroxide relaxer users visit the salon while home users tend to use the guanidine system. These differences should be considered by professionals, home users, and dermatologists involved in deciding which relaxer system is most appropriate for individual use.

Conclusions

Hair straightening treatments are popular and can be used to achieve individually desired styles. However, care must be taken to decrease the chances of overprocessing that may occur when processes and chemical treatments are performed improperly. The future of straightening processes and treatments is only limited by science and technology. History shows that even though there have been major scientific advancements, the technology to straighten hair either temporarily or permanently still involves the use of heat with mechanical stress or chemical products. Over time, incremental improvements in thermal appliances and formulations for chemical treatments will continue to occur. Despite the advances, it will remain important to understand the advantages and disadvantages and proper techniques of each method based on personal style preference, hair type, and quality to reduce adverse effects.

Appendix

Thiol procedure with heat

After the hair is washed and towel-dried, the reducing cream is applied to a small section of hair for the recommended time for a strand test. The minimum time that it takes to achieve the level of curl reduction in that section is noted and the section of hair is rinsed after that time. The hair is then saturated with the cream and gently smoothed into a straight configuration. The cream should be left on the hair for the minimum time that was noted during the strand test; however, the time should not exceed the recommended time. The hair is rinsed thoroughly with water then the hair is 80% dried. A protecting smoother is applied to the hair and then a brush in conjunction with a blow-dryer or a flat iron is used to straighten the hair in small sections. The hair should be neutralized using an oxidizing solution which should be left on the hair for the recommended time during that step. To keep from drying out, the neutralizing solution is usually reapplied (for 5 minutes) and then the hair is rinsed abundantly with warm water followed by towel drying. The hair should be conditioned with a rinse-out conditioner and styled as desired. The time for the procedure can be up to 6 hours.

References

1. Lindelöf B, Forslind B, Hedblad MA, Kaveus U. (1988) Human hair form: Morphology revealed by light and scanning electron microscopy and computer aided three-dimensional reconstruction. *Arch Dermatol* **124**, 1359.
2. Thibaut S, Gaillard O, Bouhanna P, Cannell DW, Bernard BA. (2005) Human hair shape is programmed from the bulb. *Br J Dermatol* **152**, 630.
3. De la Mettrie R, Saint-Léger D, Loussouarn G, Garcel AL, Porter C, Langaney A. (2007) Shape variability and classification of human hair: a worldwide approach. *Hum Biol* **79**, 265.
4. Wortmann FJ, Sendelbach G, Popescu C. (2007) Fundamental DSC investigations of alpha-keratinous materials as basis for the interpretation of specific effects of chemical, cosmetic treatments on human hair. *J Cosmet Sci* **58**, 311–7.
5. Marsh JM, Clarke CJ, Meinert K, Dahlgren RM. (2007) High pressure differential scanning calorimetry of colorant products. *J Cosmet Sci* **58**, 621–7.
6. Wortmann FJ, Deutz H. (1993) Characterizing keratins using high-pressure differential scanning calorimetry. *J Appl Polym Sci* **48**, 137.
7. Porter C, Diridollou S, Dixon F, Bryant H, de la Mettrie R, Barbosa VH. Comparisons of curly hair from people of different ethnicities. (in press) *Int J Dermatol*.
8. Stoves JL. (1942) The reactivity of the cystine linkage in keratin fiber. I. The action of alkalies. *Trans Faraday Soc* **38**, 254.
9. Wolfram LJ. (1981) The reactivity of human hair: a review. In: Orfanos CE, Montagna W, Stuttgen G, eds. *Hair Research*. Berlin/Heidelberg, Germany: Springer Verlag, pp. 479–500.
10. Zviak C, Sabbagh A. (2008) Permanent waving and hair straightening. In: Bouillon C, Wilkinson J, eds. *The Science of Hair Care*, 2nd edn. New York: Informa Healthcare, pp. 201.
11. Haber L, Morgan GA. (1991) *Black Pioneers of Science and Invention*. Harcourt Trade.
12. de la Guardia MJ. (1981) *Hair straightening process and hair curling process and compositions therefore*. USA: Carson Products Company.
13. Darkwa AG, Newell F. (1994) *Conditioning hair relaxing system*. USA: Johnson Products Co. Inc.
14. Nguyen NV, Cannell DW. (2003) *Hair relaxer composition utilizing complexing agent activators*. USA: L'Oreal SA.
15. Tolgyesi E, Fang F. (1981) Action of nucleophilic reagents on hair keratin. In: OrfanosCE, MontagnaW, StuttgenG, eds. *Hair Research*. Berlin/Heidelberg, Germany: Springer Verlag, p. 116.
16. Wong M, Wis-Surel G, Epps J. (1994) Mechanism of hair straightening. *J Soc Cosmet Chem* **43**, 347.
17. Loussouarn G, Rawadi C, Genain G. (2005) Diversity of hair growth profiles. *Int J Dermatol* **44**, 6.
18. Shansky A. (1963) The osmotic behavior of hair during the permanent waving process as explained by swelling measurements. *J Soc Cosmet Chem* **14**, 427.
19. Yang G, Barbosa VH. Relaxer use and side effects. (in press) *Int J Dermatol*.
20. Bryant H, Yang G, Barbosa VH. (2005) Lye vs. no-lye relaxers: comparison of laboratory results and end-user perceptions. Presented at *Ethnic Hair and Skin: Advancing the Scientific Frontier*. Chicago, IL.
21. Khumalo NP, Doe PT, Dawer RPR, Ferguson DJP. (2000) What is normal black African hair? A light and scanning electron-microscopic study. *J Am Acad Dermatol* **43**, 814–20.
22. Bernard BA, Franbourg A, Francois AM, Hallegot P. (2002) Ceramide binding to African-American hair fibre correlates with resistance to hair breaking. *Int J Cosmet Sci* **24**, 1–12.
23. Syed AN, Ayoub H, Kuhajda A. (1998) Recent advances in Treating Excessively Curly Hair. *Cosmetics & Toiletries* **113**, 47–56.

CHAPTER 31

Hair Styling: Technology and Formulations

Thomas Krause[1] and Rene C. Rust[2]

[1] Wella/Procter & Gamble Service GmbH, Darmstadt, Germany
[2] GSK/Stiefel, Brentford, Middlesex, UK

> **BASIC CONCEPTS**
> - Hair styling aids arrange and maintain hair in a groomed position and impart conditioning, shine, body, and increased manageability.
> - There are a wide variety of styling aid product forms including hairsprays, gels, mousses, creams, waxes, lotions, and brilliantines. Heated styling implements such as blow-dryers and curling or straightening irons are also used to achieve style.
> - Polymers, emollients and waxes are the main functional ingredients in styling aids. Polymers bond hair strands together to provide hold. Emollients and waxes – amongst other ingredients – increase single hair fiber intercation and smooth cuticles, imparting shine and reduced hair frizz.
> - Styling aids are in general safe for skin and hair; however, misuse can result in hair damage.
> - Styling aids may be useful in improving the appearance of hair dermatologic conditions that result in thinning hair, hair dullness, or unruliness.

Introduction

The appearance of a person's hair, its length, shine, and smoothness, is a strong indicator of general age, health, and attractiveness [1]. Additionally, hair style or link to trends may be used to express personality traits or may make a social statement. Marie Antoinette was said to have changed her iconic hairstyle to promote her French identity [2], and who can forget the long flowing hair of the rebellious 1960s flower child? However, today as in the days of Marie Antoinette, hair does not grow naturally into the wide variety of hair styles desired by men and women – manipulation through brushing, setting, and the use of styling aids is necessary to smooth and arrange the hair into the desired style that is also maintained over time. The use of hair styling products to help achieve hair styles is also not new – Ancient Egyptians were known to use castor and other oils as hair dressings and bees wax to help style and plait wigs [3].

Styling aids not only correct the hair, but can also help transform hair for those with hair loss or hair damage resulting from medical conditions or other factors – hairsprays and other products can give lift to thinning hair, smoothing creams help tame unruly frizz, and gloss serums can help restore a more youthful shine. This chapter describes the wide variety of hair styling aids – their basic chemistry, utility, and potential issues that clinicians need to be aware of in their everyday practice.

Definitions

Hair styling is the process of reshaping the hair mass to an arrangement or style that can be maintained over time. Hair, by its nature, is easily reshaped when wet and dried or through the application of heat; however, because of hair's susceptibility to atmospheric humidity, these changes require the assistance of chemical styling aids to maintain the shape over time. Styling aids with polymers can help improve hair volume and height by increasing hair strand stiffness and hair fiber interactions. Styling aids with emollients and waxes can help smooth out frizz and increase hair shine by aligning fibers and reducing friction and can also have a conditioning effect on the hair fiber (Figure 31.1). Styling products, such as sprays, gels, and waxes, modify only the surface of hair – not the structure itself. These products are not designed to be permanent, unlike permanent waves and chemical straighteners, and the majority of these products are designed for easy removal by shampooing.

Physiology

Hair strands are made up of lengths of bundles of keratin polymer chains [4]. These chains are linked by two main types of bonds: strong and weak (Figure 31.2). Strong bonds are made of cystin amino acids and can only be broken chemically (e.g.

Cosmetic Dermatology: Products and Procedures, Second Edition. Edited by Zoe Diana Draelos.
© 2016 John Wiley & Sons, Ltd. Published 2016 by John Wiley & Sons, Ltd.

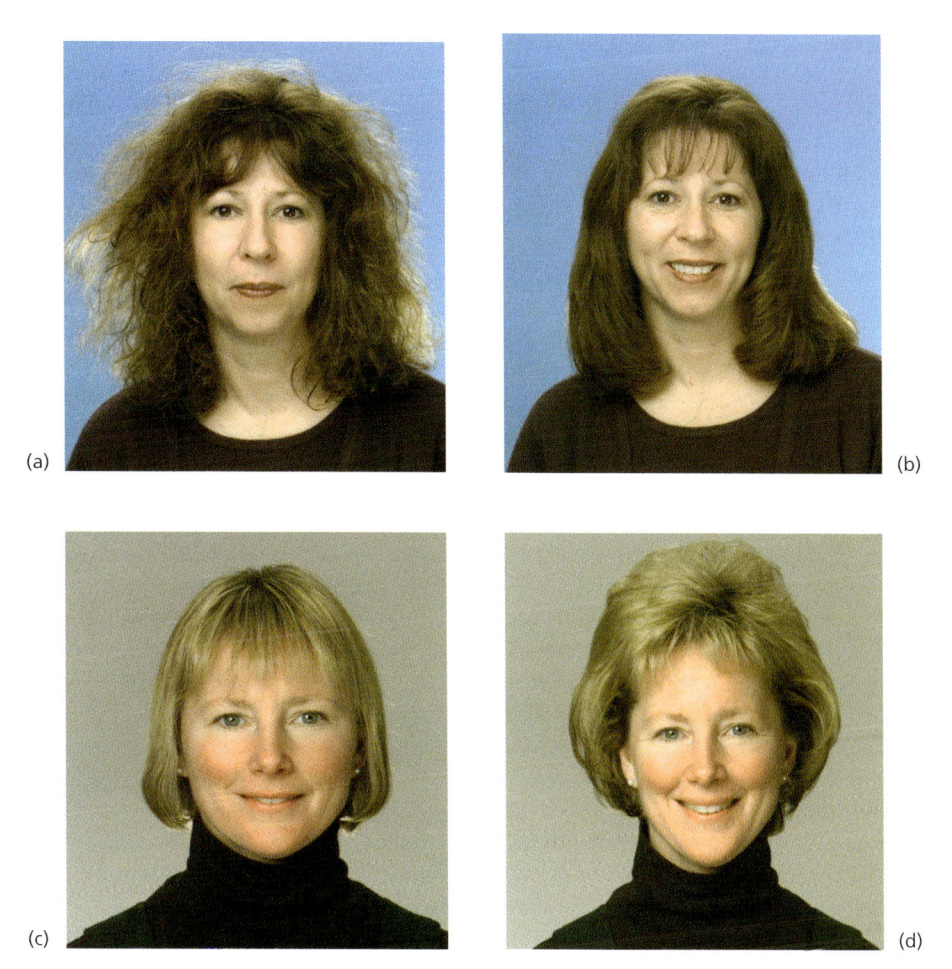

Figure 31.1 Styling aids can provide improved appearance of hair volume and smoothness. (a) Frizzy unruly hair dried without styling aids. (b) Frizzy unruly hair smoothed with application of styling aids. (c) Fine/thin hair dried without styling aids. (d) Fine/thin hair volumized through the application of styling aids.

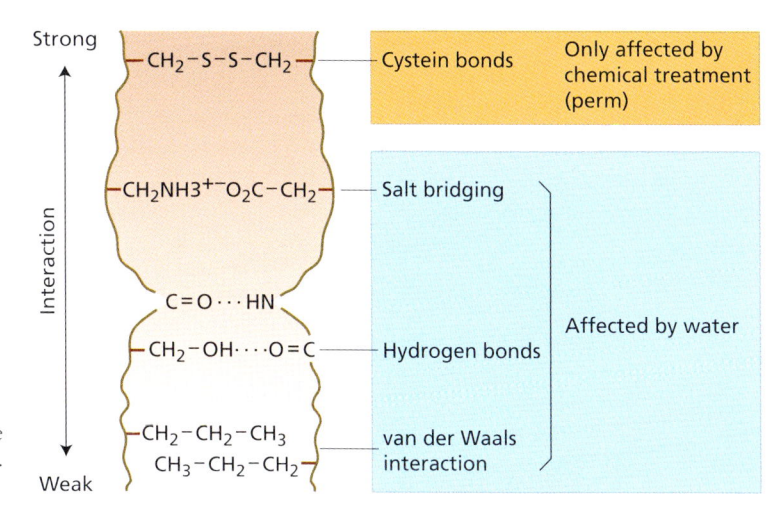

Figure 31.2 Mechanisms to stabilize hair structure and shape via keratin chain interactions. (Source: Umbach, 2004 [7]. Reproduced with permission of John Wiley & Sons.)

by permanent wave solutions). Weak bonds include van der Waals, salt bonds, and hydrogen bonds which can be affected by changes in water concentration alone [5,6].

Wet setting is the mechanism of shaping hair strands through controlled wetting and drying conditions. Hydrogen bonds can be easily opened by humidity in the air or water accessing the

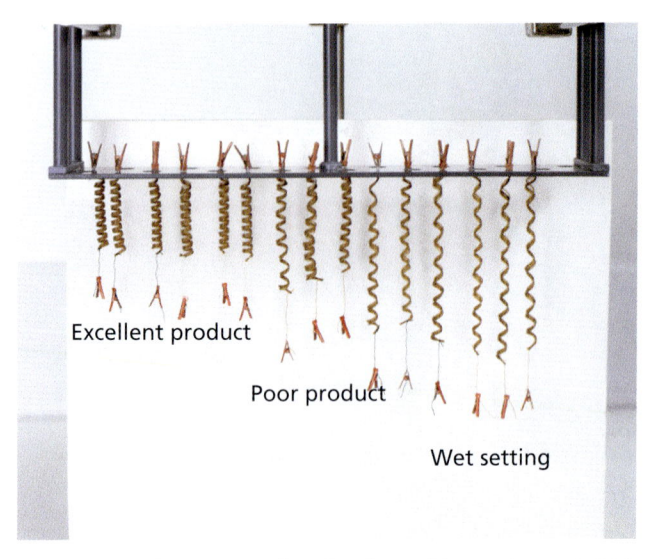

Figure 31.3 Curl retention with and without addition of spray in high humidity (85% relative humidity. (Source: Wella, 2001 [8]. Reproduced with permission of Pocter & Gamble.)

hair from the environment. Rearrangement of the hydrogen bonds will occur by removing water while drying and reformation of new bridges into a different shape by holding the hair strand in the desired shape while drying. Unfortunately, these new bonds are also susceptible to humidity from the environment and may revert back to their natural state of frizzy, curly or weak, straight hair over time.

Styling aids help make the styling process and finished style to be more independent of the molecular interactions inside the hair and more robust against environmental influences because the polymers are less affected by humidity. With the correct polymers, adequate deposition, and sufficient distribution of styling product, significant style holding power can be achieved. Figure 31.3 shows that hair treated with styling aids in a high humidity environment will keep the shape much longer than wet set hair alone.

Formulation

Because of very different hair structures, needs, and fashion trends a very broad range of styling products cover today's consumer needs and demands (Figure 31.4). Fundamentally, two different types of technology exist; both of these approaches have strong styling benefits and help to protect the hair, but have different styling properties:

1. Polymer-based formulations that cover hair with a film and form dry welds between hair strands:
   - Advantages: high mechanical strength, dry touch, gloss.
   - Disadvantages: will break with mechanical stress, cannot be reformed once broken except by rewetting.
2. Wax and emollient-based formulations that deposit hydrophobic material on hair. These hydrophobic materials do not dry over time and create fluid bonds that can be broken and reformed:
   - Advantages: no spot welds will break, interaction of single hair fibers can be opened and closed again, styling is remoldable.
   - Disadvantages: limited mechanical strength, in high concentrations can feel waxy/oily, potentially look negative on thin hair.

Polymer formulations

Hairsprays, gels, mousses, and liquid settings work on the principle of film-forming polymers. The active ingredients can be divided into three groups:

1. *Film-forming polymers:* main ingredient in application such as hairsprays and gels but also as minor ingredients in waxes.
2. *Conditioning and film-forming polymers:* usually in wet applications such as mousses to improve wet combability.
3. *Rheology modifier:* usually does not contribute to fixation but controls consistency of the product.

These film-forming active ingredients are modified to optimized performance by additional ingredients such as emollients (including silicone), solvents, plasticizers, fragrance, and preservatives. Table 31.1 provides a list of typical ingredients found in polymer-based styling aids.

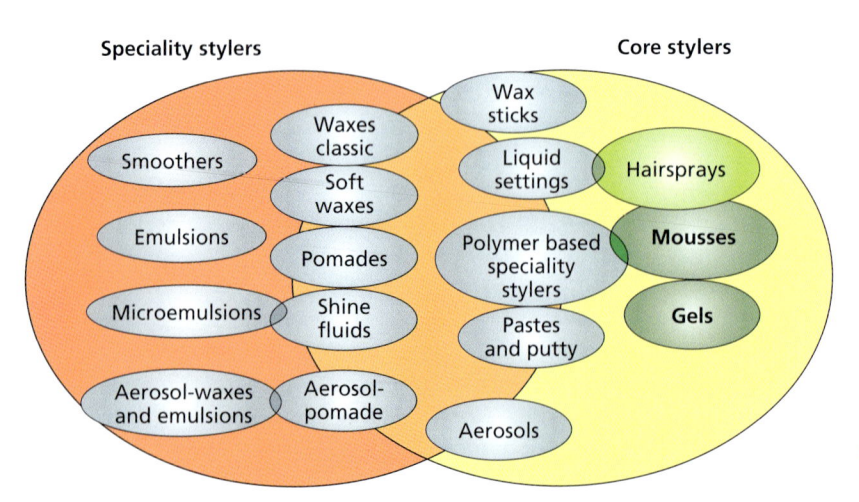

Figure 31.4 The broad range of modern styling aid forms and chemistries.

Table 31.1 Typical ingredients for polymer-based styling aids.

Ingredient (INCI)	Function	Hairspray	Gel	Mousse
PVP (polyvinylpyrrolidone)	Film former		x	x
Octylacrylamide/acrylates/butylamino-ethylmethacrylate copolymer	Film former	x		
PVP/VA copolymer (PVP/vinylacetate)	Film former	x	x	
PQ-11	Film former			x
PQ-16	Film former			x
PQ-4	Film former			x
Chitosan (derived from chitin)	Film former			x
Carbomer (cross-linked acrylic acid)	Rheology modifier		x	
Acrylates/ceteth-20-itaconate copolymer	Rheology modifier		x	
Hydroxyethylcellulose	Rheology modifier		x	
Alcohol	Solvent	x	(x)	(x)
Water	Solvent	(x)	x	x
Dimethicone	Plasticizer	x		
Panthenol	Moisturizer	x	x	x
Propane/butane	Propellant	x		x
DME (dimethylether)	Propellant	x		x
Ethylhexymethoxycinnamate	UV-absorber	x	x	x
PEG-40-hydrogenated castor oil	Emulsifier		x	x
Laureth-4	Emulsifier			x
Aminomethylpropanol	Neutralizer	x	x	
Phenoxyethanol	Preservative		x	x
Methylparaben	Preservative		x	x
Fragrance	Scent	x	x	x

Wax and emollient formulations

The area of waxes and emollients covers a broad range of products with a variety of different benefits and applications:
- *Pure waxes:* water-free formulations, often without preservatives. Mostly compact appearance, provide high hair control. Matte (i.e. low shine) derivatives are also called clay, paste, or putty.
- *Cream emulsions:* contain three main types of ingredients: water, emulsifiers, and oil/wax components. Consistency from soft lotion to rich cream.

Table 31.2 provides a list of typical ingredients found in wax and emollient-based styling aids.

Product forms, application, and uses

Hairsprays and liquid settings

Aerosol hairspray is one of the most widely used styling products. The ease of use and broad application areas make it a versatile tool for stylists and consumers. These products are usually finishing products and are applied in the very last step of styling on dry hair. Aerosol hairsprays contain a solution of polymer ingredients, alcohol, water, and liquefied propellants under pressure. The release of propellant pressure during dispensing results in a fine mist of polymer-containing liquid that deposit on the hair fibers, spreads, covers hair, and forms spot welds between the fibers (Figure 31.5).

Besides the aerosol version, hairsprays are also sold in non-aerosol sprays where distribution of the liquid to droplets is done mechanically by a pump. These sprays are perceived by consumers to be wetter than aerosol hairsprays on application because of the bigger droplet size resulting from the pump spray mechanism.

The main ingredients of hairsprays in general are:
- *Polymer:* film-forming polymer.
- *Solvents:* ethanol, water.
- *Propellant:* e.g. dimethylether (DME), propane/butane, fluorinated hydrocarbons (HF-152 A) for VOC-formulations in USA, water.
- *Additives:* e.g. silicones, UV-absorber, vitamins.
- *Fragrance*.

Non-aerosols have similar ingredients only without any propellant.

Hairsprays have been the target of regulatory restrictions ever since the banning of CFHC-based propellant compounds in the

Table 31.2 Typical ingredients in wax and emollient-based styling aids.

Ingredient (INCI)	Function	Wax	Cream
Carnauba wax	Hard wax	x	x
Paraffin liquid	Oil	x	x
PEG-60 (polyethylene glycol)	Wax	x	x
Cetyl alcohol	Wax	x	x
PEG-90M (polyethylene glycol high molecular)	Creates thread-like consistency		x
PVP (Polyvinylpyrrolidone)	Film former		x
PVP/VA copolymer (PVP/vinylacetate)	Film former		x
Carbomer	Stabilizer		x
Hydroxyethylcellulose	Stabilizer		x
Triceteareth-4-phosphate	Emulsifier	x	x
PEG-24 hydrogenated castor oil	Emulsifier	x	x
PEG-40-hydrogenated castor oil	Emulsifier		x
Dimethicone	Care/combability	(x)	x
Panthenol	Moisturizer		x
Ethylhexylmethoxycinnamate	UV-absorber	x	x
Aminomethylpropanol	Neutralizer		x
Phenoxyethanol	Preservative		x
Benzyl alcohol	Preservative		x
Fragrance	Scent	x	x

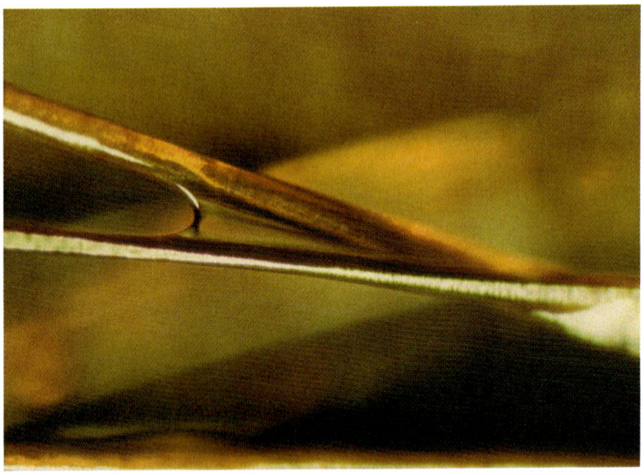

Figure 31.5 Hairspray bond – spot weld.

1970s because of concerns about the earth atmosphere's ozone layer. A more recent development has been the restriction of volatile organic compounds (VOCs) to 80/55% of hairspray formulas in the USA. Formulas have now been developed that substitute propellants judged to have a lower risk of impacting the ozone layer water (such as hydrofluorocarbon 152A or HFC 152A) and an increased proportion of water in the formulas. While initially these technology changes negatively impacted hairspray performance, more recently new polymer systems have been developed to work at these lower alcohol and higher water contents [9].

Hairsprays are safe when used as directed; however, there are some potential issues surrounding misuse. First, aerosols can create a fine mist of droplets which may be inhaled. Hairspray manufacturers carefully check the droplet size and proportion of the formulas and dispensers in order to avoid significant inhalable quantities of droplets to insure consumer safety during typical use at home or in a hair salon [10]. Additionally, hairsprays should to be removed periodically by shampooing. Hairspray polymers have been formulated to break down in the presence of shampoo surfactants. However, if hair is not shampooed frequently, hairspray and other styling aids can build up on the hair causing dullness, potential hair breakage, and polymer flaking that can be mistaken for a symptom of dandruff.

Setting lotions are a special application form of hairspray and pump-spray. The formulation is similar but the usage is different. Typically, the damp hair is prepared with rollers and the product is applied from a small bottle with a nozzle. After blow-drying the rollers are removed and the hair is brushed. The deposition of polymer increases surface friction and creates volume, the main benefit of this product type. A significant group pf users with gray hair use lotions containing blue dyes to make their hair color brighter and less yellowish. Overdosing and build-up resulting from low shampoo frequency may cause a bluish appearance of the hair in these people; however this can easily be removed by thorough washing.

Mousse

Mousses belong also to the widely used products such as hairsprays. Typically, they are wet application products for volume in combination with a blow-dryer. As combing and/or brushing are important parts of the styling procedure, good wet combability is a base requirement. Mousses in general consist of:
- Polymer: mostly quaternized, single or in combination with other cationic on non-ionic polymers ("film former").
- *Surfactants*.
- *Solvents*: water, ethanol.
- *Additives*: e.g. silicones, UV-absorber, vitamins.
- *Propellant*: e.g. propane/butane, DME.
- *Fragrance*.

Non-aerosol mousses have similar composition without propellants, but a mechanical actuator to create the mousse.

As mousses contain cationic charged polymers they may interact in special conditions (hair structure) with anionic polymers from hairsprays. The resulting complex can be hard to remove because of its poor solubility. Repeated shampooing in combination with a conditioner will remove unwanted depositions. Overdosing may contribute to weighing down the hair, residues, reduction of shine, or appearance of white flakes that might be mistaken for the symptoms of dandruff.

Gels and spray gels

In the last 20 to 30 years, gels became more popular as they allow a highly visible styling effect. Today, gels are designed to create every style from smooth hold to extreme looks with spikes to express personality or fashion trends. The use depends strongly on habits; different looks result if applied to wet hair or dry hair or when the hair is blow-dried or air-dried.

Spray gels start at the lower end of the hold scale and provide a well-groomed look. Spray gels are easy to apply evenly throughout the hair. The consistency is usually from water-thin to low viscous. Gels offered in tubes typically have a medium to high viscosity and represent the upper end of a hold scale. The amount of film-forming polymer in the gel formulation usually determines the hold level. Typical ingredients for gels include:
- *Thickener*: e.g. polyacrylates (carbomer), polysaccharides.
- *Polymer*: film former.
- *Moisturizer*: e.g. glycerin for wet look.
- *Solvents*: water, ethanol.
- *Additives*: e.g. silicones, UV-absorber, vitamins.
- *Preservatives*: e.g. paraben types, phenoxyethanol.
- *Fragrance*.

Removal of a gel requires shampooing – in some cases a second lathering is recommended in case of high level use and should the first wash not eliminate all residues. Dry, brittle gels with high hold levels may tend to generate flakes when the hair is moved, similar to hairsprays. Build-up is not usually observed with regular shampooing. Some gels are also sold in cream form and their appearance is not clear, but turbid to white and texture is richer and softer than a typical gel.

Creams, pomades, and emulsions

Creams, pomades, and emulsions are a growing segment which contains very specialized niches for texture and styling results. The common base of cream-like products is always:
- Hydrophobic base such as wax, oil, or related chemistry.
- Water, mainly as the continuous phase (oil-in-water emulsions).
- Emulsifier combination.

The composition and structure of the emulsion controls the application properties. By adding polymers, the level of hold can be modified; the texture might be changed by adding polymeric thickeners or particles such as bentonite or diathomaceous clay to provide a rough, clay-like feel with a matte effect to take away shine. The following list shows typical components:
- *Wax compound*:
  - Synthetic: e.g. paraffin type, polyethylene glycol.
  - Natural: e.g. carnauba wax, bees wax.
- *Surfactants/emulsifiers*: tridecteareth-4-phosphate.
- *Solvent water*.
- *Polymers*: if required for hold or texture.
- *Additives*: e.g. silicones, UV-filter, vitamins.
- *Particles (optional)*: e.g. bentonite, silica for special texture.
- *Preservatives*: e.g. paraben types.
- *Fragrance*.

Application is related to desired effect or style in dry or damp hair for finger styling. Usually, this procedure is part of the finishing touches to a hairstyle. The advantage over polymer-based formulations is the softer nature of hair and the remoldability of the style without the need for reapplying product. A special type of emulsion is the clear jelly-like microemulsion which is also called a "ringing gel" because of the sound effect it creates when the container is tapped with a finger.

These formulations contain a high amount of surfactants so formulators must keep in mind the potential risk for skin irritation, and especially eye irritation, in their selection of ingredients. In combination with sweat there is a possibility for the product to be dissolved on the hair and getting into contact with the eye. Good formulations contain a combination of emulsifiers and surfactant that are not irritating *in vitro* and in patch testing.

Waxes and clays

Water-free waxes are a special group of styling aides that provides strong control and bigger effects than cream-like products. Their consistency is harder and application needs more education or skills by the consumer – especially to prevent overusage and build up.
- *Wax compound*:
  - Synthetic: e.g. polyethylene glycol.
  - Natural: e.g. Carnauba wax, bees wax.
- *Surfactants/emulsifiers*: only for washability.
- *Additives*: e.g. silicones, UV-filter, vitamins.
- *Particles*: e.g. bentonite, silica for special texture.
- *Preservatives*: usually not required.
- *Fragrance*: if desired.

Table 31.3 Typical ingredients in silicone products.

Ingredient (INCI)	Function	Serum	Spray/Aerosol
Dimethicone	Shine enhancer	x	x
Dimethiconol	Shine enhancer	x	x
Cyclopentasiloxane	Shine enhancer	x	x
Alcohol	Solvent		x
Propane/butane	Propellant		x
Panthenol	Moisturizer	x	x
Ethylhexymethoxycinnamate	UV-absorber	x	x
Fragrance	Scent	x	x

Application is on damp or dry hair similar to creams. The stiff consistency requires warming in the hands before application. Shampooing and use of conditioning agents remove waxes, but in some cases may require repeated application to ensure no build-up is created after repeated usage.

Silicone serums and sprays

Silicones – mostly used as oils – are a part of many of the formulations described above to add care properties, improve combability, shine, or modify polymer-based formulations as plasticizer. Other product formulations are mainly based on silicones and therefore utilize higher levels of this versatile ingredient. The main benefit of these products is to provide pure shine or highlight strands to finish the styling process (Table 31.3).

Formulations differ from application form and heaviness of the effect:

1. *Serums*:
   ◦ oily liquids that provide long-lasting, high gloss effects;
   ◦ contain low volatile silicones and low amounts of solvents such as alcohol;
   ◦ designed to highlight strands, no fill head application;
   ◦ have to be carefully applied by hands – need expertise in use.
2. *Pump sprays*:
   ◦ are lighter in effect than serums;
   ◦ effect is less durable as the silicones are more volatile;
   ◦ contain solvents such as alcohol;
   ◦ easier to apply for consumers;
   ◦ also for full head application.
3. *Aerosol sprays*:
   ◦ are comparable to pump sprays in performance;
   ◦ designed to intensify gloss of styling for finish;
   ◦ also suitable to refresh shine.

Table 31.4 shows hair products according to categories, physical description, typical applications, and desired result.

Products designed for African hair types

Hair of people of African descent has always been treated very differently from Caucasian or Asian hair. The structure of African hair is different from other hair types, as its extreme

Table 31.4 Hair products (categories, physical description, typical applications, desired result).

Category	Physical description	Typical applications	Desired result	Typical packaging
Hairspray (aerosol)	Liquid, clear, low viscous	Spray with propellant on dry hair after styling	Hold of finished styling, invisible net	Aerosol can, aluminum or tinplate with actuator
Hairspray (non-aerosol pump spray)	Liquid, clear, low viscous	Spray without propellant on dry hair or on damp hair for blow-drying	Hold of finished styling	Bottle with mechanical actuator
Gel/gel spray	Medium to viscous, clear jelly-like consistency	Dry hair for air drying or wet hair for blow-drying	Visible styling effects, shaping of hair bundles, creating spikes, etc.	Tube or dispenser
Mousses	Soft, creamy mousse, semi-stable that breaks under mechanical stress	Wet hair with blow-drying, rollers might be used, typically brushed	Volume and hold	Aerosol can
Emulsions	Creamy consistency, typically white appearance, soft feel, and slightly fatty touch	Mostly wet hair, but also dry hair as finish product	Weight down effect, antifrizz properties, alignment, and control of shape, moldability	Jar, tube, or dispenser
Waxes	Tough to hard consistency that melts under mechanical stress	Dry hair	Visible styling effects, bundling of hair, textured looks, also matte effects desired	Jar
Silicones	Clear, oily liquids	On dry hair for styling purpose with fingers or as spray	Pure shine in addition to hold provided by styling products applied before	Small bottles

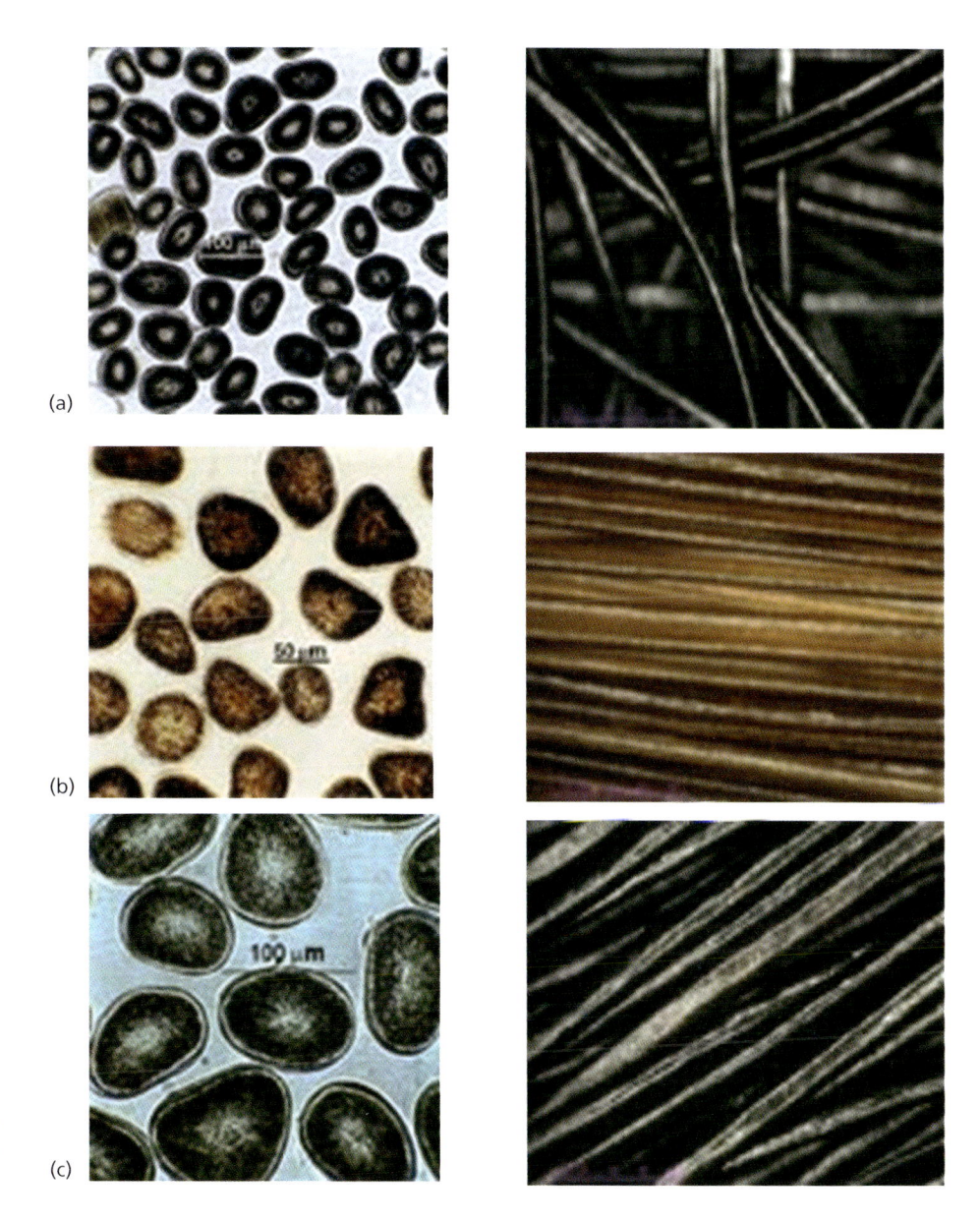

Figure 31.6 Comparison of African (a), Caucasian (b), and Asian (c) hair structure.

curvature is thought to be caused by the different profile of the hair shaft, which may be caused by differences in the morphology of the upper hair follicle. African hair has a distinctively more oval profile than Caucasian or Asian hair (Figure 31.6).

These structural characteristics go hand in hand with further challenges for styling African hair, especially as the time and effort spent on styling African hair tends to be higher than on Caucasian hair. For example: heightened brittleness of the hair shaft, regular use of relaxing chemistry, knotting, braiding, and use of extensions. Excessive braiding and the use of extensions can often cause strain on the hair shaft in the follicle and therefore can lead to temporary hair loss, which is often seen especially along the hairline of the forehead and the partings.

The majority of the African specialty styling products are targeted at helping to relax and smooth the curly African hair and make it easier to manage and maintain. Therefore, most products (such as brilliantines and pomades) contain high levels of waxes and oils and/or polymers. These ingredients deliver the hold African hair needs and are typically applied with the fingers and whole hand to achieve good coverage and maximum hold benefits. Another advantage of the high levels of oils and waxes in these products, but also in other products like oil sheens, is that they enhance the light reflected from the hair surface, which gives especially dark hair a more healthy appearance and striking shine.

Lotions are often used to protect the hair shaft and are useful for African hair as it tends to be more brittle and more prone to breakage. Lotions are mainly emulsions that offer combinations of conditioning ingredients and styling ingredients. The conditioning ingredients (such as silicones and fatty alcohols) protect the hair and enhance its appearance. Lotions are highly beneficial for African hair as they have a good efficacy as leave-in products and as they can help to counteract the negative effects of the variety of damaging styling techniques used.

As the vast majority of African specialty products tend to have higher levels of styling polymers and/or waxes/oils, it is crucial to wash the hair regularly to prevent excessive build up and associated hair negatives.

Protecting the hair structure with styling aides

One distinct benefit of styling aides – that has become a stronger focus over the last years – is their ability to protect the hair fiber from external damaging influences. As styling habits – together with chemical treatments and environmental factors – are key drivers in hair fiber structural damage, styling aides can be used successfully to reduce the damage incurred by these factors. The specific use of styling aides being applied to hair, not rinsed out, and not removed until the next wash, makes them a preferred technology option to reduce the impact of damaging factors during and after the styling process. A variety of ingredients in styling product technologies have a protective function on the hair fiber, such as silicones, polymers, waxes, and fatty alcohols. The formulation of the styling aide can be tailored to provide a homogeneous layer of these ingredients on the hair fiber which then provides protective benefits. Furthermore, additional actives such as UV filters can contribute to a reduction of hair damage due to environmental influences. This can be beneficial during the styling process, i.e. reducing friction, increasing smoothness, especially when hair is styled when it is wet and particularly vulnerable to damage. Heat protection properties offered by some styling products provide additional benefits as the polymers contained can help manage the heat transfer into the hair as well as smoothing the hair surface to reduce friction which can be particularly damaging during heat application. After the styling process, the product formulations can continue to protect the hair fiber and therefore they are often recommended to be used in combination with dedicated hair care products.

Considerations for consultations with patients about hair styling

Despite the many advantages and fundamental benefits for appearance – and consequently confidence – misuse of styling products can have an adverse effect on the hair quality and appearance [11,12]. Often, patients overuse or misuse styling products, and especially styling appliances, in their quest for a better appearance. For example, the excess use of heat styling appliances has wide consequences for the hair quality, as studies have shown [13]. Some modern heat styling appliances operate with temperatures of well over 200°C, which is beyond the temperature that the hair's molecules, especially the proteins like keratin and its amino acids, can withstand without major structural damage. Patients with high heat styling needs and habits should be advised to use tailored products that have a reduced heat output and/or tailored technology to minimize hair damage and overheating. Furthermore, modern ion technology in heat styling appliances can help to reduce some adverse effects from excessive heat styling. Mechanical stress whilst heat styling is one factor that can cause damage to the hair fiber. Therefore, the use of appliances and styling aides especially designed to reduce hair damage during the heat styling process is recommended. Design features of these include low friction styling surfaces such as ceramics, flexible plates, etc.

Other potential issues with styling products include overuse or mix of the wrong styling product technologies. Overuse of styling products without removal through proper hair hygiene can lead to negative effects on the appearance and tactile properties of hair. The polymers used as main actives can – when overused and not removed – accumulate on the hair surface and can lead to dullness, adhesion of dust and dirt, and to hair being less easy to manage and prone to tangling – creating the opposite effect to what users are trying to achieve.

Because of the character of the ingredients used, styling products are generally safe to use. However, as with other cosmetic products, in rare cases the use of some styling products may be associated with allergies or irritations if there is a history of contact allergic reactions to selected ingredients. These may stem from single ingredients in the product formulations such as fragrance ingredients. Even though the risk of this is low because of limited contact of the products with skin, in case of irritations or adverse reactions that could be associated with styling products, it is advisable to investigate the type of product used, and the ingredients contained, and the way it was used as well as to identify known allergies of the patient. In case of an identified allergic reaction, dermatologists are advised to run an allergy alert test with the patient and/or to contact the manufacturer of the product to find out about the nature of the ingredients used in the product.

In consultations with patients concerning styling-related issues, it is imperative to assess the specific hair-related issues of the patients first and then to understand what styling and haircare products were used. This should enable a good understanding of what caused the issues and the psychologic impact on the patient. The advice to patients with hair styling-related issues should be focused on the right selection, and the right amount of styling products targeted at their hair needs and used in combination with a good quality haircare regime. Often manufacturers of high quality haircare and styling products tailor their different product technologies to match and provide maximum styling benefits with minimum negative effects. A recommendation to patients who overuse or misuse styling products should include a focus on potential reduction of the use amount and frequency of the product as well as on the selection the right products.

Future of hair styling aids – trends and technologic development

As there are continuous research efforts dedicated to hair, the knowledge of hair (hair biology, hair structure, and hair biochemistry) is growing and will continue to grow in the future. Styling aides are a prime example that trends and science and technology advancements are closely interwoven. Over the course of the last 50 and more years, emerging trends demanded new technologies to be developed to enable the creation of new hair styles. Vice versa, the development of new styling technologies enabled the creation of new trends in fashion and beauty. One example is the trend for "big hair" in the 1980s which drove the development of maximum volume and hold products, which in turn allowed for the creation of even bigger hair styles and laid the foundation for the modern variety of product technologies. A key development over the years, which will continue into the future, is the focus on ease of use of the new styling products to enable everybody to create impressive styles. Also, it is likely that a key focus of future development will be on creating even longer lasting styling benefits and to further improve the protective benefits of the different styling technologies to further complement hair care product benefits.

Consequently, the current science and technology advancements will – no doubt – have a profound effect on future trends and will enable new hair styles that everybody can create and recreate, from the most advanced fashion stylists to consumers in their homes.

Conclusions

Styling aids come in a wide variety of types and are used by many to augment hair appearance. Familiarity with the range and use of hair styling aids will help a clinician not only diagnose potential problems arising from misuse or allergy, but can also help when counseling those with thinning, aging, or damaged hair. Styling products can impart the appearance of healthier hair by improving hair shine and smoothness, increasing the appearance of hair body by building in body and volume.

Acknowledgment

The authors thank Dianna Kenneally for her contributions to the first edit of this chapter.

References

1 Gray J. (2007) *Assessment of Hair Quality Using Eye Tracking Technology*. London: Royal Society of Medicine Press, p. 2.
2 Rosenthal A. (2004) Raising hair. *Eighteenth Century Studies* 38 (1), 1–16.
3 Lucas A, Harris JR. (1999) *Ancient Egyptian Materials and Industries*. Courier Dover Publications, p. 332.
4 Wella AG. (2001) The Fascination of Hair. Available from Procter & Gamble Service GmbH, Berliner Allee 65, 64274 Darmstadt, Germany, pp. 6–7.
5 Robbins CR. (2002) *Chemical and Physical Behavior of Human Hair*, 4th edn. Springer, pp. 133–4.
6 Wella AG, Schwan-Jonczyk A. (2003) *Haar umformung*, 1st edn. Pocter & Gamble Service, Darmstadt, Germany, pp. 10–11.
7 Umbach W. (2004) *Kosmetik und Hygiene*, 3rd edn. Wiley-VCH, Weinheim, Germany, pp. 264–7.
8 Wella AG. (2001) *The Fascination of Hair*. Pocter & Gamble Service, Darmstadt, Germany, p. 43.
9 Pfaffernoschke M. (2005) Formulating low VOC aerosol hairsprays. Int J Aerosol Spray Pack Technol April.
10 Zviak C. (1986) *The Science of Hair Care*. New York: Marcel Dekker, pp. 167–8.
11 Gray J. (1997) *World of Hair: A Scientific Companion*. Macmillan Press.
12 Gray J. (2000) *Human Hair Diversity*. Oxford: Blackwell Science.
13 German Wool Research Institute (2007) Study on the Effects of Heat on Human Hair Structure. Aachen, Germany: DWI.

PART IV
Anti-aging

SECTION 1 Cosmeceuticals

CHAPTER 32
Botanicals

Carl R. Thornfeldt
Episciences, Inc., Boise, ID, USA

> **BASIC CONCEPTS**
> - There are many options available to choose from in the skin care/cosmetic product arena, with an increasing interest in herbal-based products.
> - Herbal extracts may be promising therapy for photoaging.
> - Herbal products provide multiple beneficial functionalities with highly reactive molecules and compounds in stable preparations.
> - Botanicals contain terpenoids, alkaloids, and phenolics, which have been chemically characterized for their biologic effects.
> - Products using herbal ingredients must be carefully formulated. Ideally, the finished product is then tested for efficacy and safety.

Introduction

Herbs are the 14,000 species of higher plants with extracts for medicinal, fragrance or flavoring use [1]. The growing interest in herbal products has resulted in significant growth of the number of commercially available natural products in our domestic market to over 90,000. These products are based on over 1100 commercially available herbs. Six wholesale companies each market over 100 herbal extracts, with one company selling over 1000 [2].

Despite the increase in the number of herbal products, the usage rate appears to be flattening after rapid growth over the past six years. Supplement consumption rose from 33.8% in the general population in 1990, to 55% in those seeking cosmetic procedures in 2006. The incidence of supplement use in the latter population declined to 49% in 2012. Unfortunately, 60–72% of supplement users do not report these to their physician pre-operatively for cosmetic procedures [3,4].

Herb-based products provide the advantage of having multiple functionalities in stable blends of highly reactive ingredients such as antioxidants and antimicrobials. While it is difficult to create efficacious and stable cosmeceutical formulations, herbs contain blends of multiple, often unique, active ingredients that are biologically active [2,4]. Since most skin conditions and diseases are multifactorial with multiple mechanisms of action inducing the visible changes, herbal products would be expected to produce visible benefit. While 73% of women polled said it is important to have younger looking skin, the vast majority of topical botanical products promise youth but lack true clinical evidence. This evidence is defined as blinded clinical trials of statistically significant numbers, using the finished, marketed product. Studies with individual ingredients in a laboratory vehicle system are not valid due to the chemical complexity of topical formulations that impact ingredient chemistry and function [5].

Regulatory

A surprising 78.7% of women polled did not know claims made for skin care products are not regulated, evaluated, or verified by any governmental agency. Only in the USA are herbal products sold as dietary supplements which are governed by the Dietary Supplement, Health and Education Act in 1994. Such products are intended to affect the structure and function of the human body, as well as provide calories and nutrients. Topically applied herbs for treating cosmetic skin conditions are commonly referred to as cosmeceuticals. These products improve the appearance of skin like a cosmetic, but modulate surface skin morphology like a drug. Yet there is no official regulatory category for cosmeceutical ingredients.

Cosmetic Dermatology: Products and Procedures, Second Edition. Edited by Zoe Diana Draelos.
© 2016 John Wiley & Sons, Ltd. Published 2016 by John Wiley & Sons, Ltd.

Certain ingredients used in cosmeceuticals may be claimed to be therapeutic for common skin diseases. These ingredients are regulated as over the counter (OTC) drug monographs for acne, dermatitis/psoriasis, skin protectant, topical analgesia and sunscreens, by the Food and Drug Administration (FDA). Non-prescription products that list these active ingredients that are used in the specified concentration range in topical formulations may claim the finished product to be effective and safe therapy for the specific skin conditions listed. The United States has a regulatory classification for food supplement and cosmetic ingredients with proven safety, called Generally Recognized as Safe, or GRAS [5,6].

CFR Title 21 – Food Drugs & Cosmetic Act regulates skin care products and cosmetics, including cosmeceuticals. These products are not supposed to harm the public. Cosmeceuticals are actually helpful to the skin. According to this regulation, mislabeling a cosmetic is illegal. Mislabeling is defined as labeling the cosmetic with false or misleading information, or the label does not include all the information required by this Act. There are also four other statutes that do not apply to topicals. The FDA has become more aggressive in regulating topicals, thus experts are calling for revision and updating CFR Title 21. Products that claim to affect gene expression and DNA are among those under scrutiny as drugs. Recently, warning letters addressing cosmetics that make drug claims have been issued. Additionally, the FDA is monitoring social media, which resulted in a citation for using Facebook to promote unapproved "new" drugs, defined as "making therapeutic claims." Moreover, such regulatory monitoring is needed as more herbal products with actives which are known to have toxic components are being marketed. These apparently are without any basic safety data presented in any communication medium. Cosmetics can only claim to temporarily improve appearance [7].

There is no consistent definition of "natural" in US skin care products, so it is marketing jargon without functionality [9]. Recently a recommended criterion is, "Five percent or more of the ingredients are found in nature." Organic products are ones that are certified free of synthetic chemical use in the fields, and using production methods of the ingredients obtained in nature [1]. The US Department of Agriculture now has certification criteria for this designation to include certified as 100% organic, but can claim organic if 95% of components are. Organic-derived can be claimed if 70% of the components are organic [10]. There has been no decision by the FDA about genetically modified foods labeled as "natural."

Factors affecting concentration and quality of active ingredients

The skin care practitioner should select a herb for a specific desired beneficial effect based on scientific research and/or traditional medical knowledge founded on ethnobotany. As interest in phytomedicines for improving health as well as treating disease is growing rapidly, many "exotic" species with certain "fad" characteristics are being touted also for cosmeceuticals. Fortunately, most of these exotic ingredients are added at subtherapeutic doses just for the marketing story of the product. Little is known about efficacy and safety of many of these ingredients.

The active ingredients of plants used for human skincare are generally small molecules not involved in regular metabolic processes, known as secondary metabolites (SM). These ingredients are used for nutrient storage or organism protection. The goal of extraction processes is to improve consistency of SM concentration, increase SM potency, and increase product purity [1].

Herbal extracts are much more susceptible to quality variations than synthetic products due to environmental and processing factors affecting solubility, stability, pharmacokinetics, pharmacology and toxicity of the active ingredients. These include:

1. Growing conditions of the plant.
2. Health of the plant.
3. Harvesting time.
4. Care of botanical products during transport.
5. Storage time and method prior to processing.
6. Selecting the proper anatomic site on the plant.
7. Processing methods include air or oven drying, crushing, cold pressing, comminuting (fracturing) and grinding.
8. Extraction methods include solvents such as water, alcohol, glycol, glycerin, ester or oil [1,2].
9. Secondary purification including super critical fluids and column chromatography [10].

Additional details are provided in the previous edition of this book [11].

The processing of herbal extracts provides a variety of products, including:

1. Isolated pure molecules that may then be used as prescription medication such as colchicine and reserpine. Certain substances may be used in cosmetic products such as glycyrrhetic acid for skin lightening and sericoside for wrinkles.
2. Standardized extracts in dry, oily or soft (butter) forms.
3. Phytosomes such as Centinella asiatica triterpenes for wrinkles.
4. Actiphytes from cold processing in hydroglycolic, alcohol, glycerin or oil bases.
5. Organoleptics or flavorings.

Safety

Patients and clients entrust skincare professionals to create effective and safe regimens for their skin, yet there are no safety requirements for cosmeceuticals. Best corporate practices should ensure safety studies are performed on all herbal products. The incidence of dangerous adverse reactions to herbal medicines is infrequent, but is growing. The most common adverse reaction consists of 40% of US women who claim to have sensitive skin [1,6].

German chamomile (*Matricaria recutita*), cayenne (*Capsicum annuum*) and echinacea (*Echinacea angustifolia*) have been reported to produce anaphylactic reactions even to death. Taborandi (*Pilocarpus microphyllus*) induced death via cardiac arrest, while poison ivy (*Rhus toxicodendron*) induced death via coma. Fatalities have also been reported with Aloe, Aristocholia, Arnica, Black Mustard, Cascara, Cayenne, Chinese Rhubarb, Comfrey, Croton, Kava Kava, Ma Huang, Mistletoe, Oleander, Senna, Scotch pine, Spruce and Yohimbe [2,8,10].

A product labeled as "natural" does not equal a safe product. Chinese practitioners are concerned about the well-known side effects of hepatotoxicity, contact dermatitis and teratogenicity which occur in up to a third of people using topical Chinese herbal preparations. Moreover, a significant number of congenital anomalies occur when these herbs are used topically during pregnancy [12].

Another risk of herbal products is the relatively high incidence of cross-reactivity with other herbs. For example, in 106 dermatitis afflicted people, 12 were allergic to tea tree oil and all 12 had one or more patch test reactions to 10 other herbs, most commonly, lavender [13].

A preferred safety test for a cosmeceutical product would be the Repeat Insult Patch Test (RIPT) on 50 panelists to evaluate risk of contact irritant and allergic dermatitis with topical use. This is a one-month test that measures for irritant reactions in the first 10 days and allergic sensitization in the last 10 days. It will not predict systemic reactions such as gynecomastia due to widespread topically applied lavender in atopic children and teens used for prolonged periods [10,14].

Effectiveness

In the last decade a new development has been the use of blinded clinical studies to document efficacy of cosmeceutical products presented at peer-reviewed meetings or in scientific journals. This is the most convincing scientific evidence of therapeutic efficacy. A total of 16 companies have produced 50 blinded clinical trials of herbs to treat photoaging. One company who produced the first blinded trial in 2002 has accounted for 16 of these blinded trials. Twelve of the 50 trials have compared the test herbal or herbal/synthetic blend formulations to prescription products. The most prolific company accounted for seven of these trials.

Cosmeceutical efficacy claims for an herbal product being sold in your practice would ideally be supported by a double-blind clinical trial [1,5].

The true measure of a prescription or nonprescription drug's efficacy has been determined by United States regulatory agencies to be a p value of <0.05. P value is a measure of probability, also known as statistical significance. A p value of <0.05 means if you run a study 100 times, the comparable positive result will occur in at least 95% of the attempts. A highly statistically significant result is when p value is <0.001. This means running the study 1000 times produces the comparable positive result in 99.9% of the attempts [10].

A major challenge to the clinical efficacy of any herbal extract is the delivery of therapeutic concentration(s) of the desired active ingredients across the stratum corneum intact in their functional state to affect organelles, cells, receptors, metabolic and cell signaling pathways. The different solubilities, polarities, size and architecture of the several to hundreds of multiple secondary metabolites (SM) in herbal extracts creates difficulty. Moreover, the degree of biodegradability, biocompatibility, toxicity, release profile and antigenicity also vary amongst the multitude SM in one extract. Contributing to the challenge is the different SM bind to cells and receptors in different cutaneous strata.

To meet this challenge of negotiating the tortuous proteohydrolipid stratum corneum, several novel methodologies have been developed that is beyond the scope of this chapter, but thoroughly analyzed in this listed reference [10].

Mechanism of action

Plants are equipped with protective defensive mechanisms, storage, color and aroma via low molecular weight compounds called SM. These are not used in primary metabolic processes such as photosynthesis, respiration, assimilation of nutrients, transport, growth or differentiation. They usually provide protection against ultraviolet light, herbivores, parasites, pathogenic microbes, and animals. Certain fatty acids and certain carbohydrates function within both metabolic processes and as SM.

About 20% of the higher plants have been studied with spectrometry, nuclear magnetic resonance and/or x-ray diffraction which have identified about 40,000 SM [1].

SM are divided into more than 15,500 terpenoids, 12,000 alkaloids and 6000 phenolics, which have been chemically characterized from herbal extracts, as have 10 other chemical classes representing the other 6500; more extensive discussion is given in the previous edition of this book [1,11].

Cosmeceutical products

To help separate true scientifically based safe and effective herbal-based cosmeceuticals from "snake oil" products using voodoo science, and before making a decision on retailing or recommending any particular brand of skin care products, the practitioner should ask the following questions:

1. Is the herb being used in other living breathing organisms, i.e. used as a veterinary or dental medicine; or a part of traditional Asian or homeopathic medicines; or used in food technology for mammalian exposure?
2. Is the biologically active ingredient and therapeutic concentration range known and used in this cosmeceutical product?

3. The development of the formulation should include chemical, physical and photo-stability to ensure efficacy and that toxic metabolites are not formed.
4. Does the herbal SM penetrate the stratum corneum permeability barrier in its active state at a high enough concentration to manipulate its target cell, organelle, enzyme, receptor or compound? Soothing mucilage or occlusive SM function by placement upon the mucocutaneous surface.
5. When was the finished product manufactured? Freshness matters with herbal products. All cosmeceutical active ingredients including antioxidants, vitamins, and herbal SM undergo chemical reactions when combined in any formulation. This auto-oxidation reaction is affected by formulation manufacturing method. For example, heating speeds up the auto-oxidation process and destroys the activity of virtually all antioxidants [1,2].
6. Does the product really work in the skin, as determined by blinded clinical trials with the finished product you are selling?
7. Is the product safe? Are there reports of topical toxicity? Was an RIPT test performed on the product you are selling?
8. Has the skin care practitioner thoroughly evaluated the product? Patients/clients expect the practitioner to be a clearing house for accurate information for all skin products, prescriptions and treatments. The patient/client assumes the practitioner uses the same criteria to establish which prescription drugs and treatments are offered as is used to determine which cosmeceuticals are recommended and sold [15]. In this litigious society, injury can result in criminal as well as civil judgments with use of unapproved or illegal products. Ignorance provides no legal protection [6].

Specific herbs to treat or prevent photoaging

The three theories of skin aging include:
1. Reactive oxygen species.
2. Mitochondrial dysfunction via nucleic acid mutations which are much more common than nuclear nucleic acid mutations.
3. Telomere damage via telomerase upregulation [10].

Reactive oxygen species, or free radicals, are reversed by antioxidants. Humans utilize 15 antioxidants, elements and molecules. At no body site is there only high concentration of a single one; rather there exists a cycle phenomenon to pass off some of the oxidant energy among these multiple antioxidant molecules and elements [16].

To protect mitochondria and prevent their dysfunction, adequate amounts of photoprotective herbal anthocyanins such as carotenoids, and polyphenols and catechins from green tea, grape seed, resveratrol and silymarin have documented benefit.

Camptotheca acuminate (Happy tree) has been shown to downregulate telomerase [2].

About 200 herbs have anti-inflammatory functionality with 140 of these having antioxidant activity. The other 60 include anti-inflammatory natural steroids, salicylates, and other non-antioxidants. Only six herbal extracts for treating photoaging have been a sole active ingredient in tested formulations, including: coffeeberry, date palm kernel, oat, soy milk, total soy, and soy protease inhibitors. These and the other 33 herbs tested in blinded studies to treat photoaging are listed in Table 32.1.

Table 32.1 Anti-aging herbs with clinical studies in humans

Aloe (*Aloe barbadensis*)
Apple (*Malus domestica*)
Avocado (*Persea americana*)
Black cohosh (*Cimicifuga racemosa*)
Blackberry (*Rubis ursinus*)
Blueberry (*Vaccinium myrtillus*): oral only
Cat's claw (*Uncaria guianensis, U. tomentosa*)
Coffeeberry (*Coffea arabica*)*
Comfrey, or comphrey (*Symphytum officinale*)
Date palm kernel (*Phoenix dactylifera*)*
Dill (*Anethum graveolens*)
Flax (*Linum usitatissimum*)
German chamomile (*Matricaria recutita*) + oral
Goji (*Lycium barbarum*)
Grapefruit (*Citrus paradisi*): oral only
Grape seed (*Vitis vinifera*): oral only
Green tea (*Camellia sinensis*)* + oral
Lavender (*Lavandula augustifolia*)
Licorice (*Glycyrrhiza glabra, G. inflate, G. uralensis*): oral only and Glabridin topically
Mangosteen (*Garcinia mangostana*)
Meadowfoam (*Limnanthes alba*)
Mountain rose (*Rosa canina*)
Mushroom/wheat complex
Oak quercetin
Olive (*Olea europaea*)
Plum (*Prunus domestica*)
Pomegranate (*Punica granatum*) + oral
Raspberry (*Rubus idaeus*)
Safflower (*Carthamus tinctorius*)
Sakura leaf (*Prunus speciosa*)
Southern wood (*Artemesia ambrosia*)
Soy milk, total soy (*Glycine soja, G. max*), soy protease inhibitors* + oral
Spring rest-harrow (*Ononis spinosa*)
Sweet orange (*Citrus sinensis*): oral only
Tamarind (*Tamarindus indica*)
Tomato (*Lycopersicon esculentum*): oral only
White sandalwood (*Santalum album*)
White tea (*Camellia sinensis*) + oral
White willow (*Salix alba*)

* = single active in product; + oral = oral plus topical administration.

With the appreciation of multiple clinical components of photoaging that require multiple functionalities, all the herbal products published in the last three years consist of at least six active ingredients, with others containing up to 33 different actives. The contribution of each active is difficult to ascertain in such "soups."

It has now been documented that the underlying biochemical anomalies that induce cutaneous photoaging are driven by the dual pathophysiologies of disrupted or incompetent stratum corneum barrier coupled with chronic inflammation [10]. Herbs with these foundational functions are listed in Table 32.2. The lighteners/brighteners in Table 32.3 consist of 36 herbs, including three different licorice types, to lessen or reverse mottled pigmentation, melasma and/or lentigines that have been documented to effectively treat hyperpigmentation in blinded clinical trials. Another 39 are claimed to be effective lighteners/brighteners, but have non-blinded, uncontrolled, open trials, or clinical observations. A total of 130 herbs are reported to inhibit one or more melanin synthetic molecules *in vitro*.

The 16 tighteners in Table 32.4 reverse skin laxity and help reverse wrinkles. Table 32.5 lists eight herbal modulators of nucleic acids. Table 32.6 lists 16 photoprotective herbs via topical and/or oral routes. Orally administered photoprotective products should be an important lifestyle adjunct as only 40% of the population routinely wears sunscreen [15]. Incorporating active herbal extracts into mineral makeup also assists in photoprotection [17].

The herbs most commonly used for cosmeceutical extracts are listed below.

Table 32.2 Targeting aging pathogenesis

Barrier repair herbs:
Avocado (*Persea americana*)
Jojoba (*Simmondsia chinensis*)
Mallow (*Althaea officinalis*)
Oat (*Avena sativa*)
Olive (*Olea europea*)
Safflower (*Carthamus tinctorius*)
Shea (*Vitellaria paradoxa*)
+19 others
Anti-inflammatory herbs:
Apple (*Malus domestica*)
Date palm fruit (*Phoenix dactylifera*)
Flax (*Linum usitatissimum*)
Licorice (*Glycyrrhiza glabra, G. inflate, G. uralensis*)
Meadowfoam (*Limnanthes alba*)
Mountain rose (*Rosa canina*)
Olive (*Olea europaea*)
Soy (*Glycine soja, G. max*)
Teas (*Camellia sinesensis*)
Turmeric (*Curcuma longa*)
+190 others;
140 also have antioxidant activity

Table 32.3 Lighteners/brighteners

Aloesin (*Aloe barbadensis, A. carpensis, A. vera*)
Bearberry (*Arctostaphylos uva-uris*)
Black mulberry (*Morus nigra*)
Blueberry (*Vaccinium angustifolium*)
Blue skull cap (*Scutellaria lateriflora*)
Carrot (*Daucus carota*)
Citrus fruit flavonoid [Hesperidin]
Cranberry (*Vaccinium macrocarpon, V. oxycoccos, V. erythrocarpus*)
Cucumber (*Echballium elaterium*)
Curcumin (*Curcuma longa*)
Date palm fruit (*Phoenix dactylifera*)
Echinacea (*Echinacea angustifolia, E. pallida, E. purpurea*)
Feverfew (*Tanacetum parthenium*)
Flax lily (*Dianella ensifolia*)
Ginseng, American (*Panax quinquefolius*)
Ginseng, Asian (*Panax ginseng*)
Ginseng, Siberian (*Eleutherococcus senticosus*)
Gingko (*Gingko biloba*)
Grape seed (*Vitis vinifera*)
Hibiscus (*Hibiscus sabdariffa*)
Indian gooseberry (*Emblica officinalis*)
Licorice (*Glycyrrhiza glabra, G. inflata, G. uralensis*)
[ammonium glycyrrhizinate; glabridin; liquiritin]
Mangosteen (*Garcinia mangostana*)
Oat (*Avena sativa*)
Olive (*Olea europaea*)
Pear (*Pyrus communis*)
Sakura leaf (*Prunus serrulata*)
Saxifrage (*Pimpinella saxifraga*)
Soy (*Glycine soja, G. max*)
Turmeric (*Curcuma longa*)
White mulberry (*Morus alba*)
White willow (*Salix alba*)
Wormwood (*Artemisia absinthium*)
Yellow dock (*Rumex crispus, R. obtusifolius*)

Aloe (*Aloe barbadensis, A. capensis, A. vera*)

The three species of aloe may cross-react with garlic, onions and tulip allergies. Gel from the leaves is the best source for SM, which includes aloe resins, dithranol, chrysorobin, allantoin, saponins, sterols, tannins, salicylates, amino acids, flavonoids, mono- and polysaccharides, arachidonic acid, lipase and cyclo-oxygenase.

Table 32.4 Tighteners

Birch (*Betula alba*)
Cinnamon (*Cinnamomum verum*)
Flax (*Linum usitatissimum*)
Ginger (*Zingiber officinale*)
Gingko (*Gingko biloba*)
Green tea (*Camillia sinensis*)
Hops (*Humulus lupulus*)
Horse chestnut (*Aesculus hippocastanum*)
Meadowfoam (*Limnanthes alba*)
Mountain rose (*Rosa canina*)
Peppermint (*Mentha piperita*)
Red sandalwood (*Pterocarpus santalinus*)
Rosemary (*Rosmarinus officianalis*)
Sage (*Salvia lavandulae, s. folia*)
Spearmint (*Mentha spicata*)
Witch hazel (*Hamamelis virginiana*)

Table 32.5 Botanicals which modulate nucleic acids

Camptotheca acuminata	
Cat's claw (*Uncaria guianensis, U. tomentosa*)	
Mushrooms:	*Agaricus blazei*
	Cordyceps sinesis
	Coriolus (*Tremetes versicolor*)
	Maitake (*Grifolia frondosa*)
	Reishi (*Ganoderma lucidum*)
	Shiitake (*Lentinula edodes*)

Table 32.6 Photoprotective herbs

Black tea (*Camellia sinensis*)
Cocoa (*Theobroma cacao*): oral only
Feverfew (*Tanacetum parthenium*)
Golden fern (*Polypodium leukotomas*): oral only
Grapeseed (*Vitis vinifera*) + oral
Green tea (*Camillia sinensis*) + oral
Kale (*Brassica oleracea*)
Oat (*Avena sativa*)
Olive (*Olea europea*)
Pomegranate (*Punica granatum*) + oral
Ringworm bush (*Cassia lata*)
Spinach (*Spinacia oleracea*)
Strawberry (*Fragaria*)
Tamarind (*Tamarindus indica*)
Tomato (*Solanum lycopersicum*)
White sandalwood (*Santalum album*)

Aloe is antibacterial (AB) to *Helicobacter pylori*, *Bacillus subtilis*, and methicillin-resistant *Staphylococcus aureus*. This herb has anti-fungal (AF), anti-viral (AV), anti-antihistaminic (AH), anti-inflammatory (AI), vasoconstrictive, and anti-oxidant (AO) properties. It improves photoaging by increasing collagen synthesis and microcirculation. Aloe did not decrease UVB induced erythema in a human in-vivo study. As one of five herbal plus synthetic antioxidants, aloe effectively reversed the signs of photodamage in a placebo controlled trial. Aloesin extract is a potent tyrosinase inhibitor and inhibits UV induced melanogenesis but less so than kojic acid. Adverse reactions are a rare contact dermatitis. Aloe should not be used during pregnancy or lactation [2,8,18].

Charentais cantaloupe (*Melo reticulatus*)

This melon has the highest content of superoxide dismutase, the most potent AO enzyme, and it activates synthesis of two other enzymatic anti-oxidants, catalase and glutathione oxidase. It is also a rich source of vitamins A, C, B1, B3, B5, B6 and folate [2,19].

One double-blind clinical trial combining charentais cantaloupe extract combined with nine other herbs produced highly statistically significant decrease in wrinkles after one week of use compared to a growth factor product and an L-ascorbic acid/tocopherol product [pending publication].

Coffee (*Coffea arabica*)

Coffea arabica yields three commercial products: coffee beans which are the seeds, the fruit which is coffeeberry and coffee charcoal which is roasted fruit until black. The major SM include purine alkaloids such as caffeine, theobromine and theophylline, the polyphenols caffeic, chlorogenic, and ferulic acids, diterpenes, phytoestrogens, proanthocyanadins, saccharides, and magnesium. These provide AO, photo-protective and anti-tumor (AT) functions. Caffeine itself also seems to improve skin roughness and fine lines.

Coffeeberry extract is obtained from subripe coffee fruit. These beneficial molecules are preserved with new roasting techniques. A double-blind study of coffeeberry as the only active on 20 females compared to baseline revealed statistically significant 30% improvement in hyperpigmentation, 20% improvement in fine lines and wrinkles. In another 10-female trial versus placebo there was a statistically significant 25% improvement in fine lines and wrinkles and a 15% reduction of hyperpigmentation [1,2,8,20].

Adverse reactions include three deaths from rectal enemas; coma, stroke and anaphylactic IgE reactions are rare.

Cucumber (*Cucumis sativa*)

Cucumber slices applied directly on eyelid skin to relieve puffiness is due to AO, AI, AT and anti-parasitic (AP) flavonoids, curcubitacins, alkaloids, and tannins plus ascorbic acid and peptides. Inhibition of matrix metalloproteinases also occurs, likely reducing photoaging. This herb inhibits melanogenesis while improving wound healing. In a blinded clinical trial of 21 panelists, cucumber produced statistically significant decreases in sebum production but no significant decrease in melanogenesis. It should not be consumed during pregnancy and lactation [2,21,22].

Feverfew (Tanacetum parthenium)
Parthenolide is a sesquiterpene lactone that is the most active component but also the most toxic. Among the other 40 SM, are flavonoids, tanetin and apigenin, polyynes, volatile oils such as camphor, chrysanthyl acetate, linalool and melatonin. The commercially available powdered leaves lack parthenolide, yet are AI, AH, AO, AT, photoprotective, vasoconstrictor, inhibits serotonin and arachidonic acid release and gene transcription. Inhibition of TNF alpha was 35–1000 times higher than black, green, and white tea, echinacea, chamomile, aloe vera, and licorice extracts. Adverse reactions include oral ulcerations and angioedema. A double-blind study of 31 women with sensitive skin using a parthenolide free Feverfew moisturizer twice daily for three weeks produced statistically significant decrease ($p < 0.05$) in erythema, tactile roughness, and overall irritation. It was also effective therapy for shaving-induced irritation [23].

Feverfew is a member of the Compositae family, so it cross-reacts with marigold, daisy, ragweed, bromelain, milk thistle, arnica, and chamomile. Feverfew should never be used during pregnancy and lactation, or with children under two years of age [1,2,8].

German chamomile (Matricaria recutita)
The major SM of this herb are mucilages from the entire plant. Volatile oils such as bisabolol and flavonoids such as apigenin, quercetin, chalmazulene, rutin and coumarins are also extracted from the flower. Chamomile has AH, AO, AI (superior to 0.5% hydrocortisone) via inhibiting lipo-oxygenase and cyclo-oxygenase, and has estrogenic effects. It is AT, and AB against staphylococcus, AV and anti-candida yeast (ACY). Chamomile is also reported to reduce rough, xerotic, inelastic skin and signs of photodamage, and treats mucositis to 11 common chemotherapeutic agents including methotrexate and hydroxyurea.

This herb is a member of the Compositae family, and thus cross-reacts with marigold, daisy, feverfew, ragweed, arnica, milk thistle, and bromelain. There has been at least one death by anaphylactic reaction, and it uncommonly causes allergic contact dermatitis. Avoid in pregnancy and lactation [1,3,8].

Golden fern (Polypodium leucotomos)
This herb has documented therapeutic efficacy in clinical trials for vitiligo, psoriasis, sunburn and UVA induced phototoxicity when administered orally. Topical lotions reduced photodamage in vivo.

The primary SM include the polyphenols chlorogenic, ferulic and caffeic acids. This extract is AI, AH via inhibiting mast cells, and AO. This herb statistically significantly decreases erythema, sunburn cells, pyrimidine dimers, epidermal proliferation, reducing graft rejection, while reducing loss of Langerhans cells, thus stimulating humoral immunity. In a trial treating 25 panelists with polymorphous light eruption and solar urticaria with 480 mg orally each day, 41% of them improved by more than 50% compared to baseline. Photo-protection occurs with 7.5 mg/kg/day or 240 mg three times daily. Vitiligo is treated with 120 mg three times daily [2,8,24].

Grape (Vitis vinifera)
Grape SM include the flavonoids quercetin, tannins, monomeric catechins, oligomeric proanthocyanidins (OPC) polymers, resveratrol, tocopherol and fruit acids. These SM provide AT via cytotoxicity and inducing apoptosis, AH, AI, AO, and vasodilating effects. It inhibits matrix metalloproteinases (MMP), which stabilizes collagen. Grape is 50-fold more potent than AO efficacy by vitamins C or E. An oral product reduced melasma by 6 months in an open trial. When combined with six other actives in an oral anti-aging product, skin firmness improved by 6 months. Red wine has 10 times the amount of flavonoids as white wine. The most potent wine for AO and resveratrol is Granache, or garnacha, wine.

Grape extract also treats allergic rhinitis, improves wound healing, canker sores, and chronic venous insufficiency. There is one report of non-fatal anaphylactic reaction to grape skin [2,8,25,26].

Green tea
Green tea extract ointment (Veregen® by Bradley Pharmaceuticals) received FDA approval as prescription therapy for genital and perianal warts. Green tea reduced gum inflammation and premalignant leukoplakia. Topically, it reduces sunburn and puffy eyelids.

Green tea is unfermented *Camellia sinensis*. This tea is rich in polyphenols including catechins with the most potent AO being epigallo catechin gallate (EGCG), flavandiols, flavonoids and phenolic acids. Other green tea SM include sterols and anti-inflammatory estrogenic lignans and inhibit 5-alpha reductase. These polyphenols protect DNA and mitochondria. Green tea SM are AB, AI and AV.

The only blinded clinical trial proving benefit of green tea in reversing photoaging used oral and topical formulations. Another blinded study in premalignant actinic keratosis failed to show benefit with topically applied green tea.

Unlike the fermented teas of black and oolong, green tea lacks theaflavins, which also exist in chocolate. Black tea also contains gallic acid and thearubigin. These are AT and AV molecules that protect DNA [2,8].

Licorice (Glycyrrhiza glabora)
Up to 15% of licorice SM are AI triterpene saponins including glycyrrhetic acid, glycyrrhizia, and glabrolide. Isoflavonoids are AI with estrogenic properties including glabridin and glyccyrrhisoflavone. AO flavonoids such as liquiritigenin, licochalcone A and licoricidin. Sterols and coumarins are other SM. Licorice extracts are also AB, AH, anti-platelet, AT and ACY. In addition,

licorice extracts stimulate T lymphocytes, interferon gamma and are cytotoxic by stimulating NK cells. The flavonoids also increase tumor sensitivity to anti-neoplastic drugs, so licorice is classified as a chemo-preventative agent by the FDA.

At low concentrations, glabridin has estrogen receptor dependent growth promoting effects but has anti-proliferative effect at high concentrations. Licorice decreases testosterone and androstenedione. It is an abortifacient so should be avoided in pregnancy and lactation.

Licorice extract does inhibit three of the 17 steps in melanin synthesis. Two double-blinded controlled trials using formulations containing this ingredient were found to be significantly superior to hydroquinone in treating hyperpigmentation with significantly greater tolerability. A shampoo is marketed to reduce seborrhea [2,8,11].

Milk thistle (Silybum marinium)
Silybin accounts for 75% of milk thistle extract known as silymarin. It provides AI, inhibits UVB sunburn, AO, and AT activity. Other SM include fatty oils, flavonoids such as apigenin, quercetin, sterols, glucosides, fumaric acid and polyynes. Silymarin is a potent inhibitor of TNF alpha and has estrogenic activity. Its adverse reactions include pruritis, eczema, urticarial and angioedema. Avoid during pregnancy and lactation.

This herb is a member of the Compositae family, and thus cross-reacts with ragweed, feverfew, marigold, daisy, arnica, chamomile and bromelain allergy [1,2,8].

Mushrooms
The major medicinal mushrooms come from Asian traditional medicine. These include *Agoricus blazei*, *Cordyceps sinensis*, *Coriolus* (*Trametei versicolor*), Reishi in Japan, Lingzhi in China (*Ganoderma lucidum*), Maitake (*Grifola frondosa*), and Shiitake (*Leninus edodes*). Mushroom extracts contain polysaccharides such as beta glucan, peptides including adenosine, triterpenes, polyphenols, protease inhibitors and sphingolipids. MMP and activating protein-1 are inhibited by most mushrooms suggesting effectiveness for photoaging therapy. These SM have AI, AO, AT, AB, and anti-HIV effects. They also stimulate natural killer (NK) cells [1,2,8]. Six species modulate nucleic acids.

Maitake mushroom (Grifola frondosa)
An open clinical study of mushroom and wheat protein complex treated 37 women. Statistically significant improvements in photoaging epidermal parameters and pinch recoil improved by 8 weeks versus baseline occurred [1,2,8].

Shiitake mushroom (Lentinus edodes)
This fungus is also a rich source of ergocalciferol (vitamin D) and the immune stimulating AI, polysaccharide betaglucan. When combined with other herbs, the product produced highly statistically significant decrease in wrinkles compared to a growth factor serum and an L-ascorbic acid/tocopherol blend in a double-blind trial [1,2,8, unpublished by author].

Oat (Avena sativa)
This herb has proven double-blinded clinical trials for relief of pruritic skin, xerosis, and seborrheic dermatitis. The SM include polysaccharides, such as beta glucan, steroid saponins, flavonoids such as apigenin, and polyphenols such as avenathramide (comparable to 1% hydrocortisone), caffeic and ferulic acids, hydroxycinnamate, coumaric acids and tocotrienols. Oat is AI, AO, and UVA blocking.

In an open trial treating acne induced by epidermal growth factor receptor agonists, 60% achieved complete remission and 30% partial response. Oats not contaminated with barley or wheat have been proven not to aggravate celiac gluten sensitive enteropathy. Oat can be safely used in people with celiac disease. Contact dermatitis to oat occurs infrequently [2,8,27].

Oleander (Nerium oleander)
Oleander disrupts the normal calcium gradient in the epidermis and stratum corneum, thus disrupting the skin barrier and slowing its repair, producing clinically visible or subclinical cutaneous inflammation with edema, creating a perceived anti-aging result. This herb also has AP, AT and insecticidal properties.

Despite being marketed in topical products to treat skin aging, no double-blind studies proving efficacy have been published or presented at scientific meetings. A branded multinetworking product uses a patent-pending extraction technology that produces a specific extract combining aloe vera with Nerium oleander extract. An open human visualization trial showed improved photoaging parameters by 30% after 4 weeks of use, but no mention of number of panelists, comparison to placebo or baseline, or statistical significance. Safety studies of these topical products also have not been presented.

This is one of 15 herbs known to induce fatal reactions when topically applied and has resulted in at least two deaths. Toxicity is dependent on the concentration of this ingredient, the extent and frequency of application, user's age, body site and whether there is underlying skin barrier compromise. The most adverse reaction is contact dermatitis. Topical formulations must be absolutely avoided during pregnancy and lactation, as seizures occurred in a neonate after mother's use in third trimester [2,8,28].

Papaya (Carica papaya)
The SM of this herb include papain and chymopapain, lipases, alkaloids such as carpain, glycosides, glucosinolates and saponins. This herb improves wound healing, increases humoral immunity, and is AT, AP and AB.

Papaya does cross-react with latex sensitivity as well as fig and kiwi, rarely producing severe allergic systemic and contact reactions. This herb should be avoided in pregnancy [2].

Pineapple (Ananas comosus)
The proteinase enzyme bromelain used for wound, burn and ulcer debridement and to treat postoperative edema is extracted from pineapple. It has AI comparable to diclofenac, AO, AH and

AT activities. Pineapple extract SM include malic and citric acid plus vitamins A and C [2].

Pomegranate (*Punica granatum*)

Pomegranate juice and fruit contain more polyphenols and anthocyanadins than green tea, red wine, cranberry, blueberry or orange juice, with AO activity three times higher than green tea or red wine. Other SM include tannins such as ellagic acid, citric, linoleic, and tartaric acids, and phytoestrogens. This herb stimulates wound healing, melanogenesis, is anti-viral to HIV, AB to *Staphylococcus aureus*, AF, AP and photoprotective.

Pomegranate stimulates keratinocyte proliferation, inhibits MMP-1 and increases fibroblast procollagen synthesis, thus benefit for photoaging therapy is expected but not proven with topical administration [2,8]. It was effective in reducing photoaging as part of a multinutrient oral product [10].

Pumpkin (*Curcubita pepo*)

These SM are carotenoids including lutein and beta carotene, unsaturated fats including oleic, palmitic, stearic, with nearly half being linoleic acid. This oil is also rich in gamma and alpha tocopherols, sterols including cholesterol and curcubitin, which mimics dihydrotestosterone. This extract has AO and AP activity. No blinded clinical trials have been published for photoaging therapy [2].

Pycnogenol (*Pinus pinaster, P. maritima*)

The French maritime pine tree yields SM including flavonoid monomers, dimers, oligomers and polymers of catechins, epicatechin and taxifolin, which are known as oligomeric proanthocyanidins (OPC). Pycnogenol also contains phenolics such as ferulic, caffeic and coumaric acids and polysaccharides. It has AH, AI, and AO photoprotective functions. This ingested herb effectively treats chronic venous insufficiency better than horse chestnut. It is photoprotective. This herb stimulates wound healing, inhibits MMPs, stimulates cellular and humoral immunity. Clinical trials document it is effective therapy for psoriasis, atopic dermatitis and lupus.

In a 30-day open human clinical trial for melasma therapy, there was highly statistically significant ($p < 0.001$) decrease in melasma area and pigment intensity with 30 mg three times daily [2,8,29].

Rosemary (*Rosmarinus officianalis*)

This herb is also a rich source of triterpenes, especially ursolic acid, as well as camphor, flavonoids, diterpenes such as carnosolic acid and caffeic acids, including rosmarinic. Rosemary is AB AF, AT, AV, while improving vascular perfusion to accelerate wound healing. Rosemary should not be used during pregnancy [2,8].

Sage (*Salvia lavandulae, S. folia*)

These herbs are rich sources of ursolic acid, a triterpene documented to two clinical trials to reduce signs of photoaging. It also contains AO, AI flavonoids, diterpenes including carnosolic acid, caffeic acids such as rosmarinic and chlorogenic acids and camphor. It has AB, AF, AV, AT, while increasing local circulation. It should not be used during pregnancy. The toxin, thujone, must be removed during manufacturing [2,8].

Soy (*Glycine max*)

SM from the soy bean include all of the essential amino acids needed for protein synthesis as well as calcium, potassium, iron, vitamins K2, B3, and isoflavones with estrogenic effects including genistein, equol and daidzein, and AO estrogenic lignans. Other SM include phytosterols such as beta sitosterol, phospholipids such as phosphatidyl choline, and saponins including triterpenes. Soy isoflavones are AI, AO, and AT. Unfortunately, soy does inhibit synthesis of thyroid hormone.

The positive impact of soy in reversing photoaging has been documented in four double-blind controlled clinical trials using different forms of soy including whole soy, soy milk and soy isoflavones plus lignans. Success in treating acne has also been observed [2,8,30,31].

Swiss apple (*Uttwiler spätlauber*)

This apple was discovered to stay fresh-looking for up to 4 months due to longevity of its stem cells. Unfortunately, only 20 of these trees exist on a farm in Thurgau, Switzerland. Researchers have suggested that stem cells from these apples protect human skin cells from aging, yet this conclusion was only supported by a 10-panelist open, uncontrolled study which demonstrated 25% reduction of wrinkles after four weeks. Efficacy was demonstrated in a double-blind clinical study using this herb and five other actives. Safety with chronic use has not been documented [32,33,34].

Tamarind (*Tamarindus indica*)

This flavoring agent contains SM including a polysaccharide (pectin) that chemically closely resembles eye mucin. It also contains methyl salicylate, thiazole, malic and tartaric acids, protein, vitamins, minerals, pyrazines, monosaccharides, monoterpenoids, and cinnamates. These extracts are AB, AF AP and ACY. Topically, tamarind reduces parameters of photoaged skin [2].

Turmeric (*Curcuma longa, C. domestica*)

This herb is best known as the food spice, curry. Curcumin is the therapeutic component extracted that is AH, AI (greater than ibuprofen), AO, AT and stimulates wound healing. SM include volatile oils such as tumerone, the source of the aroma; curcuminoids including curcumin, the yellow pigment; and polysaccharides. Curcumin has weak estrogenic effects, prevents genetic transcription, suppresses MMPs, inhibits angiogenesis while stimulating cellular immunity. Curcumin is AB, AP, AV (against HIV).

Topical curcumin is a safe therapy for radiation dermatitis wound repair. Turmeric extracts should not be used in pregnancy [1,2,8].

The next six herbs have been combined in a commercially available blend, documented in six double-blinded, prospective, controlled clinical trials to be statistically superior ($p < 0.05$) to prescription tretinoin 0.05% and 12% ammoniated lactic acid in reversing photoaging of the skin [35,36].

Apple (Malus domestica)
SM of this fruit provide AB, AH, AI, AO, AT functionalities with flavonoids including quercetin and phloretin but also malic, succinic, lactic and citric acids, phyto steroids, B and C vitamins, carotenoids, tannins, caffeoylquinic acid and aromatic hexanal, and ethyl butyrate. It also has skin lightening properties [2,8].

Date palm fruit (Phoenix dactylifera)
This extract contains 50% saccharose and 10% oils of phytosteroids, leucoanthocyanidins, and flavonoids such as quercetin. In one screening study, this extract had the highest AI activity of all healthy food stuffs [8,10]. A blinded clinical trial demonstrated a statistically superiority to placebo in reducing periorbital fine lines [37]. Combined with meadowfoam and white willow bark, periorbital fine wrinkles were reduced by 42% in another double-blinded, prospective, controlled clinical trial compared to placebo [36].

Flaxseed (Linum usitatissimum)
Also known as linseed, flax is one of the richest sources of the omega 3 essential fatty acid, linolenic acid. It also contains lignans at a dose of 800-fold higher than in soy. These SM provide AI, AO, AT and estrogenic functions. Combined with meadowfoam oil, flax produces the ideal omega-3: omega-6 ratio for optimizing cutaneous endogenous AI activity. Used orally with borage oil in a double-blind trial of 45 panelists, flax significantly decreased erythema, roughness and scaling, while hydration and skin barrier function were improved [2,8,10].

Meadowfoam (Limnanthes alba)
This oil is a richer source of monounsaturated fatty acids than olive oil as well as a rich source of omega-3 and omega-6 fatty acids. Meadowfoam is also the richest source of phyto DHA, an essential fatty acid and a key precursor to synthesis of acetylcholine which increases skin firmness. This herb is AI and AT [10].

Mountain rose (Rosa canina)
This herb has long been used as a dietary supplement for vitamin C, malic and citric acids and pectin. Rose SM include citronellol, geraniol, nerol, linalool and citral, as well as proanthocyanidins and tannins [2,8].

Safflower (Carmathus tinctorius)
Safflower is the oil with the highest concentration of linoleic acid, one of the three physiologic stratum corneum barrier oils along with ceramide and cholesterol. Linoleic acid provides epidermal AB, AF, AI, AP effects, plus helps maintain the acid mantle. Safflower oil also inhibits MMP-2 and -9, thus reducing photoaging. Safflower seed oil was also shown to inhibit melanogenesis more potently than arbutin [2,8,38,39].

Recent herbal clinical trials

1. Plum fruit (*Prunus domestica*), sakura leaf (*Prunus speciosa*), and three synthetics to treat moderate hyperpigmentation and photoaging in 114 panelists for 8 weeks. Statistically significant improvement was seen. Dahl A, Oregajo C, Yatskayer M. 69th Annual Meeting, Amer Acad of Dermatol, February 4–8, 2011, New Orleans, LA. Poster #3209.
2. *Dianella ensifolia*, white birch, tetrahydrocurcumin, glycyrrhretinic acid statistically significantly improved hyperpigmentation. Mommone T, Muizzudin N, Declercq L, *et al*. Modification of skin discoloration by a topical treatment containing an extract of *Dianella ensifolia*, a potent antioxidant. *J Cosmet Dermatol* 2010; **9**: 89–95.
3. Review of herbal hyperpigmentation therapies. Berson D. *Pract Dermatol* 2012; **9**: 33–3.
4. *Polypodium leucotomos* statistically significantly improved photosensitivity with 480 mg and 720 mg daily doses. Tanew A, Radakovic S, Gonzalez S, *et al*. Oral administration of a hydrophilic extract of polypodium leukotomos for prevention of polymorphous light eruption. *J Amer Acad Dermatol* 2012; 66 (1): 58–62.
5. Dill, blackberry, zinc, copper. N = 33 significant improvement in some photoaging parameters. Baumann, LS, Figueras KA, Bell M, Flitter CJ. *Skin & Allergy News*, Nov 2012; **28**: 29.
6. Tetrahydrocurcumin ascorbate, glabridin and 4 synthetics for hyperpigmentation equals 4% hydroquinone in efficacy and tolerability. Makino ET, Herndon JH, Sigler ML, *et al*. Clinical efficacy and safety of a multimodality skin brightener composition compared with 4% hydroquinone. *J Drugs Dermatol* 2012; **11**: 1478–82.
7. Tibetan goji berries, Himalayan raspberry, Iceland moss, and Carob (*Ceratonia siliqua*), with Dead Sea mineral water as a base of two products. N = 10 for 4 weeks, both products reduced wrinkle depth and increased hydration. Wineman E, Portugal-Cohen M, Sorok Y, *et al*. Photodamage protective effect of two facial products containing a unique complex of Dead Sea minerals and Himalayan actives. *J Cosmet Dermatol* 2012; **11**: 183–90.
8. *Bulbinella frutecens*, Centella asiatica, oleurapeia in dimethicone enchance hydration, promote collagen-1 formation and maturation of scar compared to 100% petrolatum. N = 120. At week 2, statistically significant reduction in scar thickness, height, vascularity and itching. Kircik L. Comparative study of the efficacy and tolerability of a unique topical scar product vs. white petrolatum following shave biopsies. *J Drugs Dermatol* 2013; **12** (1): 86–90.

9. Licorice and vitamin C. Park US, Campo SO, Costa A. Thirty-five panelists treated 60 days for melasma had a MASI score reduction by a statistically significant 35.1%. 71st Annual Meeting, Amer Acad of Dermatol, March 1–5, 2013, Miami, FL. Poster #6811.
10. Oatmeal and petrolatum. Zernikow R, Nebus J, Suero M, Appa Y. Two blinded trials: $N = 11$ for 3 days on abraded skin, $n = 28$ for 14 days for winter dryness. Statistically significant improved hydration at 24 hours and TEWL improved by 14 days. 71st Annual Meeting, Amer Acad of Dermatol, March 1–5, 2013, Miami, FL. Poster #6390.
11. Dill, olive oil, a peptide and niacinamide used for 12 weeks. After 4 weeks, significantly improved uneven skin texture was noted with improved elasticity also by 12 weeks vs. negative control. There were statistically significant improved eyelid fine lines/wrinkles at 7 days. Osborne R, Reichart D, Li J, et al. 71st Annual Meeting, Amer Acad Dermatol, March 1–5, 2013, Miami, FL. Poster #7051 and #7071.
12. Twenty-one herbs with 29 synthetics in a formulation reduced facial erythema by 32.7% after 4 weeks in 44 volunteers. Dupont E, Leveille C, Gomez J, et al. Clinical efficacy of a serum integrating multiple cosmetic ingredients in the management of erythema of the face in aging skin. *J Cosmet Dermatol* 2012; **11**: 207–212.
13. A quick review of 69 herbals. Botanical Blockbusters. Tashetta-Millane M. Dayspa 2013 (Jan); **18**(1): 60–67.
14. Curcumin: a novel treatment for skin related disorders. Nguyen TA, Friedman AJ. *J Drugs Dermatol* 2013 (Oct); **12**: 1131–7.
15. Green tea, resveratrol, caffeine reduced facial erythema in all 16 panelists by 6 weeks. Ferzli G, Patel M. Phrsai N, Brody N. Reduction of facial redness with resveratrol added to topical product containing green tea, polyphenols and caffeine. *J Drugs Dermatol* 2013 (July); **12**: 770–4.
16. Grape seed extract with 2 synthetics for photoaging significantly increased collagen by 74% and dermal density as well as other photoaging parameters in 40 panelists for 60 days. Gomes-Neto A, Costa A, Arruda L, et al. 70th Annual Meeting, Amer Acad Dermatol, March 16–20, 2012, San Diego, CA, poster #4703.
17. Nebus J, Vassilatou K, Philippo U, Wallo W. Oak quercetin used for 60 days on eyelids of 32 panelists produced statistically significant improvement of wrinkling and smoothness in over 90%. 69th Annual Meeting, Amer Acad Dermatol, February 4–8, 2012, New Orleans, LA, poster #1615.
18. Anthonavage M, Saliou C, Tucker-Smaras S, Zedayko T. Southern wood (*Artemis ambrosia*) in 20 panelists to treat photoaging for 2 weeks produced statistically significant decrease in fine lines and mottled hyperpigmentation. 69th Annual Meeting Amer Acad Dermatol, February 4–8, 2012, New Orleans, LA, poster #810.
19. Spring restharrow (*Ononis spinosa*) root and a synthetic active in open trial of 48 panelists for 2 weeks reduced wrinkles and lifted skin. DeCunha A, Nkenge A, Bertin C, et al. 69th Annual Meeting, Amer Acad Dermatol, February 4–8, 2012, New Orleans, LA, poster #808.

Conclusion

The use of herbal products remains a very active area of research in cosmetic formulations. Their popularity is in part a result of the perceived safety naturally derived ingredients. Consumer perceptions of botanicals as positive ingredients also make them a welcome addition to otherwise mundane formulations. This chapter has evaluated some of the key considerations when assessing and testing herbal based cosmetic products, including the scientific basis and clinical trials of the most commonly used herbal ingredients.

References

1. VanWyk BE, Wink M. In: *Medicinal Plants of the World*. Timber Press: Portland, OR, 2004: 16–26, 371–94.
2. Jellin JM, Gregory PJ, eds. In: *Natural Medicines Comprehensive Data Base*, 13th edn. Therapeutic Research Faculty: Stockton, California, 2012: 38–42, 31, 42, 215, 255, 262, 263, 301, 443, 623–5, 768, 769, 788–93, 1009–1013, 1107, 1162, 1200–1202, 1260–62, 1295–8, 1333–5, 1356–9, 1374, 1375, 1424, 1439–50, 151215.
3. Zwiebel SJ, Lee M, Alleryne B, Guyuron B. The incidence of vitamin, mineral, herbal and other supplements use in facial cosmetic patients. *Plas Recon Surg* 2013; **132** (1): 78-82.
4. Heller J, Gabbay JS, Ghadjar M, et al. The top 10 list of herbal and supplemental medicines used by cosmetic patients. *Plas Recon Surg* 2006; **117** (2): 436–45.
5. Draelos ZD. The art and science of new advances in cosmeceuticals. *Clin Plas Surg* 2011; **38** (3): 397–407.
6. Winnington P. Skin care and medical dermatology. *Pract Dermatol* 2007; Nov: 35–44.
7. Epstein HA. Cosmetic science. *SKIN Med*, 2013; **11**: 297–9.
8. Greenwald J, Brendler T, Jaenicke C, eds. In: *PDR for Herbal Medicines*, 4th edn. Thomson Healthcare, Inc: Montvale, NJ, 2007.
9. Draelos Z. Optimizing redness reduction, part 2. *Cosmet Dermatol* 2008; **21**: 433–6.
10. Thornfeldt C, Bourne K. In: *The New Ideal in Skin Health: Separating Fact from Fiction*. Allured Books: Carol Stream, IL, 2010; 31–55, 134, 143, 144, 191, 352–67.
11. Thornfeldt C. In: DraelosZ (ed.) *Cosmetic Dermatology*, 1st edn. Wiley Blackwell Publishing Ltd, Chichester, UK, 2010; (34): 1269–80.
12. Koo J. Arain S. Traditional Chinese medicine in dermatology. *Clin Dermatol* 1999; **17**: 21–7.
13. Jancin B. Cross-sensitivity in tea tree oil allergy. *Skin Allergy News* 2002; Mar:38.
14. Henley DV, Lipson N, Korach K, Bloch C. Prepubertal gynecomastia linked to lavender and tea tree oils. *NEJM* 2007; **356**: 479–85.

15 Lewis W. Cosmeceuticals roundup. *Plastic Surg Products* 2007; Sept: 38–42.
16 *Antioxidants in Human Skin*. www.wikipedia.org (accessed 19 Jan 2014).
17 Saluja R, Yosowitz G, Goldman M. Evaluation of mineral cosmetics. *Cosmet Dermatol* 2007; **20**: 382–7.
18 Jin Y, Lee S, Chung M. Aloesin and arbutin via a different action mechanism. *Arch Pharm Res* 1999; **22**: 232–6.
19 Milesi MA, Lacan D, Brosse H, *et al*. Effect of an oral supplementation with a proprietary melon juice concentrate (Extramel®) on stress and fatigue in healthy people: a pilot, double-blind, placebo-controlled clinical trial. *Nutr J* 2009; **8**: 40.
20 Cohen J. Coffeeberry. *Skin Allergy News* 2007; **1**:32.
21 Akhtar N, Mehmood A, Ali Khan B, *et al*. Exploring cucumber extract for skin rejuvenation. *African J Biotech* 2007; **10** (7): 1206–16.
22 Baumann LS. Cucumber. Cosmeceutical Critique. *Skin & Allergy News* 2012; Oct: 21.
23 Tierney N, Liebel F, Kurtz ES, Martin K. Daily use of a topical formulation containing parthenolide-free extract of feverfew clinically reduces the appearance of erythema due to ultraviolet exposure. Poster presented at 63rd annual meeting of the American Academy of Dermatology, New Orleans, LA, 2007.
24 Middlekamp-Hup M, Puthak M, Parrado C, *et al*. Oral polypodium leukotomos extract decreases ultraviolet induced damage of human skin. *J Am Acad Dermatol* 2004; **51**: 910–8.
25 Baumann LS. Melasma and its newest therapies. *Cosmet Dermatol* 2007; **20**: 349–53.
26 Yamakoshi J, Sano A, Tokutake S, *et al*. Oral intake of proanthocyanidin-rich extract of grape seeds improves chloasma. *Phytother Res* 2004; **18**: 895–9.
27 Högberg L, Laurin P, Fälth-Magnussen K, *et al*. Oats to children with newly diagnosed coeliac disease: a randomized double-blind study. *Gut* 2004; **53**: 649–54.
28 www.cancer.org/treatments, accessed 10 January 2014.
29 Ni A, Mu Y, Gulati O. Treatment of melasma with pycnogenol. *Phytother Res* 2007; **16**: 567–71.
30 Wallo W, Nebus J, Leyden J. Efficacy of a soy moisturizer in photoaging: a double-blind, vehicle controlled, 12-week study. *J Drugs Dermatol* 2007, **6**: 917–22.
31 Baumann LS, Wu J. Cosmeceutical Critique Compendium: supplement to *Skin and Allergy News* 2008; 1–19.
32 A Swiss apple a day keeps wrinkles at bay. www.swissinfo.ch (accessed 11 Jan 2014*).*
33 www.Greenmedinfo.com/blog/science (accessed 13 May 2013).
34 Farris PK, Edison BL, Brouda I, *et al*. Swiss apple stem cells plus 4 synthetics and one peptide. Improved photoaging to statistically significant degree in 69 women for 16 weeks. A high potency multi-mechanism skin care regimen provides significant anti-aging effects: results from a double-blind, vehicle-controlled clinical trial. *J Drugs Dermatol* 2012; **11**: 1447–54.
35 Thornfeldt C, Sigler M. A cosmeceutical with novel mechanisms of action effectively reduces signs of extrinsic aging. Poster #1128, presented at: 64th Annual Meeting, Amer Acad Dermatol, San Francisco, CA, 2006.
36 Thornfeldt C, Sigler M. Comedolytic anti-inflammatory cosmeceutical reduces signs of maturity. Poster #229, presented at 64th Annual Meeting, Amer Acad Dermatol, San Francisco, CA, 2006.
37 Bauza E, Dal Farra C, Berghi A, Oberto G, Peyronel D, Domloge N. Date palm kernel extract exhibits anti-aging properties and significantly reduces skin wrinkles. *Int J Tissue React* 2002; **24**: 131–6.
38 Solanki K, Matnani M, Kale M, *et al*. Transcutaneous absorption of topically massaged oil in neonates. *Indian Pediatr* 2005; **42** (10): 998–1005.
39 Roh JS, Han JY, Kim JH, Hwang JK. Inhibitory effects of active compounds isolated from safflower (Carthamus tinctorius L.) seeds for melanogenesis. *Biol Pharm Bull* 2004; **27** (12): 1976–8.

CHAPTER 33
Antioxidants and Anti-inflammatories

Bryan B. Fuller
DermaMedics LLC, Oklahoma City, OK, USA

> **BASIC CONCEPTS**
> - An antioxidant is a molecule that prevents the oxidation of other molecules thereby protecting cells from damage caused by free radicals.
> - The most common oxygen radicals in the body are the superoxide anion ($O_2^{\bullet-}$) and the hydroxyl radical ($\bullet OH$).
> - Free radicals cause extensive and irreversible damage to proteins, DNA, and lipids, with serious consequences affecting cell survival, malignant transformation, and the development of disease.
> - Antioxidants include vitamin C, vitamin E, curcumin, green tea, carotenoids, and ubiquinone.
> - Anti-inflammatories include botanical extracts, corticosteroids, non-steroidal anti-inflammatories, and immunomodulators.
> - Endogenous antioxidants and anti-inflammatories are necessary to prevent damage that contributes to both extrinsic and intrinsic aging.

Antioxidants

Introduction

The use of oral and topical antioxidants to provide protection from and treatments for various diseases, including cancer, and to prevent aging, has gained considerable popularity over the past 25 years. While it is clear that antioxidants such as vitamins C, E and A, and carotenoids, can protect cells from free radical damage, it is not clear whether or not taking large quantities of antioxidants can prevent the occurrence of disease or slow the aging process. Some clinical studies have suggested such a role for antioxidants, while other studies have not provided clear evidence that antioxidant supplements can reduce the risk of cancer, heart disease or aging [1]. Regardless of clinical study results, the fact that antioxidants can block free radical damage to cells has led to rapidly growing markets for antioxidant nutritional supplements, antioxidant beverages, and has fueled an entire industry focused on finding foods with ever higher antioxidant potential. Most, if not all, topical skin care products manufactured today contain antioxidants such as vitamin E, vitamin C, and carotenoids, to mention a few. The question of whether or not the antioxidants in topical skin care products may provide any skin benefits will be explored in this section.

Antioxidants, free radicals and reactive oxygen species (ROS)

An antioxidant is simply a molecule that can prevent the oxidation of other molecules. Their importance in protecting cells from damage results from their ability to block the progression of oxidative damage caused by free radicals.

Free radicals are molecules or atoms with unpaired electrons. Having an unpaired electron leaves an incomplete electron shell and makes the atom or molecule more chemically reactive than those with complete electron shells. Because atoms seek to reach a state of maximum stability, they will try to fill the outer shell by "stealing" an electron from another molecule. When the target molecule loses an electron to the free radical it then, in turn, becomes a free radical and must find a "donor" it can steal an electron from. Thus, a chain reaction begins that causes considerable damage to cellular proteins, lipids, membranes and DNA. Most free radicals in biological systems are derivatives of oxygen. The most common oxygen radicals in the body are the superoxide anion ($O_2^{\bullet-}$) and the hydroxyl radical ($\bullet OH^-$). While free radicals have extremely short half-lives, in the order of nanoseconds or microseconds, this is sufficient time to attack molecules and generate new free radicals. In addition to the above oxygen radicals, there are other reactive oxygen species (ROS) which are not actually radicals, but which are reactive and which can cause extensive damage to cells and tissues. Two of the more important of these are hydrogen peroxide and hypochlorite ion [2].

Free radicals and other ROS can cause irreversible and destructive changes to proteins, DNA, and lipids and these can have serious consequences on cell survival, malignant transformation and the development of disease. One of the most damaging free radical events is lipid peroxidation to membrane lipids

---

Cosmetic Dermatology: Products and Procedures, Second Edition. Edited by Zoe Diana Draelos.
© 2016 John Wiley & Sons, Ltd. Published 2016 by John Wiley & Sons, Ltd.

which play a key role in cell signaling. In this case a hydroxyl radical may remove a hydrogen atom from the side chain of a fatty acid, thereby converting the fatty acid into a radical. The fatty acid then reacts with oxygen to form a very reactive peroxyl radical. A chain reaction begins in which one lipid radical becomes two lipid radicals. Ultimately, the lipid radicals may form covalent crosslinks with each other thereby ending the chain reaction. Unfortunately the result is crosslinked and functionally damaged lipids. A good example of this is the free radical damage to low-density lipoprotein (LDL). This damage has been shown to lead to atherosclerosis.

ROS effects on signaling pathways

Free radicals and other reactive oxygen species (ROS) can not only damage proteins, lipids and other cellular constituents, they can activate signaling pathways that lead to the increased expression of genes controlling inflammation and proliferation. Although ROS are produced constantly by normal cellular events such as respiration, or as a result of enzyme activity, e.g. NADH oxidases, they are continually being inactivated by cellular antioxidants such as superoxide dismutase (SOD), catalase, glutathione (GSH) peroxidase and GSH. However, if the "load" of ROS in a cell becomes very high due to exposure to such "insults" as UVR, ionizing radiation, chemotherapeutic drugs, or environmental factors, the endogenous antioxidant mechanisms are overwhelmed, "oxidative stress" occurs, and signaling pathways are activated. Many studies have shown that ROS can activate members of the mitogen activated protein kinases (MAPK) family, which includes the growth factor-regulated extracellular signal-related kinases (ERKs), the stress-activated MAPKs, c-jun NH2-terminal kinases (JNKs) and p38 MAPKs. Activation of these kinases leads to the enhanced expression of a number of genes including those involved in inflammation and proliferation [3]. How ROS activate the MAPK pathways is not completely understood, but evidence suggests that these free radicals may function by:

1. promoting ligand-independent clustering and activation of membrane receptors, such as the epidermal growth factor membrane receptor, which, when activated, stimulates the MAPK pathway;
2. inactivating MAPK phosphatases (MKP), which ordinarily function to dephosphorylate and inactivate MAPK thereby "dampening" the kinase mediated events;
3. altering the protein structure of receptor tyrosine kinases and MAPK and, by doing so, irreversibly activate them [4,5,6].

Regardless of the mechanism of activation, the end result of stimulating the MAPK pathway is that gene expression is altered leading to: (1) increased cellular proliferation; (2) increased inflammatory cytokine and chemokine expression; (3) increased COX-2 expression, resulting in high levels of PGE-2; (4) cell transformation/carcinogenesis; and (5) increased production of MMPs (matrix metalloproteinases), including MMP-1, MMP-2, and MMP-9, all of which can cause damage to the skin's matrix [7,8].

ROS and glycation: effects on skin aging

A large body of recent work has shown a strong link between AGEs (advanced glycation end products) and both skin aging and skin inflammation. Aging effects on skin that result from glycation include alterations in skin thickness, texture, resiliency, loss of matrix components, and a decrease in elasticity. Glycation is a non-enzymatic linkage of sugar to proteins, lipids and nucleic acids. Specifically the carbonyl group of simple sugars such as glucose and fructose binds to the amino group of amino acids (especially lysine and arginine). This initial and reversible reaction forms a Schiff base which is chemically unstable. This Schiff base then re-arranges to form a more stable ketoamine. Like the Schiff base, this intermediate is also reversible, but because it is reactive, the ketoamine can form irreversible complexes with peptides and proteins, such as collagen, resulting in the production of crosslinks which are non-reversible and, unfortunately, are resistant to even enzymatic degradation. These large complexes can also undergo additional reactions such as oxidation, polymerization, and dehydration resulting in new forms of AGEs. Since AGEs are resistant to turnover, they accumulate with age, and the skin structure becomes increasingly damaged. Extracellular matrix (ECM) proteins are known to be a major target for glycation. Type I collagen is subject to glycation as is elastin and fibronectin. Collagen is not only a key structural component in the dermis, providing mechanical support for tissues, but it plays an active role in regulating such cell functions as migration, proliferation and gene expression. Glycation of collagen causes crosslinks between molecules and thus, creates stiffness that reduces skin elasticity. In addition, glycation alters the structure of collagen to the point that it is no longer able to bind correctly to target cells. This leads to lost cell communication. Table 33.1 shows a few of the "aging" effects of glycation on skin cells [9–11].

Evidence suggests that free radicals produced by UVR can accelerate the development of AGEs, and further, in the process of glycation and AGE formation, ROS are produced. These ROS, in turn, cause more damage to proteins and lipids and also activate signaling pathways that cause inflammation. Recent

Table 33.1 Glycation mediated skin aging effects

Cell type	Action	Aging effect
Keratinocyte	Decreased proliferation	Reduced cell renewal
Keratinoycte	Increased MMPs	Matrix destruction
Keratinocyte	NFκB activation	Inflammation
Fibroblasts	Decreased proliferation	Increased senescence
Fibroblasts	MMP increase decreased collagen synthesis	Loss of matrix strength and elasticity
Fibroblasts	Increased apoptosis	Cell death, thinning skin
Fibroblasts	Increased ROS	inflammation
Vascular endothelium	Increase adhesion molecules in endothelial cells	Increase in immune cells into skin: increased cytokines and chemokines. Inflammation

studies have identified a membrane receptor for AGE, appropriately named receptor for advance glycation end products (RAGE). Upon binding to AGEs, the RAGE receptor is activated and this activation leads to the stimulation of several signaling pathway components including mitogen-activated protein kinases (MAPKs), extracellular signal-regulated kinases (ERK) 1 and 2, phosphatidyl-inositol 3 kinase, p21Ras, stress-activated protein kinase/c-Jun-N-terminal kinase and the janus kinases [33,41]. Stimulating these pathways results in activation of various transcription factors, and in particular, the activation of nuclear factor kappa-B (NF-κB). This transcription factor, activates a variety of matrix damaging genes, such as MMP-1 and MMP-9, as well as inflammatory genes, including TNF-alpha, IL-1, IL-8, and COX-2 [12,13].

Antioxidants protect cells from free radicals, ROS, and glycation

Antioxidants protect cells from free radical/ROS damage by either donating an electron to a free radical thereby stabilizing it and halting the chain reaction or by accepting the one unpaired electron, again stabilizing the free radical and preventing it from interacting with and damaging proteins, DNA and lipids. By donating an electron to the free radical to stop the chain reaction, the antioxidant itself becomes a free radical. However, because of its structure, the antioxidant is far less reactive than other radicals. If it is relatively large, the effect of the unpaired electron is "diluted" along its structure. The antioxidant "radical" may also be neutralized by another antioxidant or it may be enzymatically restored to its non-free radical form. Gluthione is one antioxidant that can donate a hydrogen atom to a hydroxyl radical thereby neutralizing it. The oxidized glutathione is converted back to its reduced form by glutathione reductase and is then ready to reduce additional free radicals.

Recent studies have shown that antioxidants can prevent free radical damage to the skin in several ways:

1. Antioxidants inactivate ROS and PREVENT the ROS mediated stimulation of signaling pathways that can lead to the activation of inflammatory and aging genes, such as TNF-alpha, IL-1, COX-2 and MMPs.
2. Antioxidants can interfere directly with receptor activation of signaling pathways that stimulate inflammatory genes.
3. Antioxidants prevent free radical induced changes to proteins and to membrane lipids that destroy their normal cellular functions.
4. Antioxidants reduce the formation of AGEs, and AGEs produced ROS thus, reducing skin aging and inflammation [14–16].

An antioxidant's "potency" may be quantified by use of ORAC assays. ORAC stands for oxygen radical absorbance capacity and is a method of measuring antioxidant capacities of different foods, vitamins and compounds [17]. The assay measures the oxidative destruction of a fluorescent molecule (for example, fluorescein) after it is mixed with a free radical producer that generates peroxyl and hydroxyl radicals. By comparing the

Table 33.2 ORAC Values of Antioxidants

Antioxidant	ORAC mole TE/100g
Olive extract	2,700,000
Clove	1,078,700
Quercetin	1,090,000
Resveratrol	620,000
Cinnamon	267,536
Vitamin C	189,000
Vitamin E	135,000
Cocoa	80,7000
Acai	38,700
Pomegranate	10,500
Blueberry (raw)	7,700
Lycopene	5,800

change in fluorescence in a reaction tube that contains only the fluorescent molecule and free radical with the change in fluorescence measured in the assay tube containing the antioxidant along with the free radical, a measure of antioxidant potential (ORAC score) can be obtained. Table 33.2 shows the ORAC scores of some representative antioxidants.

Of the many antioxidants that are now being formulated into topical products, two of the most common and most important are vitamin C and vitamin E. Vitamin C is the most prominent antioxidant in the aqueous compartment of cells. It can neutralize hydroxyl, alkoxyl and peroxyl radicals by hydrogen donation and is thus, an extremely important antioxidant for biological systems. Further, vitamin C can regenerate oxidized vitamin E and is, in turn, regenerated by glutathione. It is a useful antioxidant to incorporate into topical products, including suncare products because in the skin, vitamin C neutralizes free radicals generated by either UVA or UVB radiation. Unfortunately, vitamin C needs to be continually replaced since even a low dose of UV radiation from the sun can deplete 30–40% of the vitamin C present in the skin [18].

Vitamin E is one of nature's most important lipid antioxidants since it associates with membranes and protects the lipid environment by scavenging lipid peroxyl radicals. Vitamin E is found in the stratum corneum where it can act as a "front line" defense against UV radiation induced free radicals. As mentioned above, the vitamin E radical can be regenerated by vitamin C, and also by glutathione and ubiquinol (coenzyme Q10).

There are many other antioxidants that have been formulated into skincare products including ferulic acid, retinol, idebenone, and epigallocatechin gallate to mention a few. As discussed below, some of the skin benefits these antioxidants provide may be the result of actions on cells that go beyond their ability to simply scavenge free radicals.

Antioxidants as anti-inflammatories: effects on cell signaling pathways

Inflammatory skin disorders are common and range from occasional rashes accompanied by skin itching and redness to more chronic conditions such as atopic dermatitis, rosacea, seborrheic dermatitis, and psoriasis. As mentioned, many naturally occurring antioxidants have pronounced anti-inflammatory activities, and because of the negative side effects of many prescription anti-inflammatories (discussed below), there is increasing interest by pharmaceutical companies in identifying botanically derived compounds to treat inflammatory skin conditions. The goal is to find compounds which have excellent anti-inflammatory properties, but which do not suppress the immune system or cause other side effects, such as skin thinning.

Biology of the skin inflammatory process

Skin inflammation, which is characterized by redness, swelling, heat, itching and pain, can exist in either an acute or chronic form with acute disease frequently progressing to a more chronic condition. Acute inflammation can result from exposure to UV radiation (UVR), ionizing radiation, allergens, or to contact with chemical irritants (soaps, hair dyes, etc.). Assuming that the triggering stimulus is eliminated, this type of inflammation is typically resolved within 1 to 2 weeks with little accompanying tissue destruction. A chronic inflammatory condition, however, can last a lifetime, and cause considerable damage to the skin. Some of the cellular and biochemical events which occur in the skin in response to a triggering stimuli (e.g. UVR, chemical or antigen) and which lead to an inflammatory response are shown in Figure 33.1. Within minutes of exposure of skin to an insult there is a rapid release of inflammatory mediators from keratinocytes and fibroblasts and from afferent neurons. Keratinocytes produce a number of cytokines and chemokines including PGE-2, TNF-alpha, IL-1, IL-6 and IL-8. Dermal fibroblasts also respond to the insult and to IL-1 produced by keratinocytes by increasing production and secretion of cytokines including IL-1, IL-6, IL-8 as well as PGE-2. PGE-2 increases vasodilation and vascular permeability, facilitates the degranulation of mast cells, and increases the sensitivity of afferent neuronal endings. Increased vasodilation and vascular permeability by PGE-2 and histamine leads to increased blood flow and extravasation of fluid from blood vessels, resulting in visible redness and swelling. Increased production of TNF-alpha and IL-1, leads to the expression of intracellular adhesion molecules, such as VCAM and ICAM, on endothelial cells of the blood vessels [19–21]. These proteins, as well as P and E selectin, serve as anchoring elements for blood-borne monocytes and neutrophils. The attachment of leukocytes to the adhesion molecules slows their

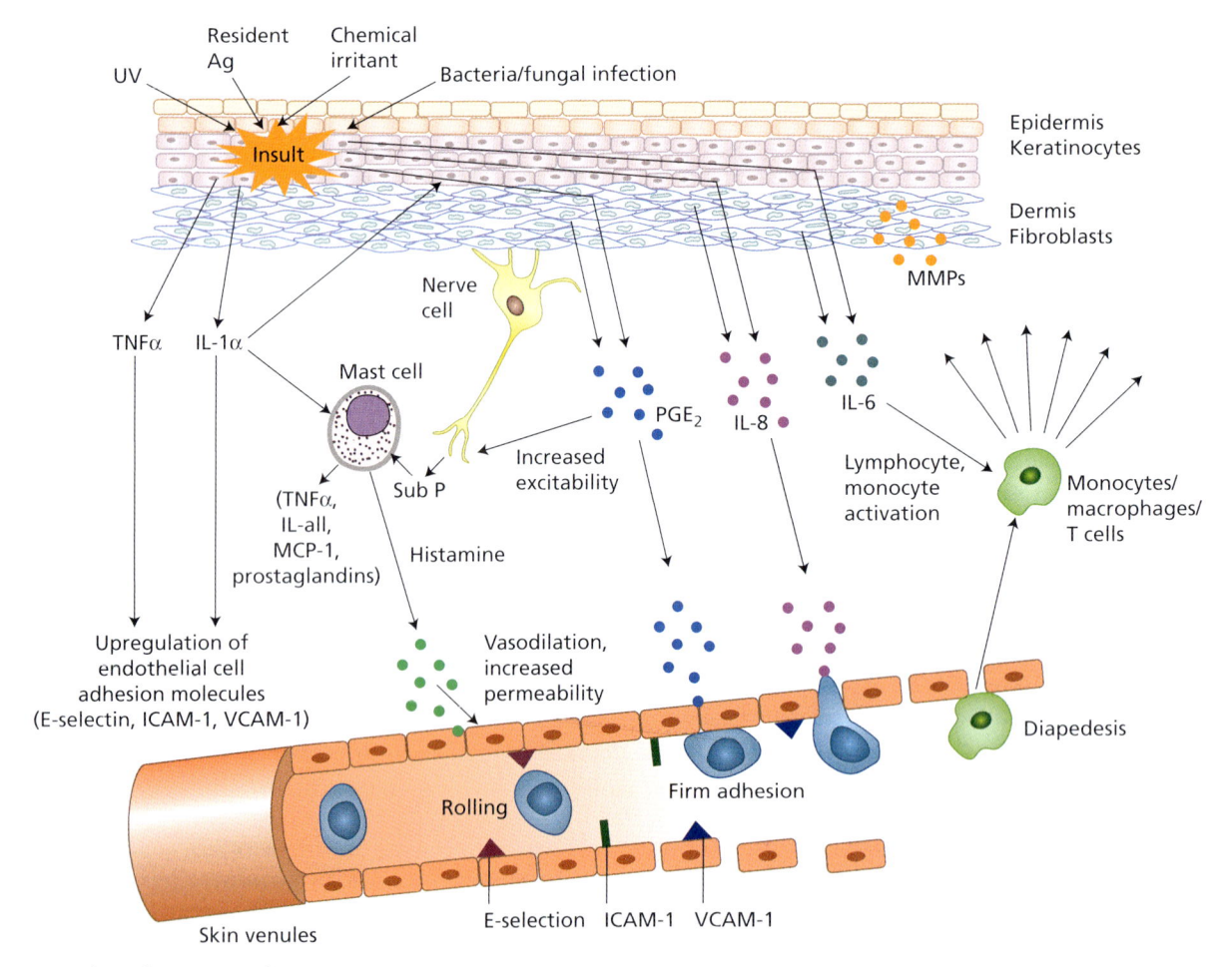

Figure 33.1 Skin inflammation pathway.

movement through the bloodstream and finally causes their adhesion to the endothelial wall. In the presence of chemokines, particularly, IL-8 produced and released by both keratinocytes and fibroblasts, the adherent leukocytes undergo chemotaxis and migrate from the blood vessel out into the skin where they act to scavenge the area of debris and also produce additional inflammatory mediators. The initial acute response occurs within minutes of the insult to the skin. The subsequent movement of neutrophils and monocytes into the "wounded" area typically takes up to 48 hours to occur. If the triggering stimulus is eliminated, inflammatory mediator production by keratinocytes, fibroblasts and mast cells ceases, the influx of leukocytes to the "wounded" area decreases and inflammation subsides [22–24].

In contrast to acute inflammation which typically resolves in 1 to 2 weeks, chronic inflammation results from a sustained immune cell mediated inflammatory response within the skin itself and is long-lasting. This response involves antigen presenting cells (APC) in the skin, called Langerhans cells in the epidermis and dendritic cells (DC) in the dermis, that, when activated, transport antigens through the lymphatics and to T lymphocytes where the antigen is "presented". The T-lymphocytes are activated and travel back to the skin where they proliferate and express a wide range of inflammatory mediators as well as matrix-eroding enzymes (MMP-1; collagenase) [25]. Cytokines produced by T-lymphocytes can stimulate fibroblasts and keratinocytes to produce additional cytokines and chemokines, and can also induce the expression of a variety of tissue-destructive enzymes by fibroblasts, including MMP-1 (collagen), MMP-3 (stomelysin-1) and MMP-9 (gelatinase B). As long as the antigen or insult stimulus persists in the skin, the inflammatory response will continue resulting in significant and serious tissue destruction.

Inflammatory processes in the skin, particularly those triggered by long-term exposure to solar radiation trigger molecular pathways that escalate the aging process. Actinic aging, or photoaging, that occurs following prolonged exposure of the skin to ultraviolet (UV) light from the sun results in increased cytokine production with attendant activation of genes in both keratinocytes and fibroblasts that cause erosion of the normal skin structure. Matrix metalloproteinases (MMPs), which break down the skin extracellular matrix causing sagging and wrinkling, are stimulated in sun-exposed skin. Furthermore, dermal fibroblast synthesis and assembly of collagen, which is required to maintain and restore the extracellular matrix, is inhibited while elastin production is over- stimulated, leading to elastosis. It is now widely accepted that sun-exposed skin in most individuals remains in a constant state of low level UV-induced inflammation, and that this "smoldering" inflammation is responsible for the signs of skin aging that appear in middle age [26,27,28].

Many antioxidants have anti-inflammatory, as well as anti-aging activities. Vitamin C, for example, not only stimulates the collagen I and III genes in dermal fibroblasts, but can also inhibit UVR-induced levels of inflammatory cytokines, chemokines and hormones including PGE-2. Further, this vitamin stimulates cell proliferation in dermal fibroblasts [29]. The major lipid soluble anti-oxidant, vitamin E, has been shown to alter the expression of cell cycle genes in human T cells and to suppress PGE-2 production [30]. This PGE-2 inhibition may explain, in part, vitamin E's ability to partially protect skin from UVR induced erythema.

One of the best anti-inflammatory antioxidants produced by nature may be curcumin. In addition to its ability to neutralize free radicals, it can also interfere with cell signaling pathways involved in inflammation. Considerable research efforts have focused on understanding how curcumin blocks inflammatory pathways [31–35]. From these studies the following picture has emerged:

1. Curcumin blocks the activation of the NF-κB transcription factor, which is responsible for the activation of a variety of inflammatory genes including TNF-alpha, IL-1, Il-8, and COX-2.
2. Curcumin blocks Nf-κB activation by preventing the phosphorylation of the NF-κB inhibitor IKB. Since phosphorylation of this factor is required for NF-κB activation, preventing its phosphorylation blocks NF-κB activation.
3. Curcumin also inhibits the activation of the inflammation related genes, ICAM and IL-12, which are controlled, at least in part, by Jak-STAT signaling pathways. This inhibition is due to curcumin's ability to block the phosphorylation and activation of the STAT transcription factor [8].
4. Curcumin can block the ligand activation of cell surface receptors. For example, curcumin blocks the activation of the EGF receptor, and since over-expression of this receptor is linked to several epithelial cell cancers, the potential use of curcumin as a cancer therapeutic has received considerable attention. Since curcumin has been shown to block the recruitment of "scaffolding proteins" to a receptor that has been "activated" by binding its ligand, it is likely that this is the mechanism by which curcumin blocks EGF activation of downstream signaling pathways.

Given all of these data, it seems likely that curcumin's ability to prevent the activation of inflammatory genes results from its ability to interfere with the initial "scaffolding" events that are required to stimulate the signaling cascade. In addition, curcumin's ability to inactivate ROS prevents the ROS mediated activation of surface receptors. A cartoon depicting the probable sites of action of curcumin, and likely other phenolic antioxidants, in preventing the activation of inflammatory (and aging) genes is shown in Figure 33.2.

In addition to curcumin, a large number of other phenolic and polyphenolic compounds derived from plants have now been shown to have direct anti-inflammatory effects on cells as well as antioxidant activity. These include quercetin, luteolin, resveratrol, ferulic acid, dihydroeugenol, apigenin, genistein, and epigallocatechin gallate [10–12]. While some of these antioxidants reduce inflammatory gene expression through interfering with NF-κB driven genes, others interfere with MAPK signaling pathways that lead to the activation of the

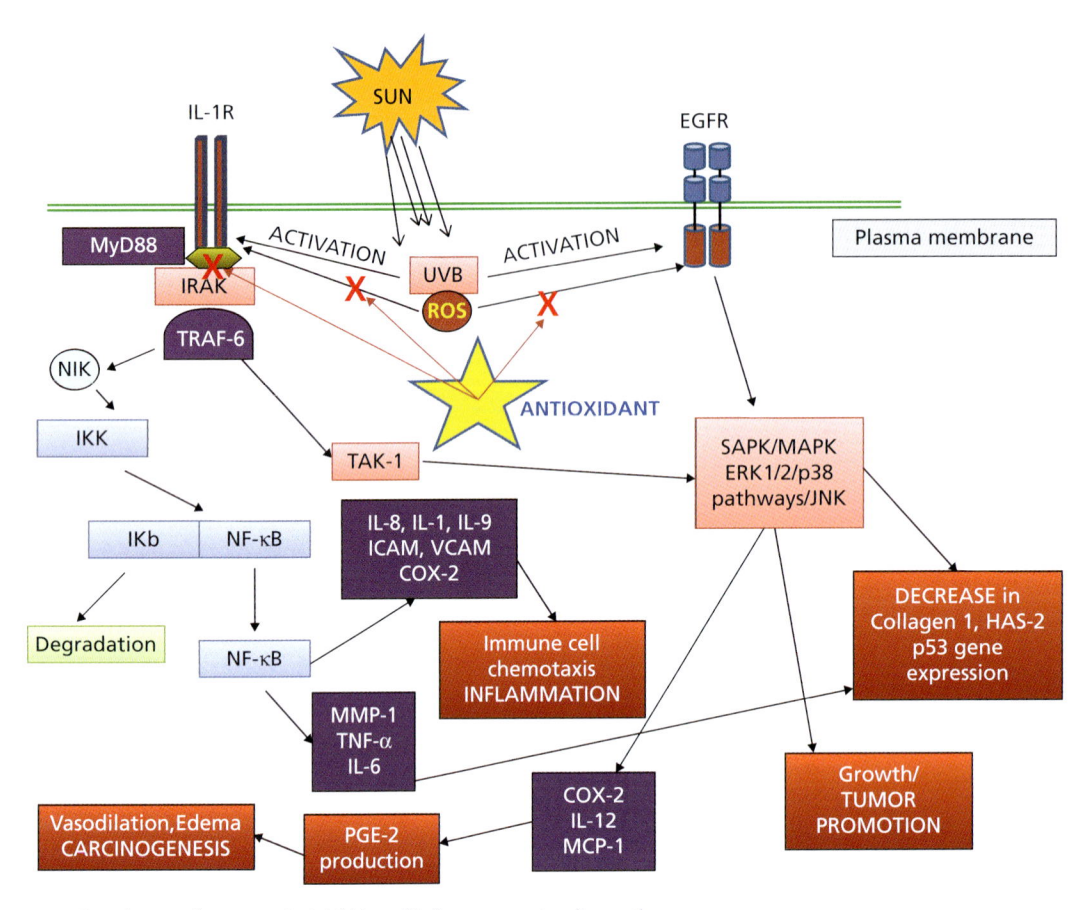

Figure 33.2 Proposed mechanism for curcumin inhibition of inflammatory signaling pathways.

transcription factor, AP-1. By interfering with the ability of AP-1 to activate target genes, these compounds, such as luteolin, prevent the activation of such inflammatory genes as IL-6, COX-2, IL-18 and MCP-1 (monocyte chemotactic protein-1) [36–39]. With regard to skin anti-aging benefits, not only can luteolin reduce the expression of inflammatory cytokines and chemokines, but it inhibits hyaluronidases and thus preserves hyaluronic acid levels in the skin [40]. A related polyphenol, genistein, blocks intracellular signaling pathways by inhibiting tyrosine kinases, and the phosphorylation of the epidermal growth factor receptor (EGF-R) [41]. A bar graph showing the effect of several antioxidants on inhibition of IL-1 induced PGE-2 levels in human dermal fibroblasts is shown in Figure 33.3a, while the effect of luteolin and ascorbyl acetate in inhibiting a variety of inflammatory cytokines in human keratinocytes induced with TPA, is shown in Figure 33.3b.

Topical formulation of antioxidants

Although it is clear that polyphenolic antioxidants as well as simpler antioxidants such as vitamins C and E can reduce inflammation in the skin, for these compounds to be effective when applied topically, they must penetrate into the skin at a sufficient concentration to exert their protective effects on target cells, such as keratinocytes, fibroblasts, and immune cells migrating in from the vasculature. Whether or not a particular compound will be able to cross the stratum corneum and penetrate down into the skin to reduce inflammatory events in the epidermis and dermis depends on two main factors: (1) size; and (2) solubility of the compound. With regard to *size*, it is well-known that molecules larger than 500 MW are too big to penetrate through the stratum corneum, at least to any significant degree [42]. Although it is theoretically possible for a large molecule, e.g. growth factors, enzymes, other protein and peptides to enter the skin through the follicle route, or through sweat glands, unfortunately these structures represent less than 1% of the skin's surface. Thus, this route of skin penetration would be of little value in addressing skin problems, such as inflammation. With regard to *solubility characteristics*, since the stratum corneum is composed largely of lipids, water soluble compounds regardless of how small they are, will not easily penetrate through this barrier. For any compound to penetrate into and through the stratum corneum, it should have a partition coefficient (Log P value) of around 2.5. Partition coefficient simply refers to the ratio between a compound's solubility in

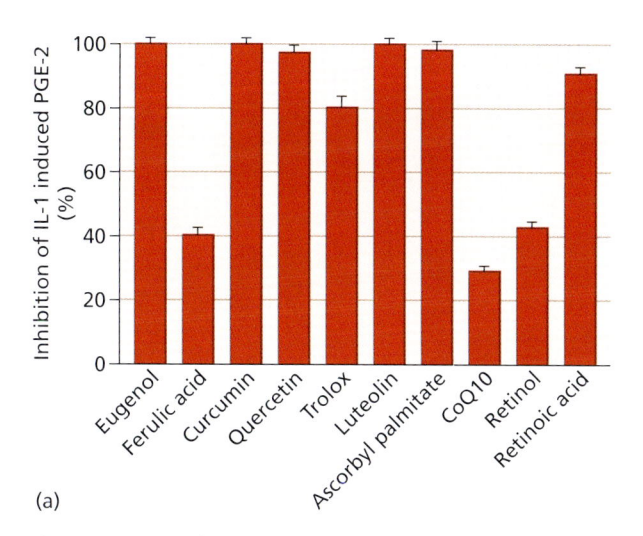

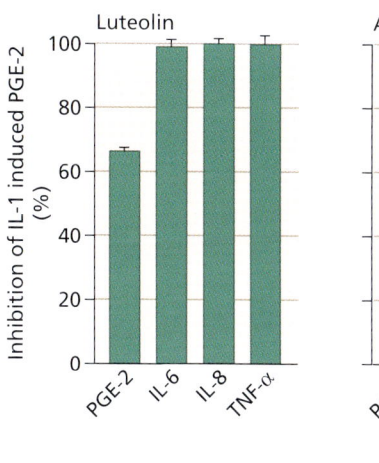

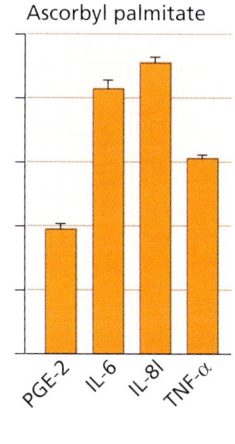

Figure 33.3 Anti-inflammatory properties of antioxidants. (a) Inhibition of the inflammatory mediator prostaglandin E 2 (PGE-2) in human keratinocytes by antioxidants. (b) Inhibition of four important skin inflammatory mediators by luteolin and vitamin C.

octanol (oil soluble) and its solubility in water. The logarithm of this ratio is called the LogP. So a compound with a LogP of 2 is much more soluble in octanol than water and will be likely to penetrate through the stratum corneum. A compound that has a LogP considerably under (e.g. −3) or over (e.g. 8) the value of 2 will likely not be a good candidate for topical use. A LogP of 8 means the compound is so hydrophobic that if it enters the stratum corneum, it will never move into the aqueous environment of the skin. Likewise, a compound with a negative LogP is too water soluble to penetrate the lipid environment of the stratum corneum. Many phenolic and polyphenolic antioxidants have exactly the properties needed for efficient topical delivery. Curcumin, luteolin, quercetin and 4-propyl guaiacol are all less than 400 molecular weight and all have a LogP of between 2 and 2.5. Unfortunately curcumin, luteolin and quercetin are yellow in color and will appear yellow when applied topically. Thus, they have not been used to any extent in topical products. The plant derived antioxidant, 4-propyl guaiacol, however, is colorless and moves through the stratum corneum with high efficiency. It also has pronounced anti-inflammatory activity.

Anti-inflammatories

Prescription medicines for inflammation and mechanism of action
Corticosteroids
Some of the most effective and commonly used prescription drugs for treating inflammation are the corticosteroids, particularly the glucocorticoid related steroids. They are effective for many forms of eczema, including atopic dermatitis and allergic contact dermatitis, and are fairly effective in ameliorating the symptoms of psoriasis. Corticosteroids can be used topically or orally. Given the efficacy of corticosteroids in treating many different types of skin inflammation and autoimmune based inflammatory diseases such as rheumatoid arthritis, asthma, lupus erythematosus, and allergic rhinitis, considerable research has been directed toward understanding their mechanism of action.

Corticosteroids act on target cells by binding to the glucocorticoid receptor present primarily in the cytosol. This binding "activates" the receptor resulting in its translocation to the nucleus. The steroid hormone receptor complex then binds, as a homodimer, to DNA regulatory elements along the promoter regions of specific genes. This binding usually results in the up-regulation of gene activity but can also cause transcriptional repression of the target gene [43]. The effectiveness of corticosteroids as inhibitors of inflammation stems from the ability of the steroid activated glucocorticoid receptor complex to interfere with the activation of genes regulated primarily by two transcription factors, NF-κB and AP-1 [44,45]. These two transcription factors are largely responsible for the transcriptional activation of a wide variety of pro-inflammatory genes including cytokines IL-1, IL-2, IL-3, IL-4, IL-6, IL-11, IL-12 and IL-13, TNF-alpha, and GM-CSF, chemokine genes IL-8, RANTES, MCP-1, adhesion molecules ICAM-1, VCAM-1 and E-selectin, the COX-2 gene, and the matrixmetalloproteinase genes, MMP-1 [46].

The transcription factors, NF-κB or AP-1 are activated by kinases which, in turn, are activated as a result of a hormone or cytokine binding to, and activation of, a surface receptor. In the case of the NF-κB activation pathway, a kinase, IκK, when activated, phosphorylates an inhibitor protein, IκB. Unphosphorylated IκB binds to and represses the activity of NF-κB, but when phosphorylated, it dissociates from NF-κB and is degraded. Once freed from the IκB, NF-κB can translocate to the nucleus where it binds to the promoter region of specific genes and activates them [47]. In regard to the AP-1 transcription factor, it

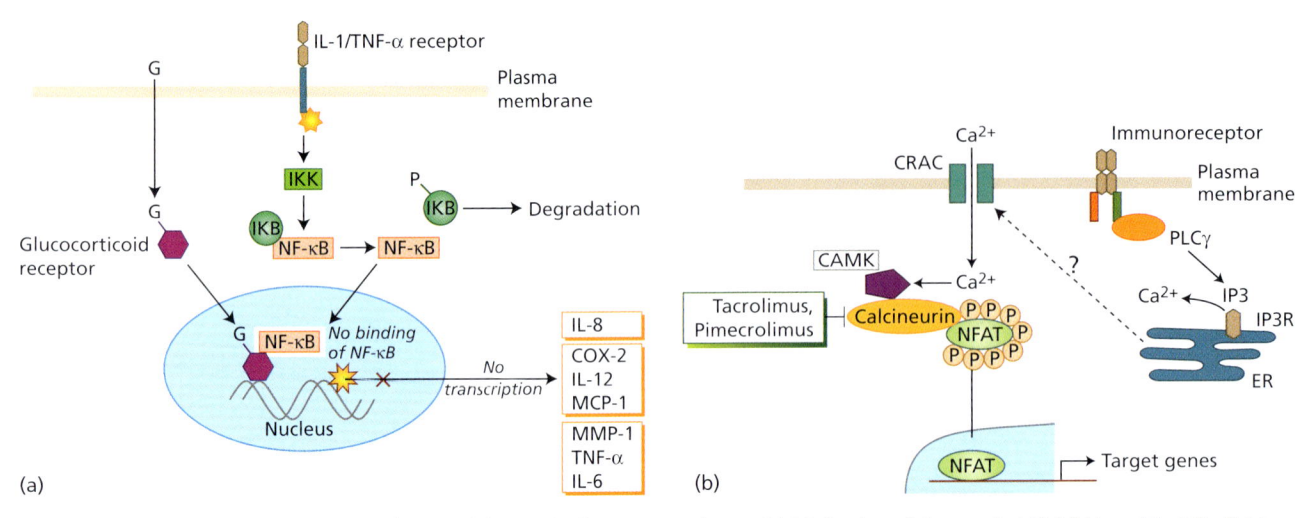

Figure 33.4 Glucocorticoid and immunomodulator inhibition of inflammatory pathways. (a) Mechanism of glucocorticoid inhibition of the NF-κB driven inflammation pathway. (b) Diagram of calcineurin and NFAT activation and inhibition by tacrolimus/pimecrolimus.

is phosphorylated and activated as a result of a kinase "signaling cascade" that begins with the binding of a hormone/cytokine, such as IL-1 or TNF-alpha to a surface receptor on target cells [45].

As mentioned, the anti-inflammatory activity of corticosteroids comes from their ability to repress either the activation or activity of the NF-κB and AP-1 transcription factors thereby suppressing transcription of genes coding for inflammatory mediators. A model showing one mechanism glucocorticoids use to block the transcriptional activity of NF-κB is shown in Figure 33.4a. When activated by hormone binding, the glucocorticoid receptor translocates to the nucleus where it can bind to NF-κB and suppress its transcriptional activity, either by preventing its binding to the promoter region of target genes or by preventing NF-κB's ability to activate the transcriptional machinery when bound to the promoter. Thus, inflammatory genes that require NF-κB for activation remained turned off. [48,49]. Similarly, the activated glucocorticoid receptor interacts with the AP-1 transcription factor and prevents it from binding to and activating target inflammatory genes.

While the glucocorticoids are very effective in suppressing the activation of pro-inflammatory genes they unfortunately produce a variety of undesirable side effects. First, due to their potent inhibition of genes involved in an immune cell driven inflammatory response, they have an overall immune suppressive effect. Prolonged use of glucocorticoids leads to a reduction in B and T lymphocyte populations, and a reduced ability to fight skin infections. Further, steroids adversely affect the ability of dermal fibroblasts to synthesize collagen and at high doses they reduce the proliferation rate of these cells. Consequently, long-term use of topical steroids leads to skin thinning and a decrease in the dermal matrix. Other potential negative side effects caused by prolonged use of steroids include altered carbohydrate metabolism, suppression of the hypothalamic-pituitary-adrenal axis, increased osteoporosis, and increased risk of developing cataracts.

NSAIDs

The most well-known of all the non-steroidal anti-inflammatory drugs (NSAIDs), aspirin, has been used for over 100 years to control various forms of inflammation. NSAIDs are available in OTC and prescription forms. Common OTC forms are ibuprofen, naproxen, and aspirin. Those available with a prescription include celecoxib (Celbrex®), diclofenac (Votaren®), etodolac (Lodine®), indomethacin (Indocid®), ketoprofen (Orudis®) and Rofecoxib (Vioxx®) to name a few. One topical prescription NSAID that has received FDA approval in the U.S. is Solareze® (diclofenac) which is indicated for the treatment of actinic keratoses [50,51].

When one examines the published data on the efficacy of topical NSAIDs in treating various inflammatory symptoms, the results show considerable disparity. A statistical analysis of clinical data from a wide number of trials with various topical NSAID preparations concluded that long-term use the effectiveness of the NSAID treated group was not significantly different from the placebo group [52]. Other studies, however, do suggest that topical NSAID treatment for joint pain provides relief beyond that observed with the placebo group [53–55]. Few studies have evaluated topical formulations that contain newer NSAIDs, including the specific COX-2 inhibitors, but it seems likely that a topical preparation of a potent NSAID that delivers adequate levels of an effective COX inhibitor through the skin would likely be effective in treating a variety of inflammatory conditions in which PGE-2 is indicated as a causative factor.

The target for NSAIDs is the enzyme cyclooxygenase (COX), which exists in two forms, COX-1 and COX-2. While most older versions of NSAIDs including aspirin and ibuprofen are not selective inhibitors of any particular form of COX, newer drugs have been designed to target primarily COX-2 [56].

Because of their ability to lower PGE-2 levels, topical NSAIDs have been evaluated for their ability to reduce the severity of a sunburn, which is largely mediated by PGE-2. Topical application of the COX-2 inhibitor, celecoxib, after UVB irradiation of skin, reduced erythema, edema, PGE-2 levels, the number of sunburn cells, and dermal infiltration of neutrophils [57]. The topical NSAID, diflofenac (branded Solareze*), which is approved for use in the U.S. to treat actinic keratoses, has been shown to reduce sunburn symptoms when applied within 4 hours of the initial onset of sunburn [51]. Interestingly, several studies implicate PGE-2 as a causative factor in skin cancer, and results from mouse experiments show that topical application of a PGE-2 inhibitor lowers the UVB induced number of papillomas detectable 12 weeks after UVB dosing [58,59].

Immunomodulators

A newer type of non-steroid anti-inflammatory drugs is represented by the immunomodulators. Two anti-inflammatory drugs that have received FDA approval for topical use are the immunomodulators, tacrolimus and the related drug, pimecrolimus. These drugs, along with cyclosporine, which exerts its effects through the same mechanism of action, had their origin as immunosuppressive agents used to prevent organ rejection after transplant surgery [60]. Both pimecrolimus and tacrolimus have been approved for topical use in treating atopic dermatitis, but not for psoriasis. As is the case with the glucocorticoids, the immunomodulators inhibit the production of inflammatory mediators but unlike the corticosteroids, both tacrolimus and pimecrolimus do not thin the skin [61–63].

Tacrolimus, pimecrolimus and cyclosporine all repress inflammatory genes in target cells through a common mechanism that involves the repression of activity of a ubiquitous calcium-activated phosphatase, calcineurin, that is involved in the activation of specific inflammatory genes [64]. A cartoon showing the calineurin pathway is shown in Figure 33.4b. When surface membrane receptors are activated by binding to a hormone or cytokine, there is an increase in intracellular calcium. The increased calcium causes the activation of calmodulin which then binds to the calcium dependent enzyme, calcineurin and activates it. The activated calcineurin enzyme is a phosphatase, which can dephosphorylate the cytosolic subunit of a transcription factor, NFATc (nuclear factor of activated T cells, cytosol). The dephosphorylation of the cytosolic NFAT subunit allows it to translocate to the nucleus where it forms a complex with the nuclear subunit of NFAT (NFATn) whose synthesis was induced by signaling cascade initiated by the antigen binding to the T-cell surface receptor. Once the NFAT dimer has formed in the nucleus, it can bind to the promoter region of several inflammatory genes including those for IL-2, IL-3, IL-4 and TNF-α [64].

When the drugs, tacrolimus, pimecrolimus or cyclosporine enter the cell they bind to a cytosol protein, either FKBP for tacrolimus or pimecrolimus or cyclophilin for cyclosporine. Once formed, this complex is able to bind to and inactivate calcineurin. The now inactive calcineurin can no longer dephosphorylate NFATc which results in the transcription factor remaining unactivated and in the cytosol. Thus, the NFATn protein in the nucleus has no binding partner and cannot bind to and activate inflammatory genes [63].

While tacrolimus and other calcineurin inhibitors are much more specific than corticosteroids in terms of the types of cells they act on, they still inhibit a wide variety of inflammatory genes and are therefore, immunosuppressive. In 2006, the FDA issued a "black box" warning that the use of either Elidel (pimecrolimus) or Protopic (tacrolimus) may be linked to an increased risk for cancer.

Another class of immunomodulators, called "biologic response modifiers (BRM)" or simply "biologics" because they are made from living organisms, have been developed over the past 5 years. These are essentially "designer" drugs because they target a specific event or mediator involved in inflammation. Most of these are "humanized" monoclonal antibodies that bind to and inactivate various inflammatory cytokines. Anti-inflammatory drugs in this category include the TNF-alpha inhibitors, Enbrel (etanercept), Remicade (infliximab) and Humira (adalimumab) [51], a fusion protein that can bind to the CD2 binding site on T-lymphocytes and prevent the antigen-mediated activation of the cell (Amevive) and finally, an antibody, Raptiva, that prevents leukocytes cells from binding to adhesion molecules on endothelial cells, thereby preventing migration of these cells into the skin.

These new protein-based "biologic" immunomodulators, although effective and useful for treating various dermatological conditions are, however, not without side effects. Because of their potent immunosuppressive effects, particularly on T-lymphocytes, the risk of infection among patients taking these medications is elevated [65].

Topical antioxidant anti-inflammatories
Determining topical efficacy

The increasing interest in using "natural" antioxidants to address, not only skin aging, but also inflammatory diseases such as eczema, atopic dermatitis, seborrheic dermatitis and even psoriasis and cancer, has led to the introduction of many products that contain botanical extracts or plant-derived compounds, which are believed to have anti-inflammatory activity [66–68]. Some of the many antioxidant botanical extracts now in topical products include green tea extracts, curry extract, jewelweed, calendula, aloe, chamomile and willow bark, and many more. Pure phenolic antioxidants with known anti-inflammatory activities that have been incorporated into topical formulations include EGCG (epigallocatechin gallate) [69], vitamin C [70] and resveratrol [71,72] to mention a few. Given the abundance of botanicals which claim anti-inflammatory activity, is there any scientific evidence to suggest that any of these can actually block the production of inflammatory mediators or the process of inflammation when applied topically? Although there are many cell culture and animal studies that have examined the anti-inflammatory activities of these compounds, there have been very few clinical studies to assess their effectiveness when applied topically. One of the easiest human studies to run to determine if topically applied antioxidants can block inflammation is a sunburn study. In the few studies that have been carried out, non-sun exposed skin (e.g. buttocks) was treated with dose of UVB equal to 3–5 times the MED dose, and the effect of a topical antioxidant in blocking the resultant sunburn (inflammation) determined. Studies with topical formulations containing either EGCG, caffeic acid, ferulic acid, or p-coumaric acid, have shown some protection from erythema. Unfortunately, all of these studies were conducted on skin that was *pre-treated* for several days with the antioxidant. Because phenolic and polyphenolic compounds can absorb UV radiation, the studies do not distinguish between the anti-inflammatory effect of the antioxidant and simply its sunscreen effect, i.e. the ability to block UV radiation from damaging the skin [73–75].

In a different study carried out with a lotion containing 2% dihydroeugenol, human subjects were irradiated in two areas on the inner forearm with an FS 20 sunlamp at a dose equal to three times the MED. However, in this study, lotions were applied only *after* the irradiation was carried out. One area of irradiated skin was treated with the lotion without the antioxidant 4-propyl guaiacol while the other irradiated spot was treated with the same lotion containing 2% 4-propyl guaiacol. Six hours later the site was photographed, and as shown in the photograph, the site treated with the phenolic antioxidant showed considerably less erythema (Figure 33.5).

Designing effective anti-inflammatory and anti-aging topicals targeting three key mediators: TNF-alpha, IL-1, and PGE-2

Since the inflammatory process in skin is extremely complex and involves the production and action of many cytokines and chemokines, as well as various paracrine and autocrine factors, how does one decide which anti-inflammatory compound to use in a topical formulation to achieve the best efficacy in treating skin problems, including aging? Although there are many inflammatory mediators that play important roles in propagating an inflammatory response, there are at least three mediators which play major roles in skin diseases, and in skin aging:

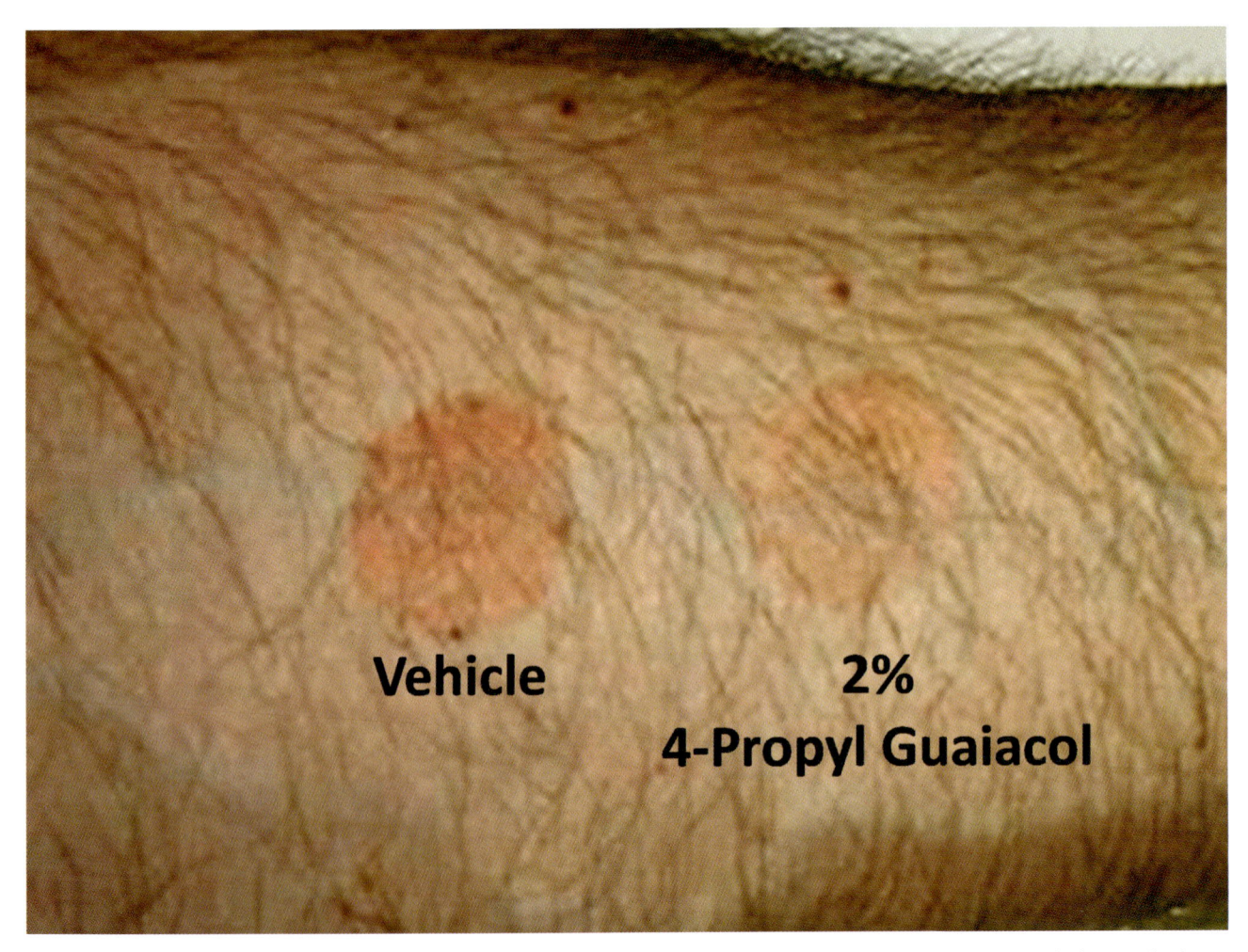

Figure 33.5 Inhibition of UVR induced erythema by post-irradiation topical application of phenolic antioxidant, 4-propyl guaiacol. Photograph taken 6 hours after UVB irradiation with 3 MED.

1. Tumor necrosis factor (TNF-alpha) is a key cytokine involved in psoriasis and in other autoimmune based diseases, including Crohn's disease. Several "biologic response modifiers" such as Enbrel, have been developed to specifically target this cytokine. They work by binding to the cytokine, thus inhibiting its ability to bind to and activate its receptor on target cells. TNF-alpha stimulates the expression of a wide number of inflammatory genes and also increases the production of cellular adhesion molecules (CAM) in vascular endothelium. These adhesion molecules act to tether immune cells to the vasculature, allowing them to leave the blood vessels and enter into the skin. Blocking either the production or action of TNF-alpha can prevent the "chemotaxis" of immune cells into the skin and markedly improve immune cell based diseases.

2. A second important cytokine that is not only pro-inflammatory but also plays a role in skin aging, is interleukin 1 (IL-1). This cytokine has been referred to as the "master cytokine" for inflammation because of its ability to activate a number of inflammatory genes including COX-2, TNF-alpha, IL-1 (autocrine effect), MCP-1, IL-6, IL-8, adhesion molecules (ICAM, e-selectin) and several others [76]. With regard to its aging effects, IL-1 (both IL-α and IL-β forms) is produced by keratinocytes upon exposure of skin to UVR or to other "insults" such as chemical irritants. Once secreted, IL-1 binds to target cells (fibroblasts and keratinocytes, immune cells) and stimulates MAPK and NF-κB pathways leading to nuclear activation of NF-κB and AP-1 transcription factors. This leads to activation of MMP genes including MMP-1 (type I collagenase), and MMP-9 (type IV collagenase, gelatinase, elastase), and may promote keratinocyte transformation leading to skin cancer [77–80].

3. The third important skin inflammatory mediator, is PGE-2. This prostaglandin is the produced by the action of prostaglandin E synthase (PGES-1) and cyclooxygenase (COX), both of which are inducible in skin cells by IL-1. The key enzyme involved in large increases in PGE-2 production in the skin is, however, COX-2, which converts arachidonic acid to the intermediate PGH2, which is then converted rapidly to PGE-2. Over 100 scientific publications have now linked high levels of PGE-2 to either initiating or stimulating proliferation in many cancers, including skin cancer [58–60]. Studies in animal models have shown that blocking PGE-2 production can reduce the formation of UVR induced tumors by almost 90%. Other published studies have shown that PGE-2 is also involved in scar formation and in poor wound healing [61,81]. Finally, PGE-2 also has aging effects by upregulating MMP genes, inhibiting collagen I gene transcription, and by increasing TNF-alpha and IL-1 production. PGE-2 can also act in an autocrine loop to stimulate COX-2 gene activity (and thus its own synthesis) in fibroblasts [82–85]. Given its role in inflammation, sunburn, matrix destruction and in promoting cancer formation, the use of topical antioxidants with the ability to block PGE-2 production in skin might be expected to reduce or prevent the formation of actinic keratoses and skin cancers if used daily. Finally, recent research has shown that exposure of skin to brief treatments with a CO_2 laser can increase PGE-2 levels nine-fold, and that even 3 weeks after the laser treatment, PGE-2 levels are still 4–5 times higher than basal [86]. What long-term damage to the skin might result from high levels of PGE-2 that remain elevated for over 3 weeks remains to be seen.

Conclusion

Although there are a wide number of potent prescription topical anti inflammatories available that are effective in treating skin inflammation, all have some side effects that negatively impact their usefulness. Topical steroids are effective for treating many dermatological diseases but can lower collagen production in dermal fibroblasts, reduce their proliferation and cause skin thinning. Topical immunomodulators are immunosuppressive and can lead to increased risk for infection and even cancer. There is a need for identifying newer, safer, anti-inflammatory technologies that can effectively treat skin disorders without having such strong immunosuppressive effects. Botanically-derived antioxidants with anti-inflammatory activities could help meet this need. Their safety profile is well-known because of their presence in common foods, their widespread use for hundreds of years in traditional medicines, and their current use as nutritional supplements. In addition, whereas prescription drugs are typically very potent and are designed to be effective in the nanomolar or even picomolar range, natural antioxidants have anti-inflammatory potencies in the micromolar range. Thus, it seems likely that when applied topically, a less potent anti-inflammatory may be effective in treating the skin problem without causing undesirable side effects, which are more likely to occur with highly potent drugs. Traditional medicine relies heavily on botanically derived therapies, and given the fact that these treatments have been passed down for hundreds of years, perhaps their value should not be discounted.

References

1 Huang WY. (2010) Natural phenolic compounds from medicinal herbs and dietary plants: potential use for cancer prevention. *Nutr Cancer* **62**, 1–20.

2 Husain N, Kumar A. (2012) Reactive oxygen species and natural antioxidants: A review. *Adv Biores* **3**, 164–75.

3 Fruehauf JP, Meyskens FL. (2007) Reactive oxygen species: a breath of life or death? *Clin Cancer Res* **13**, 789–94.

4 Finkel T. (2011) Signal transduction by reactive oxygen species. *J Cell Biol* **194**, 7–15.

5 Son Y, Cheong Y-K, Kim N-H, *et al.* (2011) Mitogen-activate protein kinases and reactive oxygen species: How can ROS activate MAPK pathways? *J Signal Transduct* **2011**, 1–6.

6. Bai XC, Lu D, Liu AL, et al. (2005) Reactive oxygen species stimulates receptor activator of NF-kappaB ligand expression in osteoblast. *J Biol Chem* **280**, 17497–506.
7. Kai S, Subbaram S, Carrico PM, Melendez JA. (2010) Redox control of matrix metalloproteinase-1: A critical link between free radicals, matrix remodeling and degenerative disease. *Respir Physiol Neurobiol* **174**, 299–306.
8. Korbecki J, Baranowska-Bosiacka I, Gutowaska I, Chlubek D. (2013) The effect of reactive oxygen species on the synthesis of prostanoids from arachidonic acid. *J Physiol Pharmacol* **64**, 409–21.
9. Gkogkolou P, Bohm M. (2012) Advanced glycation end products: Key players in skin aging? *Dermato-Endocrinol* **4**, 259–70.
10. Nedic O, Rattan SI, Grune T, Trougakos IP. (2013) Molecular effects of advanced glycation end products on cell signaling pathways, aging and pathophysiology. *Free Radic Res* **47**, 28–38.
11. Prasad, YD, Sonia S, Balvinder S, Charan CR. (2013) Advanced glycation end products: A review. *Sch Acad J Biosci* **1**, 39–45.
12. Xie J, Mendez JD, Mendez-Valenzuela V, Aguilar-Hernandez MM. (2013) Cellular signaling of the receptor for advanced glycation end products (RAGE). *Cell Signal* **25**, 2185–97.
13. Sparvero LJ, Asafu-Adjei D, Kang R, et al. (2009) RAGE (receptor for advanced glycation endproducts), RAGE ligands, and their role in cancer and inflammation. *J Transl Med* **7**, 17–38.
14. Shinde A, Ganu J, Naik PJ. (2012) Effect of free radicals and antioxidants on oxidative stress: A review. *J Dent Allied Sci* **1**, 63–6.
15. Chen L, Hu JY, Wang SQ. (2012) The role of antioxidants in photoprotection: a critical review. *J Am Acad Dermatol* **67**, 1013–24.
16. Pham-Huy LA, He H, Pham-Huy C. (2008) Free radicals, antioxidants in disease and health. *Int J Biomed* **4**, 89–96.
17. Cao G, Alessio H, Cutler R. (1993) Oxygen-radical absorbance capacity assay for antioxidants. *Free Radic Biol Med* **14**, 303–11.
18. Placzek M, Gaub S, Kerkmann U, et al. (2005) Ultraviolet B-induced DNA damage in human epidermis is modified by antioxidants Ascorbic acid and d-alpha-tocopherol. *J Invest Dermatol* **124**, 304–307.
19. Serhan CN, Ward PA, Gilroy DW. (eds) (2010) *Fundamentals of Inflammation*. New York: Cambridge University Press, 488 pp.
20. Wullaert A, Bonnet MC, Pasparakis M. (2011) NF-κB in the regulation of epithelial homeostasis and inflammation. *Cell Res* **21**, 146–58.
21. Huggenberger R, Detmar M. (2011) The cutaneous vascular system in chronic skin inflammation. *J Invest Dermatol Symp Proc* **15**, 24–32.
22. Ley K. (2003) The role of selectins in inflammation and disease. *Trends Mol Med* **9**, 263–8.
23. Esche C, de B Benedetto A, Beck LA. (2004) Keratinocytes in atopic dermatitis: inflammatory signals. *Curr Allergy Asthma Rep* **4**, 276–84.
24. . Nathan C. (2002) Points of control in inflammation. *Nature* **420**, 846–52.
25. Medzhitov R. (2008) Origin and physiological roles of inflammation. *Nature* **454**, 428–33.
26. Quan T, Qin Z, Xia W, et al. (2009) Matrix-degrading metalloproteinases in photoaging. *J Invest Dermatol Symp Proc* **14**, 20–24.
27. Debacq-Chainiaux F, Leduc C, Verbeke A, Toussaint O. (2012) UV, stress, and aging. *Dermato-Endocrinol* **4**, 236–40.
28. Jenkins G. (2002) Molecular mechanisms of skin ageing. *Mech Ageing Dev* **123**, 801–10.
29. Tajima S, Pinnel SR. (1996) Ascorbic acid preferentially enhances type I and type III collagen gene transcription in human skin fibroblasts. *J Dermatol Sci* **11**, 250–310.
30. Wu D, Hayek MG, Meydani S. (2001) Vitamin E and macrophage cyclooxygenase regulation in the aged. *J Nutr* **131**, 382S–8S.
31. Shishodia S. (2013) Molecular mechanisms of curcumin action: gene expression. *Biofactors* **39**, 37–55.
32. Aggarwal BB, Shishodia S. (2004) Suppression of the nuclear factor-[kappa]B activation pathway by spice-derived phytochemicals: reasoning for seasoning. *Ann NY Acad Sci* **1030**, 434–41.
33. Kim HY, Park EJ, Joe E-H, Jou I. (2003) Curcumin suppresses janus kinase-STAT inflammatory signaling through activation of Src Homology 2 domain-containing tyrosine phosphatase 2 in brain microglia. *J Immunol* **171**, 6072–9.
34. Sikora E, Scapagnini G, Barbagallo M. (2010) Curcumin, inflammation, ageing and age-related diseases. *Immun Ageing* **7**, 1–4.
35. Jurrmann N, Brigelius-Flohe R, Bol G-F. (2005) Curcumin blocks Interleukin-1 (IL-1) signaling by inhibiting the recruitment of the IL-1 receptor-associated kinase IRAK in murine thymoma EL-4 cells. *J Nutr* **135**, 1859–64.
36. Boots AW, Haenen GR, Bast A. (2008) Health effects of quercetin: from antioxidant to nutraceutical. *Eur J Pharmacol* **585**, 325–37.
37. Huang YT, Hwang JJ, Lee PP, et al. (1999) Effects of luteolin and quercetin, inhibitors of tyrosine kinase, on cell growth and metastasis-associated properties in A431 cells overexpressing epidermal growth factor receptor. *Br J Pharmacol* **128**, 999–1010.
38. Chen D, Milacic V, Chen MS, et al. (2008) Tea polyphenols, their biological effects and potential molecular targets. *Histol Histopathol* **23**, 487–496.
39. Vicentini FT, He T, Shao Y, et al. (2011) Quercetin inhibits UV irradiation-induced inflammatory cytokine production in primary human keratinocytes by suppressing NF-kB pathway. *J Dermatol Sci* **61**, 162–8.
40. Kuppusamy UR, Khoo HE, Das NP. (1990) Structure-activity studies of flavonoids as inhibitors of hyaluronidase. *Biochem Pharmacol* **40**, 397–401.
41. Zhang LL, Li L, Wu DP, et al. (2008) A novel anti-cancer effect of genistein: reversal of epithelial mesenchymal transition in prostate cancer cells. *Acta Pharmacol Sin* **29**, 1060–8.
42. Bos JD, Meinardi MM. (2000) The 500 Dalton rule for the skin penetration of chemical compounds and drugs. *Exp Dermatol* **9**, 165–9.
43. Uva L, Miguel D, Pinheiro C, et al. (2012) Mechanism of action of topical corticosteroids in psoriasis. *Intl J Endocrinol* **2012**, Article ID 561018, 16 pp.
44. Dostert A, Heinzel T. (2004) Negative glucocorticoid receptor response elements and their role in glucocorticoid action. *Curr Pharm Des* **10**, 2807–16.
45. De BK, Vanden BW, Haegeman G. (2003) The interplay between the glucocorticoid receptor and nuclear factor-kappaB or activator protein-1: *molecular mechanisms for gene repression Endocr Rev* **24**, 488–522.
46. Hermoso MA, Cidlowski JA. (2003) Putting the brake on inflammatory responses: the role of glucocorticoids. *IUBMB Life* **55**, 497–504.
47. Tak PP, Firestein GS. (2001) NF-kappaB: a key role in inflammatory diseases. *J Clin Invest* **107**, 7–11.
48. Almawi WY, Melemedjian OK. (2002) Negative regulation of nuclear factor-kappaB activation and function by glucocorticoids. *J Mol Endocrinol* **28**, 69–78.
49. Necela BM, Cidlowski JA. (2004) Mechanisms of glucocorticoid receptor action in noninflammatory and inflammatory cells. *Proc Am Thorac Soc* **1**, 239–46.

50 Jarvis B, Figgitt DP. (2003) Topical 3% diclofenac in 2.5% hyaluronic acid gel: a review of its use in patients with actinic keratosis. *Am J Clin Dermatol* **4**, 203–13.

51 Nelson C, Rigel D, Smith S, et al. (2004) Phase IV, open-label assessment of the treatment of actinic keratosis with 3.0% diclofenac sodium topical gel (Solaraze). *J Drugs Dermatol* **3**, 401–7.

52 Lin J, Zhang W, Jones A, Doherty M. (2004) Efficacy of topical non-steroidal anti-inflammatory drugs in the treatment of osteoarthritis: meta-analysis of randomised controlled trials. *BMJ* **329**, 324–9.

53 Vaile JH, Davis P. (1998) Topical NSAIDs for musculoskeletal conditions. *A review of the literature. Drugs* **56**, 783–99.

54 Grace D, Rogers J, Skeith K, Anderson K. (1999) Topical diclofenac versus placebo: a double blind, randomized clinical trial in patients with osteoarthritis of the knee. *J Rheumatol* **26**, 2659–63.

55 Roth SH, Shainhouse JZ. (2004) Efficacy and safety of a topical diclofenac solution (pennsaid) in the treatment of primary osteoarthritis of the knee: a randomized, double-blind, vehicle-controlled clinical trial. *Arch Intern Med* **164**, 2017–23.

56 Rainsford KD. (2007) Anti-inflammatory drugs in the 21st century. *Subcellular Biochem* **42**, 3–27.

57 Wilgus TA, Ross MS, Parrett ML, Oberyszyn TM. (2000) Topical application of a selective cyclooxygenase inhibitor suppresses UVB mediated cutaneous inflammation. *Prostaglandins Other Lipid Mediat* **62**, 367–84.

58 Brecher AR. (2002) The role of cyclooxygenase-2 in the pathogenesis of skin cancer. *J Drugs Dermatol* **1**, 44–7.

59 Muller-Decker K. (2011) Cyclooxygenase-dependent signaling is causally linked to non-melanoma skin carcinogenesis: pharmacological, genetic and clinical evidence. *Cancer Metast Rev* **30**, 343–61.

60 Zhan H, Zheng H. (2007) The role of topical cyclo-oxygenase-2 inhibitors in skin cancer: treatment and prevention. Am *J Clin Dermatol* **8**, 195–200.

61 Wilgus TA, Vodovotz Y, Vittadini E, et al. (2003) Reduction of scar formation in full-thickness wounds with topical celecoxib treatment. *Wound Repair Regen* **11**, 25–34.

62 Miyauchi-Hashimoto H, Kuwamoto K, Urade Y, et al. (2001) Carcinogen-induced inflammation and immunosuppression are enhanced in xeroderma pigmentosum group A model mice associated with hyperproduction of prostaglandin E2. *J Immunol* **166**, 5782–91.

63 Nghiem P, Pearson G, Langley RG. (2002) Tacrolimus and pimecrolimus: from clever prokaryotes to inhibiting calcineurin and treating atopic dermatitis. *J Am Acad Dermatol* **46**, 228–41.

64 Bos JD. (2003) Non-steroidal topical immunomodulators provide skin-selective, self-limiting treatment in atopic dermatitis. *Eur J Dermatol* **13**, 455–61.

65 Gupta AK, Chow M. (2003) Pimecrolimus: a review. *J Eur Acad Dermatol Venereol* **17**, 493–503.

66 Lazarous MC, Kerdel FA. (2002) Topical tacrolimus Protopic. *Drugs Today (Barc)* **38**, 7–15.

67 Hogan PG, Chen L, Nardone J, Rao A. (2003) Transcriptional regulation by calcium, calcineurin, and NFAT. *Genes Dev* **17**, 2205–32.

68 Fantuzzi F, Del Giglio M, Gisondi P, Girolomoni G. (2008) Targeting tumor necrosis factor alpha in psoriasis and psoriatic arthritis. *Expert Opin Ther* **12**, 1085–96.

69 Middleton E Jr, Kandaswami C, Theoharides TC. (2000) The effects of plant flavonoids on mammalian cells: implications for inflammation, heart disease, and cancer. *Pharmacol Rev* **52**, 673–751.

70 Berson DS. (2008) Natural antioxidants. *J Drugs Dermatol* **7**, 7–12.

71 Oresajo C, Pillai S, Manco M, et al. (2012) Antioxidants and the skin: understanding formulation and efficacy. *Dermatol Ther* **25**, 252–9.

72 Lee JH, Chung JH, Cho KH. (2005) The effects of epigallocatechin-3-gallate on extracellular matrix metabolism. *J Dermatol Sci* **40**, 195–204.

73 Murray JC, Burch JA, Streilein RD, et al. (2008) A topical antioxidant solution containing vitamins C and E stabilized by ferulic acid provides protection for human skin against damage caused by ultraviolet irradiation. *J Am Acad Dermatol* **59**, 418–25.

74 Ferzil G, Patel M, Phrsai N, Brody N. (2013) Reduction of facial redness with resveratrol added to topical product containing green tea polyphenols and caffeine. *J Drugs Dermatol* **12**, 770–74.

75 Udenigwe CC, Ramprasath VR, Aluko RE, Jones PJ. (2008) Potential of resveratrol in anticancer and anti-inflammatory therapy. *Nutr Rev* **66**, 445–56.

76 Dinarello CA, Simon A, van der Meer JWM. (2012) Treating Inflammation by blocking interleukin-1 in a broad spectrum of diseases. *Nat Rev Drug Discovery* **11**, 633–52.

77 Wang X, Zhigang B, Wenming C, Wan Y. (2005) IL-1 receptor antagonist attenuates MAPkinase/AP-1 activation and MMP1 expression in UVA-irradiated human fibroblasts induced by culture medium from UVB-irradiated human skin keratinocytes. *Intl J Mol Med* **16**, 1117–24.

78 Cataisson C, Salcedo R, Hakim S, et al. (2012) IL-1R-MyD88 signaling in keratinocyte transformation and carcinogenesis. *J Exp Med* **209**, 1689–1702.

79 Nasti TH, Timares L. (2012) Inflammasome activation of IL-1 family mediators in response to cutaneous damage. *Photochem Photobiol* **88**, 1111–25.

80 Murphy J-E, Robert C, Kupper TS. (1999) Interleukin-1 and cutaneous inflammation: A crucial link between innate and acquired immunity. *J Invest Dermatol* **114**, 602–608.

81 Wilgus TA, Bergdall VK, Tober KL, et al. (2004) The impact of cyclooxygenase-2 mediated inflammation on scarless fetal wound healing. *Am J Pathol* **165**, 753–61.

82 Korbecki J, Bosiacka-Baranowska I, Gutowska I, Chlubek D. (2013) The effect of reactive oxygen species on the synthesis of prostanoids from arachidonic acid. *J Physiol Pharmacol* **64**, 409–21.

83 Kim HH, Cho S, Lee S, et al. (2006) Photoprotective and anti-skin-aging effects of eicosapentaenoic acid in human skin in vivo. *J Lipid Res* **47**, 921–30.

84 Habib MA, Salem SAM, Hakim SA, Shalan YAM. (2014) Comparative immunohistochemical assessment of cutaneous cyclooxygenase-2 enzyme expression in chronological aging and photoaging. *Photodermatol Photoimmunol Photmed* **30**, 43–51.

85 Han JH, Roh MS, Park CH, et al. (2004) Selective COX-2 inhibitor, NS-398, inhibits the replicative senescence of cultured dermal fibroblasts. *Mech Ageing Dev* **125**, 359–66.

86 Sandulache VC, Chafin JB, Li-Korotky HS, et al. (2007) Elucidating the role of interleukin 1 beta and prostaglandin E2 in upper airway mucosal wound healing. *Arch Otolaryngol Head Neck Surg* **133**, 365–74.

CHAPTER 34

Peptides and Proteins

Karl Lintner
KAL'IDEES S.A.S. Paris, France

> **BASIC CONCEPTS**
> - Amino acids, linked in a linear chain, are the building blocks of peptides and proteins.
> - Peptides are biologically active communication tools that direct skin functioning.
> - Engineered peptides are a new category of active skin ingredients suitable for almost any cosmetic vehicle.
> - Peptide bioactivity is fully documented using gene chip array analysis, *ex vivo* protocols and vehicle controlled clinical tests.

Introduction

Peptides, proteins, and amino acids are often mislabeled and the terms applied as if they were interchangeable, yet they are different in their characteristics, uses, biological activities, and cosmetic potential [1]. An important distinction must be made between simple protein hydrolysates (often called "peptides"[2]) and synthetically engineered, specifically chosen peptide sequences. After defining peptides and proteins, the first part of the chapter discusses the specificities of these molecules and their physiologic, biological function, particularly in the skin; what can they do, what are the obstacles to their use in cosmetic products and how can these obstacles be overcome. In the four years since the first edition of this book, a great number of such peptides have been studied, developed and used for cosmetic applications and both skin and hair care benefits. In the second part, a number of concrete examples of peptides and some proteins, in particular for the "anti-aging" sector, are discussed before concluding with an outlook for the future of this ingredient category.

Definitions

It is important to understand the differences between amino acids, peptides, and proteins.

Amino acids
Amino acids are the building blocks of which peptides and proteins are made. They are small molecules, with a molecular weight of 100–200 Da, characterized by the fact that both an amino group (NH_2) and a carboxylic acid group (COOH) are attached to the central carbon atom which also carries further quite variable structures, known as side chains, by which the different amino acids are distinguished (Figure 34.1).

Of the essentially unlimited theoretical number of amino acids that can be imagined on paper, only 20 (e.g. alanine, proline, tyrosine, histidine, phenylalanine, lysine, glutamine...) are incorporated into peptides and proteins via the genetic code. With few exceptions, these amino acids in isolation have no specific intrinsic biological activity. Within cells, they exist in a pool from which they can be called upon to make peptides and proteins or, sometimes, biogenic amines, such as serotonin or dopamine. In the upper layers of the skin, they are part of the natural moisturizing factor (NMF) where they participate in the water holding capacity of the skin contributing to both osmolytic and hygroscopic properties. The result of linking two or more amino acids in a linear chain via an amide ("peptide-") bond between the carboxyl group of one and the amino group of the following amino acid is called a peptide, when the length of the chain is

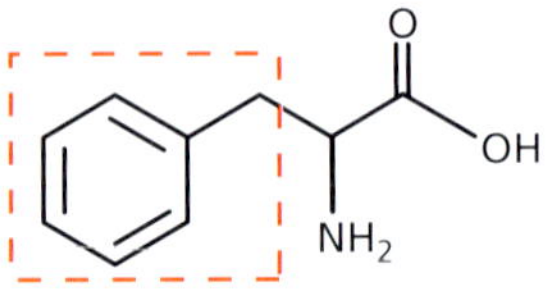

Figure 34.1 Phenylalanine, one of the 20 proteinogenic amino acids. The "side chain" which is characteristic of each amino acid (here a phenyl group) is shown in the box.

Cosmetic Dermatology: Products and Procedures, Second Edition. Edited by Zoe Diana Draelos.
© 2016 John Wiley & Sons, Ltd. Published 2016 by John Wiley & Sons, Ltd.

less than approximately 100 amino acids, or a protein when the chain is longer.

Peptides

The general terminology uses prefixes to describe the type of a peptide. For example, when the peptide is made of two amino acids, such as tyrosine and arginine written as Tyr-Arg, it is called a dipeptide. Three amino acid combinations yield a tripeptide, four amino acid combinations yield a tetrapeptide, etc. "Oligo" stands for a "few" so that oligopeptides can have 2 to ≈20 amino acids linked in a chain. The term polypeptides is used to mean many amino acids, although these latter distinctions are not strict and not governed by official rules.

The most important characteristic of a peptide, besides its length determined by the number of amino acids in the chain, is its sequence. The sequence is the precise order in which the various amino acids are linked together. Both glycyl-histidyl-lysine and glycyl-lysyl-histidine are tripeptides, composed of the three amino acids glycine, histidine, and lysine. However, the fact that these amino acids are linked in the Gly-His-Lys sequence in the former and in Gly-Lys-His sequence in the latter is crucial. The former peptide, usually abbreviated GHK, stimulates collagen synthesis in fibroblasts [3]; the latter GKH stimulates lipolysis in adipocytes [4]. The primary function of most peptides is to bring a biochemical message from place A in the body to place B allowing effective communication.

Proteins

A peptide chain of more than approximately 100 amino acids is termed a protein. However, interleukins, cytokines, and interferon are also sometimes referred to as peptides, even though they possess a much higher molecular weight. Sometimes the distinction between the two categories relies more on the function of the molecule rather than the size.

Proteins can be categorized by their function, roughly into the following:
- Structural *proteins*: building tissue, such as collagen, elastin, fibronectin and many others;
- Enzymes: very specific proteins that catalyze biochemical reactions, such as superoxide dismutase (SOD), chymotrypsin, tyrosinase;
- Transport proteins that bind to a specific substrate and carry it along in the body (e.g. hemoglobin as oxygen carrier, ferritin for iron transport, lipoprotein for lipids, including cholesterol);
- Difficult to categorize proteins with highly specific functions: receptors such as protein G, genetic regulators such as peroxisome proliferator-activated receptor (PPAR), antibodies, coagulants, histones.

Proteins with individual molecular mass of hundreds of thousands of Daltons often auto-assemble into large structures with very complex mechanisms of activity.

Biological functions of peptides and proteins in the skin

Peptides

Peptides perform many important biologic signal (hormonal) functions. The word hormone – from Greek, simply meaning messenger – applies to various classes of substances (steroids, peptides, biogenic amines…). All messenger molecules, including certain peptides, act in similar fashion: some disturbance, either internal or external, leads to the release of a small amount of peptide in a cell, blood, gland, or in some other organ. The peptide then travels in the body until it interacts with a target receptor either on the cellular surface or within the cell nucleus after having penetrated the cell wall. This interaction triggers further activity at the site, destined to respond and correct the initial disturbance.

This mechanism of action is usually characterized by three items:
1. Peptides circulate and act at their target sites at extremely low concentration levels, generally in the nanomolar (10^{-9} mol/L) level.
2. Each peptide sequence has, at its defined target, a highly selective binding affinity and carries a distinct message such that its activity is quite specific. The highly simplified concept of "key" and "lock" (i.e. peptide and receptor) interaction is used to explain this potency and specificity.
3. Peptides have short lifespans in the organism because proteolytic enzymes break them down quickly in order to avoid overload at the target site.

Well-known biological activities of peptide hormones in the human body are, for instance: regulation of blood sugar concentration (insulin); blood pressure regulation (angiotensin, bradykinin, calcitonin gene-related peptide [CGRP]); lactation and birthing (oxytocin); diuresis (vasopressin); pain repression (endorphins, enkephalin); tanning (α-MSH); radical scavenging (glutathione); other peptides include vasointestinal peptide (VIP), substance P, neurotensin, luteotropin and hundreds more. Peptides with various bioactivities have been identified in all organs of our body and the skin is no exception. An increasing volume of research is devoted to the understanding of peptide functions in the skin and consequently to find cosmetic applications of this huge category of bioactive substances.

As this section's term of "anti-aging" is not clearly defined, it shall be interpreted here in a rather broad way to represent anything that helps the skin look younger. Hence we shall discuss, in the subsequent paragraphs, a variety of cosmetic skin care activities for which peptides have been developed and used with success, such as antioxidant peptides, tissue repair peptides, skin whitening or tanning peptides, soothing and neuromodulating peptides, hair growth controlling peptides, and mention only in passing lipid metabolism mediating peptides, moisturizing and barrier repair peptides and others. These examples are, of course, far from being exhaustive. A few words about potential pitfalls are, nevertheless, in order first.

Obstacles to peptide use in cosmetic formulation

The incorporation of peptides into various galenic forms of skin care products can be challenging. Some of the hurdles confronted with peptide formulation include: skin penetration, stability, toxicity, analysis, and cost.

Skin penetration

The stratum corneum is not the primary target for peptides, as they need viable, living skin to receive their message. It is necessary for a peptide to cross the cutaneous barrier in order to reach the viable epidermis (keratinocytes), the basal layer (melanocytes, nerve cell endings), the dermis (fibroblasts), and even the hypodermis (adipocytes). Even small peptide molecules, such as the dipeptide carnosine, are too hydrophilic and electrically charged to penetrate easily any further than the first or second layer of the stratum corneum. Lintner and Peschard [5] have shown that the attachment of a lipophilic chain (fatty acid of sufficient length) to carnosine can increase the penetration rate by a factor of 100 or more. Similar effects were confirmed by Leroux et al. [4]. Goebel et al. [6] have further studied the penetration behavior of this molecule and describe various techniques of formulation to overcome the problem. This technique of vectorizing the peptides has its limits because the longer the peptide chain, the less penetration the fatty acid will produce. The larger the peptide (beyond six or seven amino acids), the less likely it is to reach the deeper layers of the skin. Thus, the long peptide sequences of CGRP, POMC, EGF, other chemokines and similar structures, do not function well as active ingredients in cosmetic formulas. Another limitation of this technique is the possible interference of biologic activity by acylation of the peptide. The N terminal ionic charge may be of importance for triggering effects at the target site or otherwise interfering with the peptide's properties. For example, the antioxidant activity of carnosine turns into pro-oxidant activity when the peptide is modified to become palmitoyl-carnosine. Recent research has discovered alternative ways of increasing transcutaneous delivery, using amphiphilic cell penetration peptides CPP [7], attaching a poly-arginine chain to the peptide [8] or designing hyaluronic acid (HA) conjugates [9] to help molecules penetrate the stratum corneum. Liposome formulations may also help carry the peptide through the barrier, but little if anything has been published in this respect.

Stability

Peptides have a reputation of limited chemical stability. While it is true that in aqueous environments, such as those frequently encountered in cosmetic applications, some degree of hydrolysis may occur, experience has shown that the right choice of excipients and stabilizers can help overcome this obstacle [10], the more so as the apparent instability (disappearance of the peptide from the cream) is often an artifact. The above mentioned long chain acylated lipopeptides have a tendency to self-associate and to form gels which simply pose a challenge to the analytical chemist [11].

Analysis

Detecting the presence of a peptide in a formulation 6–12 months after product manufacture can be difficult when the peptide is present in micromolar or lower concentrations (p.p.m. level). Special analytical techniques, such as derivatization, mass spectrometry, and fluorescence spectrometry, have to be individually developed for each peptide. This is not always possible and/or very costly and sometimes proves an insurmountable hurdle. A recent paper by Chirita et al. [12] demonstrates nevertheless both the possibility of detecting 3 to 5 ppm of a pentapeptide in a complex cream matrix and the proven long-term stability of the substance.

Toxicity

Generally, the smaller the peptide, the less likely it is to show untoward effects. Peptides, in contrast to proteins, are hardly big enough to elicit allergic reactions, but specific undesirable cellular effects may occur with unknown sequences. It is advisable to use peptides with a biomimetic amino acid sequence, as the likelihood of toxicity is close to nil when the peptide is – almost – identical to human peptides of known safety status. Nevertheless, proper safety evaluation of newly developed peptides, especially if the peptide is modified by acylation or esterification, is necessary.

Cost

Peptides of defined sequence and high purity (>90%) are relatively expensive to produce; although extraction from some protein hydrolysates is theoretically possible, most peptides used in cosmetic applications are synthetic (i.e. made in a step-by-step process from the individual amino acid building blocks). It is noteworthy that the amino acids themselves are frequently of natural plant or fermentation origin. However, the very high potency of the peptides compensates for their cost and makes it possible to employ them at efficient level in all types of skincare formulas, because they are used at the p.p.m. level (0,000x%) in finished cosmetics.

Therefore, in spite of these formulation challenges, peptides have become popular, widely used active ingredients for anti-aging skincare products, discussed next.

Antioxidant peptides
Glutathione (γ-glutamyl-cysteyl-glycine)

This tripeptide GSH is one of the "oldest" members of the peptide family, with respect to its discovery, analysis, and confirmatory synthesis. It contains an –SH bearing cystein amino acid which confers antioxidant activity to the molecule (Figure 34.2). The

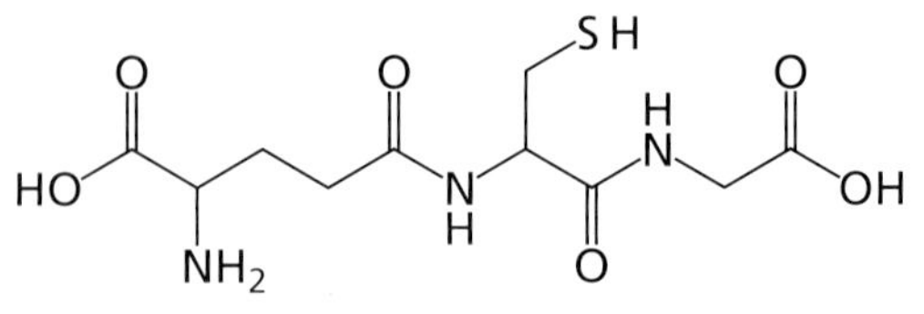

Figure 34.2 Glutathione (γ-glutamyl-cysteinyl-glycine).

Figure 34.3 The matrikine concept: A tissue protein (e.g. collagen, elastin, fibronectin) is broken into fragments by enzymatic hydrolysis, either during normal tissue renewal, or as a consequence of induced damages (free radicals, burning, mechanical wound). The breaking up of the protein does not occur randomly, nor sequentially from one or the other end; various pieces of amino acid strings are generated, which when small enough, are readily available to act as "messengers" in the surrounding tissue, and will act as chemoattractants, transport aids, and stimulants to trigger neosynthesis of the necessary tissue molecules to renew/repair the three-dimensional structure.

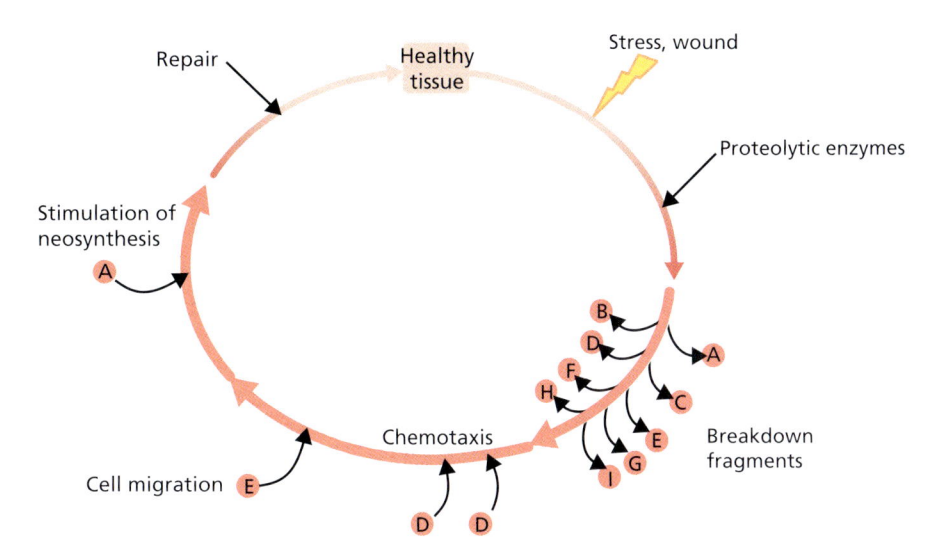

level of glutathione concentration in the body decreases notably with age, which may be a cause and a symptom of aging both at the same time [13]. Besides affording this protective, antioxidant activity, for which there is in vitro but very little documented clinical evidence of skin benefits (for a medical study, see [14]), GSH may also have so-called "skin whitening" effects, as described by Villarama and Maibach [15].

Carnosine (β-alanyl-l-histidine)

Carnosine has been proven to scavenge reactive oxygen species (ROS) formed from peroxidation of cell membrane fatty acids during oxidative stress. Carnosine is also shown to be useful to counter the effects of glycation (the non-enzymatic binding of sugars to proteins) which leads to cytotoxic advanced glycation endproducts (AGEs). A new derivative of azelaic acid and histidine (azeloyl tetrapeptide 23) also possesses antioxidant and strong anti-glycation activity [16].

Nagai et al. [17] showed that carnosine might also promote wound healing, at least indirectly, as exogenous carnosine is degraded by carnosinase into β-alanine and ultimately histamine. Whereas β-alanine was found to stimulate the biosynthesis of nucleic acids and collagen, histamine is considered to enhance the process of wound healing by stimulating effusion at the initial stage of inflammation. This example illustrates the economical side of nature using both the original substance (carnosine) and both its metabolic fragments for concurring purposes, a mechanism found particularly often with peptides.

Tissue repair peptides

One of the most popular claims of anti-aging concerns the repair or restoration of the extracellular matrix of the skin, mainly to reduce the appearance of wrinkles.

The term matrikines is used to describe naturally occurring fragments of matrix macromolecules endowed with stimulatory, tissue repair activity [18]. Schematically and very simplified, this matrikine concept of recycling breakdown fragments of macromolecules for triggering repair activity is illustrated in Figure 34.3. The concept is valid not only for proteins and peptide fragments, but also for poly- and oligosaccharides, where the term glycokine applies. The best-known matrikine peptide used in skin care is the pentapeptide Pal-KTTKS, derived from the shortest pro-collagen I fragment capable of stimulating collagen synthesis in fibroblasts (Katayama et al. [19]). A DNA array study on this molecule indicated that mostly genes implicated in the wound healing process were upregulated in cells incubated with the peptide. Furthermore, the palmitoylated peptide stimulates not only the synthesis of collagen I, but also of collagen IV, fibronectin, and glycosaminoglycanes in monolayer culture of normal and aged human fibroblasts and in full thickness skin [20]. This peptide was tested in vehicle controlled clinical trials where it proved to thicken the skin, improve the epidermal–dermal junction, and macroscopically reduce fine lines and wrinkles [20–22].

Hajem et al. [23] describe the naturally occurring Ac-Ser-Asp-Lys-Pro tetrapeptide as an angiogenic factor that contributes to repair of cutaneous injuries. A substantial amount of work has gone into studying the activities of this peptide at the level of in vitro mechanisms.

The tetrapeptide Arg-Gly-Asp-Ser (RGDS), a sequence found within the fibronectin structure responsible for the binding affinity of this protein to collagen and to cell membranes, is able to help cells migrate during the wound healing process. A cyclic RGD peptide, able to bind to integrin receptors was tested in a clinical study and found to possess anti-wrinkle properties [24].

The peptide Pal-Gly-Gln-Pro-Arg (Pal-GQPR) is a fragment of the natural circulating protein IgG and stimulates macromolecule synthesis in cell culture but also contributes to the reduction of basal and UV-induced IL-6 release in keratinocytes and fibroblasts (Table 34.1.), which leads to improved skin firmness in vivo.

Table 34.1 Variation in IL-6 levels in presence of Pal-GQPR.

Pal-Gly-Gln-Pro-Arg (ppm)	Decrease of basal IL-6 (% of baseline level)	Decrease of UVB-induced IL-6 (% of baseline)
10	−15.6 ± 8.2	−33.2 ± 12.8
15	−20.0 ± 6.6	−37.3 ± 13.0
30	−24.6 ± 17.6	−60.3 ± 8.5
45	NT	−70.6 ± 9.8
65	NT	−85.5*
85	NT	−86.5*

NT, not tested.
* n = 2.

The tripeptide Gly-His-Lys, found in different parts of broken-down collagen and in some serum proteins, also stimulates collagen synthesis in human skin fibroblasts, as found by Maquart et al. [3]. In its palmitoylated form (Pal-GHK) it can mimic the effects of retinoic acid [5]. The in vitro synergy between the tri- and tetrapeptide (Pal-GHK + Pal-GQPR) [25] led to an investigation of the combination in a clinical, vehicle controlled, blind study on 23 panelists. Twice daily application of an oil-in-water (O/W) emulsion containing 4 p.p.m. of Pal-GHK and 2 p.p.m. of Pal-GQPR against vehicle showed significant wrinkle reduction, an increase in skin firmness, and visible smoothing after 1–2 months. More recent data on this peptide combination highlight the true anti-aging potential of peptides: measuring the Subepidermal Low Echogenic Band (SLEB: Figure 34.4) by ultrasound echography, Mondon et al. [26] were able to show, based on the strong correlation between age and the thickness of the SLEB described by Querleux [27], a decrease in apparent age of the skin of ≈5 years in a panel of volunteers using the peptide containing creams for 2 months.

In another formulation, the peptide GHK was coupled to biotin, instead of palmitic acid, in order to strengthen the affinity of the peptide to hair keratin. This biotinyl-GHK peptide was then tested on hair growth in vitro (Figure 34.5) where 2 p.p.m. of the peptide increased hair length by 58%, and 5 p.p.m. achieved 120% increase. The production of the mitotic marker Ki67 and stimulation of collagen IV and laminin 5 syntheses were also investigated. Confirmation of the improved anchoring of the hair to the follicular infundibulum came from a clinical trial to study hair loss in alopecia patients where a significant improvement of the anagen: telogen ratio was observed, in line with histologic observations on plucked hairs from the panelists [28]. Loing et al. [29] describe a similar result with an undisclosed biomimetic peptide in both in vitro and in clinical studies on hair loss prevention.

Concepts derived from wound healing research are but one approach to peptide-based anti-aging treatments. Reducing senescence via p53 expression and ataxia telangiectasia mutated (ATM) as investigated by Gruber et al. [30] is another promising path. Still another idea centers on the complex process of methionine sulfoxide reductases (protein repairing enzymes). While Frechet et al. [31] present a peptidomimetic N-acetyl-methionyl-decarboxymethionin (AMDM) modulation with powerful anti-oxidant and defense properties, Mondon et al. [32] developed a doubly oxidized Pal-Lys-Met (O2)-Lys peptide that proves to increase the synthesis of the six major macromolecules in the dermis and is able, in vehicle controlled clinical studies to demonstrate the repair of wrinkles both in the eye zone and on the front, i.e. frown lines (Figure 34.6). The sulfoxidized methionine in this peptide clearly plays a significant role that needs further investigation.

Many more small peptides and their derivatives can be found with claims of tissue repair and cosmetic anti-age effects.

Neuropeptides

The skin and the brain are derived from the same initial embryonic tissues [34]; thus, it is not surprising that many peptides that are found to exist and possess activities in the brain are also found in the skin. Neurotensin, VIP, NPY, substance P, and CGRP, although endowed with potent biological activity, are not candidates for cosmetic applications because of their size and irritation potential. This is not the case for the β-endorphin, enkephalin and the kyotorphine peptide complex. The dipeptide Tyr-Arg, which is known as kyotorphine, has been shown to be analgesic via enkephalin release in mouse brain [35] (Figure 34.7). The

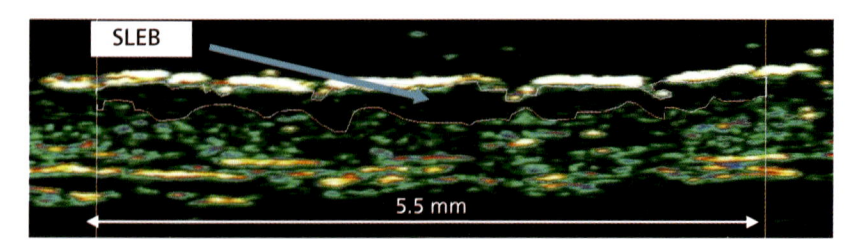

Figure 34.4 A Dermascan C (Cortex) echograph equipped with a 50 MHz frequency probe was used to obtain images approximately 6 mm wide and 3 mm thick with a resolution of 25 × 60 μm. A sequence of 100 successive images was recorded over 4 cm. Five representative images were extracted and analysed by image analysis. The SLEB is traced accurately over a width of 5.5 mm allowing its depth (in μm) and density (in Grey Scale Levels or GSL) to be calculated automatically.

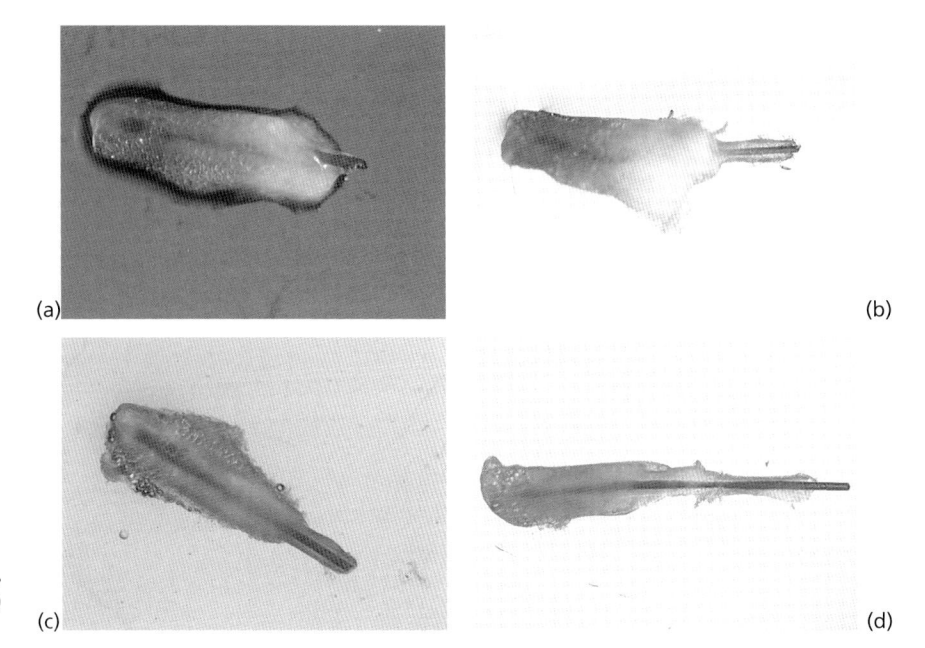

Figure 34.5 Hair follicles in survival medium, incubated 14 days; (a & b) control; (c & d) 5 p.p.m. Biot-GHK.

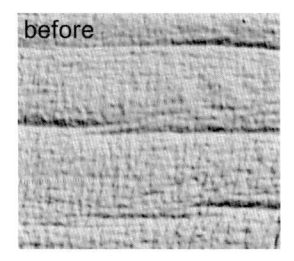

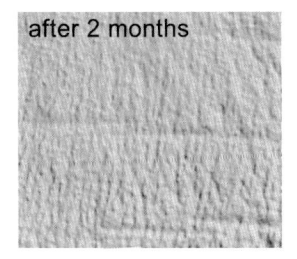

Figure 34.6 Expression lines on the front before and after treating a panelist with the Pal-KM(O$_2$)K peptide for two months.

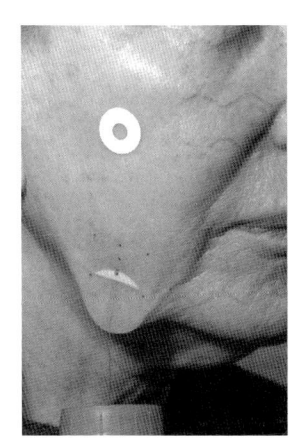

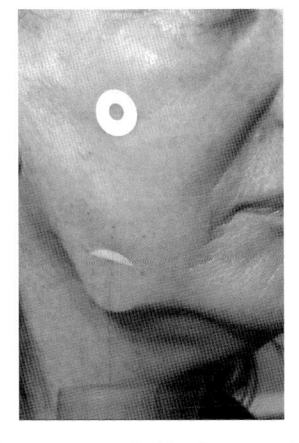

Figure 34.7 demonstration of the improvement of skin firmness after using the Ac-Tyr-Arg-hexadecylester dipeptide for one month. A weight is attached to the jowl and the skin extension is quantified. Left: before; right: after one month.

modified peptide N-acetyl-tyr-arg-hexadecylester demonstrates improved skin bioavailability and stimulates the release of β-endorphin in keratinocytes. It is also able to reduce skin sensitivity to external thermal, chemical, and mechanical stress. A double-blind, vehicle controlled study using a lie detector established that this peptide, at 300 p.p.m. in an O/W emulsion, was able to diminish skin electrodynamic response to mechanical trauma induced by wiping the skin with sandpaper [36]. Sensitivity of the skin to thermal trauma induced by a heat probe and chemical trauma induced by topical capsaicin is also decreased after application of the peptide Furthermore, the peptide also inhibits *in vitro* muscle contraction similarly to other modulators of nerve-muscle interactions, such as curare [36].

Injections of derivatives of the Botulinium neurotoxin have been approved in a number of countries to diminish glabellar wrinkles. To develop a peptide with similar effects, Blanes-Mira *et al.* [38] synthesized the hexapeptide N-Ac-Glu-Glu-Met-Gln-Arg-Arg-NH2 (N-Ac-EEMQRR-NH2), a fragment of the SNAP-25 molecule [39]. It is reported to inhibit neurotransmitter release, apparently as a result of interference with the formation and/or stability of the protein complex that is required to drive Ca^{2+}-dependent exocytosis, namely the vesicular fusion known as SNARE complex, similar to what happens with Botulinium neurotoxin injections. The authors also claim that an unspecified peptide solution, formulated at the concentration of 10% in an O/W emulsion, reduced wrinkle depth up to 30% upon 30 days treatment on a panel of 10 human female volunteers [37].

Skin elasticity

Wrinkle treatment is one of the most obvious targets in anti-age research, but not the only important one. Sagging skin (ptosis) reflecting the loss of elasticity, caused by increased elastolysis and decreased neosynthesis of the crucial elastin molecule in the dermis, has attracted much attention from the research community and peptide scientists. Acetyl-tetrapeptide 2, was specifically designed to fight flaccidity as it increases Fibulin 5 and LOXL1 activity, stimulates elastin synthesis and other processes involved in elastic fiber laydown [38], but the hexapeptide-10 and the Ac-arg-trp-diphenylglycine peptides [39], the cyclopeptide-5 and the above mentioned Ac-Tyr-Arg-hexadecylester dipeptide all show similar *in vitro* activity (protein synthesis, enzyme regulation, fiber organization and bundling, MMP inhibition…), and possess specific elasticity enhancing properties *in vivo* with sometimes spectacular clinical results (Figure 34.8).

Melanogenesis

The well-named age-spots (lentigines) are another clear sign of the advancing years; visible in the face and on many other sun-exposed areas of the body, they constitute an esthetic problem and a cosmetically treatable target. Given the fact that melanogenesis is triggered by the a-MSH peptide (a fragment of proopiomelanocortin [40]), a huge number of peptide analogs and derivatives of a-MSH have been synthesized and tested for modulating melanin synthesis and skin pigmentation. The tetrapeptide Pro-Lys-Glu-Lys (PKEK) is described as being able to exert skin-whitening effects [41]. The authors have carried out four clinical vehicle controlled studies based on the observation that *in vitro* the peptide reduces the expression of inflammatory chemokines (IL6, IL8 and TNF-a, known to contribute to hyperpigmentation) and the synthesis of POMC by keratinocytes. Whereas PKEK is inspired by the KEK motive in cathelicidin, an a-MSH derived hexapeptide analog activates the MCR-1 receptor and reduces UV induced DNA damages [Loing 42] and an acetyl pentapeptide proposed as a "bronzing" peptide actually increases melanin synthesis and tanning via stimulating the adenyl cyclase pathway [44].

These and many other examples (anti-inflammatory peptides [45,46], peptides modulating lipid metabolism in adipocytes [47–49], barrier-repair and moisture regulating peptides [50,51]) show that the field of cosmetic applications for bioactive peptides is still wide open.

Proteins

Structural proteins are building blocks for the organs and tissues of the human body. Collagen, one of the most abundant protein families, as well as keratin, elastin, fibronectin, actins, together with glycoproteins and proteoglucans, arrange themselves in finely tuned, three-dimensional structures to form muscles and skin. The use of native collagen, elastin and keratins (extracted from animal tissue) has dramatically declined since the BSE scare in the 1990s, and is only now making a slow comeback. Not much bioactivity is attached to these structural proteins given that their size makes skin penetration rather unlikely. In the dermal layer, however, these proteins undergo a constant renewal process, even in the absence of external disturbances. These structural proteins present a contrast to enzymes, which fulfill an entirely different function. Enzymes speed up biochemical reactions, which would otherwise occur too slowly for the body to function. Enzyme function is highly specific. This specificity results from the precise amino acid sequence, which not only aligns the correct atoms and side chains in the right order, but also directs the precise folding pattern of the enzyme protein, thus guaranteeing its biological function. Enzymes are catalysts acting at low concentrations. The most important families of enzymes are proteolytic, lipolytic, antioxidant, DNA repair, and those involved in protein synthesis and gene regulation. A variety of enzymes have been employed in cosmetic products, of which we shall cite only a few examples.

Proteolytic enzymes

Proteolytic enzymes are used as an alternative to α-hydroxy acids for superficial peeling of the skin surface, but care must be taken with the dosage. Figure 34.8 illustrates the proteolytic smoothing effect obtained with these enzymes.

T4 endonuclease V

T4 endonuclease V, isolated from *Escherichia coli* infected with T4 bacteriophage, has been shown to repair UV-induced cyclobutane pyrimidine dimers in DNA. Applied topically, liposomes containing T4 endonuclease V reduced the incidence of basal cell carcinomas by 30% and of actinic keratoses

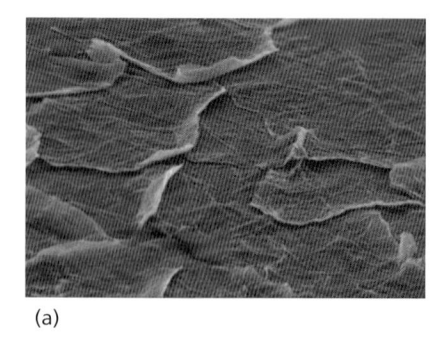

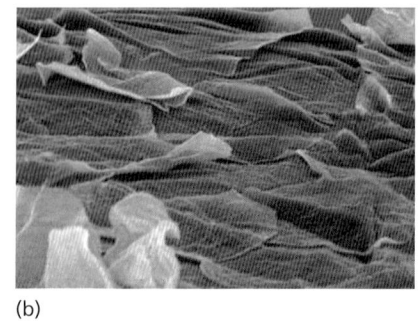

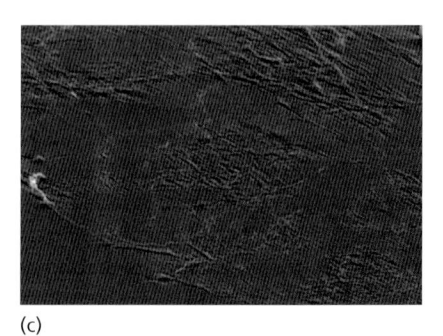

(a)   (b)   (c)

Figure 34.8 Scanning electron microscope (SEM) pictures of skin treated with an occlusive patch for 2 hours; (a) control cream pH 7; (b) cream with AHA to pH 3.5; (c) cream with 2% proteolytic enzyme solution (10 proteolytic units/mL).

by 68% without adverse effects and no evidence of allergic or irritant contact dermatitis. Although the photoprotective effect of T4N5 has been investigated only in xeroderma pigmentosum patients, it may be also be effective for normal skin [52]. Cosmetic products based on this concept are in the current marketplace.

Superoxide dismutase and catalase

Superoxide dismutase, an antioxidant enzyme, is present at the surface of the skin. Adding this enzyme to cosmetic formulations to strengthen the natural defense system is tempting, although the transmutation of the superoxide anion to hydrogen peroxide, without further detoxification of the peroxide, is not necessarily sufficient for protecting the skin. Catalase, an enzyme that reduces hydrogen peroxide to harmless water and oxygen, should work in conjunction with SOD; it is however prohibited for cosmetic use in Europe. Furthermore SOD and catalase, derived from bovine blood, from yeast or other biotechnologically useful microorganism do not guarantee sufficient stability to survive manufacturing procedures and shelf life in cosmetic consumer products.

A novel alternative is based on extremozymes (enzymes produced by extremophile bacteria, such as *Thermus thermophilus*). Mas-Chamberlin *et al.* [53] have shown that these enzymes are heat and UV stable, possessing both SOD and catalase-mimicking activity which protects the skin against UV-induced free radical damage. A 6-month clinical vehicle controlled blind trial under tropical conditions (Figure 34.9; Tables 34.2 and 34.3) on the island of Mauritius [54] demonstrated the visible and measurable benefits of protecting the skin in preventive manner. New but as yet unpublished data (Mondon P. personal communication) on this particular enzyme preparation show that the skin can also be protected against the possible damages resulting from Infrared radiation, a new target for preventive cosmetic concepts.

Other enzymes (lipase, lactoperoxidase) and transport proteins (lactoferrin, hemocyanin) are more of theoretical than practical use in cosmetic research and application.

Table 34.2 Changes in transepidermal water loss (TEWL) after exposure to tropical climate (25 panelists); group treated with extremozyme formula.

Time	Variation (g/m^{-2}/h^{-1}) (mean ± SEM)	% Change (mean)	Significance
Week 4 vs. T0	−1.0 ± 0.7	−6%	NS* ($p = 0.192$)
Week 12 vs. T0	+0.8 ± 0.9	+5%	NS ($p = 0.391$)
Week 24 vs. T0	+0.2 ± 0.9	+1%	NS ($p = 0.855$)

* NS, not significant.

Source: Soap Perfumery and Cosmetics. Reproduced with permission.

Table 34.3 Changes in transepidermal water loss (TEWL) after exposure to tropical climate (25 panelists); group treated with *placebo* formula; clearly the increase in TEWL indicates damaged skin barrier.

Time	Change (g.m^{-2}.h^{-1}) (mean ± SEM)	% change (mean)	Significance
4 weeks vs. T0	+0.9 ± 0.8	+7%	NS ($p = 0.258$)
12 weeks vs. T0	+1.3 ± 0.7	+10%	NS ($p = 0.081$)
24 weeks vs. T0	+1.4 ± 0.7	+11%	borderline ($p = 0.057$)

Source: Soap Perfumery and Cosmetics. Reproduced with permission.

Conclusion

Peptides, much more than proteins, have become an important tool for improving many aspects of the skin's appearance, as the abundant scientific and commercial literature demonstrates. This chapter presents some justification for this success. Although the list of peptides naturally occurring in the human body is long, allowing for further biomimetic peptide development for skincare, the possibility to create derivatives, analogs, and other variations on a theme is enormous and even more exciting. For example, the number of possible pentapeptides based on the 20 proteinogenic amino acids is 20^5 or 3,200,000. As our understanding of cellular mechanisms, gene regulation, receptor activity, and metabolic interactions increases, still many new peptides will appear in cosmetic products of the future, aiming to achieve even higher specificity and greater effects in ever shorter time, all the while assuring safety in use.

References

1. Lintner K. (2007) Peptides, amino acids and proteins in skin care? *Cosmet Toiletries* **122**, 26–34.
2. Anonymous (2012) Verisol®, the bioactive collagen peptides. *HPC – Household and Personal Care Today*, **1**, 35.
3. Maquart FX, Pickart L, Laurent M, *et al.* (1988) Stimulation of collagen synthesis in fibroblast cultures by the tripeptide-copper complex glycyl-L-histidyl-L-lysine-Cu^{2+}. *FEBS Lett* **238**, 343–5.
4. Leroux R, Peschard O, Mas-Chamberlin C, *et al.* (2000) Shaping up. *Soap Perfum Cosmet* **12**, 22–4.

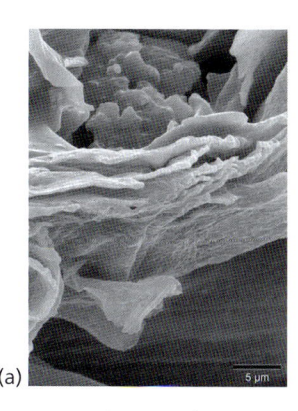

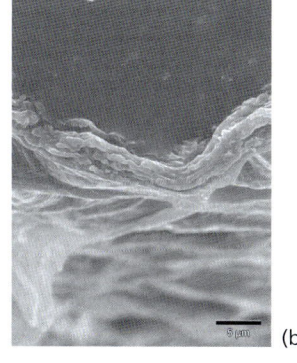

Figure 34.9 Scanning electron microscope (SEM) pictures of stratum corneum strippings: skin exposed to 6 months' tropical climate, treated with moisturizer. (a) Control formula; (b) extremozyme-containing moisturizer. (Source: Soap Perfumery and Cosmetics. Reproduced with permission.)

5 Lintner K, Peschard O. (2000) Biologically active peptides: from a lab bench curiosity to a functional skin care product. *Int J Cosmet Sci* **22**, 207–18.

6 Goebel ASB, Schmaus G, Neubert RHH, Wohlrab J. (2012) Dermal peptide delivery using enhancer molecules and colloidal carrier systems – Part I: carnosine. *Skin Pharmacol Physiol* **25**(6), 281–7.

7 Nasrollahi SA, Fouladdel S, Taghibiglou C, *et al.* (2012) A peptide carrier for the delivery of elastin into fibroblast cells. *Int J Dermatol* **51**(8), 923–9.

8 Lim JM, Chang MY, Park SG, *et al.* (2003) Penetration enhancement in mouse skin and lipolysis in adipocytes by TAT-GKH, a new cosmetic ingredient. *J Cosmet Sci* **54**, 483–91.

9 Yang JA, Kim ES, Kwon JH, *et al.* (2012) Transdermal delivery of hyaluronic acid – human growth hormone conjugate. *Biomaterials* **33**(25), 5947–54.

10 Ruiz MA, Clares B, Morales ME, *et al.* (2007) Preparation and stability of cosmetic formulations with an anti-aging peptide. *J Cosmet Sci* **58**, 157–71.

11 Palladino P, Castelletto V, Dehsorkhi A, *et al.* (2012) Conformation and self-association of peptide amphiphiles based on the KTTKS collagen sequence. *Langmuir.* **28**(33), 12209–15.

12 Chirita RI, Chaimbault P, Archambault JC, *et al.* (2009) Development of a LC–MS/MS method to monitor palmitoyl peptides content in anti-wrinkle cosmetics. *Analytica Chimica Acta* **641**, 95–100.

13 Rizvi SI, Maurya PK. (2007) Markers of oxidative stress in erythrocytes during aging in humans. *Ann NY Acad Sci* **1100**, 373–82.

14 Enomoto TM, Johnson T, Peterson N, *et al.* (2005) Combination glutathione and anthocyanins as an alternative for skin care during external-beam radiation. *Am J Surg* **189**, 627–31.

15 Villarama CD, Maibach HI. (2005) Glutathione as a depigmenting agent: an overview. *Int J Cosmet Sci* **27**, 147–53.

Guglielmini G, Rigano L, Bachietto E. (2012) Rejuvenating amino peptide fights skin aging. *Personal Care Europe*, **5**, 77–79.

17 Nagai K, Suda T, Kawasaki K, Mathuura S. (1986) Action of carnosine and beta-alanine on wound healing. *Surgery* **100**, 815–21.

18 Maquart FX, Simeon A, Pasco S, Monboisse JC. (1999) Regulation of cell activity by the extracellular matrix: the concept of matrikines. *J Soc Biol* **193**, 423–8.

19 Katayama K, Armendariz-Borunda J, Raghow R, *et al.* (1993) A pentapeptide from type I procollagen promotes extracellular matrix production. *J Biol Chem* **268**, 9941–4.

20 Lintner K. (2002) Promoting production in the extracellular matrix without compromising barrier. *Cutis*, **70** n°6S (suppl.), 13–16.

21 Mas-Chamberlin C, Lintner K, Basset L, *et al.* (2002) Relevance of antiwrinkle treatment of a peptide: 4 months clinical double blind study *vs* excipient. *Ann Dermatol Venereol* **129**: Proceedings 20th World Congress of Dermatology, Book II, PO 438, Paris.

22 Robinson LR, Fitzgerald NC, Doughty DG, *et al.* (2005) Topical palmitoyl pentapeptide provides improvement in photoaged human facial skin. *Int J Cosmet Sci* **27**, 155–60.

23 Hajem N, Chapelle A, Bignon J, *et al.* (2013) The regulatory role of the tetrapeptide ACSDKP in skin and hair physiology and the prevention of aging effects in these tissues – a potential cosmetic role. *Int J Cosm Sci* **35**(3), 286–98.

24 Graf R, Reiffen KA, Anzali S, *et al.* (2012) *In vivo* anti-aging efficacy of a cyclic peptide composition. *IFSCC Mag* **15**(1), 23–27.

25 Lintner K. (2010) Peptides: Anti-Ageing and Much More. In: ML.SchlossmanML (ed.) *Chemistry and Manufacture of Cosmetics: Cosmetic Specialties and Ingredients*. Carol Stream, IL: Allured Business Media, pp. 113–25.

26 Mondon P, Feuilloley M, Peschard O, *et al.* (2012) Evaluation of dermal ECM and EDJ modifications Using Four Methods: Histology, Maldi-MS, *In Vivo* Laser Confocal Microscopy and Echography – effect of age and peptide applications. 27th IFSCC Congress 2012. *Book of Abstracts*, Proceedings on Cd Rom, **359**, 37–38.

27 Querleux B, Baldeweck T, Diridollou S, *et al.* (2009) *Skin Res Technol* **15**, 306–313.

28 Mas-Chamberlin C, Mondon P, Lamy F, *et al.* (2005) Reduction of hair-loss: Matrikines and plant molecules to the rescue. In Proceedings of the 7th Scientific Conference of the Asian Society of Cosmetic Chemists, Bangkok, Thailand.

29 Loing E, Lachance R, Ollier V, Hocquaux M. (2013) A new strategy to modulate alopecia using a combination of two specific and unique ingredients. *J Cosm Sci* **64**, 45–58.

30 Gruber JV, Ludwig P, Holtz R. (2013) Modulation of cellular senescence in fibroblasts and dermal papillae cells *in vitro*. *J Cosm Sci* **64**(2), 79–87.

31 Fréchet M, Lafitte P, Maccario F, *et al.* (2012) Regeneration by the MSR enzymatic system potentiates the mitochondria-protective effect of a methionine-containing peptidomimetic. 27th IFSCC Congress 2012. *Book of Abstracts*, **152**, 360–62.

32 André N, Doridot E, Peschard O, *et al.* (2011) Dermis redensification *via* collagen synthesis. *Personal Care Europe* **4**(3), 33–34.

33 Misery L. (2002) Les nerfs à fleur de peau. *Int J Cosmet Sci* **24**(2), 111–6.

34 Shiomi H, Ueda H, Takagi H. (1981) Isolation and identification of an analgesic opioid dipeptide kyotorphin (Tyr-Arg) from bovine brain. *Neuropharmacology* **20**, 633–8.

35 Mas-Chamberlin C, Peschard O, Mondon P, Lintner K. (2004) Quantifying skin relaxation and well-being. *Cosmet Toiletries* **119**, 65–70.

36 Lintner K, Mas-Chamberlain C, Mondon P, *et al.* (2003) A lie-detector investigation to measure neuromodulating activity of a topically applied peptide: double blind clinical study of N-Acetyl-Tyr-Arg-cetylhexylester *vs*. placebo. *J Cosmet Sci* **54**, 98–99.

37 Blanes-Mira C, Clemente J, Jodas G, *et al.* (2002) A synthetic hexapeptide (Argireline) with antiwrinkle activity. *Int J Cosmet Sci* **24**, 303–10.

38 Chen YA, Scheller RH. (2001) SNARE mediated membrane fusion. *Nat Rev Mol Cell Biol* **2**, 98–106.

39 Rull M, Davi C, Cañadas E, *et al.* (2013) How to counteract the force of gravity. *COSSMA, English Edition Online* **14**(11), 10–12.

40 Rull M, Davi C, Cañadas E, *et al.* (2012) Reversing signs of aging in mature skin. *Personal Care Europe* **5**(4), 75–7.

41 Yamamoto K, Tanaka K, Iddamalgoda A. (2012) The potential role of alpha-MSH(1-8) as a novel melanogenesis-regulating factor. *Fragrance J Japan*, **11**, 48–53.

42 Marini A, Farwick M, Grether-Beck S, *et al.* (2012) Modulation of skin pigmentation by the tetrapeptide PKEK: *in vitro* and *in vivo* evidence for skin whitening effects. *Exp Dermatol* **21**(2), 140–6.

43 Loing E, Suere T. (2012) A new approach to protect and repair human epidermal cells from UV-induced DNA damages. 27th IFSCC Congress 2012. *Book of Abstracts*, **34**, 156–7.

44 Cruz LjJ, Acosta G, Gutiérrez-Reyes C. (2011) Neuropeptides – a new strategy for skin care. *Australasian J Cosm Sci* **24**, 5, 36–39.

45 Rull M, Davi C, Cañadas E, *et al.* (2013) Peptides working together – a relief for sensitive skin. *COSSMA, English Edition Online*, **14**, 9 (September), 14–16.

46 Rull M, Davi C, Cañadas E, *et al.* (2013) Attenuating facial redness and an exacerbated inflammatory response using a specific tetrapeptide. *SÖFW Journal*, English Edition, **139**, 7 (July), 34–41.

47 Rull M, Davi C, Cañadas E, Van Den Nest W, Delgado R. (2012) Novel proposal to ameliorate silhouette and reduce its imperfections. *Euro Cosmetics* **20**(11/12), 19–21.

48 Rull M. (2013) Managing volume for.the desired silhouette. *COSSMA, English Edition Online* **14**, 3, 10—11.

49 Nicolaÿ Jf, Fréchet M. (2012) Neuroendocrine control of lipolysis. Expression Cosmétique – The Global Information on Cosmetics and Fragrances – 2011, Hors Série – November, 278–282.

50 Mantelin J. (2011) ISP, New synthetic peptide enhances skin's natural UV defenses. Cosmetics Business – Online Newsletter by SPC – Soap, Perfumery and Cosmetics, 2011, 27 January 2011.

51 Mateu M, Davi C, Cañadas E. (2013) An integral 360° Hydration Approach. *HPC – Household and Personal Care Today*, **8**, 2 (March–April), Monographic Supplement Series, Supplement on Body Care Grooming, Protection and Hygiene.

52 Cafardi JA, Elmets CA. (2008) T4 endonuclease V: review and application to dermatology. *Expert Opin Biol Ther* **8**, 829–38.

53 Mas-Chamberlin C, Lamy F, Mondon P, *et al.* (2002) Heat and UV stable cosmetic enzymes from deep sea bacteria. *Cosmet Toiletries* **117**, 22–30.

54 Mas-Chamberlin C, Mondon P, Lamy F, *et al.* (2006) Potential preventive performance. *Soap Perfum Cosmet* **6**, 34–6.

CHAPTER 35
Cellular Growth Factors

Rahul C. Mehta[1] and Richard E. Fitzpatrick[2]
[1] SkinMedica, Inc, An Allergan Company, Carlsbad, CA, USA
[2] UCSD School of Medicine, San Diego, CA, USA

> **BASIC CONCEPTS**
> - Skin aging is like a chronic wound that does not completely heal.
> - Cellular growth factors that promote wound healing may accelerate reversal of aging.
> - High levels of active growth factors are required to produce biological effects after topical application.
> - Multiple clinical studies show efficacy of products containing physiologically balanced cellular growth factors.

Introduction

This chapter discusses cellular growth factors, which are proteins capable of stimulating cellular growth, proliferation, and cellular differentiation. Growth factors are important for regulating a variety of cellular processes. They have been best studied in wound healing models, but have been adapted as cosmeceuticals for their ability to improve the appearance of aging skin.

Physiology

Skin aging and wound healing

Extensive research on skin aging in the last decade has resulted in an improved understanding of the pathophysiology of intrinsic (age-related) and extrinsic aging (UV-mediated photoaging). Biochemical processes resulting in skin damage following exposure to UV radiation are now being identified and understood [1]. A correlation between biochemical processes following photodamage and creation of wound is emerging. Of specific interest to cosmeceutical manufacturers are the effects of growth factors in the process of wound healing. Figure 35.1 shows the stages of wound healing and role of growth factors in each stage. Growth factors are regulatory proteins that mediate signaling pathways between and within cells. After a skin damage, a variety of growth factors flood the wound site and interact synergistically to initiate and coordinate each phase of wound healing. They help recruit and activate fibroblast to rapidly produce extracellular matrix to close the wound followed by stimulation and multiplication of keratinocytes to form new epidermis. The overall process is complex and not completely understood [2].

Following skin damage, a variety of inflammatory pathways are activated including nuclear factor-κB (NF-κB) mediated activation of tumor necrosis factor-α (TNF-α) and interleukins [3]. Reactive oxygen species (ROS or free radicals) and proteolytic enzymes are generated as a result of inflammation resulting in degradation of extracellular matrix. ROS increase oxidative phosphorylation of cell surface receptors causing activation transcription factors activator protein 1 (AP-1) and NF-κB, two critical components of mitogen-activated protein (MAP) kinase signaling pathway [4]. ROS therefore have a central role in intrinsic and extrinsic aging. AP-1 stimulates transcription of matrix metalloproteinase (MMP) growth factor genes in fibroblast and keratinocytes, and inhibits type 1 procollagen gene expression in fibroblasts [5]. Multiple studies have shown that activation of the MMP secretion as a result of intrinsic and extrinsic aging produces breakdown of dermal matrix [6]

Different subtypes of MMP have different substrate proteins on which they act to produce a break in their primary sequence. MMP-1 (collagenase) produces cleavage at a single site in central triple helix of fibrillar type I and III collagen. The cleaved subunits are further degraded by MMP-3 (stromelysine 1) and MMP-9 (gelatinase). Tissue inhibitors of metalloproteinase (TIMP) decrease activity of MMPs. ROS inactivates TIMP thereby further increasing MMP activity. AP-1 mediated reduction in synthesis of procollagen appears to result from two mechanisms: interference of AP-1 with type 1 and 3 procollagen gene transcription and blocking the profibrotic effects of TGF-β by impairment of TGF-β type 2 receptor–Smad

---

Cosmetic Dermatology: Products and Procedures, Second Edition. Edited by Zoe Diana Draelos.
© 2016 John Wiley & Sons, Ltd. Published 2016 by John Wiley & Sons, Ltd.

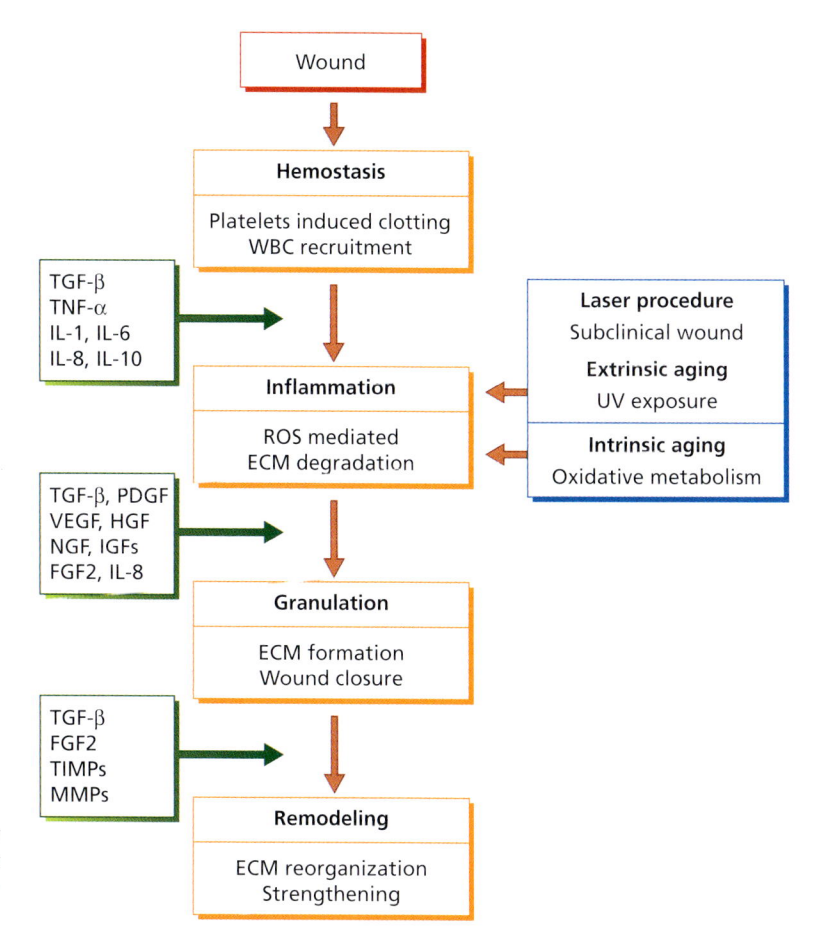

Figure 35.1 Healing and remodeling of skin damaged by the effect of intrinsic aging, extrinsic aging, wound or laser procedures. (Source: Mehta & Fitzpatrick, 2007 [2]. Reproduced with permission of John Wiley & Sons.)

pathway [3]. Activation of NF-κB stimulates transcriptions of proinflammatory cytokine genes including interleukin 1 (IL-1), TNF-α, IL-6, and IL-8 [4]. Inflammation resulting from these cytokines increases secretion of ROS and more cytokines further enhancing the effect of UV exposure.

Inflammation causes protease-mediated degradation of elastin and UV exposure causes formation of abnormal elastin by fibroblasts. UV light is also an inhibitior of leukocyte elastase thereby increasing accumulation of elastotic materials [7]. The accumulation of elastotic materials is accompanied by degeneration of surrounding collagenous network.

The overall effects of these interlinked biochemical activities is reduction of procollagen synthesis, increase of collagen degradation in the dermal extracellular matrix, and increase in irregular elastin deposition. Successful resolution of damage to skin and wound healing requires a balance between development of inflammation and its rapid resolution which includes involvement of growth factors and cytokines such as TGF-β, TNF-α, platelet-derived growth factor (PDGF), IL-1, IL-6, and IL-10 [8]. Intrinsic aging does not show the inflammatory component seen with healing of acute photodamage and wounds; instead, mitochondrial oxidative metabolism produces some of the key mediators of extracellular matrix degradation including ROS [9].

Transition from inflammatory phase of wound healing to granulation phase is mediated by a variety of growth factors and cytokines including PDGF, TGF-α, TGF-β, fibroblast growth factors (FGFs), insulin-like growth factor 1 (IGF-1), colony stimulating factors (CSF), interleukins and TNF-α [10]. The growth factors and cytokines are derived from macrophages, epidermal keratinocytes, and fibroblasts. Multiple metabolic pathways lead to formation of new collagen and repair of extracellular matrix during the granulation phase.

The final stage of skin repair after granulation and re-epithelialization or peeling of sunburned skin is the beginning of dermal tissue remodelling. During this stage, low strength, unorganized, type 3 collagen and irregular elastin structures produced during the extracellular matrix production phase are replaced by stronger type 1 collagen and structured elastin fibres to provide strength and resiliency to the dermis. This remodelling phase can last for several months and is the key to reversing the visible effects of skin aging [11].

Most studies have evaluated the role of single growth factors in controlled wound-healing environments. These studies demonstrate the importance of growth factors in the repair of damaged tissue, but research into the phases of wound healing has demonstrated that it is the interaction of multiple growth factors that is vital to tissue regeneration. Cosmeceutical manufacturers have taken notice of the positive results of clinical studies showing accelerated wound healing and have included growth factors in products designed to mitigate damage from chronologic aging and sun exposure [11].

Role of cellular growth factors in skincare

The use of growth factors and cytokines in skin rejuvenation and reversal of photoaging is fast becoming a cornerstone of antiaging treatments. Table 35.1 lists some important growth factors and cytokines that affect the proliferation of dermal fibroblasts and extracellular matrix production [12]. Growth factors, cytokines, and other agents that help rebuild the extracellular matrix are critical in the reversal of the signs of skin aging such as fine lines and wrinkles. Providing a physiologically balanced mixture of these growth factors and cytokines to cells responsible for extracellular matrix production and remodeling may benefit in rejuvenation of aging skin. Several cosmeceutical products containing either a single human growth factor or combination of multiple human growth factors and cytokines are currently marketed for skin rejuvenation. Several clinical and skin biology studies now show that human growth factors when applied topically provide beneficial effects in reducing the signs of facial skin aging [2].

Unique attributes

Growth factors produce antiaging benefits by virtue of their biologic role to maintain healthy skin structure and function. Together with cytokines, growth factors provide constant communication between cells of the immune system, keratinocytes, and fibroblasts throughout the process of wound healing and skin repair and regeneration. During the final remodeling phase of wound healing, a number of different growth factors and cytokines interact with each other and with the surrounding

Table 35.1 Partial list of growth factors and cytokines identified in active gel and their function in skin [12].

Growth factor/cytokine	Skin-related functions
Fibroblast growth factors: bFGF (FGF-2), FGF-4, FGF-6, KGF (FGF-7), FGF-9	Angiogenic and fibroblast mitogen
Hepatocyte growth factor (HGF)	Strong mitogenic activities; three-dimensional tissue regeneration and wound healing
Platelet derived growth factors: PDGF AA, PDGF BB, PDGF Rb	Chemotactic for macrophages, fibroblasts; macrophage activation; fibroblast mitogen, and matrix production
Insulin-like growth factors: IGF1, IGFBP1, IGFBP2, IGFBP3, IGFBP6	Endothelial cell and fibroblast mitogen
Transforming growth factor: TGF-β1, TGF-β2, TGF-β3	Keratinocyte migration; chemotactic for macrophages and fibroblasts
Tissue inhibitor of metalloproteinases: TIMP1 (MPI1), TIMP2 (MPI2)	Prevent enzymatic degradation of collagen and hyaluronic acid
Vascular endothelial growth factor (VEGF)	Influence vascular permeability and angiogenesis to improve tissue nutrition
Placenta growth factor (PLGF)	Promote endothelial cell growth
Bone morphogenetic protein: BMP7	Promote development of nerve cells in developing tissue
Interleukins: IL-1α, IL-1β	Early activators of growth factor expression in macrophages, keratinocytes, and fibroblasts
Interleukin: IL-2	Enhance epithelial wound healing
Interleukin: IL-6	Mediator of acute phase response to wound and has synergistic effect with IL-1
Interleukin: IL-10	Inhibits pro-inflammatory cytokines to reduce inflammation prevents scar formation
Interleukin: IL-4, IL-13	Stimulate production of IL-6
Interleukin: IL-3, IL-4, IL-5	Leukocyte maturation and degranulation during inflammatory phase
Interleukins: IL-7, IL-8, IL-15	Leukocyte activation and proliferation during inflammatory phase
Leptin	Epidermal keratinocyte proliferation during wound healing
Colony stimulating factors: GCSF, GM-CSF, M-CSF	Stimulate the development of neutrophils and macrophages

CSF, granulocyte colony stimulating factor; GM-CSF, granulocyte macrophage colony stimulating factor; M-CSF, macrophage colony stimulating factor.

cells in concert to improve the quality of extracellular matrix. Use of individual growth factors is unlikely to duplicate these complex interactions essential for remodeling of skin. Therefore, a mixture of growth factors and cytokines proven to have a role in skin remodeling should provide superior benefits than individual growth factors. Ideal growth factor products should contain this unique mixture obtained from natural sources.

Advantages and disadvantages

Clinically proven benefits in reversal of skin aging and post-procedure healing

In one of the first pilot clinical studies with a product containing a natural combination of fibroblast-derived growth factor mixture, 14 patients with Fitzpatrick class II or greater facial photodamage applied TNS Recovery Complex (SkinMedica, Carlsbad, CA, USA) twice daily for 60 days. The results show a statistically significant reduction in fine lines and wrinkles and reduction in periorbital photodamage by clinical grading and by optical profilometry. Figure 35.2 shows an example of a skin biopsy section with increased collagen after treatment with the study product. Measurements of grenz zone collagen and epidermal thickness from the biopsy show a 37% increase in grenz zone collagen and a 30% increase in epidermal thickness [11].

Vehicle controlled studies on cosmeceutical products are very difficult to conduct as topical vehicles can have benefits by virtue of skin hydration, reduced epidermal water loss, or simply providing physical barrier against the environment. Because of these effects, most vehicles cannot be classified as "inactive" and make it more difficult to achieve statistical significance in a vehicle controlled, double-blind study design. In spite of these difficulties, if the product contains any new active combinations, the study must include a reasonably matched vehicle to scientifically validate effects of the new active [13].

In a double-blind vehicle controlled study, 60 subjects were randomly assigned to receive either TNS Recovery Complex or vehicle and apply it twice daily for 6 months along with a moisturizing cleanser and sunscreen. Treatment with TNS Recovery Complex for 3 months produced greater reduction in fine lines and wrinkles than vehicle treatment as measured by optical profilometry and assessment of photographs. The results were either statistically significant ($p \leq 0.05$) or trending towards statistical significance ($p \leq 0.1$). Figure 35.3 shows improvement in facial photodamage observed in this study. The study demonstrates that even when compared with a treatment with a good moisturizer and sunscreen, the product being tested showed significant benefits of reversal of signs and symptoms of skin aging [12].

In another double-blind study, 18 patients with Fitzpatrick class II or greater facial photodamage applied Bio-Restorative Skin Cream (NeoCutis, Inc, San Francisco, CA, USA) twice daily for 60 days. The results showed that while the average facial roughness did not decrease, a significant improvement was seen in several other parameters of facial wrinkles. The measurements were conducted by a three-dimensional surface mapping technique [14].

A split-face study of 42 subjects using human cell conditioned medium CCM (Histogen Inc, San Diego, CA, USA) immediately after ablative and non-ablative laser resurfacing produced accelerated wound healing and more normal skin recovery [15].

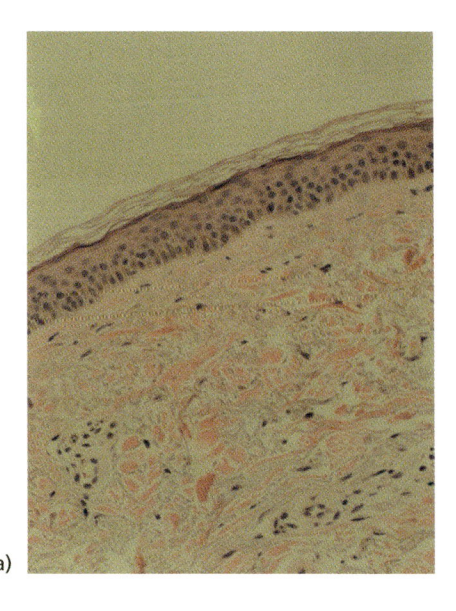

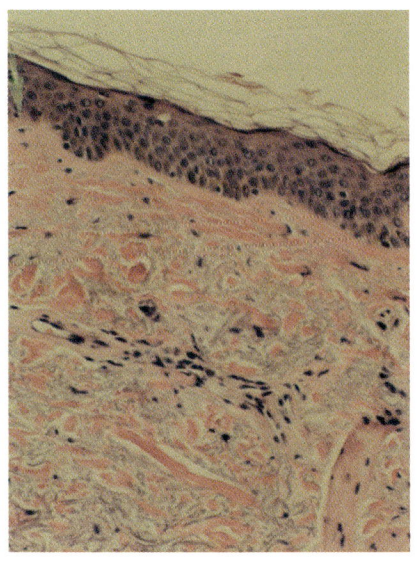

Figure 35.2 Histology of skin before (a) and after 3 months of TNS Recovery Complex (b) showing increase in grenz-zone collagen and epidermal thickness after treatment [11].

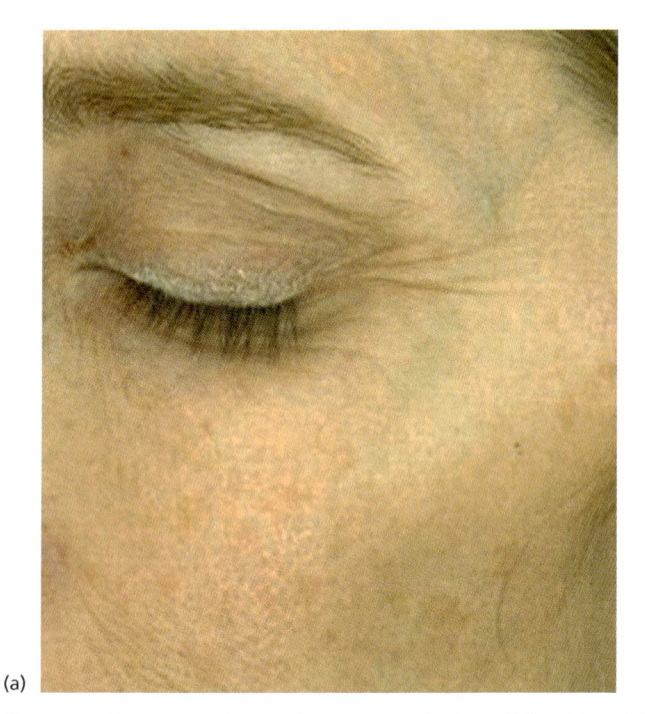

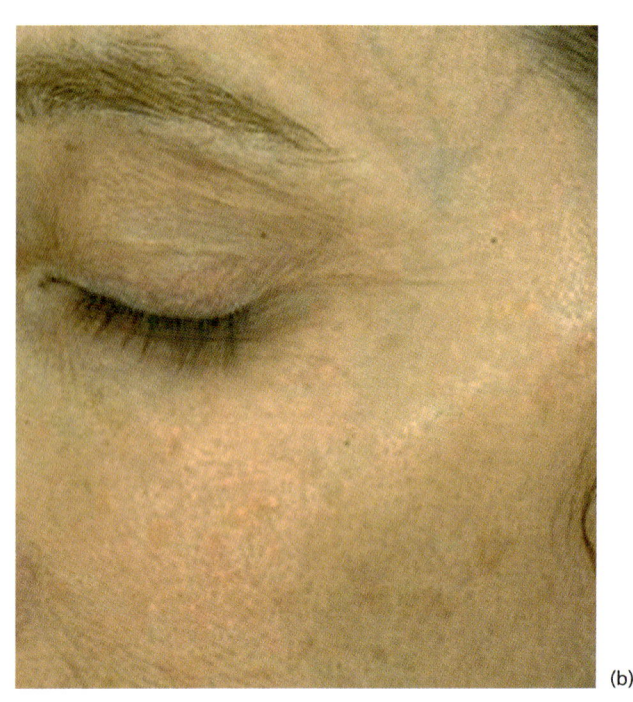

Figure 35.3 Photograph of periorbital and upper cheek area before (a) and after 6 months of TNS Recovery Complex (b) showing reduction in wrinkles and fine lines after treatment [12].

Risks associated with growth factors

Growth factors are key molecules that affect cellular proliferation and differentiation which, if unregulated, can lead to carcinogenic transformation of cells. Presence of receptors for some growth factors in melanoma cells and expression of certain growth factors by cancerous cells [16] has raised concerns about the potential for topically applied growth factors to stimulate the development of cancer. However, whether presence of receptors or increased expression contributes to tumor growth is uncertain. A recent finding suggests that chronic administration of high concentrations of PDGF directly into debrided diabetic pressure wounds may result in increased mortality from cancer. It is unlikely that growth factors applied topically to intact skin would affect tumor proliferation as the protein molecules are too large to be absorbed in large quantities [12]. In addition, it is unlikely that the levels of growth factors in skin after topical application is significantly higher than those following inflammation-causing event such as chemical peel, lasers, or skin infections.

Maintaining activity of growth factors through product shelf-life

Growth factors and other biologically active peptides are inherently unstable in non-physiologic environment, unless they are stored frozen at temperatures below −20°C. Presence of surface active additives, alcohols, and other protein denaturing excipients further decrease product stability and compromise product efficacy during the claimed shelf-life of the product. Analytical techniques have advanced to a point where presence of growth factors in simple solution or gel formulations can be easily detected by immunoassay as demonstrated by analysis of a commercial growth factor product stored at room temperature for 2 years [12,17]. While complex multiphase formulations such as creams containing combination of cellular growth factors may be difficult to analyse, a new technique for determination of biological activity of anti-aging products was recently validated and published. The study evaluates expression of extra-cellular matrix related genes in full-thickness human skin using retinoic acid as positive control. Figure 35.4 shows gene expression changes with use of a

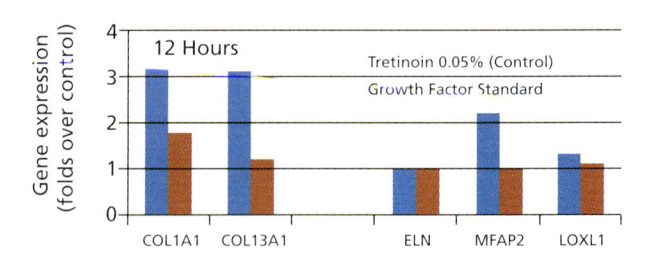

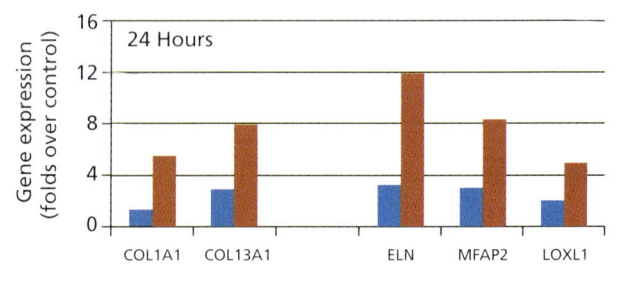

Figure 35.4 Human skin model for determining biological activity of growth factor containing products [18].

commercial growth factor product [18]. Techniques such as this must be used to verify stability and activity of growth factors during the product shelf-life period to ensure that patients receive the claimed growth factors.

Ingredients

Natural growth factors

Human growth factors may be obtained from two major sources: cultured human cells or genetically engineered microorganisms. Human cells cultured in a three-dimensional network secrete a mixture of a large number of growth factors and other proteins capable of promoting wound healing [19]. The composition of the growth factor mixture varies with cell phenotype and environmental variables. Cells growing under conditions resembling a wound are most likely to produce growth factors, cytokines, and matrix proteins that assist in wound healing.

TNS by SkinMedica is collected from a three-dimensional matrix of cultured human dermal fibroblasts induced to produce collagen, the same protein they produce during wound healing. The associated combination of growth factors and cytokines naturally secreted during the collagen production phase of the tissue culture therefore represents the most appropriate combination to induce wound healing (Table 35.1) [12]. CCM Complex by Histogen prepared from cultured human fibroblasts under embryonic-like conditions contain a mixture of growth factors appropriate for wound healing [15]. Naturally secreted growth factors can also be obtained from fibroblast and keratinocyte co-cultures. PSP by Neocutis uses a different method of collecting a mixture of growth factors and cytokines. Growth factors from cultured fibroblasts are collected by lyses followed by purification of all intracellular content present at the time of lysis. The purification process concentrates the growth factors and removes culture media but may also remove some important components of the growth factor mixture [20].

Growth factors secreting stem cells

Adipose-derived stem cells and umbilical cord mesenchymal stem cells have been studied for promotion of wound healing and anti-aging effects by virtue of their ability to secrete growth factors. Preliminary studies show that intradermal injection of adipose-derived stem cell suspension can produce increased collagen production, increase cellular antioxidant levels and reduce signs of skin aging. These preclinical results warrant further evaluation in clinical studies after adequate testing and standardization of methods to obtain autologous adipose-derived stem cells [21,22].

Synthetic growth factors

Individual growth factors and cytokines can be made via recombinant technology using bacterial or yeast cultures

Table 35.2 Synthetic growth factors registered as cosmetic ingredients [23].

INCI name	Growth factor
Human oligopeptide-1	Epidermal growth factor
Human oligopeptide-2	Insulin-like growth factor-1
Human oligopeptide-3	Basic fibroblast growth factor
Human oligopeptide-5	Keratinocyte growth factor
Human oligopeptide-7	Transforming growth factor-β3
Human oligopeptide-8	Interleukin 10
Human oligopeptide-10	Platelet derived growth factor
Human oligopeptide-11	Vascular endothelial growth factor
Human oligopeptide-12	Fibroblast growth factor 10
Human oligopeptide-13	Acidic fibroblast growth factor
Human oligopeptide-14	Transforming growth factor-α
Human oligopeptide-15	Interleukin 4
Human oligopeptide-19	Nerve growth factor
Human oligopeptide-20	Tissue inhibitor of metalloproteinases

modified to include DNA sequence for growth factors. Many growth factors of cosmeceutical interest are produced by this technique including TGF-β, vascular endothelial growth factor (VEGF), epidermal growth factor (EGF), various FGFs, PDGF, and more [23]. Table 35.2 lists various growth factors registered with International Cosmetic Ingredient Dictionary and Handbook as cosmetic ingredients. While clinical studies have shown a marginally beneficial effect for some of the individual growth factors, more studies must be carried out to understand the role of combinations of growth factors in skin rejuvenation. Combinations of growth factors that complement each other's effects is likely to be more effective as multiple growth factors are involved in most biochemical processes including wound healing [8].

Related products

Phytokinins

Kinetin, a plant-derived growth hormone discovered almost 50 years ago, has been recently used in several cosmeceutical products as an antiaging ingredient [24]. Kinetin is found in the DNA of almost all organisms tested so far, including human cells. In plants, kinetin regulates cellular differentiation by an endocrine pathway with unknown mechanism; however, its function in human cells is not known. Kinetin and other cytokinins are products of oxidative metabolism of the cell. Kinetin is formed in the nucleus by reaction of hydroxyl free radicals with DNA whereas reaction of hydroxyl radical with RNA results in formation of zeatin, another cytokinin used in cosmeceutical products.

Alternate delivery methods

Mesotherapy is the micro-injection of growth factors or other active molecules into the mesoderm with the premise that the active molecules are directly delivered to the target tissue using fine gauge short needles to a 2–5 mm depth of penetration. Multiple, close spaced injections are made to ensure adequate coverage of the treatment area. There are no clinical studies evaluating the efficacy of the procedures and safety remains a concern because of lack of availability of sterile growth factor solutions.

A variation of mesotherapy is the use of micro-needle devises or fractionated lasers to create micro-punctures into the stratum corneum before topical application of growth factors with the assumption that reduced barrier will result in greater efficacy. Again, very little clinical evidence exists to show effectiveness of these procedures.

Conclusions

Studying the role of growth factors in cutaneous wound healing has led to research demonstrating positive cosmetic and clinical outcomes in photodamaged skin. Although the topical use of growth factors is an emerging treatment approach, clinical studies demonstrate that dermal collagen production and clinical improvement in photodamage appearance are significant. Further, the increase in dermal collagen produced by topical growth factors can be measured quantitatively by biopsy. Although the functions of growth factors in the natural wound healing process are complex and incompletely understood, it appears that wound healing is dependent on the synergistic interaction of many growth factors. The most promising research suggests that multiple growth factors used in combination stimulate the growth of collagen, elastin, and glycosaminoglycans leading to reduction in fine lines and wrinkles. The use of a multiple growth factor topical formulation provides a good first line treatment for mild to moderate photodamaged skin.

References

1. Gilchrest BA. (1989) Skin aging and photoaging: an overview. *J Am Acad Dermatol* **21**, 610–3.
2. Mehta RC, Fitzpatrick RE. (2007) Endogenous growth factors as cosmeceuticals. *Dermatol Ther* **20**, 350–9.
3. Quan T, He T, Kang S, et al. (2004) Solar ultraviolet irradiation reduces collagen in photoaged human skin by blocking transforming growth factor-beta type II receptor/Smad signaling. *Am J Pathol* **165**, 741–51.
4. Fisher GJ, Talwar HS, Lin J, et al. (1998) Retinoic acid inhibits induction of c-Jun protein by ultraviolet radiation that occurs subsequent to activation of mitogen-activated protein kinase pathways in human skin in vivo. *J Clin Invest* **101**, 1432–40.
5. Schwartz E, Cruickshank FA, Christensen CC, et al. (1993) Collagen alterations in chronically sun-damaged human skin. *Photochem Photobiol* **58**, 841–4.
6. Fisher GJ, Wang ZQ, Datta SC, et al. (1997) Pathophysiology of premature skin aging induced by ultraviolet light. *N Engl J Med* **337**, 1419–28.
7. Martin P. (1997) Wound healing: aiming for perfect skin regeneration. *Science* **276**, 75–81.
8. Eming SA, Krieg T, Davidson JM. (2007) Inflammation in wound repair: molecular and cellular mechanisms. *J Invest Dermatol* **127**, 514–25.
9. Sohal RS, Weindruch R. (1996) Oxidative stress, caloric restriction, and aging. *Science* **273**, 59–63.
10. Moulin V. (1995) Growth factors in skin wound healing: review article. *Eur J Cell Biol* **68**, 1–7.
11. Fitzpatrick RE, Rostan EF. (2003) Reversal of photodamage with topical growth factors: a pilot study. *J Cosmet Laser Ther* **5**, 25–34.
12. Mehta RC, Smith SR, Grove GL, et al. (2008) Reduction in facial photodamage by a topical growth factor product. *J Drugs Dermatol* **7**, 864–71.
13. Draelos ZD. (2007) Exploring the pitfalls in clinical cosmeceutical research. *Cosmet Dermatol* **20**, 556–8.
14. Gold MH, Goldman MP, Biron J. (2007) Human growth factor and cytokine skin cream for facial skin rejuvenation as assessed by 3D in vivo optical skin imaging. *J Drugs Dermatol* **6**, 1018–23.
15. Zimber MP, Mansbridge JN, Taylor M, et al. (2012) Human cell-conditioned media produced under embryonic-like conditions result in improved healing time after laser resurfacing. *Aesthetic Plast Surg.* **36**, 431–7.
16. Liu B, Earl HM, Baban D, et al. (1995) Melanoma cell lines express VEGF receptor KDR and respond to exogenously added VEGF. *Biochem Biophys Res Commun* **217**, 721–7.
17. Sundaram H, Mehta RC, Norine JA, et al. (2009) Topically applied physiologically balanced growth factors: A new paradigm of skin rejuvenation. *J Drugs Dermatol.* **8**:s4–s13
18. Vega VL, Mehta RC, Bachelor MA, et al. (2013) Differential modulation of ECM components and GFR by retinoic acid and physiologically balanced GF formulation. *J Invest Dermatol* **133**, S155.
19. Mansbridge J, Liu K, Patch R, et al. (1998) Three-dimensional fibroblast culture implant for the treatment of diabetic foot ulcers: metabolic activity and therapeutic range. *Tissue Eng* **4**, 403–14.
20. Schütte H, Kula MR. (1990) Pilot- and process-scale techniques for cell disruption. *Biotechnol Appl Biochem* **12**, 599–620.
21. Park BS, Jang KA, Sung JH, Park JS, Kwon YH, Kim KJ, et al. (2008) Adipose-derived stem cells and their secretory factors as a promising therapy for skin aging. *Dermatol Surg* **34**, 1323–6.
22. Liu Q, Luo Z, He S, Peng X, et al. (2013) Conditioned serum-free medium from umbilical cord mesenchymal stem cells has anti-photoaging properties. *Biotechnol Lett.* **35**, 1707–14.
23. Gottscha TE, Bailey JE, eds. (2008) *International Cosmetic Ingredient Dictionary and Handbook*. Washington DC: Toiletry and Fragrance Association, pp. 1170–4.10
24. Barciszewski J, Massino F, Clark BF. (2007) Kinetin: a multiactive molecule. *Int J Biol Macromol* **40**, 182–92.

CHAPTER 36
Topical Cosmeceutical Retinoids

Olivier Sorg[1], Gürkan Kaya[2], and Jean H. Saurat[1]

[1] Swiss Centre for Applied Human Toxicology, University of Geneva, Geneva, Switzerland
[2] Department of Dermatology, Geneva University Hospital, Geneva, Switzerland

> **BASIC CONCEPTS**
> - Retinoids define a class of substances comprising vitamin A (retinol) and its naturally and synthetic derivatives.
> - Retinoids are lipophilic molecules that diffuse through plasma membranes or cross the cutaneous barrier when applied topically. Inside the cells, retinoids bind to nuclear receptors (RAR-α, -β, -γ, and RXR-α, -β, -γ), then the ligand–receptor complexes bind to a RAR-response element (RARE) DNA sequence, resulting in the modulation of the expression of genes involved in cellular differentiation and proliferation.
> - As biologically active agents given to humans, retinoids can be divided into therapeutics and cosmeceuticals.
> - The ranking order of retinoid-like activity following topical application is as follows: retinoic acid > retinaldehyde > retinol >>> retinyl esters.

Biological concepts

Therapeutic and cosmeceutical retinoids

Retinoids define a class of substances comprising vitamin A (retinol) and its naturally and synthetic derivatives. Although they were first discovered in the retina as central players of the biology of vision, they function as key regulators of differentiation and proliferation in various tissues. Retinol is produced in the small intestine either by hydrolysis of retinyl esters, or by oxidation of various carotenoids [1,2]. Retinol can be oxidized into retinaldehyde, and then into retinoic acid, the biologically active form of vitamin A. Retinol may be also esterified with fatty acids to form retinyl esters. Retinoic acid is oxidized to a less active metabolite, 4-oxoretinoic acid, or converted to retinoyl glucuronide, whereas retinol is converted to retinyl glucuronide. Two other vitamin A metabolites, 4-oxoretinol and 4-oxoretinal, are believed to be the products of oxidation of retinol and retinal, respectively, by CYP26-related hydroxylases, although this has not been demonstrated [3,4] (Figure 36.1). The two predominant endogenous retinoids are retinol and its esters. Retinol and retinyl esters account for more than 99% of total cutaneous retinoids, i.e. ≈1 nmol/g [5]. Retinoic acid is catabolized either by phase I or phase II enzymes, giving rise to retinoyl glucuronide or 4-oxoretinoic acid [6,7]. Although the latter has long been considered an inactive catabolite of retinoic acid, other oxoretinoids, i.e. 4-oxoretinol and 4-oxoretinal, have been shown to be the predominant retinoids in some models of morphogenesis [8-10], and exert some of the retinoid-like activities in mouse *in vivo* [11]. As lipophilic molecules, they can diffuse through plasma membranes or cross the cutaneous barrier when applied topically. Inside the cells, they bind to nuclear receptors (RAR-α, -β, -γ, and RXR-α, -β, -γ), then the ligand–receptor complexes bind to a RAR-response element (RARE) DNA sequence, resulting in the modulation of the expression of genes involved in cellular differentiation and proliferation [4,12–14] (Figure 36.1).

As biologically active agents given to humans, retinoids can be divided into therapeutics and cosmeceuticals.

Therapeutic retinoids are usually RAR or RXR ligands (except for isotretinoin), and are available on medical prescription to treat diseases such as acne, psoriasis, and actinic keratosis, or oncological diseases such as acute promyelocytic leukemia, cutaneous T-cell lymphoma, and squamous or basal cell carcinoma [15]. Endogenous active metabolites of retinol (vitamin A) such as all-*trans*-retinoic acid (tretinoin), 9-*cis*-retinoic acid (alitretinoin) and 13-cis-retinoic acid (isotretinoin), as well as the synthetic monoaromatic retinoids acitretin and etretinate, and the arotinoids adapalene, tazarotene and bexarotene, belong to the therapeutic retinoids [16,17] (Figure 36.2A).

Endogenous precursors of retinoic acids, i.e. retinyl esters, retinol and retinaldehyde, as well as 4-oxoretinoids (4-oxoretinol, 4-oxoretinal and 4-oxoretinoic acids), do not bind to nuclear retinoid receptors; are found in many OTC products; and constitute the group of topical cosmeceutical retinoids [4] (Figure 36.2B).

Epidermal vitamin A

Vitamin A is present in the epidermis as free and esterified retinol at an average concentration of 1–2 nmol/g [5,18]. Retinol and retinyl esters may be oxidized to retinaldehyde and then to

---

Cosmetic Dermatology: Products and Procedures, Second Edition. Edited by Zoe Diana Draelos.
© 2016 John Wiley & Sons, Ltd. Published 2016 by John Wiley & Sons, Ltd.

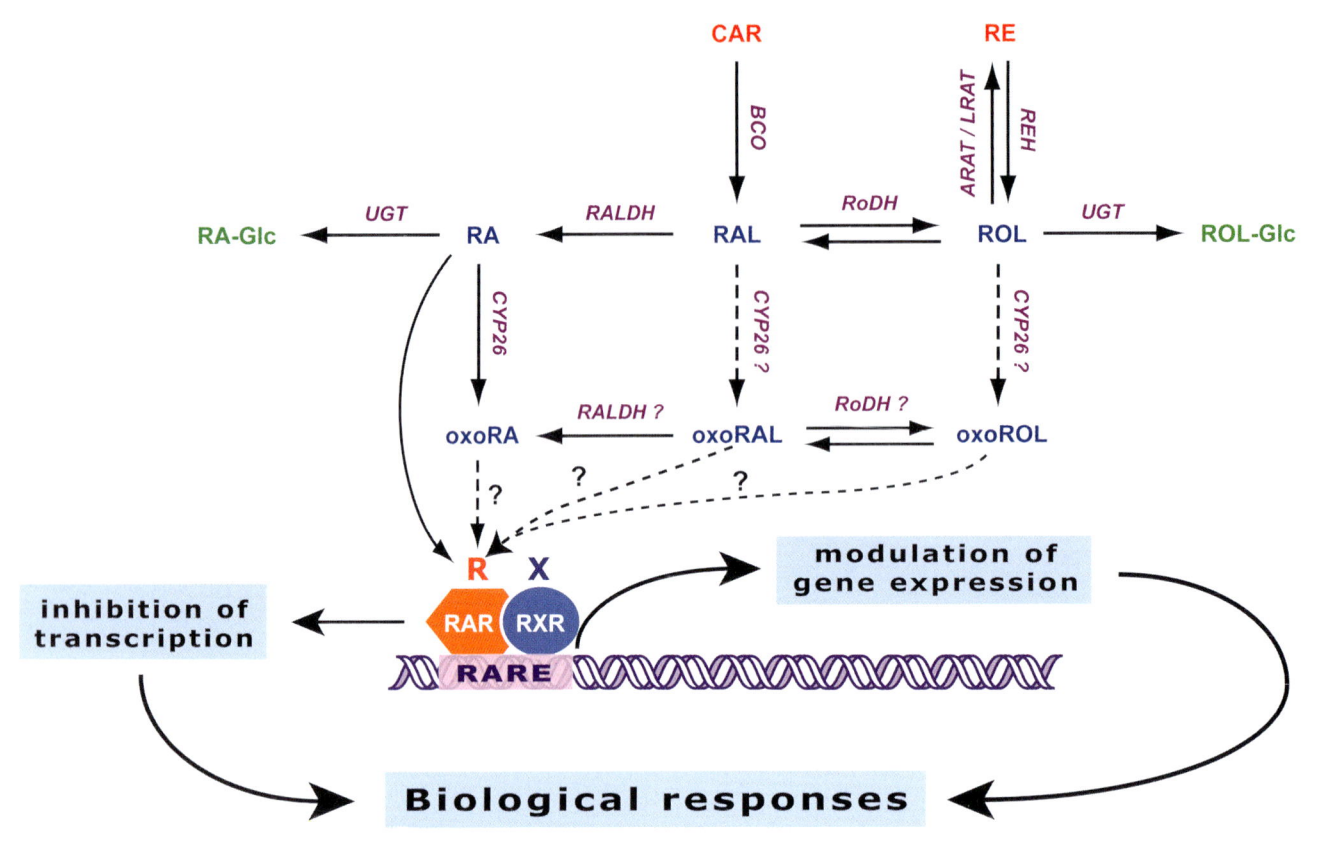

Figure 36.1 Biochemical pathways from dietary provitamins A to biological responses. Abbreviations: ARAT, acyl-coenzyme A:retinol acyltransferase; BCO, β-carotene-15,15'-monooxygenase; CAR, β-carotene; CYP26, cytochrome P450 26; LRAT, lecithin:retinol acyltransferase; oxoRA, all-*trans*-4-oxoretinoic acid; oxoRAL, all-*trans*-4-oxoretinal; oxoROL, all-*trans*-4-oxoretinol; RA, all-*trans*-retinoic acid; RA-Glu, all-*trans*-retinoyl-β-D-glucuronide; RAL, all-*trans*-retinaldehyde; RALDH, retinal dehydrogenase; RE, retinyl esters; REH, retinyl ester hydrolase; RoDH, retinol dehydrogenase; ROL, all-*trans* retinol; ROL-Glu, all-*trans*-retinyl- β-D-glucuronide; UGT, UDP-glucuronosyl transferase.

retinoic acid *cis/trans* isomers within keratinocytes [19–21]. An epidermal hypovitaminosis A may be the consequence of nutritional deficiency [22,23], acute or long term UV exposure [24], oxidative stress [18,25] and aging [26]. A deficiency of vitamin A manifests in the skin as a follicular hyperkeratosis known as phrynoderma, characterized by rough, hyperkeratotic, follicular papules on the skin of elbows and knees [27]. Vitamin A deficiency is also a risk factor for the development of skin cancers [28–32]. Retinoids increase the expression of the tumor-preventive transcription factor p53 [31,33] and decrease that of AP-1 and NF-κB [34,35], transcription factors linked to proliferation and inflammation, two events involved in tumor formation [36,37]. This defines the biochemical foundation for the use of retinoids in cancer treatment and prevention [32,38–43].

The intracrine pro-ligand concept

Chronological aging and photoaging are not only a question of aesthetics that is often accompanied by psychological problems, they also constitute the background for the development of precancerous and cancerous skin lesions, as well as severe functional skin fragility now called dermatoporosis [44,45]. Many clinical studies indicate that certain structural changes induced by excessive sun exposure can be reversed, to some extent, by the use of topical retinoids [46]. Although retinoic acid is widely used for topical therapy of several skin diseases and for improvement of skin aging, it induces irritation of the skin, which precludes its long-term use to treat extrinsic or intrinsic aging.

Irritation might be explained, at least in part, by an overload of the retinoic acid-dependent pathways with supraphysiological amounts of exogenous retinoic acid in the skin. It is still not established whether all the therapeutic activities of topical retinoids are mediated by nuclear receptors, and whether irritation is necessary for obtaining some of these activities, although most experts now consider that irritation is not mandatory for activity.

To overcome the problems encountered by topical retinoic acid, delivery can be targeted with precursors of biologically active retinoids; these "pro-ligands" are then converted in a controlled process into active ligands [47]. This *intracrine concept*, in which the active ligand is produced within the targets cells, has been explored to deliver retinoid activity to mouse and human skin topically with natural retinoids such as retinaldehyde that do not bind to nuclear receptors [5,48–52]. This might be a convenient definition of cosmeceutical topical retinoids.

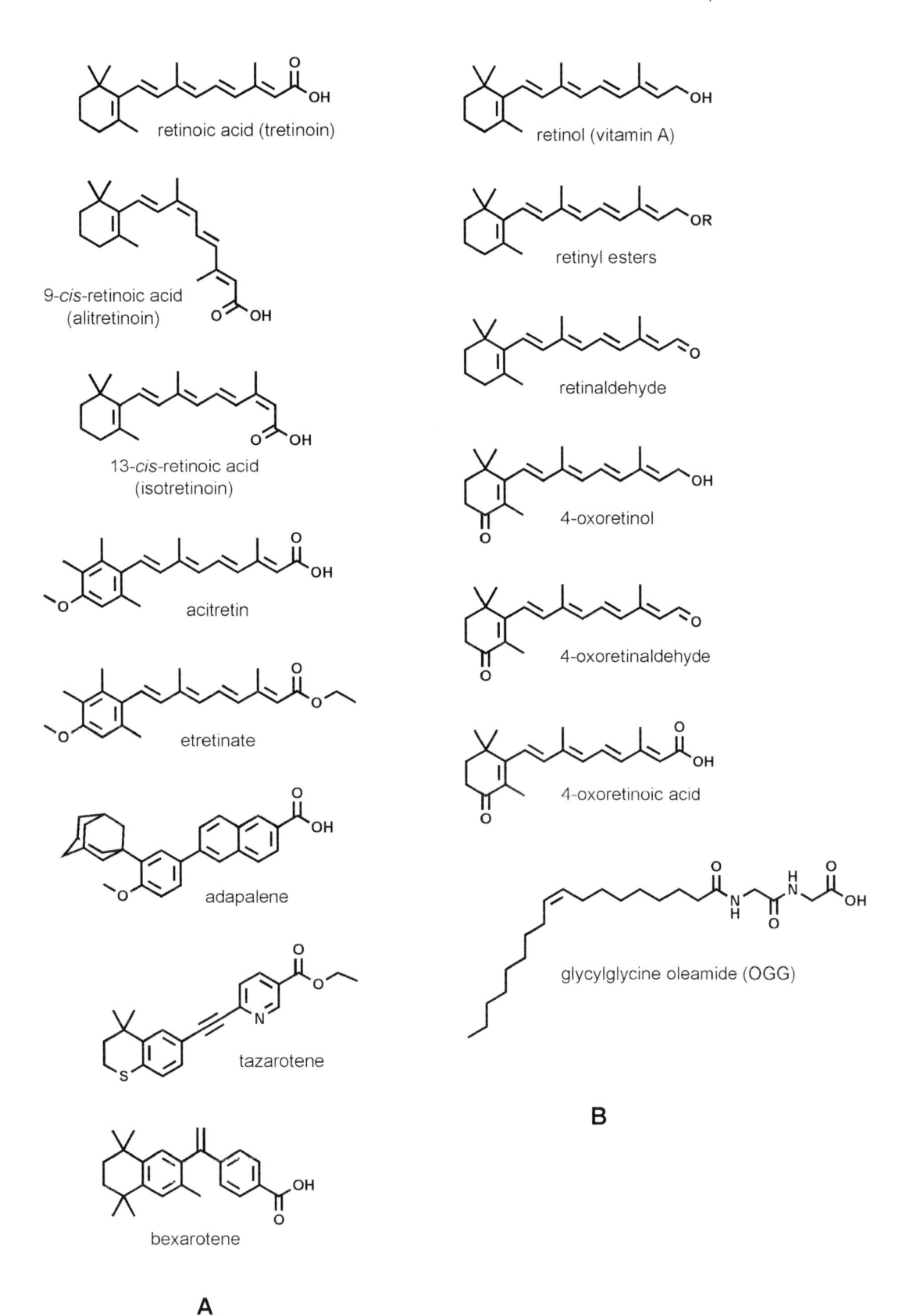

Figure 36.2 Molecular structures. The molecular structures of therapeutic (A) and cosmeceutical (B) retinoids are indicated. Notes: (1) "R" in retinyl esters represents an acyl radical; (2) 4-oxoretinoids are indicated, because they have been shown to have a "soft" retinoid action [11]; however, to our knowledge, they haven't yet been added in topical formulations; (3) OGG is not a retinoid, but, as mentioned in the text, is a potential cosmeceutical retinoid partner.

To validate this *intracrine* concept, the precursor should penetrate easily through the epidermis by topical application and be metabolized into biologically active retinoids, while the latter should be well tolerated and result in biological effects [53-55]. The ranking order of retinoid-like activity following topical application is as follows: retinoic acid > retinaldehyde > retinol >>> retinyl esters; in other words, this corresponds to the metabolic pathways: retinyl esters are hydrolysed to retinol, which is oxidized to retinaldehyde, which is in turn oxidized to retinoic acid. On the other hand, probably for the same reason, the tolerance ranking order is the opposite: retinyl esters > retinol ≥ retinaldehyde >> retinoic acid.

Genomic effects

The genomic effects of topical retinoids are the consequence of the modulation of gene expression following their binding to nuclear RAR or RXR receptors. These effects most probably explain the results obtained in reversing and preventing various hallmarks of skin aging such as the activation of matrix metalloproteinase [56,57], oxidative stress and the degradation of extracellular matrix [58]. In particular, retinoids are known to inhibit keratinocyte differentiation and to stimulate epidermal hyperplasia [11,59,60]. Heparin binding-epidermal growth factor (HB-EGF) activation of keratinocyte ErbB receptors via a RAR-dependent paracrine loop has been proposed to mediate retinoid-induced epidermal hyperplasia [61]. It has been shown that CD44v3, a heparan sulfate-bearing variant of CD44, which is a multifunctional polymorphic proteoglycan and principal cell surface receptor of hyaluronan (HA), recruits active matrix metalloproteinase 7, the precursor of HB-EGF (pro-HB-EGF) and one of its receptors, ErbB4, to form a complex on the surface of murine epithelial cells [62]. We have previously shown that topical application of retinaldehyde increases the expression of CD44 in mouse skin. The increased expression of CD44 accompanying epidermal hyperplasia induced by topical retinaldehyde is associated to an increase in epidermal and dermal HA and with increased expression of the HA synthases 1, 2 and 3 [63]. These observations indicate that the HA system is associated to the HB-EGF paracrine loop, with the transcriptional up-regulation of CD44 and HA synthases. Thus, retinaldehyde-induced *in vitro* and *in vivo* proliferative response of keratinocytes is CD44-dependent and requires HB-EGF, its receptor ErbB1, and matrix metalloproteinases [64].

Non-genomic effects

There is some evidence that retinoids might exert a biological activity independently of their binding to nuclear receptors [11,65], thus confirming the concept of cosmeceutical retinoids. Such indirect effects have been well documented, and clinical manifestations have been observed. In particular, isotretinoin (13-*cis*-retinoic acid), is the only retinoid active at inducing sebaceous gland atrophy, whereas it does not bind itself to nuclear retinoid receptors; for this reason, it is the best therapeutic treatment for severe acne [66,67].

Photobiology of topical retinoids

Owing to their side chain containing multiple double bonds, retinoids strongly absorb UV light, with molar extinction coefficients of ≈52,000 (M^{-1}. cm^{-1}) at wavelengths ranging from 325 nm for retinol to 385 nm for retinaldehyde. This property is crucial in the retina, where photoisomerization of 11-*cis*-retinaldehyde into all-*trans*-retinaldehyde is the first step in the biochemical cascade leading to the generation of nervous influx from the optic nerve to the visual cortex [68-70]. This property also enables retinoids to act as UV filters when applied topically [71]: topical retinoids have been shown to load the skin with supraphysiological epidermal concentrations [5,18,19,72].

For instance, topical retinyl palmitate 2% was as efficient as a commercial sunscreen with a sun protection factor of 20 to prevent UVB-induced erythema and DNA photodamage in the skin of healthy volunteers [73]. In mice, retinoic acid, retinaldehyde, retinol and retinyl palmitate were efficient in preventing UVB-induced apoptosis and DNA photodamage [71]. The similar potencies of these retinoids indicate a physical action mediated by their spectral properties rather than a biological action mediated by the binding to nuclear receptors. This also implies that sun exposure induces significant vitamin A depletion in the epidermis [18], which significance in term of photoaging has not been fully analysed. In particular, hypovitaminosis A is known to induce a follicular hyperkeratosis known as phrynoderma [27], and is a risk factor for cancer development [31,32].

On the other hand, the biological effects of photodegradation of vitamin A and other retinoids are less understood and may be important for sun-exposed tissues, such as the skin. Exposure of retinol or its esters to UV light generates free radicals and reactive oxygen species that can damage a number of cellular targets, including proteins, lipids and DNA [74,75]. The balance between positive, filter-like properties, and possible damage to biomolecules is difficult to assess, and might depend on several factors [76-79]. For this reason, it is still recommended to avoid UV exposure when using topical retinoids.

Antibacterial activity of retinaldehyde

Aldehydes represent a relatively unstable intermediate state of oxidation between alcohols and carboxylic acids [80-83]. Retinaldehyde may thus exert a direct biological activity by reacting non-enzymatically with many biomolecules on skin surface, as well as on bacterial flora, independently of its conversion to retinoic acid and subsequent activation of nuclear receptors [84].

The putative anti-infective property of vitamin A had already been observed in the 1920s, although its mechanism of action was not understood [85]. Retinoic acid has been shown to protect dendritic cells in mice [86] and topical retinaldehyde, owing to its better tolerance profile than retinoic acid, was successfully applied to a long period of time to patients with inflammatory dermatoses [55]. Retinaldehyde has been successfully used against Gram-positive bacteria of the cutaneous flora: two weeks of treatment with topical retinaldehyde 0.05% displayed a significant decrease in counts of viable *Propionibacterium acnes*,

Staphylococcus aureus and *Micrococcus* spp. in healthy volunteers, whereas retinaldehyde showed to be more potent than retinol and retinoic acid when assessing the minimal inhibitory concentration on various bacterial strains [87,88].

Topical cosmeceutical retinoids as antioxidants
Oxidative stress is considered to be the cornerstone of the biochemical pathways leading to both intrinsic (chronological) and extrinsic aging (photoaging) [14,89-93]. The skin, which is exposed to environmental factors and pollutants, possesses an efficient antioxidant system able to counteract the deleterious effects of occasional oxidative stress of moderate magnitude [94,95]; however, in the case of chronic or severe oxidative stress, this endogenous antioxidant network reaches its limit and irremediable tissue damage is unavoidable [93,96-100]. According to the free radical theory of aging, oxidative stress increases with age, whereas during the same time the endogenous antioxidant systems become less efficient [101-104]. It thus seems logical to provide the skin with exogenous antioxidants in order to slow the natural process of skin aging. Although many clinical trials failed to demonstrated a benefit for the use of antioxidants, this concept is still actual when analysing these studies in detail and unveiling the reasons for such a misconception about cosmeceutical antioxidants [105].

Retinoids have been shown to exert a free radical scavenging activity *in vitro* [18,106-110]. This property is most probably due to the conjugated double bond structure of the side chain and their cyclohexenyl or aromatic moiety, rather than their ability to bind nuclear retinoid receptors, indicating that topical cosmeceutical retinoids should be as good candidates as therapeutic ones to prevent or improve skin aging. Because the endogenous antioxidants act together in a functional organized network, when supplying any organ with antioxidants, this concept should be followed; this means that if cosmeceutical retinoids have a role to play in the prevention or improvement of skin aging, they should be considered as partners of other topical antioxidants, rather than as a whole antioxidant system.

In mice, the peroxidation of epidermal lipids induced by topical menadione (vitamin K3) was completely prevented by a pretreatment with either 0.25% topical α-tocopherol (vitamin E, a known efficient endogenous cutaneous antioxidant) or topical retinaldehyde 0.05% [109]. In human, topical retinol 0.075% provided a better protection of the stratum corneum against physical (UV) and chemical (sodium lauryl sulfate) threat than a cream containing α-tocopherol 1.1% [111].

Effects of topical cosmeceutical retinoids on pigmentation
It has been observed for a long time that retinoic acid had a lightening property on human skin, and for this reason it has been used, alone or in combination with hydroquinone, to treat hyperpigmented lesions [112,113]. The mechanism of this effect is not clear: depending on the cell culture model, retinoic acid inhibits tyrosinase activity – the rate-limiting step of melanogenesis – inhibits cell proliferation, decreases the melanin content or has no effect on tyrosinase, melanin content and cell growth; in particular, in monolayer cultures, there is few or no effect with retinoic acid [114–117]. This suggests that the observed *in vivo* depigmenting effect of retinoic acid, and retinoids in general, may be due to the increased rate of epidermis "turnover" rather than to a direct effect on melanin content or melanocyte growth [117,118].

The best depigmenting product containing a retinoid is the formula developed by Kligman and Willis, consisting of 0.1% tretinoin (retinoic acid), 5.0% hydroquinone, and 0.1% dexamethasone, but none of its active ingredients can be used in cosmetic products. Amongst cosmeceutical retinoids, retinaldehyde, the direct precursor of retinoic acid, is well tolerated in human skin and has been shown to have several biologic effects identical to that of retinoic acid [54,55]. In the mouse tail model of depigmentation, topical retinaldehyde 0.05% showed a higher depigmenting effect than retinoic acid 0.05%, indicating that this effect of retinaldehyde was not solely due to its bioconversion to retinoic acid, but also to a retinoid receptor-independent mechanism [118-120]. A clinical trial in which retinol 10% and lactic acid 7% replaced tretinoin 0.1% and dexamethasone 0.1% in the formula of Kligman and Willis was successfully applied to patients with hyperpigmented lesions on the face. This new formula was shown to be comparable to that of Kligman and Willis, with the advantage of preventing the steroid-induced skin atrophy [121].

Retinyl esters, in particular retinyl palmitate, are widely used in cosmetics. According to the pro-ligand concept discussed above, in order to exert a retinoid-like activity, retinyl esters have first to be hydrolysed to retinol, and then oxidized to retinoic acid, a process being less effective compared to retinol and retinaldehyde, since it requires the activation of the hydrolysing enzymes acyl:retinol acyltransferase (ARAT) and lecithin:retinol acyl transferase (LRAT) [49,52,122,123]. If a non-genomic effect is expected, the total retinoid content of the skin would be determinant. However, very few studies aimed at assessing the penetration of retinyl esters through human skin have been reported. In hairless mice, we found that topical retinol 0.05% and retinyl palmitate 0.05% loaded the epidermis with similar amounts of epidermal retinoids, i.e. a ten-fold increase compared to vehicle [71]. Thus, retinyl esters seem to deliver the skin with similar amounts of retinoids and have less genomic effects than retinol, suggesting that they should have similar depigmenting properties to retinol.

Hyaluronan as a partner for cosmeceutical retinoids

Hyaluronan (HA) is the major component of the extracellular matrix and is found in high quantities in the skin. HA is a high molecular weight non-sulfated linear glycosaminoglycan composed of repeating units of D-glucuronic acid and N-acetyl-D-glucosamine linked together via alternating β-1,4 and β-1,3 glycosidic bonds. HA chains can have as much as 25,000 disaccharide repeats, corresponding to a molecular mass of ≈8 MDa. In normal skin, HA is synthesized essentially by dermal fibroblasts and epidermal keratinocytes. Due to its negatively charged residues, HA can accommodate many water molecules, which help to maintain the normal hydration and viscoelasticity of the skin [124–126].

With increasing lifespan, the chronic cutaneous insufficiency syndrome now called *dermatoporosis* is becoming an emerging clinical problem with significant morbidity, which sometimes results in prolonged hospital stays [44,45,127]. Dermatoporosis is principally due to chronological aging and long-term and unprotected sun exposure, but it may also result from the chronic use of topical and systemic corticosteroids. Experimental evidence suggests that defective function of CD44, a transmembrane glycoprotein that acts as the main cell surface HA receptor, and the corresponding impaired HA metabolism, are implicated in the pathogenesis of dermatoporosis, and may be a target for intervention [128]. Cleavage of the high molecular weight HA polymer during tissue remodelling gives rise to lower molecular weight fragments that elicit a variety of CD44-mediated cellular responses, including proliferation, migration, HA synthesis, and cytokine synthesis [125,126]. The cellular responses elicited by topical application of HA, and specifically HA synthesis by keratinocytes, depend on the size of the HA oligosaccharides [129–131].

Topical retinoids are known to stimulate epidermal hyperplasia through the activation of a RAR-dependent HB-EGF paracrine loop [61,132]. HA production is also selectively stimulated by retinoids in mouse and human skin [133,134]. In mouse skin, topical retinaldehyde increases HA content, the expression of CD44 and HA synthases [63], and prevents UV-induced depletion of HA and CD44, an effect also observed with topical retinol and retinoic acid, although to a lesser extent [135]. In humans, topical retinaldehyde has been shown to restore the epidermal thickness and CD44 expression in lichen sclerosus and atrophic lesions [136]. The proliferative response of keratinocytes elicited by either retinaldehyde or intermediate size HA fragments (HAFi) is dependent of CD44 and requires the presence of HB-EGF, its receptor erbB1, as well as matrix metalloproteinase-7 (MMP-7) [64,137,138]. In particular, topical application of HAFi in combination with retinaldehyde caused epidermal hyperplasia by specifically stimulating the CD44 platform molecules in the keratinocytes and increased the HA content of epidermis and dermis [138,139]. Thus topical retinoids, in particular retinaldehyde, can restore epidermal functions by stimulating HA synthesis and biological functions.

Specific profiles of cosmeceutical retinoids

Retinaldehyde

Retinaldehyde is much less irritant than retinoic acid, which explains its good compliance, and has been shown to be well tolerated and effective in treating photoaging on long periods of time: in particular, retinaldehyde produced significant improvement in fine and deep wrinkles [140]. Retinaldehyde does not bind to nuclear retinoid receptors and selectively delivers low concentrations of retinoic acid at the cellular level [54,132]; this prevents an excess of retinoic acid in the skin, a condition that contributes to cutaneous irritation [5,47] and confers to retinaldehyde the required properties for the intracrine concept discussed above [18,47]. The association of retinaldehyde and δ-tocopheryl-gluco-pyranoside, a vitamin E-like precursor, improved the protection against the generation of free radicals – a condition leading to aging – as well as the skin elasticity [141]. Retinaldehyde, which possesses an aldehyde functional group, exerts direct receptor-independent biological actions not shared by other retinoids. This explains the usefulness of topical retinaldehyde 0.05% against *P. acnes* and *Staphylococcus* spp. [87,88]. As discussed above, retinaldehyde shares with other retinoids a high absorption power in the UVA range, and may decrease the fluence received in this window significantly [71]. As compared to other retinoids, retinaldehyde loads the skin with natural retinoids very efficiently, probably due to its better penetration profile through the skin, and its ability to be reduced to retinol or oxidized to retinoic acid very rapidly [142–146]. Retinaldehyde has been shown to reduce the pigmentation when applied to the skin for a couple of weeks or longer; this could be due in part to a melanosomal dilution resulting from an increase of epidermal turnover, an effect attributable to its conversion to retinoic acid. The depigmenting property of retinaldehyde could also be due to its antioxidant power, since the production of small quantities of hydrogen peroxide has been considered to be an essential step of the melanogenesis [147]. Indeed, topical retinaldehyde 0.05% decreases the melanin content by 80% and the density of active melanocytes by 75% in mouse tail skin, whereas an application of retinaldehyde 0.01% to guinea pig ear skin decreases epidermal melanin by 50% and the density of active melanocytes by 40% [118]. Owing to these properties, retinaldehyde should be considered as a key partner in topical depigmenting preparations. For instance retinaldehyde, combined to the tyrosinase inhibitor 4-(1-phenylethyl)-resorcinol and the antioxidant precursor δ-tocopherylglucopyranoside, was shown to have a good depigmentation and tolerance profile in murine melanocytes and in a three-dimensional human reconstructed epidermis [148].

Retinol and retinyl esters

Retinol and retinyl esters (mostly retinyl palmitate) have been incorporated into many skin products. Theoretically, these topical endogenous retinoids, which are natural precursors of cutaneous retinaldehyde and retinoic acids [142,149,150], could also be useful in treating skin conditions for which retinoic acid is active. However, although retinol is widely used in cosmetic formulations to improve photoaging, topical retinol has not been demonstrated to be effective to treat any skin condition, maybe because of its slow oxidation into retinaldehyde and retinoic acid [151]. It seems that the retinol concentrations required to induce a measurable biological action similar to that of retinoic acid (0.05%) induce a similar irritant dermatitis [121]. Thus, to avoid high concentrations of retinol or retinyl esters in topical formulation, the best way would be to combine them at moderate concentrations with other topical agents such as tocopherols, ascorbate and derivatives, flavonoids or other biological antioxidants [152-154]. Another useful property of retinol is its absorption spectrum: it absorbs UV light in shorter wavelengths (325 nm) than retinaldehyde (385 nm) and retinoic acid (345 nm). Therefore, topical retinol could be useful as a filter partner of many cosmetic and cosmeceutical products in the most biologically active solar UV range (290–320 nm), while delivering small amounts of retinoic acid on a relatively long period of time [71,73]. This can be expanded to retinyl esters, which have the same UV spectrum as retinol, have the better tolerance profile among topical retinoids, while being the weaker retinoic acid precursors [49].

Associations

Association with hyaluronan fragments

The molecular mechanisms underlying retinoid-induced epidermal hyperplasia are closely related to CD44-dependent pathways in keratinocytes. It is well demonstrated that retinoids synergize with the activities of hyaluronate fragments of defined size (HAFi) on cell renewal and *de novo* hyaluronate synthesis [63,138,139,155]. Accordingly, the topical application of HAFi was found to have repairing action in dermatoporosis [137]. Therefore the combination of HAFi with a retinoid is highly promising as preventive treatment in early phases of dermatoporosis.

High molecular weight HA, that does not show the topical activities of HAFi, has been widely used in cosmetic preparations [156]. Application of high molecular weight HA-containing cosmetic products to the skin is reported to moisturize and restore elasticity [157]. HA-based cosmetic formulations or sunscreens may also be capable of protecting the skin against ultraviolet irradiation due to the antioxidant properties of HA [158]. In almost all of these cosmetic formulations, the HA is associated with retinol. Scientific proof that the association of any topical retinoids with high molecular weight HA has some specific synergizing effect is currently lacking.

Association with glycylglycine oleamide

Glycylglycine oleamide (OGG, Figure 36.2B) is a small amphiphilic molecule designed to protect the connective tissue of the skin from glycation and elastosis [159]. Its ability to potentiate the esterification of retinol by retinaldehyde might make OGG a new retinoid partner in cosmeceutical formulations aimed at preventing cutaneous hypovitaminosis A [18]. In particular, a lotion containing 0.1% retinaldehyde, 0.1% OGG and 0.05% δ-tocopherylglucopyranoside improved the antioxidant capacity and decreased the lipoperoxidation in a clinical trial (manuscript in preparation).

Summary

The novelty in retinoid cosmeceutics clearly consists in the association of a retinoid with middle-size HA fragments, tyrosinase inhibitors or antioxidant precursors. Such an association seems to act synergistically to stimulate the targets of the retinoid partners, while optimizing the tolerance profile due to a decreased retinoid concentration in combined formulations. Current laboratory and clinical data indicate that retinaldehyde is the retinoid of choice for this association.

References

1. Castenmiller JJM, West CE. (1998) Bioavailability and bioconversion of carotenoids. *Annu Rev Nutr* **18**,19–36.
2. Vogel S, Gamble MV, Blaner WS. (1999) Biosynthesis, absorptiom, metabolism and transport of retinoids. In: Nau H, Blaner WS, eds. *Retinoids The biochemical and molecular basis of vitamin A and retinoid action*. Berlin: Springer.
3. Roos TC, Jugert FK, Merk HF, Bickers DR. (1998) Retinoid metabolism in the skin. *Pharmacol Rev* **50**, 315–33.
4. Sorg O, Antille C, Kaya G, Saurat JH. (2006) Retinoids in cosmeceuticals. *Dermatol Ther* **19**, 289–96.
5. Saurat JH, Sorg O, Didierjean J. (1999) New concepts for delivery of topical retinoid activity to human skin. In: NauH, BlanerWS, eds. *Retinoids The Biochemical and Molecular Basis of Vitamin A and Retinoid Action*. Berlin: Springer-Verlag, pp. 521–36.
6. Sass JO, Forster A, Bock KW, Nau H. (1994) Glucuronidation and isomerization of all-trans- and 13-cis-retinoic acid by liver microsomes of phenobarbital- or 3-methylcholanthrene-treated rats. *Biochem Pharmacol* **47**, 485–92.
7. Taimi M, Helvig C, Wisniewski J, et al. (2004) A novel human cytochrome P450, CYP26C1, involved in metabolism of 9-cis and all-trans isomers of retinoic acid. *J Biol Chem* **279**, 77–85.
8. Achkar CC, Derguini F, Blumberg B, Langston A, Levin AA, Speck J, et al. (1996) 4-Oxoretinol, a new natural ligand and transactivator of the retinoic acid receptors. *Proc Natl Acad Sci USA* **93**, 4879–84.
9. Blumberg B, Bolado J, Jr., Derguini F, Craig AG, Moreno TA, Chakravarti D, et al. (1996) Novel retinoic acid receptor ligands in Xenopus embryos. *Proc Natl Acad Sci USA* **93**, 4873–8.
10. Ross SA, De Luca LM. (1996) A new metabolite of retinol: all-trans-4-oxo-retinol as a receptor activator and differentiation agent. *Nutr Rev* **54**, 355–6.
11. Sorg O, Tran C, Carraux P, Grand D, Barraclough C, Arrighi JF, et al. (2008) Metabolism and biological activities of topical 4-oxoretinoids in mouse skin. *J Invest Dermatol* **128**, 999–1008.
12. Fisher GJ, Voorhees JJ. (1996) Molecular mechanisms of retinoid actions in skin. *FASEB J* **10**, 1002–13.
13. Napoli JL. (1996) Retinoic acid biosynthesis and metabolism. *FASEB J* **10**, 993–1001.
14. Sorg O, Antille C, Saurat JH. (2004) Retinoids, other topical vitamins, and antioxidants. In: RigelDS, WeissRS, LimHW, DoverJS, eds. *Photoaging*. New York: Marcel Dekker, pp. 89–115.
15. Dawson MI. (2004)Synthetic retinoids and their nuclear receptors. *Curr Med Chem Anticancer Agents* **4**, 199–230.
16. Sorg O, Kuenzli S, Saurat JH. (2007) Side effects and pitfalls in retinoid therapy. In: VahlquistA, DuvicM, eds. *Retinoids and Carotenoids in Dermatology*. New York: Informa Healthcare, pp. 225–48.
17. Kuenzli S, Saurat JH, Retinoids. (2003) In: Bolognia JL, Jorizzo JL, Rapini RP, eds. *Dermatology*. London: Mosby, Chapter 127, pp. 1991–2006.

18. Sorg O, Saurat JH. (2014) Topical retinoids in skin aging: A focused update with reference to sun induced epidermal vitamin A deficiency. *Dermatology* (in press).
19. Duester G. (2000) Families of retinoid dehydrogenases regulating vitamin A function: production of visual pigment and retinoic acid. *Eur J Biochem* **267**, 4315–24.
20. Jurukovski V, Simon M. (2000) Epidermal growth factor signaling pathway influences retinoid metabolism by reduction of retinyl ester hydrolase activities in normal and malignant keratinocytes. *J Cell Physiol* **183**, 265–72.
21. Kurlandsky SB, Xiao JH, Duell EA, et al. (1994) Biological activity of all-trans retinol requires metabolic conversion to all-trans retinoic acid and is mediated through activation of nuclear retinoid receptors in human keratinocytes. *J Biol Chem* **269**, 32821–7.
22. Johnson KA, Bernard MA, Funderburg K. (2002) Vitamin nutrition in older adults. *Clin Geriatr Med* **18**, 773–99.
23. Miller SJ. Nutritional deficiency and the skin. (1989) *J Am Acad Dermatol* **21**, 1–30.
24. Andersson E, Rosdahl I, Törmä H, Vahlquist A. (1999) Ultraviolet irradiation depletes cellular retinol and alters the metabolism of retinoic acid in cultured human keratinocytes and melanocytes. *Melanoma Res* **9**, 339–46.
25. Ihara H, Hashizume N, Hirase N, Suzue R. (1999) Esterification makes retinol more labile to photolysis. *J Nutr Sci Vitaminol (Tokyo)* **45**, 353–8.
26. Torras H. (1996) Retinoids in aging. *Clin Dermatol* **14**, 207–15.
27. Maronn M, Allen DM, Esterly NB. (2005) Phrynoderma: a manifestation of vitamin A deficiency?… The rest of the story. *Pediatr Dermatol* **22**, 60–3.
28. Levine N. (1998) Role of retinoids in skin cancer treatment and prevention. *J Am Acad Dermatol* **39**, S62–S6.
29. Marks R. (1991) *Retinoids in Cutaneous Malignancy*. Oxford: Blackwell Scientific.
30. Moon TE, Levine N, Cartmel B, Bangert JL. (1997) Retinoids in prevention of skin cancer. *Cancer Lett* 19;**114**, 203–5.
31. Einspahr JG, Bowden GT, Alberts DS. (2003) Skin cancer chemoprevention: strategies to save our skin. *Recent Results Cancer Res* **163**, 151–64; discussion 264–6.
32. Fields AL, Soprano DR, Soprano KJ. (2007) Retinoids in biological control and cancer. *J Cell Biochem* **102**, 886–98.
33. Mrass P, Rendl M, Mildner M, et al. (2004) Retinoic acid increases the expression of p53 and proapoptotic caspases and sensitizes keratinocytes to apoptosis: a possible explanation for tumor preventive action of retinoids. *Cancer Res* **64**, 6542–8.
34. Darwiche N, Bazzi H, El-Touni L, Abou-Lteif G, Doueiri R, Hatoum A, et al. (2005) Regulation of ultraviolet B radiation-mediated activation of AP1 signaling by retinoids in primary keratinocytes. *Radiat Res* **163**, 296–306.
35. Fanjul A, Dawson MI, Hobbs PD, et al. (1994) A new class of retinoids with selective inhibition of AP-1 inhibits proliferation. *Nature* **372**, 107–11.
36. Bayon Y, Ortiz MA, Lopez-Hernandez FJ, et al. (2003) Inhibition of IkappaB kinase by a new class of retinoid-related anticancer agents that induce apoptosis. *Mol Cell Biol* **23**, 1061–74.
37. Na SY, Kang BY, Chung SW, et al. (1999) Retinoids inhibit interleukin-12 production in macrophages through physical associations of retinoid X receptor and NFkappaB. *J Biol Chem* **274**, 7674–80.
38. Camacho LH. (2003) Clinical applications of retinoids in cancer medicine. *J Biol Regul Homeost Agents* **17**, 98–114.
39. Carr DR, Trevino JJ, Donnelly HB. (2011) Retinoids for chemoprophylaxis of nonmelanoma skin cancer. *Dermatol Surg* **37**, 129–45.
40. Ralhan R, Kaur J. (2003) Retinoids as chemopreventive agents. *J Biol Regul Homeost Agents* **17**, 66–91.
41. Saurat JH. (2001) Skin, sun, and vitamin A: from aging to cancer. *J Dermatol* **28**, 595–8.
42. So PL, Lee K, Hebert J, et al. (2004) Topical tazarotene chemoprevention reduces Basal cell carcinoma number and size in Ptch1+/− mice exposed to ultraviolet or ionizing radiation. *Cancer Res* **64**, 4385–9.
43. Zusi FC, Lorenzi MV, Vivat-Hannah V. (2002) Selective retinoids and rexinoids in cancer therapy and chemoprevention. *Drug Discov Today* **7**, 1165–74.
44. Kaya G, Saurat JH. (2007) Dermatoporosis: a chronic cutaneous insufficiency/fragility syndrome. Clinicopathological features, mechanisms, prevention and potential treatments. *Dermatology* **215**, 284–94.
45. Saurat JH. Dermatoporosis. (2007) The functional side of skin aging. *Dermatology* **215**, 271–2.
46. Stratigos AJ, Katsambas AD. (2005) The role of topical retinoids in the treatment of photoaging. *Drugs* **65**, 1061–172.
47. Saurat JH, Sorg O. (1999) Topical natural retinoids. The "Pro-lig-and-non-ligand" concept. *Dermatology* **199**, 1–2.
48. Duell EA, Derguini F, Kang S, et al. (1996) Extraction of human epidermis treated with retinol yields retro-retinoids in addition to free retinol and retinyl esters. *J Invest Dermatol* **107**, 178–82.
49. Duell EA, Kang S, Voorhees JJ. (1997) Unoccluded retinol penetrates human skin in vivo more effectively than unoccluded retinyl palmitate or retinoic acid. *J Invest Dermatol* **109**, 301–5.
50. Schaefer H. (1993) Penetration and percutaneous absorption of topical retinoids. *Skin Pharmacol* **6**, 17–23.
51. Tran C, Kasraee B, Grand D, et al. (2005) Pharmacology of RALGA, a mixture of retinaldehyde and glycolic acid. *Dermatology* **210**, 6–13.
52. Tran C, Sorg O, Carraux P, et al. (2001) Topical delivery of retinoids counteracts the UVB-induced epidermal vitamin A depletion in hairless mouse. *Photochem Photobiol* **73**, 425–31.
53. Didierjean L, Sass JO, Carraux P, et al. (1999) Topical 9-*cis*-retinaldehyde for delivery of 9-*cis*-retinoic acid in mouse skin. *Exp Dermatol* **8**,199–203.
54. Didierjean L, Tran C, Sorg O, Saurat JH. (1999) Biological activities of topical natural retinaldehyde. *Dermatology* **199**,19–24.
55. Saurat JH, Didierjean L, Masgrau E, et al. (1994) Topical retinaldehyde on human skin : biological effects and tolerance. *J Invest Dermato* **103**, 770–4.
56. Fisher GJ, Datta SC, Talwar HS, et al. (1996) Molecular basis of sun-induced premature skin aging and retinoid antagonism. *Nature* **379**, 335–9.
57. Fisher GJ, Wang ZQ, Datta SC, et al. (1997) Pathophysiology of premature skin aging induced by ultraviolet light. *N Engl J Med* **337**,1419–28.
58. Griffiths CE, Russman AN, Majmudar G, et al. (1993) Restoration of collagen formation in photodamaged human skin by tretinoin (retinoic acid). *N Engl J Med* **329**, 530–5.
59. Ponec M, Weerheim A, Havekes L, Boonstra J. (1987) Effects of retinoids on differentiation, lipid metabolism, epidermal growth factor, and Low-density lipoprotein binding in squamous carcinoma cells. *Exp Cell Res* **171**, 426–35.

60 Saurat JH. How do retinoids work on human epidermis? A breakthrough and its implications. (1988) *Clin Exp Dermatol* **13**, 350–64.
61 Xiao JH, Feng X, Di W, *et al.* (1999) Identification of heparin-binding EGF-like growth factor as a target in intercellular regulation of epidermal basal cell growth by suprabasal retinoic acid receptors. *EMBO J* **18**,1539–48.
62 Yu WH, Woessner JF, Jr., McNeish JD, Stamenkovic I. (2002) CD44 anchors the assembly of matrilysin/MMP-7 with heparin-binding epidermal growth factor precursor and ErbB4 and regulates female reproductive organ remodeling. *Genes Dev* **16**, 307–23.
63 Kaya G, Grand D, Hotz R, *et al.* (2005) Upregulation of CD44 and hyaluronate synthase by topical retinoids in mouse skin. *J Invest Dermatol* **124**, 284–7.
64 Kaya G, Tran C, Sorg O, *et al.* (2005) Retinaldehyde-induced epidermal hyperplasia via heparin binding epidermal growth factor is CD44-dependent. *J Invest Dermatol* **124**, A32.
65 Clifford JL, Menter DG, Wang M, *et al.* (1999) Retinoid receptor-dependent and -independent effects of N-(4-hydroxyphenyl)retinamide in F9 embryonal carcinoma cells. *Cancer Res* **59**, 14–8.
66 Layton A. (2009) The use of isotretinoin in acne. *Dermatoendocrinol* **1**, 162–9.
67 Wiegand UW, Chou RC. (1998) Pharmacokinetics of oral isotretinoin. *J Am Acad Dermatol* **39**, S8–S12.
68 Nakanishi K. (2000) Recent bioorganic studies on rhodopsin and visual transduction. *Chem Pharm Bull (Tokyo)* **48**, 1399–409.
69 Blomhoff R, Blomhoff HK. (2006) Overview of retinoid metabolism and function. *J Neurobiol* **66**, 606–630.
70 Schoenlein RW, Peteanu LA, Mathies RA, Shank CV. (1991) The first step in vision: femtosecond isomerization of rhodopsin. *Science* **254**, 412–5.
71 Sorg O, Tran C, Carraux P, *et al.* (2005) Spectral properties of topical retinoids prevent DNA damage and apoptosis after acute UVB exposure in hairless mice. *Photochem Photobio* **81**, 830–6.
72 Kang S, Duell EA, Fisher GJ, *et al.* (1995) Application of retinol to human skin in vivo induces epidermal hyperplasia and cellular retinoid binding proteins characteristics of retinoic acid but without measurable retinoic acid levels or irritation. *J Invest Dermatol* **105**:549–56.
73 Antille C, Tran C, Sorg O, *et al.* (2003) Vitamin A exerts a photoprotective action in skin by absorbing UVB radiations. *J Invest Dermatol* **121**(5):1163–7.
74 Dillon J, Gaillard ER, Bilski P, *et al.* (1996) The photochemistry of the retinoids as studied by steady-state and pulsed methods. *Photochem Photobiol* **63**:680–5.
75 Fu PP, Xia Q, Yin JJ, *et al.* (2007) Photodecomposition of Vitamin A and Photobiological Implications for the Skin. *Photochem Photobiol* **83**, 409–24.
76 Ferguson J, Johnson BE. (1989) Retinoid associated phototoxicity and photosensitivity. *Pharmacol Ther* **40**, 123–35.
77 Fu PP, Cheng SH, Coop L, *et al.* (2003) Photoreaction, Phototoxicity, and Photocarcinogenicity of Retinoids. *J Environ Sci Health Part C Environ Carcinog Ecotoxicol Rev* **21**, 165–97.
78 Kligman LH. (1987) Retinoic acid and photocarcinogenesis. A controversy. *Photodermatol* **4**, 88–101.
79 Fisher D, Lichti FU, Lucy JA. (1972) Environmental effects on the autoxidation of retinol. *Biochem J* **130**, 259–70.
80 Becker TW, Krieger G, Witte I. (1996) DNA single and double strand breaks induced by aliphatic and aromatic aldehydes in combination with copper(II). *Free Radic Res* **24**, 325–32.
81 Witz G. (1989) Biological interactions of alpha,beta-unsaturated aldehydes. *Free Radic Biol Med* **7**, 333–49.
82 Esterbauer H, Schaur RJ, Zollner H. (1991) Chemistry and biochemistry of 4-hydroxynonenal, malonaldehyde and related aldehydes. *Free Radic Biol Med* **11**, 81–128.
83 Feron VJ, Til HP, de Vrijer F, *et al.* (1991) Aldehydes: occurrence, carcinogenic potential, mechanism of action and risk assessment. *Mutat Res* **259**, 363–85.
84 Ambroziak W, Izaguirre G, Pietruszko R. (1999) Metabolism of retinaldehyde and other aldehydes in soluble extracts of human liver and kidney. *J Biol Chem* **274**, 33366–73.
85 Green HN, Mellanby E. (1928) Vitamin A as an anti-infective agent. *Br Med J* **II**, 691–6.
86 Halliday GM, Ho KKL, Barnetson RSC. (1992) Regulation of the skin immune system by retinoids during carcinogenesis. *J Invest Dermatol* **99**, 83S–6S.
87 Péchère M, Germanier L, Siegenthaler G, *et al.* (2002) The antibacterial activity of topical retinoids: the case of retinaldehyde. *Dermatology* **205**, 153–8.
88 Péchère M, Pechere JC, Siegenthaler G, *et al.* (1999) Antibacterial activity of retinaldehyde against *Propionibacterium acnes*. *Dermatology* **199**, 29–31.
89 Wenk J, Brenneisen P, Meewes C, *et al.* (2001) UV-induced oxidative stress and photoaging. *Curr Probl Dermatol* **29**, 83–94.
90 Yaar M, Gilchrest BA. (1998) Aging versus photoaging: postulated mechanisms and effectors. *J Investig Dermatol Symp Proc* **3**, 47–51.
91 Pinnell SR. (2003) Cutaneous photodamage, oxidative stress, and topical antioxidant protection. *J Am Acad Dermatol* **48**, 1–19; quiz 20–2.
92 Nishigori C, Hattori Y, Arima Y, Miyachi Y. (2003) Photoaging and oxidative stress. *Exp Dermatol* **12**, 18–21.
93 Sorg O, Kaya G. (2007) Oxidative stress in human pathology. *Adv Gene Mol Cell Ther* **1**, 56–67.
94 Sies H, Stahl W. (2004) Nutritional protection against skin damage from sunlight. *Annu Rev Nutr* **24**, 173–200.
95 Thiele JJ, Schroeter C, Hsieh SN, *et al.* (2001) The antioxidant network of the stratum corneum. *Curr Probl Dermatol* **29**, 26–42.
96 Halliwell B. (1994) Free radicals and antioxidants : a personal view. *Nutr Rev* **52**, 253–65.
97 Jacob RA, Burri BJ. (1996) Oxidative damage and defense. *Am J Clin Nutr* **63**, 985S–90S.
98 Kohen R, Gati I. (2000) Skin low molecular weight antioxidants and their role in aging and in oxidative stress. *Toxicology* **148**, 149–57.
99 Sorg O. Oxidative stress : a theoretical model or a biological reality? (2004) *CR Biol.* [review] **327**, 649–62.
100 Halliwell B, Gutteridge JMC. (1999) *Free Radicals in Biology and Medicine*, 3th edn. HalliwellB, GutteridgeJMC, eds. Oxford: Oxford University Press.
101 Berr C. (2000) Cognitive impairment and oxidative stress in the elderly: results of epidemiological studies. *Biofactors* **13**, 205–9.
102 Barja G. (2004) Free radicals and aging. *Trends Neurosci* **27**, 595–600.
103 Harman D. (2001) Aging: overview. *Ann NY Acad Sci* **928**, 1–21.
104 Crastes de Paulet A. (1990) [Free radicals and aging]. *Ann Biol Clin* **48**, 323–30.
105 Bast A, Haenen GR. (2013) Ten misconceptions about antioxidants. *Trends Pharmacol Sci* **34**, 430–6.
106 Singh DK, Lippman SM. (1998) Cancer chemoprevention. Part 1: Retinoids and carotenoids and other classic antioxidants. *Oncology (Williston Park)* **12**, 1643–53, 57–58; discussion 59–60.

107 Tsuchiya M, Scita G, Freisleben HJ, et al. (1992) Antioxidant radical-scavenging activity of carotenoids and retinoids compared to alpha-tocopherol. *Methods Enzymol* **213**, 460–72.

108 Tesoriere L, D'Arpa D, Re R, Livrea MA. (1997) Antioxidant reactions of all-*trans* retinol in phospholipid bilayers: effect of oxygen partial pressure, radical fluxes, and retinol concentration. *Arch Biochem Biophys* **343**, 13–8.

109 Sorg O, Tran C, Saurat JH. (2001) Cutaneous vitamins A and E in the context of ultraviolet- or chemically-induced oxidative stress. *Skin Pharmacol Appl Skin Physiol* **14**, 363–72.

110 Sorg O, Kuenzli S, Kaya G, Saurat JH. (2005) Proposed mechanisms of action for retinoid derivatives in the treatment of skin aging. *J Cosm Dermatol* **4**, 237–44.

111 Goffin V, Henry F, Piérard-Franchimont C, Piérard GE. (1997) Topical retinol and the stratum corneum response to an environmental threat. *Skin Pharmacol* **10**, 85–9.

112 Kligman AM, Willis I. (1975) A new formula for depigmenting human skin. *Arch Dermatol* **111**, 40–8.

113 Griffiths CE, Finkel LJ, Ditre CM, et al. (1993) Topical tretinoin (retinoic acid) improves melasma. A vehicle-controlled, clinical trial. *Br J Dermatol* **129**, 415–21.

114 Hoal E, Wilson EL, Dowdle EB. (1982) Variable effects of retinoids on two pigmenting human melanoma cell lines. *Cancer Res* **42**, 5191–5.

115 Edward M, Gold JA, MacKie RM. (1988) Different susceptibilities of melanoma cells to retinoic acid-induced changes in melanotic expression. *Biochem Biophys Res Commun* **155**, 773–8.

116 Fligiel SE, Inman DR, Talwar HS, et al. (1992) Modulation of growth in normal and malignant melanocytic cells by all-trans retinoic acid. *J Cutan Pathol* **19**, 27–33.

117 Yoshimura K, Tsukamoto K, Okazaki M, et al. (2001) Effects of all-trans retinoic acid on melanogenesis in pigmented skin equivalents and monolayer culture of melanocytes. *J Dermatol Sci* **27**, S68–S75.

118 Sorg O, Kasraee B, Salomon D, Saurat JH. (2013) The Potential Depigmenting Activity of Retinaldehyde. *Dermatology* **227**, 231–7.

119 Kasraee B, Tran C, Sorg O, Saurat JH. (2005) The depigmenting effect of RALGA in C57BL/6 mice. *Dermatology* **210**, 30–4.

120 Ortonne JP. (2006) Retinoid therapy of pigmentary disorders. *Dermatol Ther* **19**, 280–8.

121 Yoshimura K, Momosawa A, Aiba E, et al. (2003) Clinical trial of bleaching treatment with 10% all-trans retinol gel. *Dermatol Surg* **29**, 155–60.

122 Kurlandsky SB, Duell EA, Kang S, et al. (1996) Auto-regulation of retinoic acid biosynthesis through regulation of retinol esterification in human keratinocytes. *J Biol Chem* **271**, 15346–52.

123 Ross AC. (2003) Retinoid production and catabolism: role of diet in regulating retinol esterification and retinoic acid oxidation. *J Nutr* **133**, 291S–6S.

124 Fraser JR, Laurent TC. (1989) Turnover and metabolism of hyaluronan. *Ciba Found Symp* **143**, 41–59.

125 Laurent TC. (1987) Biochemistry of hyaluronan. *Acta Otolaryngol Suppl* **442**, 7–24.

126 Laurent TC, Fraser JR. (1992) Hyaluronan. *FASEB J* **6**, 2397–404.

127 Kaya G, Jacobs F, Prins C, et al. (2008) Deep dissecting hematoma: an emerging severe complication of dermatoporosis. *Arch Dermatol* **144**, 1303–8.

128 Kaya G, Rodriguez I, Jorcano JL, et al. (1997) Selective suppression of CD44 in keratinocytes of mice bearing an antisense CD44 transgene driven by a tissue-specific promoter disrupts hyaluronate metabolism in the skin and impairs keratinocyte proliferation. *Genes Dev* **11**, 996–1007.

129 Forrester JV, Balazs EA. (1980) Inhibition of phagocytosis by high molecular weight hyaluronate. *Immunology* **40**, 435–46.

130 West DC, Hampson IN, Arnold F, Kumar S. (1985) Angiogenesis induced by degradation products of hyaluronic acid. *Science* **228**, 1324–6.

131 Wiest L, Kerscher M. (2008) Native hyaluronic acid in dermatology–results of an expert meeting. *J Dtsch Dermatol Ges* **6**, 176–80.

132 Didierjean L, Carraux P, Grand D, et al. (1996) Topical retinaldehyde increases skin content of retinoic acid and exerts biological activity in mouse skin. *J Invest Dermatol* **107**, 714–9.

133 Margelin D, Medaisko C, Lombard D, et al. (1996) Hyaluronic acid and dermatan sulfate are selectively stimulated by retinoic acid in irradiated and nonirradiated hairless mouse skin. *J Invest Dermatol* **106**, 505–9.

134 Tammi R, Ripellino JA, Margolis RU, et al. (1989) Hyaluronate accumulation in human epidermis treated with retinoic acid in skin organ culture. *J Invest Dermatol* **92**, 326–32.

135 Calikoglu E, Sorg O, Tran C, et al. (2006) UVA and UVB decrease the expression of CD44 and hyaluronate in mouse epidermis which is counteracted by topical retinoids. *Photochem Photobiol* **82**, 1342–7.

136 Kaya G, Saurat JH. (2005) Restored epidermal CD44 expression in lichen sclerosus et atrophicus and clinical improvement with topical application of retinaldehyde. *Br J Dermatol* **152**, 570–2.

137 Kaya G, Tran C, Sorg O, et al. (2006) Hyaluronate fragments reverse skin atrophy by a CD44-dependent mechanism. *PLoS Med* **3**, e493.

138 Barnes L, Tran C, Sorg O, et al. (2010) Synergistic effect of hyaluronate fragments in retinaldehyde-induced skin hyperplasia which is a CD44-dependent phenomenon. *PLoS One* **5**, e14372.

139 Kaya G, Tran C, Sorg O, et al. (2006) Synergistic effect of retinaldehyde and hyaluronate fragments in skin hyperplasia. *J Invest Dermatol* **126**, 33.

140 Creidi P, Vienne MP, Ochonisky S, et al. (1998) Profilometric evaluation of photodamage after topical retinaldehyde and retinoic acid treatment. *J Am Acad Dermatol* **39**, 960–5.

141 Boisnic S, Branchet-Gumila MC, Nocera T. (2005) Comparative study of the anti-aging effect of retinaldehyde alone or associated with pretocopheryl in a surviving human skin model submitted to ultraviolet A and B irradiation. *Int J Tissue React* **27**, 91–9.

142 Siegenthaler G, Saurat JH, Ponec M. (1990) Retinol and retinal metabolism. Relationship to the state of differentiation of cultured human keratinocytes. *Biochem J* **268**, 371–8.

143 Kishore GS, Boutwell RK. (1980) Enzymatic oxidation and reduction of retinal by mouse epidermis. *Biochem Biophys Res Commun* **94**, 1381–6.

144 Napoli JL, Race KR. (1988) Biogenesis of retinoic acid from b-carotene. *J Biol Chem* **263**, 17372–7.

145 Raner GM, Vaz AD, Coon MJ. (1996) Metabolism of all-trans, 9-cis, and 13-cis isomers of retinal by purified isozymes of microsomal cytochrome P450 and mechanism-based inhibition of retinoid oxidation by citral. *Mol Pharmacol* **49**, 515–22.

146 Sorg O, Didierjean L, Saurat JH. (1999) Metabolism of topical natural retinoids. *Dermatology* **199**, 13–7.

147 Kasraee B. (2002) Peroxidase-mediated mechanisms are involved in the melanocytotoxic and melanogenesis-inhibiting effects of chemical agents. *Dermatology* **205**, 329–39.

148 Sorg O, Kasraee B, Salomon D, Saurat JH. (2013) The combination of a retinoid, a phenolic agent and an antioxidant improves tolerance while retaining an optimal depigmenting action in reconstructed epidermis. *Dermatology* **227**, 150–6.

149 Bailly J, Crettaz M, Schifflers MH, Marty JP. (1998) In vitro metabolism by human skin and fibroblasts of retinol, retinal and retinoic acid. *Exp Dermatol* **7**, 27–34.

150 Boehnlein J, Sakr A, Lichtin JL, Bronaugh RL. (1994) Characterization of esterase and alcohol dehydrogenase activity in skin. Metabolism of retinyl palmitate to retinol (vitamin A) during percutaneous absorption. *Pharm Res* **11**, 1155–9.

151 Connor MJ. (1988) Oxidation of retinol to retinoic acid as a requirement for biological activity in mouse epidermis. *Cancer Res* **48**, 7038–40.

152 Bruce S. (2008) Cosmeceuticals for the attenuation of extrinsic and intrinsic dermal aging. *J Drugs Dermatol* **7**, s17–s22.

153 Burgess C. (2008) Topical vitamins. *J Drugs Dermatol* **7**, s2–s6.

154 Picardo M, Carrera M. (2007) New and experimental treatments of cloasma and other hypermelanoses. *Dermatol Clin* **25**, 353–62.

155 Tammi R, Pasonen-Seppanen S, Kolehmainen E, Tammi M. (2005) Hyaluronan synthase induction and hyaluronan accumulation in mouse epidermis following skin injury. *J Invest Dermatol* **124**, 898–905.

156 Manuskiatti W, Maibach HI. (1996) Hyaluronic acid and skin, wound healing and aging. *Int J Dermatol* **35**, 539–44.

157 Brown MB, Jones SA. (2005) Hyaluronic acid: a unique topical vehicle for the localized delivery of drugs to the skin. *J Eur Acad Dermatol Venereol* **19**, 308–18.

158 Trommer H, Wartewig S, Bottcher R, *et al.* (2003) The effects of hyaluronan and its fragments on lipid models exposed to UV irradiation. *Int J Pharm* **254**, 223–34.

159 Bel A, Fort-Lacoste L, Ginestar-Gonzales J, Navarro R, inventors. (1999) Glycylglycine oleamide in dermo-cosmetology. France.

CHAPTER 37
Topical Vitamins

Donald L. Bissett, John E. Oblong, and Laura J. Goodman
Procter & Gamble Beauty Science, The Procter & Gamble Co., Sharon Woods Innovation Center, Cincinnati, OH, USA

> **BASIC CONCEPTS**
> - Vitamins are commonly used as topical active agents in skincare products designed to improve aging skin appearance.
> - With appropriate selection of vitamin form and concentration, many vitamins (e.g., A, B_3, B_5, C, E) can be safely applied topically for skin improvement effects.
> - Appropriate formulation and packaging of vitamins is required to prevent loss of activity through processes such as light inactivation or oxidation and to achieve aesthetically acceptable products.

Introduction

Vitamins are organic compounds required in small quantities for normal skin function and are typically obtained from the diet. Many materials have been described as vitamins [1]. A few have been used in topical cosmetic products, and certainly there is technical rationale for such use, in particular based on the skin consequences in individuals consuming deficient diets. For example, vitamin B3 deficiency leads to the medical condition pellagra, which encompasses a broad range of symptoms from dermatitis to dementia to death.

Since vitamins are essential nutrients, several of them functioning in a wide array of biochemical processes, they have potential to provide beneficial effects across a wide spectrum of skin problems, even in people who are nutritionally sufficient. Also, since they are well studied due to their importance in nutrition, their mechanisms and toxicology are often well understood. Additionally, with topical application and subsequent delivery into skin, they are more likely to have local meaningful effects vs. oral intake with the consequent limited delivery via the circulation to the specific skin site of interest (e.g., facial skin).

Since there are so many vitamins, this review is necessarily selective, focusing on a few, with particular emphasis on those materials for which there are available well-controlled *in vivo* human studies to illustrate skin care effects. Selected literature citations are provided to give the reader some references that can serve as a starting point to probe deeper into the available technical data.

Vitamin A

Forms
Several forms of vitamin A are used cosmetically, the most widely utilized ones being retinol, retinyl esters (e.g., retinyl acetate, retinyl propionate, and retinyl palmitate), and retinaldehyde. Through endogenous enzymatic reactions, all are converted ultimately to trans-retinoic acid, the active form of vitamin A in skin. Specifically, retinyl esters are converted to retinol via esterase activity. Retinol is then converted to retinaldehyde by retinol dehydrogenase. Finally retinaldehyde is oxidized to retinoic acid by retinaldehyde oxidase (Figure 37.1).

Mechanisms
Since trans-retinoic acid (RA) is the active form of vitamin A in skin, the abundant published literature on the former is applicable to this discussion. RA interacts with nuclear receptor proteins described as retinoic acid receptors (RAR) and retinoid X receptors (RXR), which can form heterodimer complexes. These complexes then interact with specific DNA sequences to affect transcription, to either increase or decrease expression of specific proteins/enzymes [2].

Using genomic methodology, work in our laboratories has found that the expression of over 1200 genes is significantly affected by topical retinoid treatment of photoaged human skin (unpublished observations). Many of these changes can be ascribed, at least on some level, as being normalization of the altered skin conditions that occur with aging (induced by both chronological and environmental influences such as chronic

---

Cosmetic Dermatology: Products and Procedures, Second Edition. Edited by Zoe Diana Draelos.
© 2016 John Wiley & Sons, Ltd. Published 2016 by John Wiley & Sons, Ltd.

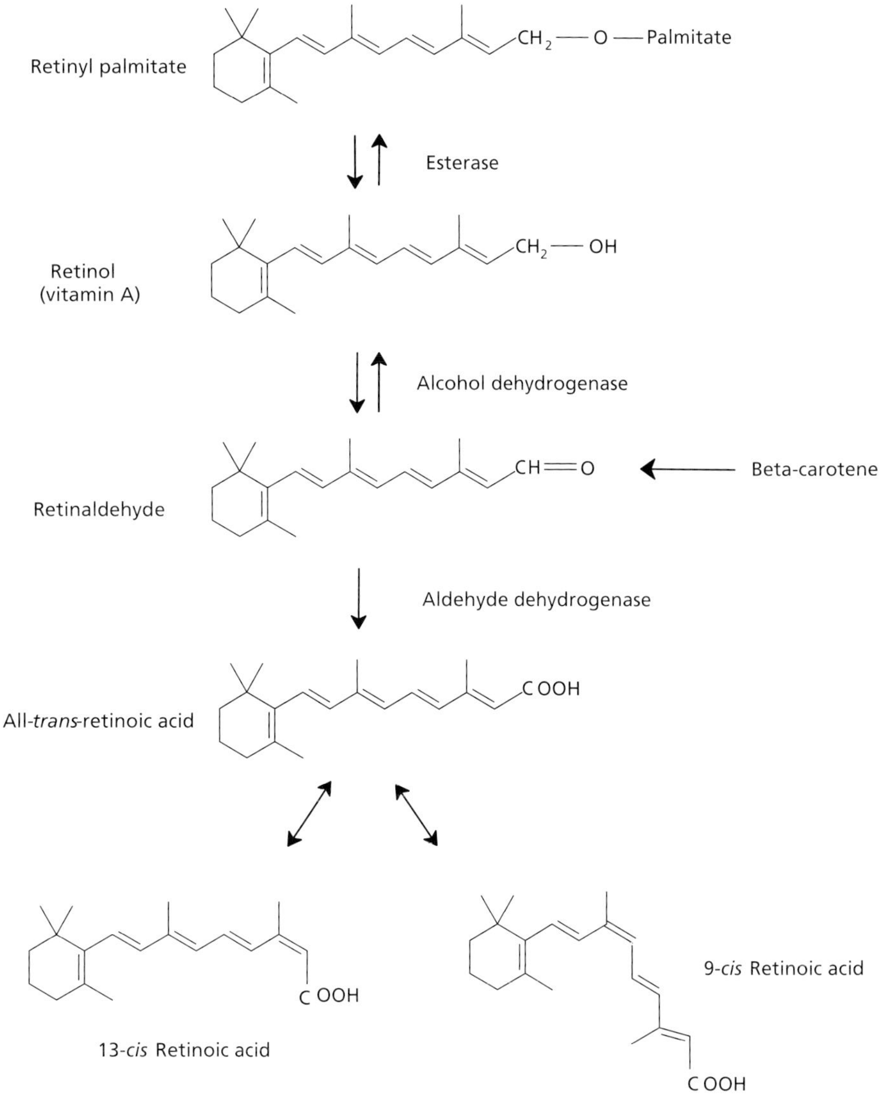

Figure 37.1 Conversion of retinyl ester into trans-retinoic acid in the skin.

sun exposure). Some specific changes induced by retinoid that are likely relevant to skin appearance effects are those that result in increased production of epidermal ground substance (glycosaminoglycans or GAGs which bind water, increasing epidermal hydration); increased dermal production of extracellular matrix components such as collagen (to increase dermal thickness and restructure the matrix); and thicker and "restored" epidermis, e.g., increased epidermal proliferation and differentiation (increased epidermal thickness and epidermal turnover). These effects would be expected to contribute to improvements in the appearance of fine lines, wrinkles, and roughness [3].

In addition to stimulation of events in skin, retinoids also have an inhibitory effect on other tissue components. For example, retinoids are reported to inhibit production of collagenase. And while retinoids will stimulate production of ground substance (GAGs) in epidermis, they have the opposite effect in dermal tissue, specifically inhibiting production of excess ground substance in the upper dermis of photoaged skin. While a low level of GAGs are required in the dermis for normal collagen structure and function, excess dermal GAGs are associated with altered dermal collagen structure and wrinkled skin appearance in the Shar Pei dog and in photoaged skin [4]. Removal of the excess dermal GAGs has been shown to be associated with improved matrix structure and reduced skin wrinkling.

Since at least some of the epidermal effects of topical retinoid (e.g., epidermal thickening and turnover) occur relatively rapidly (days) after initiation of treatment, some skin surface effects (e.g., diminution of roughness and fine line appearance) can potentially be realized quickly. The dermal effects likely occur on a much longer time frame (weeks to months) such that reduction in skin problems via this mechanism will require much longer time frames (weeks to months).

In addition to the fine line, wrinkle, and roughness effects of retinoids, they are also well known as agents to improve hyperpigmentation (e.g., hyperpigmented spots, post-inflammatory hyperpigmentation, solar lentigos, melasma), with the effect being achievement of lighter and more uniform skin color. The mechanisms by which retinoids affect the skin's pigmentary system have not been completely identified. Yet it is known that retinoids stimulate epidermal turnover, which simply could be interpreted as exfoliating pigmented stratum corneum cells from the skin surface. Retinoids also inhibit UV-induced pigmentation via reducing tyrosinase activity and melanin synthesis, by regulatory action on transcription processes in the epidermis (in melanocytes and keratinocytes) [5]. These effects would reduce hyperpigmentation, leading to lighter skin color (time frame of at least several weeks).

Topical effects

While much of the substantial literature on the improvement of skin fine lines, wrinkles, roughness, and hyperpigmentation by topical retinoids is focused on trans-retinoic acid, there are also data available on the vitamin A compounds that are used cosmetically. Since retinoids are irritating to skin, defining skin-tolerated concentrations clinically is a key step in working effectively with these materials. Retinol is better tolerated by the skin than trans-retinoic acid. In our testing we noted that retinyl propionate is milder to skin than the widely used retinol and retinyl acetate (Table 37.1) [6].

Since retinoids in general tend to be fairly potent, topical doses of less than 1% are generally sufficient to obtain significant effects. At low doses, in double-blind, split-face, placebo-controlled facial testing (12-week duration), both retinol and retinyl propionate have been shown to be significantly effective in reducing facial hyperpigmentation and fine lines/wrinkles across the study (Figure 37.2). Determination of treatment effects was based on quantitative computer image analysis and blinded expert grading of high-resolution digital images [6].

There are also clinical studies published on other retinoids. Retinyl palmitate has very low irritation potential and has been reported to be effective if tested at a very high dose, such as 2%. There are also a few studies revealing the clinical efficacy of retinaldehyde, typically at a dose of 0.05%. However, retinaldehyde has irritation potential similar to retinol [7].

Formulation challenges

There are two primary challenges in working with retinoids. One is their tendency to induce skin irritation (as noted above), which negatively affects skin barrier properties. While high doses will provide greater skin aging appearance

Table 37.1 Cumulative back irritation measures for retinol and its esters (double-blind, vehicle-controlled, randomized study; daily patching for 20 days, under semi-occluded patch, $n = 45$; 0–3 irritation grading). Equimolar doses and abbreviations used were: 0.09% RP (retinyl propionate), 0.086% RA (retinyl acetate), and 0.075% ROH (retinol). RP and RA were significantly less irritating than ROH, and RP was directionally less irritating than RA.

Topical treatment (oil-in-water emulsions)	Expert Grader Cumulative Irritation Scores	Significance of Expert Grader Cumulative Scores*	Chromameter "a" Measure (day 21)	Significance of chromameter "a" measure*
Emulsion control	3.9	a	0.4	a
0.09% Retinyl propionate	24	b	2.7	b
0.086% Retinyl acetate	39	b	3.8	bc
0.075% Retinol	164	c	7.6	d

*Treatments with the same letter codes are not significantly different from each other ($p < 0.05$).

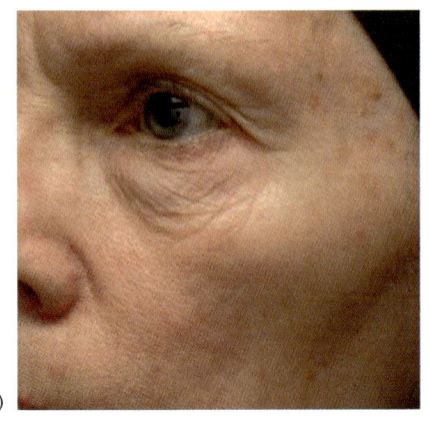

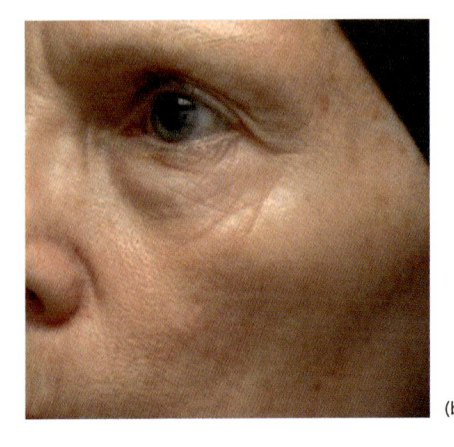

Figure 37.2 Topical retinyl propionate (RP) reduces the appearance of fine lines/wrinkles. 0.2% retinyl propionate in a stable skin care emulsion system was applied twice daily for 12 weeks. Images were taken at baseline, and weeks 4, 8, and 12.

improvement, the associated irritation tends to define an upper concentration limit where they can be used practically. While the skin may have some capacity to accommodate to retinoid treatment to respond with less irritation over time, it is not completely eliminated even with long-term use, as demonstrated by evaluation of skin barrier function. Mitigation of the irritation may be managed to some extent with appropriate formulation to meter delivery into the skin, use of retinyl esters which are less irritating than retinol (as noted above), or inclusion of other ingredients (e.g., those with anti-irritancy or anti-inflammatory activity) to counter this issue.

The second key issue is instability, especially to oxygen and light. Thus, to ensure stability of retinoid in finished product, formulation and packaging must be done in an environment that minimizes exposure to oxygen and light. The final product packaging also ideally needs to be opaque and oxygen impermeable, including use of a small package orifice to reduce oxygen exposure once the container is opened. In addition, a variety of other strategies might be employed, e.g., encapsulation of the retinoid, inclusion of stabilizing antioxidants, and unit dosing.

Vitamin B3

Forms
There are three primary forms of vitamin B3 that have found utility in skin care products: niacinamide (*aka* nicotinamide), nicotinic acid, and nicotinate esters (e.g., myristoyl nicotinate, benzyl nicotinate).

Mechanisms
Vitamin B3 serves as a precursor to a family of endogenous enzyme co-factors (Figure 37.3), specifically nicotinamide adenine dinucleotide (NAD+), its phosphorylated derivative (NADP+), and their reduced forms (NADH, NADPH). NADPH/NADP+ ratios serve as an indicator of redox status whereas NAD+/NADH ratios function as a critical cofactor in the regulation of metabolism, epigenetics, and circadian rhythms [8,9].

These co-factors are involved in many enzymatic reactions in the skin, and thus have potential to influence many skin processes as well as overall aging [10]. The ability of niacinamide to incorporate into cellular NAD+ pools and be utilized by sirtuins and poly-ADP ribose polymerases may be a key mechanistic basis for the diversity of clinical effects observed for a simple material such as niacinamide [11,12].

Recently, it has been reported that niacinamide can protect both glycolysis and oxidative phosphorylation under conditions of hydrogen peroxide-induced oxidative stress, which mechanistically involves incorporation into cellular NAD+ pools [13]. The emerging role of NAD+ in protecting cellular bioenergetics under oxidative stress conditions and as a limiting cofactor for these critical enzymatic processes may contribute to the specific actions of niacinamide have been described [14–16]. For example, topical niacinamide has the following effects:

- Niacinamide inhibits sebum production, specifically affecting the content of triglycerides and fatty acids. This may contribute to the observed reduction in skin pore size and thus improved skin texture (a component of texture being enlarged pores).
- Niacinamide increases epidermal production of skin barrier lipids (e.g., ceramides) and also skin barrier layer proteins and their precursors (keratin, involucrin, filaggrin), leading to the

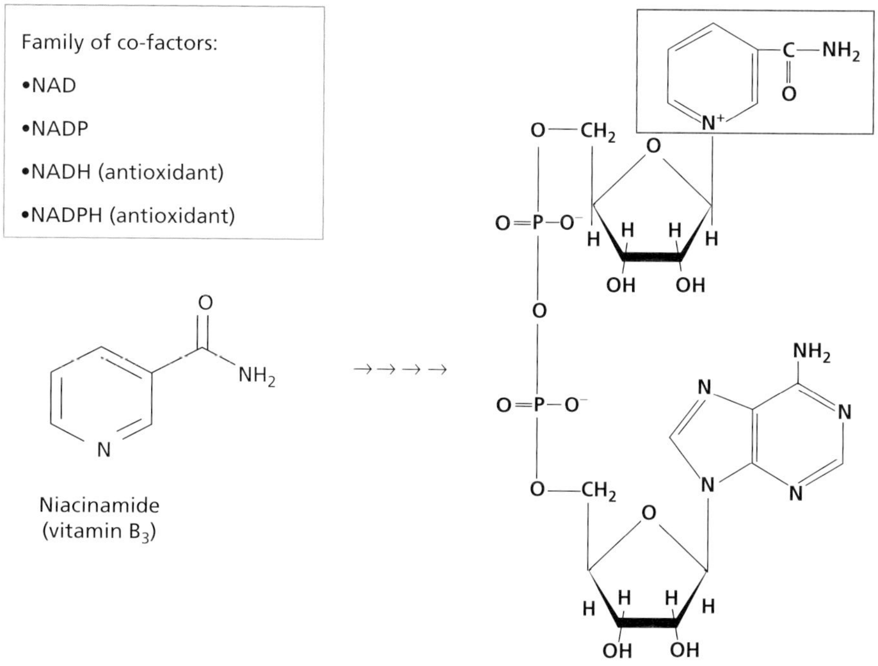

Figure 37.3 Niacinamide as precursor to energy co-factors: nicotinamide adenine dinucleotide (NAD), nicotinamide adenine dinucleotide phosphate (NADP), and their reduced forms NADH and NADPH.

observed enhancement of barrier function as determined by reduced TEWL (transepidermal water loss). This improved barrier also increases skin resistance to environmental insult from damaging agents such as surfactant and solvent, leading to less irritation, inflammation, and skin redness (e.g., facial red blotchiness). Since inflammation is involved in development of skin aging problems, the barrier improvement may also contribute to the anti-aging effects of topical niacinamide. Additionally, the anti-inflammatory and sebum reduction effects of niacinamide likely contribute to the anti-acne effect reported for this material.

- Niacinamide and its nucleotide derivatives (e.g., NAD) have anti-inflammatory properties (e.g., inhibition of inflammatory cytokines).
- Niacinamide increases production of collagen, which may contribute to the observed reduction in the appearance of skin wrinkling.
- Niacinamide reduces the production of excess dermal GAGs (glycosaminoglycans). As noted above for retinoids, this reduction is associated with dermal matrix remodeling and improved skin wrinkling.
- Niacinamide inhibits melanosome transfer from melanocytes to keratinocytes, leading to reduction in skin hyperpigmentation (e.g., hyperpigmented spots).
- Niacinamide inhibits skin yellowing. A contributing factor to yellowing is protein oxidation (glycation; Maillard reaction), which is a spontaneous oxidative reaction between protein and sugar, resulting in cross-linked proteins (Amedori products) that are yellow-brown in color. These products accumulate in matrix components such as collagen that have long biological half-lives [17]. Niacinamide has anti-glycation effects and antioxidant properties, due at least in part to its conversion to the antioxidant NAD(P)H [13].
- Niacinamide improves dermal skin elasticity, as measured by cutometry. The mechanism by which elasticity improvements occur is not defined, but dermal remodeling (as evidenced by the observed increase in skin collagen and decrease in excess dermal GAGs noted above) and prevention of dermal matrix glycation (of collagen and elastin, as discussed above) may be contributory factors.
- Niacinamide provides an ultraviolet radiation (UVR) protective effect (inhibition of broad spectrum UVR-induced immunosuppression), revealing its utility for incorporation into sunscreen products to protect against environmental insult [18]. Part of the mechanism of action for this effect has been speculated to involve modulation of cellular bioenergetics, in particular protection of glycolysis.

Since nicotinic acid and its esters are also precursors to NAD(P)H, they would be expected to provide these same effects to skin. Nicotinic acid and many (if not all) of its esters (following in-skin hydrolysis to free nicotinic acid) also stimulate blood flow, leading to increased skin redness or a flush response. While in some situations this might be a desired effect (e.g., warming sensation for body skin), it is difficult to manage for the more sensitive facial skin and can lead to irritation and itch.

Topical effects

A well-studied member of the vitamin B3 family of compounds is niacinamide. There are many published reports on its mechanisms of action, its delivery into human skin, and the diversity of clinical effects provided by topical niacinamide. The clinical observations were obtained from several double-blind, single-variable, placebo-controlled, left-right randomized studies. An example of the clinical effects is significant improvement in skin barrier [14], as measured by reduction in loss of water, i.e., lowered TEWL (Table 37.2). The niacinamide-treated skin is then more resistant to environmental damage, as determined by exposure of the skin to the surfactant SLS (sodium lauryl sulfate) and assessment of the resulting TEWL (Table 37.3).

As another example, topical niacinamide has been shown to reduce the appearance of skin fine lines/wrinkles [14,15]. The effect increases over time and is significant after 8-12 weeks of treatment. Additionally, topical niacinamide improves skin elastic properties as demonstrated for two parameters of skin elasticity, in particular R5 (measure of viscoelastic properties) and R7 (measure of elastic recovery). Topical niacinamide also improves other aspects of aging skin, such as reduction in sebaceous lipids (oil control) as shown in Table 37.4 and reduction in pore size, which likely contributes at least in part to the observed improved skin texture.

Table 37.2 Topical niacinamide strengthens forearm skin barrier as assessed by TEWL.

Topical treatment	TEWL (gram water per m²·hour)			
	Day 1	Day 12	Day 19	Day 24
Placebo	3.14	3.39	3.58	3.24
2% Niacinamide	3.22	3.05	3.09	2.58
Significance	–	$p < 0.05$	$p < 0.05$	$p < 0.05$

Table 37.3 Topical niacinamide pre-treatment reduces the barrier-damaging effects of the surfactant SLS on forearm skin.

Topical treatment	TEWL (gram water per m²·hour)		
	Day 24	1 hour post SLS patch	24 hours post SLS patch
Placebo	3.24	17.2	15.4
2% Niacinamide	2.58	14.1	12.1
Significance	$p < 0.05$	$p < 0.05$	$p < 0.05$

Table 37.4 Facial sebum excretion reduction after topical treatment with 2% niacinamide.

Topical treatment	% Change in facial sebum excretion (after 8 weeks of topical treatment)
Placebo formulation	–3.5
2% Niacinamide formulation	–23.0 ($p < 0.05$)

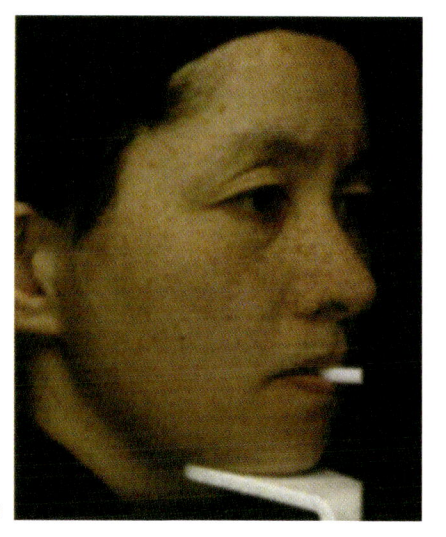

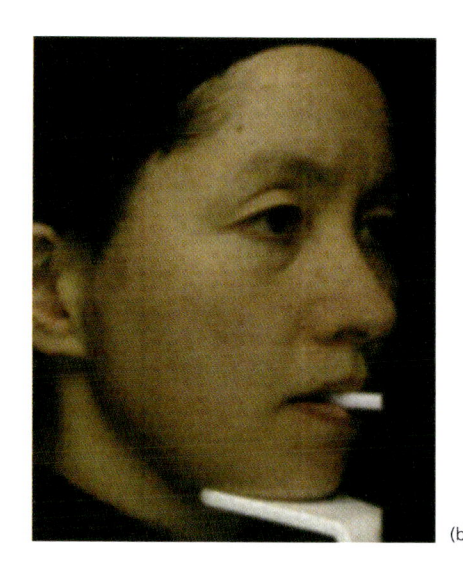

Figure 37.4 Topical niacinamide reduces hyperpigmented spots.

Beyond the above effects, there is also improvement in skin color (evening of skin tone), such as improvement in red blotchiness and skin yellowing, and in particular reduction in the appearance of hyperpigmented spots (Figure 37.4). The effect on spots has been reported in many published studies [19–21].

A key property that contributes to the ability of niacinamide to provide the wide diversity of clinical effects is its penetration into skin [19]. More than 10% of the topically applied dose penetrates into and through human skin, making the compound readily available throughout the tissue. Such a high degree of skin penetration results, at least in part, from its small size and lack of charge, permitting it to enter the skin much more readily than most other skin care active agents.

Fairly high doses (2–5%) of vitamin B3 have been used to achieve the observed clinical effects. However, since there is very high tolerance of the skin to niacinamide even with chronic usage, high doses can be used acceptably. In fact, as noted above, since topical niacinamide improves skin barrier, it actually increases the skin's resistance to irritation, damage, and environmental insult (e.g., from surfactant) and thus reduces red blotchiness.

Limited data on myristoyl-nicotinate have been presented to suggest that a similar broad array of effects may occur with this agent when used topically (1–5% doses) [22]. Clinical data for topical nicotinic acid and other esters are not available.

Niacinamide has also been tested clinically in combination with and in regimens involving other cosmetic agents (N-acetyl glucosamine, peptide, undecylenoyl-phenylalanine, vitamin A, salicylic acid). The clinical results indicate at least additive effects (reduction in the appearance of fine lines, wrinkles, texture, hyperpigmentation) of the agents used in the topical testing [21,23–25]. In mixtures with other agents (e.g., in combination with N-acetyl glucosamine), the human skin penetration of niacinamide remains unchanged, as does the delivery of the other agent [19]. Thus, the observed additive clinical effect is not the result of altered permeation into skin, but rather is due to the combined effects of the active agents.

Formulation challenges

The key challenge for working with niacinamide and nicotinate esters on the face is avoiding hydrolysis to nicotinic acid. Nicotinic acid, even at low doses, can induce an intense skin reddening (flushing) response. While a little skin redness (increased skin "pinkness") may be a desired effect for the face, the flushing response among individuals is highly variable in terms of dose to induce it, time to onset of the response, and duration of response. Additionally, the flushing can also have associated issues such as facial burn, sting, and itch, particularly under cold and/or dry environmental conditions. To avoid hydrolysis to nicotinic acid, formulating in the pH range of 5–7 is preferred. This flushing issue also requires that the purity of the raw material (e.g., niacinamide) be very high to minimize any contaminating free acid.

For the nicotinate esters, there are several commercial options. Many of them unfortunately are readily hydrolyzed to nicotinic acid on or in the skin such that flushing responses occur rapidly (within seconds-minutes) even at very low concentrations (<<1% in some cases). The longer chain esters (e.g., myristoyl-nicotinate) apparently are more resistant to this hydrolysis and thus appear to be more suitable for chronic use topically.

Vitamin B5

Forms

Pantothenic acid is the active vitamin. A precursor is panthenol or pro-vitamin B5 which is also known as pantothenol or pantothenyl alcohol. The widely used D optical isomer of panthenol is termed dexpanthenol. Panthenol is water soluble, stable, and low molecular weight (readily penetrates the stratum corneum).

Mechanisms

Panthenol has been used topically to treat wounds, bruises, scars, pressure and dermal ulcers, thermal burns, postoperative incisions/distention, and dermatoses [26,27]. The specific mechanisms for these effects are not known. However, dexpanthenol is a precursor to pantothenic acid (vitamin B5). Pantothenic acid is a component of co-enzyme A which functions in acyl group transfer during fatty acid biosynthesis and gluconeogenesis. By increasing skin lipid synthesis, improved barrier should occur, resulting in improved wound healing. In addition, panthenol promotes fibroblast proliferation and epidermal re-epithelialization, effects that promote wound healing. Furthermore, panthenol has found utility for skin penetration enhancement.

Topical effects
Topical panthenol is extremely well tolerated by the skin, leading to wide topical use of this material and many reported skin effects [26–28]. Among those are hydration and the associated improvement in roughness, scaling, and epidermal elasticity; improved skin barrier function; protection against skin irritation and SLS-induced damage; skin soothing; and anti-inflammatory and anti-pruritic effects.

Hydration
Panthenol's hydration effect likely derives from its hygroscopic properties. Panthenol is an effective moisturizer of stratum corneum and is even more effective when combined with glycerol. In addition, it improves the dryness, roughness, scaling, pruritus, and erythema associated with a wide variety of skin problems such as atopic dermatitis, ichthyosis, psoriasis, and contact dermatitis [26]. It also reduces the cutaneous side effects associated with retinoid therapy [29]. This hydration effect has further led to its use in hair care, promoting improved elasticity, softening, and easier combing.

Barrier and irritation
Panthenol protects against irritation via improvement in skin barrier function [26,28,30]. Topical pre-treatment with panthenol was observed to increase skin's resistance to visible irritation upon subsequent exposure to the surfactant SLS (Table 37.5). Since panthenol is the precursor to pantothenic acid which is a co-factor in barrier layer lipid biosynthesis, this could account for the noted barrier effect.

Some consumers are sensitive to specific components (e.g., certain preservatives, fragrances, sunscreen actives, etc.) in cosmetic

Table 37.5 Prevention of sodium lauryl sulfate (SLS)-induced erythema by topical 1% panthenol.

Time point post SLS treatment	Erythema score (0–6 scale) for skin treated with:	
	SLS	Panthenol then SLS
2 days	4.0	2.4
3 days	3.4	1.7
4 days	2.7	1.4

Table 37.6 Reduction in negative kinesthetic effects of formulation containing panthenol vs. formula not containing 1% panthenol.

Visible or kinesthetic attribute	Reduction in attribute by panthenol (0–6 scale)
Redness	−1.4
Burning	−2.4
Tingling	−5.7
Stinging	−4.9
Itching	−4.9
Warming	−5.7

formulations, leading to induction of negative kinesthetic irritation effects such as burn, sting, itch, and tingling. Topical panthenol incorporated into such formulations can reduce those negative effects (Table 37.6). The mechanism for this may be related to the reported soothing or anti-inflammatory effect of panthenol [26].

Formulation challenges
Panthenol at high concentrations can yield sticky/greasy feeling formulations. Thus, doses greater than approximately 1% may require appropriate formulation adjustment.

Vitamin C

Forms
Of the many forms of this vitamin, some of the more commonly used are ascorbic acid, ascorbyl phosphate (as the magnesium and sodium salts), and other ascorbate derivatives (e.g., ascorbyl palmitate, ascorbyl glucoside).

Mechanisms
Vitamin C is well known as an antioxidant and has been utilized as a skin lightener (e.g., via tyrosinase inhibition and/or its antioxidant effect). It also has been reported to have anti-inflammatory properties since it reduces the erythema associated with postoperative laser resurfacing [31]. In addition, ascorbic acid also serves as an essential co-factor for the enzymes lysyl hydroxylase and prolyl hydroxylase, both of which are required for post-translational processing in collagen (Types I and III) biosynthesis. Thus, by stimulating these biosynthetic steps, ascorbic acid has the potential to increase the production of collagen which could lead to wrinkle reduction (as discussed above for vitamins A and B3).

While the ascorbic acid derivatives may possess some properties of the free acid (e.g., antioxidant), hydrolysis of the derivatives would be required for the increased collagen production effect since the acid is the active co-factor. Demonstration of the hydrolysis of all these derivatives in skin has not been well documented.

Topical effects
There are several published studies discussing the anti-skin aging effect of ascorbic acid, such as reduced UVA-induced oxidation and reduction in skin aging appearance parameters (skin

surface replicas, dermatologist grading, algorithm-based facial image analysis, and histological assessment of biopsy specimens of dermal matrix, such as collagen). For example, topical 5% ascorbic acid for 6 months [32] improved photodamaged forearm and upper chest skin based on dermatologist scores, skin surface replicas, and biopsy specimen analysis (specifically improvements in elastin and collagen fiber appearance). At a high dose (23.8%), topical ascorbic acid for two weeks improved surface roughness, fine lines, and dyspigmentation [33].

Formulation challenges
The key challenge with vitamin C compounds in general is stability (oxygen sensitivity), particularly with ascorbic acid. Not only does oxidation lead to loss of the active material, there is also rapid product yellowing (an esthetic negative for the consumer). Various stabilization strategies can be attempted to address the issue, such as exclusion of oxygen during formulation, oxygen impermeable packaging, encapsulation, low pH, minimization of water, and inclusion of other antioxidants. In spite of all those approaches, in general ascorbate stability remains a challenge, and some of these approaches (e.g., very low pH) can lead to unwanted aesthetic skin effects such as irritation.

For the ascorbyl phosphates (Mg and Na salts), the resulting high content of salt in product can dramatically impact the thickener system, requiring increased use of thickener ingredients or other formulation approaches. These ascorbate derivatives are also considerably more expensive than other ascorbate compounds.

Vitamin E

Forms
This vitamin is also commonly known as tocopherol. There are several isomers based, for example, on number and position of substituents on the phenyl ring. Thus, there are α, β, γ, δ, and ε isomers of tocopherol. There are also several esters. A widely used form of vitamin E is α-tocopherol acetate.

Mechanism
Vitamin E is an antioxidant. The various isomeric forms have varying potencies as antioxidants. The active form is free tocopherol, so topical use of esters such as α-tocopherol acetate would require enzymatic hydrolysis to the free vitamin on or in the skin for maximal activity. Since it is lipid soluble, its site of action is more likely to be in lipid-rich environments (e.g., cell membranes).

Topical effects
While vitamin E is often used as a preservative/stabilizer in formulation, at relatively high topical doses it is quite effective in preventing oxidative damage to skin, such as preventing acute and chronic ultraviolet (UV) radiation damage. For example, in an *in vivo* model of UV radiation damage, topical tocopherol reduced by approximately 50% the visible skin damage (e.g., skin wrinkling) induced by chronic UV exposure [34]. There are also some clinical data describing improved skin moisturization and reduced skin roughness effects with topical vitamin E [35]. Since antioxidants are the topic of another chapter in this volume, the discussion here has been kept brief.

Formulation challenges
Tocopherol has some oxidative stability concerns, thus esters such as α-tocopherol acetate are most often used. Both tocopherol and its alkyl esters are oils, so high doses can be greasy/sticky, requiring formulation to address the esthetic impact.

Other vitamins

Vitamin D
There are several vitamin D compounds, and many synthetic variations. The active vitamin is 1,25-dihydroxyvitamin D3. Dehydrocholesterol (pro-vitamin D) is a cosmetically used material which can be converted into active vitamin D upon exposure to UV. Due to the effects of vitamin D compounds on epidermal growth and differentiation, there has been discussion of their skin barrier and photodamage mitigation activities, as seen in *in vivo* model testing [36,37]. Vitamin D compounds, like vitamin A materials, are often very potent, requiring caution in selecting specific compounds and topical doses.

Vitamin K
There are several forms of vitamin K, such as phylloquinone and menaquinone. Vitamin K compounds function in blood clotting, and there are data showing effects for mitigating bruising [38] and reducing purpura [39], which often occurs as a side effect to laser therapy for telangiectasia. There is also much speculation about the use of them in improving other skin problems such as under-eye dark circles. However, there appear to have not been any controlled studies presented to support that latter use. Oxidative stability is a concern with at least some of the vitamin K compounds.

Vitamin P (flavonoids)
This family of plant-derived and synthetically prepared chemicals encompasses a huge diversity of compounds. Some of the many types of flavonoids are flavons, isoflavones, flavanones, chalcones, coumarins, and chromones. Activities associated with flavonoids include antioxidant, anti-inflammatory, and phytoestrogen effects [40–42]. They are appearing in cosmetic products, often as components of natural extracts. Additionally, topical effects of a few specific compounds are emerging in the published literature [43,44]. This is a fertile area for identification of materials active in improving aging skin.

Discussion

While oral vitamins are well studied due to their importance in nutrition, the entire spectrum of possible effects from topical vitamins has not been thoroughly studied for the potential to improve skin. As the information presented in this chapter shows, at least some vitamins used topically can provide appearance-improving effects to aging skin, even in nutritionally normal individuals. With the wide array of vitamin materials, additional effects from their topical use are likely to emerge in the future.

A vitamin alone is not likely to be highly potent, although the high tolerance by skin for some vitamins provides opportunity to use high topical doses to achieve greater effects. A key to achieving that is development of esthetic formulations, to provide elegant product forms containing those high levels that the consumer will use on a regular basis to achieve the skin benefits. Also, combinations of different vitamins or vitamins plus other effective agents have potential to achieve considerably more dramatic effects. For example, combining a vitamin B3 with a vitamin A or with a peptide leads to greater effects than the individual materials. There is certainly opportunity to continue to explore this avenue of combinations.

As an individual compound, the vitamin B3 compound niacinamide is probably the most clinically studied agent in the cosmeceutical arena, based on the large number of peer-reviewed published studies. Interestingly, an independent review [3] of materials used widely in cosmetic products concluded that there is sufficient data on niacinamide, in particular, to support its accurate definition as a cosmeceutical ingredient: a material with substantial published robust data on skin permeability, mechanisms of action, and effectiveness in controlled clinical testing. In contrast, other widely used materials lack the depth of these technical elements to meet the criteria to be designated as a cosmeceutical ingredient. For niacinamide, the volume of controlled clinical data continues to expand in the peer-reviewed published literature, adding to the strength of its technical foundation and broadening the array of skin care benefit effects attributable to this multi-functional vitamin.

References

1. Newstrom H. (1993) Part 1: vitamins. In: NewstromH (ed.) *Nutrients Catalog*. McFarland & Company: Jefferson, NC, pp. 1–121.
2. Varani J, Fisher GJ, Kang S, *et al.* (1998) Molecular mechanisms of intrinsic skin aging and retinoid-induced repair and reversal. *J Invest Dermatol Symp Proc* **3**, 57–60.
3. Levin J, Del Rosso JQ, Momin SB. (2010) How much do we really know about our favorite cosmeceutical ingredients? *J Clin Aesthet Dermatol* **3**, 22–41.
4. Kligman AM, Baker TJ, Gordon HL. (1975) Long-term histologic follow-up of phenol face peels. *Plast Reconstruct Surg* **75**, 652–9.
5. Ortonne JP. (2006) Retinoid therapy of pigmentation disorders. *Dermatol Ther* **19**, 280–88.
6. Oblong JE, Saud A, Bissett DL, *et al.* (2005) Topical retinyl propionate achieves skin benefits with favorable irritation profile. In: Elsner P & MaibachHI (eds) *Cosmeceuticals and Active Cosmetics*. Taylor & Francis: Boca Raton, FL, pp. 441–463.
7. Fluhr JW, Vienne MP, Lauze C, *et al.* (1999) Tolerance profile of retinol, retinaldehyde, and retinoic acid under maximized and long-term clinical conditions. *Dermatol* **199S**, 57–60.
8. Canto C, Auwerx J. (2011) NAD+ as a signaling molecule modulating metabolism. *Cold Spring Harb Symp Quant Biol* **76**, 291–8.
9. Sassone-Corsi P. (2012) NAD+, a circadian metabolite with an epigenetic twist. *Endocrinol* **153**, 1–5.
10. Xu P, Sauve AA. (2010) Vitamin B3, the nicotinamide adenine dinucleotides and aging. *Mech Ageing Dev* **131**, 287–98.
11. Jacobson EL, Giacomoni PU, Roberts MJ, *et al.* (2001) Optimizing the energy status of skin cells during solar radiation. *J Photochem Photobiol B* **63**, 141–147.
12. Guarente L. (2011) Sirtuins, aging, and metabolism. *Cold Spring Harb Symp Quant Biol* **76**, 81–90.
13. Rovito HA, Oblong, JE. (2013) Nicotinamide preferentially protects glycolysis in dermal fibroblasts under oxidative stress conditions. *Brit J Dermatol* **168** (S2), 1–10.
14. Bissett DL, Oblong JE, Saud A, *et al.* (2003) Topical niacinamide provides skin aging appearance benefits while enhancing barrier function. *J Clin Dermatol* **32S**, 9–18.
15. Bissett DL, Miyamoto K, Sun P, *et al.* (2004) Topical niacinamide reduces yellowing, wrinkling, red blotchiness, and hyperpigmented spots in aging facial skin. *Int J Cosmet Sci* **26**, 231–8.
16. Berson DS, Oblong JE, Osborne RM, *et al.* (2014) Niacinamide: a topical vitamin with wide ranging skin appearance benefits. In: Farris PK (ed.) *Cosmeceuticals and Cosmetic Practice*. John Wiley & Sons: Oxford, (in press).
17. Odetti P, Pronzato MA, Noberasco G, *et al.* (1994) Relationships between glycation and oxidation related fluorescence in rat collagen during aging. *Lab Invest* **70**, 61–7.
18. Sivapirabu G, Yiasemides E, Halliday GM, *et al.* (2009) Topical nicotinamide modulates cellular energy metabolism and provides broad-spectrum protection against ultraviolet radiation-induced immunosuppression in humans. *Brit J Dermatol* **161**, 1357–64.
19. Bissett DL, Robinson LR, Raleigh PS, *et al.* (2007) Reduction in the appearance of facial hyperpigmentation by topical N-acetyl glucosamine. *J Cosmet Dermatol* **6**, 20–26.
20. Kimball AB, Kaczvinsky JR, Li J, *et al.* (2010) Reduction in the appearance of facial hyperpigmentation after use of moisturizers with a combination of topical niacinamide and N-acetyl glycosamine: results of a randomized, double-blind, vehicle-controlled study. *Brit J Dermatol* **162**, 435–41.
21. Bissett DL, Robinson LR, Raleigh PS, *et al.* (2009) Reduction in the appearance of facial hyperpigmentation by topical N-undecyl-10-enoyl-L-phenylalanine and its combination with niacinamide. *J Cosmet Dermatol* **8**, 260–66.
22. Jacobson MK, Kim H, Coyle WR, *et al.* (2007) Effect of myristyl nicotinate on retinoic acid therapy for facial photodamage. *Exp Dermatol* **16**, 927–35.
23. Robinson LR, Fitzgerald NC, Doughty DG, *et al.* (2005) Topical palmitoyl pentapeptide provides improvement in photoaged human facial skin. *Int J Cosmet Sci* **27**, 155–60.
24. Fu JJ, Hillebrand GG, Raleigh P, *et al.* (2010) A randomized, controlled comparative study of the wrinkle reduction benefits of a cosmetic niacinamide/peptide/retinyl propionate product regimen vs. a prescription 0.02% tretinoin product regimen. *Brit J Dermatol* **162**, 647–54.
25. Kaczvinsky JR, Li JX, Mack CE, *et al.* (2014) Effectiveness of a salicylic acid-niacinamide regimen for improvement in the appearance of facial skin texture and pores in post-adolescent women. *J Drugs Dermatol* submitted.

26 Ebner F, Heller A, Rippke F, *et al.* (2002) Topical use of dexpanthenol in skin disorders. *Am J Clin Dermatol* **3**, 427–33.

27 Stozkowska W, Piekos R. (2004) Investigation of some topical formulations containing dexpanthenol. *Acta Polon Pharm* **61**, 433–7.

28 Camargo FB, Gaspar LR, Maia Campos PM. (2011) Skin moisturizing effects of panthenol-based formulations. *J Cosmet Sci* **62**; 361–70.

29 Draelos ZD, Ertel KD, Berge CA. (2006) Facilitating facial retinization through barrier improvement. *Cutis* **78**, 275–81.

30 Biro K, Thaci D, Ochsendorf FR, *et al.* (2003) Efficacy of dexpanthenol in skin protection against irritation: a double-blind, placebo-controlled study. *Contact Derm* **49**, 80–84.

31 Alster TS, West TB. (1998) Effect of topical vitamin C on postoperative carbon dioxide laser resurfacing erythema. *Dermatol Surg* **24**, 331–4.

32 Humbert PG, Haftek M, Creidi P, *et al.* (2003) Topical ascorbic acid on photoaged skin: clinical, topographical and ultrastructural evaluation: double-blind study vs. placebo. *Exptl Dermatol* **12**, 237–44.

33 Xu T-H, Chen JZS, Li Y-H, *et al.* (2012) Split-face study of topical 23.8% L-ascorbic acid serum in treating photo-aged skin. *J Drugs Dermatol* **11**, 51–56.

34 Bissett DL, Chatterjee R, Hannon DP. (1990) Photoprotective effect of superoxide-scavenging antioxidants against ultraviolet radiation-induced chronic skin damage in the hairless mouse. *Photodermatol Photoimmunol Photomed* **7**, 56–62.

35 Yenilmez E, Yazan Y. (2010) Release of vitamin E from different topical colloidal delivery systems and their *in vitro-in vivo* evaluation. *Turk J Pharm Sci* **7**, 167–88.

36 Mitani H, Naru E, Yamashita M, *et al.* (2004) Ergocalciferol promotes in vivo differentiation of keratinocytes and reduces photodamage caused by ultraviolet irradiation in hairless mice. *Photoderm Photoimmun Photomed* **20**, 215–23.

37 Reichrath J, Lehmann B, Carlberg C, *et al.* (2007) Vitamins as hormones. *Hormone Med Res* **39**, 71–84.

38 Shah NS, Lazarus MC, Bugdodel R, *et al.* (2002) The effects of topical vitamin K on bruising after laser treatment. *J Am Acad Dermatol* **47**, 241–4.

39 Lee Cohen J, Bhatia AC. (2009) The role of vitamin K oxide gel in the resolution of post-procedural purpura. *J Drugs Dermatol* **8**, 1020–24.

40 Vaya J, Tamir S. (2004) The relation between the chemical structure of flavonoids and their estrogen-like activities. *Cur Med Chem* **11**, 1333–43.

41 Kim HP, Park H, Son KH, *et al.* (2008) Biochemical pharmacology of bioflavonoids: implications for anti-inflammatory action. *Arch Pharm Res* **31**, 265–73.

42 Amic D, Davidovic-Amic D, Beslo D, *et al.* (2007) SAR and QSAR of the antioxidant activity of flavonoids. *Cur Med Chem* **14**, 827–45.

43 Tsai Y-H, Lee K-F, Huang Y-B, *et al.* (2010) In vitro permeation and in vivo whitening effect of topical hesperetin microemulsion delivery system. *Int J Pharm* **388**, 257–62.

44 Wolfle U, Esser PR, Simon-Haarhaus B, *et al.* (2011) UVB-induced DNA damage, generation of reactive oxygen species, and inflammation are effectively attenuated by the flavonoid luteolin *in vitro* and *in vivo*. *Free Rad Biol Med* **50**, 1081–93.

CHAPTER 38
Clinical Uses of Hydroxyacids

Barbara A. Green,[1] Eugene J. Van Scott,[2] and Ruey J. Yu[3]
[1]NeoStrata Company, Inc., Princeton, NJ, USA
[2]Private Practice, Abington, PA, USA
[3]Private Practice, Chalfont, PA, USA

> **BASIC CONCEPTS**
> - Hydroxyacids are low pH substances that exfoliate the stratum corneum and modulate the process of keratinization.
> - The hydroxyacids include alpha-hydroxyacids (AHAs), beta-hydroxyacids (BHAs), polyhydroxy acids (PHAs), aldobionic acids (bionic acids), and aromatic hydroxyacids (AMAs).
> - Effects of hydroxyacids include increased thickness of epidermis and papillary dermis; improved barrier properties; increased amounts of hyaluronic acid in the dermis and of other dermal glycosaminoglycans which correspond to increased skin thickness measured micrometrically; improved histologic features of dermal collagen; increase in total skin thickness which in turn diminishes clinical wizened appearances; and diminished dyspigmentation.
> - PHAs and bionic acids can be distinguished from AHAs in that they are gentle, moisturizing and provide skin protective benefits including MMP inhibition, antioxidant/chelation effects and reduced non-enzymatic glycation.
> - Hydroxyacids are effective skin peeling agents.

Introduction

Research on aging today is motivated by the belief that innate degenerative processes of aging, and aging itself, can be modulated, prevented, and perhaps reversed. Even though a complete understanding of the mechanisms of aging may not be known, improvement in clinical appearance and function of the skin with anti-aging measures is a signal that modulation of aging and/or degenerative processes has probably occurred.

After many years of research and clinical use, hydroxyacids (HAs) have been shown to have biologic importance and clinical value for both younger skin and older skin with a variety of hyperkeratotic and aging-related conditions. This chapter covers HAs, including alpha-hydroxyacids (AHAs), beta-hydroxyacids (BHAs), polyhydroxy acids (PHAs), aldobionic acids (bionic acids), and aromatic hydroxyacids (AMAs). These compounds positively impact skin morphology and function, naturally playing physiologic roles in promoting normalcy and defending the skin against endogenous and exogenous adversities. They provide measurable clinical and anti-aging benefits that can be considered both preventative and corrective over the course of time.

Chemical categorization and natural occurrence of hydroxyacids

Hydroxyacids may be divided into five groups based on their chemical structures: AHAs, BHAs, PHAs, bionic acids, and AMAs.

Alpha-hydroxyacids

The AHAs are the most widely studied and commercialized ingredients within the HA family. They are the simplest of the HAs, consisting of organic carboxylic acids with one hydroxyl group attached to the alpha position of the carboxyl group. Both the hydroxyl and carboxyl groups are directly attached to an aliphatic or alicyclic carbon atom. As a result, the hydroxyl group in the AHA is neutral and only the carboxyl group provides acidity to the molecule, a property that distinguishes the AHAs from aromatic hydroxyacids such as salicylic acid as described below.

Many AHAs are present in foods and fruits, and therefore are called fruit acids (Table 38.1). Glycolic acid, the smallest AHA, occurs in sugar cane and citric acid is found in lemon juice at a concentration of 5–8%. Some AHAs contain a phenyl group as a side chain substituent; this changes the solubility profile of the AHA providing increased lipophilicity over conventional

Table 38.1 Examples of hydroxyacids.

Category	Example	Occurrence/source	Antioxidant
Alpha-hydroxyacid (AHA)	Glycolic	Sugar cane	No
	Lactic	Sour milk, tomato	No
	Methyllactic	Mango	No
	Citric	Lemon, orange	Yes
	Malic	Apple	Yes
	Tartaric	Grape	Yes
Beta-hydroxyacid (BHA)	Beta-hydroxybutanoic	Urine	No
	Tropic	Plant	No
Polyhydroxy acid (PHA)	Gluconic	Skin, commercially derived from corn	Yes
	Gluconolactone	Skin, commercially derived from corn	Yes
Aldobionic acid (bionic acid)	Lactobionic	Lactose from milk	Yes
	Maltobionic	Maltose from starch	Yes
Aromatic hydroxyacid (AMA)	Salicylic	Ester form in wintergreen leaves	No

water-soluble AHAs and can be used to target oily and acne-prone skin. Examples include mandelic acid (phenyl glycolic acid) and benzilic acid (diphenyl glycolic acid).

Beta-hydroxyacids

The BHAs are organic carboxylic acids with one hydroxyl group attached to the beta position of the carboxyl group. Both the hydroxyl and carboxyl groups are attached to two different carbon atoms of an aliphatic or alicyclic chain rendering the hydroxyl group neutral in nature. Some BHAs are present in body tissues as metabolic intermediates and energy source. For example, β-hydroxybutanoic acid is produced by the liver and utilized by skeletal and cardiac muscle as an energy source. In contrast to the water-soluble β-hydroxybutanoic acid, tropic acid is derived from a plant source, and is a lipid-soluble BHA. For the most part, BHAs have yet to be commercialized in skincare mainly because of a lack of commercial supply and high cost.

Some AHAs are also BHAs when the molecule contains two or more carboxyl groups. In this case, the hydroxyl group is in the alpha position to one carboxyl group, and at the same time is in the beta position to the other carboxyl group. For example, malic acid (apple acid) with one hydroxyl group and two carboxyl groups is both an AHA and a BHA. In the same manner, citric acid contains one hydroxyl group relative to three carboxyl groups and is both an AHA to one carboxyl group and a BHA to the other two carboxyl groups. These ingredients have been commercialized in skincare formulations to adjust pH and to deliver antioxidant and anti-aging benefits.

Polyhydroxy acids

The PHAs are organic carboxylic acids that possess two or more hydroxyl groups in the molecule. The hydroxyl and carboxyl groups are attached to the carbon atoms of an aliphatic or alicyclic chain. All the hydroxyl groups in the PHA are neutral, and only the carboxyl group accounts for its acidity. Although hydroxyl groups may be attached to several positions of the carbon chain, in order to be both an AHA and PHA it is essential that at least one hydroxyl group be attached to the alpha position.

Many PHAs are endogenous metabolites or intermediate products from carbohydrate metabolism in body tissues. Both galactonic acid and galactonolactone are derived from galactose, which is an important component of glycosaminoglycans. Gluconic acid and gluconolactone are important metabolites formed in the pentose phosphate pathway from glucose during the biosynthesis of ribose for ribonucleic acid. Gluconolactone is the most widely studied and commercialized skincare ingredient among the PHAs.

Aldobionic acids or bionic acids

The aldobionic acids, also called bionic acids, consist of one carbohydrate monomer chemically linked to a PHA via a stable ether linkage; examples are lactobionic acid (galactose/gluconic acid) and maltobionic acid (glucose/gluconic acid) (Figure 38.1). The bionic acid is commonly obtained from its disaccharide through chemical or enzymatic oxidation. For example, lactobionic acid is obtained from lactose and maltobionic acid from maltose. In general, the bionic acids have a larger molecular size and weight than most PHAs because of the additional sugar unit; however, at 358 Da (lactobionic acid and maltobionic acid) these molecules remain small enough to penetrate skin.

Aromatic hydroxyacids

AMAs such as salicylic acid and gallic acid are derived from benzoic acid, which has been used in combination with salicylic acid

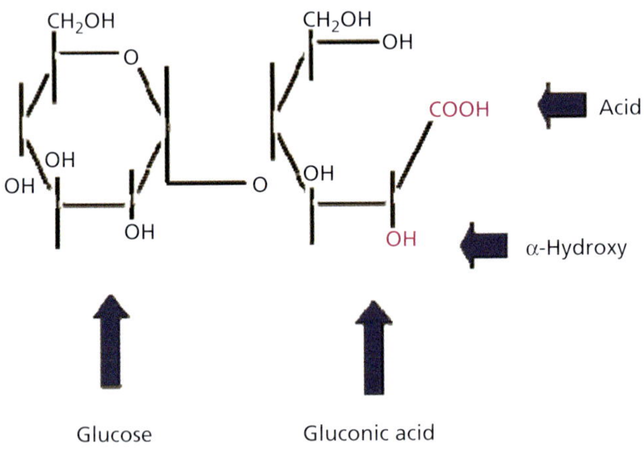

Figure 38.1 Maltobionic acid, a bionic acid.

as Whitfield's ointment (e.g., 6% benzoic acid/3% salicylic acid) for hyperkeratotic conditions and fungal infections. Salicylic acid is 2-hydroxybenzoic acid and may be called an HA within a broad definition; however, its effects on skin differ from those of the AHAs, BHAs, PHAs, and bionic acids. Salicylic acid is a conventional keratolytic agent which desquamates corneocytes, layer by layer from the top downward [1]. In contrast, AHAs and BHAs appear to act at the innermost layers of the stratum corneum, the stratum compactum, near the junction with stratum granulosum [2,3]. Moreover, AHAs, PHAs, and bionic acids have been shown to stimulate biosynthesis of dermal components and increase dermal skin thickness upon topical application, whereas salicylic acid has been shown to decrease dermal skin thickness [3–7]. Salicylic acid is an approved topical drug for the treatment of acne in accordance with the United States Food and Drug Administration Over-the-Counter (OTC) acne drug products monograph. Its use in cosmetics may be less desirable relative to other HAs due to dermal thinning effects.

Physicochemical and biological properties distinguishing HAs

As individual compounds, HAs differ broadly in physicochemical properties. Some HAs are very small molecules such as glycolic acid and lactic acid, and some are larger molecules such as lactobionic acid. Most HAs are white crystalline at room temperature such as glycolic acid, malic acid, tartaric acid, citric acid, mandelic acid, and benzilic acid, but a few are liquid such as lactic acid. Most HAs are soluble in water, but some are also soluble in lipid solvents. Some HAs are soluble only in lipid solvents. Certain physicochemical properties of HAs are discussed herein.

Water binding properties/gel matrix formation

In contrast to AHAs and BHAs, PHAs and bionic acids are strongly hygroscopic and can attract and bind water similarly to other polyol compounds such as glycerin. The bionic acids are so strongly hygroscopic that they form a gel matrix when their aqueous solution is evaporated at room temperature. The transparent gel thus obtained retains certain amounts of water, forming a clear gel matrix. The amount of water retention depends on the individual bionic acid. For example, maltobionic acid can form a clear gel film containing 29% water complexed with maltobionic acid molecules. The formation of a gel matrix provides moisturization and may add protective and soothing properties for inflamed skin. PHAs and bionic acids are gentle and non-irritating, and can be used to provide anti-aging benefits to sensitive skin including patients with rosacea and atopic dermatitis, and following cosmetic procedures that weaken skin barrier function and increase skin sensitivity [8–11].

Antioxidant properties

Most PHAs, bionic acids, and some AHAs and BHAs with one hydroxyl group and two or more vicinal carboxyl groups have been found to be antioxidants. The antioxidant property is readily determined by using any one of the following test methods: prevention or retardation from air oxidation of: (a) anthralin, (b) hydroquinone, or (c) banana peel. A freshly prepared anthralin solution or cream is bright yellow, and an air-oxidized one is brownish or black. A hydroquinone solution or cream is colorless or white color, and an air-oxidized one is brownish or black. A freshly peeled banana peel is light yellow in color, and an oxidized one ranges in color from tan, dark tan, brown to brownish black. Known antioxidants such as vitamin C and N-acetylcysteine may be used as the positive control in these screen tests. Based on these tests, all the PHAs and bionic acids tested are antioxidants, which include ribonolactone, gluconolactone, galactonolactone, lactobionic acid, and maltobionic acid [11]. Among AHAs and BHAs, malic acid, tartaric acid, citric acid, and isocitric acid have been shown to be antioxidants.

Another method to determine antioxidant, free radical scavenging properties utilizes an *in vitro* model of cutaneous photoaging. Compounds are assessed to determine their ability to prevent UV-induced activation of the elastin promoter gene in skin via free radical scavenging activity. An increase in the expression of this gene causes the abnormal production of poorly structured elastin in skin, resulting in the condition known as solar elastosis – a hallmark of photoaging. In this model, free radical scavengers can reduce elastin promoter gene activation by approximately 50%; the balance of gene activation is reportedly caused by direct UV damage to cells and cellular DNA, and can only be prevented with agents that protect the skin against UV penetration such as sunscreens. Results of the study indicate that the PHA, gluconolactone, provides up to 50% reduction of gene activation, the maximum effect afforded by antioxidant/free radical scavengers. Gluconolactone is not a significant UV absorbing compound (i.e., sunscreen) and the results were therefore attributed to the compound's ability to chelate oxidation-promoting metals and possibly via direct free radical scavenging effects [12].

It is interesting to note that lactobionic acid is an important antioxidant chelator used in organ transplantation preservation solutions to suppress tissue damage caused by hydroxyl radicals during organ storage and blood reperfusion. In this regard, lactobionic acid reportedly inhibits hydroxyl radical production by forming a complex with Fe(II) [13]. Furthermore, both lactobionic acid and maltobionic acid have been shown to function as hydroxyl radical scavengers in the *in vitro* lipid peroxidation antioxidant model [14–16]. Inhibition of lipid peroxidation is vital for maintaining cell membranes and mitochondria, protecting cells against sun damage and oxidative stress, and is a measure of a substance's antioxidant capacity.

Antiglycation effects of PHA and bionic acids

Non-enzymatic protein glycation is one of many detrimental aging processes that occurs in skin over time. It is a chemical reaction that results from the non-enzymatic joining of a reducing sugar (e.g., glucose) and a primary amino group found on dermal structural proteins (e.g., collagen and elastin). This reaction yields glycation intermediates that are further oxidized to form irreversible advanced glycation end-products (AGEs). An increase in AGEs compromises the skin's integrity and functionality due to unintended and permanent protein cross-linking. Ultimately, this manifests morphologically as dermal inelasticity and collagen degradation and, cosmetically, as visual wrinkling and loss of firmness [17–20]. In addition, AGEs have been shown to impart a yellow color and sallow appearance, another common symptom associated with skin aging [21].

Anti-glycation is considered an important anti-aging approach in the maintenance of healthy, youthful skin. Compounds that inhibit non-enzymatic glycation interfere in various steps in the Maillard reaction pathway (Figure 38.2). In order to prevent the formation of AGEs, some cosmetic compounds interfere in the last step of the Maillard pathway by functioning as antioxidants and/or chelators of oxidation-promoting metals [17,20,22,23]. The bionic acids, including lactobionic and maltobionic acids, and the polyhydroxy acid, gluconolactone, are oxidized sugar acids with antioxidant and metal chelation properties. An *in vitro*, antiglycation test was performed with these compounds (0.05%–0.5%) to evaluate their ability to modulate the process of non-enzymatic glycation between glucose and serum albumin (protein). Experimental findings revealed a significant, dose-dependent inhibitory effect of non-enzymatic glycation compared with the water control ($p < 0.05$), with similar efficacy to the positive control, aminoguanidine (0.01%) [24] (Figure 38.3). Previous studies have demonstrated the ability of the PHA/bionic acid compounds to improve the appearance of sallowness up to 36% when applied topically twice daily over 12 weeks, $p < 0.05$. (Table 38.2) [5,25]. This may in part be due to an anti-glycation effect and the resultant formation of morphologically correct matrix protein relative to dysfunctional glycated protein.

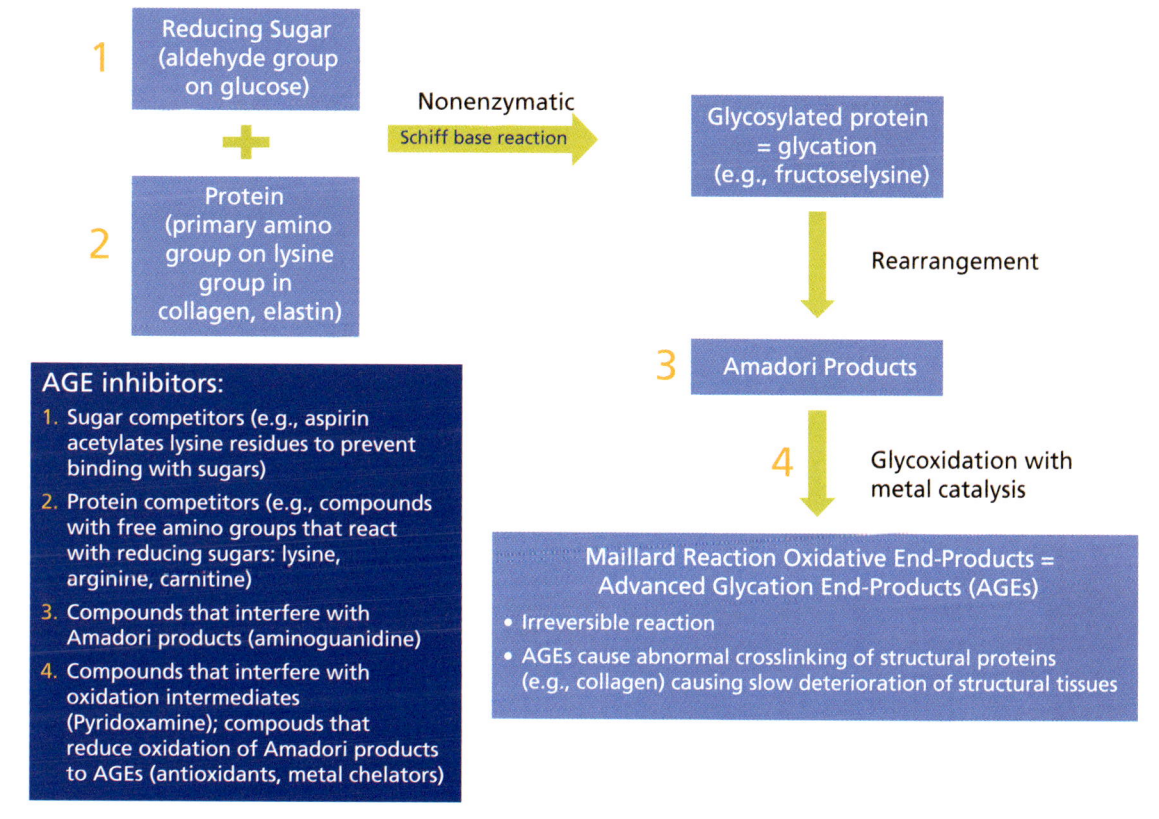

Figure 38.2 Reduction of advanced glycation end-products (AGEs) by targeting specific steps in the Maillard reaction.

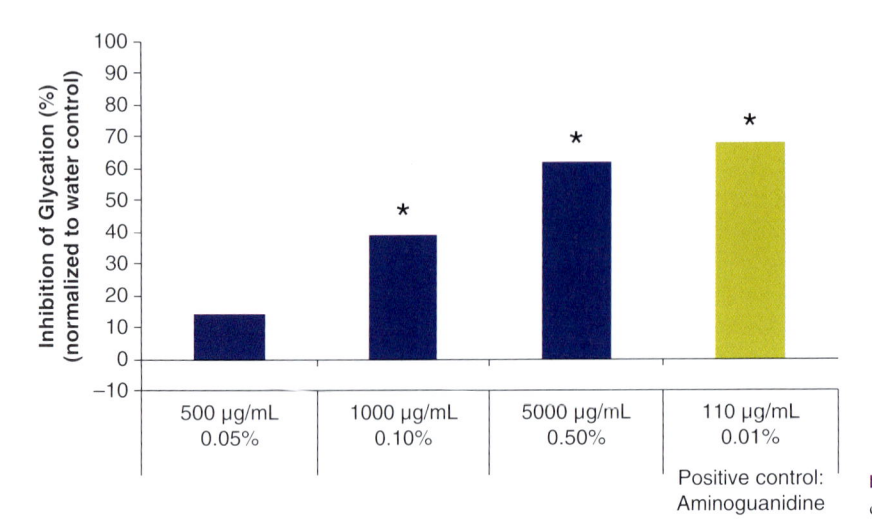

Figure 38.3 Percent inhibition of non-enzymatic glycation by maltobionic acid *p < 0.05.

Table 38.2 Clinical grading results for subjects treated with maltobionic acid 8% cream: baseline versus week 12.

Variable	Grading site	Mean baseline score (n = 28)	Mean 12-week score (n = 28)	Mean change	Standard deviation	Statistical difference (p < 0.05)[4]	Change from baseline (%)[5]
Pore size[1]	Cheek	4.77	4.01	−0.76	0.37	↓	−20.2
Roughness[1]	Cheek	4.29	1.51	−2.78	1.08	↓	−65.9
Laxity[1]	Cheek	5.43	4.51	−0.92	0.35	↓	−18.2
Fine lines[1]	Eye	4.57	3.29	−1.29	0.40	↓	−29.7
Coarse wrinkles[1]	Eye	5.22	4.12	−1.11	0.40	↓	−22.0
Mottled pigmentation[1]	Face	4.54	3.32	−1.22	0.40	↓	−28.1
Sallowness[1]	Face	3.79	2.60	−1.20	0.34	↓	−33.4
Clarity/radiance[1]	Face	3.79	7.13	3.35	0.90	↑	92.4
Pinch recoil[2]	Face	1.66	1.42	−0.24	0.11	↓	−14.2
Erythema[3]	Face	0.18	0.20	0.02	0.32	ns	0.6
Dryness[3]	Face	0.38	0.00	−0.38	0.52	↓	−12.5
Stinging[3]	Face	0.00	0.11	0.11	0.42	ns	3.6

[1] Visually graded by a trained assessor using an anchored 0–10 point scale with 0.25 point increments. 0 = low extreme, 10 = high extreme.
[2] Measurement collected in triplicate by a trained evaluator using a stopwatch in hundreths of a second; a decrease in pinch recoil time indicates an increase in skin firmness.
[3] Visually graded by a trained assessor using an anchored 0–3 point scale (none, mild, moderate, severe) with 0.5-point increments.
[4] Arrow indicates statistically significant increase or decrease from baseline; ns = not significant.
[5] Percent change from baseline, mean calculated on an individual basis and then averaged.

Sun sensitivity

AHAs and PHAs have been evaluated to determine whether daily application alters the sensitivity of normal human skin to UVB radiation. A change in UV sensitivity resulting from enhanced transmission of UVB can be monitored by the formation of sunburn cells (SBCs). Treatment with glycolic acid has been shown to increase the formation of SBCs in skin [26]; this effect can be prevented with use of low level sunscreens [26,27].

Importantly, pretreatment with gluconolactone (PHA) does not lead to an increase in sunburn cells following UVB irradiation, presumably due to its antioxidant effects [12].

Sensory responses

One of the distinguishing benefits of the PHAs and bionic acids is their gentleness on skin. When compared with glycolic acid and lactic acid, PHAs and bionic acids are non-stinging and non-burning. A 14-day cumulative irritation test of a 12% PHA/bionic acid cream formulation at pH 3.8 conducted under full occlusion revealed no difference in irritation potential from the negative control (normal saline), thereby validating the non-irritating nature of these compounds even at high strength and bioavailable pH [11]. Accordingly, product use studies have demonstrated compatibility with sensitive skin, including clinically sensitive skin such as rosacea and atopic dermatitis [8–10]. Furthermore, PHAs and bionic acids are gentle enough to be applied to the skin immediately following cosmetic procedures such as microdermabrasion and non-ablative laser procedures, providing complementary anti-aging benefits while helping to reduce redness [11,28].

MMP inhibition effects of bionic acids

Matrix metalloproteinase enzymes (MMPs) provide a vital metabolic function by digesting the skin's degraded and aged extracellular matrix components. Naturally occurring inhibitors of MMPs protect the skin from excessive degradation caused by these enzymes. With aging and exposure to ultraviolet light, there is an increase in MMP activity along with a decrease in natural MMP inhibitors that contributes to elevated MMP activity. This shifts the metabolic balance in favor of protein catabolism which ultimately contributes to the negative clinical manifestations of aging including wrinkles, skin laxity, and telangiectasia [29]. Research has shown that the bionic acid, lactobionate, is an inhibitor of MMP enzymes obtained from human liver effluents during organ transplantation procedures [30]. Similarly, topical lactobionic acid has been shown to inhibit MMPs via skin histopathology which may help protect skin against deterioration from photodamage [5]. *In vitro* evaluation of maltobionic acid and lactobionic acid (0.0001%–0.1% solutions) demonstrated significant inhibition of the MMP collagenase, with nearly complete inhibition at the highest concentration (0.1%) (Figure 38.4) [15,16]. In cosmetic anti-aging formulations, these compounds may be used to help preserve existing collagen in skin.

Effects of HAs on skin – similarities and differences

Clinical and histologic observations on the biofunctionality of HAs, both in connection with therapeutic performance on numerous skin disorders and in the course of investigative studies on normal skin, confirm that AHAs, PHAs, and bionic acids have favorable effects on the stratum corneum, epidermis, and dermis. These effects appear to modulate form and function toward more normal or optimal states (Table 38.2). Because of these effects such compounds may be categorized as *eudermatrophic* agents (i.e. agents that nourish the skin toward normalcy).

Stratum corneum and epidermis

The initial response to AHA application on ichthyotic skin is a sheet-like, disjunctive desquamation of the thick, compact stratum corneum. With continued daily use of AHA formulations, the stratum corneum becomes histologically normal in thickness and in appearance, and the hyperplastic acanthotic underlying epidermis returns to more normal thickness [31]. The opposite occurs in the treatment of atrophic skin of the elderly wherein the stratum corneum and epidermis are both thin. After daily applications of AHAs for several weeks, histologic examination reveals both the stratum corneum and keratinocyte layer to have regained more normal thickness [5,32], with a more even distribution of pigmentation [4]. Other studies have shown AHAs improves barrier function with continued use; this finding has been particularly notable with the PHAs that possess antioxidant properties [33].

Dermis

Significant dermal remodeling occurs with daily application of AHAs to the skin. In studies on forearm skin where AHAs were applied daily, micrometrically measurable increases in dermal thickness occurred, which were correlated histologically with increased amounts of hyaluronic acid and other glycosaminoglycans

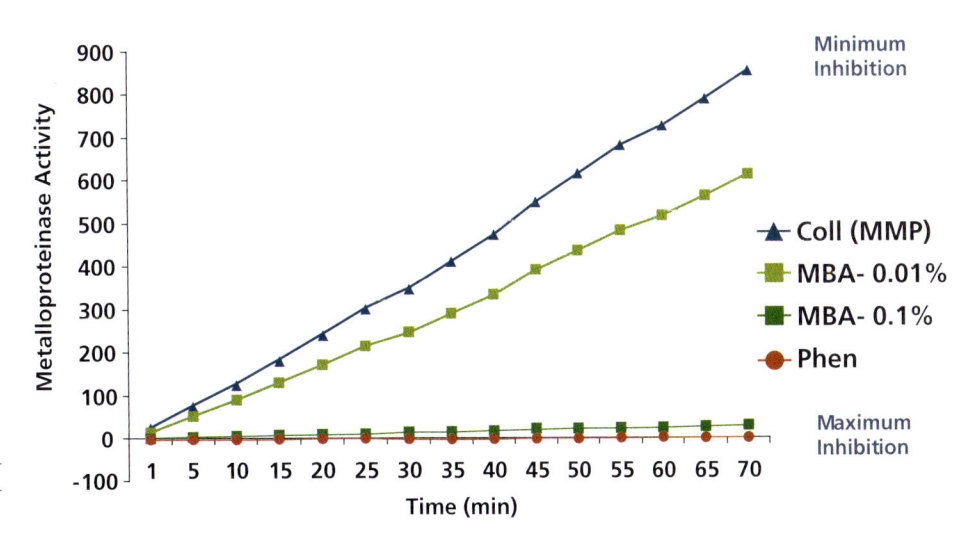

Figure 38.4 Inhibition of matrix metalloproteinase (MMP) activity by maltobionic acid *in vitro*.

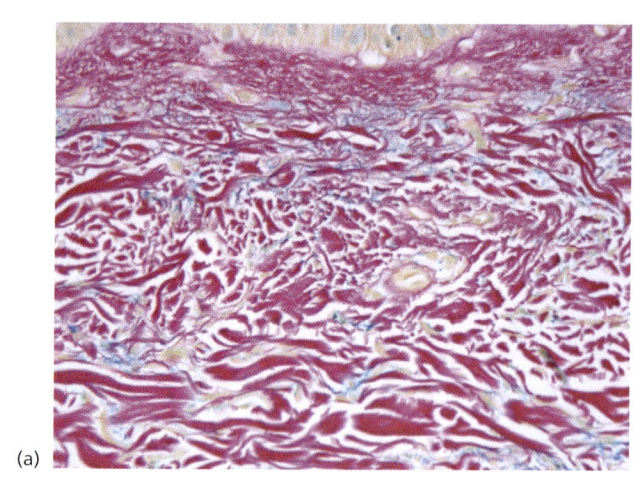

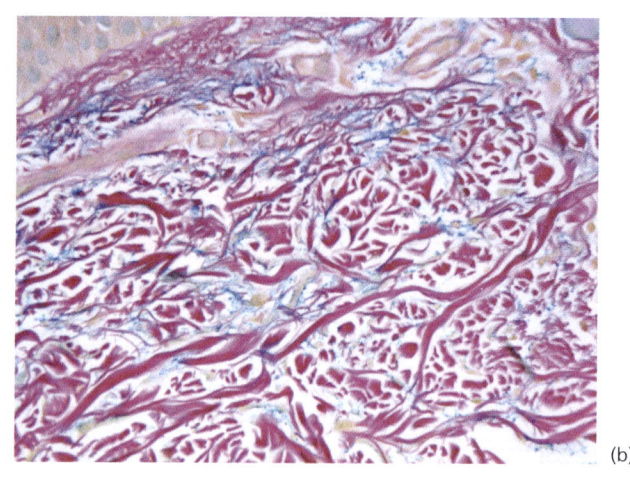

Figure 38.5 Histologic staining for acid mucopolysaccharides/glycosaminoglycans (GAGs): ×400. (a) Specimen shows staining of untreated control forearm skin. (b) Specimen shows staining following topical application of 8% maltobionic acid cream (pH 3.8) for 12 weeks. Increased density of blue colloidal iron stain demonstrates an increase in GAGs. (Source: Green & Briden, 2009 [11]. Reproduced with permission of Elsevier.)

(Figure 38.5) [4,5,7,34], and with qualitative improvements in collagen fibers and improved fibrous quality of elastic fibers [4]. Additionally, the papillary dermis increased in thickness, with increased prominence of dermal papillae thus increasing the dermal-epidermal junction surface area. Measurable increases in skin thickness without further topical applications persisted for months which further demonstrates a eudermatrophic matrix building effect [35]. Consistent with these clinical histologic findings are *in vivo* and *in vitro* observations by other researchers showing the AHA glycolic acid to increase fibroblast proliferation and production of collagen [36].

Clinical uses of HAs

HA effects on skin morphology and functionality are manifold, spanning all of the skin's layers. As a result, numerous clinical benefits have been observed with use of HAs as described herein.

Dry skin and hyperkeratinization

Previous studies demonstrated that the stratum corneum of xerotic skin was thicker and more compact than that of non-xerotic controls, and the epidermis often atrophic. Topical use of AHA formulations on xerotic skin restored the stratum corneum and epidermis to a more normal state both clinically and histologically. This restoration was accompanied by substantial reduction of clinically evident xerosis, and upon discontinuance of the topical AHA treatment the skin remained relatively normal for up to about 2 weeks when the thick compact stratum corneum again reformed [11,31,32,35].

Today we find that efficacy of HA formulations for problem dry skin conditions is improved by incorporating into the formulation combinations of AHAs, PHAs, and bionic acids selected for their efficiency in restoring and maintaining a more normal stratum corneum and epidermis. The PHAs and bionic acids, because of water-binding capabilities and inherent gentleness to the skin, offer special advantages in this regard. Combination HA formulations are found to have unparalleled efficacy for treating xerosis [37], and for treating otherwise treatment-resistant conditions such as callused fissured plantar and palmar skin (Figure 38.6). This combination also proved effective in descaling psoriatic plaques when applied twice daily for two weeks. In a double-blind clinical study, the 20% AHA/PHA/bionic acid formulation provided more efficient descaling versus the prescription comparator (6% salicylic acid cream) after one week of use. Both formulations were equally well tolerated. Since HAs may counter dermal thinning effects

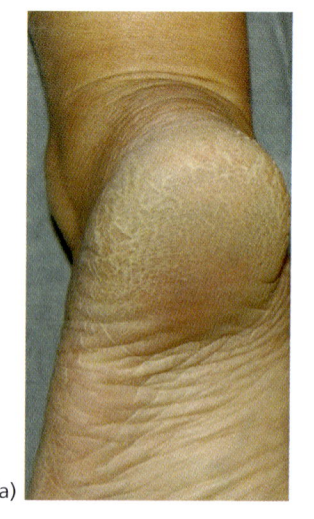

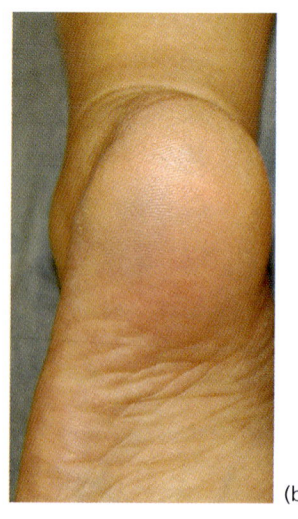

Figure 38.6 Hyperkeratotic feet treated once nightly with a cream containing an AHA/PHA/bionic acid blend (20% total) for 3 weeks. (a) Before treatment. (b) After treatment.

of topical corticosteroids, these agents may be preferred for psoriatic descaling relative to salicylic acid, which has been shown to decrease dermal thickness [38].

Keratoses and dyspigmentation

Markers of advancing years are a variety of localized hyperkeratotic lesions that include seborrheic keratoses, actinic keratoses, lentigines, age spots, and mottled pigmentation. HAs exfoliate hyperkeratotic pigmentation spots and AHAs have been shown to aid in the even disbursement of melanin [4]. PHAs and bionic acids chelate metals such as copper, an essential co-factor in the production of melanin, and have been shown to reduce melanin production in cultured murine B16 melanoma cells in a dose responsive manner [15,16]. HAs can be useful alone or in combination with skin lightening agents to lighten dyspigmentation [2,34].

Wrinkles and photoaging

AHAs, PHAs, and bionic acids are now used widely as topical anti-aging substances. They are used for superficial peeling to initiate accelerated epidermal turnover and to initiate dermal regenerative events in both therapeutic formulations under physicians' guidance and in a multitude of consumer cosmetic formulations ranging from traditional creams and lotions to home peels. The reason for this wide use is because of what may be their eudermatrophic properties, demonstrated in studies described earlier herein where effective concentrations applied to human skin have been found to normalize photoaged skin (Table 38.2). Such changes include increased thickness of epidermis and papillary dermis; improved barrier properties; increased amounts of hyaluronic acid in the dermis and of other dermal glycosaminoglycans, which correspond to increased skin thickness measured micrometrically; improved histologic features of dermal collagen; increase in total skin thickness which in turn diminishes clinical wizened appearances (Figure 38.7); and diminished dyspigmentation [3–5].

Uses as a peeling agent

Several substances have been used to date as peeling agents; these include phenol, trichloroacetic acid (TCA), salicylic acid, and AHAs. Phenol, weakly acidic in aqueous solution, is actually phenylic acid and is quite distinct from AHAs, as is TCA. Both phenol and TCA have a long history of use as peeling agents. Both are caustic, corrosive, powerful denaturants. Both cause rapid chemical destruction of skin. Neither of these agents is nutritive, and their benefits derive from post-injury replacement of destroyed epidermis and upper dermis through mechanisms of wound repair. Salicylic acid (SA), 2-hydroxybenzoic acid, a phenolic acid, is in use today as an agent for superficial peeling mainly for acne.

Of the HAs, lactic acid and glycolic acid are the most common peeling agents. Many of the AHAs are nutritive and physiologic, giving them an advantage over phenol, TCA, and SA. In high concentrations of up to 70%, lactic or glycolic acid can be applied to the skin for short times (i.e., approximately 5 minutes) to achieve substantial desquamation and initiate accelerated epidermal and dermal renewal. One of the distinguishing safety features of AHA peels is the enhanced control afforded by the ability to neutralize and terminate the action of AHA peels when desired during the peeling procedure. A neutralizing solution of sodium bicarbonate reacts with AHAs generating carbon dioxide gas bubbles. The foaming thus generated provides a visual endpoint enhancing the safety and control of these peels. To date, AHAs have been used primarily as superficial peeling agents in the adjunctive treatment of photoaging, acne, rosacea and dyspigmentation, where they offer the benefit of safety and effectiveness over the course of a series of peels [6]. (Figures 38.8, 38.9) Sensitive skin and those prone to post-inflammatory hyperpigmentation may benefit from application of lower strength peel formulations (e.g., 20%, 35%) in order to avoid provoking irritation. AHA peels can also be safely combined with other cosmetic procedures to optimize treatment results including non-ablative laser, light treatments, and with injectable fillers and botulinum toxin type A [28,39,40].

Synergy with topical drugs

Enhancement of efficacy can be observed in many conditions by the combined presence of AHAs in formulations that contain active drug ingredients for particular treatments. Examples of active ingredients whose efficacy is enhanced include retinoids,

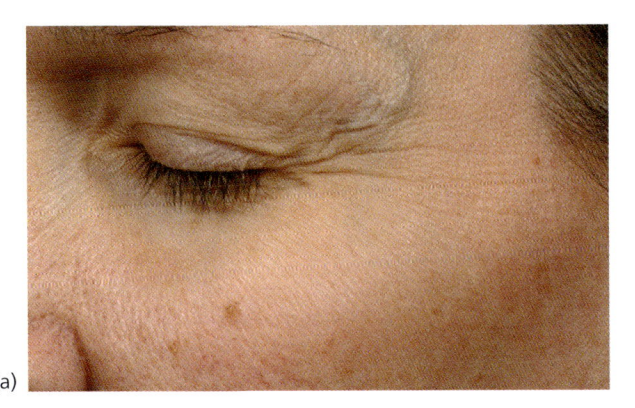

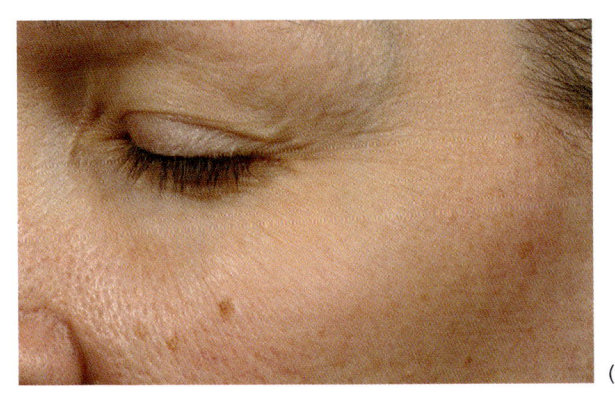

Figure 38.7 Periocular wrinkling is reduced on this 49-year-old female following twice daily application of 8% maltobionic acid cream (pH 3.8) for 12 weeks. (a) Before treatment. (b) After treatment.

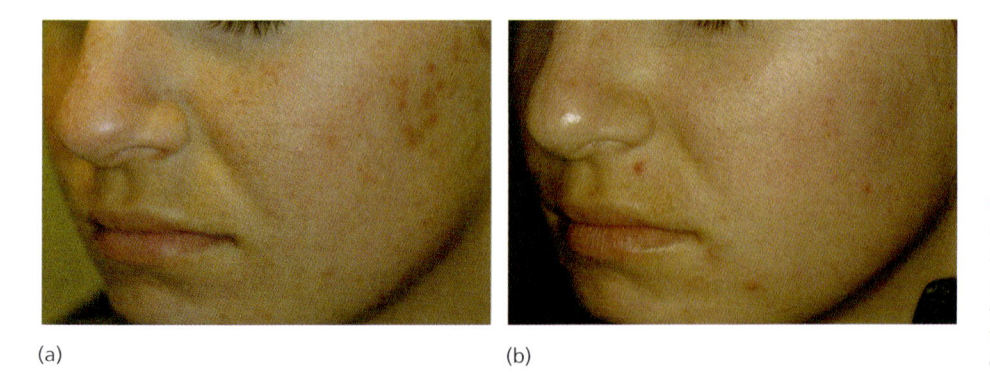

Figure 38.8 Improvement in acne and superficial acne scarring following application of five glycolic acid peels (35%, 50%, 50%, 50%, 70%) with use of adjunctive home care products containing AHAs, PHAs, bionic acids and other benefit ingredients.

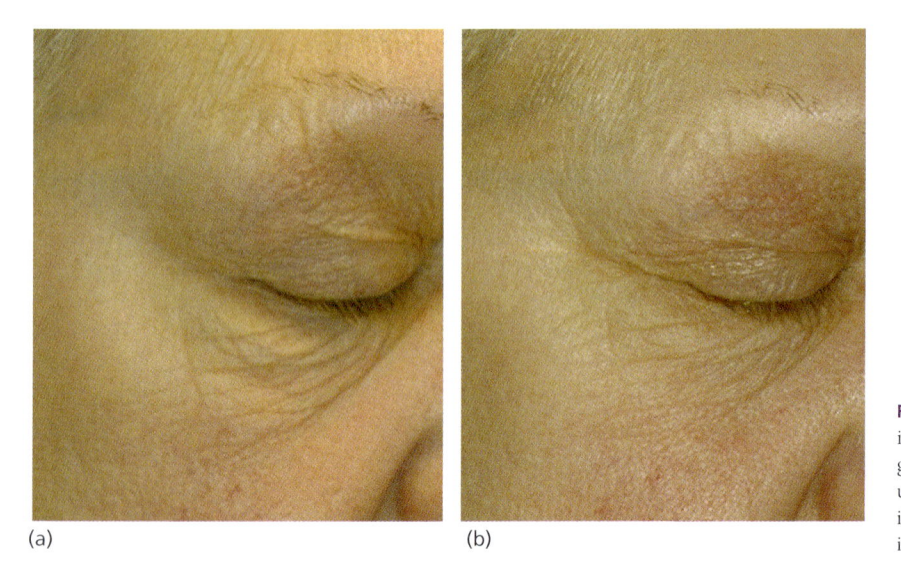

Figure 38.9 Improvement in periocular rhytides in a rosacea patient following application of four glycolic acid peels (35%, 50%, 70%, 70%) with use of adjunctive home care products containing AHAs, PHAs, bionic acids and other benefit ingredients.

antibacterials, antifungals, antipruritics, and corticosteroids. Mechanisms by which HAs complement or amplify the activity of another substance can be suspected in some instances, for example with retinoids and antibacterials in topical treatment of acne where activities of ingredients join to normalize intrafollicular keratinization and allow more efficient access of the medication into the pilosebaceous unit. The HAs also may enhance therapeutic effect of drugs by providing complementary cosmetic effects. For example, concurrent use of the PHA, gluconolactone, with azelaic acid has been shown to improve therapeutic outcomes for rosacea by reducing skin redness and diminishing the appearance of telangiectasia presumably by increasing overall skin thickness, while also improving the tolerability of the medication [41] (Figure 38.10).

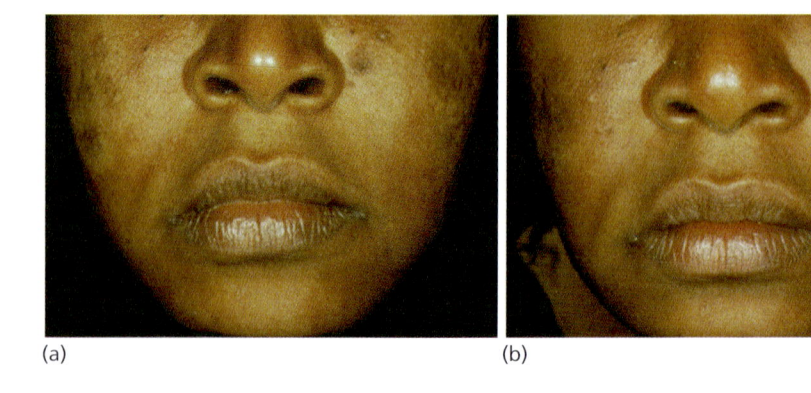

Figure 38.10 Improvement in post-inflammatory hyperpigmentation in an eczema patient following application of two glycolic acid peels (35%, 50%) with use of adjunctive PHA-containing home care products (cleanser, day cream SPF 15 and night cream) in conjunction with a 2% hydroquinone + PHA/bionic acid cream applied to areas of hyperpigmentation and a topical corticosteroid applied to eczema lesions.

Conclusions

In the quest to reverse the clinical signs of aging and improve overall skin health, the HAs (AHA, BHA, PHA, and bionic acids) have emerged as important ingredient technologies owing to their eudermatrophic effects. That is, HAs have the unique ability to nourish the skin towards normalcy, imparting meaningful cosmetic and therapeutic benefits in the process. Many of these compounds provide significant protective benefits including antioxidant, MMP-inhibition, barrier repair and anti-glycation effects, while also helping to reverse existing signs of aging including wrinkles, dyspigmentation and skin laxity. HAs can be used alone or in combination with other topicals to target the symptoms of photoaging and the myriad conditions of hyperkeratosis. HAs continue to be a mainstay in dermatology because they offer significant epidermal and dermal benefits while being safe for skin and the body, even following full body application over long periods of time such as when treating ichthyosis. As time marches forward, it is our expectation that more scientific data will lead to greater uses of HAs alone and in combination with cosmetics, drugs, and devices in dermatology.

References

1. Briden ME, Green BA. (2006) Topical exfoliation: clinical effects and formulating considerations. In: Draelos ZD, Thaman LA, eds. *Cosmetic Formulation of Skin Care Products*. New York: Taylor & Francis Group, pp. 237–50.
2. Van Scott EJ, Yu RJ. (1982) Substances that modify the stratum corneum by modulating its formation. In: Frost P, Horwitz S, eds. *Principles of Cosmetics for the Dermatologist*. St. Louis: CV Mosby, pp. 70–4.
3. Yu RJ, Van Scott EJ. (2005) α-Hydroxyacids, polyhydroxy acids, aldobionic acids and their topical actions. In: Baran R, Maibach HI, eds. *Textbook of Cosmetic Dermatology*, 3rd edn. New York: Taylor & Francis Group, pp. 77–93.
4. Ditre CM, Griffin TD, Murphy GF, et al. (1996) Effects of alpha-hydroxyacids on photoaged skin: a pilot clinical, histologic and ultrastructural study. *J Am Acad Dermatol* **34**, 187–95.
5. Green BA, Edison BL, Sigler ML. (2008) Anti-aging effects of topical lactobionic acid: results of a controlled usage study. *Cosmet Dermatol* **21**, 76–82.
6. Van Scott EJ, Ditre CM, Yu RJ. (1996) Alpha hydroxyacids in the treatment of signs of photoaging. *Clin Dermatol* **14**, 217–26.
7. Bernstein EF, Underhill CB, Lakkakorpi J, et al. (1997) Citric acid increases viable epidermal thickness and glycosaminoglycan content of sun-damaged skin. *Dermatol Surg* **23**, 689–94.
8. Bernstein EF, Green BA, Edison B, Wildnauer RH. (2001) Poly hydroxy acids (PHAs): clinical uses for the next generation of hydroxy acids. *Skin Aging* **9** (Suppl), 4–11.
9. Rizer R, Turcott A, Edison B, et al. (2001) An evaluation of the tolerance profile of a complete line of gluconolactone-containing skincare formulations in atopic individuals. *Skin Aging* **9** (Suppl), 18–21.
10. Rizer R, Turcott A, Edison B, et al. (2001) An evaluation of the tolerance profile of gluconolactone-containing skincare formulations in individuals with rosacea. *Skin Aging* **9** (Suppl), 22–5.
11. Green BA, Briden ME. (2009) PHAs and bionic acids: next generation hydroxy acids. In: Draelos Z, Dover J, Alam M, eds. *Procedures in Cosmetic Dermatology: Cosmeceuticals*, 2nd edn. Philadelphia, PA: Saunders Elsevier, pp. 209-215.
12. Bernstein EF, Brown DB, Schwartz MD, et al. (2004) The polyhydroxy acid gluconolactone protects against ultraviolet radiation in an *in vitro* model of cutaneous photoaging. *Dermatol Surg* **30**, 1–8.
13. Charloux C, Paul M, Loisance D, Astier A. (1995) Inhibition of hydroxyl radical production by lactobionate, adenine, and tempol. *Free Radical Biol Med* **19**, 699–704.
14. Ogura R, Sugiyama M, Nishi J, Haramaki N. (1991) Mechanism of lipid radical formation following exposure of epidermal homogenate to ultraviolet light. *J Invest Dermatol* **97**(6), 1044–7.
15. Brouda I, Edison BL, Weinkauf RL, Green BA. (2010) Maltobionic acid, a powerful yet gentle skincare ingredient with multiple benefits to protect and reverse the visible signs of aging. *Am Acad of Dermatol Poster Exhibit*: Chicago, August 2010.
16. Brouda I, Edison BL, Weinkauf RL, Green BA. Lactobionic acid anti-aging mechanisms: antioxidant activity, MMP inhibition, and reduction of melanogenesis. *Am Acad of Dermatol Poster Exhibit*: Chicago, August 2010.
17. Dyer D, Dunn J, Thorpe S, et al. (1993) Accumulation of maillard reaction products in skin collagen in diabetes and aging. *J Clin Invest* **91**, 2463–9.
18. Bucala R, Cerami A. (1992) Advanced glycosylation: chemistry, biology and implications for diabetes and aging. *Adv Pharmacol* **23**, 1–4.
19. Nomoto K, Masayuki Y, Seizaburo A, et al. (2012) Skin accumulation of advanced glycation end products and lifestyle behaviors in Japanese. *J Anti-Aging Med* **9**, 165–73.
20. Schmid D, Muggli R, Zülli F. (2002) Collagen glycation and skin aging. *Cosmetics and Toiletries Manufacture Worldwide*, 1–6.
21. Ohshima H, Oyobikawa M, Tada A, et al. (2009) Melanin and facial skin fluorescence as markers of yellowish discoloration with aging. *Skin Res and Tech* **15**, 496–502.
22. Fu M, Wells-Knecht K, Blackledge J, et al. (1994) Glycation, glycoxidation, and cross-linking of collagen by glucose: kinetics, mechanisms, and inhibition of late stages of the maillard reaction. *Diabetesjournals.org*. **43**, 676–83.
23. Edelstein D, Brownlee M. (1992) Mechanistic studies of advanced glycosylation end product inhibition by aminoguanidine. *Diabetes-journals.org*. **41**, 26–9.
24. Green BA, Edison BL, Bojanowski K, Weinkauf RL. (2014) Anti-aging bionic and polyhydroxy acids reduce non-enzymatic protein glycation and skin sallowness. *J Amer Acad Dermatol* **17**(5), AB22.
25. Edison BL, Green BA, Wildnauer RH, Sigler ML. (2004) A polyhydroxy acid skin care regimen provides anti-aging effects comparable to an alpha-hydroxyacid regimen. *Cutis* **73** (suppl 2), 14–17.
26. (1998) 34th Report of the CIR expert panel: safety of alpha hydroxy acid ingredients. *Int J Toxicol* **17** (Suppl 1).
27. Johnson AW, Stoudemayer T, Kligman AM. (2000) Application of 4% and 8% glycolic acid to human skin in commercial skin creams formulated to CIR guidelines does not thin the stratum corneum or increase sensitivity to UVR. *J Cosmet Sci* **51**, 343–9.
28. Rendon MI, Effron C, Edison BL. (2007) The use of fillers and botulinum toxin type A in combination with superficial glycolic acid (AHA) peels: optimizing injection therapy with the skin-smoothing properties of peels. *Cutis* **79** (Suppl 1), 9–12.

29 Thibodeau A. (2000) Metalloproteinase inhibitors. *Cosmet Toil* **115**, 75–6.
30 Upadhya GA, Strasberg SM. (2000) Glutathione, lactobionate, and histidine: cryptic inhibitors of matrix metalloproteinases contained in University of Wisconsin and histidine/tryptophan/ketoglutarate liver preservation solutions. *Hepatology* **31**, 1115–22.
31 Van Scott EJ, Yu RJ. (1974) Control of keratinization with α-hydroxy acids and related compounds. *Arch Dermatol* **110**, 586–90.
32 Van Scott EJ, Yu RJ. (1984) Hyperkeratinization, corneocyte cohesion, and alpha hydroxyacids. *J Am Acad Dermatol* **11**, 867–79.
33 Berardesca E, Distante F, Vignoli GP, *et al.* (1997) Alpha hydroxyacids modulate stratum corneum barrier function. *Br J Dermatol* **137**, 934–8.
34 Grimes PE, Green BA, Wildnauer RH, Edison BL. (2004) The use of polyhydroxy acids (PHAs) in photoaged skin. *Cutis* **73** (Suppl 2), 3–13.
35 Van Scott EJ, Yu RJ. (1995) Actions of alpha hydroxy acids on skin compartments. *J Geriat Dermatol* **3** (Suppl A), 19–24.
36 Kim SJ, Park JH, Kim DH, *et al.* (1998) Increased in vivo collagen synthesis and *in vitro* cell proliferative effect of glycolic acid. *Dermatol Surg* **24**, 1054–8.
37 Kempers S, Katz HI, Wildnauer R, Green, B. (1998) An evaluation of the effects of an alpha hydroxy acid-blend skin cream in the cosmetic improvement of symptoms of moderate to severe xerosis, epidermolytic hyperkeratosis, and ichthyosis. *Cutis* **61**, 347–50.
38 Akamine KL, Gustafson CJ, Yentzer BA, *et al.* (2013) A double-blind, randomized clinical trial of 20% alpha/poly hydroxy acid cream to reduce scaling of lesions associated with moderate, chronic plaque psoriasis. *J Drugs Dermatol* **12**(8), 855–9.
39 Effron C, Briden ME, Green BA. (2007) Enhancing cosmetic outcomes by combining superficial glycolic acid (AHA) peels with nonablative lasers, intense pulsed light, and trichloroacetic acid peels. *Cutis* **79** (Suppl 1), 4–8.
40 Briden E, Jacobsen E, Johnson C. (2007) Combining superficial glycolic acid (AHA) peels with microdermabrasion to maximize treatment results and patient satisfaction. *Cutis* **79** (Suppl 1), 13–6.
41 Draelos ZD, Green BA, Edison BL. (2006) An evaluation of a polyhydroxy acid skincare regimen in combination with azelaic acid 15% gel in rosacea patients. *J Cosmet Dermatol* **5**, 23–9.

CHAPTER 39

The Contribution of Dietary Nutrients and Supplements to Skin Health

Helen Knaggs, Steve Wood, Doug Burke, Jan Lephart, and Jin Namkoong
Nu Skin and Pharmanex Global Research and Development, Provo, UT, USA

> **BASIC CONCEPTS**
> - Diet and oral supplementation can influence skin appearance.
> - Nutrients effective in minimizing UV skin damage include carotenoids, vitamin E (tocopherols), flavonoids, vitamin C (ascorbate) and n-3 fatty acids.
> - Selenium, zinc, and copper protect against UV-induced damage.
> - Diets containing high amounts of refined sugars may predispose skin to premature aging through the formation of advanced glycation end products (AGEs).

Introduction

The skin is one of the largest organs in the body and is exposed to many environmental factors affecting its appearance and health. Additionally, there are changes occurring over time in skin, determined by our genes and hormones. It is often said that the appearance of the skin can predict overall health or is a window to health inside of the body and there is much interest in maintaining a healthy skin appearance and function. One approach to achieve an optimal skin appearance is through the use of topical products, such as cosmetics. However, there is now a growing body of research indicating that diet and/or oral supplementation can also influence skin appearance as is reviewed in this chapter.

Historically, dietary deficiency of many of the essential nutrients (e.g. thiamine, zinc, and vitamins A and C) was first noted as a result of disruption of skin integrity or by a change in the skin's appearance [1]. Many nutrients are important co-factors in biochemical processes occurring within skin cells and therefore deficiencies are manifested by changes in the skin. For example, vitamin C was first discovered for its role in preventing scurvy and is an important co-factor for collagen synthesis [2]. Another example is riboflavin, which, when deficient, causes cracks in the corner of the mouth (angular cheilitis) as well as reddening and cracking of the lips, tongue, and mouth. Zinc deficiency may be noted in poor wound healing [3], and niacin and vitamin A deficiencies can cause dry skin or, in more extreme cases, dermatitis.

Conversely, published studies seem to show that supplementation of some of these key nutrients can result in an improvement in skin condition and this has fueled the use of vitamins and other nutrients as benefit agents in cosmetic preparations. There is obvious interest in whether dietary supplementation of these key agents can also provide benefit to skin and how this compares with providing these actives via the topical route. For example, higher intakes of vitamin C have been associated with a lower likelihood of a wrinkled appearance and skin dryness, independent of age, race, education, body mass index (BMI), and supplement use [4,5], while use of vitamin C in topical products is fraught with challenges presented by the instability of the vitamin in skincare formulations. Vitamin C has a number of different biologic roles in skin, including participating in collagen synthesis, skin regeneration, and wound healing [6].

Many nutrients are required by the skin for different functions and this chapter aims to describe some of the key nutrients and discusses the data describing the use of these nutrients when provided orally for skin benefits (Table 39.1). Below is a description of several aspects of skin health and studies of nutrients or dietary supplements that have been shown to improve skin health and appearance.

Nutrients and their role in protecting against UV-induced damage

One of the leading consumer skin concerns is skin aging, and products to delay or reverse the signs of aging are in high demand. A major contributing factor to skin aging is UV radiation, mostly from

---

Cosmetic Dermatology: Products and Procedures, Second Edition. Edited by Zoe Diana Draelos.
© 2016 John Wiley & Sons, Ltd. Published 2016 by John Wiley & Sons, Ltd.

Table 39.1 Nutrients and their skin health benefits.

Nutrient groups	Specific nutrients	
Antioxidants	Vitamin C	Vitamin C is necessary for collagen synthesis, and higher intakes are associated with better skin appearance [4]. Supplemental vitamin C and E for 3 months significantly reduced the sunburn reaction to UVB irradiation and skin DNA damage [25]
	Vitamin E	Vitamin E is a fat-soluble antioxidant that accumulates in skin cells. It protects against free radical damage. However, if cell membranes are oxidized they become more rigid leading to skin wrinkle formation. Studies have shown that supplemental vitamin E reduced levels of malondialdehyde (MDA, a marker of oxidative stress) in the skin upon exposure to UV rays [19]. Skin healing is also affected by supplemental vitamin E. In 57 patients with pressure ulcers, administration of 400 mg/day oral vitamin E promoted faster healing than the placebo [23]
	β-carotene	β-carotene can be used in the body as a source of vitamin A, which is important for skin maintenance and repair. Several studies have also demonstrated that supplemental carotenoids improve skin health
	Lycopene	Lycopene is depleted from the skin faster than β-carotene upon UV exposure [5]. Ten weeks of supplementation of tomato paste, high in lycopene, provided protection against erythema formation following UV irradiation [11,12]
	Lutein/zeaxanthin	Supplemental lutein/zeaxanthin has produced decreased UV damage and increased skin hydration and elasticity [17,18]
	Astaxanthin	Subjects given astaxanthin have shown significant improvements in elasticity, moisture content, and wrinkles [34], and those consuming astaxanthin and vitamin E exhibited significant reductions in fine wrinkles and pimples, and increased moisture levels, after 4 weeks of supplementation [35]
	CoQ10	An important antioxidant necessary for energy metabolism. Supplementation of 60 mg CoQ10 for 3 months significantly reduced wrinkle grade (depth and area of wrinkles) and improved skin properties [40]
	α-lipoic acid	A potent antioxidant that has benefit to water-soluble and fat-soluble portions of cells. In a preclinical study, α-lipoic acid has been shown to reduce advanced glycation end products (AGEs) [41]
	Combinations of antioxidants	Subjects given β-carotene, lycopene, vitamin E, vitamin C and experienced significant protection from sun damage [50]. Consumption of lycopene, lutein, β-carotene, α-tocopherol and selenium improved skin surface [8]
Fish oil/omega-3 fatty acids	Eicosapentaenoic acid (EPA) and docosahexaenoic acid (DHA)	Dietary consumption of fish oil is known to modulate the lipid inflammatory mediator balance and therefore is valuable in the treatment of inflammatory skin disorders. Consumption of EPA and DHA totalling 3–4 g/day for up to 3 months reduced erythema upon UV exposure in several studies [5]
Polyphenol and flavonoids	Green tea polyphenols	Polyphenols protect against free radical damage. Forty-one women aged 25–75 years given 300 mg (green tea extract containing 97% pure polyphenols) twice daily for 2 years experienced fewer fine wrinkles and telangiectasias and overall less solar damage compared with baseline and the control group [37]
	Grape seed extract and resveratrol	When subjects received 100 mg oligomeric proanthocyanidins along with vitamin C and SiO_2 and were then exposed to UV rays, they experienced less erythema and increased skin hydration [51]
	Pycnogenol	A French maritime pine bark extract with a potent free radical scavenger, which contains 65–75% procyanidins, increased skin hydration and improved skin elasticity [45]
Vitamin D		Vitamin D is a compound that is formed/activated in the skin upon sun exposure [52]. Unfortunately, there have not yet been any studies on skin health and supplementation
Minerals	Zinc	Zinc serves as a co-factor for many important enzymes in the body. Some of the best known are important for skin healing [3, 53]
	Copper	Copper is an important co-factor for elastin, the support structure for skin
	Selenium	Selenium is a component of the antioxidant enzyme glutathione peroxidase. Supplemental selenium and copper have shown significant protection (versus placebo) against UV-induced cell damage [30]
Negative nutritional components	Diet high in fats and carbohydrates	Diets high in fats and carbohydrates have been shown to increase the likelihood of a wrinkled appearance [4]

the sun. Both UVA and UVB rays generate harmful free radicals in the skin contributing to photodamage, leading to the production of fine lines and wrinkles, and, in extreme cases of sun exposure, sunburn and skin cancers. With sun exposure and no or inadequate sun protection, the skin depends solely on its internal or endogenous defenses such as melanin for protection. Dietary micronutrients which act as antioxidants can help to protect against the free radical formation induced by UV irradiation. Some of the most widely studied nutrients that have been effective in minimizing UV damage occurring within skin include carotenoids, vitamin E (tocopherols), flavonoids, vitamin C (ascorbate), and n-3 fatty acids [7,8].

Currently, there is perhaps the most evidence to support the role of carotenoids in providing skin benefits, especially for UV damage. Topically, vitamin A has been shown to reduce the signs of photodamage and is most effective in the acid form available on prescription as Retin A® (Ortho Dermatologics, USA) (retinoic acid). β-carotene, lycopene, lutein, and zeaxanthin are major carotenoids in human blood and tissues, and are highly effective at quenching singlet molecular oxygen formed during photooxidative processes. In fact, carotenoids from a normal, unsupplemented diet accumulate in the skin [9] and confer a measurable photoprotective benefit (at least in lightly pigmented Caucasian skin) that is directly linked to tissue concentrations [10]. Dietary intake of tomato paste, which contains a number of carotenoids, including β-carotene, lycopene, lutein, and zeaxanthin, has been shown to provide photo-protective activity [11,12]. Dietary supplementation with 25 mg total carotenoids a day for 12 weeks to healthy volunteers significantly diminished erythema upon UV irradiation given at week 8. This effect was enhanced when the same regimen was given with 335 mg/day (500 IU) RRR-α-tocopherol [13]. A 12-week supplementation of β-carotene from *Dunaliella* algae was also effective in suppressing UV-induced erythema given at a dose of 25 mg/day to healthy volunteers [13]. It is thought that other carotenoids such as lycopene act synergistically with β-carotene to protect the skin from UV irradiation [5]. In humans, it was shown that lycopene is depleted from the skin faster than β-carotene upon UV exposure [14], suggesting a primary role of lycopene in mitigating oxidative damage in tissues, and an important role in the defense mechanism against adverse effects of UV irradiation on the skin. In fact, when a single UV light exposure of three times minimal erythemal dose (MED) was administered to human skin, lycopene concentrations decreased rapidly but skin β-carotene concentrations declined slowly.

Lutein and zeaxanthin (LZ) are found in dark, leafy, green and yellow vegetables, and there is evidence that they can provide protection against UV-induced damage. The presence of these carotenoids in the skin following dietary and oral supplementation has been demonstrated [15,16], along with a benefit in reducing UV damage. Forty female subjects aged 25–50 years were assigned to receive one of the following groups: placebo, oral only, topical only or both oral and topical, twice daily for 12 weeks. Dosage for oral supplementation was 5 mg lutein, 0.3 mg zeaxanthin; and dosage for topical application was 50 ppm lutein and 2 ppm zeaxanthin. All active treatments reduced UV-light induced malondialdehyde (MDA: a measure of lipid peroxidation) production, with the topical and oral and topical treatments producing similar results, and the combined treatment producing the greatest reduction. Other benefits were also noticed in this study-there were measurable increases in skin lipids produced by all treatments, with the oral regimen producing significantly greater increases than the topical treatment. Additionally, hydration was increased similarly by oral and topical treatments, and significantly more with the combination treatment. All differences were significant for all treatments at week 12 compared with placebo, and for all time points after week 2 [17,18].

The benefit of tocopherols in photoprotection has also been studied. Vitamin E is commonly associated with protecting cell membranes from oxidative damage and administration of oral 400 IU/day vitamin E significantly reduced MDA production but no other measures of oxidative stress in the skin or sensitivity to UV damage [19]. The production of sebum containing dietary vitamin E by the sebaceous glands was shown to be the primary delivery route for sources of tocopherols to the skin surface [20].

Researchers have found that supplemental flavonoids for 10–12 weeks in humans protects against UV-induced erythema [21], although this is related to dose, with high doses appearing necessary to provide benefits. In one study, a cocoa supplement with 329 mg total flavanols produced an increased microcirculation in the skin, while the same cocoa drink containing 27 mg/day total flavanols had no benefit. Another study compared two groups of women ingesting either a high (329 mg/day) or low (27 mg/day) flavanol cocoa powder dissolved in 100 mL water for 12 weeks. The production of erythema following a 1.25 MED UV ray dose was reduced significantly by 15% and 25% at 6 and 12 weeks, respectively, in the high dose supplemented group. No such benefit was observed for the group receiving the lower dose of flavanols. In addition, in the high dose group, but not the low-flavanol group, increases in blood flow to cutaneous and subcutaneous tissues were observed, as well as increases in skin thickness, skin density, and skin hydration, along with a significant decrease in skin roughness and scaling [22].

Antioxidant combinations can provide added protection beyond single antioxidants alone in preventing UV damage. For example, in healthy volunteers given a carotenoid blend (25 mg/day) for 12 weeks there was a significant decrease in skin reddening following blue light exposure to the skin, whereas combining this with 500 IU vitamin E had an even more dramatic decrease after only 8 weeks of consumption [8]. Interestingly, in healthy individuals on a normal diet, little benefit was shown with individual antioxidants like vitamin E in preventing UV-induced skin damage [23]. Data show that a combination of supplemental antioxidants that most closely mimics a diet rich in antioxidants can provide a photoprotective effect against sun damage [24]. Administration of 1 g vitamin C and 500 mg vitamin E (as D-α-tocopherol) for 3 months to human volunteers significantly reduced the sunburn reaction to UVB irradiation as measured by a reduction in thymine dimer formation by 43% indicating a reduction in skin DNA damage, and an increased in MED by 41% [25].

Oral intake of lipids and lipid-soluble vitamins has long proved beneficial for skin. One study observed a photoprotective effect of a diet higher in olive oil on the skin [26]. Some evidence suggests that n-3 fatty acids (FA) may also be effective in protection against UV-induced skin cancers and photoaging, in part brought about by the reduction of UV-induced release of cytokines and other inflammatory mediators in a variety of skin cell types [27,28]. In humans, supplemental omega-3 FA have been shown to significantly increase the UVR-mediated erythema threshold and reduce the level of proinflammatory, immunosuppressive prostaglandin E2 levels from UVB irradiation [29]. Fish oil supplements, which provide eicosapentaenoic and docosahexanoic acid, have also shown a photoprotective effect [5, 7].

Selenium, zinc, and copper have also been shown to provide benefit and protect against UV-induced damage. This could be because these nutrients are critical components for the activity of several enzymes associated with skin repair following UV irradiation (e.g. matrix metalloproteinase) [30]. A combination of 200 µg selenium and 4 mg copper alone, or with 14 mg vitamin E, 3.6 mg niacin, 0.4 mg pyridoxine, 0.12 mg thiamine, 0.08 mg riboflavin plus 9000 IU retinol per day during meals for 3 weeks gave significant protection (versus placebo) against UV-induced cell damage in the form of sunburn cells, but did not reduce UV-induced erythema. This study was performed on 16 healthy Caucasian subjects aged 20–37 years and the combined supplements gave the strongest effect [30].

Nutrients and their role in improving skin appearancwe

The benefit of nutrients in protecting the skin from damage was discussed in the previous section [4–33]. Cumulative photodamage results in the appearance of fine lines and wrinkles on the face, as well as changes in pigmentation and skin dryness and roughness. There is also evidence to support the use of oral nutrients in improving the signs of photodamage, once formed, and in improving overall skin condition.

The carotenoid astaxanthin is found in plants and algae and provides pink-orange color to shellfish and salmon. Supplementation of astaxanthin produced significant improvements in pre-existing skin wrinkles, and also improved skin elasticity and transepidermal water loss (TEWL) [34]. Another study with 16 female subjects (mean age 40 years) with dry skin conditions were given either 2 mg astaxanthin (as 40 mg AstaReal®, Fuji, Toyama, Japan) and 4 mg natural tocotrienols or a control supplement for 4 weeks. Treated subjects exhibited significant reductions in fine wrinkles and pimples, and had increased skin moisture levels. These parameters contributed to the individual assessments that reported reduced swelling under the eyes, improved elasticity, and "better skin feel." Subjects on the placebo did not improve and generally worsened during this time [35].

Vitamin C is an important co-factor for the enzymes involved in collagen synthesis and it has also been shown to provide benefit in protecting against signs of photodamage. Using data from the National Health and Nutrition Examination Survey (NHANES I), associations between dietary nutrient intakes and signs of skin aging in 4025 women aged 40–74 years were compared. High dietary intakes of vitamin C were associated with a lower likelihood of senile skin dryness and a reduced wrinkled appearance. In fact, an increase consumption of vitamin C, by 1 log unit, was associated with an 11% reduction in the odds of a wrinkled appearance and a 7% reduction in the odds of senile dryness, independent of age, race, education, BMI, other supplement use, sun exposure, menopausal status, family income, energy intake, or physical activity [4]. This was an important study as it was the first to directly relate dietary intakes, rather than supplementation, of vitamin C with skin aging and showed that a diet high in foods supplying vitamin C can lead to a lower prevalence of an aged appearance. Other dietary factors were also studied: a lower intake of vitamin A, lower protein, and higher thiamine intakes were also linked to a wrinkled appearance. Conversely, higher intakes of fat and carbohydrates were associated with an increased chance of wrinkled skin appearance and skin atrophy. Thus, it appears that one's appearance may be an indicator of overall health status because balanced nutrition is essential, not only to prevent chronic diseases such as cardiovascular disease, certain cancers, and diabetes [31], but also to maintain skin health and ensure normal cellular function. It is a bold statement, but this evidence suggests that looking "old for one's age" may also reflect and/or be associated with an increased risk of disease and mortality [32,33].

Similarly, soy isoflavones have been shown to provide a significant improvement in fine wrinkles and skin elasticity, compared with a placebo group [36] after 12 weeks' supplementation. This study showed that the benefits were evident in women in their late thirties and early forties. Another study examined the effect of green tea on skin condition. Forty-one women aged 25–75 years were given 300 mg of a proprietary green tea extract containing 97% tea polyphenols or a placebo twice daily for 2 years. At 24 months, fine wrinkles were significantly reduced compared to baseline, and at 12 months, telangiectasias were significantly reduced in the green tea supplemented group, but not the placebo group. At 24 months compared with 12 months, overall solar damage was reduced over time for the green tea supplemented group but not in the placebo group [37].

Sun damage to skin does not need to have been severe for it to respond to oral supplements within a relatively short period of time. Eight weeks is common for topical treatments to produce a noticeable difference in skin condition, which includes an improvement in moderate photodamage with 8 weeks' supplementation with key nutrients. For example, one study investigated 30 dry-skinned women aged 48–59 years with moderate xerosis and photoaging. The group was randomized to receive either a topical nanocolloidal gel containing 0.5 mg α-lipoic acid and 15 mg melatonin/emblica along with a nutritional supplement containing 3 mg lutein, 2.5 mg α-lipoic acid, 45 mg ascorbic acid, and 5 mg tocopherol. All treatments were given twice daily for 2 months. Dietary supplements, but not the placebo, significantly reduced blood free radical activity compared with baseline. Skin hydration was significantly increased in all groups compared with baseline and placebo. An increase in superficial skin lipids was found for the treatments, with all being significantly different from baseline. Significantly greater effects were seen with the combined versus individual treatments, and all treatments than the placebo. Lipid peroxidation at weeks 2, 4, and 8 on the skin was significantly greater with the control group [38].

A study of topical application of coenzyme Q10 (CoQ10) for 3 months showed reduced depth and area of wrinkles around the eye area of 20 elderly volunteers, compared with the vehicle, which was applied around the opposite eye. There was a 27% reduction in mean peak to valley depth of the skin and a 26% reduction in Rq values measured on the PRIMOS, compared with controls [39]. Similar findings were reported following daily oral supplementation of 60 mg CoQ10 for 3 months [40].

Diets containing high amounts of refined sugars may predispose skin to premature aging through the formation of advanced glycation end products (AGEs). Glycation is a non-enzymatic reaction between amino groups on proteins (i.e. lysine) and reducing sugars (i.e. fructose). This reaction creates cross-links in the skin and once these reactions occur they disrupt normal function and predispose skin to oxidation or premature aging in the extracellular matrix of the dermis. For example the cross-linkages between dermal molecules cause the loss of elasticity or other properties of the dermis observed during aging. Some preclinical studies have shown that supplemental nutrients such as α-lipoic acid may prevent the detrimental effects AGEs to the skin [41]. Interestingly, some researchers have shown that AGEs may actually be photosensitizers to cause more severe DNA damage to the skin from phototoxicity which ultimately causes accelerated skin aging and increased risk of skin cancer. Future studies will help establish nutritional strategies to prevent the formation and detrimental effects of AGEs. Carnosine is a naturally occurring antioxidant, which has been shown to inhibit AGE formation *in vitro*. In a recent clinical trial, significant improvements in the skin were observed by a combination of dietary supplements which included carnosine and vitamin E [42]. After 3 months of supplementation, skin surface structure improved and showed more smoothing.

In summary, there is a growing body of literature that demonstrates that oral nutrients not only protect the skin from UV damage and reduce free radical damage, but also can improve skin condition after the effects of sun damage has formed.

Nutrients shown to provide additional skin benefits

As well as protecting from UV and improving photodamage, data exist to show that diet and nutritional supplementation can provide many other benefits for skin. Ingestion of 5 mg lutein and 0.3 mg zeaxanthin twice daily for 12 weeks was shown to improve skin moisture and elasticity [17,18] and this may have resulted from an increase in skin lipids which was demonstrated during the study. Increases in skin lipids and improvements in skin smoothness and elasticity have been reported from previous studies of orally ingested antioxidants [38, 43].

Another nutritional supplement with improved skin elasticity and hydration is pycnogenol. Pycnogenol is an extract of French maritime pine bark, with a potent free radical scavenging activity. It is also known to regenerate the active forms of vitamin C and E [44]. Oral supplementation which included 75 mg pycnogenol for 12 weeks resulted in increased skin hydration at 6 weeks and improved skin elasticity in 6 and 12 weeks [45].

A combination of nutrients was also found to provide significant skin changes. Thirty-nine healthy people with normal skin were divided into three groups and given 3 mg lycopene, 3 mg lutein, 4.8 mg β-carotene, 10 mg α-tocopherol, and 75 μg selenium per day, a similar supplement with double the amount of lycopene without lutein, or a placebo. A significant increase of skin density and thickness, as determined by ultrasound, along with improved skin surface of decreased roughness and skin scaling (evaluated by Visioscan) was found for both antioxidant groups but not the placebo [8]. In a 14-week study with a blend of soy isoflavone, lycopene, vitamin C, vitamin E and fish oil also demonstrated the skin improvement, such as reduced skin roughness [46]. Further evaluation with skin biopsies indicated increase in collagen quantity and quality in some individuals.

Nutrients and their potential in improving dermatologic disorders and wound healing

Skin disorders that have an inflammatory component (e.g. psoriasis and eczema) and are manifested by dry and flaky skin have responded to topical omega-3 polyunsaturated fatty acid supplementation [47] and these nutrients may therefore offer a therapeutic benefit when given orally.

There is also evidence to show that oral supplementation can assist in healing. In 57 patients with pressure ulcers, administration of 400 mg/day vitamin E provided faster healing of the ulcer compared with placebo. When 10 females with lichen sclerosis took 300–1200 IU/day vitamin E, five improved markedly, two moderately, and three slightly [23]. Zinc deficiency has been associated with delayed wound healing and roughness of the skin [3, 24, 48]. Mixtures of tocopherol and CoQ10 have proved to be beneficial for skin healing [49].

Conclusions

An individual's appearance has been regarded as an indicator of overall health, wellbeing, and age. In fact, it might perhaps be an indicator of life expectancy [32,33]. Nutrients provided in the diet or through dietary supplements can provide benefits to overall skin health and appearance, and in some cases can reverse a wrinkled or aged appearance. There is also evidence that providing several nutrients together is more beneficial than providing single nutrients in isolation. The benefits of nutrients, such as carotenoids, flavonoids, CoQ10, α-lipoic acid, minerals, and omega-3 fatty acids are related to their antioxidant potential, but significant other benefits are also provided, for example nutrients often serve as co-factors for key metabolic enzymes in skin (e.g. vitamin C and collagen production).

References

1 Boelsma E, van de Vijver LP, Goldbohm RA, et al. (2003) Human skin condition and its associations with nutrient concentrations in serum and diet. *Am J Clin Nutr*; 77, 348–55.
2 Miller SJ. (1989) Nutritional deficiency and the skin. *J Am Acad Dermatol* 21: 1–30.
3 Corbo MD, Lam J. (2013) Zinc deficiency and its management in the pediatric population: a literature review and proposed etiologic classification. *J Am Acad Dermatol* 69, 616–624 e611.
4 Cosgrove MC, Franco OH, Granger SP, et al. (2007) Dietary nutrient intakes and skin-aging appearance among middle-aged American women. *Am J Clin Nutr* 86, 1225–31.
5 Boelsma E, Hendriks HF, Roza L. (2001) Nutritional skin care: health effects of micronutrients and fatty acids. *Am J Clin Nutr* 73, 853–64.
6 Catani MV, Savini I, Rossi A, et al. (2005) Biological role of vitamin C in keratinocytes. *Nutr Rev* 63, 81–90.
7 Sies H, Stahl W. (2004) Nutritional protection against skin damage from sunlight. *Annu Rev Nutr* 24, 173–200.
8 Heinrich U, Tronnier H, Stahl W, et al. (2006) Antioxidant supplements improve parameters related to skin structure in humans. *Skin Pharmacol Physiol* 19, 224–31.
9 Darvin ME, Patzelt A, Knorr F, et al. (2008) One-year study on the variation of carotenoid antioxidant substances in living human skin: influence of dietary supplementation and stress factors. *J Biomed Opt* 13, 044028.
10 Stahl W, Heinrich U, Aust O, et al. (2006) Lycopene-rich products and dietary photoprotection. *Photochem Photobiol Sci* 5, 238–42.
11 Stahl W, Heinrich U, Wiseman S, et al. (2001) Dietary tomato paste protects against ultraviolet light-induced erythema in humans. *J Nutr* 131, 1449–51.
12 Sies H, Stahl W. (2003) Non-nutritive bioactive constituents of plants: lycopene, lutein and zeaxanthin. *Int J Vitam Nutr Res* 73, 95–100.
13 Stahl W, Heinrich U, Jungmann H, et al. (2000) Carotenoids and carotenoids plus vitamin E protect against ultraviolet light-induced erythema in humans. *Am J Clin Nutr* 71, 795–8.
14 Ribaya-Mercado JD, Garmyn M, Gilchrest BA, et al. Skin lycopene is destroyed preferentially over beta-carotene during ultraviolet irradiation in humans. *J Nutr* (1995) 125, 1854–9.
15 Wingerath T, Sies H, Stahl W. (1998) Xanthophyll esters in human skin. *Arch Biochem Biophys* 355, 271–4.
16 Lee EH, Faulhaber D, Hanson KM, et al. (2004) Dietary lutein reduces ultraviolet radiation-induced inflammation and immunosuppression. *J Invest Dermatol* 122, 510–17.
17 Palombo P, Fabrizi G, Ruocco V, et al. (2007) Beneficial long-term effects of combined oral/topical antioxidant treatment with the carotenoids lutein and zeaxanthin on human skin: a double-blind, placebo-controlled study. *Skin Pharmacol Physiol* 20, 199–210.
18 Roberts RL, Green J, Lewis B. (2009) Lutein and zeaxanthin in eye and skin health. *Clin Dermatol* 27, 195–201.
19 Thiele JJ, Ekanayake-Mudiyanselage S. (2007) Vitamin E in human skin: organ-specific physiology and considerations for its use in dermatology. *Mol Aspects Med* 28, 646–67.
20 Thiele JJ, Weber SU, Packer L. (1999) Sebaceous gland secretion is a major physiologic route of vitamin E delivery to skin. *J Invest Dermatol* 113, 1006–10.
21 Stahl W, Sies H. (2007) Carotenoids and flavonoids contribute to nutritional protection against skin damage from sunlight. *Mol Biotechnol* 37, 26–30.
22 Neukam K, Stahl W, Tronnier H, et al. (2007) Consumption of flavanol-rich cocoa acutely increases microcirculation in human skin. *Eur J Nutr* 46, 53–6.
23 Tebbe B. (2001) Relevance of oral supplementation with antioxidants for prevention and treatment of skin disorders. *Skin Pharmacol Appl Skin Physiol* 14, 296–302.
24 Richelle M, Sabatier M, Steiling H, et al. (2006) Skin bioavailability of dietary vitamin E, carotenoids, polyphenols, vitamin C, zinc and selenium. *Br J Nutr* 96, 227–38.
25 Placzek M, Gaube S, Kerkmann U, et al. (2005) Ultraviolet B-induced DNA damage in human epidermis is modified by the antioxidants ascorbic acid and D-alpha-tocopherol. *J Invest Dermatol* 124, 304–307.
26 Purba MB, Kouris-Blazos A, Wattanapenpaiboon N, et al. (2001) Skin wrinkling: can food make a difference? *J Am Coll Nutr* 20, 71–80.
27 Jackson MJ, Jackson MJ, McArdle F, et al. (2002) Effects of micronutrient supplements on u.v.-induced skin damage. *Proc Nutr Soc* 61, 187–9.
28 Rhodes LE, Durham BH, Fraser WD, et al. (1995) Dietary fish oil reduces basal and ultraviolet B-generated PGE2 levels in skin and increases the threshold to provocation of polymorphic light eruption. *J Invest Dermatol* 105, 532–5.
29 Black HS, Rhodes LE. (2006) The potential of omega-3 fatty acids in the prevention of non-melanoma skin cancer. *Cancer Detect Prev* 30, 224–32.
30 la Ruche G, Cesarini JP. (1991) Protective effect of oral selenium plus copper associated with vitamin complex on sunburn cell formation in human skin. *Photodermatol Photoimmunol Photomed* 8, 232–35.
31 Willett WC. (2002) Balancing life-style and genomics research for disease prevention. *Science* 296, 695–8.
32 Purba MB, Kouris-Blazos A, Wattanapenpaiboon N, et al. (2001) Can skin wrinkling in a site that has received limited sun exposure be used as a marker of health status and biological age? *Age Ageing* 30, 227–34.
33 Christensen K, Iachina M, Rexbye H, et al. (2004) "Looking old for your age": genetics and mortality. *Epidemiology* 15, 251–2.
34 Tominaga K, Hongo N, Karato M, et al. (2012) Cosmetic benefits of astaxanthin on humans subjects. *Acta Biochim Pol* 59, 43–7.
35 Yamashita E. (2002) Cosmetic benefit of dietary supplements containing astaxanthin and tocotrienol on human skin. *Food Style 21* 216, 112–17.
36 Izumi T, Saito M, Obata A, et al. (2007) Oral intake of soy isoflavone aglycone improves the aged skin of adult women. *J Nutr Sci Vitaminol (Tokyo)* 53, 57–62.

37 Janjua R, Munoz C, Gorell E, *et al.* (2009) A two-year, double-blind, randomized placebo-controlled trial of oral green tea polyphenols on the long-term clinical and histologic appearance of photoaging skin. *Dermatol Surg* **35**, 1057–65.

38 Morganti P, Bruno C, Guarneri F, *et al.* (2002) Role of topical and nutritional supplement to modify the oxidative stress. *Int J Cosmet Sci* **24**, 331–9.

39 Hoppe U, Bergemann J, Diembeck W, *et al.* (1999) Coenzyme Q10, a cutaneous antioxidant and energizer. *Biofactors* **9**, 371–8.

40 Ashida Y, Kuwazuru S, Nakashima M, *et al.* (2004) Effect of coenzyme Q10 as a supplement on wrinkle reduction. *Food Style 21* **8**, 1–4.

41 hirunavukkarasu V, Nandhini AT, Anuradha CV. (2004) Fructose diet-induced skin collagen abnormalities are prevented by lipoic acid. *Exp Diabesity Res* **5**, 237–44.

42 Babizhayev MA, Deyev AI, Savel'yeva EL, *et al.* (2012) Skin beautification with oral non-hydrolized versions of carnosine and carcinine: Effective therapeutic management and cosmetic skincare solutions against oxidative glycation and free-radical production as a causal mechanism of diabetic complications and skin aging. *J Dermatolog Treat* **23**, 345–84.

43 Segger D, Schonlau F. Supplementation with Evelle improves skin smoothness and elasticity in a double-blind, placebo-controlled study with 62 women. *J Dermatolog Treat* (2004) **15**, 222–6.

44 Draelos ZD. (2010) Nutrition and enhancing youthful-appearing skin. *Clin Dermatol* **28**, 400–408.

45 Marini A, Grether-Beck S, Jaenicke T, *et al.* (2012) Pycnogenol(R) effects on skin elasticity and hydration coincide with increased gene expressions of collagen type I and hyaluronic acid synthase in women. *Skin Pharmacol Physiol* **25**, 86–92.

46 Jenkins G, Wainwright LJ, Holland R, *et al.* (2014) Wrinkle reduction in post-menopausal women consuming a novel oral supplement: a double-blind placebo-controlled randomized study. *Int J Cosmet Sci* **36**, 22–31.

47 Henneicke-von Zepelin HH, Mrowietz U, Farber L, *et al.* (1993) Highly purified omega-3-polyunsaturated fatty acids for topical treatment of psoriasis. Results of a double-blind, placebo-controlled multicentre study. *Br J Dermatol* **129**, 713–17.

48 Lansdown AB, Mirastschijski U, Stubbs N, *et al.* Zinc in wound healing: theoretical, experimental, and clinical aspects. *Wound Repair Regen* (2007) **15**, 2–16.

49 de Luca C, Deeva I, Mikhal'Chik E, *et al.* (2007) Beneficial effects of pro-/antioxidant-based nutraceuticals in the skin rejuvenation techniques. *Cell Mol Biol (Noisy-le-grand)* **53**, 94–101.

50 Cesarini JP, Michel L, Maurette JM, *et al.* (2003) Immediate effects of UV radiation on the skin: modification by an antioxidant complex containing carotenoids. *Photodermatol Photoimmunol Photomed* **19**, 182–9.

51 Hughes-Formella B, Wunderlich O, Williams R. (2007) Anti-inflammatory and skin-hydrating properties of a dietary supplement and topical formulations containing oligomeric proanthocyanidins. *Skin Pharmacol Physiol* **20**, 43–9.

52 Holick MF, Chen TC, Lu Z, *et al.* (2007) Vitamin D and skin physiology: a D-lightful story. *J Bone Miner Res* **22** Suppl 2, V28–33.

53 Rostan EF, DeBuys HV, Madey DL, *et al.* (2002) Evidence supporting zinc as an important antioxidant for skin. *Int J Dermatol* **41**, 606–611.

SECTION 2 **Injectable Anti-aging Techniques**

CHAPTER 40
Botulinum Toxins

J. Daniel Jensen,[1] Scott R. Freeman,[2] and Joel L. Cohen[3,4]
[1]Scripps Clinic, Bighorn Mohs Surgery and Dermatology Center, La Jolla, CA, USA
[2]Sunrise Dermatology, Mobile, AL, USA
[3]AboutSkin Dermatology and DermSurgery, Englewood, CO, USA
[4]University of Colorado at Denver, Aurora, CO, USA

BASIC CONCEPTS

- Botulinum toxins are high molecular weight protein complexes that are secreted by clostridial bacteria. These neuromodulator agents exert their effects by binding to and cleaving specific proteins in the presynaptic nerve terminus, thus preventing release of acetylcholine and focally preventing nerve conduction.
- Currently, there are three type A botulinum toxins approved in the USA for cosmetic use. Botox® is FDA approved for use in the glabella and crow's feet. Dysport® and Xeomin® are approved for treatment of the glabellar frown lines.
- In many other anatomic areas, injectable botulinum toxins have a favorable safety profile and are effective in treating the upper, mid, and lower face, as well as several regions of focal hyperhidrosis (axillary, palmar, plantar, facial). They have all been used worldwide to treat other medical conditions including strabismus, blepharospasm, and cervical dystonia.
- Injection-related complications for esthetic regions can frequently be avoided with good technique and a detailed understanding of the regional anatomy.

Introduction

Botulinum toxins are produced by the Gram-positive, spore-forming anaerobe *Clostridium botulinum*, and cause chemical denervation by suppressing the release of the neurotransmitter acetylcholine from the axon terminals of peripheral nerves. There are seven distinct subtypes of botulinum toxin (A–G), with types A and B being the only clinically relevant subtypes at this time. Currently, there are three botulinum neurotoxin type A (BoNTA) and one botulinum neurotoxin B (BoNTB) toxins available for human use in the USA. Botox® (onabotulinumtoxinA, Allergan, Inc., Irvine, CA, USA), Dysport® (abobotulinumtoxinA, Medicis Pharmaceuticals Corp., Scottsdale, AZ, USA), and Xeomin® (incobotulinumtoxinA, Merz, Frankfurt, Germany) comprise the type A toxins currently available.

Botox is currently US Food and Drug Administration (FDA) approved for several non-cosmetic therapeutic indications (including blepharospasm, strabismus and axillary hyperhidrosis), as well as for cosmetic use for temporary improvement of moderate to severe glabellar lines (approved 2002) and lateral canthal rhytides/crow's feet (2013). Dysport® is FDA approved for treatment of cervical dystonia and has cosmetic indication for temporary improvement of moderate to severe glabellar frown lines (2009). Xeomin®, the newest to market type A toxin in the US, is FDA indicated for treatment of cervical dystonia and blepharospasm, as well as for temporary improvement of moderate to severe glabellar frown lines (2011). Myobloc® (Rimabotulinum toxin, Solstice Pharmaceuticals, South San Francisco, CA, USA), a type B botulinum toxin, is currently only approved for the therapeutic treatment of cervical dystonia (2000).

While the various type A botulinum toxins are FDA approved for cosmetic use in the glabella (all) and crow's feet (Botox only), they are used off-label in various other facial sites as well. Additionally, while Botox is also FDA approved for axillary hyperhidrosis, Botox as well as Dysport and Xeomin are also used off-label for hyperhidrosis of the palms, soles, face, and scalp. Treatment doses are not interchangeable for any of the botulinum products (even among the strains of type A toxin) and all references to BoNTA dose, unless otherwise stated in this chapter, refer to and are specific for Botox.

Cosmetic Dermatology: Products and Procedures, Second Edition. Edited by Zoe Diana Draelos.
© 2016 John Wiley & Sons, Ltd. Published 2016 by John Wiley & Sons, Ltd.

Clostridial bacteria secrete high molecular weight protein complexes that include three key proteins: a 150-kDa toxin, a non-toxin hemagglutinin protein, and a non-toxin non-hemagglutinin protein. The non-toxin proteins may provide the toxin complex protection against temperature or enzymatic denaturation [1], or at least that has been a historical perspective by some of the formulators. The 150-kDa toxin is cleaved by bacterial proteases to form a di-chain composed of a 100-kDa heavy chain and a 50-kDa light chain. Disulfide and non-covalent bonds link the heavy and light chains, and both chains are required for neurotoxicity [1].

In 1987, Canadian ophthalmologist Jean Carruthers recognized the cosmetic potential of BoNTA. While treating patients for benign essential blepharospasm, Dr. Carruthers noted that several patients treated for blepharospasm had significant improvement of dynamic rhytides in the periocular region. Following this observation, the husband and wife team of Drs. Alastair and Jean Carruthers began more systematic studies of BoNTA for cosmetic indications. In 1991, the Carruthers reported their initial findings of cosmetic treatment with BoNTA at North American dermatology and ophthalmology meetings. After initiating clinical trials, their first publication on this topic was in 1992, demonstrating the safe and effective treatment of dynamic rhytides in the glabella with BoNTA [2]. After over a decade of off-label cosmetic use in the USA, BoNTA (Botox) was approved specifically for the treatment of glabellar rhytides in 2002. Currently, off-label cosmetic uses continue to expand with regions of treatment encompassing not only the forehead and periocular areas, but also the mid-face, lower face, neck and décolleté.

Botox and other BoNTA toxins are also widely used worldwide for medical and therapeutic purposes, including the treatment of hyperhidrosis, headaches, spasticity disorders, and depression. This chapter highlights both traditional and newer cosmetic applications of BoNTA.

Mechanism of action

The process of chemical denervation requires that the neurotoxin heavy chain bind the synaptic vesicle glycoprotein 2 (SV2) on the presynaptic nerve terminal. This process leads to toxin–receptor complex endocytosis with subsequent toxin light chain release through vesicle lysis [3]. All toxins cause chemical denervation by suppressing the release of acetylcholine from the axon terminals of peripheral motor nerves. After vesicle lysis occurs within the axon terminus, toxin light chains ultimately prevent neurotransmission by cleaving specific protein isoforms necessary for the docking, fusion, and release of acetylcholine from this nerve terminus. Toxins A, C, and E cleave synaptosomal-associated protein 25 (SNAP-25) and toxins B, D, F, and G cleave vesicle associated membrane protein (VAMP, also known as synaptobrevin) [1]. Muscle paralysis typically occurs within approximately 3–7 days, and synaptic regeneration reverses the paralytic effect within 3–6 months [3].

Neurotoxin physical characteristics

The neurotoxin-protein complex size of Botox is approximately 900 kDa and the most common vial size used is 100 units, though it is available in 50 units as well. One vial contains 5 ng of toxin. One unit (U) is standardized to equal the median amount necessary to kill 50% of female Swiss-Webster mice after intraperitoneal injection (LD50) [3,4,5]. Botox is a vacuum-dried product, and in addition to 100 U of toxin, each vial contains 500 µg albumin and 900 µg sodium chloride [1,5]. Typical cosmetic doses of Botox range from 10 to 60 units, depending on the number of areas treated in one session. The complex size of Dysport ranges from 500–900 kDa, and one vial contains 300 units of freeze-dried abobotulinum toxin. In addition, each 300 unit vial contains 125 µg of human serum albumin and 2.5 mg lactose. Xeomin is a vacuum-dried 150 kDa toxin protein free from biologically inert complexing proteins. Xeomin is packaged in 50 and 100 unit vials, and in addition to the active toxin, each 100 unit vial also contains 1 mg human serum albumin and 4.7 mg sucrose [6]. Product characteristics of Botox compared with the other FDA-approved neurotoxins are provided in Table 40.1.

Product stability

Package inserts indicate that Botox and Dysport should be stored at 2–8 °C and away from light. Xeomin is stable at room temperature (20 to 25°C), but may also be stored at refrigerator (2 to 8°C) or freezer (−20 to −10°C) temperatures for up to 36 months. Once a vial of Botox or Xeomin has been reconstituted, product should be stored at 2–8°C and should be used within 24 hours. Dysport, once reconstituted, should be stored at 2–8°C

Table 40.1 Botulinum toxin comparison.[1]

	Botox[3]	Dysport[4]	Xeomin[5]	Myobloc[6]
Serotype	A	A	A	B
Molecular weight (kDa)	900	500–900	150	700
FDA[2] approved for cosmetic use?	Yes	Yes	Yes	No
Protein weight per vial (ng)	5	5		25, 50, or 100
Units per vial	100	300	50, 100	5000
pH (after reconstitution)	7.4	7.4	7.4	5.6
Target	SNAP-25[7]	SNAP-25	SNAP-25	VAMP[8]

[1]Dosages are not equivalent between products.
[2]Food and Drug Administration.
[3]Allergan, Inc., Irvine, CA, USA.
[4]Medicis, Scottsdale, AZ, USA
[5]Merz, Frankfurt, Germany
[6]Solstice Pharmaceuticals, South San Francisco, CA, USA. Marketed as Neurobloc outside of the USA.
[7]Synaptosomal-associated protein 25 (SNAP-25).
[8]Vesicle-associated membrane protein (synaptobrevin).

and administered within 4 hours. However, recent studies suggest that botulinum toxin products product may be viable for much longer when properly handled. A double-blind, randomized study of 30 patients showed no significant difference in the treatment of canthal lines between those treated with Botox reconstituted with sterile, non-preserved saline immediately prior to injection compared with toxin reconstituted 1 week prior to injection [7]. Furthermore, another study demonstrated that Botox reconstitution at times ranging 1–6 weeks prior to injection produced statistically similar results in patients treated for glabellar rhytides compared with product reconstitution 1 day prior to injection [8]. While none of these three agents should be shaken, they are often lightly swirled upon reconstitution – and it is recommended that Xeomin actually be inverted to most effectively reconstitute the product.

Safety and contraindications

Botulinum toxinA has a large margin of safety, with an estimated human median lethal dose of 1.3–2.1 ng/kg when injected intramuscularly or intravenously. This correlates to a LD50 of approximately 26–42 U/kg, making its cosmetic use a relatively safe endeavor at recommended cosmetic doses [9,10]. Care should be taken to use the necessary dosing ranges in a given region in order to optimize patient satisfaction and preserve a natural result. Injectors should possess excellent knowledge of facial anatomy, especially considering the close proximity of adjacent musculature that may not be part of the intended area of treatment.

Contraindications to BoNTA are few and are listed in Table 40.2 along with several medications that require caution when administering BoNTA [11].

Table 40.2 Precautions and contraindications.

Precaution	Mechanism
Cyclosporine	Has been reported to cause neuromuscular blockade, possibly through calcium channel blockade
Aminoglycoside antibiotics	Large doses can prevent release of acetylcholine from neurons
D-penicillamine	May cause formation of antibodies targeting acetylcholine receptor
Contraindication	
Myasthenia gravis	Autoantibodies targeting acetylcholine receptor
Lambert–Eaton syndrome	Paraneoplastic, antibodies targeting calcium channels
Amyotrophic lateral sclerosis	Neurodegenerative disease
Pregnancy or breastfeeding	Insufficient safety data
Allergy to any constituent of BoNTA	Potential for anaphylaxis

Standard injection techniques

General considerations

Prior to treatment, patients should be informed that the typical duration of efficacy is likely to be 3–4 months, and potential side effects should be discussed. Duration studies comparing the duration of efficacy for the various type A toxins have yielded mixed results and it is not clear which toxin, if any, has the most long-lasting effect. The mean onset of action for BoNTA should also be discussed with the patient, as some patients may have misperceptions and expect immediate results. While it has been published that Dysport onset often starts by Day 1, a recent Botox study demonstrated that approximately half of patients experience initial onset by post-injection day 1 and nearly all patients will experience onset of action by day 4 [12].

Informed consents should clearly indicate that treatment of areas other than those approved by the FDA constitute off-label use. Consent should be in the form of an oral discussion as well as a signed, written document. Pretreatment asymmetries and scars should always be discussed, documented, and we also recommend photography prior to treatment.

Patient satisfaction may be improved by the application of ice packs to the intended treatment areas prior to injection of toxin. This serves a two-fold purpose by providing mild anesthesia to the treatment area as well as causing vasoconstriction, thereby potentially decreasing the risk of bruising.

While we provide suggested doses (herein listed in Botox units) for various injection techniques, it must be remembered that these should serve as guidelines for the practitioner and not as a "cookbook." Treatment doses should be patient specific and be primarily based on prominence of individual muscles as well as patient preference. For example, the corrugator supercilii of the typical male patient are larger and more prominent than those of the average female. Additional consideration for the patient's desired result should be made and addressed during the pretreatment interview, as some patients prefer little to no movement in the treated muscles, while others may prefer a gentle softening of movement of treated area. The forehead, for example, is an area where it is very important to discuss this difference with patients.

Additionally, we caution against attempts to apply "conversion factors" to equate Botox, Dysport, and Xeomin. While they may provide a general guide for the beginner, we recommend that that the injector become familiar with the use and properties of each neuromodulator agent they choose to employ in their practice.

Treatment of the upper face

Photodamage and overactive musculature can cause changes in the upper face that convey a fatigued or angry look that is often discordant with reality. Treatment of the upper face with BoNTA can lead to a more youthful, relaxed, and rested appearance [13,14]. Data also support the use of BoNTA in multiple areas of the upper face in a single treatment session [15].

Forehead

The frontalis muscle is contiguous with the galea aponeurotica of the scalp superiorly, and inserts inferiorly into the skin of the brow. Its configuration varies between individuals but it is generally considered to be either a uniform band across the forehead or V-shaped with a relative absence of fibers medially (Figure 40.1). Fibers of the frontalis are oriented vertically, and thus when they contract the brows elevate and horizontal forehead lines become imprinted in the skin over time. The lateral fibers of the orbicularis oculi muscle pull down on the lateral brow, and thus directly oppose the upward forces of the frontalis. This muscular interaction allows for the creation of a neurotoxin lateral brow lift (discussed below).

A recent Botox consensus article addressed treatment of horizontal forehead lines caused by the frontalis [16]. The authors recommended ranges of 6–15 U and 6 to <15 U BoNTA for females and males, respectively (Table 40.3), and agreed that doses over 20 U are more likely to lead to complications or patient dissatisfaction (e.g. eyebrow ptosis and patient complaints of immobility and unnatural appearance). Forehead injections of BoNTA are generally placed over 4–9 injection sites. In order to avoid eyebrow ptosis, the injections should generally not be placed any closer than 1–1.5 cm above the bony orbital rim (Figure 40.2). Patients with tall foreheads may benefit from 2-3 rows of injections, and patients with wider foreheads may also require more injection sites. Attention to the shape and positioning of the patients baseline brow is essential,

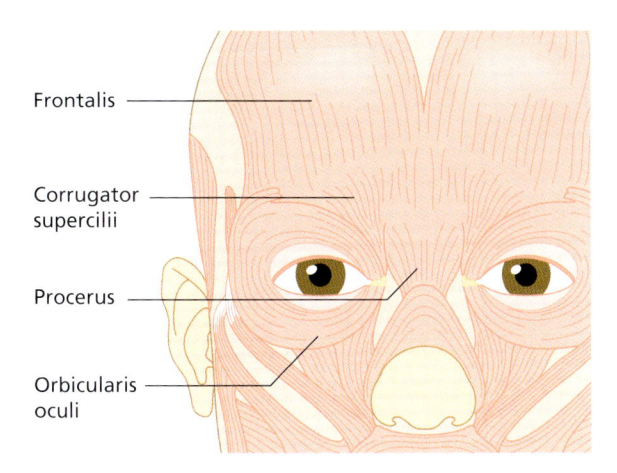

Figure 40.1 Relevant musculature of the upper face. (Source: Sommer B, Sattler G, eds. (2001) *Botulinum Toxin in Aesthetic Medicine*. Blackwell Science, Boston, MA. Reproduced with permission of John Wiley & Sons.)

and often injection sites in women are performed in an arch to try to preserve the arch of the brow below. Patients with dermatochalasis or low-set brows should be evaluated carefully prior to injection as they represent the population most at risk for significant eyebrow ptosis and/or complaints of "heaviness" after treatment. Accordingly, older patients who are more dependent upon their frontalis for brow elevation will typically not tolerate (or at least not like) the higher doses that younger patients will

Table 40.3 Treatment recommendations by site (Botox units).

Treatment site	Muscles	Typical number of injection points	Typical total Botox units* Women	Typical total Botox units* Men
Upper face				
Horizontal forehead lines	Frontalis	4–9	6–15	6 to >15
Glabellar complex	Procerus, depressor supercilii, orbicularis oculi	5–7	10–30	20–40
Crow's feet	Orbicularis oculi	2–5 per side	10–30	20–30
Narrow palpebral aperture	Pretarsal fibers of orbicularis oculi	1 per side	2	2
Lateral brow lift	Superolateral fibers of orbicularis oculi	1–2 per side	8–12	8–12
Mid face				
Bunny lines	Nasalis	1 per side	3–5	3–5
Gummy smile	Levator labii superioris alaeque nasi	1 per side	1–2	1–2
Lower face				
Perioral lines	Orbicularis oris	4–6 per lip	4–12	4–12
Dimpled chin	Mentalis	1–2	4–8	4–8
Downturned smile	Depressor anguli oris	1–2	6–8	6–8
Platysmal bands	Platysma	2–12 per band	20–35	20–35
Nefertiti lift	Platysma	7 per side	28–42	28–42
Masseter hypertrophy	Masseter	5–6 per side	50–60	50–60

*Suggested doses are based on Botox units in this table. All sites other than glabellar complex (Botox, Dysport, Xeomin) and crow's feet (Botox) are currently "off label" in the USA.

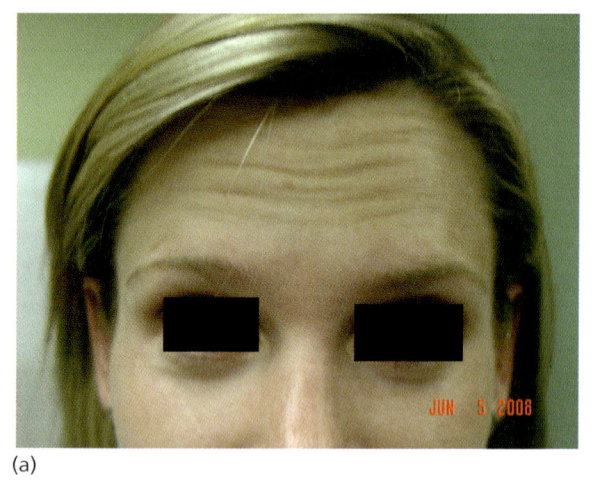

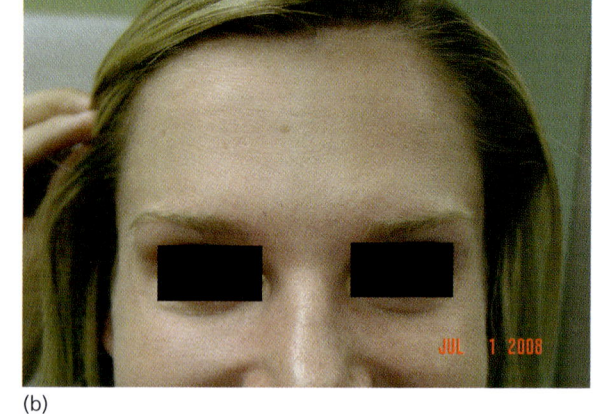

Figure 40.2 Horizontal forehead lines before (a) and after (b) Botox injection.

tolerate, and thus are most frequently treated with lower doses. Patients with significant etched-in lines immediately superior to their lateral brows are also patients who may frequently be advised not to have BoNTA treatment as they depend on the baseline action of the lower frontalis fibers to hoist the brow upward and away from their eyelid. These patients may benefit from other treatments including tightening devices, lifting devices, filler agents to occupy volume, or surgical correction with brow lift techniques.

Additionally, it is recommended that the frontalis be treated usually in conjunction with the glabella (discussed below). The frontalis is the only elevator of the brow, and when rendered less functional by treatment by BoTNA in the context of active glabellar muscles (which are depressors), this will result in an overall lowering of the brow. This will have the tendency to cause an unacceptable cosmetic (forehead heaviness and brow downward repositioning, or flat brow instead or arched), and sometimes functional (brow ptosis), result.

Glabella

The glabellar complex (Figure 40.1) represents the site most commonly treated with BoNTA. The glabella is the only cosmetic site for which all three type A botulinum toxins currently on the US market have FDA approval. It is one of the easiest sites to treat, and thus is a good place for novice injectors to begin. Both the corrugator supercilii and the depressor supercilii originate on the nose and insert into the mid-brow. These muscles draw the brow medially and downward, creating vertical lines in the glabella. Treatment of these brow depressors with BoNTA leads to relaxation of these muscles, which usually results in a medial lift of the brow to some extent. The procerus muscle originates on the nasal bridge and inserts into skin of the mid-glabella. Contraction of the procerus also pulls the medial brow down, but with the pure vertical orientation of this muscle a horizontal line becomes etched in the skin with contraction over time.

Glabellar doses of Botox typically range from 10–30 total U in women and 20–40 U in men, with the FDA approval pivotal study showing efficacy of 20 units in most patients. Injections are most commonly placed in five specific sites: one injection in the procerus, one in each of the medial corrugators, and one in each of the lateral corrugators (Figure 40.3). Sometimes, in patients who display significant medial recruitment above the mid-brow, 1–2 additional injection sites can be helpful to avoid this central pulling. Other patients who have smaller corrugator supercilii may be adequately treated with a total of 3 injection sites. Again, this highlights the need for individualization of treatment plans from patient to patient to determine not only dose but also injection points. Some injectors choose to literally "thread" small droplets of neuromodulators along a muscle to limit injection points and target more of the muscle. Anatomically, patients can have different orientations of the corrugator muscles from vertically-oriented to horizontally-oriented to more of a diagonal-in between-pattern [17], and thus injection targets may be different. In most circumstances, these agents are not placed any closer than about 1 cm above the bony orbital rim in the mid-pupillary line in order to try to avoid lid ptosis. Lid ptosis can occur from migration of the toxin through the orbital septum to knock out the function of the levator palpebrae superioris muscle (which functions to elevate the lid upwards).

Periorbital

The orbicularis oculi muscle is a circular, sphincter-like muscle that surrounds the eye and functions in eyelid closure. The circularity of this muscle creates an anatomical structure composed of fibers running in multiple directions. The muscular diversity of the orbicularis oculi creates functional diversity in animation of the periorbital area. For example, the lateral and superolateral fibers of the orbicularis oculi immediately below the brow function as brow depressors. Treatment of the lateral canthal rhytides (commonly described as crow's feet) is often satisfying for the novice injector and the patient. Because of the

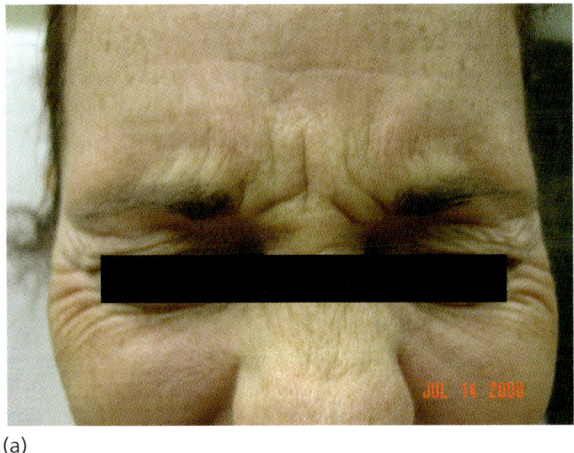

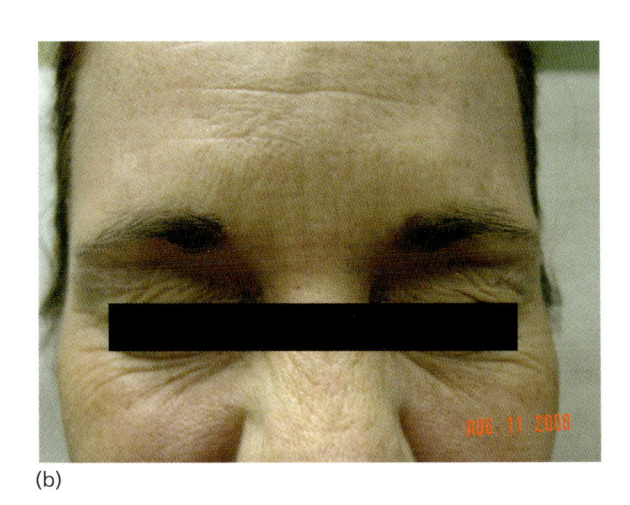

Figure 40.3 Glabellar frown lines before (a) and after (b) Botox injection.

presence of many small vessels in the lateral periocular area, it is often recommended to place BoNTA injections superficially (even intradermally) in this region, usually creating a wheal at the injection site. For treatment of lateral canthal rhytides, the injector typically chooses 2–5 injection points per side, depending on the prominence of the musculature of the area. The reality is that orbicularis oculi muscle prominence varies between patients, making individual assessment of anatomy and patterns of dynamic muscular lines helpful prior to treatment of each patient [18]. Typically, 5–15 units of Botox are injected into each side (Figure 40.4). Care should be taken to inject no closer than 0.5–1 cm to the lateral orbital rim in order to avoid migration of toxin causing unintended paralysis of ocular muscles. In many circumstances, the needle can be inserted medially, so that the tip of the needle is pointing lateral – thereby focusing on softening the lateral canthal musculature while trying to avoid medial migration which could rarely affect the eye lubrication or extra-ocular musculature.

In a small minority of patients, pretarsal bands of the orbicularis oculi muscle can be hypertrophic at the lower lid. A hyperfunctional, pretarsal orbicularis oculi muscle can cause unsightly bands (also known as "jelly rolls") around the lower eyelid and narrowing of the palpebral aperture which are especially evident when smiling. If treating this infraorbital type of hyperfunctional musculature, it is recommended to first evaluate lower lid laxity with a "snap-test" to ensure lid competency after the muscle is weakened. Typically, 1–2 units of Botox are used in this pretarsal area for patients who complain of significant muscle prominence of this area, or those who desire changing the shape of their eye from an almond-type shape to that of a more rounded eye with a widened palpebral aperture. Injections are placed carefully from a lateral approach subdermally, about

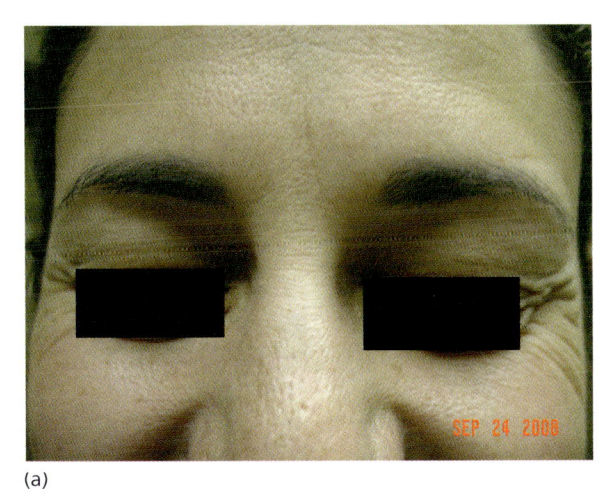

Figure 40.4 "Crow's feet" before (a) and after (b) Botox injection.

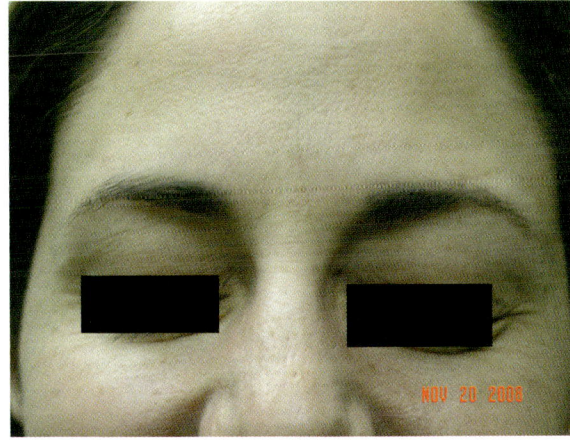

3 mm below the ciliary margin in the mid-pupillary line [16]. A lateral approach in this area helps to ensure a superficial injection, and to allow the non-injecting hand to pull down the lower lid and protect the patient from movement. The patient should be lying back against a solid headrest, and the needle is usually oriented purely horizontally and placed very shallow.

Lateral brow lift

In patients with downturned or ptotic lateral brows, either from dermatochalasis, overactive lateral orbicularis oculi activity pulling down on the tail of the brow, or inadvertent paralysis of the most inferior fibers of the frontalis after aggressive forehead BoNTA treatment, partial correction can sometimes be achieved with a BoNTA chemical brow lift. This lateral brow lift can be obtained by injection into the superolateral fibers of the orbicularis oculi muscle. This technique relaxes the specific aspect of the orbicularis oculi that is pulling the lateral brow downward, and carefully tries to avoid some of the adjacent inferolateral frontalis fibers just superior to the brow – as these frontalis fibers can be helpful to try to pull the lateral brow upward. To accomplish this effect, the injector places 3–6 units of Botox just below the lateral infrabrow [19]. Identification of this injection site requires that the patient first elevate their brows to find the lateral margin of the frontalis muscle (known as the temporal fusion plane). Second, the patient must close their eyes forcefully in order to localize the area where the orbicularis oculi exerts maximal medial and downward pull on the lateral brow. The proper injection point is just inferior to the point of maximal pull downward on the brow, but making sure this site is at least 1–1.5 cm inferior to the most lateral fibers of the frontalis muscle (Figure 40.5). Avoiding these trailing lateral frontalis fibers allows for the preservation of the lift the lateral frontalis normally provides at baseline. Patients with more significant brow redundancy can sometimes be improved with a combination of BoNTA in conjunction with small volumes of fillers (e.g. 0.1–0.2 mL of a hyaluronic acid product) placed just below the lateral brow (often facilitated by using a blunt-tipped cannula) or an energy based lifting device such as focused ultrasound or radiofrequency, but clearly those with more severe dermatochalasis can really only be effectively treated with surgical intervention.

Treatment of the mid-face
Bunny lines

Contraction of the nasalis muscle creates diagonal lines along the proximal nasal sidewall. This area is becoming a more common area for BoNTA treatment. Patients seeking treatment of these lines often have experienced the benefits of BoNTA softening the forehead, glabella, and crow's feet and are looking to extend a more relaxed look to the mid-face. Identification of the muscle is straightforward and accomplished by having the patient "scrunch" their nose. Three to five units of Botox can be placed superficially into the muscle at the medial aspect of the proximal nasal sidewall on each side of the nose. Placement of BoNTA too far laterally can lead to unwanted paralysis of the adjacent levator labii superioris alaeque nasi (LLSAN), resulting in elongation or drooping of the upper lip. The final cosmetic result can often be enhanced with concomitant treatment of the procerus in some patients with more significant bunny lines that seem to be most bulky on the midline proximal nasal dorsum.

Softening of the nasolabial fold and "gummy smile"

An overactive LLSAN can be a component of an accentuated or prominent superior nasolabial fold. Treatment of the LLSAN can be an option for young patients looking to soften the superior aspect of the nasolabial fold without using fillers or at a lower cost than fillers. A total of 1–2 units of Botox can often achieve a softening of the top of the nasolabial fold, and a 1992 anatomic study by Pessa illustrated that the LLSAN is actually the more important muscle contributing to the prominence of the nasolabial fold. Higher doses (typically 3–5 units) of BoNTA are usually used at the same location for patients with significant gummy smiles. Injection of 3–5 units per side of BoNTA into the belly of LLSAN at the pyriform aperture can elongate the upper cutaneous lip and partially correct the excessive gingival display [20]. Doses of 5–7.5 units of Botox in patients with very severe gummy smiles have been reported [20].

In cases of a prominent nasolabial fold or a gummy smile, injection of the LLSAN is primarily a treatment for younger patients who can compensate for the resulting pronounced elongation of the cutaneous lip with other musculature. In addition to the LLSAN, the muscles responsible for the elevation of the upper lip, particularly in younger individuals, are the levator labii superioris, levator anguli oris, zygomaticus major and minor, and the depressor septi nasi. Older patients seem to be more reliant on primarily the levator labii muscles alone.

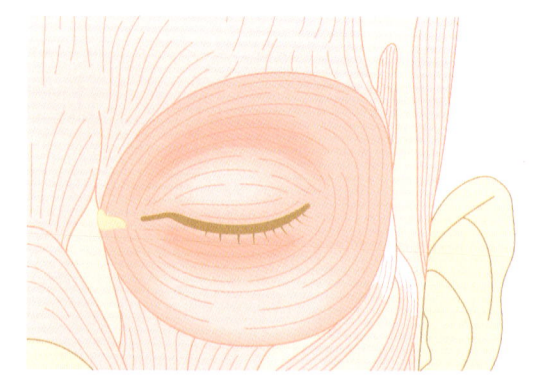

Figure 40.5 The lateral bow lift can be obtained by injection into the superolateral fibers of the orbicularis oculi muscle. This technique relaxes the specific aspect of the orbicularis oculi that is pulling the lateral brow downward. (Source: Sommer B, Sattler G, eds. (2001) *Botulinum Toxin in Aesthetic Medicine*. Blackwell Science, Boston, MA. Reproduced with permission of John Wiley & Sons.)

Treatment of the lower face

Treatment of the perioral area, and lower face in general, can have an increased risk of adverse side effects given that muscles around the mouth play an important functional role for speaking, eating, and drinking. Therefore it is best that the clinician gain experience with injection of BoNTA on other, more forgiving areas of the face (i.e., glabella, crow's feet) before attempting injections on the lower face.

Perioral lines

The lips are the cosmetic focal point of the lower face and careful, conservative corrections can often dramatically improve aspects of an aging face. Vertical "etched in" lines of the perioral skin are common and are caused by years of contraction of the orbicularis oris muscle, a sphincter-like muscle that encircles the mouth. Etched-in lines are preceded by years of vertical muscle columns in women, leading eventually to imprinting of the perioral skin. The skin in this area is highly innervated and vascular, and therefore injections into this region are generally associated with more discomfort and can be associated with bruising or swelling. Topical anesthetics and/or the application of ice-packets can be very beneficial.

Tenants of injecting BoNTA into the lip musculature include: use of low doses with frequent follow-up for retreatment, preservation of symmetry utilizing photography and carefully placed injections, treatment of both upper and lower lips at the same time, and avoidance of midline injections to preserve the desirable Cupid's bow. Injection technique varies depending on individual anatomy, but typical treatments include four superficial injection sites in the upper lip (two points on each side of the upper lip) just above the vermillion border. In patients with more significant vertical muscle columns (taller, bulkier, deeper) sometimes an additional site on each side of the upper lip (often 1 cm above the vermillion border placed between the lower injection sites) can be helpful. For the lower lip, usually 2–4 superficial injection sites are performed as well (two sites on each side of midline approximately 1.5 cm apart). It is important to inject superficially and use lower dosages, especially for a patient's first treatment. Follow-up 2 weeks later will typically allow the injector to see if additional units may be helpful. Some have advocated doses for perioral injection to be in a range of 4–5 units of Botox [16], while another recent study demonstrated equivalent reduction in hyperdynamic perioral lines with a total of 7.5 units versus 12 units using four injection sites [21].

Dimpled chin

The mentalis muscle originates in the incisive fossa and inserts into the skin of the chin. Contraction of this muscle can create a dimpled appearance of the chin that has been termed "pebbled chin," "golfball chin," "peau d' orange chin," and "apple dumpling chin." A total of 4–8 U of Botox, placed as a single midline injection (or sometimes in two points 0.5 cm lateral to midline at the bony part of the chin), can be very effective. Product placed too far laterally risks paralysis of the depressor labii inferioris and can cause speech problems.

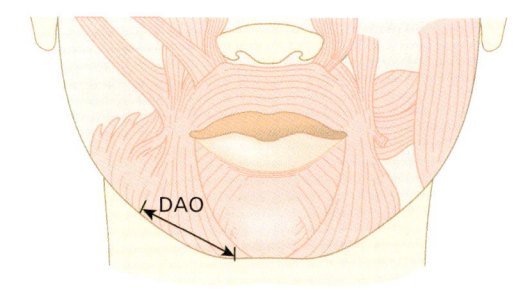

Figure 40.6 Treatment of a downturned smile is accomplished by injection into the posterior fibers of the depressor anguli oris (DAO) muscles. (Source: Sommer B, Sattler G, eds. (2001) *Botulinum Toxin in Aesthetic Medicine*. Blackwell Science, Boston, MA. Reproduced with permission of John Wiley & Sons.)

Downturned smile

Descent of the lateral commissures of the mouth can result from gravity and volume loss and sometimes from hypertrophy of the depressor anguli oris (DAO) muscle. Injection of Botox (3–4 units per side) into the posterior aspect of the DAO in a single injection site can sometimes partially correct this appearance of a downturned smile (Figure 40.6). Complications associated with medial diffusion or injection of BoNTA into the depressor labii inferioris are discussed below. DAO prominence is often associated with volume loss of the lower face, and in our experience combination treatment with fillers and BoNTA is more consistently effective than BoNTA alone.

Platysmal bands

The platysma is a thin, superficial muscle that can create vertical bands in the neck which are displeasing to many patients. Patient selection is key to successful treatment of this condition, and the most appropriate candidates are those with prominent vertical bands at rest. A typical treatment session includes injection of 2–3 bands with 20–35 U of BoNTA total (2–12 injection points per band). Dysphagia is a rare complication that has been reported with cosmetic use of BoNTA in higher doses for treatment of platysmal bands [22]. Conservative treatment, with low dosages and superficial injections, is recommended in order to avoid this very rare and disturbing complication that can persist for weeks. Marking injection points and pinching the band between the thumb and forefinger can aid in the precise superficial placement of BoNTA in small aliquots at approximately 1.5 cm intervals.

In addition to the treatment of platysmal bands, placement of toxin along the inferior margin of the mandible and in the superior aspect of the posterior platysmal band may redefine the mandibular border. This procedure has been termed the "Nefertiti lift" and was described by Levy in a study of 130 patients [23]. Patients were treated with 2–3 units of Botox per injection site, with five sites being along the margin of the mandible and two sites being in the superior aspect of the posterior platysmal band. It was hypothesized that the resultant sharpening of the mandibular border was secondary to partial reversal of the chronic downward pull on the cheeks by the platysma. At present, placement of fillers along the mandibular margin has helped to achieve a more consistent recontouring of the jawline.

Masseter hypertrophy

Prominent masseter bulk over the posterior mandible can create a squared-off shape to the face which is not desirable to some people. A study of 45 patients with masseter hypertrophy were treated with BoNTA and followed for 10 months [24]. Total doses of 25 to 30 units of Botox were injected into each masseter in 5–6 injection points. The maximum reduction in masseter thickness as measured by ultrasound was seen at 1 month, and CT scan found continued reduction of masseter muscle thickness up to 3 months after treatment. Eighty-two percent of patients were satisfied with the treatment. Local adverse effects included masticatory difficulties (44% of patients) and speech disturbance (16% of patients). All side effects were transient.

A study specifically measuring bite force in patients treated with 25 units of Botox per masseter (50 units total) reported significant bite-force reduction at 2, 4, and 8 weeks post-injection ($p < 0.05$) [25]. Difference in bite-force reduction was not statistically significant at the 12-week measurement, and while bite-force measurements trended upward, they still did not achieve preinjection values at the end of 12 weeks. So while injection can beneficially alter the shape of the masseter, it may alter mastication. Further study is needed to better define the duration and significance of the observed bite-force reduction.

Combination of botulinum toxin with fillers

While BoNTA treatment works well for dynamic rhytides, resting lines and volume loss are not corrected by neurotoxin placement alone. Combination treatment consisting of hyaluronic acid and BoNTA often yield impressive results and may double the duration of response compared with filler treatment alone in some areas [26]. Combination therapy can be useful in the glabella, periorbital area, perioral, mentalis, jawline and sometimes the nasolabial creases. Placement of filler prior to BoNTA treatment may decrease untoward migration of same-day toxin caused by massage of the filler molding and the common practice of confirming placement of the filler product after injection.

Complications and management

Bruising, swelling, and mild asymmetry are commonly encountered issues. Less common is migration of toxin to adjacent but unintended musculature, which can result in significant asymmetry. Eyebrow ptosis can occur from toxin placement too close to the brow in the frontalis muscle, poor patient selection and use of higher dosages in the forehead. In fact, a 2008 consensus publication recommended using about half the frontalis dose of BoNTA previously suggested in an earlier statement by the same group [16].

In a double-blind, placebo-controlled, glabellar study, headache occurred in 20% of patients in the placebo group vs. 11.4% in the BoNTA treated group, leading authors to conclude that headache was likely related to trauma from the injection needle itself [27]. A non-blinded case series of 320 patients treated for cosmetic reasons with BoNTA reported the occurrence of severe, debilitating headaches in 1% of patients treated [28]. In this study, these headaches occurred within 2 days of injection with BoNTA and persisted at a high level for 2 weeks to 1 month after injection.

It is best to wipe off the patient's make-up prior to injection (particularly in the lateral canthal area) in order to best identify little veins in the area and avoid them. This also reduces the risk of introducing foreign make-up material into the skin. Ice prior to injection to facilitate vasoconstriction is also very helpful in helping to reduce the mild pain of the injections themselves. If patients are on prophylactic medications or supplements that may have an anticoagulant effect, it may be helpful if they discontinue these agents a few days prior to injection. An example of such an agent would be the use of aspirin as a preventive measure in patients lacking a history of atherosclerotic disease, stroke, clot, or atrial fibrillation. However, patients on anticoagulant therapies for specific purposes (i.e., prior deep vein thrombosis, valvular disease, etc) should generally avoid modifying the dose or discontinuing their medication for these small cosmetic injectable procedures.

Immunogenicity to BoNTA has been reported in the literature but is very rare in patients treated with the newer (post-1997) formulation of Botox. The newer formulation of Botox has only 20% of the protein content that the older batch had (pre-1997), and presumably has made the product significantly less immunogenic. One case report, however, describes neutralizing antibody formation to the post-1997 formulation of Botox in a patient treated cosmetically for masseter hypertrophy [29]. Presence of neutralizing antibody was supported by two positive mouse protection assays and by ELISA testing [29]. Risks associated with immunogenicity are very large doses of toxin (more frequent in therapeutic uses of BoNTA) and short intervals (less than 3 months) between high-dose injections [30].

Generalized reactions have been reported related to toxicity and include headache, nausea, malaise, fatigue, flu-like symptoms, and rashes distant to injection sites. These reactions have arisen from improper dosages and the use of "experimental strains of botulinum toxin" [31]. In studies measuring complications in patients treated with legitimate BoNTA, adverse events occurred in similar frequencies in both treatment and placebo groups. Most post-injection issues are transient in nature and resolve spontaneously, requiring no intervention other than reassurance.

Upper face

Injection into the frontalis muscle can lead to brow ptosis, and patients can develop a quizzical look (raising of the lateral brow because of residual non-treated frontalis fibers pulling upward) if only medial fibers of the frontalis are treated. This "Mr. Spock" look can usually be easily treated with placement of 1–2 units in each side of the lateral functional frontalis. In addition, patients can rarely experience painful electric shock-like sensations if the supraorbital or supratrochlear sensory nerves are inadvertently hit with the injection needle.

Eyelid ptosis is also uncommon (less than 1% of patients in the hands of experienced injectors) and presumably occurs when injecting the lateral corrugator area, with migration of toxin through the orbital septum leading to the paralysis of the levator palpebrae superioris. This is a transient event (generally resolving by 2–3 weeks) and can be treated to some extent, but often not fully, by using ophthalmic drops such as Naphcon (Alcon, Fort Worth, TX, USA; can be purchased over-the-counter) which exert mild adrenergic effects, or prescription Iopidine (Alcon, Fort Worth, TX, USA) drops [22]. The mechanism of both treatments is adrenergic stimulation and contraction of the adjacent Mueller's muscle which can partially raise the eyelid. Iopidine may mask underlying glaucoma so this treatment should be reserved for short periods of treatment such as 3–5 weeks [32].

Lower face

Treatment of the orbicularis oris muscle for correction of vertical lip lines can very rarely lead to drooling or difficulty with phonation. Thus, when treating vertical muscle columns caused by a hyperfunctional orbicularis oris muscle, care should be taken to use lower dosages and avoid overtreatment. In addition, medial placement of these injections can help avoid unintended musculature being affected, especially near the oral commissure. However, care should be taken to not place injections to closely to the philtrum and cupid's bow area, as this may produce an undesirable flattening effect and loss of lip definition.

Correction of downturned smile is best accomplished with careful BoNTA placement in the posterior aspect of the depressor anguli oris muscle. This posterior placement helps avoid unintended medial migration and effect on the depressor labii inferioris, a complication that can cause slurred speech and drooling and lasts weeks to months [33]. Similar to injection of the lateral canthus, consider introducing the needle medially and pointing it laterally to try to avoid medial spread from the DAO. Injection of BoNTA into the neck for softening of platysmal bands has in one report led to prolonged dysphagia secondary to paralysis of the deeper strap muscles requiring placement of nasogastric tube [22]. This event can be best avoided by following the recently revised recommendations presented in this chapter.

Even the most experienced of injectors may observe asymetric treatment effect, despite consistent technique, especially when treating many patients. This unbalanced appearance is usually easily corrected with additional enhancement injections. Finally, temporary strabismus or diplopia are extremely rare and infrequently reported, and likely occur by either large diffusion or direct injection of toxin into the extraocular muscles.

On the horizon

A topical formulation of BoNTA (RT001, Revance Therapeutics, Inc., Newark, CA, USA) is currently in Phase 3 clinical trials and is being investigated for various cosmetic and non-cosmetic applications. Cosmetic use for topical formulations of BoTNA will likely be limited to areas where skin is thin, underlying musculature lies superficially, and extremely accurate placement of toxin is not necessary. Currently, RT001 is being tested for treatment of lateral canthal lines [34], but may also have use for hyperhidrosis.

Notably, a novel alternative to neurotoxins for temporary reduction of dynamic rhytides on the forehead has recently gained approval in Europe. The device, called iovera° (Myoscience, Redwood City, CA, USA), uses focused cold therapy to temporarily inhibit motor nerve conduction in the temporal branch of the facial nerve. This results in inhibition of voluntary contraction of the frontalis and glabella muscle groups [35].

References

1. Huang W, Foster JA, Rogachefsky AS. (2000) Pharmacology of botulinum toxin. *J Am Acad Dermatol* **43**, 249–59
2. Carruthers JDA, Carruthers JA. (1992) Treatment of glabellar frown lines with C. botulinum exotoxin. *J Dermatol Surg Oncol* **18**, 17–21.
3. Sadick NS, Matarasso SL. (2004) Comparison of botulinum toxins A and B in the treatment of facial rhytides. *Dermatol Clin* **22**, 221–6.
4. Ting PT, Freiman A. (2004) The story of Clostridium botulinum: from food poisoning to Botox®. *Clin Med* **4**, 258–61.
5. Matarasso SL. (2003) Comparison of botulinum toxin types A and B: a bilateral and double-blind randomized evaluation in the treatment of canthal rhytides. *Dermatol Surg* **29**, 7–13.
6. Dressler D, Benecke R. (2007) Pharmacology of therapeutic botulinum toxin preparations. *Disabil Rehabil* **29**, 1761–8.
7. Lizarralde M, Gutierrez SH, Venegas A. (2007) Clinical efficacy of botulinum toxin type a reconstituted and refrigerated 1 week before its application in external canthus dynamic lines. *Dermatol Surg* **33**, 1328–33.
8. Hexsel DM, Trindade de Almeida A, Rutowitsch M, *et al*. (2003) Multicenter, double-blind study of the efficacy of injections with botulinum toxin type A reconstituted up to 6 consecutive weeks before application. *Dermatol Surg* **29**, 523–9.
9. Scott AB, Suzuki D. (1988) Systemic toxicity of botulinum toxin by intramuscular injection in the monkey. *Mov Disord* **3**, 333–5.
10. Arnon SS, Schechter R, Inglesby TV, Henderson DA, Bartlett JG, Ascher MS, Eitzen E, Fine AD, Hauer J, Layton M, Lillibridge S, Osterholm MT, O'Toole T, Parker G, Perl TM, Russell PK, Swerdlow DL, Tonat K; Working Group on Civilian Biodefense. (2001) Botulinum toxin as a biological weapon: medical and public health management. *JAMA* **285**, 1059–70.
11. Cote TR, Mohan AK, Polder JA, *et al*. (2005) Botulinum toxin type A injections: adverse events reported to the US Food and Drug Administration in therapeutic and cosmetic cases. *J Am Acad Dermatol* **53**, 407–15.

12 Beer KR, Boyd C, Patel RK, *et al.* (2011) Rapid onset of response and patient-reported outcomes after onabotulinumtoxinA treatment of moderate-to-severe glabellar lines. *J Drugs Dermatol* **10**, 39–44.

13 Cox SE, Finn JC, Stetler L, *et al.* (2003) Development of the Facial Lines Treatment Satisfaction Questionnaire and initial results for botulinum toxin type A-treated patients. *Dermatol Surg* **29**, 444–9; discussion 449.

14 Finn JC, Cox SE, Earl ML. (2003) Social implications of hyperfunctional facial lines. *Dermatol Surg* **29**, 450–5. Review.

15 Flynn TC. (2006) Update on botulinum toxin. *Semin Cutan Med Surg* **25**, 115–21.

16 Carruthers J, Fagien S, Matarasso SL, and the Botox Consensus Group. (2008) Advances in facial rejuvenation: botulinum toxin type a, hyaluronic acid dermal fillers, and combination therapies: consensus recommendations. *Plast Reconstr Surg* **121** (Suppl), 5–30S.

17 de Almeida AR, da Costa Marques ER, Banegas R, Kadunc BV. (2012) Glabellar contraction patterns: a tool to optimize botulinum toxin treatment. *Dermatol Surg* **38**, 1506–15.

18 Kane MA. (2003) Classification of crow's feet patterns among Caucasian women: the key to individualizing treatment. *Plast Reconstr Surg* **112**(Suppl), 33–9S.

19 Cohen JL, Dayan SH. (2006) Botulinum toxin type A in the treatment of dermatochalasis: an open-label, randomized, dose-comparison study. *J Drugs Dermatol* **5**, 596–601.

20 Kane MA. (2003) The effect of botulinum toxin injections on the nasolabial fold. *Plast Reconstr Surg* **112** (Suppl), 66–72S; discussion 73–4S.

21 Cohen JL, Dayan SH, Cox SE, *et al.*. (2012) OnabotulinumtoxinA dose-ranging study for hyperdynamic perioral lines. *Dermatol Surg* **38**, 1497–505.

22 Carruthers J, Carruthers A. (1999) Practical cosmetic Botox techniques. *J Cutan Med Surg* **3** (Suppl 4), S49–52.

23 Levy PM. (2007) The "Nefertiti lift": a new technique for specific re-contouring of the jawline. *J Cosmet Laser Ther* **9**, 249–52.

24 Park MY, Ahn KY, Jung DS. (2003) Botulinum toxin type A treatment for contouring of the lower face. *Dermatol Surg* **29**, 477–83.

25 Ahn KY, Kim ST. (2007) The change of maximum bite force after botulinum toxin type a injection for treating masseteric hypertrophy. *Plast Reconstr Surg* **120**, 1662–6.

26 Carruthers J, Carruthers A. (2003) A prospective, randomized, parallel group study analyzing the effect of BTX-A (Botox) and nonanimal sourced hyaluronic acid (NASHA, Restylane) in combination compared with NASHA (Restylane) alone in severe glabellar rhytides in adult female subjects: treatment of severe glabellar rhytides with a hyaluronic acid derivative compared with the derivative and BTX-A. *Dermatol Surg* **29**, 802–9.

27 Carruthers JD, Lowe NJ, Menter MA, Gibson J, Eadie N, Botox Glabellar Lines II Study Group. (2003) Double-blind, placebo-controlled study of the safety and efficacy of botulinum toxin type A for patients with glabellar lines. *Plast Reconstr Surg* **112**, 1089–98.

28 Alam M, Arndt KA, Dover JS. (2002) Severe, intractable headache after injection with botulinum a exotoxin: report of 5 cases. *J Am Acad Dermatol* **46**, 62–5.

29 Lee S. (2007) Antibody-induced failure of botulinum toxin type A therapy in a patient with masseteric hypertrophy. *Dermatol Surg* **33** (1 Spec No.), S105–10.

30 Naumann M, Carruthers A, Carruthers J, *et al.* (2010) Meta-analysis of neutralizing antibody conversion with onabotulinumtoxinA (BOTOX®) across multiple indications. *Mov Disord* **25**, 2211–8.

31 Bootleg Botox sentences. New York Times January 27, 2006. Available at: http://www.nytimes.com/2006/01/27/national/27brfs.html?pagewanted=print&_r=0. Accessed August 5th, 2015.

32 Klein AW. (2003) Complications, adverse reactions, and insights with the use of botulinum toxin. *Dermatol Surg* **29**, 549–56.

33 Cohen JL. (2007) Botulinum neurotoxin clinical update. *Cosmet Dermatol* **20**, S3.

34 Glogau R, Blitzer A, Brandt F, *et al.* (2012) Results of a randomized, double-blind, placebo-controlled study to evaluate the efficacy and safety of a botulinum toxin type A topical gel for the treatment of moderate-to-severe lateral canthal lines. *J Drugs Dermatol* **11**, 38–45.

35 Hsu M, Stevenson FF. (2014) Reduction in muscular motility by selective focused cold therapy: a preclinical study. *J Neural Transm* **121**, 15–20.

CHAPTER 41
Hyaluronic Acid Fillers

Mark S. Nestor, Emily L. Kollmann, and Nicole Swenson
Center for Clinical and Cosmetic Research, Aventura, FL, USA

> **BASIC CONCEPTS**
> - Hyaluronic acid fillers are used for 86% of the volume enhancing procedures performed in the USA.
> - Hyaluronic acid filler are popular because they are non-permanent but long-lasting, have few allergic aspects, minimal side effects, are relatively painless to inject, and can be reversible.
> - Hyaluronic acid is a polysaccharide, specifically a glycosaminoglycan, that is formed from repeating D-glucuronic acid and D-N-acetylglucosamine disaccharide units. The disaccharide units are linked together in a linear chain forming a large polymer with a total molecular weight of greater than 10 MDa.
> - The different hyaluronic acid fillers possess various hyaluronic acid concentrations, sizes of particles, gel consistencies, type of cross-linking, degree of cross-linking, and the degree of gel hardness.
> - Hyaluronic acids are injected in the deep dermis for optimal volume replacement.

Introduction

The appearance of the aging face is a compilation of intrinsic aging; our genetics causing the preprogrammed loss of fat, muscle, and bone as well skin elasticity changes, and extrinsic aging; primarily photodamage that affects collagen, elastin, and accelerates the intrinsic aging process [1]. One of the hallmarks of the aging face is the loss of tissue volume and as well as the accentuation of lines and folds [2]. While many procedures can be used to improve the appearance of the aging face, the use of soft tissue, dermal fillers has become one of the most popular ways of filling lines and wrinkles as well as replacing volume in the aging face [3].

According to recent statistics of the American Society of Aesthetic Plastic Surgeons, the use of dermal fillers is only second to Botox as one of the most popular non-surgical cosmetic procedures performed in 2013. Of all the dermal fillers used in the United States, hyaluronic acid fillers accounted for over 88% of fillers used. Also, an increased use of hyaluronic acid fillers of 31.5% over the previous year was reported [4]. While hyaluronic acid fillers may not be "the perfect" filler in all aspects, they come very close to what most patients and physicians look for in the ideal filler, namely non-permanent but long-lasting, having few if any allergic aspects, minimal side effects, relatively painless to inject, and finally safe because of the reversible nature of hyaluronic acid fillers.

This chapter will outline the science and use of hyaluronic acid fillers including:
1. The chemical composition and physical properties of hyaluronic acid fillers.
2. The indications for the variety of FDA approved fillers.
3. Injection techniques, both beginner and advanced.
4. Complications of filler injections and their solutions.
5. Future uses and indications for hyaluronic acid fillers.

Chemical composition and properties of hyaluronic acid fillers

At this time, there are eight marketed FDA approved hyaluronic acid fillers used in the United States. These are listed in Table 41.1. All hyaluronic acid fillers are formed from either bacterial based or animal-based hyaluronic acid. Hyaluronic acid is a polysaccharide, specifically a glycosaminoglycan that is formed from repeating D-glucuronic acid and D-N-acetylglucosamine disaccharide units. The disaccharide units are linked together in a linear chain forming a large polymer with a total molecular weight of greater than 10 MDA. While both animal based and bacterial-based hyaluronic acid fillers are on the market, the vast majority of utilized fillers are based on bacterial production. Native hyaluronic acid would break down very quickly if injected into the skin and needs to be altered and stabilized primarily by

---

Cosmetic Dermatology: Products and Procedures, Second Edition. Edited by Zoe Diana Draelos.
© 2016 John Wiley & Sons, Ltd. Published 2016 by John Wiley & Sons, Ltd.

Table 41.1 Food and Drug Administration (FDA) approved hyaluronic acid (HA) fillers.

- Allergan
  - Juvéderm™ Ultra/Juvéderm™ Ultra Plus
  - Juvéderm Voluma™ XC
- Galderma
  - Restylane®
  - Perlane®
  - Restylane Silk®
  - Restylane Lyft®
- Mentor
  - Prevelle™ Silk (phased out)
- Merz
  - Belotero Balance®

[1] No esthetic indication.

cross-linking to have a long resident life in the skin. Since the basis of all bacterial-based dermal fillers is the same, the difference of the fillers and their properties depend upon the type and degree of cross-linking as well as the manufacturing process that forms the ultimate filler [5].

The important chemical and physical properties of the different filler substances include as noted, the type and degree of cross-linking, the total hyaluronic acid concentration, the size of the particle and/or the consistency of the gel, and the degree of gel hardness or G prime.

The most commonly used hyaluronic acid products in the United States use BDDE (1,4-butanediol diglycidyl ether) as cross-linking agents. This includes Juvederm, Perlane, Restylane and now Juvederm Voluma and Belotero which are the most commonly used hyaluronic acid products in the US. Belotero has a unique cohesive polydensified matrix which has a high concentration of non-cross-linked molecules and the degree to which the filler is cross-linked is not uniform, creating areas of greater and lesser density, thus polydensified [6].

The degree of cross-linking indicates the percentage of hyaluronic acid disaccharide monomer units that are bound to a cross-linking molecule. For hyaluronic acid fillers, some feel that when all factors are equal, a higher degree of a cross-linking agent may translate into a longer persistence of the filler. There are questions, however, about the effect that the cross-linking has on biocompatibility, namely setting the filler as a foreign substance. Therefore, there may be an optimal degree of cross-linking that may give the longest term residence in the skin without causing biocompatibility issues.

Total HA concentration refers to the amount of hyaluronic acid per ml in a product. It generally measures both cross-linked hyaluronic acid and free hyaluronic acid in a product. Free hyaluronic acid or uncross-linked hyaluronic acid is generally added in varying amounts to some products to improve lubrication or product flow. The most widely used hyaluronic acid products are of similar concentration but may vary as to the degree of free or uncross-linked hyaluronic acid, gel hardness, and hyaluronic acid gel consistency. The two most popular hyaluronic acid product lines, namely the Restylane product line and the Juvederm product line, are produced by different mechanical means. The Restylane product line is sieved, thus it is pressed through screens to split the molecules into different size particles; the smallest in Restylane Silk and the largest in Restylane Lyft. The Juvederm line is manufactured in a way that homogenizes the particles in a blender-type apparatus. Juvederm Voluma is created with a combination of low and high molecular weight hyaluronic acid, creating a more mobile fiber network which facilitates cross-linking to 1,4 butanediol.

Belotero Balance is non-sieved, meaning no particle sizing occurs and the product consists of homogeneous masses of both cross-linked and non-cross-linked hyaluronic acid molecules with variable shapes and sizes [7]. Belotero Balance begins with longer strands that are not cross-linked creating softer areas with less cross-linking and firmer areas with more cross-linking.

The different formulations and production strategies yield different gel hardness or G prime to the variety of different products. Clinically, G prime can be thought of both as the amount of force that is necessary to inject a product through a specific-sized needle, as well as the lifting capacity of the filler. In general, fillers that are thicker are more difficult to inject through smaller needles, but based on their properties can act to bring in more water and thus cause more tissue lifting in a given area. This is critical to the product's *in vivo* behavior and clinical indication and the reason that products are not easily interchangeable.

Indications

Most HA fillers are FDA approved to fill "moderate to severe lines and folds" such as the nasolabial fold. Juvederm Voluma and Restylane Lyft are approved for mid face volumization (Restylane Lyft is also known as Perlane so that it is also approved for moderate to severe lines and folds such as the nasolabial fold). Restylane is also approved for lip augmentation and Restylane Silk is approved for lip augmentation as well as perioral lines.

Historically, fillers such as collagen were used to fill fine lines and wrinkles including those in the perioral and periorbital regions. Collagen fillers were injected in the mid-dermis and usually had a clinical life in the skin of approximately three to six months. Hyaluronic acid fillers are generally injected deeper in the skin, most often below the dermis in the superficial subcutaneous layer and traditionally have primarily been indicated for deeper lines and folds [8,9]. Prior to the availability of Belotero Balance, and to a lesser extent Restylane Silk, hyaluronic acid fillers could not be injected superficially because of the risk of the Tyndall effect; whereby the filler appears as a blue hue directly under the skin [10]. This occurs because the hyaluronic acid implanted into the superficial dermis scatters the light striking it so that blue light, which has a shorter wavelength, is reflected back to an observer's eye. Belotero Balance, which has been available in Europe for several years, is now available in the United States and has been used to inject superficial lines in the perioral, periorbital, and cheek areas. Tyndall effect has not been noted with Belotero Balance, even when the product is injected very superficially in the dermis [11]. The majority of hyaluronic acid fillers used to date were initially used in the nasolabial fold, mesiolabial fold as well as other similar lines and folds in the face. More recently, the use of hyaluronic acid fillers has also eclipsed into volume replacement. Thicker hyaluronic acid fillers such as Juvederm Voluma and Restylane Lyft are now are FDA approved for the indication of volume deficit replacement in the midface, with reports of durability of Juvederm Voluma of up to 2 years after initial volume replacement [12].

Hyaluronic acid fillers may be used to augment areas such as the lips by both replacing lost volume with aging and enhancing lip volume and Restylane Silk has also been shown to significantly improve perioral lines. Additionally, fillers are used to replace volume in areas such as the hands and resculpt and act as reshaping agents in areas such as the nose and the chin [13,14]. Hyaluronic acid fillers have significant advantage for these indications because of their longevity and overall low incidence of inflammation and significant swelling.

Injection techniques

Fillers in general are injected using three basic techniques:
1. Droplet injection.
2. Linear threading either antegrade or retrograde.
3. Fanning.
4. Volumizing.

As noted, the majority of hyaluronic acid are injected either in the deep dermis or superficial subcutaneous layer and studies have shown that the vast majority of injections are in the sub cutaneous layer [9]. Most injectors use a combination of injection techniques depending upon the specific area that is being injected. Studies have shown that slower injection techniques tend to decrease side effects and swelling as well as decrease patient discomfort [15].

Patients are usually prepared by cleansing the area either with alcohol or another anti-infective topical cleansing substance. A topical anesthethic is often used either in the form of topical lidocaine, or compounded topicals that may include lidocaine and Betacaine. Many injectors also use cooling methods to both decrease pain of injection, as well as decrease swelling and bruising. Finally, although many HA fillers incorporate lidocaine in the filler product, many injector mix lidocaine with epinephrine into the filler prior to injection to decrease pain and bruising. As the injector gets more comfortable, advanced injection techniques, specifically with regard to volume, may utilize the use of large volumes of hyaluronic acid filler to replace and sculpt volume in areas of loss and these injections may take place in the deeper subcutaneous tissue or under the muscle layer. When volumizing, injections should create a network of scaffolding with small bolus, limiting complications such as biofilms. Injection sites that may be under the muscle include the tear troughs and malar regions [12].

Complications

Possible complications of hyaluronic acid fillers include unevenness of the filler substance, inflammation, swelling, and bruising, injection of the hyaluronic acid filler too superficially in the dermis, and rarely vascular events and abscesses, both bacterial and sterile [16]. Swelling and bruising can be thought of by some as complications, but are usually normally associated with any filler injection. Depending upon the injection technique, swelling and bruising may be common but can often be mitigated by the use of ice as well as the use of a slow injection technique. Patients should be warned that they certainly can experience some swelling and bruising for at least the first 48 hours after injection. The most common type of complication is the unevenness of hyaluronic acid fillers. The clinician needs to evaluate a patient and understand very clearly the needs of that patient and proper injection technique to minimize unevenness. Patients are not symmetrical and they often may need differing amounts of hyaluronic acid on one aspect of the face versus the other. It is also very important that the filler is massaged and the clinician can feel whether the various areas of the face are even upon completion of the injection of the filler. If a patient comes back in or is referred for unevenness, there are two methods of correcting this complication. The first is to simply inject more filler to correct the imbalance, and the second is the use of hyaluronidase to dissolve the uneven filler. Most unevenness can be adjusted by injecting small amounts of filler in the contralateral side to even, however, when bumps and areas are too apparent or uneven, hyaluronidase, usually in 25 to 200 units can be injected and within 48 hours the area of unevenness or of bulging can be dissolved [17].

When a filler is injected too superficially and a tindle effect occurs, oftentimes it can be extruded by making a small puncture with a #25 gauge needle and massaging the filler through the opening. If this fails, hyaluronidase can be used to dissolve the filler. Finally, in those rare cases of sterile abscess or long-term inflammation, topical anti-inflammatories can be used somewhat successfully and when they fail, the use of clarithromycin may also be effective. Rarely vascular events occur including necrosis, embolization and retinal occlusion. If vascular events occur physicians should have a minimum of the following: hyaluronidase to hydrolyze the hyaluronic acid and increase tissue permeability, warm compresses and Sildenafil to increase vasodilation, aspirin, Heparin, and Nitropaste [18].

The development of biofilms after injection of fillers is a newly recognized complication. It is very rare with HA fillers but may be more of a risk with longer acting volumizing fillers such as Juviderm Voluma. Biofilms are defined as an aggregate of microorganisms comprising cells adhering to each other to a surface and embedded within a self-secreted extracellular polymeric substance [19,20]. A biofilm occurs in the filler substance after bacteria from the skin surface is introduced to the product during the injection and this may occur without a significant host response [21–23]. Biofilms present weeks to months after injection as erythematous, persistent, mildly tender nodules and more commonly occur after the injection of long lasting fillers versus hyaluronic acid fillers. Several bacterial strains have been cultured in animal models and because of the properties of the biofilm in the filler, substrate often has antibiotic resistant properties making successful treatment a challenge [24]. Treatment options for biofilms include the use of hyaluronidase, or passing a small gauge needle back and forth through the nodule allowing dispersion. The use of antibiotics such as macrolides and fluoroquinolones have also been suggested for the treatment of biofilms [25,26].

Treatment optimization: persistence of dermal fillers and *in vivo* collagen stimulation

Hyaluronic acid fillers injected as a single treatment in the nasolabial fold, with or without one touch-up 1–2 weeks later usually just for the initial treatment, persists in a subset of patients for up to 12 months or longer [27]. It has generally been hypothesized that the prolonged efficacy of stabilized hyaluronic acid fillers versus injectable substances such as collagen is attributed to the sustained persistence of the product in the skin due to the effect that cross-linking has on limiting breakdown from *in vivo* hyaluronidase. However, new data may indicate that, in addition to residual product left at each reinjection that provides a base, hyaluronic acid fillers can stimulate collagen synthesis and inhibit collagen breakdown, which can contribute to their persistence and correlates with physician observations that patients require less overall filler over time to retain optimal correction. A landmark study by Narins *et al.* [28] which is the basis for a new FDA approval for Restylane for up to 18 months, may provide a key piece of evidence to show that full correction followed a single optimizing treatment can not only optimize longevity and in turn patient satisfaction, but also may enhance the patient's *in vivo* collagen stimulation. This paper is an 18-month interim analysis of a 30-month study to evaluate efficacy and persistence of non-animalized, stabilized hyaluronic acid 100000 gel particles/mL filler based on different re-treatment schedules. The results in this study seem to indicate initial full correction of the nasolabial folds, followed by an optimizing treatment at an interval somewhere between 4 and 9 months, causes improved long-term persistence of the filler and may indicate that full correction followed by retreatment at optimum treatment intervals may enhance the patient's own in vivo collagen stimulation. This hypothesis is supported by *in vivo* studies by Wang *et al.* [29] who demonstrated that NAHSA 100000 gel particles/mL hyaluronic acid filler can induce synthesis of type-I collagen probably by stretching fibroblasts. The effect of optimizing treatments intervals to enhance *in vivo* collagen stimulation is consistent with Wang's data and is further supported by data with other types of treatments that cause collagen stimulation *in vivo*, namely laser, light and radiofrequency devices. The data by Narins *et al.*, as well as Wang *et al.*, leads to a new paradigm in the use of dermal hyaluronic acid fillers. Up until now, the standard for aesthetic correction using hyaluronic acid dermal fillers has been to inject fillers to replace lost volume and to replace the fillers as they slowly degraded. These data may indeed indicate a new treatment approach. Optimizing initial treatment by achieving full correction and thereby stretching fibroblasts and maximally stimulating collagen synthesis, followed by a second optimizing treatment, perhaps at an interval of 4 to 9 months may lead to long-term benefit and a continued enhancement effect by the hyaluronic acid filler. It is possible that with each touch-up injection set the product builds up on a base already there, the metabolism of filler degradation decreases, and collagen production is continually stimulated.

Summary

The use of dermal fillers and hyaluronic acid fillers specifically has become a mainstay in the treatment of the aging face. Hyaluronic acid fillers can be used safely and effectively in treating a variety of aspects of the aging face including folds and wrinkles as well as replacing lost volume. Hyaluronic acid fillers can also be used to sculpt areas such as the chin, the nose, tear troughs, and the eyebrows to enhance features in a non-invasive and completely reversible procedure. Recently approved for use in the United States are Restylane Silk, Restylane Lyft, Belotero Balance, and Juvederm Voluma, which add new indications and possibilities for facial rejuvenation. Finally, new treatment paradigms such as initial treatment followed by an optimization treatment within 6 months may cause long-term improvements and optimize *in vivo* collagen synthesis. Hyaluronic acid fillers will continue to be the mainstay of treatment for static folds, lines, and wrinkles and volume replacement in the near future.

References

1. Chung J, Soyun C, Sewon K. (2004) Why does the skin age? Intrinsic aging, photoaging, and their pathophisiology. In: Rigel DS, Weis RA, Lim HW, Dover JS, eds. *Photoaging*. New York: Marcel Dekker, Inc, pp. 1–13.
2. Rohrich RJ, Pessa JE. (2008) The fat compartments of the face: anatomy and clinical implications for cosmetic surgery. *Plast Reconstr Surg* **121**, 1061.
3. Brandt FS, Cazzaniga A. (2008) Hyaluronic acid gel fillers in the management of facial aging. *Clin Interv Aging* **3**, 153–9.
4. (2013) Statistics: American Society of Aesthetic Plastic Surgery.
5. Tezel A, Fredrickson GH. (2008) The science of hyaluronic acid dermal fillers. *J Cosmet Laser Ther* **10**, 35–42.

6 Lorenc ZP, Fagien S, Flynn TC, Waldorf HA. (2013) Clinical application and assessment of Belotero: a roundtable discussion. *Plast Reconstr Surg* **132**, 69S–76S.

7 Stocks D, Sundaram H, Michaels J, Durrani MJ, Wortzman MS, Nelson DB. (2011) Rheological evaluation of the physical properties of hyaluronic acid dermal fillers. *J Drugs Dermatol* **10**, 974–80.

8 Narins RS, Brandt F, Leyden J, et al. (2003) A randomized, double-blind, multicenter comparison of the efficacy and tolerability of Restylane® versus Zyplast® for the correction of nasolabial folds. *Dermatol Surg* **29**, 588–95.

9 Arlette JP, Trotter MJ. (2008) Anatomic location of hyaluronic acid filler material injected into nasolabial fold: a histologic study. *Dermatol Surg* **34**, S56–S63.

10 Narins RS, Jewell M, Rubin M, et al. (2006) Clinical conference: management of rare events following dermal fillers – focal necrosis and angry red bumps. *Dermatol Surg* **32**, 426–34.

11 Kühne U, Imhof M, Kirchmeir M, Howell DJ. (2012) Five-year retrospective review of safety, injected volumes, and longevity of the hyaluronic acid Belotero Basic for facial treatments in 317 patients. *J Drugs Dermatol* **11**, 1032–5.

12 Callan P, Goodman GJ, Carlisle I, Liew S, Muzikants P, Scamp T, Halstead MB, Rogers JD. (2013) Efficacy and safety of a hyaluronic acid filler in subjects treated for correction of midface volume deficiency: a 24 month study. *Clin Cosmet Invest Dermatol* **6**, 81–9.

13 Gold MH. (2007) Use of hyaluronic acid fillers for the treatment of the aging face. *Clin Interv Aging* **2**, 369–76.

14 Beer KR. (2006) Nasal reconstruction using 20 mg/ml cross-linked hyaluronic acid. *J Drugs Dermatol* **5**, 456–65.

15 Glogau RG, Kane MA. (2008) Effect of injection techniques on the rate of local adverse events in patients implanted with nonanimal hyaluronic acid gel dermal fillers. *Dermatol Surg* **34**, S105–S109.

16 Cohen JL. (2008) Understanding, avoiding, and managing dermal filler complications. *Dermatol Surg* **34**, S92–S99.

17 Cavallini M, Gazzola R, Metalla M, Vaienti L. (2013) The role of hyaluronidase in the treatment of complications from hyaluronic acid dermal fillers. *Aesthet Surg J* **33**, 1167–74.

18 Lorenc AP, Fagien S, Flynn TC, Waldorf HA. (2013) Clinical application and assessment of Belotero: a roundtable discussion. *Plast Reconstr Surg* **132**, 69S.

19 Lear G, Lewis GD, eds. (2012) *Microbial Biofilms: Current Research and Applications*. Norwich, United Kingdom: Caister Academic Press.

20 Parsek MR, Singh PK. (2003) Bacterial biofilms: An emerging link to disease pathogenesis. *Annu Rev Microbiol* **57**, 677–701.

21 Christensen LH. (2009) Host tissue interaction, fate, and risks of degradable and nondegradable gel fillers. *Dermatol Surg* **35**, 1612–9.

22 Narins RS, Coleman WP III, Glogau RG. (2009) Recommendations and treatment options for nodules and other filler complications. *Dermatol Surg* **35**, 1667–71.

23 Rohrich RJ, Monheit G, Nguyen AT, Brown SA, Fagien S. (2010) Soft-tissue filler complications: The important role of biofilms. *Plast Reconstr Surg* **125**, 1250–624.

24 Alhede M, Er O, Eickhardt S, et al. (2014) Bacterial biofilm formation and treatment in soft tissue fillers. *Pathog Dis* **70**, 339–46.

25 Kanoh S, Rubin BK. (2010) Mechanisms of action and clinical application of macrolides as immunomodulatory medications. *Clin Microbiol Rev* **23**, 590–615.

26 Lewis K. Riddle of biofilm resistance. (2001) *Antimicrob Agents Chemother* **45**: 999–1007.

27 Lupo MP, Smith S, Thomas J, et al. (2008) Effectiveness of Juvederm ultraplus dermal filler in the treatment of severe nasolabial folds. *Plast Reconstr Surg* **121**, 289–97.

28 Narins RS, Dayan SH, Brandt FS, Baldwin EK. (2008) Persistence and improvement of nasolabial fold correction with nonanimal-stabilized hyaluronic acid 100000 gel particles/mL filler on two retreatment schedules: results up to 18 months on two retreatment schedules. *Dermatol Surg* **34**, S2–S8.

29 Wang F, Garza LA, Kang S, et al. (2007) In vivo stimulation of de novo collagen production caused by cross-linked hyaluronic acid dermal filler injections in photodamaged human skin. *Arch Dermatol* **134**, 155–63.

CHAPTER 42
Calcium Hydroxylapatite for Soft Tissue Augmentation

Stephen Mandy
Department of Dermatology, University of Miami, Miami, FL, and Private Practice, Miami Beach, FL, USA

> **BASIC CONCEPTS**
> - Calcium hydroxylapatite is a fibroplastic filler in which volume correction is achieved in part through the biologic response of the host.
> - Calcium hydroxylapatite is approved for correction of moderate to severe wrinkles and folds, treatment of HIV-associated lipoatrophy, and vocal fold insufficiency.
> - The injectable filler is composed of microspheres of calcium hydroxylapatite suspended in an aqueous carrier gel.
> - Ideal areas for correction with calcium hydroxylapatite are the malar eminences, center of the cheek, nasolabial and nasojugal (tear trough) folds, prejowl sulcus/marionette, and chin and jawline regions. It is also very suitable for rejuvenation of the hands.
> - Filler duration is documented for as long as 12 months, although some loss of correction may occur.

Introduction

Facial volume loss leads to dramatic changes in appearance resulting from aging, disease, or hereditary conditions. The deflation from lipoatrophy causes skin redundancy, which is compounded by loss of elasticity and collagen degeneration from solar radiation and oxidative damage. Skeletal bone resorption further leads to deflation, enlargement of the ocular orbit, and shrinkage of the jaw. These visual signs of aging cannot be corrected by surgical tightening without volumization as this procedure alone leads to a skeletal, windswept appearance.

Replacement of volume through soft tissue augmentation can often offer facial rejuvenation with or without surgery. A variety of suitable materials for soft tissue augmentation exists. Natural fillers, such as collagen, hyaluronic acid, and calcium hydroxylapatite (CaHA), are synthesized to mimic, or are derived from biologic materials. Synthetic fillers may be permanent, such as acrylates and silicone, or biodegradable, such as poly-L-lactic acid [1].

Physiology and pharmacology

CaHA is a new type of fibroplastic filler in which volume correction is achieved in part through the biologic response of the host. Radiesse® (Merz Aesthetics, Inc, USA) is an injectable filler composed of microspheres of 30% CaHA suspended in an aqueous gel consisting of water, glycerin, and sodium carboxymethylcellulose. Once injected, the gel carrier is soon absorbed. The remaining microspheres are 25–45 μm in diameter, which facilitates injection but resists immediate phagocytosis. These bioceramic spheres have no antigenicity, foreign body or giant cell response, and cause a minimal inflammatory reaction. They do not stimulate ossification. Although visible on X-ray images and magnetic resonance imaging scans, they are radiolucent, appearing somewhat like frosted glass, and pose no impediment to radiologic analysis [2]. The CaHA microspheres form a scaffold for the fibroplastic proliferation, which provides the natural tissue feel of the implant. The local fibroplastic response results in the fibrous encapsulation of the particles and their gradual dissolution into calcium and phosphate ions (Figures 42.1, 42.2, and 42.3) [3]. Calcium hydroxylapatite requires no allergy testing which allows for immediate injection.

Indications and techniques

CaHA is a thick, white, clay-like, cohesive material intended for subdermal injection. The density of the material would make intradermal injection difficult because of poor tissue intrusion into the dermal stroma. It is not intended or suitable for fine lines, superficial injection, or injection into highly mobile areas such as the lip or above the orbital rim, where accumulation of material from movement might result in nodule formation. Because of its density the filler is most easily injected through a 27-g standard needle or a 28-g wide bore (Exel®) needle. It is most commonly injected in a linear retrograde fashion following penetration of the dermis at a 45° angle and then fully

---

Cosmetic Dermatology: Products and Procedures, Second Edition. Edited by Zoe Diana Draelos.
© 2016 John Wiley & Sons, Ltd. Published 2016 by John Wiley & Sons, Ltd.

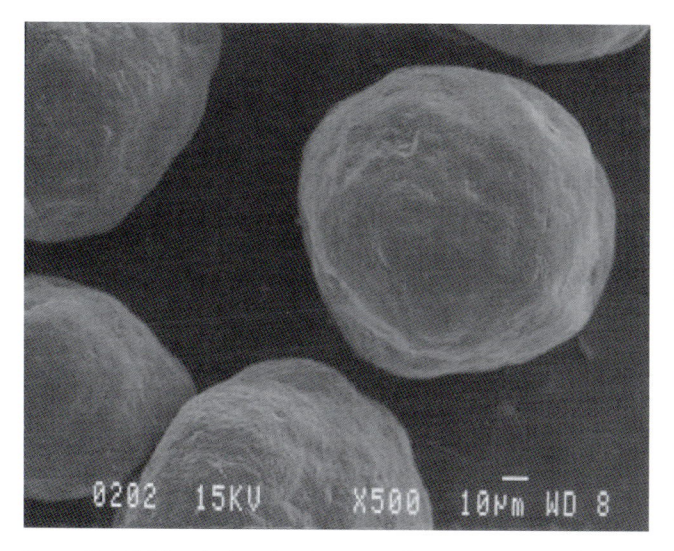

Figure 42.1 Calcium hydroxylapatite microspheres, 25–45 μm in diameter. (Source: BioForm Medical, San Mateo CA. Reproduced with permission.)

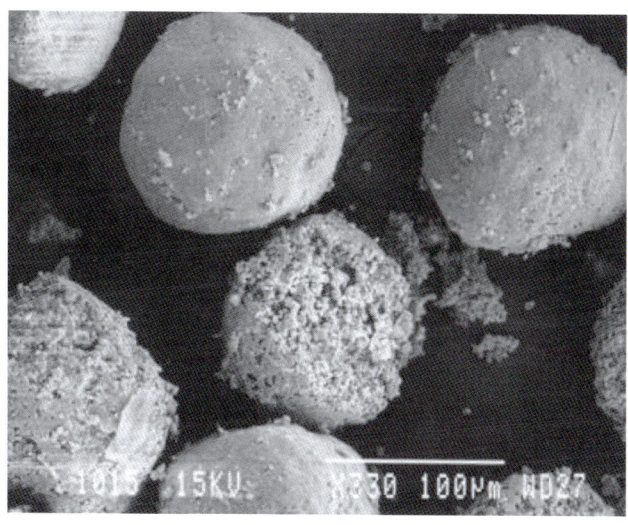

Figure 42.2 Gradual dissolution of microspheres. (Source: BioForm Medical, San Mateo CA. Reproduced with permission.)

(a)

(b)

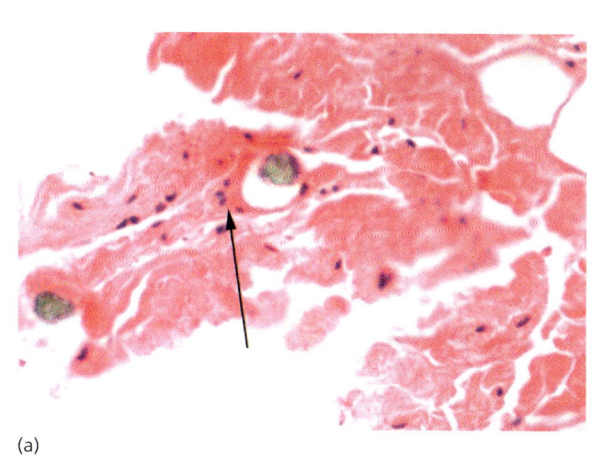

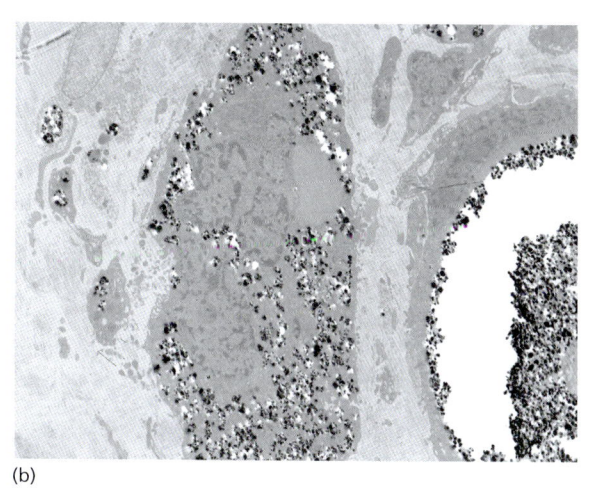

Figure 42.3 (a) Light microscopic section at 1 month post-injection showing microspherules at the dermal subcuticular junction and a slight increase in histiocytes (arrows). (Illustration courtesy of Drs. David J. Goldberg and Ellen Marmur.) (b) Electron microscopic section at 6 months showing both an intact microspherule and one undergoing a histiocytic derived catabolic process into smaller particles of calcium (black particles). The phosphate ions are not seen because they are dissolved in the processing of tissue for electron microscopy analysis. (Source: David J. Goldberg and Ellen Marmur. Reproduced with permission.)

inserting the needle in the subcutaneous plane parallel to the surface. The material is then extruded upon withdrawal of the needle in a threadlike manner. Multiple parallel or layered repeat injections may be utilized to achieve correction of a soft tissue contour. Injection through a blunt 27 gauge cannula may afford single port injection of the entire mid face and help avoid vascular injury and bruising [4].

Fanning and cross-hatching are utilized to achieve greater volume by smooth even injections of 0.1–0.2 mL per pass, followed by massage to avoid lumps and irregularities. One of the advantages of CaHA is its immediate "moldability" by massaging the injected area firmly against underlying structures or bimanually between the injector's fingers. Supraperiosteal placement is used to correct bony deformity.

Several comparative studies have demonstrated that lesser volumes of CaHA are required for full correction than with collagen or hyaluronic acid [5]. Ideal areas for correction are the malar eminences, center of the cheek, nasolabial and nasojugal (tear trough) folds, prejowl sulcus/marionette, and chin and jawline regions. Reinflation of the midface, including the malar, cheek, nasolabial, tear trough areas, yields a facelift-like effect and a far more dramatic rejuvenation than simple "line filling" (Figures 42.4 and 42.5) [5,7]. CaHA is a structural, volumetric filler analogous to the concrete foundation of facial

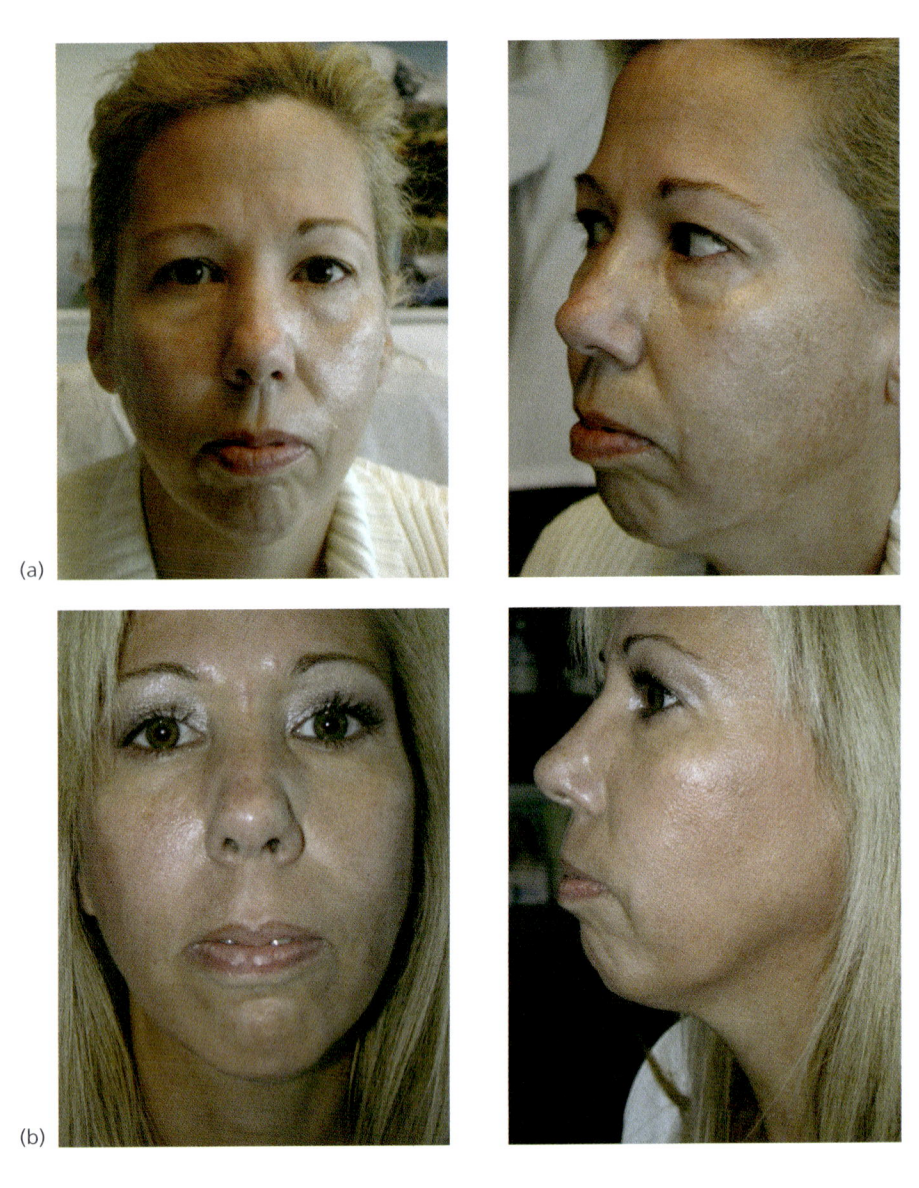

382 ANTI-AGING Injectable Anti-aging Techniques

Figure 42.4 Preinjection (a) and post-injection (b) of 2.6 mL CaHA.

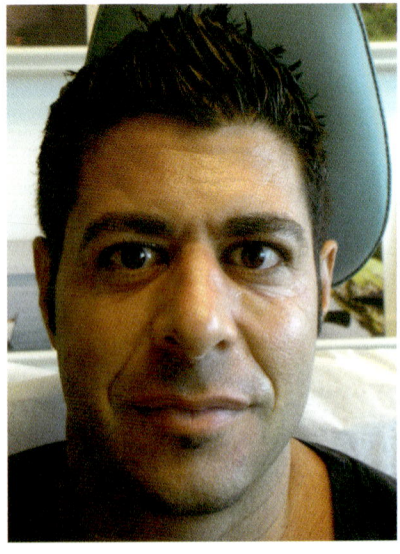

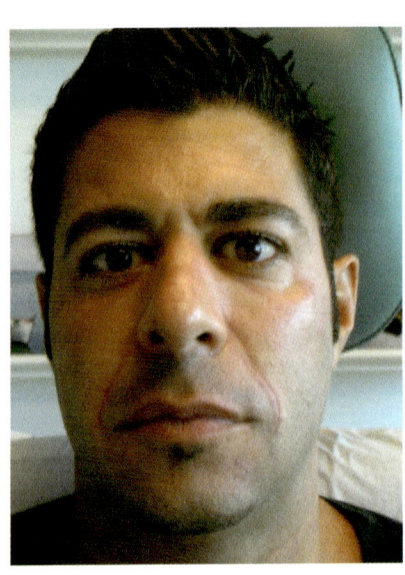

Figure 42.5 Preinjection (a) and immediately post-injection (b) of 2.6 mL CaHA.

restructuring. It is compatible with other more superficial fillers that can be overlaid for fine line smoothing, and with use in conjunction with radiofrequency and laser devices.

Preinjection topical anesthesia, 20–30 minutes pretreatment, is very important to insure patient comfort. A popular, FDA-approved means of achieving anesthesia is to mix CaHA with lidocaine via sterile syringe transfer [5]. CaHA is transferred via a female–female connector into a syringe containing 0.02–1.0 mL lidocaine and then the two are mixed by repeatedly passing the emulsion back and forth (Figure 42.6) [8]. Avoidance of aspirin, non-steroidal anti-inflammatory drugs (NSAIDs), and other medications or supplements that *promote* bruising are advisable. Pre- and post-treatment viral prophylaxis is recommended in patients with a history of herpes simplex. Merz recently (January 2015) released a new form of calcium hydroxylapatite which has lidocaine incorporated in the syringe (Radiesse L).

The first indication for calcium hydroxylapatite was for vocal fold correction. In 2006, it was approved for correction of moderate to severe facial wrinkles and folds, and restoration or correction of signs of lipoatrophy in patients with HIV [2,6]. In comparative studies of nasolabial fold treatment with CaHa versus collagen or hyaluronic acid, implants with CaHA gave significantly greater and more persistent correction with lower volumes at all time points [5,9].

Duration is documented for as long as 12 months, although some loss of correction may occur prior to that. Off label, non-FDA approved applications include correction of nasal defects, chin augmentation, and filling of the hands. Injection of a full syringe (1.3 mL) into each dorsal hand is accomplished through several bolus deposits in the subcutaneous space and between veins and tendons, followed by massage evenly over the entire hand to provide a full, more youthful appearance (Figure 42.7) [9,10].

All injections are performed percutaneously. Although some authors suggest intraoral approach to the tear trough area, this approach needlessly creates the opportunity to introduce bacteria into the implant with potentially serious consequences [11]. Glabellar injections are probably ill-advised because of the risk of vascular occlusion by embolization or compression, which has been reported with nearly all previous fillers. Calcium hydroxylapatite has been demonstrated to be safe and effective in skin of color [12].

Complications

Edema, erythema, pain, and ecchymosis are the most common complications, comparable to collagen and hyaluronic acid injections. Too superficial an injection can yield a visible white papule or plaque, which is slow to resolve. Too much material in one placement, or failure to massage, can result in palpable or visible nodules. Many of the complications, in the experience of this author, seem to be reduced when lidocaine is mixed with the CaHA prior to injection in the method described earlier.

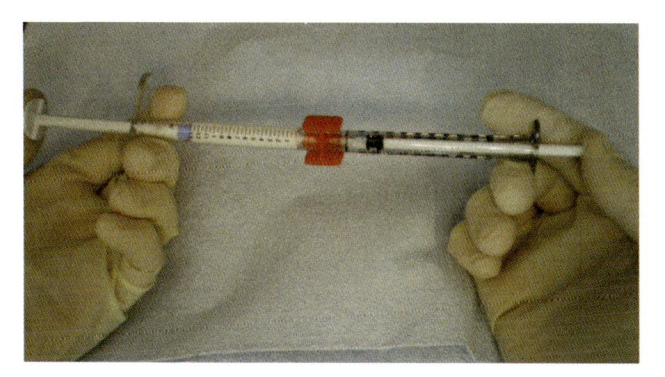

Figure 42.6 Radiesse mixed with lidocaine, using a female–female connector.

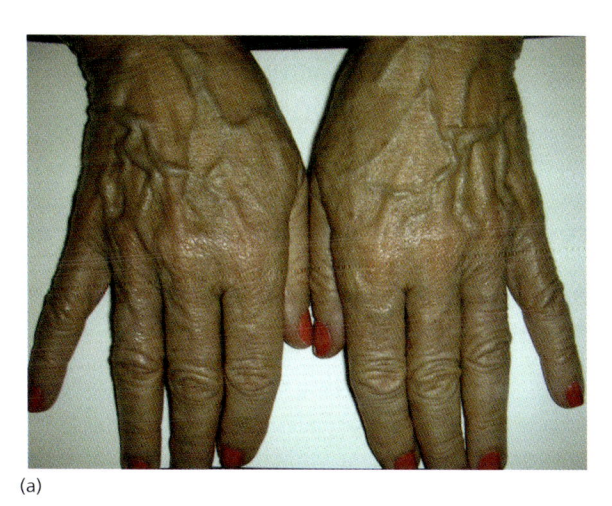

Figure 42.7 Preinjection (a) and post-injection (b) of CaHA into the hand.

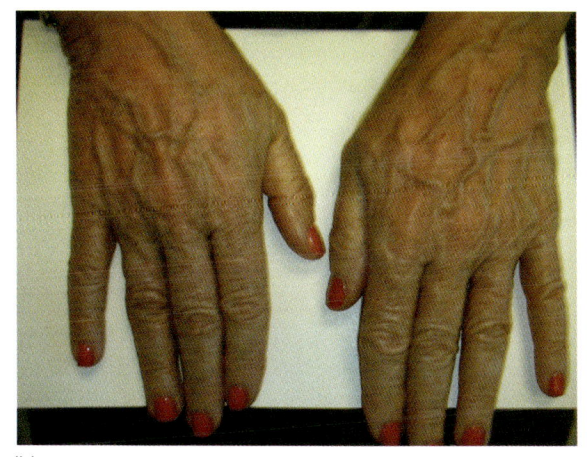

Conclusions

Substantial facial volume restoration with facelift-like effect can be achieved with the injection of CaHA. Large volume correction can be accomplished in a practical fashion because of the greater volumizing effect of CaHA in contrast to other filling agents. Success is technique-dependent; complications are infrequent and comparable to other agents. Durability of this fibroplastic filler may be up to 1 year.

References

1 Mandy SH. (2008) Fillers that work by fibroplasia: poly-L-lactic acid. In: CarruthersA, CaruthersJ, eds. *Soft Tissue Augmentation*, 2nd edn. Saunders Elsevier, pp. 101–4.
2 Carruthers A, Liebeskind M, Carruthers J, Forster B. (2008) Radiological and computed tomographic studies of calcium hydroxylapatite for treatment of HIV-associated facial lipoatrophy and correction of nasolabial folds. *Derm Surg* **34**, 578–84.
3 Marmur ES, Phelps R, Goldberg D. (2004) Clinical histologic and electron microscopic findings after injection of calcium hydroxylapatite filler. *J Cosmet Laser Ther* **6**, 223–6.
4 Niamtu J. (2009) Filler Injection with micro-cannula instead of needles. *Derm Surg* **35**, 2005–2008.
5 Moers-Carpi MM, Tufet JO. (2007) Calcium hydroxylapatite versus nonanimal stabilized hyaluronic acid for correction of nasolabial folds. *Dermatol Surg* **34**, 210–5.
6 Graivier M, Bass L, Busso M, Jasin ME, Narins RS, Tzikas TL. (2007) Calcium hydroxylapatite for correction of mid and lower face. *Plast Reconstr Surg* **120**(6), 55–66S.
7 Rohrich RJ, Pessa JE, Ristow B. (2008) The youthful cheek and the deep medial fat compartment. *Plast Reconst Surg* **121**(6), 2107–12.
8 Marmur E, Green L, Busso M. (2009) A controlled randomized study of pain levels in subjects treated with calcium hydroxylapatite premixed withlidocaine for correction of nasolabial folds. *Derm Surg* **36**, 1–7.
9 Busso M, Applebaum D. (2007) Hand augmentation with Radiesse® (calcium hydroxylapatite). *Dermatol Ther* **20**, 385–7.
10 Smith S, Busso M, McClaren M, Bass LS. (2007) A randomized, bilateral, prospective comparison of calcium hydroxylapatite microspheres versus human-based collagen for the correction of nasolabial folds. *Dermatol Surg* **33**, S112–21.
11 Wolcott R, Ehrlich G. (2008) Biofilms and chronic infection. *JAMA* **299**, 2682–4.
12 Marmur E, Taylor S, Grimes P, Boyd C, *et al.* (2009) Six month safety results of calcium hydroxylapatite for treatment of nasolabial folds in Fitzpatrick skin types IV to VI. *Derm Surg* **35**, 1641–5.

CHAPTER 43
Autologous Skin Fillers

Amer H. Nassar,[1] Andrew S. Dorizas,[1] and Neil S. Sadick[1,2]
[1]Sadick Dermatology, New York, NY, USA
[2]Department of Dermatology, Weill Medical College of Cornell University, New York, NY, USA

> **BASIC CONCEPTS**
> - Autologous fillers are a novel group of dermal fillers using the patients' own cells or tissue.
> - Autologous fillers can be divided into: platelet-rich plasma, autologous fibroblast cell therapy and adipose-derived stem cells.
> - Platelet-rich plasma has been studied most extensively from the group, while adipose-derived stem cells the least.
> - Autologous fillers can be used for volume correction, facial contouring and filling of dermal defects.

Introduction

Dermal fillers have been utilizes for decades, and recently their demand for cosmetic purposes has increased significantly. Although the desired outcome remains the same, the materials used to achieve facial contouring and correct volume loss have changed dramatically. The recent introduction of autologous dermal fillers in the field of cosmetic dermatology has shifted the focus into yet a new direction, one that possibly enhances many of the desired effects, while abolishing the adverse ones. Although autologous fillers are new and have a promising future, they are yet to be studied on a large scale.

Platelet-rich plasma

Introduction

Platelets were first described by Max Schulze in the mid 1800s, and their role in coagulation and blood clotting was discovered a short while later when Giulio Bizzozero noted the relationship between their adhesion, aggregation and the subsequent fibrin deposition [1]. The wide role platelets play in a multitude of other processes have since been described, one of which is the healing process. Platelets release a number of growth factors (Table 43.1) including transforming growth factor beta (TGF) and platelet-derived growth factor (PDGF), both closely involved in wound healing and the repair and regeneration of tissues. Platelet-rich plasma (PRP) is a concentrated source of autologous platelets, prepared from whole blood, containing roughly five times the amount of platelets as the baseline blood platelet count. These features make PRP a great source of growth factors, and its capabilities in assisting in wound healing and tissue regeneration has attracted considerable interest from the medical community [2].

Recently, the dermatological possibilities of PRP for skin rejuvenation were recognized, and its ability to serve as an autologous dermal filler was comprehended. The cocktail of growth factors released from the α-granules of platelets, serve to regulate cell migration and proliferation as well as the promotion of extracellular matrix (ECM) accumulation. This eventually led to angiogenesis stimulation which promoted activation of regional fibroblasts, thus inducing the synthesis of collagen, leading to skin rejuvenation [2].

Although robust evidence exists for the use of PRP in the fields of odontology, orthopedics, and traumatology, it was only recently that positive effects have been apparent in cosmetic dermatology. Sclafani has shown that as little as a single treatment with autologous platelet rich fibrin matrix (a similar product to PRP), has positive outcomes on deep nasolabial folds (NLF). In the past several years, PRP has received wide attention and considerable homage as an autologous filler not only for the treatment of deep NLF's, but also facial rhytids, dermal depressions and scars [3].

Moreover, PRP therapy as a possible treatment for hair loss has also been researched extensively, and it appears that fibroblast growth factor released from activated platelets plays a role as a potent stimuli for hair growth. Results appear promising for both androgenetic alopeccia as well as alopecia areata [4].

Preparation of platelet-rich plasma

The preparation of PRP is a relatively simple and quick task, usually occurring without any complications with a wide variety of preassembled PRP preparation kits are available in the market (Figure 43.1). Initially, approximately 9 cc of blood is

---

Cosmetic Dermatology: Products and Procedures, Second Edition. Edited by Zoe Diana Draelos.
© 2016 John Wiley & Sons, Ltd. Published 2016 by John Wiley & Sons, Ltd.

Table 43.1 Growth Factors released from platelets during PRP treatment.

Growth factor name	Effect
Platelet derived growth factor – AA, AB, BB (PDGF)	• Deposition of ECM • Stimulates the production of collagen, hyaluronic acid, proteoglycans, and fibronectin • Production and secretion of collagenase by fibroblasts • Contraction of collagen matrices • Chemotaxis of fibroblasts and smooth muscle cells [8]
Transforming growth factor – β 1,2 (TGF)	• Chemotaxis of macrophages and fibroblasts • Stimulation of ECM production • Inhibition of proteolytic enzymes • Formation of new granulation tissue [9]
Vascular endothelial growth factor (VEGF)	• Stimulation of angiogenesis • Chemotaxis of macrophages and neutrophils
Insulin-like growth factor 1	• Stimulation of collagen production • Stimulation of cell proliferation [10]
Basic-fibroblast growth factor (bFGF)	• Stimulation of proliferation of mesenchymal stromal cells • Stimulation of angiogenesis [11]
Epidermal growth factor (EGF)	• Stimulation of proliferation of endothelial cells
Platelet factor-4	• Chemotaxis of neutrophils and fibroblasts

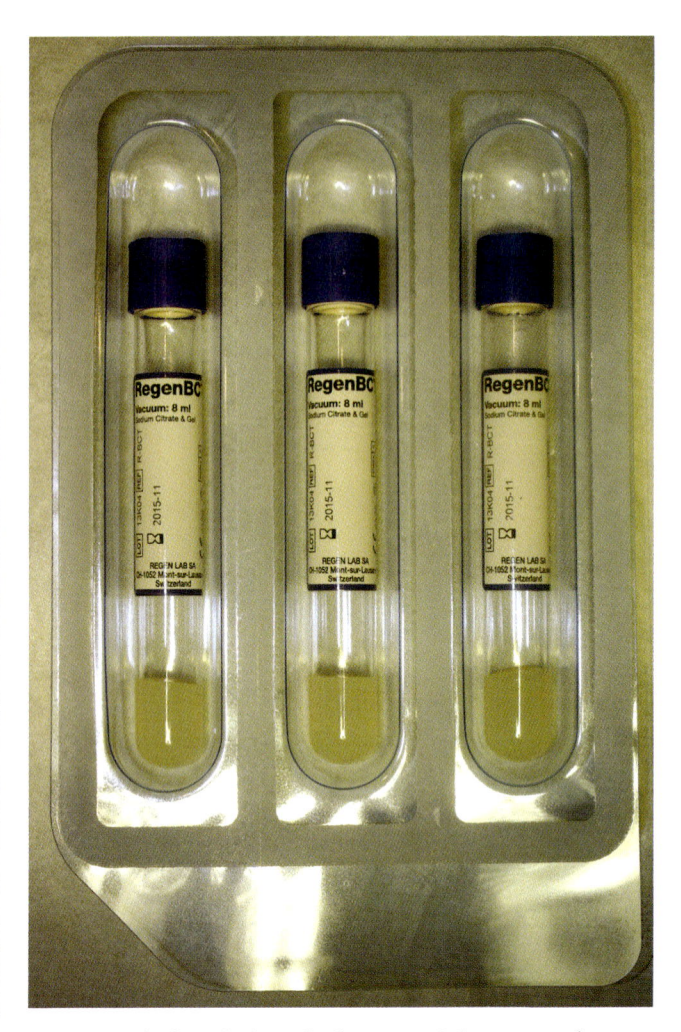

Figure 43.1 Platelet-rich plasma kit from Regen Lab containing three vacuum tubes, using a thixotropic gel for cell separation and sodium citrate as an anticoagulant.

collected into a tube containing an anticoagulant, most commonly citrate dextrose-A. After collection of the whole blood, either a single centrifugation or a 2-step centrifugation process follows. Although both processes are capable of producing PRP, the 2-step centrifugation process allows for a higher concentration for platelets and is therefore preferable. The initial step will separate the plasma containing the buffy coat from the red blood cells beneath. The second round of centrifugation accumulates the platelets at the bottom, which are used to create the PRP [2,5].

Before injection, the PRP must be activated using either thrombin or calcium chloride. This will allow exocytosis and the release of growth factors from α-granules, and facilitate the processes which will eventually lead to tissue regeneration [6].

Techniques for PRP injection

It is important to mention that injection techniques vary between physicians. A local anesthetic either in the form of a topical anaesthetic cream or simple topical ice should be used to minimize discomfort and pain. Alternatively, for correction of deep NLFs, infraorbital nerve blockade could be utilized for further pain control. All injections should be done using a 27 or 30-gauge needle. For NLF injections, a linear threading technique has proven most successful with correction performed from the alar crease to the level of the oral commissure, in the subdermal or intradermal plane. Intradermal injections should be used for fine rhytids, whereas a subscision followed by a subdermal injection using the "abundant ponfi" technique are best for treating acne scars [6,7]. Other methods of injection include the "micro ponfi" technique in the forehead and neck and the "linear retrograde technique in the cheek area [7].

Sclafani has contemplated that initial overcorrection of the dermal defects is desirable when using PRP, as much of the filler is plasma volume, which is quickly absorbed within the first 3–12 hours after the procedure [8].

Adverse reactions

As with any medical intervention, adverse reactions should always be acknowledged, and the risk minimized, when performing a procedure. Prior to the use of autologous fillers, injectable dermal fillers posed a risk of immunogenetic hypersensitivity reactions, as well as granuloma formation or chronic infections when using permanent fillers [6,8]. Since PRP is prepared from the patient's own blood, the aforementioned adverse reactions have been eliminated. The most observed side effects observed after PRP injections were mild and transient in nature.

Mild bruising was experienced by most patients, which lasted between one and three days. In a minority of patients, bruising lasted considerably longer, up to 14 days, usually with injections in the periorbital area.

There have been no reports of other adverse reactions from the use of PRP as an autologous dermal filler. Redaelli *et al.* have reported that in a group of 23 patients, none experienced any serious side effects including infections and haematomas [7]. This similar lack of adverse reactions was mentioned in another study of 15 patients by Sclafani [6].

Autologous fibroblast cell therapy

Introduction

Collagen is the primary protein found in the dermis and serves multiple functions, which provide strength and elasticity for the skin, as well as a structural scaffold for cells. With aging, the proportions of collagen in the human skin begin to vary. Certain factors, such as the levels of matrix metalloprotcinases and UV radiation, play a central role in the degradation of dermal collagen, leading to the development of rhytids, folds and accentuation of dermal defects. Thus, the replacement of dermal collagen became a major player for the rejuvenation and revitalization of aged skin. Historically, collagen has been widely used as a dermal filler. However, reports of as many as six percent of healthy patients experience localized hypersensitivity reactions, while others report the occurrence of granulomatous foreign body reactions, erythematous nodules at the injection site as well as other side effects. These adverse reactions coupled with the temporary corrective measure of collagen as a dermal filler, have limited its use and left much room for improvement [13].

Fibroblasts, being the major source of collagen production, have drawn much interest for their capabilities in cosmetic dermatology. Furthermore, the use of autologous fibroblasts sparked even greater interest, as it would eliminate problems procured from the use of allogenic substances. Fibrocell Science, Inc. formerly known as Isolagen Inc., was one of the first biotech companies focused on developing autologous fibroblasts for esthetic applications. Their production of Azfibrocel-T (brand name Laviv™), an autologous form of fibroblast cell therapy, has been the subject of numerous clinical trials for its potential use as a dermal filler [13–16]. This method involves the acquirement of small skin biopsies from the patient to develop an autologous fibroblastic cell line. Once the cell line is created and fibroblasts are multiplied, they are reinjected in the desired areas, acting as a dermal filler. After reintroduction, fibroblasts will undergo a process of collagen production and protein repair that helps sustain the long-term corrective effect of the treatment. The results are an increase in thickness as well as density of dermal collagen.

Preparation

The nature of autologous cell treatment require collection of patient tissue in order to develop a patient-specific cell line. In the case of autologous fibroblasts, a simple skin biopsy is the preferred method of tissue sampling. Three separate 3–4 mm punch biopsies are obtained, preferably from the postauricular crease. The tissue samples are then sent to a laboratory overnight, where they are isolated, cultured and expanded by tissue culture techniques over a 6-week period. Once a sufficient amount of fibroblasts has been reached, they are returned for initiation of treatment. The procedure should be undertaken within 24 hours of receiving the autologous fibroblasts. This allows for optimal results and ensures the autologous fibroblasts remain viable. Culturing will produce anywhere between 500–600 million cells, approximately 20 million cells for every 1 mL of injectable product. It is important to note that cryopreservation is an available method to store the autologous cell lines for future use, preserving viability for up to three years [16].

Techniques for autologous fibroblast injection

Once the product arrives, treatment can begin immediately with no need for further preparation. The expanded fibroblast suspension can be injected in various areas, depending on the patient's demands. Autologous fibroblasts have shown great results as a dermal filler for NLFs as well as depressed acne scars. However, it maybe be used for other wrinkles, fine lines and dermal defects as well [14,16].

One should not underestimate the importance of pain control before the start of such a procedure. It is much easier to delineate the areas of wrinkling or defects in a relaxed and calm patient. Local anesthesia can be achieved either by cold ice application, local nerve block, or topical injections of lidocaine.

Thereafter, visual delineation of the facial contour deformities should pursue, followed by the injection of the filler into the upper and middle dermal layers. The injection technique requires multiple passes and careful depth penetration so as to create transient blanching of the skin surface. This ensures that the injection was given in the right plane and in sufficient amounts. Usually, 0.1 mL per linear centimeter is to be given. A retrograde threading technique has been most commonly used, giving positive results especially with nasolabial and melolabial folds [14]. Injections into the papillary dermal plane have also been noted to be reliable when depressed or distensible acne scars are being treated [15]. It is of note that volumetric correction of the dermal deformities should not be considered an efficacy endpoint. Autologous fibroblastic cell therapy is not designed for immediate volumetric correction, instead it is intended to provide cells capable of collagen production, providing results within weeks to months.

Patients should receive a total of three treatments, separated by two to three week intervals for optimal results. One should inform patients of the delayed results and long-term correction of such a treatment, as to not provide them with unrealistic expectations of immediate results.

Adverse reactions

There have been very few documented adverse reactions from autologous fibroblast cell therapy. Self-limiting erythema, swelling and bruising might occur and are usually mild and transient in nature. Furthermore, they are most likely attributable to the procedure itself rather than the injectable used.

As with any autologous treatment, the risk of adverse reactions from hypersensitivity is low. However, injection of small amounts of autologous cells into the patients forearm, days to weeks prior to the procedure, with absence of evidence of an allergic skin reaction further minimizes the risk. Boss *et al.* reported an absence of allergic adverse effects during a two and a half year study [17].

It must be mentioned that the limited amount of studies and small patient group sizes are insufficient for excluding the possibility of short term or long-term adverse events.

Adipose-derived stem cells

Introduction

Autologous fat transplantation has been used for decades throughout the fields of medicine, and in recent years has become more popular for facial recontouring. When used for aesthetic purposes as a dermal filler, transplanted autologous fat has the tendency to fibrose [18], and even with the newer "lipostructure technique", the survivability of transplanted fat remains relatively low [19]. The lack of neovascularization is an issue that plays a major role in the survivability of transplanted autologous adipocytes. However, it soon became evident that stem cells located within adipose tissue could have a beneficial effect on transplanted fat. Adipose-derived stem cells (ASC), are mesenchymal multipotent stem cells which have the capability of differentiating into multiple cell lines. Recent studies have shown that when combined with autologous fat transfer, improve the outcome of a procedure, with up to 60% increase in fat survival [20]. The proposed mechanism is believed to be related to growth factors secreted by ASC which promote neovascularization and minimize the inflammatory response [21]. Moreover, it has been suggested that ASC alone are not capable of producing soft-tissue fill [22]. Therefore, the most promising use of ASC as a filler would be its incorporation and supplementation into a matrix formed from autologous fat [23].

Due to the relatively novel nature of ASC, there has been a lack of clinical trials based in the US. Some studies abroad have shown that ASC produce an anti-wrinkle effect as well as an increase in dermal thickness [24].

Preparation

ASCs can be acquired in large quantities with a simple surgical procedure. Initially for fat extraction, conventional techniques may rupture a high amount of extracted adipocytes due to high pressures. It is therefore advised to place cells under minimal trauma using a 3-mm cannula connected to a 10-cc syringe and using manual suction. Once the fat grafts have been obtained, isolation of ASC may commence.

Techniques for adipose-derived stem cell injection

Intradermal injections of 20% to 30% of ASCs incorporated into a matrix of autologous fat, may be used as the injectable filler. It is important to note that a large surface area contact between the graft and the vascularized tissue should be achieved in an attempt to minimize the amount of graft undergoing ischemic necrosis. This may be facilitated by incorporating the "fanning technique" which allows multiple tunnels of fat particles to be injected in the desired location.

Adverse reactions

It is also important to evaluate the safety of ASC treatment before its use increases in everyday clinical treatment. Certain reports have demonstrated a neoplastic and tumorigenic effect of ASC, especially when subculturing the cells [25]. Furthermore, there may be an association between ASC and an increased recurrence rate of certain hematologic malignancies [26].

Nevertheless, it is clear that much effort and research is yet to be done in order to achieve a full understanding in this subject. Although our current knowledge of ASC as a dermal filler is limited, it remains both promising and exciting.

Conclusion

The practice of using dermal fillers in cosmetic dermatology has been around for decades, with newer and more novel fillers entering the market occasionally. The success of platelet-rich plasma and autologous fibroblast cell therapy in recent years has proven that autologous products have a place in facial contouring and that the science of dermal fillers has much room for expansion and innovation. Moreover, the promising nature of ASCs incorporated into an adipocyte matrix is evidence that many more therapies are to be expected in the near future.

Autologous fillers are time and time again proving that they too can play a vital role in this increasingly complex field of medicine, bringing their own benefits along. It is uncertain as of yet, as to what extent they will be game-changing innovative therapies and if they will revolutionize dermal fillers and facial contouring procedures.

References

1. Brewer DB. (2006) Max Schultze (1865), G. Bizzozero (1882) and the discovery of the platelet. *Br. J. Haematol* **133**, 251–8.
2. Kim DH, Je YJ, Kim CD, *et al.* (2011) Can platelet-rich plasma be used for skin rejuvenation? Evaluation of effects of platelet-rich plasma on human dermal fibroblast. *Ann Dermatol* **23**, 424–31.
3. Sclafani AP, Romo T III, Parker A, *et al.* (2000) Autologous collagen dispersion (Autologen) as a dermal filler: clinical observations and histologic findings. *Arch Facial Plast Surg* **2**, 48–52.
4. Trink A, Sorbellini E, Bezzola P, *et al.* (2013) A randomized, double-blind, placebo- and active-controlled, half-head study to evaluate the effects of platelet-rich plasma on alopecia areata. *Br J Dermatol* **169**, 690–4.
5. Arora NS, Ramanayake T, Ren YF, Romanos GE. (2009) Platelet-rich plasma: a literature review. *Implant Dent* **18**, 303–10.
6. Sclafani AP. (2010) Platelet-rich fibrin matrix for improvement of deep nasolabial folds. *J Cosmet Dermatol* **9**, 66–71.
7. Redaelli A, Romano D, Marcianó A. (2010) Face and neck revitalization with platelet-rich plasma (PRP): clinical outcome in a series of 23 consecutively treated patients. *J Drugs Dermatol* **9**, 466–72.
8. Sclafani AP. (2011) Safety, efficacy, and utility of platelet-rich fibrin matrix in facial plastic surgery. *Arch Facial Plast Surg* **13**, 247–51.
9. Heldin CH, Westermark B. (1999) Mechanism of action and in vivo role of platelet-derived growth factor. *Physiol Rev* **79**, 1283–316.
10. Sporn MB, Roberts AB. (1989) Transforming growth factor-beta. Multiple actions and potential clinical applications. *JAMA* **262**, 938–41.
11. Lyras DN, Kazakos K, Agrogiannis G, *et al.* (2010) Experimental study of tendon healing early phase: is IGF-1 expression influenced by platelet rich plasma gel? *Orthop Traumatol Surg Res* **96**, 381–7.
12. Chieregato K, Castegnaro S, Madeo D, *et al.* (2011) Epidermal growth factor, basic fibroblast growth factor and platelet-derived growth factor-bb can substitute for fetal bovine serum and compete with human platelet-rich plasma in the ex vivo expansion of mesenchymal stromal cells derived from adipose tissue. *Cytotherapy* **13**, 933–43.
13. Watson D, Keller GS, Lacombe V, *et al.* (1999) Autologous fibroblasts for treatment of facial rhytids and dermal depressions. A pilot study. *Arch Facial Plast Surg* **1**, 165–70.
14. Weiss RA, Weiss MA, Beasley KL, Munavalli G. (2007) Autologous cultured fibroblast injection for facial contour deformities: a prospective, placebo-controlled, Phase III clinical trial. *Dermatol Surg* **33**, 263–8.
15. Munavalli GS, Smith S, Maslowski JM, Weiss RA. (2013) Successful treatment of depressed, distensible acne scars using autologous fibroblasts: a multi-site, prospective, double blind, placebo-controlled clinical trial. *Dermatol Surg* **39**, 1226–36.
16. Smith SR, Munavalli G, Weiss R, *et al.* (2012) A multicenter, double-blind, placebo-controlled trial of autologous fibroblast therapy for the treatment of nasolabial fold wrinkles. *Dermatol Surg* **38**, 1234–43.
17. Boss WK, Marko O. (1998) Isolagen. In: KleinAW, ed. *Tissue Augmentation in Clinical Practice*. Marcel Dekker Inc 335–47.
18. Watson DKG, Keller GS, Lacombe V, *et al.* (1999) Autologous fibroblasts for treatment of facial rhytids and dermal depressions. A pilot study. *Arch Facial Plast Surg* **1**, 165–70.
19. Coleman SR. (1997) Facial recontouring with lipostructure. *Clin Plast Surg* **24**, 347–67.
20. Yoshimura K, Suga H, Eto H. (2009) Adipose-derived stem/progenitor cells: roles in adipose tissue remodeling and potential use for soft tissue augmentation. *Regen Med* **4**, 265–73.
21. Beeson W, Woods E, Agha R. (2011) Tissue engineering, regenerative medicine, and rejuvenation in 2010: the role of adipose-derived stem cells. *Facial Plast Surg* **27**, 378–87.
22. Moseley TA, Zhu M, Hedrick MH. Adipose-derived stem and progenitor cells as fillers in plastic and reconstructive surgery. *Plast Reconstr Surg* 2006) **118**, 121S–128S.
23. Woo YI, Park BJ, Kim HL, *et al.* (2010) The biological activities of (1,3)-(1,6)-beta-d-glucan and porous electrospun PLGA membranes containing beta-glucan in human dermal fibroblasts and adipose tissue-derived stem cells. *Biomed Mater* **5**, 044109.
24. Kim WS, Park BS, Sung JH. (2009) Protective role of adipose derived stem cells and their soluble factors in photoaging. *Arch Dermatol Res* **301**, 329–36.
25. Rubio D, Garcia-Castro J, Martin MC, *et al.* (2005) Spontaneous human adult stem cell transformation. *Cancer Res* **65**, 3035–9.
26. Ning HYF, Yang F, Jiang M, *et al.* (2008) The correlation between cotransplantation of mesenchymal stem cells and higher recurrence rate in hematologic malignancy patients: outcome of a pilot clinical study. *Leukemia* **22**, 593–9.

CHAPTER 44
Polylactic Acid Fillers

Kenneth R. Beer[1] and Jacob Beer[2]
[1]General, Surgical and Esthetic Dermatology, West Palm Beach, FL, USA
[2]Department of Dermatology, University of Pennsylvania, PA, USA

> **BASIC CONCEPTS**
> - Polylactic acid filler (PLLA) is a volume stimulator rather than a direct volume replacement.
> - PLLA is best suited for areas that are concave.
> - PLLA results are dependent on techniques such as dilution and injection.
> - Complications from PLLA are different from those from other fillers and include subcutaneous papule formation.
> - PLLA results (both good and bad) may last for years.

Introduction

Poly-L-lactic acid is the active ingredient found in Sculptra® (also known as New-Fill; Valeant, Laval, Canada). Each bottle of material also contains sodium carboxymethylcellulose (USP) and non-pyrogenic mannitol [1]. The sodium carboxymethylcellulose and mannitol act to stabilize the PLLA and have no biologic effect on the volume stimulation. The material comes as a freeze-dried powder that must be reconstituted with sterile water [2]. At the present time, Sculptra is the only product of its kind and as such is unique. In the United States, Europe and Canada, a variety of materials are available for long term or permanent volume correction. These include Radiesse, Perlane, silicone and Juvederm Voluma in many of these markets. Sculptra differs from these materials in several key respects, the most significant of which is the fact that Sculptra is not a direct volume replacement. Rather, it stimulates the production of collagen and elastin to replace volume. Its replacement is gradual and dependent on the patient's ability to make connective tissue.

Although the amount of PLLA in a bottle of Sculptra is fixed at 367.5 mg, the methods of reconstitution and thus the volumes used for injections are variable. The ability to add different amounts of water, lidocaine and epinephrine is one opportunity for physicians to vary the use of this material and may contribute to differing reports of success and complications. Unlike other filling agents, the product injected is not standardized and the package insert does not reflect the way that the product is presently used. Initial reports of product use in Europe utilized dilutions of 3 mL pf sterile water per bottle [3]. The duration of reconstitution for these early studies was 4 hours. The package insert for the product recommends a reconstitution time of 4 hours; however, many PLLA injectors advocate longer periods, with some recommending that water imbibe for at least 24 hours, with longer periods of up to 3 weeks also touted. At the present time, there is no uniform consensus or any clinical trial data to suggest what is the optimal dilution or reconstitution time. Since the product has been used for several years, growing numbers of physicians are increasing the volume used to dilute and also increasing the amount of time for the PLLA to soak prior to injection. At the present time, many injectors are using 7–9 mL of water for at least 48 hours of imbibing time. Many expert injectors prefer to have the product imbibe for at least week and will add water and then refrigerate the product. When injecting areas other than the face, including the chest, knees and arms, dilutions above 10 mL per bottle are being utilized.

In addition to the 7–9 mL water, various anesthetic agents and epinephrine are added to the mixture. The anesthetic added to the product varies depending on injector preferences and experiences. Among the alternatives used, 1% lidocaine with 1:100 k epinephrine added is perhaps the most frequently used. Lidocaine without epinephrine (1%) and 2% lidocaine is also used.

Volumes of anesthetic added to the reconstituted material also vary based on the location of each injection and the experience of the injector. At the present time, many skilled injectors utilize 7–9 mL water for at least 24 hours and immediately before injection add 1–2 mL of 1% lidocaine with epinephrine. When injecting areas such as the back of the hands, this dilution may require additional water and the total reconstitution volume for these areas is 10 mL for many injectors. For the 10-mL dilution, the authors suggest the use of 9 mL water and 1 mL 1% lidocaine with 1:100000 epinephrine.

Once reconstituted, the bottle should be signed and dated and the material should be stored in a refrigerator. Before injection,

---

Cosmetic Dermatology: Products and Procedures, Second Edition. Edited by Zoe Diana Draelos.
© 2016 John Wiley & Sons, Ltd. Published 2016 by John Wiley & Sons, Ltd.

it should be left out so that it can warm to room temperature. Whether or not gently heating it to body temperature before injecting improves outcomes is another area of controversy. At the present time, it seems reasonable to inject material that is at room or body temperature, but not to heat the product beyond these temperatures. There is a paucity of data to suggest what the optimal injection temperature for this product is.

Advantages and disadvantages

PLLA has many unique properties and strengths and weaknesses. Among the strengths of the product are its long-lasting nature, ability to correct large volume losses, and ease of injection. Weaknesses of the product include the formation of subcutaneous papules, multiple injection visits, expense, and, most importantly, there is no way to predict the degree of improvement that will result from any given injection. This latter point means that unlike the hyaluronic acids (HA) or calcium hydroxylapatite, there is no way for a physician to correct a given area with a 1:1 defect to product replacement ratio. Instead, the injector must wait to see the extent to which new collagen will form. Interims of approximately four weeks should separate injections.

One of the advantages of this product is its ability to produce collagen, providing a correction that lasts for more than 1 year [4]. The only products that are able to provide this type of long-term correction are those that are permanent (such as Artefill or silicone) or the highly cross-linked hyaluronic acids such as Voluma. Another advantage of Sculptra is the fact that it is easily enhanced when the volume begins to subside. Typically, patients may return for an annual enhancement with 1–2 bottles of material. Despite the initial high cost of injection, the degree and duration of the PLLA correction makes it cost effective. Volume replacement for moderate lipoatrophy costs $3000–4000. When compared with the cost of other fillers for the same time interval, PLLA correction is reasonably priced. Newer, more cross-linked hyaluronic acid fillers such as Juvederm Voluma may provide corrections that are of comparable duration.

PLLA is technically easy to inject. In fact, the difficulty associated with this product lies more with poor patient selection, inappropriate and inadequate volume reconstitution and injections into areas that should not be injected with this product (e.g. the lips). The very nature of the product as it is injected (it is a suspension rather than a solution or gel) means that even with the best technique, particles of PLLA will migrate following injection. In addition, density differences both in the syringe and in the patient as the PLLA particles settle provide non-homogeneous product dispersion even with the best technique.

One additional advantage of the product is its utility in various parts of the face. It has been successfully used in the prejowl sulcus, temples, malar area, nasolabial creases, pre-auricular region, tear trough and mandibular border. Patient satisfaction with PLLA is high, with 99.1% of patients in one study reporting satisfaction with the procedure [4].

Standard injection techniques

Beginners should not have technical problems injecting this product as long as they select the right patients and locations to treat. The most common problem encountered by novice injectors is clogging of material in the needle, resulting in sporadic injections of product under high pressure and placement of the product at the wrong plane.

Rapid injection is the best technique for injecting PLLA. This avoids needle clogs producing high pressure injections and areas of high and low concentration product placement. Injection needles should be either 25 or 26 gauge and 0.5–1 inch in length. Smaller bore and longer needles may result in difficulty extruding the product into the tissue. However, the advantage of longer needles are that they can get to a wide area with fewer injection sites and less theoretical trauma. Cannulas may also be used for the insertion of Sculptra but should be 25 G to avoid clogging. One advantage of cannulas is that they enable the injector to deposit Sculptra across a wide area of the face with far fewer punctures than a traditional needle.

Injections of PLLA require deep product placement. Thus, the needle should be at the level of the deep dermis or dermal–subcutaneous junction. Superficial placement will increase the probability of visible papule formation. Various methods of injecting including serial puncture, linear threading, and fanning have been described and espoused. Standard injection techniques should try to include aspects of each because the goal of the injection is to obtain a homogeneous distribution of product at the plane where it will do the most good. Which technique predominates for a given individual depends on the area being injected and the amount of product being placed. Following any technique, it is essential to massage the product vigorously to distribute it. When massaging, deep pressure adequate to move product from discrete pearls into a contiguous plane is required.

One disadvantage of the product is the need for multiple injections. This need substantially increases the risk of bleeding and trauma from injections. It is not clear whether or not the use of epinephrine in the dilution decreases this risk, but it is likely that this is the case. As with other injections, bruising resulting from PLLA injections may be treated with pulse dye laser to help resolution. There is anecdotal evidence that injections that utilize more than one bottle in a session will provide faster volume replacement. Most injectors do not favor decreasing the interval between injections for fear of creating subcutaneous papules.

The most frequently injected areas are the cheeks, jawline, and temples. For the cheeks, it is helpful to inject half a bottle (4.5 mL) per session into each cheek. Experienced injectors may increase the amount injected per session to two bottles to accelerate the process. Each injection should be accomplished such that approximately 0.05 mL is inserted and the space between injections is about 0.5 cm. Serial puncture and fanning may be combined to produce a spoke-like network of injections (Figure 44.1). Typical

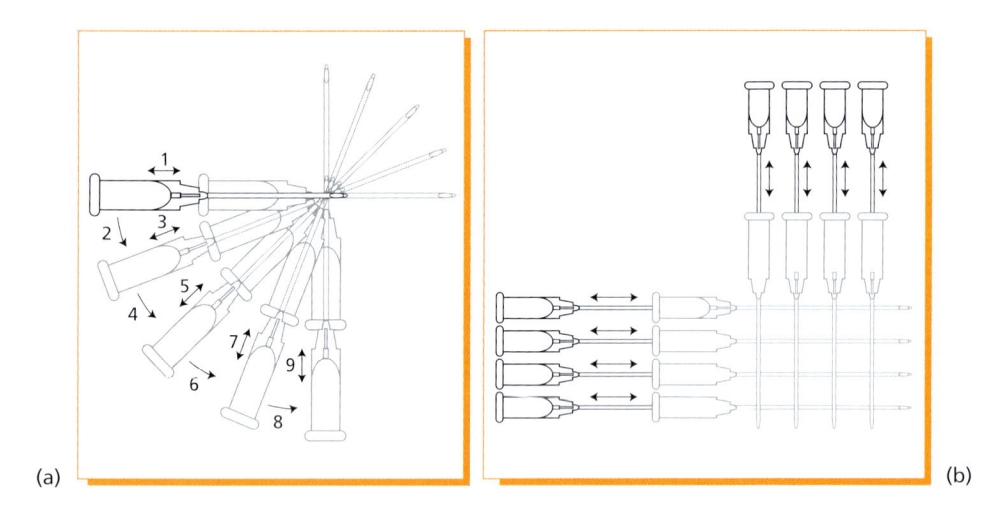

Figure 44.1 Serial puncture and fanning techniques. (a) Fan technique. (b) Cross-hatching technique.

injection schedules for the cheeks include three injections spaced at least 1 month apart. In many patients, one bottle of product will be used for each injection. However, many physicians have recently increased the number of bottles injected per session to two. Patients with severe lipoatrophy may require more injections and more material per injection. It is acceptable to advise these patients that between 4–6 sessions will be required until full volume restoration is accomplished. However, it is not advisable to decrease the time interval between sessions.

Correction of jawline volume loss may be required following loss of subcutaneous tissue and bone resorption. Loss of bony support is one hallmark of facial aging. As the support structure for the skin is lost, the skin and soft tissue sag. PLLA injections may be performed to stimulate collagen in this area with outstanding results. Standard injection techniques for this area are serial puncture and fanning. Needle insertion for this location should be at the level of the deep tissue (subcutaneous or just above the periosteum). As with other locations, deep massage is necessary to move the product into a homogeneous plane.

Needle orientation for the jawline is typically at 45° to the skin. Moderate volume loss may be treated with 3–4 bottles of the 9 mL dilution of PLLA and can be completed in three visits for many patients. Severe volume loss may be treated with four or bottles spanning 4–8 sessions.

Temporal wasting is one of the hallmarks of facial aging. Although other products may be used to treat this, PLLA is exceptionally well suited for this application. Injections in this location have several potential pitfalls that need to be avoided. The plethora of blood vessels in this area provides one potential pitfall for injection of any product and the particulate nature of PLLA is no exception. When injecting the temples with PLLA, it is important to aspirate prior to inserting product. Needle placement should be deep and at the level just superficial to the periosteum. Placement at this level will also help avoid formation of visible subcutaneous papules. Recent articles highlight the efficacy of PLLA for temporal volume restoration and describe optimal techniques for treatment [5]. These authors also advocate the use of lasers to rejuvenate the skin of the area for a comprehensive approach to this region. Average injection volume per side is 4.5 mL using the 9 mL volume dilution. The technique for injecting PLLA in this area is predominantly the fanning method, but serial puncture is also used. Restoration of temporal volume may require 3–4 sessions, requiring 3–4 bottles for most patients.

Treatment of lipoatrophy remains one of the best uses for PLLA. Injections of PLLA in patients with lipoatrophy are associated not only with improvements in the appearance of their face, but also improvements in the quality of their lives [6]. In a review of 230 HIV patients treated with up to five sessions of injections, 64% had improvements in their quality of life measured at 2 months and 58.8% had improvements at 12–18 months. As more patients live with lipodystrophy from HIV therapy, it is important to offer treatments that help relieve the visual stigmata associated with this disease.

PLLA may be safely used in skin of color to treat signs of aging as well as for the treatment of lipoatrophy. However, it has been suggested that this population may require increased intervals between treatments to minimize the potential for adverse events [7].

Advanced techniques

Perhaps the most important consideration when performing advanced techniques is to change the dilution and volume to accommodate the different areas being treated. Advanced techniques for injecting PLLA may be utilized to treat areas such as the tear troughs and the dorsum of the hands. When treating these areas, it is worthwhile to dilute each bottle with at least 10 mL of total volume rather than with 9 mL.

Tear troughs are one of the areas that should not be injected with Sculptra except by advanced injectors. Each injection should place a small amount of material (about 0.05 mL).

Injections should be about 3–5 mm apart. Following placement, each should be massaged to avoid discrete nodule formation. Despite perfect technique, injections of PLLA may result in the delayed formation of nodules and patients should be aware of this possibility prior to treatment [9].

Dorsal hand lipoatrophy and photoaging are hallmarks of aging that are frequently left untreated because of the lack of effective modalities. The use of PLLA for this location is a technique utilized by advanced injectors with very good results. As with injections of the tear trough, the dorsal hands are covered with skin that is typically thin and translucent. Thus, dilution of each bottle of Sculptra with 9 mL liquid is appropriate.

Longer needles or cannulae may be used to treat the dorsal hands. The needle may be inserted proximally and advanced parallel to the tendons and material inserted as the needle is withdrawn. Photoaged hands typically have prominent veins and care must be taken to avoid injections into these structures. Each hand will require about half a bottle per treatment session and approximately 9–10 injection sites to cover the entire hand.

Complications

The most common complications related to injections of PLLA are injection site related [2]. These include bruising, erythema, and site-related discomfort. More serious complications include nodule formation known as subcutaneous papules. These nodules are typically foreign body type granulomas mixed in with collagen matrix [10]. The subcutaneous nodules may be treated with injections of intralesional cortisone and it is reasonable to begin treatments with 2.5–5 mg/mL triamcinolone acetonide. Injections may be performed on a monthly basis until the nodule resolves. In the event that the nodule does not resolve after multiple injections it is possible to remove it surgically using a small incision. The rate of formation of these papules is approximately 4.7% [4].

More serious complications are possible with injections of PLLA (or any material) and these include necrosis of the skin. This could result from intravascular injection of PLLA and it is wise to aspirate prior to injections near major vascular structures. Inadvertent excursions of the needle into the globe may also occur with PLLA injections (or those of any product) when the periorbital area or tear troughs are injected. The injector should take care to use the non-dominant hand to palpate the infraorbital ridge and to orient the needle away from the eye so that if the patient makes a sudden movement, the needle will not jab them. As is the case with most injected agents, orbital necrosis and loss of vision secondary to embolization has been reported following injections with Sculptra [11]. The patient reported in this case had undergone injections of Sculptra in the periorbital region immediately followed by symptoms. Angiography revealed findings consistent with embolic phenomena.

PLLA compared with other fillers

With the advent of calcium hydroxylapatite, and new forms of hyaluronic acid, one question asked by some physicians is when PLLA should be used and what patients should be treated with it. PLLA is not a direct volume replacement material and instead causes the body to replace collagen. Thus, it is not a substitute product for the various fillers. Many patients that need discrete line filling will have volume loss associated that can be treated with PLLA. Patients that only require volume replacement of the malar, temporal, or jaw areas may also obtain optimal results

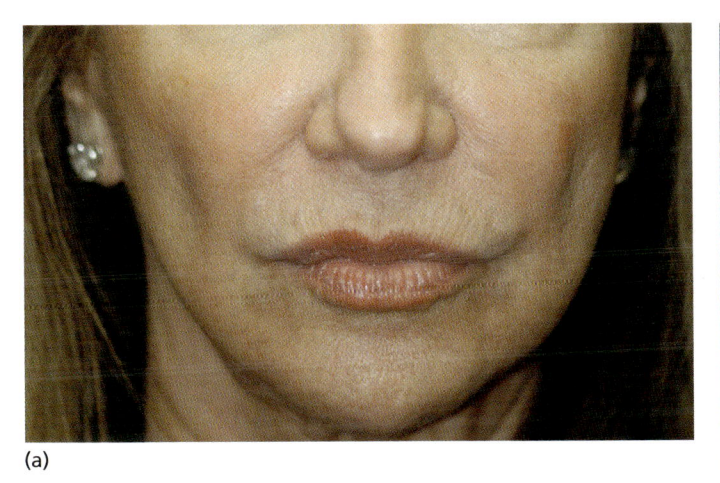

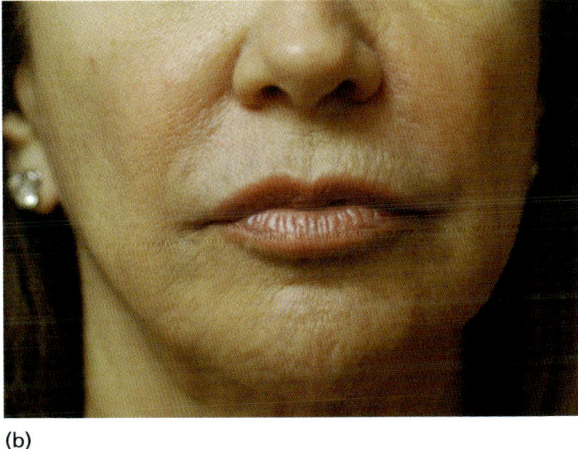

(a) (b)

Figure 44.2 (a) Before and after Sculptra injections: this is the result of three sessions, each with one bottle of Sculptra. This is typical of a three bottle correction with excellent volume restoration of the cheek area. The correction was durable for more than 18 months. (b) This is the result of three bottles initially with an excellent response that lasted for several years.

with PLLA, highly cross-linked HA or calcium hydroxylapatite. The advent of highly cross-linked HA fillers such as Juvederm Voluma provides the ability to afford immediate as well as delayed volume restoration.

Deciding where PLLA fits into one's practice is as much a patient selection issue as a technical one. Patients who have the temperament and budget to accept a gradual volume replacement should be treated with this product. Patients demanding a single visit correction should not. In addition, because there is no way to anticipate fully how any given individual will manufacture collagen, patients who will not tolerate a treatment program should be avoided.

Conclusions

PLLA is a unique molecule capable of restoring significant amounts of subcutaneous volume for long periods of time. It causes the body to make collagen and other extracellular matrix proteins. Unlike other products used in cosmetic dermatology, PLLA cannot produce exactly predictable results and it requires multiple treatment sessions to achieve its planned correction. Used judiciously, it can correct deficits that would otherwise be difficult to correct. PLLA has some unique complications that should be understood before it is used and patient selection is perhaps more important with this product than any other. However, its unique properties offer cosmetic dermatologists unique opportunities and this product should be embraced by injectors who understand its strengths and weaknesses.

References

1 Beer K. (2007) Optimizing patient outcomes with collagenic stimulators. *J Drugs Dermatol Suppl* **6**.
2 Sculptra Package Insert. Bridgewater, NJ: Sanofi-Aventis.
3 Vleggar D, Bauer U. (2004) Facial enhancement and the European experience with Sculptra. *J Drugs Dermatol* **3**, 542–7.
4 Schierle CF, Casas LA. (2011) Nonsurgical rejuvenation of the aging face with injectable poly-L-lactic acid for restoration of soft tissue volume. *Aesthet Surg J* **31**(1), 95–109.
5 Rose AE, Day D. (2013) Esthetic rejuvenation of the temple. *Clin Plast Surg* **40**(1), 77–89.
6 Duracinsky M, Leclercq P, Armstrong AR, Dolivo M, Mouly F, Chassany O. (2013) A longitudinal evaluation of the impact of a polylactic acid injection therapy on health related quality of life amongst HIV patients treated with anti-retroviral agents under real conditions of use. *BMC Infect Dis.* **20**(13), 92.
7 Hamilton TK, Burgess CM. (2010) Considerations for the use of injectable poly-L-lactic acid in people of color. *J Drugs Dermatol.* **9**(5), 451–6.
8 Burgess C, Quiroga R. (2005) Assessment of the safety and efficacy of poly-L-lactic acid for the treatment of HIV associated facial lipoatrophy. *J Am Acad Dermatol* **52**, 233–9.
9 Beer K. (2009) Delayed formation of nodules from PLLA injected in the periorbital area. **Dermatol Surg 35** Suppl 1, 399–402.
10 Lombardi T, Samson J, Plantier F, Husson C, Küffer R. (2004) Orofacial granulomas after injection of cosmetic fillers: histopathologic and clinical study of 11 cases. *J Oral Pathol Med* **33**, 115–20.
11 Roberts SA, Arthurs BP. (2012) Severe visual loss and orbital infarction following periorbital aesthetic poly-(L)-lactic acid (PLLA) injection. *Ophthal Plast Reconstr Surg* **28**(3).

SECTION 3 Resurfacing Techniques

CHAPTER 45
Superficial Chemical Peels

M. Amanda Jacobs[1] and Randall Roenigk[2]
[1] Geisinger Health Systems, Danville, PA, USA
[2] Department of Dermatology, Mayo Clinic, Rochester, MN, USA

BASIC CONCEPTS
- Chemical exfoliating agent causes destruction of the epidermis (to varying degrees) with subsequent repair and rejuvenation.
- Factors that influence the depth of a peel.
- Specific peeling agents, chemical action, and results.
- Standard and advanced techniques for superficial chemical peels.
- Complications.

Definition

Superficial chemical peels involve the application of a chemical peeling agent to the skin, resulting in destruction of the epidermis. The peel may have effects anywhere from the stratum corneum to the basal cell layer. There are many factors that affect the depth of the peel including the peeling agent and the technique of application. Chemical peels create a controlled wound which the body then heals. Permanent histologic changes can be seen after a series of superficial peels.

Physiology

Indications
Superficial chemical peels are generally safe and can be used on all Fitzpatrick skin types. The peeling agent only affects the epidermis and so this procedure is only indicated for superficial processes such as mild photoaging, superficial dyschromias (melasma, lentigines, post-inflammatory hyperpigmentation [PIH]), acne, and actinic keratoses [1]. Typically, a series of peels is required for the best clinical response.

Depth of peel
Multiple factors influence the depth of a given peel, including chemical agent selection and technique of application (Table 45.1). Each of these factors should be considered when selecting a superficial peel for a patient.

Table 45.1 Variables that affect the depth of a superficial peel.

Peeling agent and concentration
Technique of application (number of coats and pressure of application)
Duration of contact with the skin (prior to neutralization)
Anatomic location
Pretreatment regimen

Histologic changes
Superficial chemical peels injure and rejuvenate the epidermis; however, histologic changes can also be seen in the dermis, including collagen formation in the papillary dermis. Repeated application of alfa-hydroxy acids to the skin surface resulted in a 25% increase in epidermal thickness as well as increased acid mucopolysaccharides and increased density of collagen in the papillary dermis [2].

Formulation

In a superficial peel, chemical agents are applied to the skin to create a wound by destroying the epidermis. There are multiple different chemicals that fall into this category (Table 45.2).

Alfa-hydroxy acids (glycolic, lactic, malic, oxalic, tartaric, and citric acid)
These acids have been used on the skin for centuries. Ancient Egyptian women would bathe in sour milk (containing lactic

---

Cosmetic Dermatology: Products and Procedures, Second Edition. Edited by Zoe Diana Draelos.
© 2016 John Wiley & Sons, Ltd. Published 2016 by John Wiley & Sons, Ltd.

Table 45.2 Characteristics of various chemical peeling agents.

Peeling agent	Activity	Neutralization	Frosting	Unique properties	Side effects
Alfa-hydroxy acid	Diminishes corneocyte adhesion/desquamation	+	–		Deeper peel may be achieved with prolonged skin contact
Pyruvic acid	Keratolytic, sebostatic, antimicrobial	+	–	Intense burning with application	Newer formulation used for superficial peels
Jessner's solution	Stratum corneum separation, dermal edema	–	–*	Intense burning with application 2–3 coats applied	
TCA (10–25%)	Coagulation of epidermal proteins	–	+	True frost forms, intensity correlates with depth of injury	Burning with application Erythema for several days
Salicylic acid	Keratolytic, comedolytic, desquamation of upper SC Enhances other peeling agents	–	–*	Burning with initial application, then acid becomes an anesthetic	Transient salicylism may occur
Tretinoin	Not destructive Increases cell turnover	–	–	Painless Discolors skin (yellow) Must remain on skin for 6 hours Decomposed by UV light	Produces strong erythema Fine white flakes with peeling
Resorcinol	Weakens hydrogen bonds of keratin	–	–	Daily application for 3 days Time consuming	Irritant or contact allergy possible Continued use associated with thyroid dysfunction
Solid carbon dioxide	Freezes and destroys epidermis			Block of dry ice dipped in acetone/ethanol solution Used to treat acne	Cold sensitivity

*White precipitate can occur as vehicle evaporates, does not represent true frost.

acid) to smooth the skin [3,4]. They are naturally occurring in sugarcane, sour milk, and various fruits. When applied to the skin, they decrease corneocyte adhesion above the granular layer, reduce the number of desmosomes, and result in desquamation [2,4]. The application is typically painless, although some mild stinging may occur. These acids require neutralization with sodium bicarbonate or dilution with water. Prolonged contact with the skin may result in uneven penetration and deeper peel depths being achieved [1].

Pyruvic acid (alfa-keto acid)

This product has keratolytic, antimicrobial, and sebostatic properties. It is a small molecule with a low pKa which allows deep penetration in the skin. Typical formulations fall into the category of medium depth peels. This potent acid carries a high risk for scarring. Application is associated with an intense burning sensation and neutralization is required with a 10% sodium bicarbonate solution [1,3].

Berardesca et al. [3] describe the efficacy of a 50% pyruvic acid preparation with dimethyl sulfone. This buffered solution has a lower pH value. The overall result is a superficial peel with mild burning on application and mild erythema following the peel.

Jessner's solution (resorcinol 14%, lactic acid 14%, and salicylic acid 14% in alcohol)

The penetration of this solution is limited to the epidermis. The peel results in separation of the stratum corneum and upper epidermal edema [1]. Application is best with a sable hair brush. Wrung-out gauze pads may also be used. Typically, two to three coats are applied. The skin will first become erythematous and then a white, powdery appearance will emerge. This is caused by precipitation of the chemical compounds onto the skin with vehicle evaporation. This is not equivalent to a "frost" which indicates depth of peeling in a trichloroacetic acid (TCA) peel. Complications are rare with this type of peel because of the limited penetration of the peeling solution.

Trichloroacetic acid

TCA is a much stronger acid than alfa-hydroxy acid (AHA), and higher concentrations produce medium and deep peels. Superficial peels can be achieved using concentrations of 10–25%.

TCA is an inorganic compound that occurs naturally in the crystalline form. It is dissolved in distilled water to form an aqueous solution of the desired concentration. It is stable for a long time (23 weeks) and is not heat or light sensitive. Use and storage may affect the concentration of the solution and care should be taken to handle appropriately [1]. Cotton tip applicators and debris can contaminate the solution.

The mechanism of action for TCA is coagulation of epidermal proteins and necrosis of the cells. The skin gradually turns whitish gray, creating a "frost" as the epidermal proteins coagulate and precipitate (Figure 45.1) [5]. This is a self-neutralizing acid. Histologically, the epidermis and upper papillary dermis are destroyed along with new collagen deposition [1,4,6].

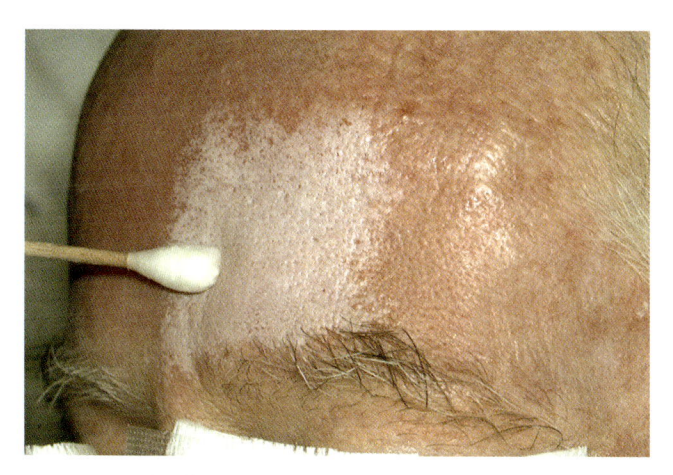

Figure 45.1 White frost seen with a trichloroacetic acid (TCA) peel indicating epidermal protein coagulation. The intensity of the frost corresponds with the peel depth.

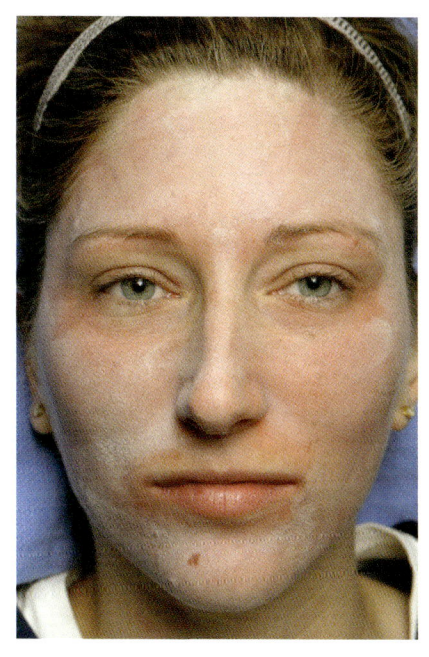

Figure 45.2 White discoloration of the skin seen during a salicylic acid peel caused by evaporation of the vehicle and precipitation of salicylate on the skin.

TCA must be applied in a controlled setting. Analgesia and/or sedation are typically required. Cotton-tipped applicators are dipped in a container with TCA solution and rolled on the edge to prevent dripping of solution. The acid is then painted on the skin, typically along cosmetic units until the desired level of frosting is achieved [6]. Multiple coats may be needed and depth of the peel correlates to the intensity of the frost. Cool compresses can be used to ease burning sensation, but do not neutralize the solution. Patients should expect several days of erythema followed by desquamation over 7 days.

This peel is operator dependent and potential for error and complications are high. The greatest risk exists for peeling more deeply than originally intended.

Salicylic acid (ortho-hydroxybenzoic acid)

This is a beta-hydroxyl acid. It is a lipophilic acid that allows desquamation of the upper layers of the stratum corneum without inflammation [1,6]. This peeling agent can be safely used on all skin types, even those prone to PIH. This agent also has keratolytic and comedolytic qualities making it ideal for acne patients. It also enhances the penetration of other acids and is often used in combination peels (such as Jessner's solution).

A mild–moderate burning sensation occurs on application. Typically, this is easily managed with a cool fan. The acid causes superficial anesthesia and so this quickly dissipates after a minute or more. The acid should be left on the skin for about 3–5 minutes. This is a self-neutralizing acid, but is typically washed off the skin after 5 minutes with plain water. A white precipitate will be seen on the skin after about 1 minute from evaporation of the vehicle (Figure 45.2). This is not a true frost and does not indicate depth of penetration. Desquamation will begin 2–3 days after the peel and continue for 7 days [1,4,6].

Salicylism is possible with this peel, although unlikely. Care should be taken to avoid peeling large areas at the same time. Patients may experience tinnitus, dizziness, and headache. The symptoms are transient and self-resolving [7]. Increased water intake may improve symptoms more quickly.

Tretinoin peel

Tretinoin applied in high concentration (1–5%) in propylene glycol is used for peeling. The solution is canary yellow and discolors skin on application. Tretinoin decomposes on UV exposure and should be applied late in the day. The application is painless and the peeling agent must be left on the skin at least 6 hours. This is a safe peel and the desquamation consists only of fine white flakes. It typically produces strong erythema and the risk for prolonged erythema is increased with this type of peel [6].

Tretinoin cream is typically used as part of a pre-peeling regimen to help improve penetration of peeling agent and improve healing time. Most practices advocate at least 2 weeks of pre-treatment prior to the peel [7].

Resorcinol (m-hydroxybenzene)

Resorcinol is structurally and chemically related to phenol and acts as a potent reducing agent. It disrupts the weak hydrogen bonds of keratin and is therefore a keratolytic. It remains stable in water, ethanol, and ether.

Typically, the peeling agent is applied as a paste in concentrations of 10–50%. It is applied daily for three consecutive days and the skin contact time is slowly increased daily [1,7]. The paste is then wiped off the skin. Water and creams must be avoided for up to 1 week.

Resorcinol is not typically used as a peeling agent. The process is time-consuming and the results can be achieved by other methods. It also can cause a non-specific irritant reaction or contact allergy. Additionally, there are reports of thyroid dysfunction with continued use (over months to years) [7]. More recent reviews indicate no danger when used in the standard fashion (as described above) [8].

Solid carbon dioxide (dry ice)
This modality has been used to treat acne for over 60 years. Brody describes a technique using a block of dry ice wrapped in a hand towel and dipped in a 3:1 solution of acetone and alcohol. Acetone dissolves sebum and lowers the temperature of the carbon dioxide. Individual lesions or segments of the face can be treated then using slow even strokes. The depth of injury is modified with pressure of application. Brody reports 5–8 seconds of moderate pressure as sufficient to freeze comedones. This is less destructive than liquid nitrogen which is more than twice as cold (−186 °C) compared to dry ice (−78 °C) [7].

Advantages and disadvantages

Superficial chemical peels are generally very safe procedures with a minimal risk profile. They can safely be performed on all Fitzpatrick skin types [4]. Patient discomfort is typically minimal and local anesthesia is not typically needed. Patients usually tolerate the erythema and desquamation following the peel quite well.

Appropriate management of patient expectations is critical with superficial peels. Patients must be aware that a series of peels is required for maximum benefit. In addition, patients should be selected appropriately, based on the degree of skin disease to ensure a successful peel candidate.

Standard technique

Initial consult
The initial consult is essential. This allows the treating physician to determine if the patient is an appropriate candidate for a chemical peel. They should have a dermatologic condition that is amenable to this therapy. A history of recent isotretinoin use, hypertrophic scarring, facial radiation, or significant psychologic disorder may make the patient a less desirable candidate. Also, a history of oral contraceptive use or hormonal agents should be noted as this may increase the chance of PIH [4]. Photographs should be obtained at this visit. Perhaps the most important aspect of this consult is managing the patient's expectations and preparing him or her for the procedure. The peel is superficial in nature and the need for serial treatments should be emphasized. Also, adherence to priming and post-treatment recommendations is essential to treatment success.

Priming
Pretreatment is important for peeling. It allows for melanocyte suppression, uniform penetration of the peeling agent, and decreased healing time. Ideally, priming occurs for 2–3 weeks prior to the peel procedure. The regimen can be customized to the patient but often includes glycolic acid products (around 10%), tretinoin, hydroquinone, and sunscreen on a regular basis. The regimen (except sunscreen) should be discontinued 3 days prior to the procedure [4,5]. Hydroquinone 2% cream has been shown to be a superior priming agent to tretinoin cream when treating patients with melasma with superficial chemical peels [9]. This is likely due to hydroquinone inhibiting melanin production by blocking tyrosinase while tretinoin may stimulate new melanin production secondary to inflammation.

Peel procedure
The depth of the chemical peel is determined by multiple variables; however, the key factors are amount and concentration of peeling agent used, pressure used with application, and duration of contact with the skin.

Basic peel protocol is similar for all types of superficial peels (Table 45.3). The procedure begins with cleansing and defatting the skin. Defatting is achieved by applying acetone or isopropyl alcohol to remove excess oil and sebum and allow for even penetration of the peeling agent. Occlusive ointment can be used to protect the lips and eyes; hair should be tied back away from face. Ideally, the office should be equipped with an eyewash station or have access to water for flushing [10].

All of the materials needed should be gathered prior to beginning. This includes a neutralization solution if needed. Patients may be more comfortable with a fan blowing cool air during the peel. Applications with either cotton-tip applicators or gauze are typically used (Figures 45.3 and 45.4).

There are inherent errors that can occur with peeling and care should be taken to avoid these situations. One error is incorrect formulation, either secondary to error in compound-

Table 45.3 Standard procedure for a superficial peel.

Initial consult
Includes pre-peel photographs
Priming
2–3 weeks prior to peel
Pre-treatment with glycolic acid, tretinoin, hydroquinone, sunscreen
Peel
Degreasing with acetone or alcohol
Application of peeling agent
Desired exposure to skin
Rinse skin or neutralize with appropriate material
Application of sunscreen and possibly anti-inflammatory agent
Post-peel
Cool compresses
Sunscreen/sun avoidance
Creams/lotions as recommended

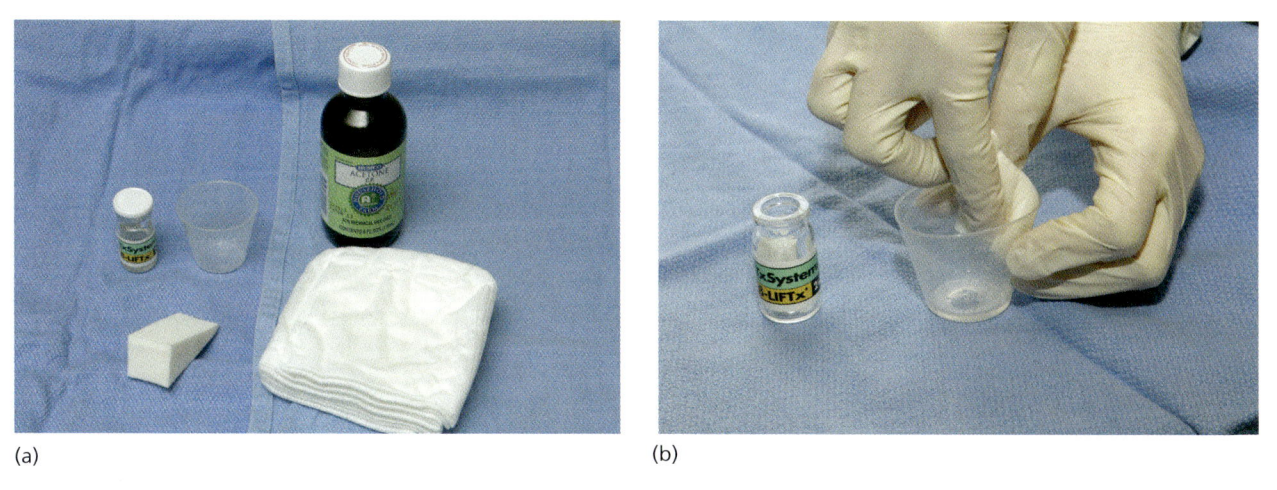

Figure 45.3 (a) Typical tray set-up for a salicylic acid peel. (b) Excess peel solution is removed from sponge prior to application.

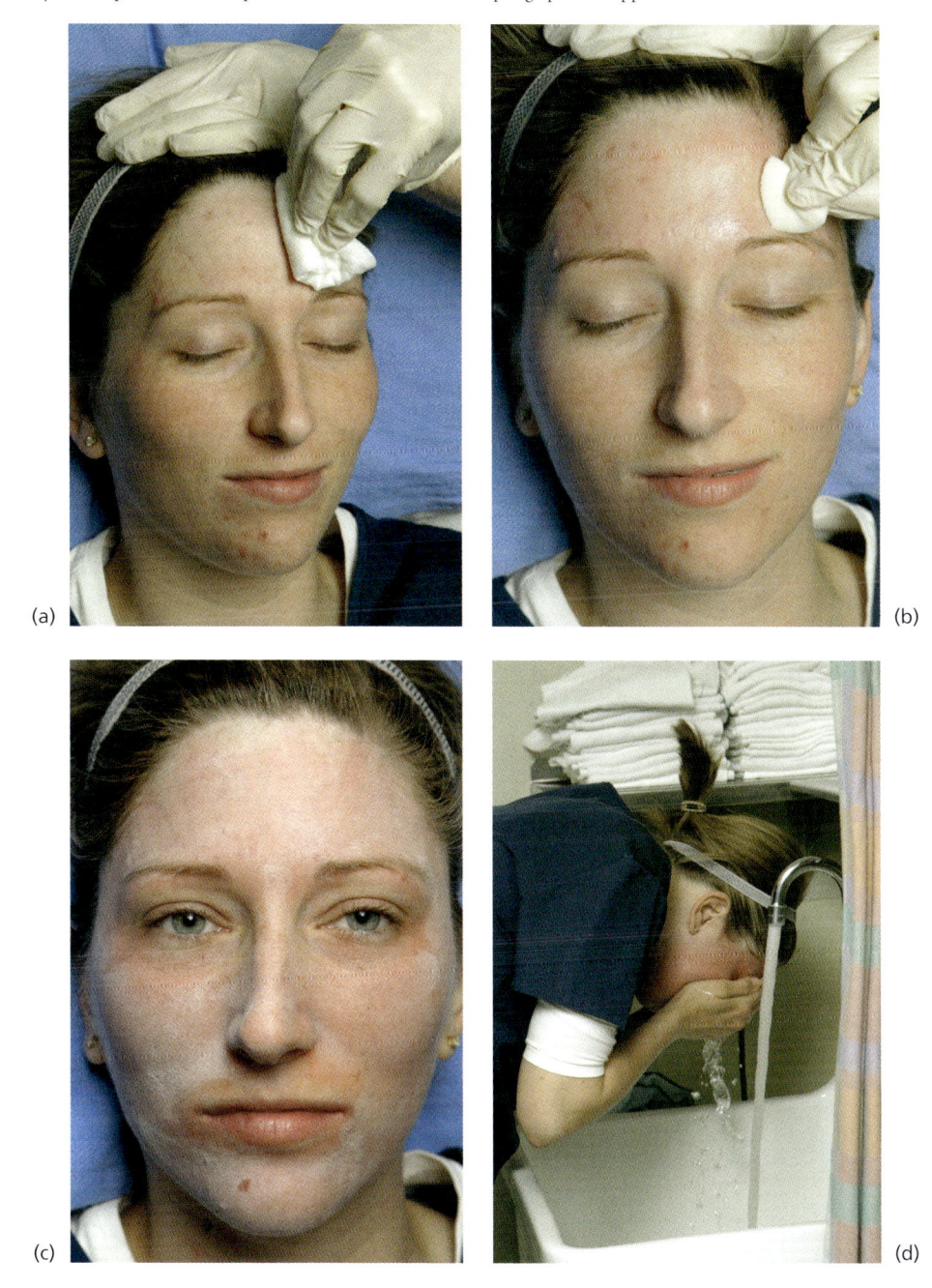

Figure 45.4 Standard peel procedure for a salicylic acid peel. (a) Face is degreased with acetone; (b) peel solution is applied; (c) erythema and white precipitate form on skin; (d) patient rinses face with water.

ing or incorrect storage leading to evaporation of alcohol/water vehicle. The latter results in a stronger peeling solution than intended. Careful labeling and storage of peeling agents is essential. If greater than one strength is being used at a time, it is recommended that only one solution be on the tray at any given time and this should be clearly marked with concentration [8].

Post-care
Post-peel care includes gentle cleansing. Light moisturizing lotions can be used 24 hours after the peel procedure (Figure 45.5). Sun protection (avoidance or sunscreen) is essential for 1 month following the peel. It is critical in the first week after the peel.

Advanced techniques/specific uses

Depth controlled TCA peel
Consistent results with TCA peels can be difficult to achieve and potential complications can occur more frequently depending on physician skill level and patient selection. A recent product, the TCA Blue Peel, offers a depth controlled TCA peel with more standardization in acid absorption [11]. The fixed concentration (15% or 20%) of TCA is mixed with the Blue Peel base (glycerin, saponins, and a non-ionic blue color). This base increases the surface tension of the solution and results in slower penetration of TCA into the skin. The blue color allows the physician to easily identify the areas that have been treated. Frosting occurs more slowly which allows the physician to control the depth of peel more consistently. Several coats may be applied depending on the desired depth of peeling.

Fluor-hydroxy pulse peel
This peel combines 5-flurorouracil with glycolic acid (70%) peels to treat actinically damaged skin. The two agents appear to have synergistic effects. One randomized study showed this combination cleared 91% of actinic keratoses, compared with 19% when treated with glycolic acid alone. The peel was repeated once weekly for 8 weeks [12].

Chemical reconstruction of skin scars
Chemical reconstruction of skin scars (CROSS) is a technique to address acne scars while minimizing the risks of deeper peels (such as scarring and pigmentary changes). The CROSS technique involves focal application of high concentration TCA (65–100%) to atrophic acne scars. Each scar is pressed firmly with a sharpened wooden applicator. Variable improvement can be seen with this technique but typically it requires a series of treatments [13].

Treatment of acne vulgaris
Chemical peels are often used as adjuvant therapy in both inflammatory and non-inflammatory acne. Recent studies reviewed the evidence supporting this practice [14]. The most beneficial effect of superficial chemical peels was on comedonal acne. One study showed a 75% reduction in lesion count using salicylic acid peels 30% alone [15]. A significant benefit in comedonal acne was seen with both glycolic acid and salicylic acid peels [14].

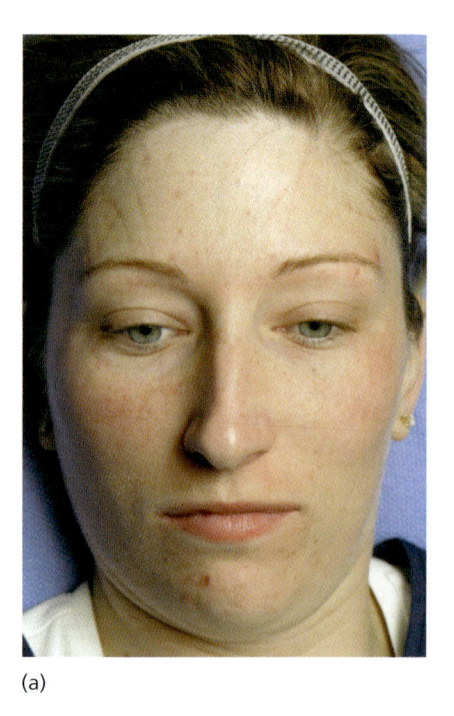

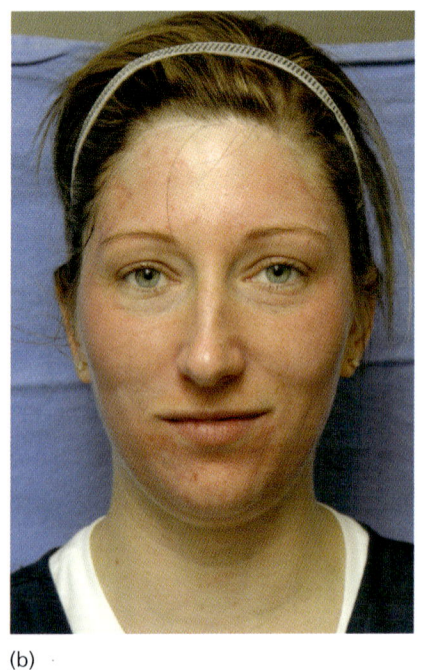

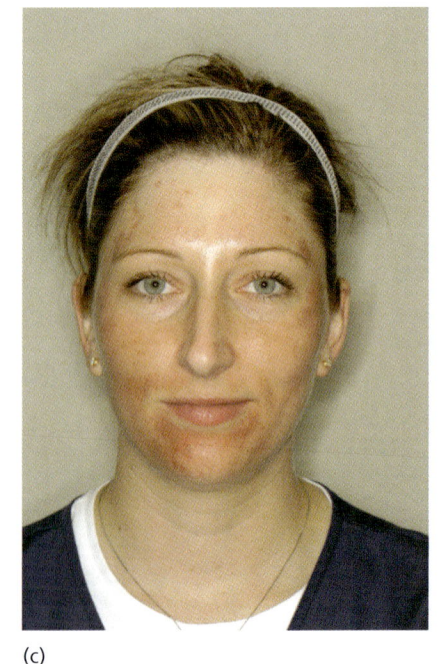

Figure 45.5 (a) Pre-peel; (b) immediately post-peel; (c) 24 hours after a salicylic acid peel.

Table 45.4 Potential complications associated with superficial peels.

Pigmentary changes
Infection
Reactivation of herpes
Prolonged erythema/pruritus
Contact dermatitis
Lines of demarcation
Transient textural changes (enlarged pores)
Milia
Cold sensitivity (CO_2)

Results for treating inflammatory acne are less clear cut. Peels, particularly glycolic acid peels, can result in flares at the beginning of treatment in 15–20% of patients [16]. Overall lesion counts did improve in these patients with continued treatments.

Treatment of post-inflammatory hyperpigmentation/melasma

Superficial peels can benefit patients with post-inflammatory hyperpigmentation. Both gylcolic acid peels and salicylic acid peels have shown benefit. Salicylic acid peels are non-inflammatory and therefore safer in patients with darker skin tones [14,17,18].

Epidermal melasma responds better to topical therapies such as chemical peels. Use of a Wood's lamp to determine the depth of pigment prior to treatment may help determine which patients will achieve the best results. Epidermal melasma shows enhancement of color contrast under Wood's light as compared to visible light. Dermal melasma does not show such change [19]. Various peels have shown benefit in treating melasma including salicylic acid, glycolic acid and TCA (10–20%) [20].

Complications

Complications arising from superficial chemical peels are relatively rare (Table 45.4) [9]. Post-inflammatory hyperpigmentation can occur, particularly in darker skin types. Technical errors (dripping of acid in the eyes) or incorrect formulation must also be avoided.

Conclusions

Superficial chemical peels wound the epidermis with destruction or desquamation. This leads to increased epidermal thickness and new collagen formation in the papillary dermis with repeated application. They are indicated for superficial processes such as superficial dyschromias, mild photoaging, acne, and actinic keratoses. They can safely be performed on all skin types and complications are rare. A series of peels is often required for the best clinical outcome.

References

1 Zakopoulou N, Kontochristopoulos G. (2006) Superficial chemical peels. *J Cosmet Dermatol* **5**, 246–53.
2 Ditre CM, Griffin TD, Murphy GF, et al. (1996) Effects of alpha-hydroxy acids on photoaged skin: a pilot clinical, histologic, and ultrastructural study. *J Am Acad Dermatol* **34**, 187–95.
3 Berardesca E, Cameli N, Primavera G, Carrera M. (2006) Clinical and instrumental evaluation of skin improvement after treatment with a new 50% pyruvic acid peel. *Dermatol Surg* **32**, 526–31.
4 Roberts WE. (2004) Chemical peeling in ethnic/dark skin. *Dermatol Ther* **17**, 196–205.
5 Roenigk RK. (1998) Facial chemical peel. In: Baran R, Maibach HI, eds. *Textbook of Cosmetic Dermatology*, 2nd edn. Malden, MA: Blackwell Science, pp. 585–94.
6 Landau M. (2008) Chemical peels. *Clin Dermatol* **26**, 200–8.
7 Brody HJ. (1992) Superficial peeling. In: *Chemical Peeling*. St. Louis, MO: Mosby Year Book, pp. 53–73.
8 Brody HJ. (2001) Complications of chemical resurfacing. *Dermatol Clin* **19** (3).
9 Nanda S, Grover C, Reddy BS. (2004) Efficacy of hydroquinone (2%) versus tretinoin (0.025%) as adjunct topical agents for chemical peeling in patients with melasma. *Dermatol Surg* **30**, 385–9.
10 Drake LA, Dinehart SM, Goltz RW, et al. (1995) Guidelines of care for chemical peeling. Guidelines/Outcomes Committee: American Academy of Dermatology. *J Am Acad Dermatol* **33**, 497–503.
11 Obagi ZE, Obagi S, Alaiti S, Stevens MB. (1999) TCA-based blue peel: a standard procedure with depth control. *Dermatol Surg* **25**, 773–80.
12 Marrero GM, Katz BE. (1998) The new fluor-hydroxy pulse peel: a combination of 5-fluorouracil and glycolic acid. *Dermatol Surg* **24**, 973–8.
13 Lee JB, Chung WG, Kwahck H, Lee KH. (2002) Focal treatment of acne scars with trichloroacetic acid: chemical reconstruction of skin scars method. *Dermatol Surg* **28**, 1017–21.
14 Dreno B, Fischer TC, Perosino E, Poli F, Viera MS, Rendon MI, et al. (2011) Expert opinion: Efficacy of superficial chemical peels in active acne management – what can we learn from the literature today? Evidence based recommendations. *JEADV* **25**, 695–704.
15 Hashimoto Y, Suga Y, Mizuno Y et al. (2008) Salicylic acid peels in polyethylene glycol vehicle for treatment of comedogenic acne in Japanese patients. *Dermatol Surg* **34**, 276–9.
16 Wang CM, Huang CL, Hu CT, Chan HL. (1997) The effect of glycolic acid on the treatment of acne in Asian skin. *Dermatol Surg* **23**, 23–9.
17 Grover C, Reddu BS. (2003) The therapeutic value of glycolic acid peels in dermatology. *Indian J Dermatol Venereol Leprol* **69**, 148–50.
18 Grimes PE. (1999) The safety and efficacy of salicylic acid chemical peels in darker racial-ethnic groups. *Dermatol Surg* **25**, 18–22.
19 Asawanonda P, Taylor CR. (1999) Review: Wood's light in dermatology. *Internat J Dermatol* **38**, 801–807.
20 Cotellessa C, Peris K, Onorati MT, et al. (1999) The use of chemical peelings in the treatment of different cutaneous hyperpigmentations. *Dermatol Surg* **25**, 450–54.

CHAPTER 46
Medium Depth Chemical Peels

Gary D. Monheit and Virginia A. Koubek

Total Skin & Beauty Dermatology Center, PC, and Departments of Dermatology and Ophthalmology, University of Alabama, Birmingham, AL, USA

> **BASIC CONCEPTS**
> - Indicated both for therapeutic field treatments of precancerous skin lesions and for various cosmetic indications.
> - Induce controlled chemical damage through the epidermis and variable portions of the dermis in order to promote the regrowth of new skin with improved surface characteristics.
> - Pretreatments including even cleansing, degreasing, and subsequent application of Jessner's solution will open the epidermal barrier for more even and deep penetration of trichloracetic acid.
> - Affords the patient a single procedure with healing time within 1 week to 10 days.
> - Considered safe and effective when used by experienced dermatologists.

Introduction

A number of acidic and basic chemical agents have been used to produce the varying effects of light, medium, or deep chemical peels, mediated by differences in their ability to penetrate and damage epidermal and dermal skin components. The level of penetration, destruction, and inflammation determines the level of peeling. The stimulation of epidermal growth through the removal of the stratum corneum without necrosis characterizes light superficial peels. Through exfoliation, it thickens the epidermis with qualitative regenerative changes. Destruction of the epidermis defines a full superficial chemical peel inducing the regeneration of the epidermis. Further destruction of the epidermis and induction of inflammation within the papillary and upper portions of the reticular dermis constitutes a medium depth peel. Further inflammatory response in the medium reticular dermis induces new collagen production and ground substances constituting a deep chemical peel [1].

Formulations

Trichloracetic acid

Trichloracetic acid (TCA) has become the gold standard of chemical peeling agents, based on its long history of usage, its versatility in peeling, and its chemical stability. Its first documented use for skin rejuvenation dates back as far as 1882, when German dermatologist Paul Gerson Unna described the properties of salicylic acid, resorcinol, phenol, and TCA [1]. TCA has since been used in many concentrations because it has no systemic toxicity and can be used to create superficial, medium, or even deep wounds in the skin. TCA is naturally found in crystalline form and is mixed weight-by-volume with distilled water. It is not light sensitive, does not need refrigeration, and is stable on the shelf for over 6 months. The standard concentrations of TCA should be mixed weight-by-volume to assess the concentration accurately. TCA crystals weight 30 g are mixed with 100 mL distilled water to give an accurate 30% weight-by-volume concentration. Any other dilutional system – volume dilutions and weight-by-weight – are inaccurate in that they do not reflect the accepted weight-by-volume measurements cited in the literature.

Because TCA, at concentrations of 50% or above, has a high potential to be scarring, the use of higher concentrations has fallen out of favor [2]. Therefore, combined applications using an initial modifying treatment followed by a 35% TCA formula were developed to better control the level of damage and minimize the risk of side effects [3].

Brody [4] first developed the use of solid CO_2 applied with acetone to the skin as a freezing technique prior to the application of 35% TCA. The preliminary freezing appears to break the epidermal barrier for a more even and complete penetration of the 35% TCA. Monheit [5] then introduced the use of Jessner's solution prior to the application of 35% TCA (Table 46.1). The Jessner's solution was found to be very effective in destroying the epidermal barrier by breaking up individual epidermal cells. This allows a deeper penetration of the 35% TCA and a more even application of the peel solution. Similarly, Coleman and

---

Cosmetic Dermatology: Products and Procedures, Second Edition. Edited by Zoe Diana Draelos.
© 2016 John Wiley & Sons, Ltd. Published 2016 by John Wiley & Sons, Ltd.

Table 46.1 Jessner's solution (Combes' formula).

Resorcinol	14 g
Salicylic acid	14 g
85% Lactic acid	14 g
95% Ethanol (q.s.ad.)	100 mL

q.s.ad, a sufficient quantity up to.

Table 46.2 Agents used for medium depth chemical peeling.

Agent	Comment
40–50% TCA	Not recommended
Combination 35% TCA + solid CO2 (Brody)	The most potent combination
Combination 35% TCA + Jessner's solution (Monheit)	The most popular combination
Combination 35% TCA + 70% glycolic acid (Coleman)	An effective combination
88% phenol	Rarely used

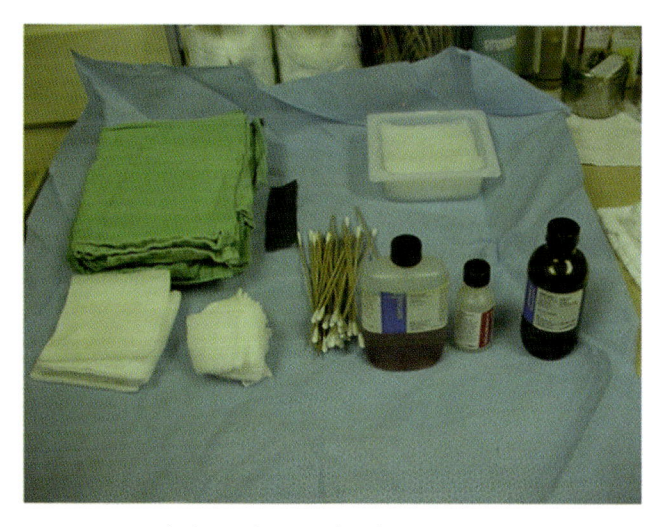

Figure 46.1 Standard setup for Jessner's and trichloracetic acid (TCA) combination peel. The standard setup includes a facial cleanser such as Septisol, acetone, Jessner's solution, 35% TCA, cotton-tipped applicators, 2 × 2 inch and 4 × 4 inch gauze pads, and cool-water soaks for patient comfort.

Futrell [6] have demonstrated the use of 70% glycolic acid prior to the application of 35% TCA. Its effect has been very similar to that of Jessner's solution.

All three combinations have proven to be as effective as the use of 50% TCA; however, with a greater safety margin. The application of acid and resultant frosting are better controlled with the combination so that the "hot spots" with higher concentrations of TCA can be controlled, creating an even peel with less incidence of dyschromias and scarring (Table 46.2).

Advantages and disadvantages

The advantages of chemical peeling compared with other modalities used to treat photoaging or precancerous lesions include the low cost, the ease of a single application, and reliable efficacy. Additionally, chemical peeling may be performed in any office setting with routine dermatologic supplies such as 2 × 2 or 4 × 4 inch gauze pads and cotton-tipped applicators, and does not require special equipment (Figure 46.1). When performed properly on the correctly chosen patient, a medium depth peel will reliably improve the appearance of photoaged skin and produce sustained clearing of most precancerous skin lesions for a period of several months to several years.

Indications

While superficial peels may improve conditions such as acne and skin texture, and deep peels may help improve moderate rhytides and acne scarring, current indications for medium depth chemical peeling include Glogau type II photoaging (Table 46.3), epidermal lesions such as actinic keratoses, pigmentary dyschromias, mild acne scarring, as well as blending the effect of deeper resurfacing procedures (Table 46.4) [7].

The Jessner's–35% TCA peel is particularly useful for the improvement of mild to moderate photoaging. It freshens sallow, atrophic skin and softens fine rhytides, with minimal risk of textural or pigmentary complications. Deep furrows, however, are not eliminated with this peel and there is no significant skin retraction as is seen with ablative fractional laser resurfacing. When used in conjunction with a retinoid, bleaching agent and sunscreens, a single Jessner's–35% TCA peel lessens pigmentary

Table 46.3 Glogau's classification of photoaging.

Group	Severity	Age Group (Years)	Features
I	Mild	Usually 28–35	Mild pigmentary change
			No keratoses
			Minimal wrinkles
II	Moderate	Usually 36–50	Early senile lentigines
			Keratoses palpable but not visible
			Parallel smile lines beginning
III	Advanced	Usually 51–65	Obvious dyschromia, telangiectasias
			Visible keratoses
			Wrinkles even when not moving facial muscles
IV	Severe	Usually 66–75	Yellow-gray color of skin
			Prior skin malignancies
			Wrinkled throughout with no normal skin

Table 46.4 Major indications for medium depth chemical peels.

Destruction of premalignant epidermal lesions – actinic keratoses
Resurfacing moderate to advanced photoaged skin (Glogau Levels II, III)
Improving pigmentary dyschromias
Improving mild acne scars
Blending laser, dermabrasion, or deep chemical peeling in photoaged skin (transition from treated to non-treated area)

Table 46.5 Contraindications to medium-depth chemical peeling.

Absolute contraindications
Poor physician–patient relationship
Unrealistic expectations
Poor general health and nutritional status
Isotretinoin therapy within the last 6 months
Complete absence of intact pilosebaceous units on the face
Active infection or open wounds (e.g. herpes, excoriations, or open acne cysts)
Pregnant or nursing patients
Relative contraindications
Medium depth or deep resurfacing procedure within the last 3–12 months
Recent facial surgery involving extensive undermining, such as a rhytidectomy
History of abnormal scar formation or delayed wound healing
History of therapeutic radiation exposure
History of certain skin diseases (e.g. rosacea, seborrheic dermatitis, atopic dermatitis, psoriasis, or vitiligo) or active retinoid dermatitis
History of autoimmune connective tissue diseases (e.g. cutaneous lupus, scleroderma)
Fitzpatrick skin types IV, V and VI

dyschromias and lentigines as well as or even more effectively than repetitive superficial peels. Epidermal growths such as actinic keratosis also respond well to this peel. In fact, the Jessner's—35% TCA peel has been found to be as effective as topical 5-fluorouracil chemotherapy in removing both grossly visible and clinically undetectable actinic keratosis, but has the advantages of lower morbidity and greater improvement in associated photoaging [8].

Another indication for the Jessner's–35% TCA peel is to blend the effects of other resurfacing procedures with the surrounding skin. It is important to note that when used in combination with other resurfacing procedures such as laser ablation and dermabrasion, the peel should be performed first, in order to avoid accidental application of the peeling agent onto previously abraded areas of skin which may lead to scarring [9].

Contraindications

Several contraindications exist when choosing a medium depth chemical peel (Table 46.5). Because patient compliance during the recovery period is essential to avoiding permanent negative sequelae, a medium depth peel should not occur in the setting of a poor physician–patient relationship. Likewise, a frank discussion of what the peel can and cannot accomplish is necessary, and unrealistic expectations on the part of the patient must be recognized. Furthermore, poor general health and nutritional status will compromise wound healing and should dissuade a procedural approach. Moreover, isotretinoin therapy within the previous 6 months has been associated with increased risk of scarring, and a medium depth chemical peel should be delayed until the patient is beyond 6 months of finishing a course of isotretinoin. Additionally, active infections or open wounds such as herpes simplex vesicles, excoriations, or open acne cysts should postpone the treatment until such conditions resolve. All patients with a history of herpes simplex virus I of the facial area should be premedicated with an antiviral agent such as acyclovir or valacyclovir and remain on prophylactic therapy for 10 days.

While not absolute contraindications, patients with overly sensitive, hyperreactive, or koebnerizing skin disorders such as atopic dermatitis, seborrheic dermatitis, psoriasis, or contact dermatitis may find their underlying disease exacerbated by a chemical peel. In particular, patients with rosacea typically develop an exaggerated inflammatory response to the peeling agents, which serves as a trigger factor for symptoms. Caution should also be exercised for patients with autoimmune connective tissue diseases (e.g. cutaneous lupus, scleroderma) as the trauma of the chemical peeling may activate the disease [9]. A history of keloid formation should be screened for prior to chemical peeling. Likewise, patients with a recent history of extensive or major facial surgery, or those who have recently had a medium depth peel in the preceding months should be evaluated closely with regard to risks and benefits. The collagen remodeling phase of wound healing due to prior treatments is still underway in such patients, and an altered wound healing response may occur. Another important relative contraindication is a history of radiation therapy to the proposed treatment area. An absence of pilosebaceous units should serve as a harbinger that the area does not have the reserve capacity of follicular epidermal cells with which to repopulate. While Fitzpatrick skin types I and II are at low risk for post-resurfacing hyperpigmentation or hypopigmentation, types III–VI are at greater risk for these complications [10].

Standard technique

Jessner's TCA peel procedure after Monheit

1. The skin should be cleaned thoroughly with Septisol® (Vestal Laboratories, St. Louis, MO, USA) to remove oils.
2. Acetone or acetone alcohol is used to further debride oil and scale from the surface of the skin.
3. Jessner's solution is applied.
4. 35% TCA is applied until a light frost appears.

5. Cool saline compresses are applied to dilute the solution.
6. The peel will heal with 0.25% acetic acid soaks and a mild emollient cream.

Informed consent

A thorough pretreatment discussion is imperative. It allows the opportunity to discuss the risks and benefits, as well as to educate the patient on the expected time frame and course of recovery. It also allows the surgeon to assess the patient's goals and expectations so that the procedure is performed only on appropriate candidates. Those who are not willing to tolerate an acute event followed by 7–10 days of desquamation and 2–3 weeks of erythema are best served by other treatments. The patient must fully understand the potential benefits, limitations, and risks of the procedure, and an informed consent form must be signed. Pretreatment photographs are also highly recommended to allow for post-treatment comparison.

Setup

All necessary reagents for a Jessner's + 35% TCA medium depth peel may be obtained in bulk for multi-application use from leading dermatologic suppliers. When ordering TCA, one must ensure that the strength of the acid is as intended by the physician. While both weight-to-weight and volume-to-volume methods of calculating acid concentration may be used, the authors prefer the more common method of weight-to-volume calculations. When changing vendors or ordering new products, the distributor's method of calculation should be confirmed so as to avoid application of a more highly concentrated or less highly concentrated formulation than intended product. The standard setup includes a facial cleanser such as Septisol, acetone, Jessner's solution, TCA, cotton-tipped applicators, 2 × 2 inch and 4 × 4 inch gauze pads, and cool-water soaks for patient comfort (Figure 46.1).

Patient preparation

All patients with a history of oral or facial herpes simplex virus (HSV) infection should be pretreated with antiherpetic agents to prevent herpetic activation during the post-peel period. Because a negative history of HSV infection does not always correspond with actual prior exposure, and because antiviral medications are extremely safe, it is prudent to place all patients undergoing medium depth peels on a post-procedural course of medication. Recommended prophylaxis consists of acyclovir 400 mg three times daily, valacyclovir 500 mg twice daily or famciclovir 250 mg twice daily, beginning on the day of the procedure. All antiherpetic agents act by inhibiting viral replication in the intact epidermal cell, such that the skin must be re-epithelialized before the agent has its full effect. Thus, the antiviral agent must be continued after a medium depth peel for at least 10 to 14 days.

Almost every patient desiring facial rejuvenation for cutaneous photoaging would benefit from botulinum toxin injections to alleviate dynamic wrinkles. When administered preoperatively in patients undergoing medium-depth chemical peels, botulinum toxin injections enhance the results of the peel by immobilizing the muscles implicated in the development of dynamic rhytides during the critical time of postoperative collagen remodelling. Another important preoperative adjunctive therapy is topical tretinoin applied on a nightly basis prior to the procedure. Retinoids increase epidermal proliferation and presumably lead to more rapid re-epithelialization after the chemical peel. Additionally, the use of topical retinoids enhances penetration of the chemical peel by decreasing the thickness of the stratum corneum. However, the chemical peel should be delayed in cases of active retinoid dermatitis, as this condition may lead to a prolongation in postoperative erythema [9].

Analgesia and sedation

Medium depth peels may be performed without anesthesia, with preceding topical anesthesia, with local nerve blocks, with mild preoperative sedation, or anxiolytic medications, or a combination of any of the above. For full-face peels in anxious patients, it is useful to give preoperative sedation (5–10 mg diazepam orally) along with mild analgesia in the form of 50 mg meperidine (Demerol, Winthrop, New York, USA) and a mild sedative such as 25 mg hydroxyzine hydrochloride intramuscularly (Vistaril, Lorec, New York, USA). The discomfort from this peel is not long-lasting, so short-acting anxiolytics and analgesics are all that are usually recommended [10].

Application technique

Vigorous cleansing and degreasing of the skin prior to application of the active peeling agent represents a crucial and often overlooked step in the protocol. The removal of skin surface lipids deriving from sebum and epidermal lipids, scale and thickened stratum corneum is particularly important for even penetration of the solution. The face is first washed with an antibacterial cleanser in glycerin (Septisol) applied with 4 × 4 inch gauze pads, then rinsed with water. Acetone is then applied with 4 × 4 inch gauze pads to remove residual oils and debris. The skin is thus débrided of stratum corneum and excessive scale. The necessity for thorough degreasing in order to achieve reliable and even penetration cannot be overemphasized. Prior to application of the active peeling agent, one should assess the thoroughness of degreasing. If oil or scale is felt, the degreasing step should be repeated. Particular attention should be focused on the hairline and nose. Thorough and uniform degreasing conditions the skin to ensure an even peel over the entire face.

Next, Jessner's solution is evenly applied, either with cotton-tip applicators or 2 × 2 inch gauze pads. Jessner's solution alone constitutes a very light peel, and thus will open the epidermal barrier for a more even and more deeply penetrating TCA application. Only one coat of Jessner's solution is usually necessary to achieve a light, even frosting with a background of erythema. The expected frosting is much lighter than that produced by the TCA. The face is treated in sequential segments progressing inferiorly from the hairline. Even strokes are used to apply the solution to the forehead first then each cheek, the nose, and the chin. The perioral area should follow, and the eyelids are treated last, creating the same erythema with blotchy frosting.

As with the application of Jessner's solution, cosmetic units of the face are then peeled sequentially with TCA from forehead to temple to cheeks, and finally to the cutaneous lips and eyelids. The 35% weight-to-volume TCA is applied evenly with 1–4 cotton-tipped applicators rolled over different areas with lighter or heavier doses of the acid. Four well-soaked cotton-tipped applicators are used with broad strokes over the forehead and the medial cheeks. Two mildly soaked cotton-tipped applicators can be used across the lips and chin, and one damp cotton-tipped applicator on the eyelids. The amount of acid delivered is thus dependent upon both the saturation of an individual cotton-tipped applicator and the number of cotton-tipped applicators used. In this manner the application is titrated according to the cutaneous thickness of the treated area.

The white frost from the TCA application, which represents the keratocoagulated endpoint, should appear on the treated area within 30 seconds to 2 minutes after application (Figure 46.2). An even application should eliminate the need for a second or a third pass, but if frosting is incomplete or uneven, the solution should be reapplied. TCA takes longer to frost than a deep phenol peel, but less time than the superficial peeling agents. After a single application to an area, the surgeon should wait at least 3–4 minutes to ensure that frosting has reached its peak. The thoroughness of application can then be analyzed, and a touch up, or less commonly another pass, can be applied as needed. Areas of poor frosting should be retreated carefully with a thin application of TCA.

The physician should seek to achieve a level II–III frosting. Level II frosting is defined as white-coated frosting with a background of erythema [11]. A level III frosting, which is associated with penetration to the reticular dermis, is solid white enamel frosting with no background of erythema. A deeper level III frosting should be restricted only to areas of heavy actinic damage and thicker skin. Although heavily damaged actinic skin may require a level III frosting, most medium depth chemical peels should strive to obtain no more than a level II frosting. This is especially true over eyelids and areas of sensitive skin. Those areas with a greater tendency to scar formation, such as the zygomatic arch, the bony prominences of the jawline, and chin, should only receive up to a level II frosting. Over coating TCA with multiple passes or highly saturated cotton-tipped applicators will increase its penetration, so that a second or third application will create further damage. One must be extremely careful to retreat only areas where the amount of solution taken up was not adequate or the skin is much thicker. One should never overcoat a fully frosted area.

Certain facial features require special attention. Careful feathering of the solution into the hairline and around the rim of the jaw and brow conceals the line of demarcation between peeled and non-peeled areas. The perioral area has fine, radial rhytides that require a complete and even application of solution over the lip skin to the vermilion border. This is best accomplished with the help of an assistant who stretches and fixates the upper and lower lips as the peel solution is applied. Alternatively, the TCA may be applied along the rhytid to the vermilion border with the wooden end of a cotton-tipped applicator. It should be noted that deeper furrows such as expression lines will not be eradicated by a medium depth peel and thus should be treated like the remaining skin.

Thickened keratoses should stand in contrast to the frosted background because they do not pick up peel solution evenly and thus do not frost evenly. Additional applications rubbed vigorously into these lesions may be needed for penetration.

Eyelid skin must be treated delicately and carefully. A damp, rather than saturated, applicator should be used. This is accomplished by draining the excess TCA on the cotton tip against the rim of the bottle or onto a dry gauze pad before using it for application. The patient should be positioned with the head elevated at 30° and the eyelids closed. The applicator is then rolled gently on the lids and periorbital skin within 2–3 mm of the lid margin. Never leave excess peel solution on the lids, because the solution can roll into the eyes. Dry tears with a separate, dry cotton-tipped applicator during peeling because they may wick peel solution to the puncta and eyes by capillary attraction.

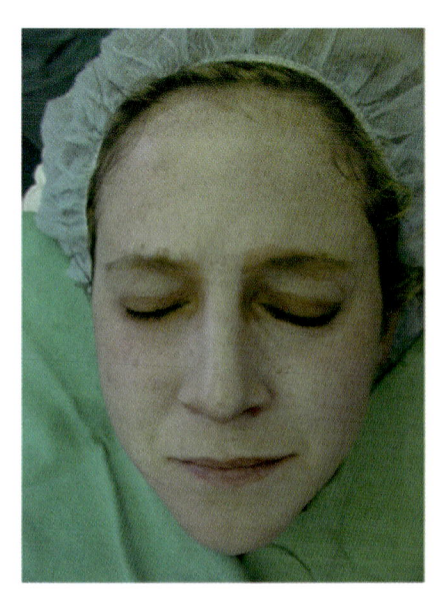

Figure 46.2 Frosting observed immediately after combined Jessner's and TCA peel. Typical opaque white frosting with mild erythema observed 2 minutes after TCA application.

The patient will experience an immediate burning sensation as the TCA is applied, but this subsides as frosting is completed. A circulating fan may be placed beside the patient for comfort. Cool saline or water compresses also offer symptomatic relief for a peeled area. The compresses are placed over the face for 5–6 minutes after the peel until the patient is comfortable. The burning subsides fully by the time the patient is ready to be discharged. At that time, most of the frosting has faded and a brawny desquamation is evident.

Table 46.6 Potential complications of medium-depth chemical peeling.

Inadvertent exposure of vulnerable structure to peeling agent
Dyspigmentation
Infection (bacterial, viral or fungal)
Persistent erythema
Scarring
Textural abnormalities
Milia
Eruptive keratoacanthomas

Post-procedure

Postoperatively, edema, erythema, and desquamation are expected. With periorbital peels and even forehead peels, eyelid edema can be severe enough to close the lids. For the first 2–4 days, the patient is instructed to soak four times a day with a 0.25% acetic acid compresses made of 1 tablespoon white vinegar in 1 pint warm water. A bland emollient is applied to the desquamating areas after soaks. After 4 days, the patient can shower and clean gently with a mild facial cleanser. The erythema intensifies as desquamation becomes complete within 4–5 days. Thus, healing is completed within 7–10 days. At this time the bright red color has faded to pink and has the appearance of a sunburn (Figure 46.3). This erythema may be covered by cosmetics and will fade fully within 2–3 weeks.

Complications

Despite proper patient and procedure selection, perfect surgical technique, and appropriate management before and after the procedure, true complications can occur with medium depth chemical peels (Table 46.6). Many of the complications seen in peeling can be recognized early on during healing stages. The cosmetic surgeon should be well acquainted with the normal appearance of a healing wound in its time frame for medium depth peeling. Prolongation of the granulation tissue phase beyond 1 week may indicate delayed wound healing. This could be the result of viral, bacterial, or fungal infection, contact irritants interfering with wound healing, or other systemic factors. A red flag should alert the physician that careful investigation and prompt treatment should be instituted to forestall potential irreparable damage that may result in scarring. Thus, it is critically important to understand the stages of wound healing in reference to medium depth peeling. The physician then can avoid, recognize, and treat any and all complications early (Figure 46.4).

During chemical peeling, intraoperative exposure of vital structures to the resurfacing agent may occur and have serious adverse consequences. The moistened applicator should never be passed over the central face, in order to avoid inadvertent exposure of the eyes to the solution. There should always be appropriate fluids readily available to rinse the area in case such an exposure does occur. Saline is used to dilute TCA.

The most common complication of chemical peeling is abnormal pigmentation. The risk for hyperpigmention is higher in patients whose Fitzpatrick skin type is IV or higher, so an extra measure of caution is necessary. Exogenous estrogens, photosensitizing medications, and direct sun exposure during the first 6 weeks after peels increase the risk of hyperpigmentation. It is best prevented and/or treated with a topical retinoid, a 4–8% hydroquinone preparation and strict photoprotection.

Infection is an uncommon complication that develops during the postoperative period and may be caused by bacterial, viral or fungal organisms. Factors contributing to post-peel bacterial infections include improper wound hygiene and the use of thick, occlusive ointments that may promote staphylococcal and streptococcal folliculitis. *Escherichia coli*, *Pseudomonas* spp. or candida infections may also occur. Medium depth chemical peeling may activate a HSV during the postoperative period with the potential for dissemination and scarring. An outbreak can even occur in patients on the recommended 10–14 day prophylactic antiviral regimen. The sudden onset of facial pain or severe scarring may herald the onset of diffuse facial HSV. Frequent postoperative visits are helpful to assure rapid recognition and aggressive treatment of any infection so that scarring does not result.

Persistent erythema beyond 2 months after a medium-depth procedure may be precipitated by the use of topical or systemic retinoid therapy, contact with various allergens and irritants, an underlying skin condition or genetic susceptibility or the presence of active infection. Persistent erythema may indicate the impending development of scar formation. Management includes massage, topical, intralesional or systemic corticosteroids, silicone gel sheeting, and pulsed dye laser therapy.

Scarring is perhaps the most feared complication of chemical resurfacing procedures. The risk of scarring increases proportionately with the depth of the peel. Factors that increase the risk of post-peel scarring include the use of TCA at concentrations greater than 50% or a history of any of the following: isotretinoin within a 6-month period, facial surgery or resurfacing within a 6-month period, or any previous radiation exposure. Of note, the risk of scarring is greater on

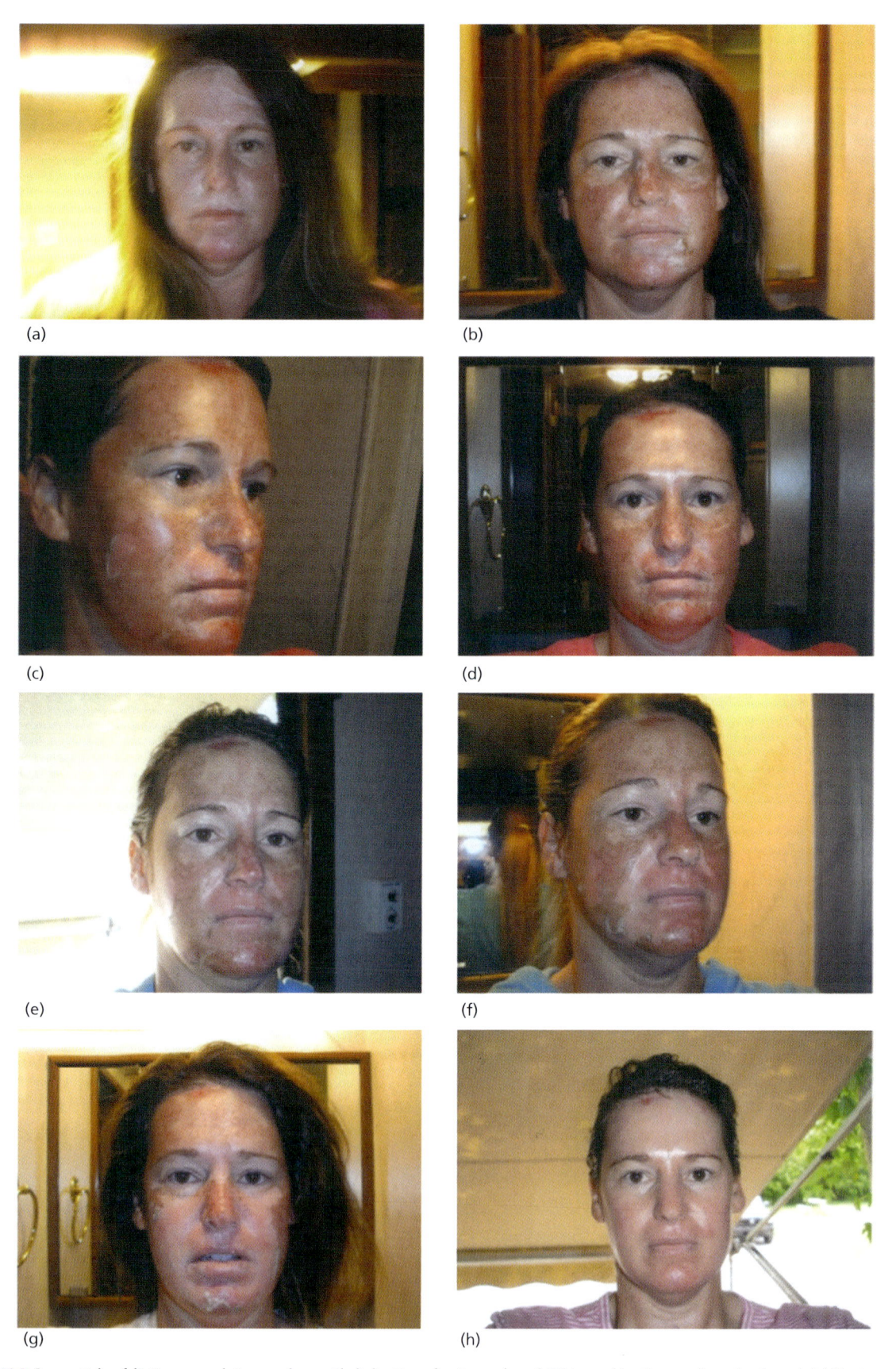

Figure 46.3 Sequential exfoliation, granulation, and re-epithelialization after Jessner's and TCA combination medium depth peel. (a) Postoperative day 1: inflammation with edema, erythema; (b) day 2: early epidermal separation with hyperpigmentation; (c, d) day 3 morning; and (e, f) day 3 afternoon: dermal inflammation with granulation tissue and early re-epithelialization; (g, h) days 5 and 6, respectively: full desquamation with regeneration of new epidermis and beginning dermal remodeling.

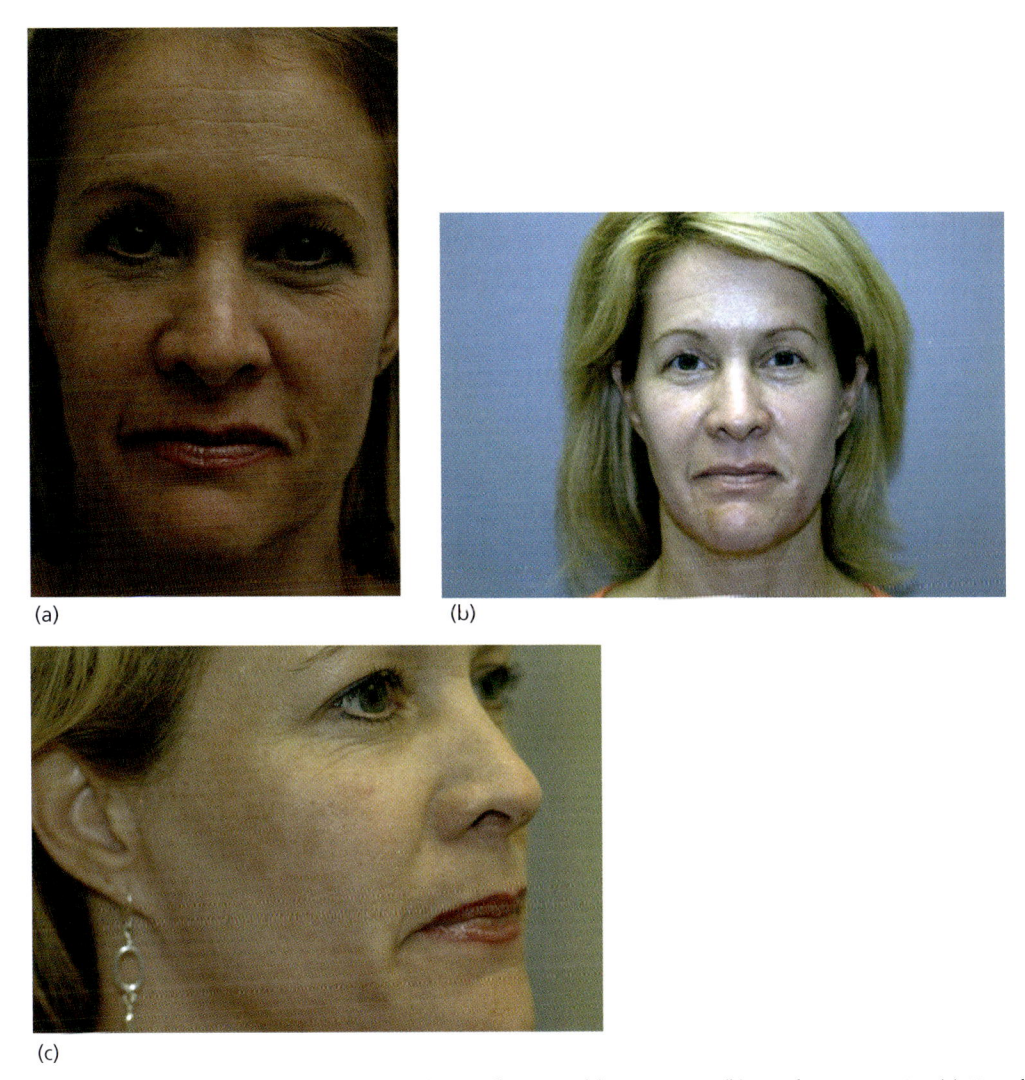

Figure 46.4 Jessner's TCA peel performed for photoaging skin and actinic keratoses. (a) Preoperative; (b) 5 weeks postoperative; (c) 10 weeks postoperative.

non-facial skin. Presumably, this is due to a relative decrease in adnexal structure when compared to the face, which impairs wound healing. Thus, when peeling non-facial skin, such as for actinic keratoses of the arms and hands, it is prudent to use lower concentrations of acids and serial treatments. In addition to scarring, medium depth chemical peeling of the dorsal arms and hands has been reported to trigger eruptive keratoacanthomas [12].

Adverse systemic effects related to medium depth chemical peels are exceedingly rare. The use of Jessner's solution poses a theoretical risk of systemic salicylate or resorcinol toxicity, but this is probably not clinically significant when application is limited to the face and neck. Additionally, a growing number of studies linking long-term systemic TCA exposure in laboratory mice to the development of liver cancer have raised concern over the potential carcinogenicity of TCA in humans. However, this link has not been demonstrated in any human studies. Further, it is unlikely that the amount of TCA exposure a person receives during a medium depth chemical peel, only 3-4 minutes before the acid is washed off, would pose a significant risk of carcinogenesis [13].

Long-term care

Long-term care of peeled skin includes sunscreen protection for up to 6 months along with reinstitution of medical treatment such as low strength hydroxy acid lotions and topical tretinoin formulations. Repeeling areas should not be performed for 6 months from the previous peel. If any erythema or edema persists, the peel should not be performed as the reinjury may create complications. Medium depth peels should not be performed on undermined skin such as facelift or flap surgery performed up to 6 months prior to the peel [14].

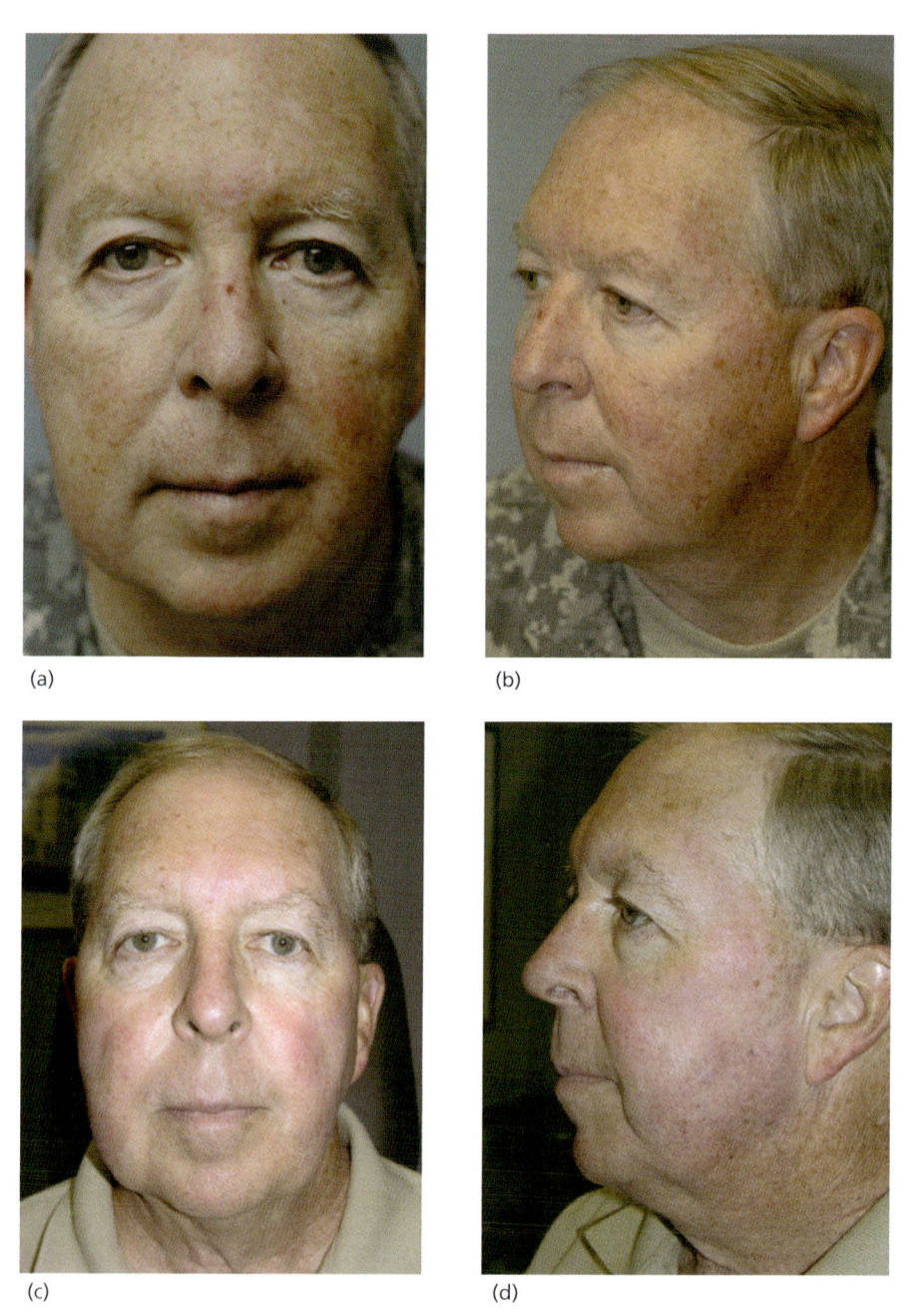

Figure 46.5 Jessner's 35% TCA peel for actinic keratoses. (a & b) Preoperative diffuse actinic keratoses and seborrheic keratoses; (c & d) 9 months postoperative.

Conclusions

The evolution of medium depth chemical peeling has changed the face of cosmetic surgery. It has introduced new techniques into the armamentarium of the cosmetic surgeon to treat problems that previously have been approached with tools inadequate to obtain the results for moderate photoaging skin or with overly aggressive treatment using deep chemical peeling agents. The combination peels have provided some of the more popular tools needed to approach a burgeoning population with photoaging and photocarcinogenesis.

The presented medium depth peel will produce excellent results for a variety of skin conditions, including actinic keratoses (Figure 46.5). Medium depth combination peels thus provide an effective, safe, and simple single procedure that can be used as both a therapeutic and cosmetic procedure to counteract cutaneous photodamage.

References

1. Brody HJ, Monheit GD, Resnik SS, Alt TH. (2000) A history of chemical peeling. *Dermatol Surg* **26**, 405–9.
2. Brody HJ. (1989) Variations and comparisons in medium depth chemical peeling. *J Dermatol Surg Oncol* **15**, 960–3.
3. Monheit GD. (2004) Chemical peels. *Skin Ther Lett* **9**, 6–11.
4. Brody HJ. (1997) *Chemical Peeling and Resurfacing*. Mosby, p. 110.
5. Monheit GD. (1989) The Jessner's + TCA peel: a medium depth chemical peel. *J Dermatol Surg Oncol* **15**, 945.
6. Coleman WP, Futrell JM. (1994) The glycolic acid + trichloroacetic acid peel. *J Dermatol Surg Oncol* **20**, 76–80.
7. Glogau RG. (1994) Chemical peeling and aging skin. *J Geriatr Dermatol* **2**, 30–5.
8. Lawrence N, Cox SE, Cockerell CJ, *et al.* (1995) A comparison of efficacy and safety of Jessner's solution and 35% trichloracetic acid vs. 5% fluorouracil in the treatment of widespread facial actinic keratoses. *Arch Dermatol* **131**, 176–81.
9. Monheit, GD, Chastain, MA. Chemical and mechanical skin resurfacing. In Bolognia JL, Jorizzo JL & Schaffer JV (eds.) *Dermatology*, 3rd edn. Elsevier: 2012: 2494–506.
10. Monheit GD. (1995) The Jessner's trichloracetic acid peel. *Dermatol Clin* **13**, 277–83.
11. Rubin M. (1995) *Manual of Chemical Peels*. Philadelphia, PA: Lippincott, pp. 120–1.
12. Mohr B, Fernandez MP, Krejci-Manwaring J. (2013) Eruptive keratoacanthomas after Jessner's and trichloroacetic acid peel for actinic keratosis. *Dermatol Surg* **39**, 331–3.
13. Zheng, L. (2011) Toxicological Review of Trichloroacetic Acid. U.S. Environmental Protection Agency.
14. Monheit GD. (1994) Advances in chemical peeling. *Facial Plast Surg Clin North Am* **2**, 7–8.

CHAPTER 47
CO_2 Laser Resurfacing: Confluent and Fractionated

Mitchel P. Goldman[1,2] and Ana Marie Liolios[1]
[1]Cosmetic Laser Dermatology, San Diego, CA, USA
[2]Private Practice, Fairway, Kansas, MO, USA

> **BASIC CONCEPTS**
> - Fractionated laser resurfacing with ablative lasers gives better results than with non-invasive lasers.
> - Confluent ablative laser resurfacing gives better results than fractionated laser resurfacing.
> - More "down-time" correlates with better results.
> - Cold air cooling and advanced topical and local anesthesia provides optimal pain control.
> - Fractionated ablative resurfacing has minimal adverse effects.

Introduction

Carbon dioxide (CO_2) lasers are currently available in two forms: confluent and fractionated. The differences between the results, adverse effects, and down-time are compared and contrasted in this chapter.

CO_2 laser resurfacing

The modern era of CO_2 laser resurfacing began in 1994 with the development of the UltraPulse CO_2 laser by Coherent Medical (now Lumenis, Inc., Santa Clara, CA, USA). This laser delivers peak fluence above the ablation threshold of cutaneous tissue (5 J/cm^2) with tissue dwell times shorter than the 1 ms thermal relaxation time of the epidermis. These new generation CO_2 lasers limited tissue dwell time by either shortening the pulse duration (i.e. UltraPulse) or using scanning technology to rapidly sweep a continuous wave CO_2 laser beam over the tissue such that the laser beam does not remain in contact with any particular spot on the tissue for longer than 1 ms (i.e. SilkTouch, Sharplan Laser Corporation, now Lumenis Inc., Santa Clara, CA, USA). These high peak-power, short-pulsed, and rapidly scanned CO_2 laser systems allow laser surgeons to precisely and effectively ablate 20–30 μm of skin per pass while leaving in its wake a considerably smaller residual zone of thermal damage (up to 150 μm) than left behind by the previous generation of continuous wave CO_2 lasers (up to 600 μm). Clinically, this technologic advancement translates into superior clinical results and a much more favorable safety profile than seen previously with the continuous wave CO_2 lasers.

The thermal effect of the CO_2 laser acts on dermal collagen stimulating neocollagenesis and tightening of facial skin. Successful ablation maximizes thermal stimulation of the dermis while limiting non-specific thermal damage. Another method used to decrease thermal damage is to follow a session of CO_2 laser ablation with the erbium:yttrium aluminum garnet (Er:YAG) laser. With this technique, the residual non-specific thermal damage left from the CO_2 laser is vaporized by subsequent passes with an Er:YAG laser which leaves little if any non-specific thermal damage.

Given the impressive clinical results achieved with the high peak power, short pulsed, and rapidly scanned CO_2 lasers, they quickly replaced chemical peels and dermabrasion as the treatment of choice for cutaneous resurfacing. However, the impressive results achieved with these new generation CO_2 lasers were not without drawbacks. Re-epithelialization can take 5–14 days and postoperative erythema and/or post-inflammatory hyperpigmentation can last 1–6 months depending on the depth of laser ablation, amount of residual non-specific thermal damage, and patient's skin type. Finally, there is a risk of fungal, viral, and bacterial infections on the denuded skin as well as delayed permanent hypopigmentation from destruction of melanocytes and resultant scarring. Minimizing these potential adverse effects requires excellent postoperative care and is time-consuming for both the patient and physician.

These side effects, as well as the significant "down-time" typically associated with CO_2 laser resurfacing and extensive postoperative care, are unacceptable to many patients and significantly dampened the initial enthusiasm associated with their use.

Cosmetic Dermatology: Products and Procedures, Second Edition. Edited by Zoe Diana Draelos.
© 2016 John Wiley & Sons, Ltd. Published 2016 by John Wiley & Sons, Ltd.

Because the CO_2 laser typically operates near its tissue ablation threshold (5 J/cm^2) in most resurfacing applications, a large fraction of its energy is invested in heating rather than ablating tissue. Consequently, the CO_2 laser produces relatively large residual thermal damage zones and causes significant desiccation of the target tissue after only a few passes. With each subsequent pass, the amount of vaporized tissue decreases while thermal damage increases and a "plateau" of ablation is typically reached after the fourth pass. Non-specific thermal damage has a negative impact, not only on the CO_2 laser's ablative capacity, but also on its side effect profile. Our research suggests that the relatively large thermally induced residual zone of necrosis (up to 150 μm) left behind by the CO_2 laser is one of the main factors contributing to its adverse sequelae including prolonged erythema, postoperative pain, delayed healing, infection, hypopigmentation, and scarring.

To minimize the issues resulting from a large residual thermal zone the Er:YAG laser was introduced for resurfacing. While it was successful in reducing thermal damage it was unable to penetrate beyond papillary dermis as a result of its high absorption by water. A multimode Er:YAG system, the Tunable Resurfacing Laser (TRL), was developed (Sciton, Inc., Palo Alto, CA, USA) which allows the user to blend a variety of ablation and thermal coagulation depths by extending the pulse duration of the Er:YAG laser which is typically less than 0.5 ms. Extending the pulse duration to 4–10 ms allowed for less flash vaporization and more prolonged thermal heating to occur. The TRL can be tuned for pure ablation or CO_2-like thermal injury, or any point in between.

Modifications of technical protocols have continued to improve clinical outcomes. Combination therapy with CO_2 immediately followed by Er:YAG lasers allow cosmetic surgeons to capitalize on the unique benefits of each laser system and to minimize their disadvantages. Er:YAG laser treatment can be used to bypass the ablation "plateau" characteristic of CO_2 resurfacing to ablate deeper into the dermis. Improved postoperative healing can also be attained when the short-pulsed Er:YAG laser is used to remove the residual zone of thermal necrosis left behind after CO_2 resurfacing (Figures 47.1 and 47.2).

Additionally, the ablative lasers have turned out to be extremely versatile therapeutic tools. Cosmetic surgeons now regularly combine ablative laser resurfacing with other problem-specific non-ablative technologies to address multiple cosmetic concerns for the patient in a single treatment session. The efficacy of Q-switched lasers in the treatment of pigmented lesions is enhanced when these lasers are used after ablative resurfacing. Treatment of vascular lesions with the pulsed dye laser, other vascular lasers, or the intense pulsed light has been shown to be extremely successful when performed prior to skin resurfacing with an ablative laser. Despite early reports advising against it, full-face laser resurfacing is now safely being combined with rhytidectomy, autologous fat transfer and/or the use of dermal filler or biostimulatory agents like Sculptra™ to achieve a more comprehensive approach to facial rejuvenation. To enhance collagen deposition we utilize a variety of neuromodulator agents like Botox™, Dysport™, or Xeomin™ usually a day or longer prior to laser resurfacing to decrease facial muscular movement.

Pre-treatment and post-treatment protocols have also improved. Although some controversy remains surrounding the topic of antibiotic prophylaxis, a number of studies in the last decade have provided relevant information on common pathogens, effective antibiotic prophylaxis regimens, and clinical situations at increased risk for infection after cutaneous laser resurfacing. Improved laser wound care regimens have reduced recovery time and decreased morbidity after laser skin resurfacing. The benefits of occlusive dressings in accelerating laser wound healing have been well established in a number of studies. Timely institution of topical medications in the postoperative

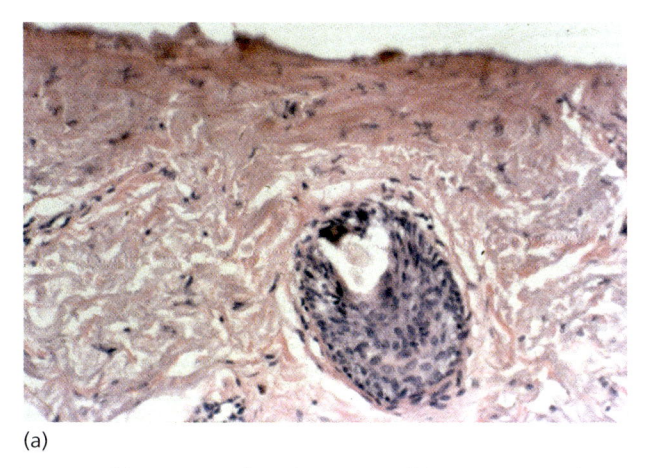

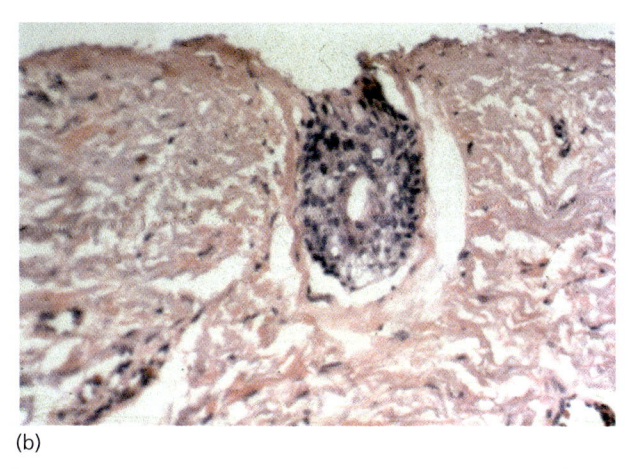

Figure 47.1 (a) Two passes of CO_2 laser at 7 J/cm^2 leaves approximately 70 μm of residual thermal necrosis. (b) Two passes of Er:YAG laser at 10 J/cm^2 results in removal of approximately 50 μm of this necrotic tissue. (Source: Carcamo & Goldman, 2006; Skin resurfacing with ablative lasers. In: Goldman MP, ed. *Cutaneous and Cosmetic Laser Surgery*. London: Mosby-Elsevier. Reproduced with permission.)

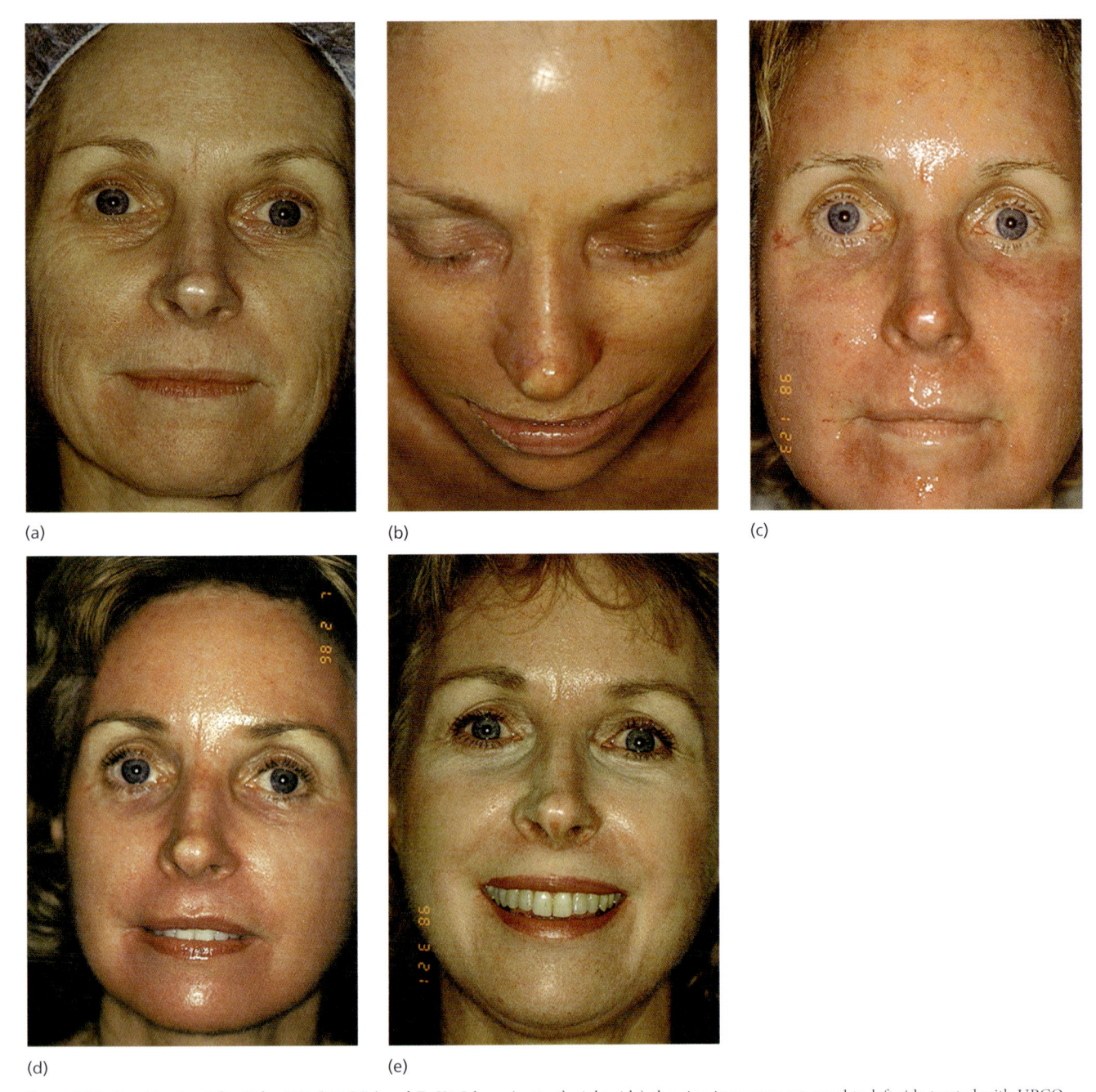

Figure 47.2 Combination UltraPulse CO₂ (UPCO₂) and Er:YAG laser (patient's right side) showing improvement equal to left side treated with UPCO₂ alone. (a) Before treatment; (b) immediately after treatment; (c) 7 days after laser resurfacing; (d) 3 weeks after laser resurfacing; (e) 2 months after resurfacing. (Source: Carcamo & Goldman, 2006; Skin resurfacing with ablative lasers. In: Goldman MP, ed. *Cutaneous and Cosmetic Laser Surgery*. London: Mosby-Elsevier. Reproduced with permission.)

period is now allowing surgeons to effectively address a number of expected postoperative symptoms and complications including postoperative erythema and edema, pruritus, and post-inflammatory hyperpigmentation. We are presently evaluating a variety of growth factors and biologic wound dressings to further enhance wound healing.

Fractionated CO₂ laser resurfacing

Because of the prolonged and meticulous postoperative care in addition to potential adverse effects, as well as the advancement in minimally invasive procedures with rapid healing times, confluent CO₂ and/or Er:YAG ablative resurfacing is rarely necessary for the full face and if performed is only utilized in the perioral and/or periorbital regions. Physicians and patients find it easier to have minimally invasive procedures performed at the expense of efficacy. The current consensus among patients is to embrace a treatment modality that delivers maximum results with minimal down-time. Unfortunately, the promises by most laser companies who have developed and are promoting these minimally invasive, non-ablative lasers have not lived up to their stated efficacy in improving photodamage. The development of fractionated lasers that treat a percentage of the skin while leaving the intervening areas untreated, allows for the more dramatic results of a variety of laser wavelengths including the 10600 nm CO_2 laser to be associated with quicker healing times and fewer postoperative sequelae.

Initially, fractional lasers were introduced in a non-ablative format. This technology was developed to overcome the homogeneous thermal damage typically created after treatment with standard CO_2 and/or Er:YAG lasers and instead creates microscopic thermal wounds which spares the tissue surrounding each wound. Initial studies showed a 2.1% linear shrinkage of periorbital rhytides was noted at 3 months with this non-ablative fractionated laser which is much less than that achieved with standard ablative CO_2 and/or Er:YAG laser resurfacing. With the disappointment of the fractionated non-ablative lasers, it did not take long for fractional photothermolysis to be applied to ablative lasers, allowing for a more aggressive treatment option. Our recommendation is that non-ablative fractionated lasers be reserved for patients who cannot accept any "down-time" and are willing to wait at least 6 months and have 4–6 treatments to see definite improvement in wrinkles and/or scarring.

Interestingly, physicians have had the ability to perform fractionated CO_2 laser resurfacing since the development of the scanning UltraPulse hand-piece in 1995. This scanner was developed to deliver precisely overlapped laser pulses that occurred in a Gaussian distribution uniformly to ablate and/or vaporize the epidermis. Recognition that one could use this scanner with a negative 10% overlap along with the development of smaller laser spot sizes (0.1 and 1.2 mm) produced the first fractionated CO_2 laser.

There are an ever-increasing variety of both fractionated CO_2, Er:YAG, and Er:YSGG lasers to assist in facial rejuvenation. Table 47.1 summarizes most of the available lasers by company, wavelength, spot size, density, frequency, power, and maximal depth (if known). Due to the ever increasing number of devices available, below is a discussion of some of the most commonly used devices at the time of this writing (early 2014). Because we have not been able to evaluate each system and little if anything is currently available in the peer-reviewed medical literature, we are thankful to our colleagues for sharing their experience.

Active and Deep FX-Lumenis

The Active and Deep FX fractionated CO_2 laser delivers the equivalent of 240 W to the tissue compared to the other 30 and 40 W systems. The nature of the 240 W square wave pulse of the UltraPulse makes it about eight times the power of competitive CO_2 laser systems. This is said to result in a cleaner ablation.

Table 47.1 Summary of available lasers by company, wavelength, spot size, density, frequency, power, and maximal depth.

Company	Product	Wavelength (nm)	Spot size (µm)	Max Depth (µm)	Density	Frequency (Hz)	Power (W)
Lumenis	Deep FX	10,600	120	4000	5–45%	300	60
Lumenis	Active FX	10,600	1300	300	55–100%	600	60
Solta	Fraxel Re:pair	10,600	120	1600	10–70%	2100 MTZ/s	40
Alma	Pixel CO_2	10,600	250	300	15–20%		70
Lasering	MiXto SX	10,600	180/300	500	20–100%		30
DEKA	SmartXide DOT	10,600	350	350	5–100%	5–100	30
Lutronic	Mosaic eCO_2	10,600	120/30/1000	2400	5–130%	200	30
Candela	CO_2RE	10,600	180				60
Cynosure	SmartSkin	10,600	350				30
Palomar	Lux 2940	2940	300	600			
Sciton	Profractional	2940	250	1500	1.5–60%	2.3 cm²/s	
Sciton	Profractional XC	2940	430	1500	5.5 or 11%		
Alma	Pixel	2940	150	<300	49 or 81	2	
Cutera	Fractionated Pearl	2790	300	200–1000			

MTZ, microthermal zone.

416 ANTI-AGING Resurfacing Techniques

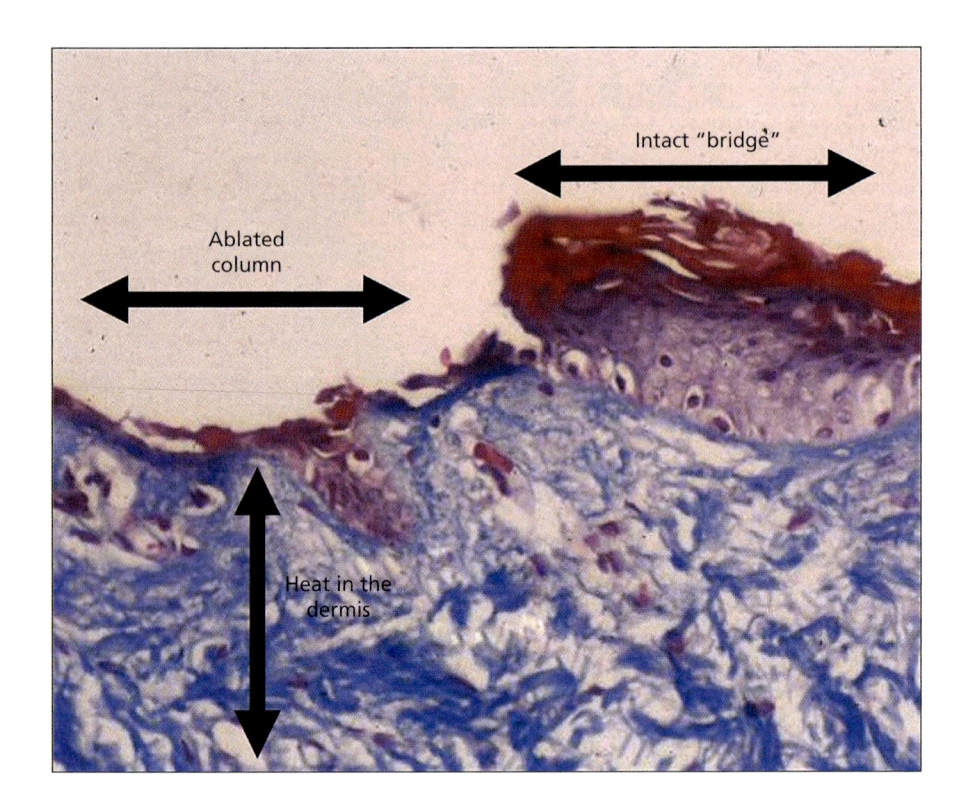

Figure 47.3 Histology of Active FX laser impulse at 100 mJ.

The Active FX hand-piece has a spot size of 1.3 mm and ablates up to 300 μm of tissue (Figure 47.3). The Deep FX hand-piece has a 120 μm diameter spot size which can ablate tissue from superficial to up to 2 mm depending on the power density chosen as well as whether the individual pulses occur as a single, double, or triple pulse (Figure 47.4). The Deep FX is used to treat individual scars and/or wrinkles. This is followed by the Active FX which is used to treat the entire face, rejuvenating the epidermis. The Total FX mode combines the Active/Deep FX modes simultaneously. In 2012, Lumenis introduced SCAAR FX which is a higher energy, shorter pulse duration treatment option which penetrates up to 4 mm in depth. This mode uses coagulation and ablation to treat complex and deep skin lesions and scars.

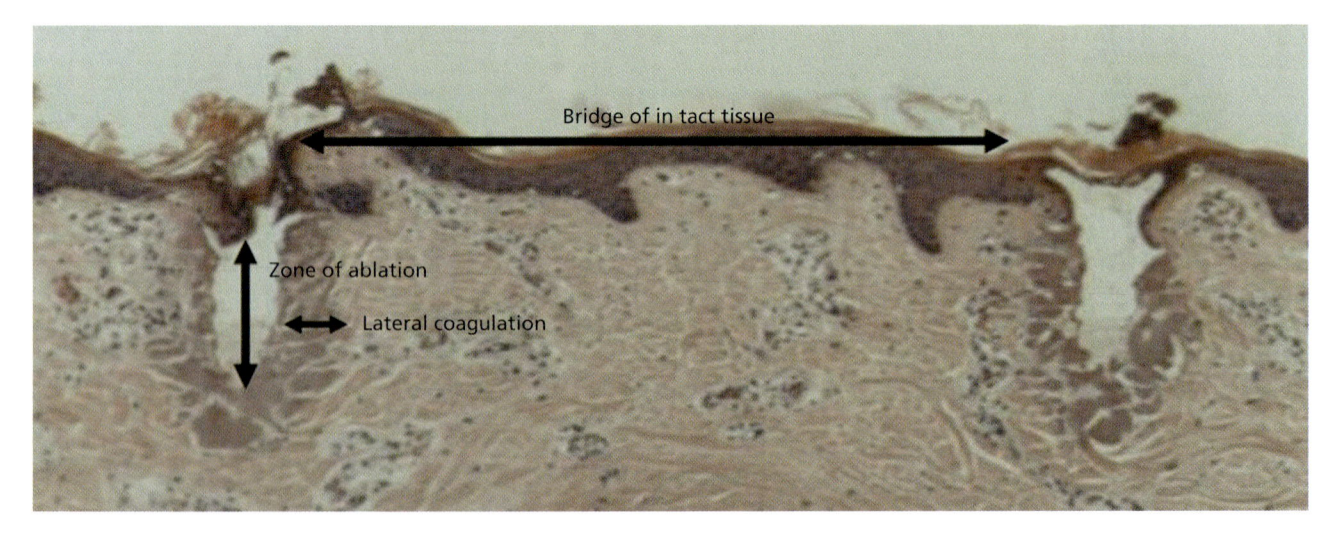

Figure 47.4 Histology of Deep FX laser impulse at 17.5 mJ. Zones of ablation are created, leaving bridges of intact tissue to aid in regeneration. Lateral and vertical coagulation stimulate a tissue regeneration response between the ablated columns.

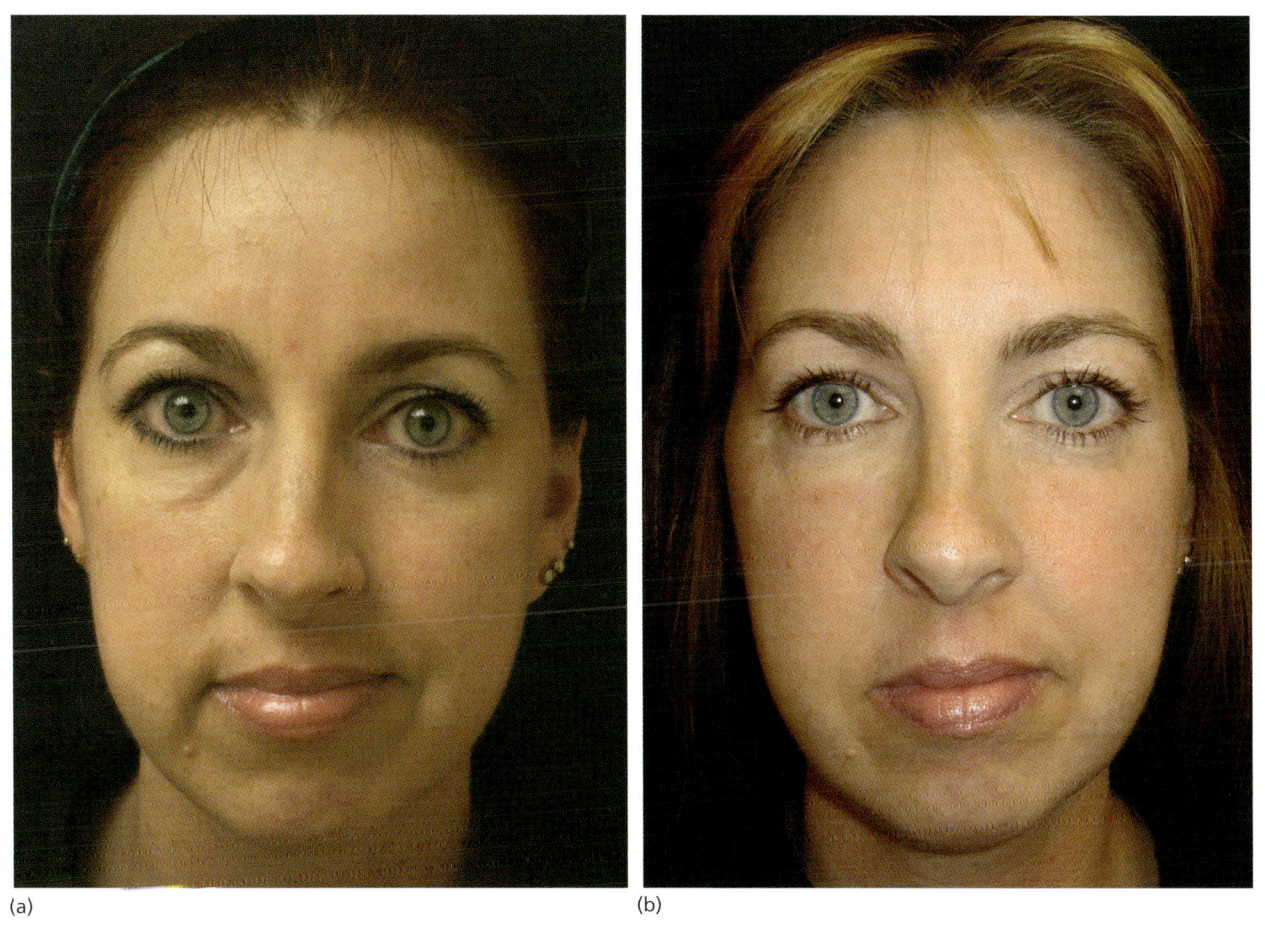

Figure 47.5 Forty-year-old female treated with Active FX fractionated CO$_2$ laser with a 1.3 mm diameter spot size, density 2, 100 mJ: (a) before; (b) two months after treatment.

We have evaluated the histologic and clinical effects of varying pulse energies and densities on ex vivo tissue as well as in vivo with the fractionated CO$_2$ laser (UltraPulse Encore Active FX™, Lumenis, Santa Clara, CA, USA). A distinct, stippled grey, fractional epidermolysis pattern is apparent during the procedure followed by erythema. Erythema lasts for about 3 days for patients treated with −10% overlap and increases by approximately 1 day for each increased density setting. Edema persists for a little more than 1 day (Figure 47.5). The level of satisfaction at 1 month is relatively high, averaging 6 on a 1–10 scale.

We find that it may take two to three separate treatments with the fractionated CO$_2$ laser to achieve the same results as non-fractionated CO$_2$ laser resurfacing (Figures 47.6 and 47.7). The advantage of the fractionated approach is that the procedure can be performed entirely under topical anesthesia and supplemented with cold air cooling and field/nerve blocks as opposed to standard CO$_2$ laser resurfacing which requires general anesthesia or the use of a large number of nerve blocks and/or tumescent anesthesia. In addition, postoperative healing is far easier with the fractionated approach. Patients do not require a Silon TSR dressing (Bio Med Sciences, Inc., Bethlehem, PA, USA) and do not have to be as diligent with vinegar water soaks. There is minimal serous exudate or crusting. Finally, patients are able to wear make-up 4–7 days post-procedure and are usually completely healed and look good without make-up within 5–7 days (Figure 47.8).

Ciocon *et al.* conducted a split-faced study to evaluate the efficacy of the Deep FX compared to the Fraxel Re:Pair (Solta Medical, Hayward, CA) for the treatment of photodamaged facial skin in eight patients. Topical benzocaine, lidocaine and tetracaine ointment was used for 1 hour prior to treatment [1]. The Deep FX was used at 20–25 mJ with a density of 2 (10%), two passes without pulse stacking were done for an overall density of 20%. For the Fraxel Re:Pair the energy was 25–40 mJ with a treatment level of 7–9 with four passes and an overall density of 25–35%. Results showed that both modalities were equally efficacious in improving wrinkles,

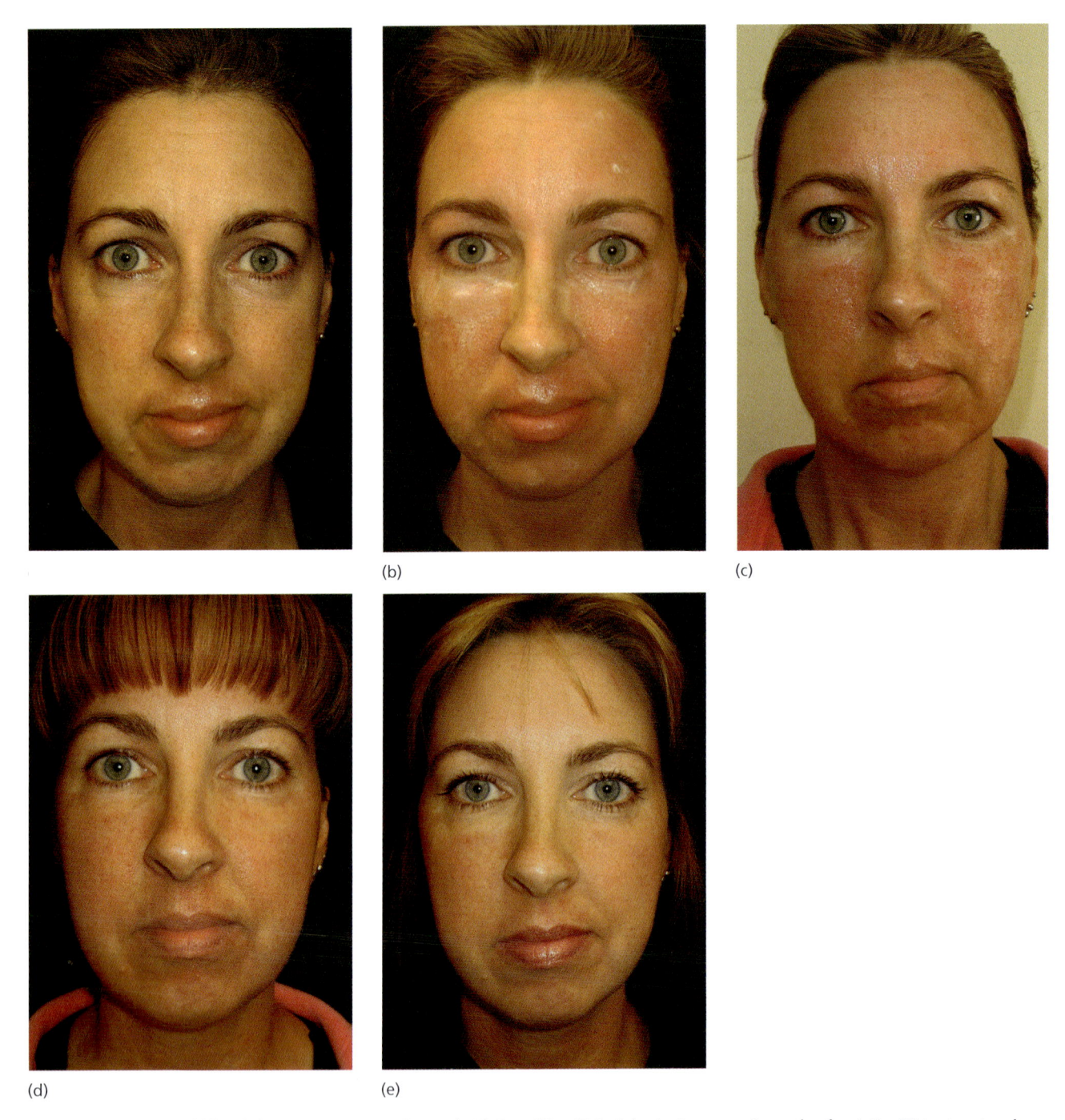

Figure 47.6 Forty-year-old female (same as in Figure 47.5) treated with Deep FX at 17.5 mJ density 1, one pass 3 months after Active FX treatment as above. (a) Immediately before; (b) immediately after treatment; (c) 1 day after treatment; (d) 2 days after treatment; (e) 2 months after treatment.

pigmentation, laxity and overall appearance at 3 months after treatment. Intraoperative pain was rated significantly higher with the Deep FX compared to the Fraxel Re:Pair in this study.

A more recent study was performed comparing four ablative fractional lasers for photodamage in a randomized, controlled quadrant study. The study compared Fraxel Re:Pair, Active and Deep FX, Quadralase (Candela, Wayland, MA), and Pearl Fractionated (Cutera, Brisbane, CA). Each subjects face was divided into four quadrants and each quadrant was randomly assigned a treatment with one of the four lasers. Settings were chosen based on clinical experiences of

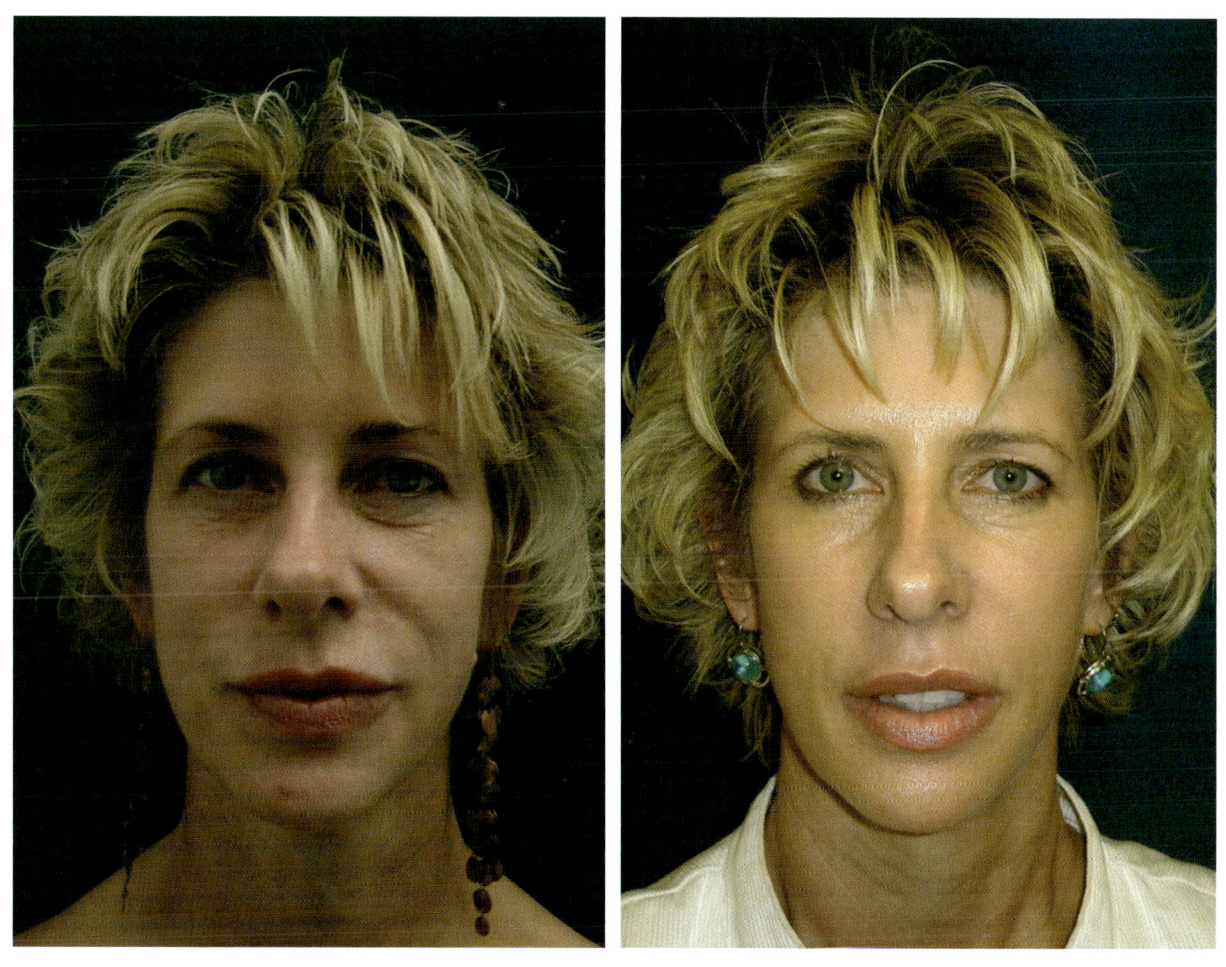

Figure 47.7 Fifty-one-year-old women treated with Deep FX at 15 mJ, density 1, one pass in the periorbital and perioral area followed by Active FX to the entire face at 100 mJ, density 2, one pass. Before and 2 months after treatment.

the investigator to optimize outcomes. Results show that all four devices showed statistical improvement in photoaging (rhytides, lentigines, skin texture and pore size), but none was significantly better than the others. Patient satisfaction and pain was not significantly different between the four lasers, but the Active and Deep FX patients healed quicker with less postoperative erythema and operative pain. Two subjects agreed to submit biopsies for histologic comparison and no significant difference was found in the depth/width of evaporative zones and total thermal injury between the four lasers.

Fraxel Re:Pair – Solta Medical

Fraxel Re:Pair (Solta Medical, Hayward, CA) is a fractionated ablative 10600 nm CO_2 laser that delivers 5–70 mJ of energy, a 350 μm spot size and a 15 × 15 mm treatment tip. This laser provides 5–70% coverage based on the treatment level chosen. Depth of penetration at 70 mJ is reported at 1.6 mm.

In 2009, Rhaman *et al.* provided a study using Fraxel Re:Pair technology to treat inner forearms initially and then photodamage of the face and neck in 30 subjects. Rhaman found that treatment with the Re:Pair was well tolerated with no serious adverse events. He reported 83% of patients had 50–100% overall improvement in photodamage as judged by blinded investigators 3 months following treatment (Figure 47.9) [2].

In 2010, Karsai *et al.* reported a randomized controlled double blind split face trial comparing fractional ablative CO_2 (Fraxel Re:Pair) and Er:YAG (MCL30 Dermablate, Ascleption Laser Technologies, Jena, Germany) laser for treatment of periorbital rhytides [3]. Rhytides were evaluated with profilometric measurement of depth and using the wrinkle score. Patient satisfaction and assessment of side effects were also done. Both lasers showed reduction in depth of rhytides and

420 ANTI-AGING Resurfacing Techniques

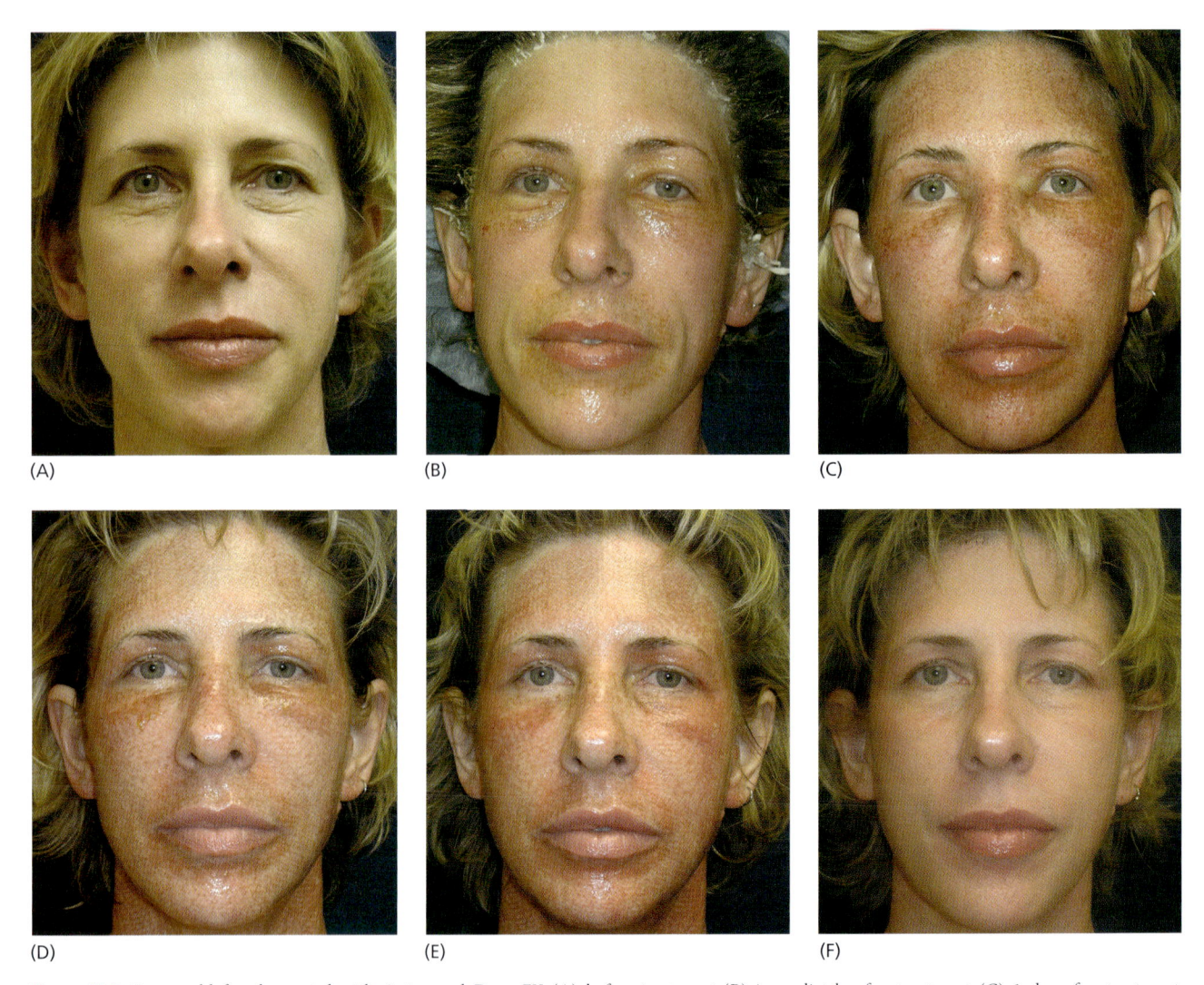

Figure 47.8 52-year-old female treated with Active and Deep FX (A) before treatment (B) immediately after treatment (C) 1 day after treatment (D) 2 days after treatment (E) 3 days after treatment (F) 1 week after treatment.

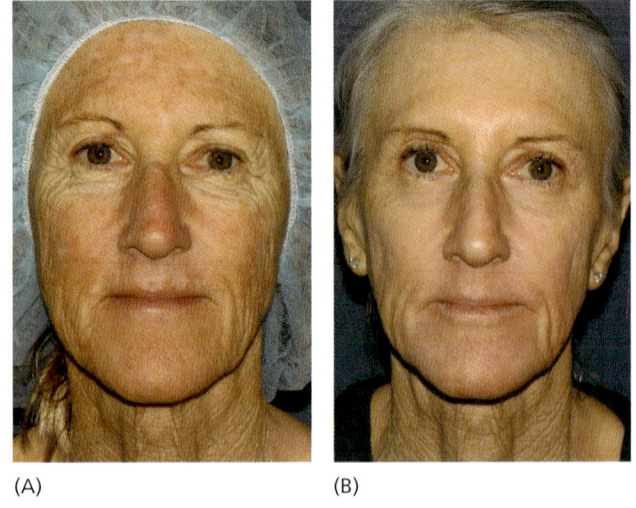

Figure 47.9 63-year-old female (A) before treatment (B) 4 months after Fraxel Re:Pair full face and neck, UPCO$_2$/Erbium periorbital/periocular, VBeam and topical Sculptra applied with Alma. (Source: Dr. Richard Fitzpatrick. Reproduced with permission.)

improvement in Fitzpatrick wrinkle scores, with no significant difference between the two lasers. Early in recovery patients reported more discomfort with the Er:YAG treatment, but later in the healing process more discomfort was reported with the CO$_2$ treatments. Overall patients did not have a preference for one laser over the other and the majority stated they would undergo the procedure again. One treatment with either fractional ablative laser that was studied showed small, but noticeable improvement in periocular rhytides, leading one to assume that multiple treatments will likely be necessary for more dramatic improvement.

MiXto SX – Lasering USA

This is a low-powered fractionated CO$_2$ laser with energy output between 0.5–30 W. This device is usually used at a power between 8 and 15 W. Variable spot sizes (180 μm or 300 μm) are available with a focusing handpiece. Depth of ablation is reported at 200 μm with an additional 300 μm of thermal damage (Tierney-Derm Therapy, 2011) [4,5.] This low-energy system has the advantage of causing only 1 day of erythema and fine, pinpoint crusting up to a week. No topical anesthesia or cold air cooling is recommended. Pain is reported as minimal and "easily tolerated" with one pass (Figure 47.10).

A split-face study comparing the Mixto SX with a microfractional Er:YAG laser (MCL30 Dermablate, Asclepion Laser Technologies, Jena, Germany), with both systems using an energy density of 15 J/cm^2 without any anesthesia, showed a slightly higher improvement (15%) with the CO_2 as opposed to the Er:YAG systems without any difference in satisfaction scores. Microcrusting lasted 1 day less with the Er:YAG system.

This laser can also be used in a continuous mode at 30 W for cutting. In fractional mode, the scanner is delivered alternatively into four quadrants to produce thermal relaxation between impact spots.

Mosaic eCO$_2$™ – Lutronic

The Mosaic eCO$_2$ is a multifunctional microfractional CO_2 laser with pulse energy that ranges from 2–240 mJ, a density of 25–400 spots/cm^2, and utilizes a fractional scanner handpiece. The eCO$_2$ allows the user to select between several scan shapes and sizes, a sequential beam pattern or a non-linear randomized

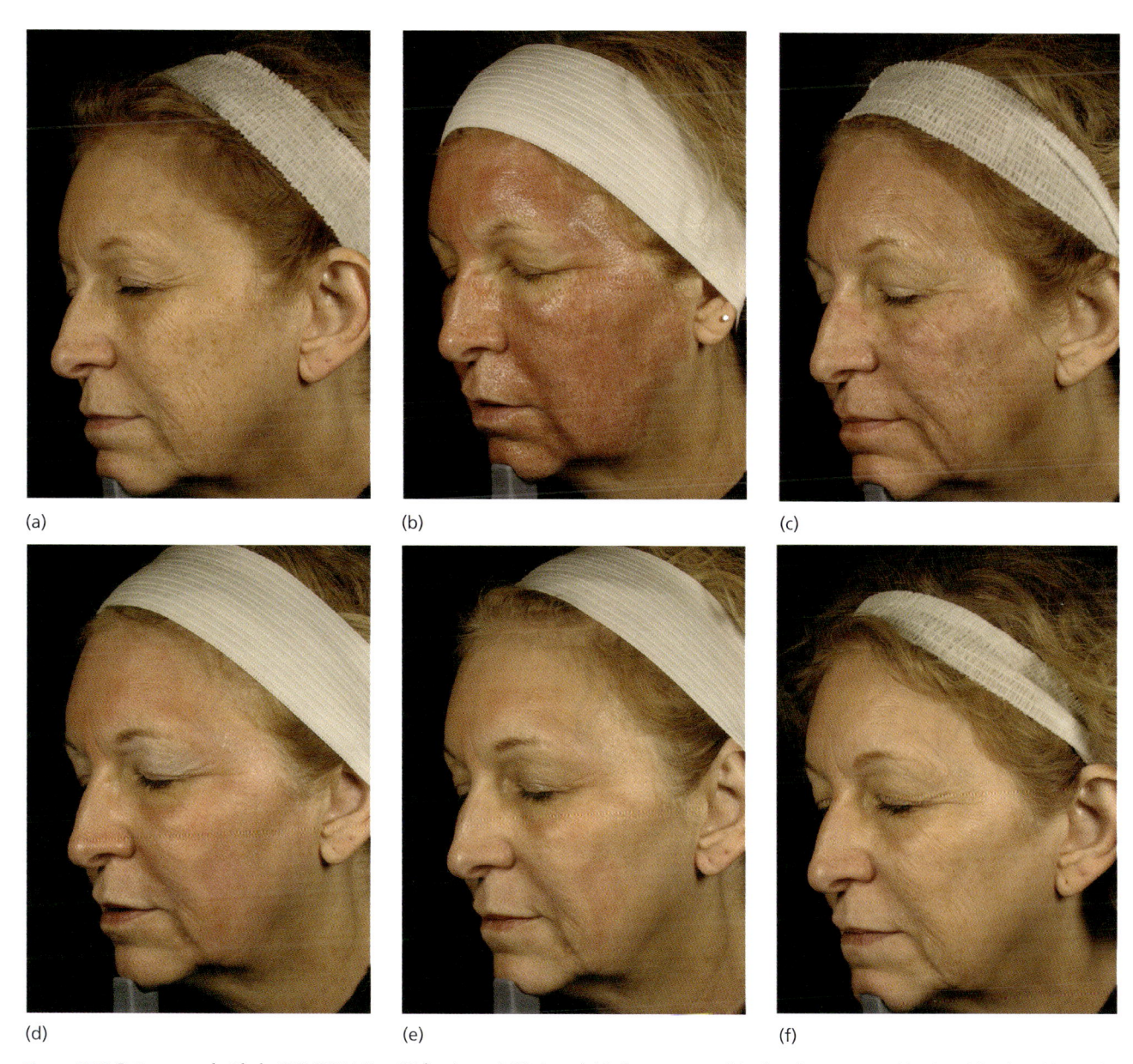

Figure 47.10 Patient treated with the SLIM E30 Mixto SX fractionated CO_2 laser. (a) Before treatment; (b) 1 day after treatment; (c) 3 days; (d) 7 days; (e) 2 weeks; (f) 8 weeks. (Source: Dr. Jeffery Hsu. Reproduced with permission.)

422   ANTI-AGING Resurfacing Techniques

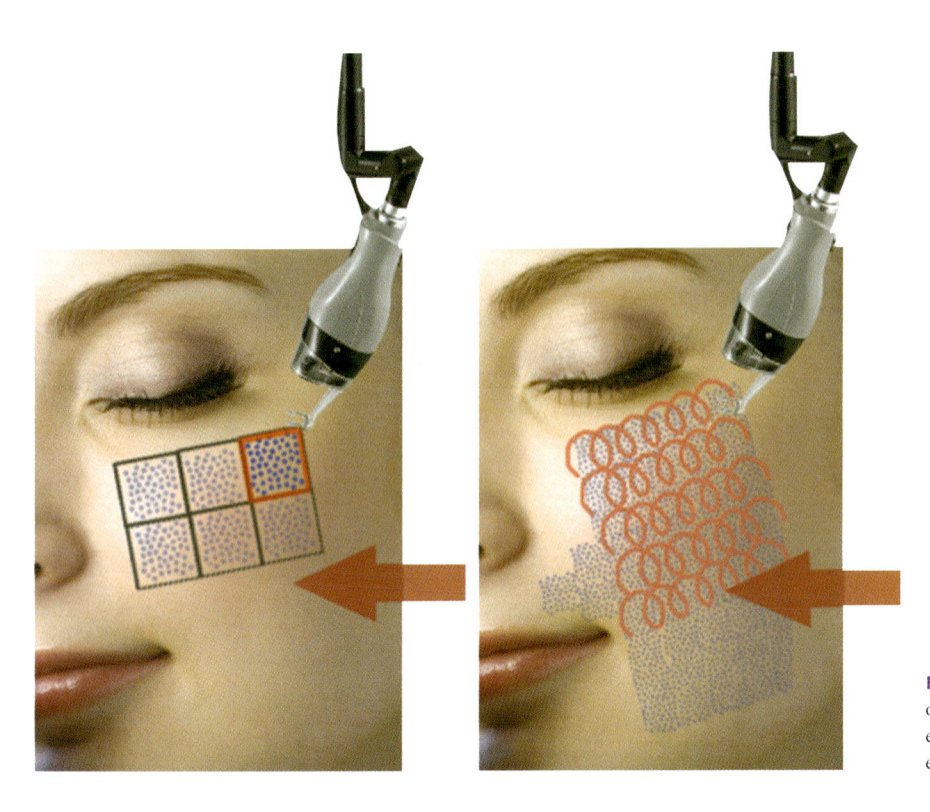

Figure 47.11 The Controlled Chaos Technology minimizes thermal damage by spacing each beam further apart to reduce the collateral thermal effect of the laser beams.

microbeam delivery pattern (known as Lutronic's Controlled Chaos Technology™ – a spray paint-like approach). The Controlled Chaos Technology minimizes thermal damage by spacing each beam further apart to reduce the collateral thermal effect of the laser beams and creates a more natural post-treatment look by non-sequentially placing the beams. There are dual operation modes, the Static Mode (a pulsed operating mode) and the Dynamic Mode (a continuous operating mode) used to "feather" the treatment to reduce the "checkerboard" appearance that is common with currently available fractional CO_2 devices (Figure 47.11). A Multiple Repetition Mode (also on the Lumenis Deep FX) enables even deeper penetration (successive shots of two to five) to create subdermal damage without the superficial damage for greater skin tightening ability. The eCO_2 laser has a variable microbeam delivery speed, skin sensing treatment tips (safety feature that prevents laser firing without skin contact), and user-friendly treatment interfaces that enable real-time tracking of microbeam delivery (automatic total density counter) in dynamic mode.

There are three interchangeable treatment tips (120, 300, and 1000 µm), which include a pinpoint beam tip for traditional ablative skin resurfacing. The 120 µm beam size has a deep penetration depth (up to 2.4 mm) (Figure 47.12). There are no consumable tips for the eCO_2 laser. Patients are usually healed within 3–5 days post-treatment at 140 mJ of pulse energy (Figure 47.13).

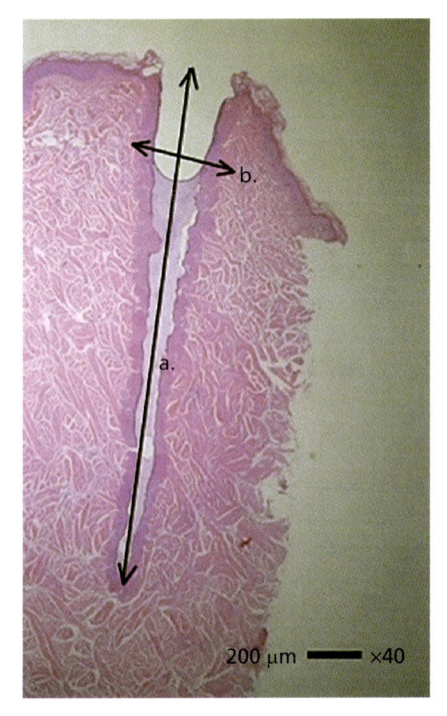

Figure 47.12 The 120 µm beam size has a deep penetration depth (up to 2.4 mm).

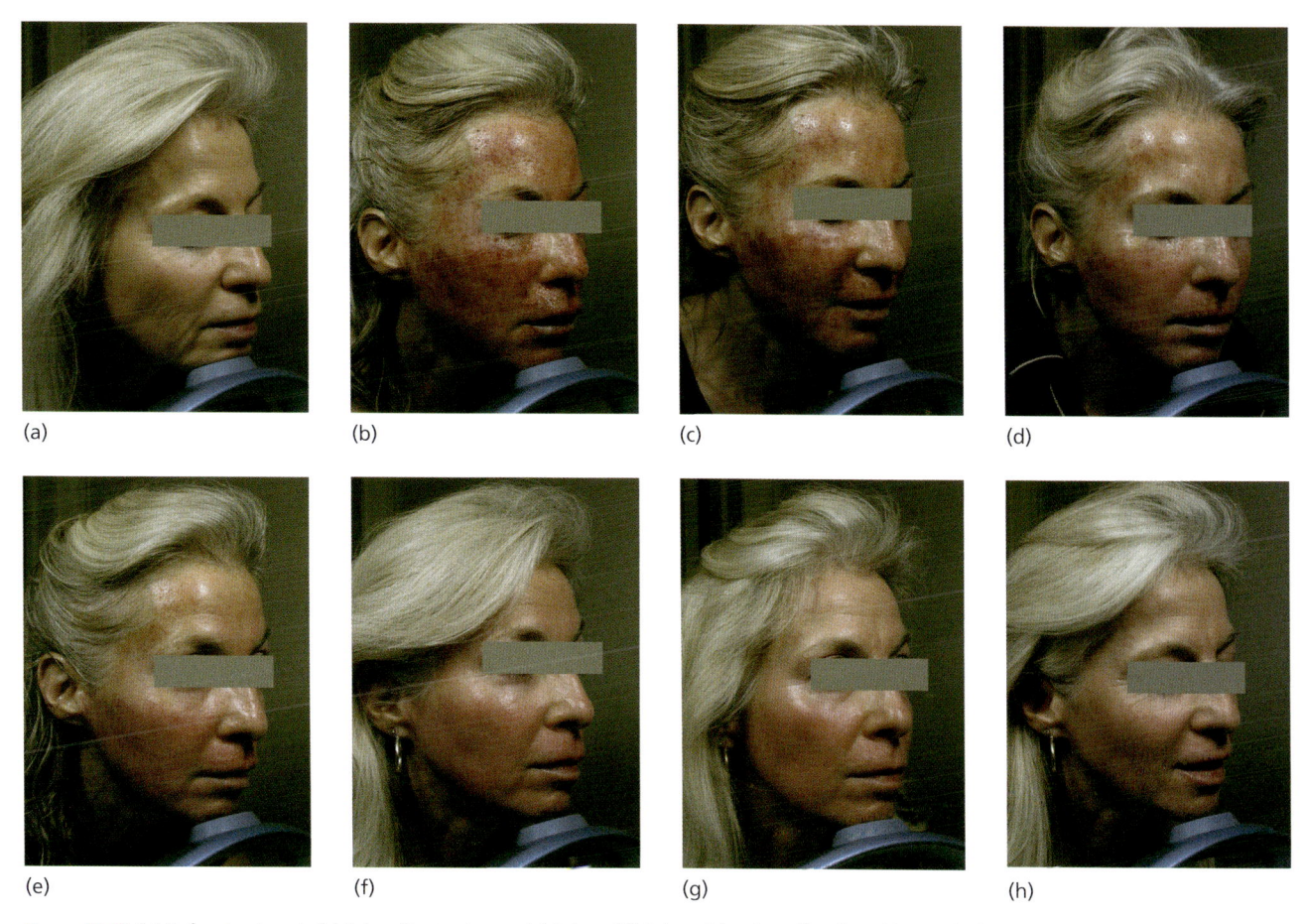

Figure 47.13 (a) Before treatment; (b) 1 day after treatment; (c) 2 days; (d) 3 days; (e) 4 days; (f) 5 days; (g) 1 week; (h) 4 weeks.

Pixel CO₂ – Alma Lasers

The Pixel CO₂ fractionated laser (Alma Lasers Ltd., Caesarea, Israel) is a 70 W fractional CO₂ laser that utilizes a patented Pixel® microoptics lens. There are three available tip options – 7 × 7, 9 × 9 and 1 × 7. With the 7 × 7 tip, 49 250 μm pixels (spots) are created. The micro-injury sites comprise approximately 15–20% of the treatment area. Thermal effect goes approximately 300 μm deep at maximal energy. A burning sensation on the skin is said to last 1–3 hours. Re-epithelialization requires 8–10 days and patients may remain erythematous for 6 weeks to 3 months.

The Pixel® CO₂ OMNIFIT hand-piece is a separate device that can fit on to nearly any existing CO₂ laser designed for skin ablation or resurfacing. It converts any pulsed or continuous wave CO₂ laser into a fractionated skin resurfacing laser.

SmartXide DOT – DEKA, Italy

The SmartXide DOT is a fractional CO₂ laser. While power up to 30 W accounts for depth of ablation of approximately 300–350 μm, dwell time (0.2–2.0 ms in microablative mode; 0.2–20.0 ms in standard mode) controls the width of the thermal pulse that is delivered directly after the microablation occurs.

A third setting space between laser impacts can be adjusted from 0.0 to 2.0 mm in order to change the laser from fractionated to fully ablative. The scan mode defines how each of the spots are laid out on the scanned surface. The "normal" option will sequentially place each spots. The "interlaced and autofill" options are especially programmed to minimize tissue overheating. In the interlaced mode, odd lines are scanned first followed by the even ones. In the autofill mode, the spots are randomly placed on the scanned area.

In 2009, Tierney *et al.* reported the use of this fractionated technology for treatment of photoaging on the neck. One to three treatments were done on 10 patients at 6–8 week intervals. Blinded evaluations were completed 2 months after last treatment. Improvement in skin laxity, texture, rhytides and overall cosmetic appearance were seen [6].

Tierney went on to publish further studies of the use of the SmartXide DOT (30 W, 500 μm pitch, and 1000–1500 μs) in 45 patients for the treatment of photoaging of the face. Blind evaluations were done 6 months after treatment and significant improvements were seen in skin texture, laxity, dyschromia and overall cosmetic result. Mild post-treatment side effects of pin-point bleeding, edema, moderate/severe erythema, mild crusting, and skin bronzing were reported, but all resolved by post-procedure day 7.

Tierney has continued to study this device, and in 2012, characterized the histologic findings and effects on photoaging of the face with the SmartXide DOT [7]. The effects on photoaging were similar to those mentioned in the above study. Authors also comment on a trend of patients that were treated with pulse durations equal or greater than 1500 μs showing greater improvement in skin textures, laxity and rhytides. Also important to note was that this study reported no long term adverse events. Histologic evaluation showed increased depth of ablation with increased pulse duration.

CO₂RE – Syneron–Candela

CO₂RE laser is a CO_2 device that provides six different modes, four fractional ablative, one traditional resurfacing, and one excision mode. The four fractional ablative modes are referred to as light, mid, deep and fusion. The depth of ablation corresponds to the mode name, with the fusion mode being a combination treatment at multiple depths. The ability to treat superficial for rejuvenation and deeper for remodelling at the same time is a beneficial feature of this laser.

SmartSkin – Cynosure

The SmartSkin is a fractional CO_2 laser offering 30 W of power, a 15 × 15 mm treatment area with a 350 μm spot size. In microablative mode the pulse duration is 0.2–2 ms and in standard mode 0.2–20 ms. Gold *et al.* report a study using this laser for treatment of acne scars and photoaging in 12 patients each receiving two treatments at 3–5 week interval. Both physicians and patients note improvement in all aspects of photodamage (hyperpigmentation, skin laxity, fine lines and wrinkles, and enlarged pores) at both 1 and 3 months post-procedure [8]. The authors also comment that acne scarring was improved, but not graded as a part of this study.

ProFractional and ProFractional-XC – Sciton

Sciton's ProFractional 2940 nm wavelength allows the user to optimize treatment depth, area coverage, and the ratio of ablation and thermal zone. The ProFractional module can selectively treat – in a single pass – from 1.5 to 60% of the skin area and from 25 to 1500 μm in depth. ProFractional-XC provides the same treatment depths and two fixed densities – 5.5 and 11% – and offers two additional features: superfast treatment speed and user-controlled thermal coagulation for increased collagen production. Thermal coagulation is achieved by using a long, low-power pulse that heats but does not vaporize tissue, immediately following a short, high-energy pulse for tissue ablation. ProFractional-XC allows the user to select and control the degree of the thermal damage independent of the ablation depth. With this tunable flexibility the user can adjust settings for different skin types and patient expectations and can emulate the thermal profile of CO_2 or other lasers (Figures 47.14–47.16).

Pixel 2940 – Alma

This fractionated Er:YAG delivers the laser via a hand-piece that splits the beam into various microbeams 150 μm in diameter using the same technology as the Pixel CO_2 laser. The 7 × 7 matrix with 49 microbeams with 150 μm in diameter yields energy density of up to 51 mJ/pulse per pixel in an area of 11 × 11 mm². The 9 × 9 matrix produces 81 microbeams 150 μm in diameter, with 31 mJ/pulse per pixel which covers 11 × 11 mm². The laser operates at energy of up to 2500 mJ/pulse and multiple passes are required to produce epidermal ablation and dermal effects. The degree of thermal effects is determined by the number of stacks (stationary technique) or passes (non-stationary technique). No Zimmer or other cooling means is required during the procedure. An unpublished study found that erythema lasts 2–10 days (mean 3.6 days). An evaluation of 28 patients treated 1–4 times demonstrated excellent (21) and good (7) results.

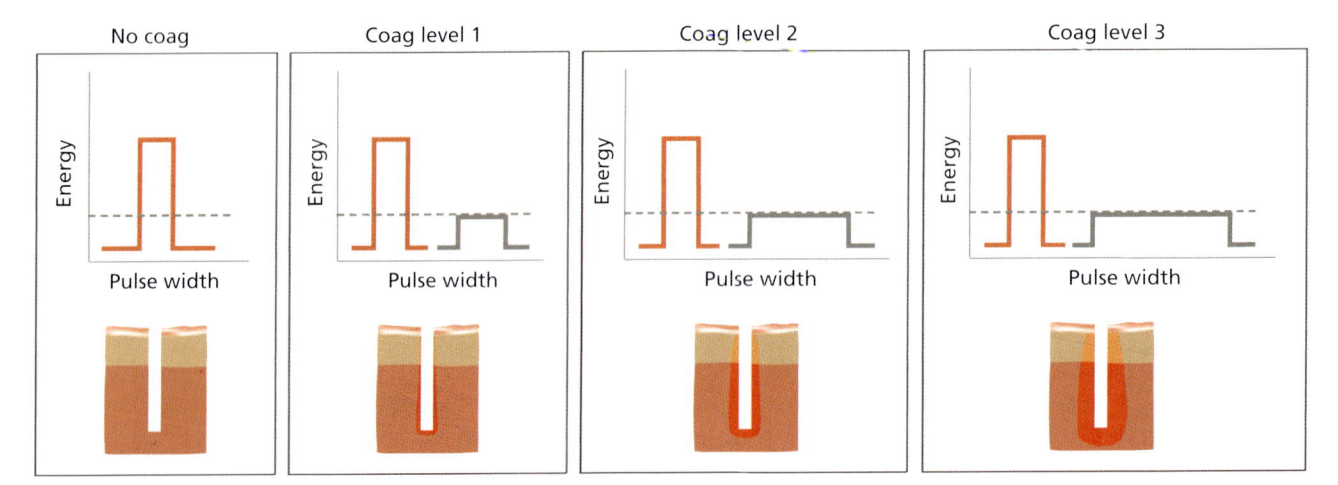

Figure 47.14 Diagrammatic representation of non-specific thermal damage by controlling the pulse width of the Sciton Er:YAG laser. (Source: Sciton, Inc., Palo Alto, CA. Reproduced with permission.)

(a)   (b)

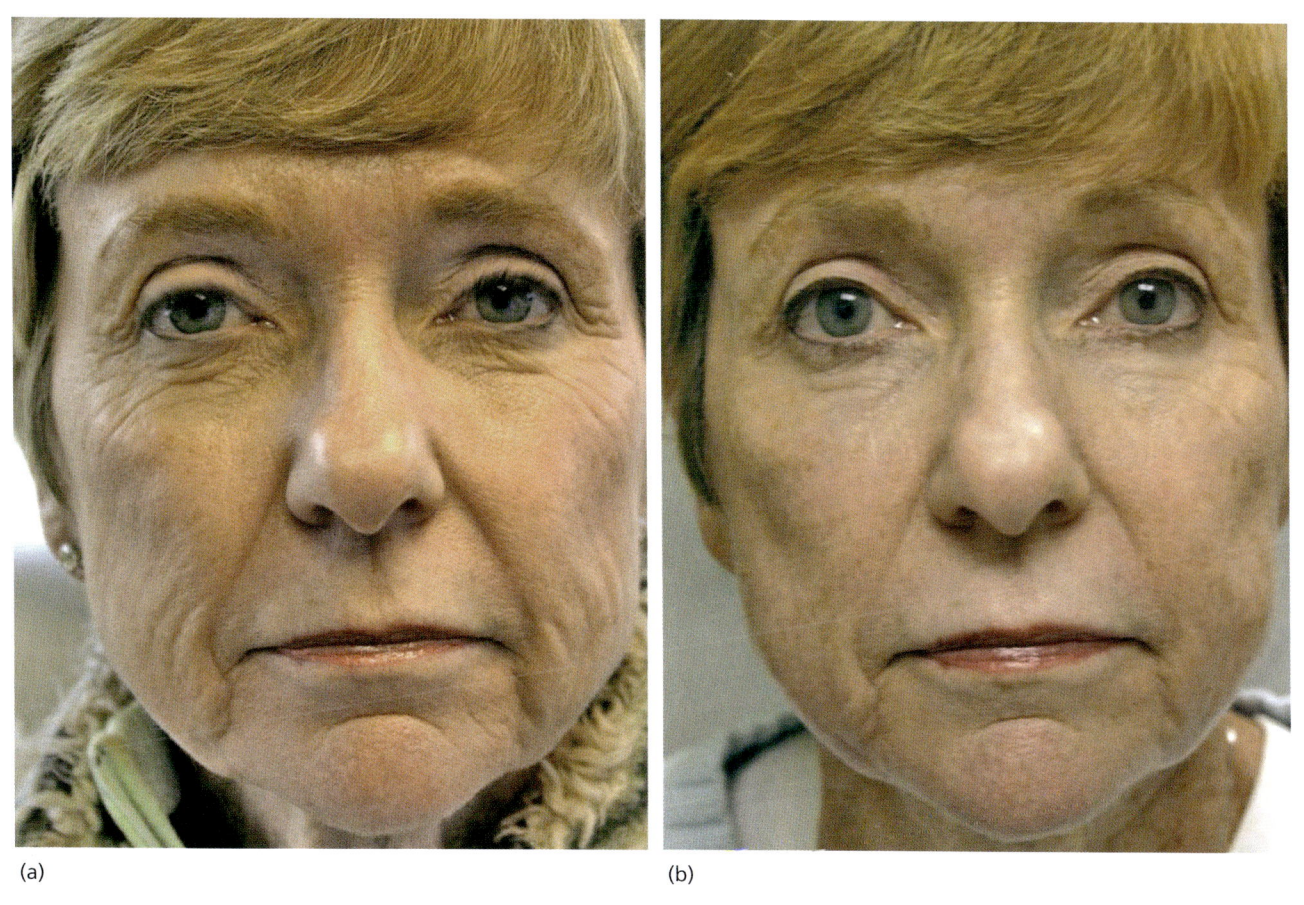

Figure 47.15 Patient treated with the Sciton Profractional at 150 μm, 1.9%. (a) Before; (b) 4 weeks after treatment. (Source: Dr. Michael Gold. Reproduced with permission.)

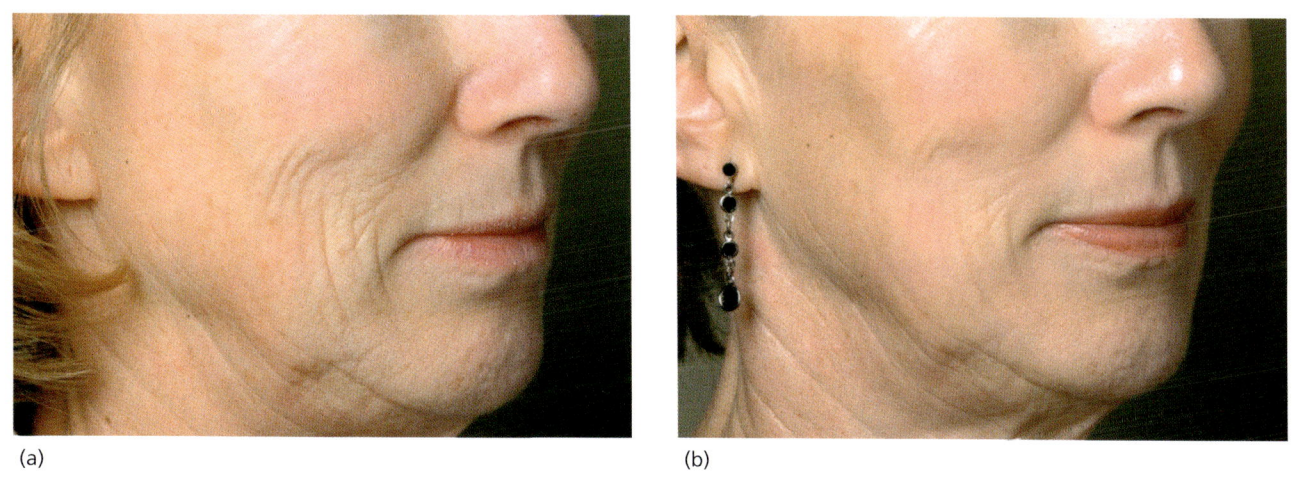

(a)   (b)

Figure 47.16 Patient treated with the Sciton Profractional-XC at 100 μm, 11%, two passes. (a) Before treatment; (b) 4 weeks after three treatments. (Source: Dr. Kent Remington. Reproduced with permission.)

Lux 2940 – Cynosure

The Lux2940 microlens array handpiece utilizes the Palomar StarLux 500 platform and is a fractionated Er:YAG laser that splits the laser beam into microbeams 300 μm in diameter. This technology utilizes a Groove Optic insert which generates a five line pattern, 6 mm long, and each 1.35 mm apart. Energy parameters are 2–5.5 mJ/0.1 mm and pulse duration ranges from 0.25–5 ms. Biopsy demonstrates ablated columns extending 600 μm below the epidermis with an approximate 20 μm coagulation area. Re-epithelialization occurs by 12 hours with a mild inflammatory response persisting for 1 month (Figure 47.17).

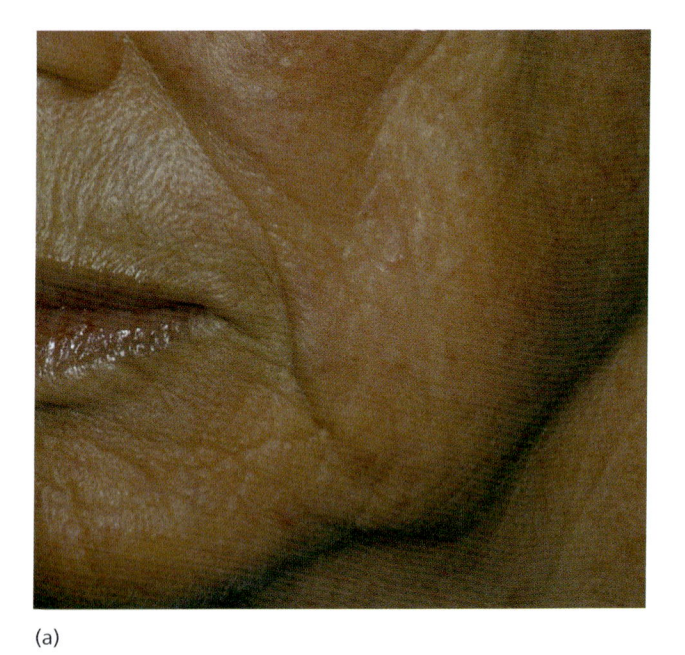

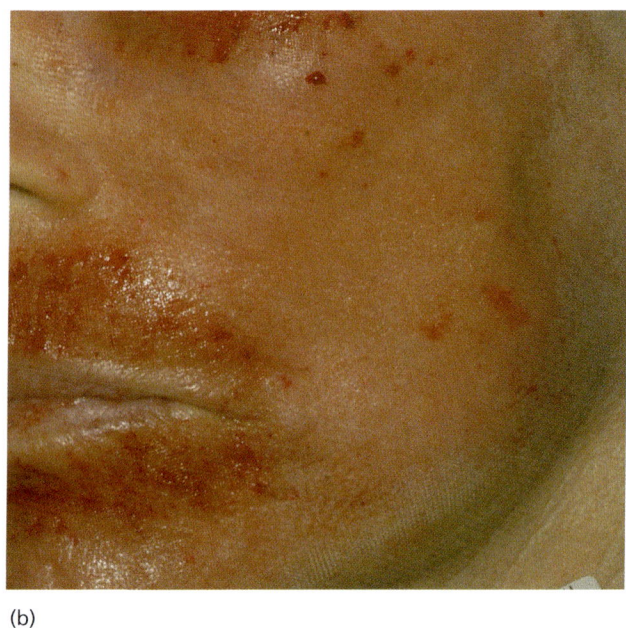

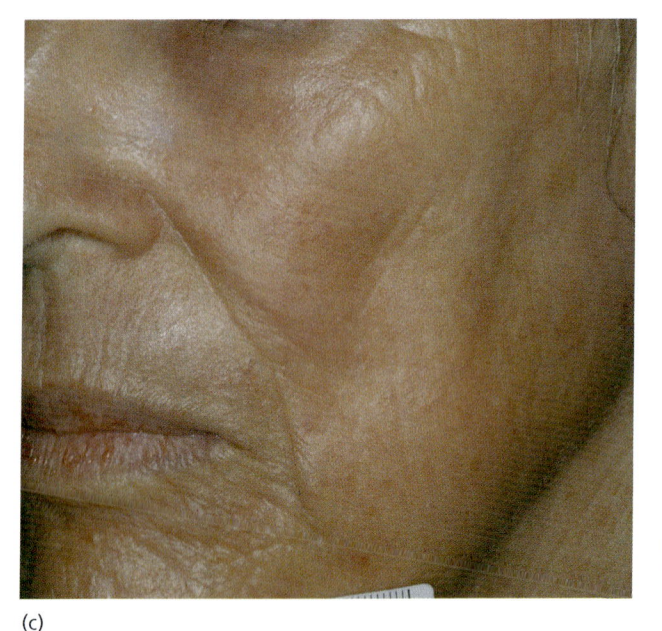

Figure 47.17 Patient treated with the Palomar fractionated 2940 nm Er:YAG laser 6 mm diameter spot, 300 µm depth, 120 µm crater diameter, 40–60% coverage. (a) Before treatment; (b) immediately after treatment; (c) 3 months after treatment. (Source: Dr. E. Vic Ross. Reproduced with permission.)

Xeo Pearl Fractionated – Cutera

This is a fractionated Er:YSGG laser with 2790 nm wavelength. Energy ranges from 60–320 mJ/microspot. The spot size is 300 microns and pulse duration is 600 microseconds. At the higher energies, depth of ablation is reported to be greater than 1 mm.

Technique and procedures for fractionated laser treatment (Active/Deep FX)

Preoperative

Our experience with full-face ablative laser resurfacing has proven that preoperative treatment with topical retinoids, glycolic or depigmenting agents such as hydroquinones are not required to enhance treatment efficacy. At best, by pretreating the skin, both patient and physician can determine what products are easily tolerated and/or irritating to the skin. This may be beneficial if and when the physician prescribes the medical creams post-laser to treat hyperpigmentation or an acneiform eruption. It does make sense to ensure that patients have adequate nutrition and vitamin stores to enhance healing and promote new collagen formation. We regularly recommend oral antioxidants and a multivitamin. No controlled clinical studies have yet to be performed to demonstrate the efficacy of this recommendation.

We have found that treating areas of hyperactive muscle movement, such as the lateral canthus, with a botulinum toxin neuromodulator 1 week before laser treatment will allow for uniform lamellar collagen deposition to occur. We do not recommend performing these injections at the same time as laser treatment because the resulting inflammation and edema from the laser may inactivate and/or promote migration of the neuromodulator from the intended site of injection.

Before treatment, patients wash their faces with a neutral cleanser. A topical anesthetic cream (lidocaine 23% and tetracaine 7% in petrolatum) is applied to the face for 30 minutes and wiped off just before treatment. We use the UltraPulse Encore™ Fractional CO_2 Laser System (Active/Deep FX, Lumenis Inc., Santa Clara, CA, USA), which emits a wavelength of 10600 nm, with spot sizes of 1.3 and 0.12 mm in diameter. We always treat the face with a 5°C cold air cooler (Zimmer) set at maximum flow. We initially use the Deep FX hand-piece with its 120 μm spot size at 15–25 mJ to treat areas of skin laxity and/or wrinkles and scars at a density of 10–15% with one to two passes. The entire face is then treated with one pass of the Active FX hand-piece with its 1.3 mm spot size at a fluence of 125 mJ, frequency of 125 Hz, pattern of 3 (square), size 7 mm, and density of 1–3. We always use the Cool Scan setting, which produces a randomized spot pattern allowing for extra cooling to occur between laser impacts and a repeat delay of 0.3 Hz. The mean duration for the entire procedure is 10–15 minutes.

Postoperative

Patients apply cold, wet compresses immediately post-treatment. They use Restorative Ointment (SkinMedica® Allergan, Irvine, CA) for 3 days until epithelial healing is complete and then a bland moisturizer such as Cetaphil cream (Galderma, Fort Worth, TX, USA) or aquaphor ointment until erythema has resolved. Approximately day 3–4 we start a mid-potency topical corticosteroid that is used by patients at night until approximately day 7. The use of the topical corticosteroid is thought to help reduce inflammation and possible risk of hyperpigmentation. Patients wear a broad spectrum, zinc oxide containing sunscreen during the day under a mineral based make-up. At 3–4 weeks, when epidermal regeneration is complete with formation of an intact epidermal barrier, patients then use a topical antioxidant growth factor serum (TNS Essential Serum, SkinMedica® Allergan, Irvine, CA) to further stimulate fibroblastic formation of new collagen and elastic fibers. Sun protection with UVA and UVB blockers is continued.

Patients are seen 1 day, 1 week, and 1 month after the procedure and then every 3 months. A botulinum toxin neuromodulator is recommended to relax hyperactive muscles and allow continued collagen deposition every 3–4 months. If patients do not achieve the degree of improvement they would like, repeat treatments are scheduled every 6 months. Histologic studies of non-fractionated CO_2 and Er:YAG laser resurfacing patients demonstrated continued collagen production and improvement lasting up to 2 years after treatment. It is not known how long fibroblastic stimulation occurs after fractionated laser resurfacing, but 6 months seems to be a reasonable estimate.

Ortiz *et al.* reported a long-term follow-up study of patients treated with fractionated CO_2 (Fraxel Re:Pair) for acne scarring and photodamage and found that at 1 and 2 years post-treatment, subjects maintained 74% of their overall improvement compared to their 3-month follow-up visits. This helps to show that fractional ablative resurfacing does offer long-term results for patients, but additional treatments in the future may be warranted to further improve their long term results [9].

Identification and management of complications

We recently performed a retrospective evaluation of 490 treatments on 374 patients with the Active/Deep FX in our office. We found 5.3% incidence acneiform eruption, 2.2% incidence of herpes simplex outbreak, 1.8% incidence bacterial infection, 1.2% incidence of yeast infections, 1.2% incidence of hyperpigmentation, 0.8% incidence of erythema lasting longer than 1 month and 0.8% incidence of contact dermatitis. There were no reports of scarring or hypopigmentation in our patient population. The average follow-up in our population was 2.18 months. It is known that with traditional CO_2 that late findings (hypopigmentation) beginning nine months or more after the procedure can occur, while we don't expect this to occur with fractional CO_2, as it has never been reported in the literature, it is possible that due to the range of follow-up times longer term side effects were missed.

Conclusions

Fractional ablative technology has truly transformed the nonsurgical resurfacing arena. Fractional ablative technology has proven time and again to offer good patient results with a favorable safety profile and minimal downtime compared to older technology.

References

1 Ciocon DH, Engelman DE, Hussain M, *et al.* (2011) A split-face comparison of two ablative fractional carbon dioxide lasers for the treatment of photodamaged facial skin. *Dermatol Surg* **37**, 784–90.

2 Rhaman Z, MacFalls H, Jiang K, *et al.* (2009) Fractional deep dermal ablation induces tissue tightening. *Lasers Surg Med* **41**, 7–86.

3 Karsai S, Czarnecka A, Junger M, *et al.* (2010) Ablative fractional lasers (CO_2 and Er:YAG): a randomized controlled double-blind split-face trial of the treatment of peri-orbital rhytides. *Lasers Surg Med* **42**, 160–67.

4 Tierney EP, Hanke CW. (2011) Fractionated carbon dioxide laser treatment of photoaging: prospective study in 45 patients and review of literature. *Dermatol Surg* **37**, 1279–90.

5 Tierney EP, Eisen RF, Hanke CW. (2011) Fractionated CO_2 laser skin rejuvenation. *Dermatol Therapy* **24**, 41–53.

Preissig J, Hamilton K, Markus R. (2012) Current laser resurfacing technologies: a review that delves beneath the surface. *Semin Plast Surg* **26**, 109–116.

6. Tierney EP, Hanke CW. (2009) Ablative fractionated CO_2 laser resurfacing for the neck: prospective study and review of the literature. *J Drugs Dermatol* **8**, 723–31.
7. Tierney EP, Hanke CW, Petersen J. (2012) Ablative fractionated CO_2 laser treatment of photoaging: a clinical and histologic study. *Dermatol Surg* **38**, 1777–89.
8. Gold MH, Heath AD, Biron JA. (2009) Clinical evaluation of the Smart Skin fractional laser for the treatment of photodamage and acne scars. *J Drugs Dermatol* **8**(11 suppl), s4–8.
9. Ortiz AE, Tremaine AM, Zachary CB. (2010) Long-term efficacy of a fractional resurfacing device. *Lasers Surg Med* **42**, 168–70.

Further reading

Alexiades-Armenakas MR, Dover JS, Arndt KA. (2012) Fractional laser skin resurfacing. *J Drugs Dermatol* **11**(11), 1274–87.

Bjorn M, Stausbol-Gron B, Braae Olesen A, *et al.* (2013) Treatment of acne scars with actional CO_2 laser at 1-month versus 3-month intervals: An intra-individual randomized controlled trial. *Lasers Surg Med* Sept 9.

Cohen JL, Ross EV. (2013) Combined fractional ablative and nonablative laser resurfacing treatment: a split-face comparative study. *J Drugs Dermatol* **12**(2), 175–8.

Goldman MP, Fitzpatrick RE, Ross EV, *et al.* (2013) *Lasers and Energy Devices for the Skin*, 2 nd edn. Boca Raton, FL: CRC Press, Taylor and Francis Group, pp. 110–77.

Helou J, Maatouk I, Moutran R, *et al.* (2013) Efficacy and safety of 10600-nm carbon dioxide fractional laser on facial skin with previous volume injections. *J Cutan Aesthet Surg* **6**(1), 30–32.

Kohl E, Meierhofer J, Koller M, *et al.* (2013) Fractional carbon dioxide laser resurfacing of rhytides and photoaging: a prospective study using profilometric analysis. *Br J Dermatol* Dec 26 (epub ahead of print).

LaTowsky BC, Abbasi H, Dover JS, *et al.* (2012) A randomized, controlled trial of four ablative fractionated lasers for photoaging: a quadrant study. *Dermatol Surg* **38**, 1477–89.

Marqa MF, Mordon S. (2014) Laser fractional photothermolysis of the skin: Numerical simulation of microthermal zones. *J Cosmet Laser Ther* Jan 10 (epub ahead of print).

Oh IY, Kim BJ, Kim MN *et al.* (2013) Efficacy of light-emitting diode photomodulation in reducing erythema after fractional carbon dioxide laser resurfacing: a pilot study. *Dermatol Surg* **39**(8), 1171–6.

Sattler EC, Poloczek K, Kastle R, *et al.* (2013) Confocal laser scanning microscopy and optical coherence tomography for the evaluation of the kinetics and quantification of wound healing after fractional laser therapy. *J Am Acad Dermatol* **69**(4), e165–73.

Serowka KL, Saedi N, Dover JS, *et al.* (2013) Fractionated ablative carbon dioxide laser for the treatment of rhinophyma. *Lasers Surg Med.* Oct 5.

Shamsaldeen O, Peterson JD, Goldman MP. (2011) The adverse events of deep fractional CO_2: a retrospective study of 490 treatments in 374 patients. *Lasers Surg Med* **43**, 453–6.

CHAPTER 48
Nonablative Lasers

Adam S. Nabatian[1] and David J. Goldberg[2]
[1]Albert Einstein College of Medicine, Bronx, NY, USA
[2]Mount Sinai School of Medicine, New York, NY, and Skin Laser & Surgery Specialists of New York and New Jersey, USA

> **BASIC CONCEPTS**
> - Nonablative laser systems are used for rejuvenation of photodamaged skin.
> - The lasers cause a dermal wounding response that results in collagen remodeling and production, while protecting the epidermis from harm.
> - There are numerous laser, light sources, and radiofrequency devices used for nonablative resurfacing with variable results on rhytides, scarring, dyschromia, and vascular change.
> - Side effects are mild and rare with nonablative devices.
> - Exciting new advances in nonfacial rejuvenation are also being made with the nonablative systems discussed.

Introduction

In recent years there has been a progressive movement towards nonsurgical interventions for facial rejuvenation. Ablative resurfacing with CO_2 and erbium-doped yttrium aluminum garnet (Er:YAG) lasers were first used to treat photodamaged skin in the 1980s and remain the gold standard today [1–5]. Yet despite their effectiveness at treating photoaging, there has been a recent push for nonablative treatment modalities with less downtime and fewer side effects.

Nonablative lasers have been used to successfully treat rhytides, dyspigmentation, vascular changes, skin texture, laxity, and scarring [1,5,6]. The main goal of these systems is to selectively induce dermal damage, resulting in collagen remodeling and production while sparing the epidermis [1,3,6–8]. Many different systems have been used with this endpoint in mind (Table 48.1), and they will be discussed in detail below.

Pathophysiology

Nonablative rejuvenation systems are composed of lasers, light sources, and radiofrequency devices. Laser systems use energy in the infrared or near infrared spectrum to target specific dermal chromophores, such as water, melanin, and hemoglobin. In contrast, radiofrequency devices produce heat in the dermis and subcutaneous tissue as a result of resistance to current flow through the tissue. Although the mechanisms of action are different, the end result is the same. Both the light sources and radiofrequency devices effectively heat the dermis eliciting a wound healing response without disturbing the integrity of the epidermis [1,5,9–11].

One of the main effects of photodamage and aging is a reduction in dermal collagen, and this is the target of nonablative rejuvenation. It has been proven that thermal induced injury to the dermis causes local release of inflammatory cytokines leading to the proliferation of fibroblasts which results in collagen synthesis [7,12–15]. *In vivo* mouse studies have been performed to evaluate collagen composition after treatment with various lasers, and they have all demonstrated a significant change in collagen and extracellular matrix [7,13].

A study by Liu *et al.* compared the dermal collagen composition after treatment with various laser systems [7]. This study confirmed that collagen I production is predominantly increased after nonablative treatment with the pulse dye laser (PDL), 1320 nm Nd:YAG laser, and the long pulsed 1064 nm Nd:YAG laser. On the other hand, collagen type III was more significantly increased in those treated with the Q-switched 1064 nm Nd:YAG laser. These results not only support the theory regarding neocollagenesis, but it also provides specific data on collagen composition and differences in laser systems. This study suggests that because of the predominant increase in collagen type III after treatment with the Q-switched Nd:YAG laser, it may be more effective in increasing the elasticity of the skin and giving a more youthful appearance.

Cosmetic Dermatology: Products and Procedures, Second Edition. Edited by Zoe Diana Draelos.
© 2016 John Wiley & Sons, Ltd. Published 2016 by John Wiley & Sons, Ltd.

Table 48.1 Lasers for Facial Rejuvenation

Laser type	System name
Pulsed KTP	Gemini (Laserscope)
	Aura (Laserscope)
	Versapulse (Coherent/Lumenis)
	Diolite (Iridex)
Pulsed dye 585 nm	Cbeam (Candela)
	SPTL-1B (Candela)
	Photogenica V (Cynosure)
595 nm	Cynosure V-star (Cynosure – 585/595)
	V-beam (Candela)
Intense pulse light (IPL)	Quantum SR (Lumenis)
	Palomar Starlux (Palomar)
	Vasculight (Lumenis)
	Estelux/Medilux (Palomar)
	Aurora DS/Aurora SR (Syneron)
1320 nm Nd:YAG	Cool Touch I, II, and III (Cooltouch)
1064 nm QS- Nd:YAG	Medlite IV Continuum (Biomedical)
	VersaPulse VPC (Lumenis)
1450 nm diode	Smoothbeam (Candela)
Er:glass 1540 nm	Aramis-Quantel (Quantel Medical)
Infrared light (1100–1800 nm)	Titan (Cutera Inc.)
Radiofrequency devices monopolar unipolar and bipolar	Thermacool TC(Thermage) Accent (Alma Laser)

Nonablative modalities

Many nonablative systems have been evaluated for efficacy in facial rejuvenation. Results have been variable and often times require multiple treatments in order to appreciate clinical improvement. The most effective treatment regimens are still being determined for facial rejuvenation, and the corresponding studies for each laser will be discussed below. The most common lasers and parameter settings used today are outlined in Table 48.2.

Potassium titanyl phosphate (KTP) 532 nm laser

The 532 nm KTP laser is one of the many modalities used in facial rejuvenation. It is absorbed more intensely by melanin and hemoglobin, and so it is thought that fewer treatments are needed when targeting these components of photodamaged skin [2]. This laser has been shown to effectively target vascular and pigmentary change, skin texture, tightening, acne scars, and rhytides [5,15].

Lee performed a 150-person study to compare the efficacy of the KTP laser alone, the long pulsed Nd:YAG alone, or the two modalities combined on collagen enhancement and photorejuvenation [15]. After 3–6 treatments, all three groups showed statistically significant improvement in rhytides, skin toning and texture, reduction in redness, and improvement in dyschromia. Overall, the KTP laser treated patients showed more improvement than the LP Nd:YAG laser, but the combined treatment group was superior to either group alone. The combined group had a 70–80% improvement in redness and pigmentation, 40–60% improvement in skin texture, tone and tightening, and a 30–40% improvement in rhytides. In addition to these findings, it was also noted that collagen remodeling continues for up to 6–12 months post-treatment, with slow regression in benefit thereafter. Although further studies are necessary, these results suggest that combined modalities may be superior at targeting various factors involved in photodamage and more effectively stimulate collagen production.

A recent study by Ho and colleagues compared the effectiveness and safety of using the 532 nm LP KTP laser, 595 nm long pulse dye laser (LPDL), 755 nm LP Alexandrite laser, and 532 nm QS Nd:YAG laser for the treatment of freckles or lentigines in Fitzpatrick skin type III and IV Asian patients [16]. Forty patients were enrolled in the study and each patient attended between one and four treatments at 4–6 weeks intervals depending on the clinical response. The laser parameters included a fluence of 12–14 J/cm^2 and spot size of 2 mm for the LP KTP laser, a fluence of 11–13 J/cm^2 and spot size of 7 mm for the LPDL, a fluence of 20–35 J/cm^2 and spot size of 10 mm for the LP Alexandrite laser, and a fluence of 0.6 J/cm^2 and spot size of 2 mm for the QS Nd:YAG laser. Statistically significant improvement of global and focal facial pigmentation was found after treatment with LP KTP, LPDL, and QS Nd:YAG lasers. No significant improvement was found after treatment with LP Alexandrite laser. Post-inflammatory hyperpigmentation was absent after LP KTP and LPDL treatment, but was seen in 20% of patients after LP Alexandrite treatment and 10% of patients after QS Nd:YAG treatment. The 532 nm LP KTP and 595 nm LPDL lasers appear to be more effective with less complications compared to the 532 nm QS Nd:YAG and 755 nm LP Alexandrite lasers for the treatment of freckles and lentigines in Fitzpatrick type III and IV skin. The authors also concluded that a long pulse laser and small spot size appear to reduce the risks of lentigines treatment in darker skin types.

Pulse dye laser (PDL) 585 nm or 595 nm

The PDL is a yellow light that targets oxyhemoglobin and melanin. It has been used to treat vascular changes and induce new collagen formation. It has been hypothesized that wavelengths targeting hemoglobin disrupt vascular endothelial cells resulting in cytokine release and subsequent collagen remodeling and production [5,17,18].

A group of 10 female patients, Fitzpatrick types I–IV, were treated in the periorbital area with the 595 nm flash lamp PDL [18]. One side of the face was treated with the following laser

Table 48.2 Nonablative lasers

Laser type	Wavelength (nm)	Fluences (J/cm^2)	Pulse duration	Spot sizes (mm)	Target
KTP (pulsed)	532	7–15	20–50 ms	2, 4, 10	Hemoglobin, melanin
Pulsed dye laser (PDL)	585	3–6.5	350, 450 ms	5, 7, 10	
	595	6–12	6–10 ms	7, 10	Hemoglobin, melanin
IPL	550–1200	25–28	2.4, 4.0 ms		Hemoglobin, melanin, water (weak)
Nd:YAG	1320	17–22	200 or 350 ms	6, 10	Water
Nd:YAG (QS)	1064	2.5–7	5 ns	6	Hemoglobin, melanin, water
Diode	1450	8–14	160–260 ms	4, 6	Water
Er:glass	1540	Up to 126	3.3	4, 5	Water
Infrared light	1100–1800	30–40	170–200 pulses		–
Radiofrequency					
RF, monopolar	RF bipolar current	61.5–63.5 (adjusted for pain)	300–400 pulses	0.25 cm, 1.0 cm, 1.5 cm, 3 cm	–
RF, unipolar	RF electromagnetic radiation	50–250			–
RF, bipolar	RF bipolar current	40–100			

settings: 1.5 msec pulse, fluences of 5–6 J/cm^2, and a spot size of 7 mm. The contralateral side was treated with a 40 msec pulse duration, fluences of 8–11 J/cm^2, and a 7 mm spot size. Cryogen cooling was administered for 30 msec with a delay of 30 msec before treatment. Subjects were treated 1–2 times, and at their 6-month follow-up, 70% treated had mild to moderate improvement overall. Sixty percent had equal improvement on both sides despite the different settings. Histologic and electron microscopic evaluation showed a significant increase in papillary dermal collagen, mainly type I.

Another study performed by Bernstein evaluated the effects of treatment of sun damaged skin with a 595 nm long pulse duration PDL [17]. Ten subjects were treated with 10 ms pulse duration, fluences of 8–10 J/cm^2, and a 10 mm spot size. Improvements were evaluated 8 weeks after treatment with photograph comparison. Blinded physician evaluation of pre- and post-photographs rated improvement in wrinkles in 50%, facial veins improved in 82%, overall redness improved 80%, pigmentary change 61.4%, and a 25% improvement in pore size.

A small clinical trial was performed on 10 patients comparing the efficacy of a long-pulse PDL (LPDL) versus an intense pulsed light (IPL) on photodamaged facial skin. [19]. When compared to the IPL, the LPDL showed greater improvement in lentigines (81% versus 62%), no significant difference in wrinkle reduction between the two groups, and fewer treatments were needed with the LPDL when compared to the IPL (3 versus 6).

In addition to using the PDL laser as a single agent in photorejuvenation, recent trends have shown effective combination with aminolevulinic acid (ALA) in treatment of photodamaged skin. It is believed that PDL at 595 nm activates protoporphyrin IX, a photosensitizer, which accumulates in photodamaged cells, causing destruction of the cells, release of cytokines, and collagen repair [1]. This is a new and exciting area of research that offers another effective treatment modality for photorejuvenation.

Intense pulsed light (IPL)

The IPL system emits light, with wavelengths of 550–1200 nm, which effectively targets melanin, hemoglobin, and water, to a lesser degree. The IPL device has been used in photorejuvenation to target vascular changes, pigmentary alteration, and mild rhytides [1,2,5,19,20]. Filters may be used with the IPL to target specific chromophores. Rapid improvement in overall appearance after IPL treatment is secondary to rapid and effective improvement of vascular and pigmentary change, rather than improvement in wrinkles [5]. As per Weiss et al., shorter pulse duration and lower cut off filters when using the IPL system, results in significant improvement in pigmentary alteration [2].

Although not thought to be the most effective treatment modality for rhytides, some studies using the IPL have shown improvement [1,3,4,19,20]. Goldberg et al. evaluated the treatment of facial rhytides with an IPL system using a 645 nm cutoff filter [3,20]. Thirty patients, skin type I–III, were treated 1–4 times over a 10-week period. Treatments were delivered using fluences of 40–50 J/cm^2, through bracketed cooling device with triple 7 ms pulses, and interpulse delay of 50 ms. At 6 months follow-up, approximately 53% showed some improvement, 30% showed substantial improvement, and 17% showed no improvement.

Hedelund et al. also performed a study looking at the efficacy of IPL treatment for perioral rhytides in comparison to CO$_2$ ablative resurfacing [4]. Twenty-seven females, skin type II, with perioral rhytides were randomly treated with 3-monthly IPL sessions or one CO_2 laser ablation. The results showed a higher degree of patient satisfaction and significant improvement in rhytides with CO_2 laser resurfacing when compared to IPL rejuvenation. In addition to the more dramatic improvement seen with CO_2 resurfacing, side effects were also found to be significantly higher in this group. Patients treated with the CO_2 laser experienced milia, dyspigmentation, and persistent erythema, while the IPL group wasn't noted to have any side effects. Both groups showed longterm improvement in skin elasticity, although no significant improvement in wrinkles was seen in the IPL treatment group. Many physicians today advocate 3–6 treatments for significant improvement, which implies that the treatment course may not have been sufficient to produce notable results.

As with PDL lasers, recent trends have shown effective combination of IPL with aminolevulinic acid (ALA) in treatment of photodamaged skin [21–24]. Patients treated with this combinational therapy demonstrated greater improvement in global photodamage, mottled pigmentation, and fine lines compared to those patients treated with IPL alone [21]. Combinational treatment is well tolerated with little difference in the incidence of adverse effects with or without 5-ALA pretreatment.

1320 nm Neodymium yttrium aluminium garnet (Nd:YAG)

One of the first laser systems to be developed for nonablative rejuvenation was the Nd:YAG 1320 nm laser [25]. At this wavelength, energy is able to penetrate into the papillary and mid reticular dermis, and it is absorbed by water associated with dermal collagen. There is a high water absorption and strong scattering in the dermis which allows for extensive dermal wounding [25]. This accelerates the productive capacity of fibroblasts as seen in its promotion of the two major secretory factors they produce: basic fibroblast growth factor (bFGF) and inhibiting transforming growth factor β1 (TGF-β1) [26,27]. This is followed byt the stimulation of collagen types I, III, and VII, and tropoelastin production [27,28]. The surface cooling systems are present to protect the epidermis from involvement.

The 1320 nm Nd:YAG laser has been used to target acne scarring, photoaging, and rhytides with variable results [1-3,25,29]. As a result of its poor absorption by melanin, it can be used in all skin types without fear of pigmentary change [29]. When treating mild rhytides or acne scars, Weiss *et al.* recommends using a fluence of 17–19 J/cm^2, a total of 25 ms of cooling (pre and post cooling at 10 ms and midcooling at 5 ms), with a fixed pulse duration of 50 ms, and 2–3 passes [2]. When treating acne scars with this regimen, 30–50% improvement has been observed in about four of five patients, while 20% show no significant response.

According to a study done by Rogachefsky *et al.*, the 1320 nm Nd:YAG laser is an effective modality to treat atrophic and mixed pattern facial acne scars [29]. After treating 12 patients with three monthly sessions, optimal improvement was noted in atrophic acne scars; however, mixed acne scars also showed softening of sclerotic and shallow pitted scars. Sadick *et al.* also confirms significant improvement in acne scars after treatment with the 1320 nm Nd:YAG, but he proposes that six sessions is more effective than three laser sessions [25].

Q-switched (QS) Nd:YAG 1064 nm laser

The QS Nd:YAG 1064 nm laser has not only proven to be successful for treatment of tattoos, vascular, and pigmented lesions, but it has recently been used to treat rhytids, photodamage, and acne scars [3,8,11,30]. This laser system is poorly absorbed by water, making deeper collagen damage more likely when compared to systems with other wavelengths [30]. It has been hypothesized that when compared to other nonablative systems, the 1064 nm QS Nd:YAG laser is able to cause the most severe dermal damage and thus produce the greatest amount of collagen remodeling. This was confirmed in a mouse study done which showed greatest improvement in skin elasticity after treatment with the QS Nd:YAG 1064 nm laser [13].

Another small study involving eight patients was performed to evaluate the effects of the QS 1064 nm Nd:YAG laser on facial wrinkles [30]. Treatments were performed monthly, for a total of three months, with a fluence of 7 J/cm^2, a 3 mm spot size, and two passes, with petechiae as the desired endpoint. In the end, six of the eight subjects demonstrated clinical improvement in rhytides.

The QS 1064 nm Nd:YAG laser has also been used to treat atrophic acne scars with notable success. In eleven patients who completed five treatment sessions with the QS 1064 nm Nd:YAG laser, significant improvement in facial acne scars was demonstrated [8]. After completing all five treatments, improvement was seen as early as 1 month, the greatest percentage improvement was noted at 3 months, and improvement had reached a plateau at 6 months. Another similar study used three dimensional topography to quantify the efficacy of five QS 1064 nm Nd:YAG treatments on facial wrinkles and acne scars [11]. At 3 months post-treatment, a 61% improvement in surface topography was recorded, and it was maintained at the six-month follow-up. These results and others, have suggested that collagen remodeling and repair continues to occur for an extended period of time following the last treatment [1,3,8,11].

Erbium:glass 1540 nm

The erbium:glass (Er:glass) 1540 nm laser has been used to treat perioral and periorbital rhytides with mild to moderate end results [1,3,12,31]. Fournier *et al.* studied the effects of the Er:glass laser on 42 patients treated at 6-week intervals for a total of five sessions [31]. Profilometry, ultrasound, and photography were used to rate clinical improvement after the final treatment. All patients reported improvement in quality and appearance of their skin at 6 months. Notable findings showed an increase in dermal thickness by 17%, a reduction of anisotropy by 44.8%, and an overall improvement in clinical appearance.

An additional 35-month study was conducted to assess the long-term benefits of treatment with the Er:glass 1540 nm laser on facial rhytides [12]. Eleven patients with periorbital and perioral rhytides were treated with a series of five treatments at six-week intervals. Approximately half of the patients also received two additional maintenance treatments at 14 and 20 months. Treatments were performed with settings of 8 J/cm^2, three stacked pulses at 2 Hz repetition rates for periorbital and five stacked pulses for perioral sites, and a 4 mm spot size. It was demonstrated that for all 11 patients treated, the improvement in collagen anisotropy measurements showed a reduction in rhytides of 51.7% at 14 months, and 29.8% at 35 months. Overall patient satisfaction was 70% at approximately 2.5 years. Based on both of the aforementioned studies, the Er:glass 1540 nm laser appears to effectively stimulate collagen remodeling with long-term results.

1450 nm diode laser

The 1450 nm diode laser targets water containing tissue to stimulate collagen remodeling and production. It has been used to treat periorbital and perioral rhytides, and facial acne scars [1–3,32,33].

A previous study was performed with the 1450 nm diode laser to assess the efficacy of treatment on facial rhytides and the associated side effects [33]. Twenty patients underwent 2–4 monthly treatment sessions focusing on perioral and periorbital wrinkles. Each session consisted of treatment of one side of the face with laser and cryogen and the other side with cryogen alone. The laser settings were: frequency of 0.5–1.0 Hz, pulse width of 160–260 ms, pre-, post- and intermediate cryogen cooling of 40–80 ms total, and a 4 mm spot size. At 6 months after the final treatment, 13 of the 20 laser/cryogen treated sites showed some improvement, while none of the cryogen only sites showed any improvement. It also showed that periorbital wrinkles showed greater improvement when compared to the perioral sites.

In addition to wrinkles, the 1450 nm diode has been used to treat atrophic acne scars with minimal side effects [32,34]. Tanzi *et al.* performed a comparison study treating 20 patients with mild to moderate atrophic acne scars with the 1320 nm Nd:YAG on half of the face and the 1450 nm diode laser on the contralateral side. Three monthly treatments were performed, and only modest improvement in facial scarring was seen among both groups at 6 months. Yet, greater overall clinical improvement and patient satisfaction was seen in the 1450 nm diode laser sites. Increase in dermal collagen and improvement in skin texture was found in both groups. Minimal side effects were reported.

Infrared light devices (1100–1800 nm)

A new nonablative broad spectrum infrared device, emitting wavelengths from 1100–1800 nm, has been recently introduced for the treatment of photoaged skin. Improvement in skin laxity and rhytides is believed to result from volumetric heating of water in the dermis which leads to tissue contraction [1,35,36]. A large component of facial aging is the development of skin laxity. With this in mind, a study was conducted to evaluate the efficacy of a filtered infrared light device in the treatment of skin laxity with ptosis of the lower face and neck [36].

Thirteen females, a mean age of 64 years old, were treated from the nasolabial folds to the preauricular area, and from the malar prominence to the clavicle. The parameters used were: fluences of 30–36 J/cm^2, 230–440 pulses per session, pulse duration up to 11 seconds, a spot size of 1.5 × 1.0 cm, and cooling of the epidermis to 40C. Treatments were administered monthly for a total of two treatments. Improvement was seen clinically in 11 of 12 patients who completed the study. Significant improvement in submental and submandibular definition was noted. The most dramatic improvement was seen in those with loss of definition due to excess skin hanging separately from deeper soft tissue. Continued improvement was noted beyond the 1-month follow-up visit. Mild erythema was the only side effect seen, and it resolved within 30 minutes after treatment.

A recent small study was performed on nine women, skin types III–IV, with variable photodamage [35]. Half of the subjects received a one time treatment to the face, while the other group had 2-monthly treatments. The laser parameters were: fluences of 30–40 J cm^2 and 170–200 pulses. Overall, both subjects' and investigators' assessments of pre and post procedural appearances found significant improvement in elasticity, pore size, dyschromia, wrinkles, and overall texture. Also, the improvement in elasticity, rhytides, and skin texture were more evident in the group treated twice. This study showed promising results but was limited to an 8-week time span and small study population. More studies will need to be performed to determine the role of new infrared light devices in the field of facial rejuvenation.

Radiofrequency devices (RF)

RF devices have become another widely accepted method of nonablative rejuvenation. The FDA has approved the RF devices for the treatment of periorbital rhytides [10]. The mechanism of action differs from nonablative lasers which use selective photothermolysis to induce collagen remodeling. As a result of the resistance to current flow through the tissue, uniform volumetric heat is produced at controlled levels of the reticular dermis and subcutaneous fat [1,9,10]. Tissue tightening is believed to result from the breaking of hydrogen bonds in the collagen triple helix. The disruption of the molecular structure of collagen causes contraction that begins immediately and continues for approximately 6 months [9]. In addition, heated fibroblasts are associated with new collagen synthesis and therefore tissue remodeling [37]. Contact cooling is used to protect the epidermis from damage.

In an early study performed, 17 patients, skin types II–IV, were treated in 20 areas with the Thermacool T (Thermage Inc) RF device to assess the efficacy and safety of treatment of facial laxity [10]. Areas of primary focus were the jowls and the brow. Treatments were performed at settings of 14.5–16.0 (125–144 J/cm^2). Tightening was found to occur gradually over 4 months, and subtle improvements were at times difficult for subjects to appreciate without seeing pre and post photography. After viewing photos, approximately 90% admitted to seeing improvement. Mild erythema was noted in all subjects but resolved within hours. There were no burns seen with this treatment, and this was thought to be due to close monitoring and adjustment of energy level based on patient pain level.

There continues to be much debate over the most successful treatment protocol for RF devices. Recent studies have looked at the efficacy of using lower energies with multiple passes and more pulses [1,9]. Sixty-six patients with moderate laxity of the lower face and neck were treated with the Thermacool RF device (Thermage Corp) [9]. Treatments were performed with a 1.5 cm tip, average treatment level was 62 (83 J/cm^2) and was titrated for level of pain, and approximately 556 pulses were administered per treatment. A maximum of five passes was performed. Patients were assessed at 4 and 6 months post treatment, and were found to have 95% and 92% improvement in facial skin laxity. In addition to standardized assessments, subject satisfaction when comparing pre- and post-treatment photographs was 70% at six months. Among these patients who had a measurable response, there was a significant improvement seen among those with both cutaneous and subcutaneous laxity versus those with subcutaneous laxity only. The investigators hypothesized that radiofrequency devices cause contraction of dermal fibrils and fibrous septae of subcutaneous fat. Treatment of areas with laxity involving both the dermis and subcutaneous tissue, such as the cheeks and jowls, may have a more significant response to tightening. Although additional trials need to be performed, this study shows good results and minimal side effects when performing multiple passes with low/moderate temperatures.

A more recent study by el-Domyati and colleagues evaluated the clinical effects and objectively quantified the histologic changes of the nonablative RF device in the treatment of photoaging [38]. Six individuals with mild to moderate wrinkles underwent 3 months of treatment (six sessions at 2-week intervals) using a monopolar RF device (Biorad, Shenzhen GSD Tech CO, Guangdong, China). Skin biopsy specimens were obtained at baseline, at 3 and 6 months after the start of treatment. Two initial passes of 150 J each were performed over the entire face and three to six additional passes of 200 J were performed to targeted treatment regions. Patients had noticeable clinical results, with high satisfaction and corresponding facial skin improvement. Compared with the baseline, there was a statistically significant increase in the mean of collagen types I and III, and newly synthesized collagen, while the mean of total elastin was significantly decreased, at the end of treatment and 3 months post-treatment. This study shows good results and histologically confirms significantly increased levels of collagen in patients treated with RF with multiple passes.

Improvements in RF systems have been seen not only with multiple pass treatments but also with new tip size availability [1,9]. There are now multiple sizes ranging from the commonly used 1.0 cm^2 or 1.5 cm^2, the 0.25 cm^2 tips for smaller treatment areas like eyelids, and the larger 3cm tips for treatment of larger surface areas.

Newer combined approaches with RF systems and nonablative lasers are currently being studied to determine if more effective facial rejuvenation can be obtained with both optical and electrical energy combined. Improvement of rhytides and photodamaged skin has been seen when using bipolar radiofrequency with infrared lasers, IPLs, or diode lasers [1,39,40]. Kim *et al.* performed sequential combination treatment using bipolar RF-based IPL, IR light, and diode laser safely in one session 3 weeks apart for four sessions [41]. The study demonstrated that a combination of three different energy sources, with bipolar RF, in one session is effective without further downtime for solving multiple problems including tone, texture, and laxity in photoaged Asian skin. Further studies need to be conducted to determine the most effective treatment regimen. In addition to combined electrical and optical modalities, newer RF devices are also emerging, such as the Accent Device (Alma Laser) which offers both unipolar and bipolar modes. This device is theoretically supposed to improve both laxity and fine lines by providing greater flexibility in penetration depths [1]. The unipolar mode targets the reticular dermis and subcutaneous junction, while the bipolar mode targets the papillary and mid dermis. There are trials underway at this time to determine effectiveness of treatment of facial laxity and cellulite.

Advanced approaches

In addition to facial rejuvenation, several of these devices have also been evaluated for use in photoaging and tightening of other anatomical sites [35,42–45] (Table 48.3). Early studies and preliminary results have suggested that nonablative resurfacing may play a significant part in nonfacial rejuvenation and tightening. Yet, further results are necessary to determine how big their role will be in this rapidly growing field.

For example, a small case series was performed using the 1320 nm Nd:YAG laser to treat photoaging hands [42]. After 6-monthly treatments, four of the seven patients showed mild to moderate improvement in smoothness, reduced wrinkles, and more even pigmentation. Subjective improvement was reported by six of the seven patients at 6 months. Although this study was small, the results showed statistically significant, although mild, improvement in photoaged hands. Radiofrequency and infrared light devices have also been used in an attempt to treat skin laxity in nonfacial areas with variable findings [36,37,40,43,44]. Although nonablative tightening results may not be as effective as surgical interventions, significant improvement has been found. A small trial using an infrared light device showed improvement in neck contour and excess skin in 11 of the 12 patients who completed

Table 48.3 Advanced nonablative resurfacing

Laser/RF device	Treatment locations	Fluence	Pulse duration/pulse number	Spot size
1320 nm Nd:YAG	Photodamaged dorsal hands	13–18 J/cm^2	50 msec macropulse (stacked 350 ms micropulses)	10 mm
Infrared light device (1100–1800 nm)	Neck skin laxity	30–36 J/cm^2 (adjusted for pain level)	11 seconds total pulses 230–440	1.5 cm
Monopolar radiofrequency (Thermacool)	Upper arm skin laxity			3 cm
Monopolar radiofrequency (Pellevé)	Hand wrinkles			2 cm
Unipolar RF device (Accent XL)	Upper thigh, buttocks, abdominal cellulite	150–170 Watts	30 seconds	

Table 48.4 Side effects of nonablative laser resurfacing

Transient erythema and edema (most common)
• Pain/discomfort
• Purpura (KTP and PDL)
• Temporary hyperpigmentation
• Petechiae/pinpoint bleeding (1064 nm QS-Nd:YAG)
• Burning and vesiculation (rare,)
• Crusting
• Edematous papules- 1–7 days (1450 nm diode)

the study [36]. Early results from the use of a monopolar radiofrequency device on upper arm contouring have shown improvement in circumferential size of 36 of 70 patients treated at a 4-month follow-up [39]. Further longterm results are still expected to follow. Other trials have demonstrated that radiofrequency devices are effective in improving the appearance of cellulite with cirumferential reduction of the buttocks, thighs, and abdomen [37,46].

Complications

One of the major benefits of all nonablative rejuvenation modalities is the low risk of potential complications involved with treatments. The most common side effect found among all nonablative lasers, light devices, and RF devices is mild transient erythema and edema which commonly resolves within hours to days [1–3,6,8–10,12,16,17,25,31–33]. Although complications are rare, temporary side effects have been recorded and are listed in Table 48.4.

Conclusions

Nonablative rejuvenation is a relatively new and exciting field in aesthetic dermatology. Many different devices are currently being used to treat changes associated with photoaging, such as rhytides, skin laxity, vascular changes, and pigmentary alterations. Although ablative resurfacing and surgical intervention remain the gold standard, nonablative systems offer an alternative option with less downtime and risk of complications. These devices selectively target the dermis, inciting a wound healing response locally, while sparing the epidermis from harm. Dermal collagen remodeling, production, and repair are upregulated as a result of this selective targeting. Multiple lasers, light sources, and radiofrequency devices have been used to induce significant neocollagenesis with measurable success. Yet despite the significant histological changes noted, the clinical enhancement is often subtle with mild to moderate improvement over time. As a result, it is important to give patients realistic expectations when performing nonablative rejuvenation. The most effective devices and treatment parameters for photorejuvenation have yet to be determined, but continued enthusiasm in this field gives hope for continued research and success.

References

1. Alexiades-Armenakas MR, Dover JS, Arndt KA. (2008) The spectrum of laser skin resurfacing: Nonablative, fractional, and ablative laser resurfacing. *JAAD* **58**, 719–37.
2. Weiss RA, Weiss MA, Beasley KL, Munavalli G. (2005) Our approach to nonablative treatment of photoaging. *Lasers Surg Med* **37**, 2–8.
3. Goldberg DJ. (2003) Lasers for facial rejuvenation. *Am J Dermatol* **4**, 225–34.
4. Hedelund L, Bjerring P, Egekvist H, Haedersdal M. (2006) Ablative versus nonablative treatment of perioral rhytides. A randomized controlled trial with long-term blinded clinical evaluations and non-invasive measurements. *Lasers Surg Med* **38**, 129–36.
5. Sadick NS. (2003) Update on nonablative light therapy for rejuvenation: A review. *Lasers Surg Med* **32**, 120–28.
6. Bosniak S, Cantisano-Zilkha M, Purewal BK, Zdinak LA. (2006) Combination Therapies in Oculofacial rejuvenation. *Orbit* **25**, 319–26.
7. Liu H, Dang Y, Wang Z, Chai X, Ren Q. (2008) Laser induced collagen remodeling: A comparative study in vivo on mouse model. *Lasers Surg Med* **40**, 13–19.
8. Friedman PM, Jih MH, Skover GR, Payonk GS, Kimyai-Asadi A, Geronemus RG. (2004) Treatment of atrophic facial acne scars with the 1064 nm Q-switched Nd:YAG laser. *Arch Dermatol* **140**, 1337–41.
9. Bogle MA, Ubelhoer N, Weiss RA, Mayoral F, Kaminer FS. (2007) Evaluation of the multiple pass, low fluence algorithm for radiofrequency tightening of the lower face. *Laser Surg Med* **39**, 210–17.

10. Narins DJ, Narins RS. (2003) Non-surgical radiofrequency facelift. *J Drug Dermatol* **2**, 495–500.
11. Friedman PM, Skover GR, Payonk G, Kauvar AN, Geronemus RG. (2002) 3D in-vivo optical skin imaging for topographical quantitative assessment of nonablative laser technology. *Dermatol Surg* **28**, 199–204.
12. Fournier N, Lagarde JM, Turlier V, Courrech L, Mordon S. (2004) A 35-month profilometric and clinical evaluation of nonablative remodeling using a 1540 nm Er:glass laser. *J Cosmet Laser Ther* **6**, 126–30.
13. Dang Y, Ren Q, Li W, et al. (2006) Comparison of biophysical properties of skin measured by using non-invasive techniques in the KM mice following 595 nm pulsed dye, 1064 nm Q-switched Nd:YAG and 1320 nm Nd:YAG laser nonablative rejuvenation. *Skin Res Technol* **12**, 119–25.
14. Keller R, Belda Junior W, Valente NY, Rodrigues CJ. (2007) Nonablative 1064 nm Nd:YAG laser for treating atrophic facial acne scars: Histologic and clinical analysis. *Dermatol Surg* **33**, 1470–76.
15. Lee MW. (2003) Combination 532 nm and 1064 nm lasers for noninvasive skin rejuvenation and toning. *Arch Dermatol* **139**, 1265–76.
16. Ho SG, Chan NP, Yeung CK, et al. (2012) A retrospective analysis of the management of freckles and lentigines using four different pigment lasers on Asian skin. *J Cosmet Laser Ther* **14**, 74–80.
17. Bernstein EF. (2007) The new-generation, high-energy, 595 nm, long pulse-duration pulsed-dye laser improves the appearance of photodamaged skin. *Lasers Surg Med* **39**, 157–63.
18. Goldberg DJ, Sarradet D, Hussain M, et al. (2004) Clinical, histologic, and ultrastructural changes after nonablative treatment with a 595-nm flashlamp-pumped pulsed dye laser: Comparison of varying settings. *Dermatol Surg* **30**, 979–82.
19. Kono T, Groff WF, Sakurai H, et al. (2007) Comparison study of intense pulsed light versus a long-pulse pulsed dye laser in the treatment of facial skin rejuvenation. *Ann Plast Surg* **59**, 479–83.
20. Goldberg DJ, Cutler KB. (2000) Nonablative treatment of rhytids with intense pulsed light. *Lasers Surg Med* **26**, 196–9.
21. Alster TS, Tanzi EL, Welsh EC. (2005) Photorejuvenation of facial skin with topical 20% 5-aminolevulinic acid and intense pulsed light treatment: a split face comparison study. *J Drugs Dermatol* **4**, 35–38.
22. Marmur ES, Phelps R, Goldberg DJ. (2005) Ultrastructural changes seen after ALA-IPL photorejuvenation: a pilot study. *J Cosmet Laser Ther* **7**, 21–24.
23. Dover JS, Bhatia AC, Stewart B, Arndt KA. (2005) Topical 5-aminolevulinic acid combined with intense pulsed light in the treatment of photoaging. *Arch Dermatol* **141**, 1247–52.
24. Gold MH, Bradshaw VL, Boring MM, et al. (2006) Split-face comparison of photodynamic therapy with 5-aminolevulinic acid and intense pulsed light versus intense pulsed light alone for photodamage. *Dermatol Surg* **32**, 795–801.
25. Sadick NS, Schecter AK. (2004) A preliminary study of utilization of the 1320 nm Nd:YAG laser for the treatment of acne scarring. *Dermatol Surg* **30**, 995–1000.
26. Zhenxiao Z, Aie X, Yuzhi J, et al. (2011) Exploring the role of a nonablative laser (1320 nm cooltouch laser) in skin photorejuvenation. *Skin Res Technol* **17**, 505–9.
27. Preissig J, Hamilton K, Markus R. (2012) Current laser resurfacing technologies: a review that delves beneath the surface. *Semin Plast Surg* **26**, 109–16.
28. El-Domyati M, El-Ammawi TS, Medhat W, et al. (2011) Effects of the Nd:YAG 1320 nm laser on skin rejuvenation: clinical and histological correlations. *J Cosmet Laser Ther* **13**, 98–106.
29. Rogachefsky AS, Hussain M, Goldberg DJ. (2003) Atrophic and a mixed pattern of acne scars improved with a 1320 nm Nd:YAG laser. *Dermatol Surg* **29**, 904–8.
30. Goldberg DJ, Silapunt S. (2000) Q-switched Nd:YAG laser: rhytid improvement by nonablative dermal remodeling. *J Cutan Laser Ther* **2**, 157–60.
31. Fournier N, Dahan S, Barneon G, et al. (2002) Nonablative remodeling: a 14 month clinical ultrasound imaging and profilometric evaluation of a 1540 nm Er:glass laser. *Dermatol Surg* **28**, 926–31.
32. Tanzi EL, Alster TS. (2004) Comparison of a 1450 nm diode laser and a 1320 nm Nd:YAG laser in the treatment of atrophic facial scars: a prospective clinical and histologic study. *Dermatol Surg* **30**, 152–7.
33. Goldberg DJ, Rogachefsky AS, Silapunt S. (2002) Nonablative laser treatment of facial rhytides: a comparison of 1450 nm Diode laser treatment with dynamic cooling as opposed to treatment with dynamic cooling alone. *Lasers Surg Med* **30**, 79–81.
34. Wada T, Kawada A, Hirao A, et al. (2012) Efficacy and safety of a low-energy double-pass 1450-nm diode laser for the treatment of acne scare. *Photomed Laser Surg* **30**, 107–11.
35. Ahn JY, Han TY, Lee CK, et al. (2008) Effect of a new infrared light device (1100–1800 nm) on facial lifting. *Photodermatol Photoimmunol Photomed.* **24**, 49–51.
36. Goldberg DJ, Hussain M, Fazeli A, et al. (2007) Treatment of skin laxity of the lower face and neck in older individuals with a broad-spectrum infrared light device. *J Cosmet Laser Ther* **9**, 35–40.
37. Belenky I, Margulis A, Elman M, et al. (2012) Exploring channeling optimized radiofrequency energy: a review of radiofrequency history and applications in esthetic fields. *Adv Ther* **29**, 249–66.
38. El-Domyati M, el-Ammawi TS, Medhat W, et al. (2011) Radiofrequency facial rejuvenation: evidence-based effect. *J Am Acad Dermatol* **64**, 524–35.
39. Sadick NS, Alexiades-Armenakas M, Bitter P, et al. (2005) Enhanced full-face skin rejuvenation using synchronous intense pulsed optical and conducted bipolar radiofreqwuency energy (ELOS): introducing selective radiophotothermolysis. *J Drugs Dermatol* **4**, 181–86.
40. Alexiades-Armenakas M. (2006) Rhytides, laxity, and photoaging treated with a combination of radiofrequency, diode laser, and pulsed light and assessed with a comprehensive grading scale. *J Drugs Dermatol* **5**, 731–8.
41. Kim JE, Chang S, Won CH, et al. (2012) Combination treatment using bipolar radiofrequency-based intense pulsed light, infrared light and diode laser enhanced clinical effectiveness and histological dermal remodeling in Asian photoaged skin. *Dermatol Surg* **38**, 68–76.
42. Sadick N, Schecter AK. (2004) Tilization of the 1320 nm Nd:YAG laser for the reduction of photoaging of the hands. *Dermatol Surg* **30**, 1140–44.
43. Goldberg DJ, Hussain M, Fazeli A, et al. (2007) Monopolar radiofrequency tightening of upper arm skin laxity: a multicenter study. *Laser Surg Med* (suppl 19), 19.
44. Vega JM, Bucay VW, Mayoral FA. (2013) Prospective, multicenter study to determine the safety and efficacy of a unique radiofrequency device for moderate to severe hand wrinkles. *J Drugs Dermatol* **12**, 24–6.
45. Kassim At, Goldberg DJ. (2013) Assessment of the safety and efficacy of a bipolar multi-frequency device in the treatment of skin laxity. *J Cosmet Laser Ther* **15**, 114–7.
46. Del Pino E, Rosado RH, Azuela A, et al. (2006) Effect of controlled volumetric tissue heating with radiofrequency on cellulite and the subcutaneous tissue of the buttocks and thighs. *J Drugs Dermatol* **5**, 714–22.

CHAPTER 49
Dermabrasion

Christopher B. Harmon and Daniel P. Skinner

Surgical Dermatology Group, Birmingham, AL, USA

> **BASIC CONCEPTS**
> - Dermabrasion involves mechanically removing the epidermis and papillary dermis, creating a newly contoured open wound to heal by second intention.
> - The most common indications for dermabrasion are for the improvement of cystic acne scarring, post-surgical scar revision, and enhanced contouring of partial thickness Mohs defects.
> - Patients must have realistic expectations of the anticipated improvement, possible side effects, and potential complications of dermabrasion prior to treatment.
> - Proper technique is paramount in order to avoid intraoperative complications.
> - Vigilance during the postoperative period is important in order to recognize complications at an early stage and prevent long-term sequelae.

Definition and history

Dermabrasion is a skin resurfacing technique that surgically abrades or planes the epidermis through the use of a rapidly rotating wire brush or diamond fraise [1]. The wire brush or diamond fraise is used as the abrading tip to create an open wound that will heal by second intention. An irregular or scarred cutaneous surface may be surgically abraded in order to achieve a more regular plane, or a more gradual transition between different planes, thereby improving skin contour and appearance.

In its simplest form, dermabrasion was practiced by ancient Egyptians in circa 1500 BC, who employed the abrasive characteristics of pumice and alabaster to treat skin blemishes [2]. Kurtin presented the first series of patients who underwent dermabrasion to Mount Sinai Hospital in 1953. Kurtin described the use of high-speed rotary abraders, intraoperative freezing, and a variety of abrasive end pieces [3]. Later publications further refined Kurtin's technique, including the use of the diamond fraise and the wire brush [4–7]. Since the introduction of modern dermabrasion by Kurtin growing interest in the technique has culminated in its application to a variety of lesions including most commonly, facial scars secondary to acne, trauma and surgery. The growing number of applications of dermabrasion has been accompanied by evolution of the technique from the use of common sandpaper in the mid-twentieth century to electrically powered devices with wire brush tips or diamond fraises of varying sizes, shapes and textures that can achieve speeds of over 33,000 revolutions per minute [8].

Mechanism of action

Fundamentally, the skin can be subdivided into three layers – epidermis, dermis, and subcutaneous tissue. The dermis is further subdivided into the more superficial papillary dermis, containing both a finely woven meshwork of collagen interdigitating with the epidermal rete as well as the superficial vascular plexus, and the deeper reticular dermis, composed of thick bundles of predominantly Type I collagen [9]. Resurfacing, by definition, involves iatrogenic removal of one or multiple layers of the skin to create a cutaneous wound. Dermabrasion mechanically removes the epidermis and papillary dermis, creating a partial thickness wound to heal by second intention. The well-characterized, yet complex, wound healing response is triggered, involving transforming growth factor beta 1 (TGF-β1)-driven myofibroblastic deposition of new Type I and Type III collagen and subsequent remodeling in the dermis [10]. Additionally, TGF-1β and epidermal growth factor (EGF) as well as other growth factors and matrix metalloproteinases (MMPs) stimulate re-epithelialization from both underlying skin appendages and adjacent epithelialized skin [10]. Defined ultrastructural and molecular alterations accompany the clinically visible changes apparent in the dermabraded area. These include increased collagen bundle density and size with a tendency toward unidirectional orientation of collagen fibers parallel to the epidermal surface, as well as altered levels of α6- and β4-integrin expression in the stratum spinosum [11].

Cosmetic Dermatology: Products and Procedures, Second Edition. Edited by Zoe Diana Draelos.
© 2016 John Wiley & Sons, Ltd. Published 2016 by John Wiley & Sons, Ltd.

When properly performed, the irregularly contoured or actinically damaged epidermal and papillary dermal layers are removed, and second intention wound healing occurs. The clinical result is a smoother, more evenly contoured surface, with fewer irregularities in the form of acne scars, rhytides, keratoses, or step-off transitions.

Indications

The most common indications for dermabrasion are desired improvement of acne scars, traumatic and surgical scars, rhinophyma, deep rhytides, and partial-thickness Mohs defects (Figure 49.1) [12]. However, it has also been described for improvement of actinic keratoses, seborrheic keratoses, angiofibromas, syringomas, solar elastosis, epidermal nevi, tattoo removal and more recently, vitiligo [13–15].

With regard to acne scarring, even in the era of laser devices, fractionated delivery approaches, and non-invasive "tissue-tightening" procedures, dermabrasion remains an important tool in the combination approach to the improvement of cystic acne scarring. While the shallow and wide, undulating, or "rolling" type acne scars are better treated with subcision, dermal grafts, fillers, or fractionated laser devices, the slightly deeper and narrower "box-car" type acne scars that demonstrate step-off vertical borders respond best to mechanical dermabrasion. Additionally, the deepest and narrowest "ice-pick" type acne scars respond best to dermabrasion subsequent to punch excisions, punch grafts, or TCA cross destruction. Dermabrasion allows a skilled practitioner to selectively plane off "hilltops" surrounding atrophic scars which are so prominent in moderate to severe acne scarring. Chemical peels and laser treatments in contrast, produce an injury of equivalent depth in both areas. Fractional CO_2 resurfacing does have the advantage of creating skin contraction through the deep penetration causing microthermal zones, which in some cases can produce improvement in acne scarring equivalent to dermabrasion [16–17].

For traumatic and surgical scars, the thickness, contour, and overall appearance is routinely improved with postoperative dermabrasion (Figure 49.2). Also known as "scarabrasion", this procedure is best performed 6–8 weeks after the initial surgery or wounding event [18]. When performed during this 6–8 week window, the late proliferative and early remodeling phases of wound healing are interrupted and partially "reset", resulting in an improved final cosmetic result.

While several modalities, including wire loop electrosurgery and CO_2 laser resurfacing, have been described for the treatment of rhinophyma, dermabrasion remains unmatched in the operator's ability to re-establish the complex contour of the many cosmetic subunits of the nose. Furthermore, although fractionated laser resurfacing has largely replaced dermabrasion for full face treatment of facial rhytides, dermabrasion can be as efficacious or more efficacious at removal of both fine and moderate facial rhytides. However, with patient preferences moving

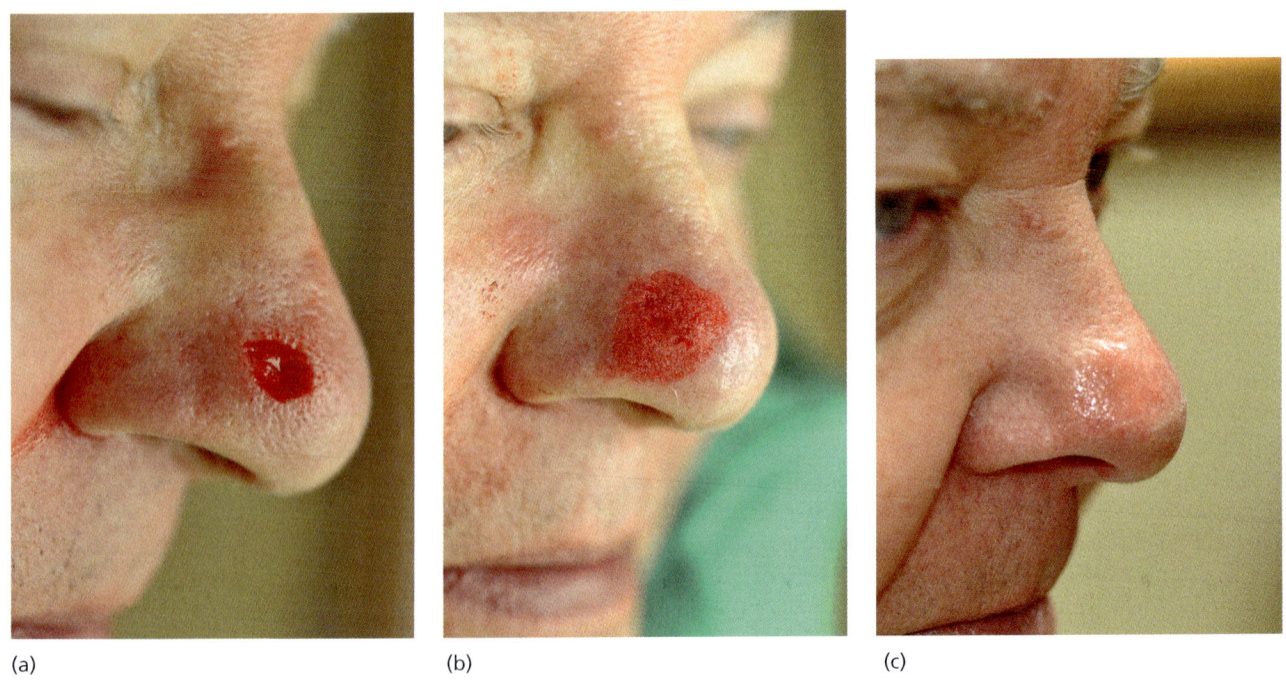

(a)　　　　　　　　　　　(b)　　　　　　　　　　　(c)

Figure 49.1 Dermabrasion after partial thickness Mohs layer on the nose (a) Male patient with a partial thickness defect after 1 stage of Mohs micrographic surgery for the removal of basal cell carcinoma (b) Immediately after spot dermabrasion to blend the surgical defect with the surrounding skin (c) 2 weeks after Mohs and dermabrasion.

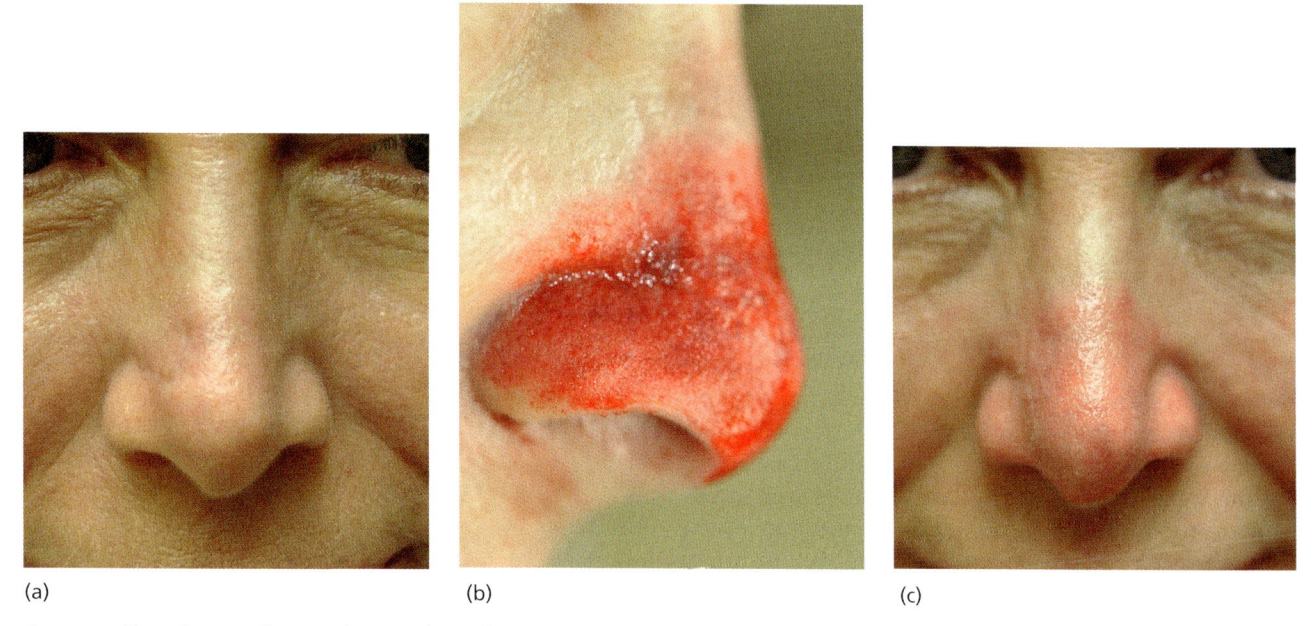

Figure 49.2 Dermabrasion of scar on the nose after Mohs surgery and reconstruction (a) Female patient with a scar on the right nasal sidewall and lateral tip 6 weeks after Mohs surgery and flap reconstruction. (b) Immediately after dermabrasion to multiple cosmetic subunits of the nose. Feathering the border of the dermabraded area (arrows) helps to minimize the color differences between the treated and untreated areas. (c) 2 weeks after dermabrasion with significant improvement in the appearance and texture of the scar.

in the direction of less invasive procedures with shorter downtime, full face dermabrasion for rhytides is unlikely to return to widespread use in the foreseeable future.

Finally, dermabrasion proves to be an incredibly useful technique in the armamentarium of the Mohs surgeon. Thin carcinomas in cosmetically sensitive or high-risk areas can often be completely removed with a shallow Mohs layer to the level of the superficial reticular dermis. After clearance, these partial-thickness defects, particularly on the nose and scalp, may lend themselves to healing by second intention rather than primary closure, yet with slightly increased risk of an evident contour discrepancy or sharp pigmentary transition. Dermabrasion of the edges surrounding the partial-thickness Mohs defect greatly improves the final contour by replacing the steeply beveled wound edge with a more gradual slope. Additionally, dermabrading the remainder of an involved cosmetic subunit of the nose results in a less obvious scar by placing the pigmentary demarcation lines at the less perceptible subunit boundaries.

Advantages and disadvantages

As compared to fully ablative resurfacing with the CO_2 and Er:YAG lasers, dermabrasion demonstrates similar or greater efficacy for the treatment of scars, rhytides, and precancerous lesions, with less postoperative erythema and more rapid re-epithelialization. While newer, fractionated delivery protocols result in even less erythema and quicker re-epithelialization than dermabrasion, their efficacies for the improvement of scars, rhytides, and precancerous lesions do not currently match that seen with mechanical dermabrasion. However, a recent study comparing fractionated CO_2 laser and mechanical dermabrasion for post-Mohs scars did show the same efficacy for both treatment modalities, with less bleeding erythema and edema in the group treated with CO_2 laser [19]. Dermabrasion has also been shown to be more efficacious than 5-fluorouracil for the treatment of actinic keratosis [20].

The major disadvantage of dermabrasion as compared to the above modalities is that it is much more operator dependent. Unlike laser and light devices, the depth of penetration is not pre-programmed. Successful treatment relies not only on the physician's knowledge of the modality and application settings, but also on his or her skilled execution. In the novice's hands, dermabrasion exhibits a narrower window or buffer between effective treatment depth and inappropriate scarring depth. However, this is quickly overcome with experience.

Patient selection and preoperative consultation

The most important components of the preoperative consultation are determining the patient's specific motivation for resurfacing and establishing realistic expectations regarding

(a) (b) (c)

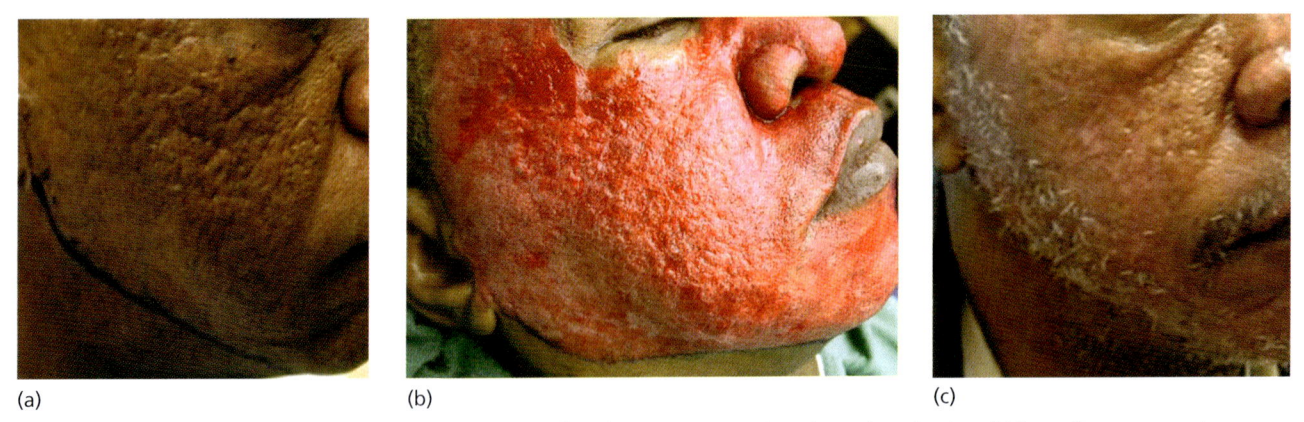

Figure 49.3 Dermabrasion of acne scars (a) African-American male with severe acne scarring prior to dermabrasion. (b) Immediate postoperative appearance of the treated area. (c) Appearance 4 weeks after dermabrasion.

the treatment outcome. The ultimate goal of any resurfacing treatment should be an improvement of the given defect rather than a complete eradication. Dermabrasion consistently achieves 30–50% improvement in the appearance of deep acne scars and rhytides (Figure 49.3), but the patient who seeks and expects the elimination of all scars and rhytides will rarely be satisfied. Reviewing before and after photographs with the patient during consultation, particularly when considering full cosmetic unit or full-face dermabrasion, may foster realistic expectations for improvement.

The preoperative consult should also include a complete history addressing bleeding disorders, prior herpes simplex infection, impetigo, keloidal or hypertrophic scarring, koebnerizing conditions, prior isotretinoin therapy, and immunosuppression. The risk/benefit ratio of an iatrogenically induced wound is unfavorable in patients who are immunosuppressed, who have a history koebnerizing conditions such as lichen planus and psoriasis, or who demonstrate a propensity towards keloidal or hypertrophic scar formation. Due to an increased risk of scarring in patients on isotretinoin, dermabrasion should be delayed until six months after finishing an oral retinoid course [21]. Caution should also be exercised when planning to dermabrade patients who have recently undergone extensive procedures involving the area to be dermabraded, such as a facelift, as a robust blood supply is necessary for appropriate wound healing. Many surgeons prefer to wait six months after a facelift before subsequent dermabrasion.

Antiviral prophylaxis should be instituted in those with a history of herpes simplex outbreak in the area to be spot dermabraded or in those who are undergoing full face or multiple cosmetic unit dermabrasion. The antiviral agents acyclovir or valacyclovir may be used, and patients should remain on prophylactic therapy for ten days after the procedure (valacyclovir 500 mg BID × ten days). Similarly, antibacterial prophylaxis with an anti-staphylococcal agent should be instituted in those with a history of impetigo.

Particular attention should also be paid to the Fitzpatrick Skin Type of the patient. Fitzpatrick Skin Types IV, V, and VI are much more prone to both postoperative hyperpigmentation and permanent, clinically significant hypopigmentation, the latter of which may not appear for several months following the procedure.

Preoperative photographs are highly recommended, and should include a frontal view, 45 and 90-degree views from both sides, and a close up view of the areas to be treated. Additionally, all preoperative and postoperative expectations should be discussed. The patient should particularly be made aware of the nature of the postoperative recovery routine, which includes extensive facial dressings with multiple changes over several days, and clinically apparent erythema for several weeks.

Instrumentation

With mechanical dermabrasion, a diamond fraise or wire brush abrading tip is driven by a handheld engine at speeds of 15,000 to 30,000 rotations per minute (RPMs). Some of the most commonly used hand engines and handpieces include the Bell, Osada, and Acrotorque.

Diamond fraises come in a range of shapes and sizes, such as pears, cones, bullets, and wheels, and also vary in coarseness from fine to extra-coarse. Alternatively, the wire brush is a 3.0–5.0 mm wide × 17.0 mm diameter wheel with steel bristles radiating from the center in a clockwise fashion when viewed from the shaft. The wire brush is the most aggressive type of end piece and can be more technically difficult to master, yet it is considered more efficacious by those experienced with its use. The microlacerations created with the wire brush are the most efficient means of removing the nodules of rhinophyma, the thick plaques of hypertrophic scars, and deep acne scars. Wire brushes are no longer being manufactured and must be purchased as a used piece of equipment from a third party.

Standard technique

Treating surgical scars, rhinophyma, and partial-thickness Mohs defects provides an excellent point of entry into the practice of dermabrasion prior to practicing advanced techniques such as full face dermabrasion. If the treatment area is limited in size, local anesthesia (1% lidocaine with epinephrine 1:100,000) or tumescent technique is adequate. When treating the entire nose, a ring block may achieve an appropriate degree of anesthesia as well. Prior to abrasion, the area to be treated is cleansed with a 4% chlorhexidine solution.

The body of the hand engine is grasped in the palm of the dominant hand with four fingers, allowing the thumb to project along the neck for stabilization. Finger position is similar to a "thumbs-up" sign or to that seen when gripping a golf club, yet the hand and instrument are pronated, with the palm facing downward (Figure 49.4a). The area of skin to be dermabraded can be tumesced with local anesthesia to provide a firm and anesthetic are of skin to abrade.

An alternate method of anesthesia for full face dermabrasion utilizes a spray refrigerant to provide topical anesthesia and a firm substrate to dermabrade. Topical refrigerant spray, Frigi-derm containing Freon 114 is applied to the treatment area in an amount necessary to achieve a 5–10 second thaw time, during which time abrasion is performed on the frozen area. Although not required in every case, refrigerant spray accomplishes two important functions: decreasing pain by cryoanesthesia and a providing a firm substrate upon which to achieve re-contouring. Concerns regarding potential harm to the environment from cryogenic sprays have limited the availability of topical refrigerant sprays in several countries, including the US. Liquid nitrogen or other agents that cryopreserve tissue create a colder temperature that can lead to scarring and/or hypopigmentation and their use is not recommended [1].

Immediately after freezing, three-point retraction is obtained by the two hands of the surgical assistant and the non-dominant hand of the surgeon. The frozen skin is thus stabilized by retraction, and the lesion is re-contoured with the wire brush rotating in a counter-clockwise direction (with the angle of the radiating bristles) as determined from the point of view of the body of the hand engine (Figure 49.4b).

For abrasive resurfacing the wire brush is passed over the treatment area in an arciform motion with the long axis perpendicular to the rotating handpiece, parallel to the body of the hand engine (Figure 49.4c). Counter-clockwise rotation of the wire brush offers a less aggressive technique of wire brush surgery that is especially well suited for spot dermabrasion of Mohs defects or surgical scars without cryoanesthesia. With counter-clockwise rotation, the radiating bristles are less prone to gouge unfrozen skin. This counter-clockwise direction of rotation is also useful when dermabrading free margins of the face such as the lips and nasal alae, in order to prevent the inadvertent "grabbing" of tissue by the rotating wire brush when dermabrading from the right side with the dominant right hand.

Regular pinpoints of bleeding signal abrasion to the level of the papillary dermis. As depth increases to the reticular dermis, the bleeding foci become larger, and frayed collagen bundles become apparent. Surgical scars will frequently disintegrate upon abrasion, which is a desirable endpoint. Contouring should often include "feathering" or graduating zones of treatment around the central scar to provide a smooth transition between different planes and improved pigment transition (Figure 49.2c). Alternatively, the treatment zone may be stopped at the border of a cosmetic unit or carried to an inconspicuous endpoint such as 1.0 cm beyond the mandible.

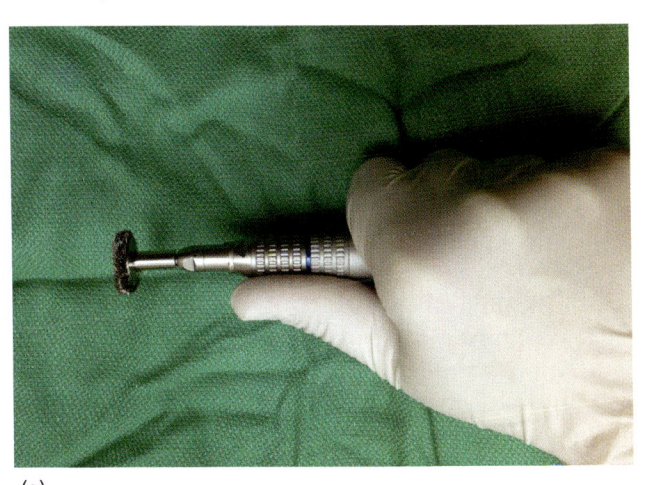

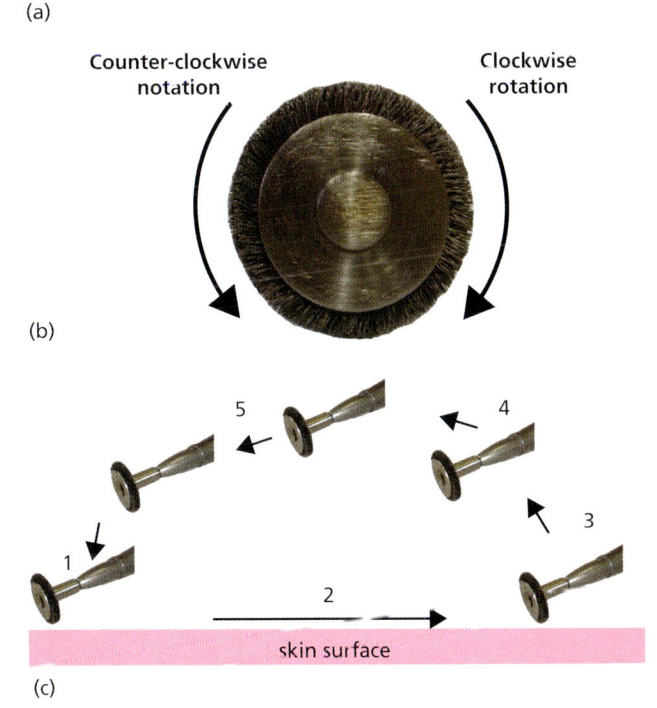

Figure 49.4 Technical considerations (a) Proper grasp of the hand engine. (b) Clockwise rotation (against the angle of the rotating bristles) of the wire brush results in removal of a thicker plane of tissue with each pass than counter-clockwise rotation (with the angle of the bristles) (c) The treatment stroke. After the wire brush comes in contact with the skin (1), it is pulled across the treatment area in in a unidirectional fashion perpendicular to the direction of the rotating wire brush (2). Following completion of the treatment stroke, the wire brush is lifted from the skin surface (3), and in an arciform fashion (4–5) is moved to a new area.

Advanced technique

While local or tumescent anesthesia may be adequate for scar or spot dermabrasion, full face abrasion of acne scarring or rhytides is best accomplished with a combination of oral (p.o.) or intramuscular (i.m.) light sedation, nerve blocks, and cryoanesthesia. A standard regimen consists of 50–75 mg i.m. meperidine, 25 mg i.m. hydroxyzine, and 5–10 mg p.o. or sublingual diazepam 30–60 minutes prior to the start of the procedure. After a chlorhexidine prep, nerve blocks to the supratrochlear, supraorbital, infraorbital, and mental nerves may also be performed.

In contrast to the counterclockwise rotation typically utilized for less aggressive dermabrasion, more experienced practitioners may opt to use a clockwise rotation of the abrasive wire brush, especially in areas of deeper scarring like mid-cheeks or with thick papules of rhinophyma. Rotation in a clockwise direction occurs against the angle of the radiating wire bristles and causes the tip to pull away from the thumb rather than driving toward it. Deeper planing and re-contouring are possible with clockwise rotation, but this direction is much less forgiving. Additionally, clockwise rotation utilized by a dominant right hand increases the risk that free margins of the face, such as lips and nasal alae, will be "grabbed" by the rotating bristles rather than brushed away, resulting in unintentional, deeper abrasion in these areas.

When performing full face dermabrasion, beginning at the periphery of the cheek or mandible and working toward the center of the face allows the practitioner to avoid gravity dependent bleeding as the procedure progresses. A surgical towel, surgical cap, or petrolatum may also be used to help prevent entanglement of hair at the periphery of the treatment area. Surgical towels are also preferable to cotton gauze as sponges on the surgical field, as gauze becomes more easily entangled in the wire brush and hand engine.

Postoperative wound care

Gauze or a non-adherent dressing soaked with 1% lidocaine with 1:100,000 epinephrine may be immediately applied to the post-abraded area for a period of 5–10 minutes to assist with hemostasis. A closed-technique, layered bandage is then applied, composed of a semi-permeable hydrogel dressing (Vigilon, Second Skin) in contact with the wound, a non-adherent dressing (Telfa) above, and paper tape or surgical netting to secure the bandage in place. Semi-permeable hydrogel dressings provide two important advantages over other types of dressings: decreased patient discomfort in the postoperative period and decreased time to re-epithelialization by up to 40% [22]. The dressing should be changed daily for 3–5 days. If full face dermabrasion has been performed, it is usually most convenient to have the patient return to the office for dressing changes during this period. For smaller areas, the patient may change the bandage at home. After 3–5 days, the patient begins an open wound care technique at home. Acetic acid soaks (0.25%: 1 tablespoon white vinegar into 1 pint of warm water) are followed by topical petrolatum ointment until re-epithelialization is complete, usually 7–10 days after the procedure. Strict adherence to this regimen reduces the risk of both secondary infection and scarring.

If full face dermabrasion is performed, a short course of oral or intramuscular steroids may also be given immediately after the procedure to help reduce facial swelling. Swelling is an anticipated consequence of full face dermabrasion and may be expected to resolve over several weeks to a few months. All previously prescribed antivirals and antibacterials should be instituted or continued, and patients should be given a prognosis and expected recovery timeframe. Once re-epithelialization has occurred, sunscreens and sun avoidance should be strictly adhered to for several weeks in order to minimize post-procedure pigment alteration. Makeup may be used to cover erythema after re-epithelialization as well.

The most common complications encountered after dermabrasion are milia and acne flares. These minor side effects should be anticipated, and may be treated by comedone expression, topical tretinoin, and oral antibiotics.

Infection, pigment alteration, and scarring are the more portentous complications that may be encountered after dermabrasion. Vigilance in the immediate postoperative period is necessary to identify these complications at an early stage and institute treatment. Herpes simplex infection may still occur while the patient is on a prophylactic antiviral dose, and clinically manifests as painful (out of proportion to healing phase), erythematous lesions 7–10 days post-procedure. Larger doses of antiviral medications are then necessary for treatment (valcyclovir 1 gram, three times per day for 7–10 more days). Bacterial and fungal infections may likewise produce persistently painful, erythematous lesions. Lesions should be cultured and empiric therapy with an anti-staphylococcal or anti-candidal agent, or both, should be implemented as warranted by clinical suspicion.

Transient, postoperative hyperpigmentation is a common complication, usually beginning 4–6 weeks after dermabrasion. Hydroquinone (4–8%), or formulations containing hydroquinone, tretinoin, and a mild steroid, should be implemented at the earliest signs of hyperpigmentation and continued for 4–8 weeks. A more difficult complication to treat is hypopigmentation. While not quite as common as with fully ablative CO_2 laser resurfacing, nearly one-third of patients will develop permanent hypopigmentation after full face wire brush dermabrasion. Furthermore, such hypopigmentation often does not develop until several months post-procedure. Female patients may camouflage such hypopigmentation with makeup, but male patients have fewer options for improvement. The 308-nm excimer laser has been shown to improve hypopigmented scars and vitiligo, and may be an option for improvement after dermabrasion as well [23]. True hypopigmentation should be differentiated from the pseudo-hypopigmentation seen when resurfaced skin without actinic damage simply appears lighter than the surrounding actinically damaged skin.

Finally, persistent erythema in the absence of infection is the harbinger of scar formation. Scars should be treated early and proactively in order to minimize sequelae. Flat, erythematous scars may be managed by topical steroids, or steroid-impregnated tape worn nightly. However, indurated scars also require intralesional corticosteroid injections and/or pulsed dye laser treatments on a regular basis. These may be repeated every few weeks until stabilization and improvement occur.

Summary

With the armamentarium of resurfacing modalities increasing, mechanical dermabrasion remains an important dermasurgical procedure, particularly for the improvement of cystic acne, post-surgical scars, and partial-thickness Mohs defects. Selecting appropriate patients and establishing realistic treatment goals are prerequisites. Small areas may be easily and safely treated with proper technique, and these demonstrate a rapid recovery. Although experience and skill are necessary in order to avoid serious complications with full face dermabrasion, its efficacy for the treatment of acne scarring and deep rhytides currently remains unmatched for the patient who is willing to endure the resultant recovery period. Close follow-up during the postoperative period is important in order to recognize and treat the most serious potential complications of infection and scarring at the earliest stages. While new technologies continue to emerge, mechanical resurfacing will likely remain an essential and unmatched modality for scar improvement into the foreseeable future.

Table 49.1 Complications of dermabrasion with suggested treatment.

Complication	Comment	Treatment
Milia and acne flare	Most common	Expression, topical retinoids, oral antibiotics
HSV "breakthrough" infection	Intensely painful erythematous lesions at 7–10 days	Increase antiviral dose (valcyclovir 1 g, 3× day for 7–10 more days)
Bacterial infection	Persistently painful erythematous lesions	Culture and begin empiric therapy with anti-staphylococcal antibiotic
Fungal infection	Persistently painful erythematous lesions	Culture and begin empiric therapy with anti-candidal agent
Hyperpigmentation	Usually transient	4–8% hydroquinone for 4–8 weeks
Hypopigmentation	Delayed onset, usually permanent	Camouflaging makeup, possibly 308-nm excimer laser
Scarring	Persistent erythema in the absence of infection	Treat early and repeatedly Topical steroids Intralesional steroids Pulsed dye laser

Table 49.2 Pearls and pitfalls

Pearls	Pitfalls
• Preoperative application of petroleum jelly, aquaphor or K-Y jelly along the hair line minimizes entanglement of the hair with the spinning tip of the hand engine.	• Avoid using gauze for blotting and retracting during these procedures since these can easily become entangled in the rapidly rotating end piece. Cotton towels are preferable.
• Thicker scars are more efficiently treated with the wire brush rotating in a clockwise direction (against the angle of the radiating bristles), and counter-clockwise rotation (with the angle of the bristles) offers a less aggressive approach.	• Dermabrasion produces aerosolized particles and could potentially result in exposure of the surgeon and staff to pathogens. Therefore preoperative planning should include evaluation for HIV and hepatitis.
• In patients who have undergone a prior procedure involving the area to be dermabraded, e.g. surgical excision, grafting or other procedures requiring extensive undermining, at least 6–8 weeks should elapse before dermabrasion is considered.	• Pseudohypopigmentation is seen when normally repigmented abraded skin has a slightly lighter tone and appearance than adjacent sun-damaged, non-abraded skin. This condition responds to superficial- or medium-depth chemical peels, nonablative lasers and intense pulsed light to blend the treated and untreated areas.
• Noticeable pigmentary differences between treated and untreated skin can be minimized by feathering the borders of the treatment area.	• Patients with unrealistic expectations will be disappointed with any outcome, regardless of the degree of improvement. Prior to surgery, extensive discussion with patients should be had regarding expected improvement.

References

1 Monheit GD. (2012) Chemical and mechanical skin resurfacing. In: Bolognia JL, et al., eds. *Dermatology,* 3rd edn. Oxford: Elsevier, pp. 2493–508.
2 Lawrence N, Mandy S, Yarborough J, et al. (2000) History of dermabrasion. *Dermatol Surg* **26**, 95–101.
3 Kurtin A. (1953) Corrective surgical planing of skin; new technique for treatment of acne scars and other skin defects. *AMA Arch Derm Syphilol* **68**, 389–97.
4 Burks JW, Thomas CC. (1956) *Wire Brush Surgery.* Springfield, IL: Charles C. Thomas.
5 Orentreich D, Orentreich N. (1987) Acne scar revision update. *Dermatol Clin* **5**, 359–68.
6 Alt TH. (1987) Technical aids for dermabrasion. *J Dermatol Surg Oncol* **13**, 638–48.
7 Yarborough JM Jr. (1987) Dermabrasion by wire brush. *J Dermatol Surg Oncol* **13**, 610–5.
8 Padilla RS, Yarborough JM. (1998) Dermabrasion. In: *Dermatologic Surgery.* Ratz JL, ed. Philadelphia: Lippincott-Raven, pp. 473–84.
9 Murphy GF. (1997) Histology of the skin. In: Elder D, et al., eds. *Lever's Histopathology of the Skin,* 8th edn. Philadelphia: Lippincott, pp. 42–3.

10 Kirsner RS. (2012) Wound healing. In: Bolognia JL, *et al*., eds. *Dermatology*, 3rd edn. Oxford: Elsevier, pp. 2313–325.
11 Harmon CB, Zelickson BD, Roenigk RK, *et al.* (1995) Dermabrasive scar revision. Immunohistochemical and ultrastructural evaluation. *Dermatol Surg* **21**, 503–508.
12 Campbell RM, Harmon CB. (2008) Dermabrasion in our practice. *J Drugs Dermatol* **7**, 124–8.
13 Roenigk HH Jr. (1977) Dermabrasion for miscellaneous cutaneous lesions (exclusive of scarring from acne). *J Dermatol Surg Oncol* **3**, 322–8.
14 Quezada N, Machado Filho CA, *et al.* (2011) Melanocytes and keratinocytes transfer using sandpaper technique combined with dermabrasion for stable vitiligo. *Dermatol Surg* **37**, 192–8.
15 Awad SS. (2012) Dermabrasion may repigment vitiligo through stimulation of melanocyte precursors and elimination of hyperkeratosis. *J Cosmet Dermatol* **11**, 318–22.
16 Manstein D, Herron GS, Sink RK, *et al.* (2004) Fractional photothermolysis: a new concept for cutaneous remodeling using microscopic patterns of thermal injury. *Lasers Surg Med* **34**, 426–38.
17 Ong MW, Bashir SJ. (2012) Fractional laser resurfacing for acne scars: a review. *Br J Dermatol* **166**, 1160–9.
18 Yarborough JM Jr. (1988) Ablation of facial scars by programmed dermabrasion. *J Dermatol Surg Oncol* **14**, 292–4.
19 Jared Christophel J, Elm C, Endrizzi BT, *et al.* (2012) A randomized controlled trial of fractional laser therapy and dermabrasion for scar resurfacing. *Dermatol Surg* **38**, 595–602.
20 Coleman WP 3rd, Yarborough JM, Mandy SH. (1996) Dermabrasion for prophylaxis and treatment of actinic keratoses. *Dermatol Surg* **22**, 17–21.
21 Rubenstein R, Roenigk HH Jr, Stegman SJ, Hanke CW. (1986) Atypical keloids after dermabrasion of patients taking isotretinoin. *J Am Acad Dermatol* **5**(2 Pt 1), 280–85.
22 Pinski JB. (1987) Dressings for dermabrasion: new aspects. *J Dermatol Surg Oncol* **13**, 673.
23 Alexiades-Armenakas MR, Bernstein LJ, Friedman PM, Geronemus RG. (2004) The safety and efficacy of the 308-nm excimer laser for pigment correction of hypopigmented scars and striae alba. *Arch Dermatol* **140**, 955–60.

SECTION 4 Skin Modulation Techniques

CHAPTER 50
Laser-assisted Hair Removal

Keyvan Nouri,[1] Voraphol Vejjabhinanta,[2] Nidhi Avashia,[3] and Jinda Rojanamatin[2]

[1] University of Miami Miller School of Medicine, Miami, FL, USA
[2] Institute of Dermatology, Bangkok, Thailand
[3] Boston University School of Medicine, Boston, MA, USA

> **BASIC CONCEPTS**
>
> - Current options for hair removal include shaving, epilation, depilatories, electrolysis, and, more efficiently, lasers.
> - Lasers are fast, safe, and effective when used appropriately.
> - Selective photothermolysis is the key concept in laser hair removal.
> - By varying specific parameters such as wavelength, pulse duration, and fluence, certain specific chromophores may be targeted while protecting other tissues.
> - Melanin is the main endogenous chromophore in hair follicles.
> - In permanent hair reduction, heat from the laser must spread from the hair shaft to the bulb and the bulge of the hair.
> - Adverse effects reported after laser-assisted hair removal including erythema, perifollicular edema, crusting, vesiculation, hypopigmentation, and hyperpigmentation.

Introduction

The use of lasers for hair removal, or photoepilation, is becoming increasingly popular. According to the American Society for Aesthetic Plastic Surgery (ASAPS), nearly 11.7 million cosmetic surgical and non-surgical procedures were performed in the USA in 2007. ASAPS, which has been collecting multispecialty procedural statistics since 1997, notes the number of cosmetic procedures has increased 457% [1]. Laser hair removal is one of the top, non-surgical, cosmetic procedures with 1 412 657 performed in 2007.

Hair removal is of great interest because excess hair, especially in those with hypertrichosis or hirsutism, can be socially and psychologically troubling [2]. The psychosocial importance of hair is great, as noted by patient distress over both hair loss and excess hair [3]. Current options for hair removal include shaving, epilation, depilatories, electrolysis, and, more efficiently, lasers [4]. All of these hair removal methods possess side effects, yet lasers are fast, safe, and effective when used appropriately. The concept of laser hair removal was defined in 1998 by the US Food and Drug Administration (FDA). Following this, manufacturers were given permission to use the term "permanent hair reduction" in their materials. The FDA definition of permanent hair reduction included "long-term, stable reduction in the number of hairs regrowing after a treatment regimen." Thus, permanent hair removal does not imply the total elimination of hairs [5], but rather a significant reduction in growth rate. Complete hair loss is defined as a lack of regrowing hairs, which can be temporary or permanent. However, permanent hair loss is defined as lack of regrowing hair indefinitely. Hair removal with lasers produces complete but temporary hair loss for 1–3 months [6].

Biology of hair follicles

Hair is a skin appendage, present on the entire body except for the palms and soles. There are approximately 5 million hair follicles on the adult body with a density of 40–800/cm^2. They are made of keratin fibers supported by specialized dermal structures. Hair is formed from the matrix epithelial cells at the base of the hair follicle. The hair matrix is contained in the hair bulb, which is the deep bulbous portion of the hair follicle that surrounds the dermal papilla. The bulge of the hair is the reservoir for hair stem cells. In permanent hair reduction, heat from the laser must spread from the hair shaft to the bulb and the bulge of the hair. Heating only the hair matrix is not sufficient for permanent hair reduction.

Cosmetic Dermatology: Products and Procedures, Second Edition. Edited by Zoe Diana Draelos.
© 2016 John Wiley & Sons, Ltd. Published 2016 by John Wiley & Sons, Ltd.

Table 50.1 Hair cycles for various body sites.

Body site	Anagen (%)	Telogen (%)	Anagen duration (months)	Telogen duration (months)	Follicular depth (mm)
Scalp	85	15	24–72	3–4	3–5
Upper lip	65	35	3–4	1–2	1–2
Axillae	30	70	3–4	2–3	3–4
Arms	20	80	2–4	2–4	2–3
Legs	20	80	5–7	3–6	3–4
Bikini area	30	70	1–3	2–3	3–4

There is no formation of new hair follicles throughout life, so, as the body expands, the density decreases. Hair changes throughout our lifetime. A single follicle can form several different types of hairs ranging from lanugo in preterm newborns to vellus hairs in children to terminal hairs in adults. Lanugo is fine, non-pigmented hairs present at birth. Vellus hairs are fine, short, non-pigmented hairs known as "peach fuzz." Terminal hairs are the thick, usually pigmented, hairs of the scalp and secondary sexual areas. Terminal hairs are the targets of photoepilation.

Hair does not grow continuously, but instead grows in three phases: anagen, catagen, and telogen. The anagen phase is known as the growth phase. Catagen is the transition phase. Telogen is the resting phase. The cycle for scalp hairs is not only asynchronous but lasts 3–5 years. The duration of the hair cycle varies depending on body location (Table 50.1). Photoepilation is most effective during certain phases of the hair growth cycle.

The regulation of hair growth is influenced by genetic factors and hormones, particularly androgens. The function of hair, while primarily psychosocial, serves to protect from mechanical, thermal, and UV damage [3]. Thus, hair removal is important for appearance and not functional reasons. The basic concepts of laser-assisted hair removal are discussed next.

Basic concepts of laser-assisted hair removal

Selective photothermolysis is the key concept in laser hair removal, known as photoepilation. Photoepilation causes thermal destruction of the hair follicle and its associated stem cells at the hair bulge. By varying specific parameters such as wavelength, pulse duration, and fluence, certain specific cutaneous chromophores may be targeted while protecting other tissues [7]. Whether the hair is in telogen at the time of removal is important, because only anagen hairs are sensitive to photothermolysis. Because melanin is the main chromophore in hair follicles, the corresponding wavelength spectrum would range from UV to near-infrared light. Longer wavelengths are preferred, because the chromophore lies deep in the skin and the penetration of light increases with wavelength.

The specific target in laser hair removal is melanin and the light emitted must be within the absorption spectrum of melanin, which is 250–1200 nm [8]. Melanin is an endogenous chromophore found in the hair bulb, bulge, and shaft. Thus, in the range of 600–1100 nm, deep dermal melanin absorption may be used for selective photothermolysis of hair follicles [9].

A drawback to the use of lasers for hair removal, especially in those with darker skin, is that melanin resides in the epidermis. This is problematic because epidermal melanin can interfere with photoepilation by distracting the laser energy, but can also lead to certain side effects, such as epidermal damage and pigmentation. Thus, proper preoperative management is essential to achieving superior results.

Preoperative management

Discrepancy can exist between patient expectations for laser-assisted hair removal and the actual effects of such a treatment. Open communication must exist between the care provider and the patient. Preoperative management for laser hair removal consists of three main steps: history and physical examination, counseling, and preparatory instructions (Table 50.2). First, an accurate patient history must be taken focusing on patient's expectations, current medications, scarring risk, and local infection including history of herpes virus infection in the area of treatment. Along with a complete history, a thorough physical examination is vital. The physical examination should assess the aspects of the patient's skin color, health condition, hair color, hair diameter, and hair density.

Following the workup of the patient, a counseling session is necessary. The patient must be advised that 4–6 weeks prior to laser treatment no plucking or other hair removal methods can be used in the treatment areas. Shaving and depilatory creams may be used as these methods do not remove the hair root, which is targeted by the laser. In addition, sun exposure and tanning should be limited. Bleaching of the skin with retinoic acid or hydroquinone can lighten the skin prior to laser treatment. Topical anesthetic creams or cryogenic sprays may be applied to the treatment area to reduce discomfort during the procedure. Cold compresses are also effective in reducing discomfort, erythema, and edema at the treatment area.

Table 50.2 Preoperative and postoperative procedures for hair removal.

History	Preoperative care (4 weeks prior to treatment)	Preoperative care (day before treatment)	Day of treatment	Postoperative care
Conditions that may cause hypertrichosis: hormonal, familial, drug, tumor	Sunscreen application	Shave area to be treated	Clean and remove make-up from area to be treated	Ice packs
History of HSV perioral and genitalis	Bleaching cream (hydroquinone) to those with darker skin	When indicated, start prophylactic antiviral	Apply topical anesthetic cream to treatment area 1–2 h prior to treatment	Avoid sun exposure and trauma
History of keloids/ hypertrophic scarring	No plucking, waxing, or electrolysis	When indicated, start prophylactic oral antibiotic		Mild topical steroid creams (if necessary)
Previous treatment modalities	Shaving or depilatory creams may be used			Prophylactic antiobiotics/ antivirals completed
Current medications				

HSV, herpes simplex virus infection.

The skin surface must be thoroughly cleansed of all makeup, anesthetic creams, and other applicants immediately prior to laser treatment. This may be done with a gentle cleanser, followed by a cloth, and should be allowed to dry completely.

Laser systems are dangerous hazards to the eye. Because there are high concentrations of melanin in the iris and in the retina, these areas are highly susceptible to damage by laser light. Every person in the room during laser treatment should wear protective eyewear that is certified for the wavelength of the laser in use. Because the patient usually lies supine, he or she may require full occlusive eye protection to prevent laser light from entering underneath a sunglasses or goggle type of protective eyewear [6].

Description of techniques

Long pulsed 694 nm ruby laser

The long pulsed ruby laser was the first widely used laser for hair removal (Table 50.3). This laser has the shortest wavelength at 694 nm of all the available lasers for hair reduction. It is absorbed the best by melanin but has the shortest penetration depth. Thus, this would mean that the ruby laser is the most effective at hair removal, but has the greatest potential for epidermal injury. A cooling hand-piece is used concomitantly during treatment to reduce the risk of injury by lowering the skin's temperature. This laser is ideal for those with light skin and dark hair, and penetrates the skin by only 1–2 mm. This laser is not recommended in darker skin types.

In a study demonstrating the efficacy of the ruby laser, 48 areas of unwanted facial and body hair from 25 patients with blonde, brown, or black hair were treated with the long pulsed ruby laser at fluences of 10–40 J/cm^2. Hair regrowth was measured at 4 weeks after the first treatment, 4 weeks after the second treatment, 4 weeks after the third treatment, and 16 weeks after the third treatment by counting the number of terminal hairs compared with baseline pretreatment values. The mean percent of regrowth after the first treatment was 65.5%, 41% after the second treatment, and 34% after the third treatment. Overall, regardless of skin type or targeted body region, patients who underwent three treatment sessions demonstrated an average 35% regrowth in terminal hair count [10].

Long pulsed 755 nm alexandrite laser

The long pulsed alexandrite laser has a wavelength of 755 nm. This longer wavelength allows deeper penetration into the dermis with less absorption by epidermal melanin. This causes less adverse side effects such as pigmentation in darker skin patients. This laser is still typically used for patients with lighter skin types, but can also be used in those with darker skin. The adverse effects of this laser, when used on patients with darker skin types, can include blistering, crusting, and alterations of

Table 50.3 Step-by-step technique for hair removal.

Skin preparation	Visibility	Treatment fluence	Technique	Cooling
Remove anesthetic cream, makeup	Treatment grid or Seymour light in order to prevent skipped areas and double treatment	Ideal treatment parameters individualized for each patient, increase fluence carefully while monitoring for adverse effects	Slightly overlapping laser pulses are delivered with a predetermined spot size and highest tolerable fluence to obtain best results	Cooling gel applied prior to pulses if device is not equipped with cooling feature

pigment, even when skin cooling devices are used. In patients classified as having the darkest skin, residual hypopigmentation or hyperpigmentation is the rule with the alexandrite laser.

Long pulsed 800 nm diode laser

The 800 nm diode laser is comparable to the 755 nm alexandrite laser, and has become more popular along with the neodymium:yttrium aluminum garnet (Nd:YAG) laser for treating patients with darker skin types. The diode laser is more effective for laser-assisted hair removal in patients with dark skin because of the higher absorption by melanin than is seen with the Nd:YAG laser. Still, temporary adverse effects have been reported with the use of the diode laser in the form of postinflammatory hyperpigmentation when used on individuals with dark skin.

A retrospective study of 313 consecutive laser-assisted hair removal treatments was conducted on a total of 23 patients (22 women, 1 man) with 58 anatomic areas by means of an alexandrite laser. The long pulsed alexandrite system was used at a 755 nm wavelength to deliver fluences ranging 17–25 J/cm^2 through a 10 mm spot size. The results showed that patients who undergo more treatment sessions achieve a higher rate of hair reduction; although this may be concomitant with an increase in the incidence of adverse effects. The benefit of more laser treatments should be balanced with the risk of occurrence of side effects in each patient [11].

1064 nm Nd:YAG laser

The 1064 nm Nd:YAG has the longest wavelength and deepest penetration amongst the aforementioned laser systems available. It is not very well absorbed by melanin, but is sufficient in achieving selective photothermolysis and has superior penetration. This laser is able to penetrate the skin to 5–7 mm, a depth at which most of the target structures lay. Furthermore, the combination of a low melanin absorption and deep penetration leads to less collateral damage to the melanin-containing epidermis. These features make this particular laser the safest method to treat all skin types, especially darker skinned patients (Figure 50.1). Unfortunately, while this laser may be the safest, it is not the most effective. In a study by Bouzari et al. [12], hair reduction by the long pulsed Nd:YAG, alexandrite, and diode lasers were compared. They found that after 3 months, the Nd:YAG was the least effective of the three.

Intense pulsed light

The intense pulsed light (IPL) system is not a laser, but has recently entered the hair removal realm as a competent contender. It has been used for virtually all of the same indications as laser systems. IPL systems utilize a xenon bulb as a light source, which produces polychromatic light with wavelengths of 515–1200 nm. This is in contrast to laser light sources, which produce monochromatic light of a specific wavelength. Light emitted by the bulb passes through a filter that excludes shorter wavelengths which may severely damage skin. The ability to "tune" the wavelength of light emitted by these systems gives IPL systems the advantage of versatility. Using different filters, a pulsed light system could mimic any number of laser systems, allowing the operator to treat many different conditions amenable to light therapy, including, of course, the removal of unwanted hair (Figure 50.2).

Radiofrequency combinations

Radiofrequency devices have been combined with both IPL and diode lasers to provide optimal hair removal treatments to a wider range of skin types. The combinations are considered safe for patients with darker skin types because the radiofrequency energy is not absorbed by melanin in the epidermis. This technology, termed electro-optical synergy (ELOS) has a dual mechanism of heating the hair follicle with electrical energy (radiofrequency) and heating the hair shaft with optical energy.

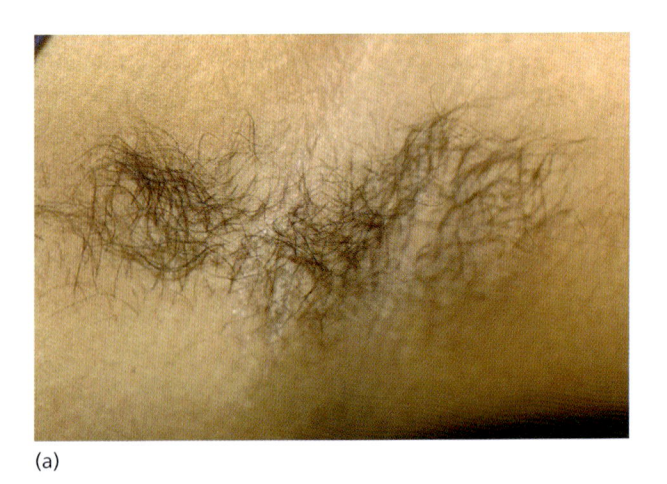

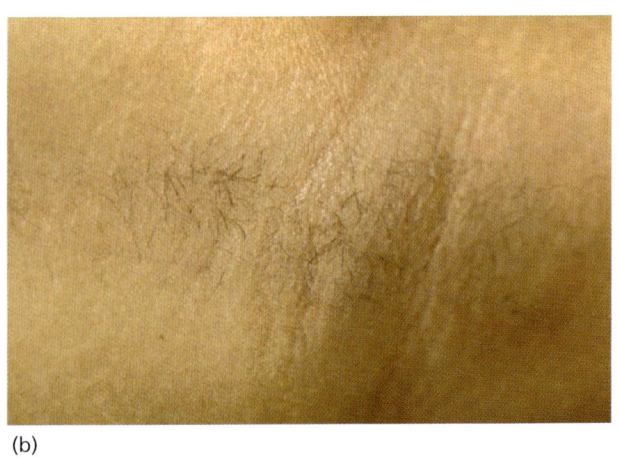

Figure 50.1 (a) Pretreatment of the right axillary area with coarse hair. (b) Only fine hair exists after 3 months after five treatments with a 1064 nm Nd:YAG laser.

(a) (b)

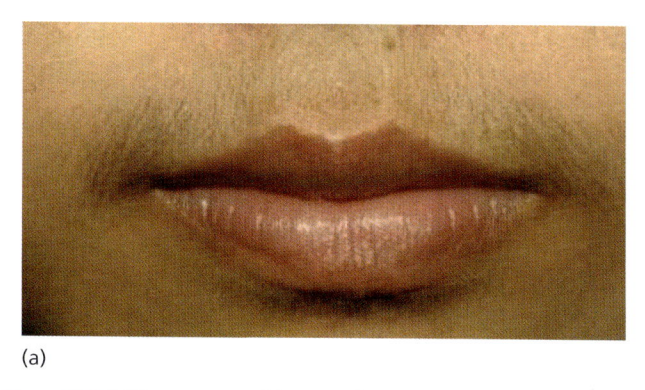

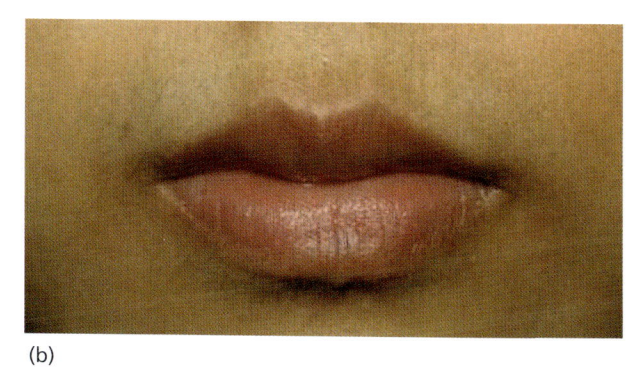

Figure 50.2 (a) Pretreatment of the upper lip area. (b) Seven weeks after two treatments with intense pulsed light (IPL) system.

Other removal methods for non-pigmented hair

Meladine, a topical melanin pigment, has been studied in Europe with interesting results. The liposome solution dye, which is sprayed on, is selectively absorbed by the hair follicle and not the skin. This in turn gives the follicles a temporary boost of melanin to optimize laser hair removal treatments. Clinical studies in Europe have shown vast permanent hair reduction in patients who used meladine prior to treatment. However, other studies have found meladine to only offer a delay of hair growth as opposed to permanent hair reduction [6].

Another option for non-pigmented hair removal is photodynamic therapy. A photosensitizer such as 5-aminolevulinic acid (5-ALA) is used because non-pigmented hair lacks a natural chromophore. In a study conducted to compare the 6-month hair removal efficacy of a combined pulsed light bipolar radiofrequency device with and without pretreatment using topical 5-ALA, researchers found that an average terminal white hair removal of 35% was observed at 6 months after treatment with the combined pulsed light bipolar radiofrequency device. When pretreatment with topical 5-ALA was provided the average hair removal of terminal white hairs was found to be 48%. This finding can be explained by the fact that light exposure activates the 5-ALA, which leads to the formation of reactive oxygen elements and slows for hair follicle destruction [13].

Postoperative management

Postoperative management consists of reducing pain and minimizing edema. This can be done using ice packs. Mild topical steroid creams can also be used to decrease redness. Antibiotics should be given if epidermal injuries occur during the procedure.

Complications

Although there is no obvious advantage of one laser system over another in terms of treatment outcome (except the Nd:YAG laser, which is found to be less efficacious, but more suited to patients with darker colored skin), laser parameters may be important when choosing the ideal laser for a patient. Adverse effects reported after laser-assisted hair removal including erythema and perifollicular edema, which are common, and crusting and vesiculation of treatment site, hypopigmentation, and hyperpigmentation (depending on skin color and other factors) (Figure 50.3).

Most complications are generally temporary. The occurrence of hypopigmentation after laser irradiation is thought to be related to the suppression of melanogenesis in the epidermis (which is reversible), rather than the destruction of melanocytes. Methods to reduce the incidence of adverse effects include lightening of the skin and sun avoidance prior to laser treatment, cooling of the skin during treatment, and sun avoidance and protection after treatment. Proper patient selection and tailoring of the fluence used to the patient's skin type remain the most important factors in efficacious and well-tolerated laser treatment. While it is generally believed that

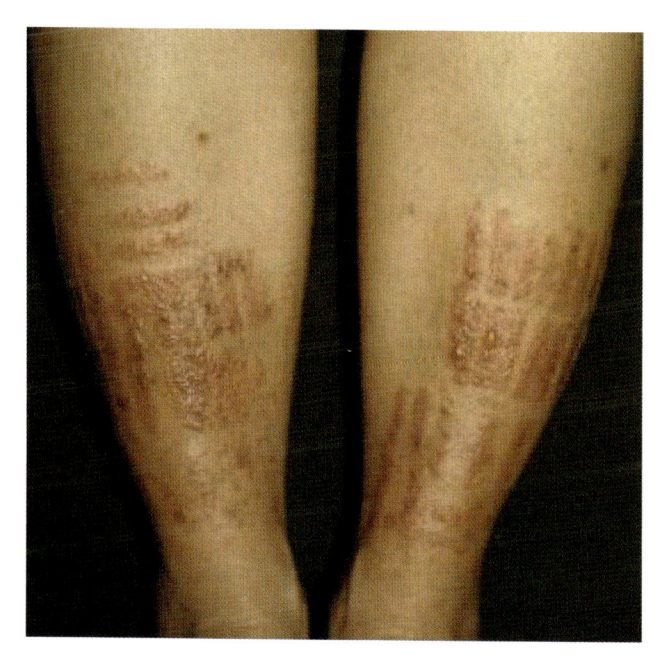

Figure 50.3 Blister formation 3 days after treatment with IPL system.

hair follicles are more responsive to treatment while they are in the growing (anagen) phase, conflicting results have also been reported. There is also no consensus on the most favorable treatment sites [14]. In addition, patients should be cautious and not use numbing agents on large areas of their body for prolonged periods of time as this can lead to methemoglobinemia.

Future directions

Laser hair removal is not FDA approved to be marketed as a permanent hair removal treatment. Further, manufacturers may not claim that laser hair removal is either painless or permanent unless the FDA determines that there are sufficient data to demonstrate such results. Several manufacturers received FDA permission to claim, "permanent reduction," not "permanent removal" for their lasers. This means that although laser treatments with these devices will permanently reduce the total number of body hairs, they will not result in a permanent removal of all hair.

There are many new laser hair removal systems that the FDA has approved for at home use and over-the-counter sales. These devices are diode laser, IPL, IPL+RF based technologies. Available data from uncontrolled clinical trials indicates short-term hair removal efficacy [15,16].

Conclusions

Up to 22% of women in North America have excessive or unwanted facial hair. Men also feel compelled to rid themselves of unwanted body hair, as dictated by popular culture and appearance anxieties. Excessive facial hair can negatively impact on one's quality of life. Prior options to hair removal have been painful, tedious, resulted in frustrated clients, and caused short-term effects. With the advent of laser technology, laser and light systems have becomes some of the most popular procedures. While this is still not a permanent solution to hair removal, is a safe, fast, and effective method for hair reduction.

References

1 American Society for Aesthetic Plastic Surgery (ASAPS). (2007) ASAPS 2007 Cosmetic Surgery National Data Bank Statistics. www.surgery.org/download/2007stats.prf Accessed 2008 Aug 20.
2 Nouri K, Trent JT. (2003) Lasers. In: NouriK, Leal-KhouriS, eds. *Techniques in Dermatologic Surgery*. St. Louis: Mosby, pp. 245–58.
3 Rassner G. (2004) *Atlas of Dermatology*. Philadelphia, PA: Lea & Febiger, pp. 224–6.
4 Olsen EA. (1999) Methods of hair removal. *J Am Acad Dermatol* **40**, 143–55.
5 Food and Drug Administration. (1998) FDA docket K980517. July 21.
6 Dierickx C, Crossman M. (2005) Laser hair removal. In: Golderg DJ, ed. *Lasers and Lights*, Vol. **2**. China: Elsevier-Saunders, pp. 61–76.
7 Anderson RR, Parrish JA. (1983) Selective photothermolysis: precise microsurgery by selective absorption of pulsed radiation. *Science* **220**, 524–7.
8 Battle EF, Hobbs LM. (2003) Lasers in dermatology: four decades of progress. *J Am Acad Dermatol* **49**, 1–31.
9 Mandt N, Troilius A, Drosner M. (2005) Epilation today: physiology of the hair follicle and clinical photoepilation. *J Investig Dermatol Symp Proc* **10**, 271–4.
10 Williams R, Havoonjian H, Isagholian K, *et al.* (1998) Clinical study of hair removal using the long-pulsed ruby laser. *Dermatol Surg* **24**, 837–42.
11 Bouzari N, Nouri K, Tabatabai H, Abbasi Z, Firooz A, Dowlati I. (2005) The role of number of treatments in laser-assisted hair removal using a 755-nm alexandrite laser. *J Drugs Dermatol* **4**, 573–8.
12 Bouzari N, Tabatabai H, Abbasi Z, *et al.* (2004) Laser hair-removal: comparison of long-pulsed Nd:YAG, long-pulsed aleandrite, and long-pulsed diode lasers. *Dermatol Surg* **30**, 498–502.
13 Goldberg DJ, Marmur ES, Hussain M. (2005) Treatment of terminal and vellus non-pigmented hairs with an optical/bipolar radiofrequency energy source: with and without pretreatment using topical aminolevulinic acid. *J Cosmet Laser Ther* **7**, 25–8.
14 Liew SH. (2002) Laser hair removal: guidelines for management. *Am J Clin Dermatol* **3**, 107–15.
15 Wheeland RG. (2012) Permanent hair reduction with a home-use diode laser: Safety and effectiveness 1 year after eight treatments. *Lasers Surg Med* **44**, 550–7.
16 Thaysen-Petersen D, Bjerring P, Dierickx C, *et al.* (2012) A systematic review of light-based home-use devices for hair removal and considerations on human safety. *J Eur Acad Dermatol Venereol* **26**, 545–53.

CHAPTER 51
Radiofrequency Devices

Vic Narurkar

Bay Area Laser Institute, San Francisco, CA, and University of California Davis Medical School, Sacramento, CA, USA

> **BASIC CONCEPTS**
> - Radiofrequency devices have been introduced for non-surgical skin tightening of facial and non-facial skin.
> - The mechanism of action of these devices involves an initial immediate collagen contraction and a secondary wound healing response producing collagen deposition and remodeling with skin tightening over time.
> - Radiofrequency devices can be divided into monopolar and bipolar categories.
> - Monopolar radiofrequency utilizes an electrical current passed from the radiofrequency energy source through a monopolar electrode in the hand-piece and the current continues through the patient to the grounding pad, which completes the circuit.
> - Bipolar radiofrequency in conjunction with light and vacuum offer more superficial treatments, and, most recently, a combined unipolar and bipolar radiofrequency device has been introduced with control of depths of radiofrequency energies.

Introduction

Radiofrequency devices have been introduced for non-surgical skin tightening of facial and non-facial skin. The mechanism of action of these devices involves an initial immediate collagen contraction and a secondary wound healing response producing collagen deposition and remodeling with skin tightening over time. There has been a great deal of controversy surrounding the use of these devices when they were first introduced for non-surgical skin tightening. With the advent of newer protocols utilizing lower energies and multiple passes, the safety and efficacy of radiofrequency devices is increasing. New directions include introduction of radiofrequency energy through cannulas and the expanded use of these technologies in combination with injectables.

Radiofrequency devices

Radiofrequency devices can be divided into monopolar and bipolar categories (Table 51.1). Monopolar radiofrequency utilizes an electrical current passed from the radiofrequency energy source through a monopolar electrode in the hand-piece and the current continues through the patient to the grounding pad, which completes the circuit. The Thermage device is an example of monopolar radiofrequency. Bipolar radiofrequency devices employ a closed system and are usually combined with other sources. Examples include systems using bipolar radiofrequency and light (electro-optical synergy systems), bipolar radiofrequency and vacuum, and a combination of unipolar and bipolar radiofrequency to deliver different depths of radiofrequency current to the skin.

Table 51.1 Examples of radiofrequency devices.

Mechanism	Examples of commercial devices
Monopolar RF	Thermage CPT(Solta), Exilis (BTL), Vanquish (BTL), Pellefirm (Ellman), TruSculpt (Cutera)
Mono/bipolar RF	Accent (Alma)
Bipolar RF	E-prime (Syneron), E-matrix (Syneron)
Tripollar RF	Apollo (Pollogen)
Multipolar RF	Venus Freeze, Swan and Legacy (Venus)
Bipolar RF/vacuum	Velashape (Syneron), Reaction (Viora)
Temperature control RF	ThermiRF (Thermiaesthetics)

Monopolar radiofrequency

Monopolar capacitive radiofrequency was the first commercially available device to be introduced for non-surgical skin tightening and is the most widely studied. The generation of heat occurs because of natural tissue resistance to the movement of electrons within a radiofrequency field which creates heat relative to the amount of current and time. The different

---

Cosmetic Dermatology: Products and Procedures, Second Edition. Edited by Zoe Diana Draelos.
© 2016 John Wiley & Sons, Ltd. Published 2016 by John Wiley & Sons, Ltd.

components of skin (dermis, fat, subcutaneous tissue, muscle, and fibrous tissue) have varying resistance to the movement of radiofrequency energy. For example, the fibrous septa are heated more than the surrounding subcutaneous tissue.

Controlled radiofrequency pulses selectively heat zones of the dermis and deeper tissue with the use of cryogen delivery to protect and cool the epidermis. A pressure-sensitive tip prevents the non-uniform application of energy to the skin and the cryogen delivery minimizes epidermal compromise and assists in comfort of the procedure.

The initial approach to utilize monopolar radiofrequency for skin tightening employed very high fluencies with one to two treatments. The discharge time was slow and the protocol was to utilize the highest tolerable fluence with a single pass over the entire treated area. With this protocol, the results were modest at best with significant pain. Moreover, the discharge time of the tip was slow at 5–6 seconds. In addition to significant discomfort and high variability in efficacy, infrequent reports of subcutaneous tissue depressions were reported (Figure 51.1). As a result, the treatment received much skepticism and criticism.

The Thermacool device utilizes monopolar radiofrequency energy with a maximal output of 225 J/cm^2 with a peak temperature 2–3 mm beneath the surface. Upon activation of the device, a cooling system which uses a cryogen spray is activated and internally precools the electrode. The cryogen continues to be delivered during (parallel cooling) and after (post-cooling) the energy delivery. The initial treatment cycle consisted of 6 seconds but the newer protocol is about 2 seconds.

A new protocol was developed to overcome these limitations based on observations and studies demonstrating that low fluence delivery with multiple passes of monopolar radiofrequency can produce a more reproducible clinical endpoint. Histologic correlations to these findings demonstrated greater collagen denaturation at multiple passes using lower energies. In addition, lower energies produced less discomfort and greater patient satisfaction. A consensus panel published these findings with the following criteria:

1. Use of patient feedback about heat sensation as a valid and preferred method for selecting the optimal amount of energy;
2. Use of multiple passes at moderate energy settings to yield consistent efficacy; and
3. Treatment to a clinical endpoint of visible tightening and contouring for maximizing predictability and long-term results.

With the original treatment protocol (single pass and high fluence) 26% of patients showed immediate tightening and 54% showed delayed tightening. With the new protocol, 87% showed immediate tightening and 92% noted tightening after 6 months, with 94% of patients of the patients showing satisfaction.

The largest studied areas for monopolar radiofrequency are the midface, lower face, and neck. The technique with the new protocol utilizes a tip that can deliver up to 900 pulses using multiple low fluence passes (typically 450 per each side of the face and neck). Treatments are administered without any topical anesthesia or intravenous sedation, as patient feedback is critical for outcomes. Up to 10 passes are performed using this algorithm.

The greatest challenge in all skin tightening modalities is patient selection and setting expectations. Because three-dimensional changes are often difficult to capture in two-dimensional photography, it is imperative to have a detailed and thorough consultation to set realistic expectations. In our practice, we perform a detailed consultation to discuss the realistic goals of monopolar radiofrequency and emphasize the variability in results. Standardized photography is absolutely critical with standardized lighting and angles to capture subtle changes. Our criteria for patient selection include the following:

1. Patients who are absolutely averse to any surgical procedures for laxity such as rhytidectomy.
2. Patients who have had rhytidectomy and are showing signs of laxity.
3. Patients who are not surgical candidates because of risks associated with surgery.
4. Post-surgical patients who still show some laxity.
5. Off face loose skin, for which there are no other options.

We also offer this procedure to candidates who seek subtle body contouring, with emphasis on the word subtle.

Complications

Complications with monopolar radiofrequency are rare. With the old protocol, subcutaneous depressions were seen. Common transient side effects include mild erythema and edema. Slight tenderness post-treatments have been reported. Lack of proper contact with the skin can produce burns. With the new protocol, there have been no reports of permanent complications. All skin types can be treated, as radiofrequency is truly color blind and does not compete with melanin chromophores. There have been no reports of postinflammatory hyperpigmentation.

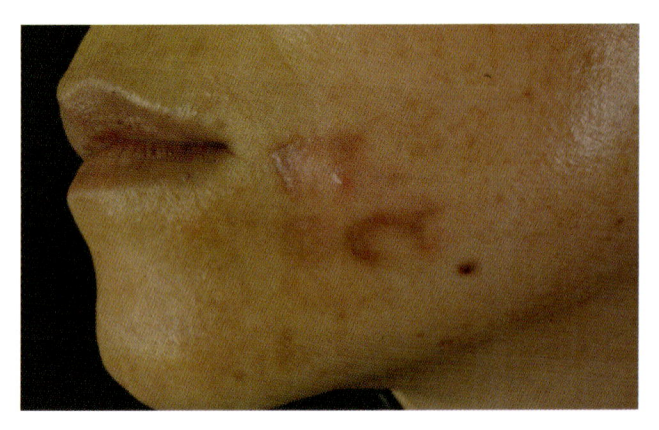

Figure 51.1 Subcutaneous atrophy from unipolar radiofrequency using old protocol with high fluencies.

Future directions

New directions for monopolar radiofrequency are the introduction of several new tips to address specific areas. These include tips for eyelid rejuvenation and large area body contouring. Eyelid rejuvenation has been one of the most exciting and innovative developments in monopolar radiofrequency tips. A shallow 0.25 cm^2 tip is utilized which delivers heat more superficially than the medium depth tips utilized for facial and body areas. Plastic corneoscleral shields are placed prior to treatment. Ideal candidates for eyelid treatment include patients with mild to moderate dermatochalasis and good skin tone and patients who have previously had blepharoplasty and show signs of skin laxity. With low fluence and multiple pass protocol, upper eyelid tightening and reduction of hooding has been seen in over 80% of patients. The newest addition to the tip armamentarium is the large diameter deep tip for large body areas. One of the limitations of treating large body areas has been the amount of time required for treatments. Recently, a 16 cm^2 deep tip was introduced which has shortened the treatment time by 50%. This allows for more efficient treatments of large body areas such as abdomen, buttocks, and flanks.

Summary

Monopolar radiofrequency, in summary, is the most widely studied modality for non-surgical skin tightening. The initial protocol has been modified with a low energy multiple pass algorithm to reduce discomfort and achieve more predictable outcomes. While midface and lower neck were the initial areas for treatments, the advent of varying depth tips has expanded the use for the treatment of eyelids and off face areas such as the abdomen, buttocks, and flanks. The biggest challenge in treatment outcomes is predictability of results, which are variable. Therefore, a thorough consultation setting realistic patient expectations and "underpromising" results are key for optimal outcomes. It is imperative to emphasize that these procedures are not a substitute for surgery and will not address severe laxity.

To further enhance outcomes of monopolar radiofrequency treatments, combination therapy approaches are being investigated. Most recently, we have initiated combining non-ablative fractional resurfacing, monopolar radiofrequency, and dermal fillers. Combination therapy is becoming the mainstay of treatments for a variety of non-surgical procedures. The combined non-ablative fractional resurfacing and monopolar radiofrequency procedure has been coined "Thermafrax," with the fractional resurfacing addressing dyschromia, superficial rhytids, and the monopolar radiofrequency addressing laxity. The treatments can be performed on the same day or as staged procedures. The radiofrequency treatments are performed first, as patient feedback is necessary and anesthesia cannot be used. This is followed by non-ablative fractional resurfacing. Dermal fillers are performed last for any volume depletion. Facial and non-facial skin can be effectively treated with this approach. Hand rejuvenation with combination of monopolar radiofrequency, non-ablative fractional resurfacing, and dermal fillers is becoming increasingly popular, with each modality complementing the other – radiofrequency addressing laxity, fractional resurfacing addressing dyschromia and photodamage, and fillers addressing volume loss (Figure 51.2).

Bipolar radiofrequency and light

The second commercially introduced modality for non-invasive skin tightening employed the combination of bipolar radiofrequency and light energy devices (900 nm diode laser in a single pulse or broadband light in the 700–2000 nm wavelength in a single pulse). The theory behind the use of two technologies is the safer delivery of radiofrequency energy, with the optical component enabling the bipolar radiofrequency energy to concentrate where the optical energy has selectively heated the target. Optical energy levels of 30–50 J/cm^2 with radiofrequency levels of 80–100 J/cm^2 are utilized in this mode. Three to four

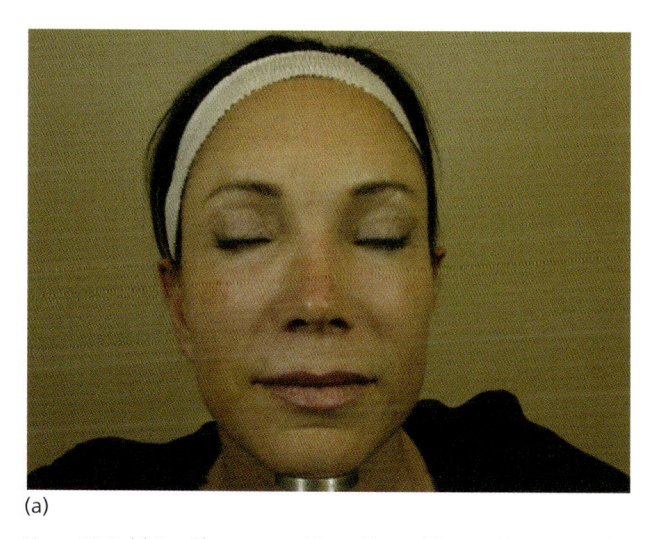

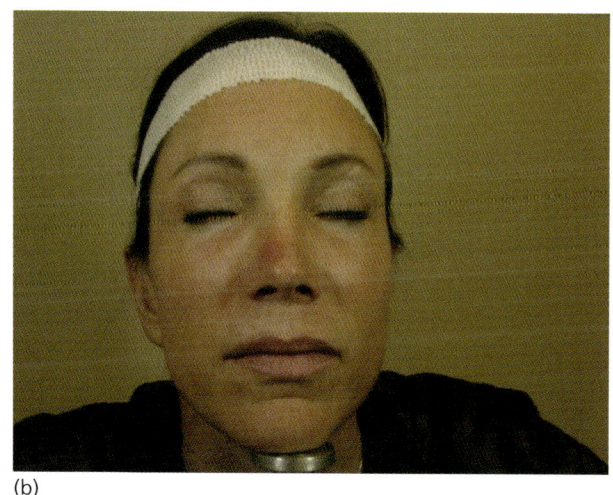

Figure 51.2 (a) Pre-Thermage and Fraxel laser. (b) Post-Thermage and Fraxel laser.

passes are usually performed and, unlike monopolar radiofrequency, 3–5 treatment sessions are necessary, as opposed to a single treatment.

The main indication for bipolar radiofrequency and light combination devices is diminution of superficial rhytids. There may be some subtle tissue tightening. There is much controversy regarding the synergistic effects of light and radiofrequency energies. The use of lower optical energies makes this a safe device in all skin types. However, because the radiofrequency energy does not penetrate very deep into the skin, tissue arcing can occur with improper technique, resulting in scar formation.

The majority of published clinical studies using these devices have focused on the treatment of mild to moderate rhytids with modest improvement. The amount of energy penetration with these devices does not produce deep volumetric heating and subsequent tightening compared with monopolar radiofrequency.

Bipolar radiofrequency and vacuum

Bipolar radiofrequency with vacuum was introduced to reduce discomfort associated with radiofrequency devices. The bipolar radiofrequency energy with an accompanying vacuum apparatus allows the tissue into the vacuum and targets the radiofrequency energy to the deep dermis. Less energy is necessary for treatment efficacy, as the vacuum brings the electrodes closer to the dermis, with the additional benefit of reducing pain. The main indications for this technology are subtle improvement of fine rhytids and tissue tightening.

Unipolar and bipolar radiofrequency device

Different depths of radiofrequency energy can be delivered to the skin – bipolar for more superficial heating and unipolar for deeper heating. It is a closed system and does not require grounding, as monopolar radiofrequency. Published data are limited and there is some evidence in the reduction of the appearance of cellulite and subtle tissue tightening.

Subdermal radiofrequency

Subdermal radiofrequency is a minimally invasive procedure which evolved from the use of radiofrequency for nerve ablation to treat glabellar furrows. A small probe is inserted underneath the skin through a needle hole. Radiofrequency is emitted through an electrode at the tip of the probe. In addition, there is a temperature gauge on the probe which monitors the exact temperature that will reach the target and a thermal camera for measurement of the surface skin temperature to avoid burns. At this time, the device is being used off label for skin tightening and there is nothing published in the literature of long term safety and efficacy.

Conclusions

Non-surgical tissue tightening has evolved considerably since its first introduction. Monopolar radiofrequency using a new treatment algorithm remains the gold standard of radiofrequency, with the largest series of published papers, longest clinical experience, and modifications for optimal outcomes. Bipolar radiofrequency in conjunction with light and vacuum offers more superficial treatments, and, most recently, a combined unipolar and bipolar radiofrequency device has been introduced with control of depths of radiofrequency energies.

The greatest challenge in all modalities of radiofrequency treatments is predictability of outcomes. Patient selection with a thorough consultation reviewing realistic expectations is key for successful outcomes. The development of newer algorithms with standardized protocols is allowing for more reproducible outcomes in using these devices for non-surgical skin tightening.

Future directions of radiofrequency include the use of minimally invasive probes that can deliver radiofrequency energy subdermally with precise temperature monitoring which may give more consistent and predictable outcomes for skin tightening.

Further reading

Alster TS, Tanzi E. (2004) Improvement of neck and cheek laxity with a nonablative radiofrequency device: a lifting experience. *Dermatol Surg* **30**, 503–7.

Biesman B, Baker SS, Carruthers J, et al. (2006) Monopolar radiofrequency treatment of human eyelids: a prospective multicenter efficacy trial. *Lasers Surg Med* **38**, 890–8.

Chipps LK, Bentow J, Prather HB, et al. (2013) Novel nonablative radiofrequency rejuvenation device applied to the neck and jowls: clinical evaluation and 3 dimensional image analysis. *J Drugs Dermatol* **12**(11), 1215–8.

Doshi SN, Alster TS. (2005) Combination radiofrequency and diode laser for treatment of facial rhytids and skin laxity. *J Cosmet Laser Ther* **7**, 11–5.

Dover JS, Zelickson BD. (2007) 14 physician multispecialty consensus panel. Results of a survey of 5700 patient monopolar radiofrequency facial skin tightening treatments: assessment of a low energy multiple pass technique leading to a clinical endpoint algorithm. *Dermatol Surg* **33**, 900–7.

Emilia del Pino M, Rosado RH, Azuela A, et al. (2006) Effect of controlled volumetric tissue heating with radiofrequency on cellulite and the subcutaneous tissue of the buttocks and thighs. *J Drugs Dermatol* **5**, 714–22.

Fitzpatrick R, Geronemus R, Goldberg D, et al. (2003) Multicenter study of noninvasive radiofrequency for periorbital tissue tightening. *Lasers Surg Med* **33**, 232–2.

Fritz M, Counters JT, Zelickson BD. (2004) Radiofrequency treatment for middle and lower face laxity. *Arch Facial Plast Surg* **6**, 370–3.

Gold MH. (2007) Tissue tightening: a hot topic utilizing deep dermal heating. *Drugs Dermatol* **6**, 1238–42.

Gold MH, Goldman MD, Rao J, et al. (2007) Treatment of wrinkles and elastosis using vacuum assisted bipolar radiofrequency heating of the dermis. *Dermatol Surg* **33**, 303–9.

Jacobson LG, Alexiades-Armenakis M, Bernstein L, Geronemus RG. (2003) Treatment of nasolabial folds and jowls with a noninvasive radiofrequency device. *Arch Dermatol* **139**, 1371–2.

Kassim AT, Goldberg DJ. (2013) Assessment of the safety and efficacy of a bipolar multifrequency radiofrequency device in the treatment of skin laxity. *J Cosmet Laser Ther* **15**(2), 114–17.

Lack EB, Rachel JD, D'Andrea L, Corres J. (2005) Relationship of energy settings and impedance in different anatomic areas using a radiofrequency device. *Dermatol Surg* **31**, 1668–70.

Sadick NS. (2005) Combination radiofrequency and light energies: electro-optical synergy technology in esthetic medicine. *Dermatol Surg* **31**, 1211–7.

Weiss RA, Weiss MA, Munavalli G, Beasley KL. (2006) Monopolar radiofrequency facial tightening: a retrospective analysis of efficacy and safety in over 600 treatments. *J Drugs Dermatol* **5**, 707–12.

Yu CS, Yeung CK, Skek SY, Tse RK, Kono T, Chan HH. (2007) Combined infrared light and bipolar radiofrequency for skin tightening in Asians. *Lasers Surg Med* **39**, 471–5.

CHAPTER 52

LED Photomodulation for Reversal of Photoaging and Reduction of Inflammation

David McDaniel,[1] Robert Weiss,[2] Roy Geronemus,[3] Corinne Granger,[4] and Leila Kanoun-Copy[5]

[1]McDaniel Institute of Anti Aging Research, Virginia Beach, VA, Eastern Virginia Medical School, Norfolk VA and Old Dominion University Norfolk VA, USA
[2]Maryland Laser Skin & Vein Institute, Hunt Valley, MD, and Johns Hopkins University School of Medicine, Baltimore, MD, USA
[3]Laser & Skin Surgery Center of New York, NY, and New York University Medical Center, New York, NY, USA
[4]L'Oreal Research, Asnieres, France
[5]L'Oréal Research, Chevilly Larue, France

> **BASIC CONCEPTS**
> - Photomodulation uses non-thermal, photobiochemical mechanism based treatments to regulate the activity of cells rather than photothermal wound healing mechanisms.
> - Photomodulation stimulates cells to perform certain functions using light packets that are low energy and modulate cell metabolism.
> - LED arrays for photomodulation are useful for collagen stimulation, textural smoothing, and reduction of inflammation.
> - Photomodulation research has recently expanded to include new therapeutic areas such as scarring, pigment disorders, hair growth, nerve regeneration and other innovative applications.

Introduction

Photorejuvenation encompasses many procedures using light or laser-based technology to reverse the effects of photoaging. Photoaging, of which dermal collagen degeneration comprises a large component, is compounded by environmental damage including smoking, pollutants, and other insults causing free radical formation. Non-ablative photorejuvenation refers to the controlled use of thermal energy to accomplish skin rejuvenation without disturbance of the overlying epidermis and with minimal to no down-time. Currently employed non-ablative modalities include primarily intense pulsed light (IPL), visible wavelengths including 585nm pulsed dye laser (PDL), and 532 nm [CH1] green light (KTP laser) [1]. Various infrared wavelengths with water as the target are used for remodeling dermal collagen. Because absorption by melanin is negligible, these devices can be used for all skin types and these include 1064, 1320, 1450, and 1540 nm [2,3]. The primary mechanism of action is thermal injury either by heating the dermis to stimulate fibroblast proliferation or by heating blood vessels for photocoagulation [4,5,6]. The newest way to deliver these wavelengths is by fractionating the dose through microlenses that allow microthermal zones surrounded by normal skin [7].

A non-thermal mechanism, which represents a fundamental change in thinking, is the theory of photomodulation. This concept involves the stimulation of cells to perform certain functions using light packets that are low energy and stimulate or inhibit various cellular processes. This novel approach to photoaging uses non-thermal light treatments to regulate activity of cells rather than to invoke thermal wound healing mechanisms [8,9]. This incurs far less risk for patients than other light modalities. The first written report on using photomodulation to improve facial wrinkles was in 2002 [10].

Photomodulation was first discovered from use of LED and low energy light therapy (LILT) in stimulating growth of plant cells [11]. The belief that cell activity can be upregulated or downregulated by low energy light had been discussed in the past, but consistent or impressive results had been lacking [12,13]. Some promise had been shown with wound healing for oral mucositis [13]. Wavelengths previously examined included a 670 nm LED array [13], a 660 nm array [14], and higher infrared wavelengths [15]. Fluence and duration of exposure were variable in these studies with high energy required for modest results [13].

To investigate LED light for rejuvenation purposes, a fibroblast culture model was utilized in conjunction with clinical testing. Particular packets of energy with specific wavelengths combined with using a very specific propriety pulse sequencing

Cosmetic Dermatology: Products and Procedures, Second Edition. Edited by Zoe Diana Draelos.
© 2016 John Wiley & Sons, Ltd. Published 2016 by John Wiley & Sons, Ltd.

"code" were found to upregulate collagen I synthesis in fibroblast culture using reverse transcription polymerase chain reaction (RT-PCR) to measure collagen I [10]. The upregulation of fibroblast collagen synthesis correlated with the clinical observation of increased dermal collagen on treated human skin biopsies [16]. Curiously, both in the fibroblast and clinical model, collagen synthesis was accompanied by reduction of matrix metalloproteinases (MMP). In particular, MMP-1 (collagenase) was greatly reduced with exposure to 595–870 nm (in a 75%:25% ratio) low energy light. Use of very low energy, narrow band light with specific pulse code sequences and durations was termed LED photomodulation by McDaniel et al. [10]. A device that utilizes pulsed code sequences of LED light to induce photomodulation was termed Gentlewaves®.

Clinical applications

LED photomodulation can be used both alone and in combination with a variety of common, non-ablative, rejuvenation procedures in an office setting. Several anti-inflammatory and wound healing applications are also possible. Treatments were delivered using the yellow/infrared light LED photomodulation unit with a full face panel. Energy density was set at 0.15 J/cm2 and 100 pulses were delivered with a pulse duration of 250 ms and an off interval of 100 ms. Treatment time was approximately 35 seconds.

Photorejuvenation

This technique was evaluated on 6000+ patients over the last 6 years. Of these treatments, 10% were LED photomodulation alone and 90% were concomitant with a thermal-based photorejuvenation procedure. Using specific pulsing sequence parameters, which are the basis for the LED photomodulation "code," the original multicenter clinical trial was conducted with 90 patients receiving a series of eight LED treatments over 4 weeks [17,18,19,20]. This study showed positive results, with over 90% of patients improving by at least one Fitzpatrick photoaging category and 65% of the patients demonstrating global improvement in facial texture, fine lines, erythema, and pigmentation. Results peaked at 4–6 months following completion of a series of eight treatments [20]. Another retrospective study, using the same 590–870 nm LED array (Gentlewaves®), demonstrated similar results (Figure 52.1). These results were confirmed by digital microscopy [21].

Most recently, the 595/870 nm LED array was used in an independent clinical laboratory confirming the findings (data on file, L'Oréal Research, France). An additional clinical trial involving 65 subjects used silicone replica impressions of lateral canthal wrinkles (crow's feet). These replicas, illuminated by reproducible lighting both parallel and perpendicular to each wrinkle, were analyzed with image-analysis software (Quantirides, Monaderm, Monaco). The analysis showed a significant reduction in the number of wrinkles 2–4 months after treatment accompanied by a significant reduction in the length of wrinkles at 5 months post-treatment. Subject self-assessment showed significant improvement in skin wrinkles, texture, softness, and radiance"Most recently, the 595(870 nm LED array was used in an independent clinical laboratory confirming the findings (data on file, L'Oréal Research, France). An additional clinical trial involving 65 subjects used silicone replica impressions of lateral canthal wrinkles (crow's feet). These replicas, illuminated by reproducible lighting both parallel and perpendicular to each

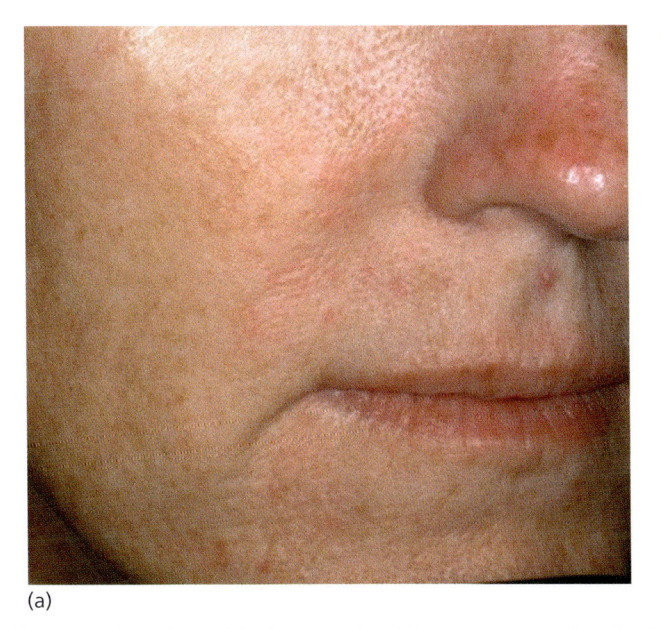

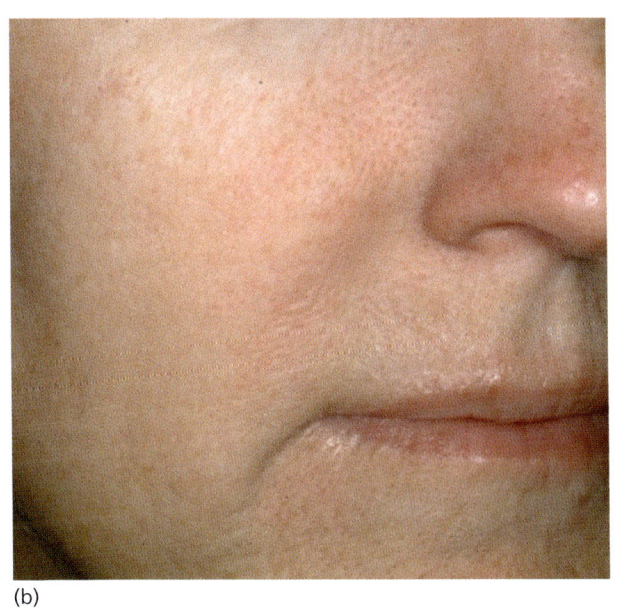

(a) (b)

Figure 52.1 Smoothing of the skin seen after eight treatments over 4 weeks of Gentlewaves® photomodulation (Gentlewaves, Inc., Charlotte, NC, USA) (a) Before treatments. (b) Eight weeks after baseline. Reduction in wrinkles, pigmentation and improvement of texture are noted.

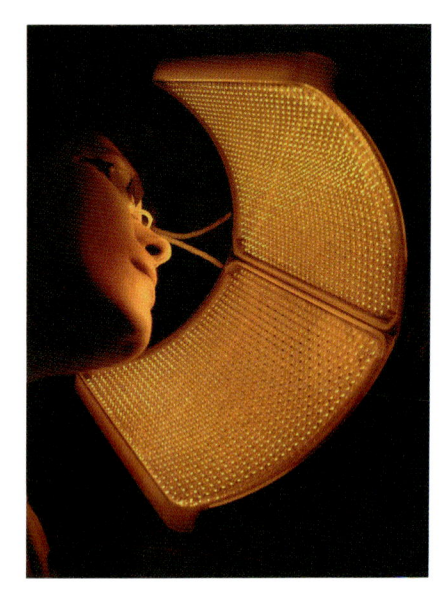

Figure 52.2 Gentlewaves LED photomodulation device. Array of LEDs.

wrinkle, were analyzed with image-analysis software (Quantirides, Monaderm, Monaco). The analysis showed a significant reduction in the number of wrinkles 2–4 months after treatment accompanied by a significant reduction in the length of wrinkles at 5 months post-treatment. Subject self-assessment showed significant improvement in skin wrinkles, texture, softness, and radiance."> [CM2]

Others have confirmed that additional wavelengths of LED light, using red and infrared wavelengths, may be effective for skin texture improvement. Although these treatments were longer in duration, 36 patients receiving nine treatments over a 5-week period showed improvement in skin softness [22]. Each treatment was administered in continuous mode, without pulsing, with a treatment time of 20 minutes using 633 and 830 nm as an LED array (Omnilux™, Phototherapeutics, Altrincham, Cheshire, UK). Another recent report using this system studied 31 subjects with facial rhytids who received nine light therapy treatments using combined wavelengths of 633 and 830 nm. Fluences were relatively high utilizing 126 J/cm2 for 633 nm and 66 J/cm2 for 830 nm. Improvements to the skin surface were reported at weeks 9 and 12 by profilometry performed on periorbital replicas. Results showed that 52% of subjects showed a 25–50% improvement in photoaging scores [23].

In the USA, the first Food and Drug Administration (FDA) cleared LED device to be used in the reduction of periocular wrinkles was in 2005 (Gentlewaves®; Figure 52.2). Other devices (Omnilux™, Photo Therapeutics Ltd., Altrincham, Cheshire, UK) then followed.

Anti-inflammatory effects

Photomodulation can also be used for the reduction of erythema from a variety of causes. Erythema may be induced from wide ranging skin injuries including but not limited to thermal laser treatments, UV burns, radiation therapy, blunt trauma, and skin disease. Treatment of atopic eczema in patients withdrawn from all topical medications led to resolution with 3–4 treatments over 1–2 weeks (Figure 52.3).

Use of LED photomodulation in combination with other laser modalities may results in faster erythema resolution. The enhanced erythema resolution may be a result of the anti-inflammatory effects of LED photomodulation. The complete mechanisms have not yet been elucidated but downregulation of inflammatory mediators from lymphocytes or macrophages is possible. Studies on human skin fibroblasts treated with LED photomodulation have shown a reduction in interleukins IL-1B1 and IL-6 [24].

A recent study looked at whether LED photomodulation therapy could accelerate resolution of post-intense pulsed light (IPL) erythema [25]. Fifteen subjects were randomized to receive LED treatment to one side of the face immediately following a single IPL treatment for photodamage. Results showed

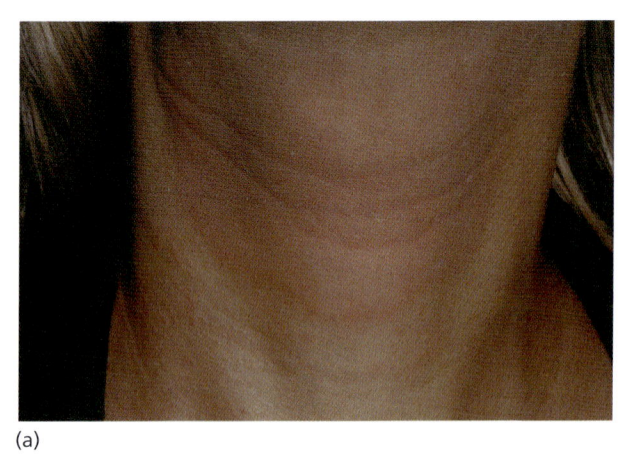

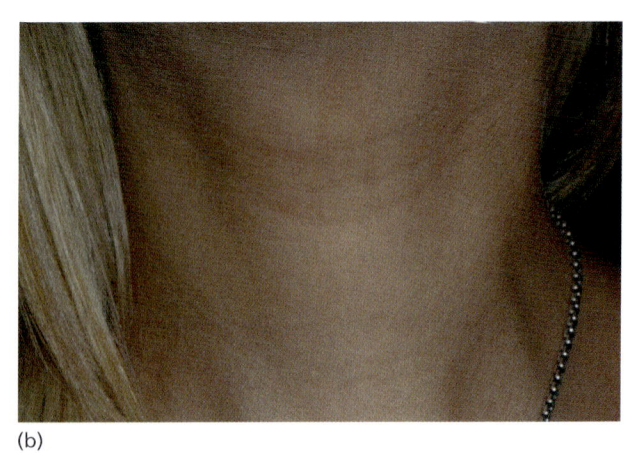

(a)   (b)

Figure 52.3 (a) Before shows flare of eczema following withdrawal of all therapy. (b) Atopic eczema after three treatments with Gentlewave LED photomodulation. The after image (b) shows effects of reduction of inflammation by LED photomodulation within 10 days.

mean erythema scores on the first visit were statistically significantly lower on the LED-treated side. This led the authors to conclude that LED photomodulation treatment may accelerate resolution of erythema following IPL treatment [25].

A study on radiation dermatitis examined whether LED photomodulation could alter and improve the outcome of intensity-modulated radiation treatments (IMRT) on overlying breast skin. Nineteen patients with breast cancer were treated with LED photomodulation immediately after every radiation session. Treatments were administered to post-lumpectomy patients receiving a full course of IMRT [26]. Skin reactions were monitored weekly using National Cancer Institute (NCI) criteria for grading. Age-matched controls ($n = 28$) received IMRT without LED photomodulation. The results of this study showed that LED treatment had a significantly positive effect. Of the LED treated patients, 94.7% (18) had grade 0 or 1 reaction and 5.3% (1) had a grade 2 reaction. Among controls, 4 (14.3%) had a grade 1 reaction and 24 (85.7%) had a grade 2 or 3 reaction. Of the non-LED treated group, 67.9% had to interrupt treatment because of side effects of skin breakdown with moist reactions but only 5% of the LED treated group had interrupted treatment. The authors concluded that not only did LED photomodulation treatments delivered immediately after each IMRT reduce the incidence of adverse NCI criteria skin reactions, but also allowed the full course of treatment and resulted in a final smoother skin texture with improved skin elasticity post-radiation treatment. Another study, focused on sensitive skin, demonstrated a significant decrease in the Erythema Index after an average of 9.9 treatments and a cumulative dose of 71.3 J/cm^2. Furthermore, the study utilized cultured human keratinocytes treated with a nontoxic dose of sodium lauryl sulphate to cause irritation prior to exposure to low level light. The resulting assay demonstrated a reduction in the release of VEGF from cells treated with low level light further indicating the anti-inflammatory capacity of photomodulation as well as indicating possible mechanism(s) of action [27].

Wound healing research of one type or another has quickly become one of the primary research foci for photomodulation's future. Literature searches will quickly turn up a variety of articles involving light and the potential benefits to wound healing of all types of injuries. One such study examined the effects of wavelengths of light on the wound healing of partial thickness dermal abrasion models in mice. 635, 730, 810 and 980 nm wavelengths were tested at equal fluence for evaluation via collagen accumulation, re-epithelialization, wound area size, and cytokeratin 14 and proliferating cell nuclear antigen staining. The results indicated biological response based on wavelength used as only 635 and 810 nm light showed any wound healing stimulation, with 810nm being most efficacious [28]. The wound healing research has begun to include lesions caused by herpes simplex labialis (HSL) as well as traditional wounding models. In a randomized, placebo controlled study examining the effect of 1072 nm IR light on time to re-epithilialization, where 87 patients suffering from HSL lesions were given 3 minutes of 1072 nm light therapy or sham treatment, the average time to complete re-epithilialization was decreased by 30% in photomodulated subjects [29].

Additional data indicates anti-inflammatory effect for LED photomodulation following UV-induced erythema. Using a solar simulator, findings indicate a photoprotective effect when delivered after UV radiation [24]. This concept is a rescue from UV damage even after inadvertant UV radiation has occurred. We have observed a reduction in UV erythema when LED photomodulation was supplied within hours after UV exposure. The use of 590–870 nm LED photomodulation produced significant downregulation of dermal matrix degrading enzymes, which were stimulated by the UV exposure [24]. Additionally, a pilot study with precise CO2 laser epidermal destruction has shown promise with using this device for accelerated wound healing.

Parallel to wound healing, use of photomodulation has been extended to a protective or preventative effect following several types of toxic injury. Experiments using LED light to protect the retina against the toxic actions of methanol-derived formic acid in a rodent model of methanol toxicity have been successful. In a recent study, LED treatment protected the retina from the histopathologic changes induced by methanol on mitochondrial oxidative metabolism in vitro and retinal protection in vivo [30]. Photomodulation may enhance recovery from retinal injury and other ocular diseases in which mitochondrial dysfunction is postulated to have a role.

Human retinal pigment epithelial (RPE) cells were treated with LED photomodulation produced by acute injury from blue light wavelengths [31]. The results showed reduction of cell death at 24 hours from 94% to 10–20%. Another in vitro test on human RPE cells showed a sevenfold reduction in vascular endothelial growth factor (VEGF) expression at 24 hours post-LED exposure using LED photomodulation at 590–870 nm delivered at 0.1 J/cm2 [32]. The RPE research has also included *in vivo* studies using a diabetic rodent model. The diabetes induced retinal abnormalities were assessed functionally and histologically in the animals and biochemically in a parallel RPE cell culture. The study demonstrated that daily treatments of 670 nm light at 6 J/cm^2 can significantly reduce the death of retinal ganglion cells, improved the photopic b wave response by 50%, and prevented diabetes induced overexpression of leukostasis and ICAM-1. In the cell culture model, the increased superoxide production, inflammatory biomarker expression and cell death were all inhibited by photobiomodulation [33]. The ability for 670 nm light to assist in prevention of retinopathy was confirmed in a second study, using not a diabetic, but a hyperoxia induced rat model. 9 J/cm^2 of 670 nm light therapy reduced neovascularization, vaso-obliteration and branching of retinal vessels caused by hyperoxia induced retinopathy [34].

Photodynamic therapy

LED red light (630 nm) has been used in combination with a sensitizer (levulinic acid) for photodynamic therapy (PDT) [30]. When exposed to light with the proper wavelength, the sensitizer produces an activated oxygen species, singlet oxygen, that oxidizes the plasma membrane of targeted cells. As a result of a lower metabolic rate, there is less sensitizer in the adjacent normal tissue, thus less of a reaction. One of the absorption peaks of the metabolic product of levulinic acid, protoporphyrin, absorbs strongly at 630 nm red. A red LED panel emitting at 630 nm (Omnilux PDT™, Phototherapeutics, Altrincham, Cheshire, UK) has been used for this purpose in Europe and Asia [31]. A full panel 590 nm LED array has also been used for facilitating PDT. This therapy is delivered by application of levulinic acid (Levulan™, DUSA, Wilmington, MA, USA) for 45 minutes and exposure to continuous (non-pulsed) 590–870 nm LED for 15 minutes for a cumulative dose of over 70 J/cm2. The results show reduction in actinic damage including improvement of skin texture and reduction of actinic keratoses [35]. While not directly PDT, as previously mentioned, photomodulation is being studied in combination with drugs for the treatment of many skin disorders like dermatophagoides farinae (Df) induced atopic dermatitis. 850nm LED treatment in conjunction with Tacrolimus (FK-506) in a Df induced mouse model demonstrated reduction in the severity of the lesions, increased serum levels of IgE and Nitric Oxide, reduced inflammatory infiltrate and recovery of skin barrier function [36].

One of the means for photomodulated upregulation of cell activity for collagen synthesis by LED is the activation of energy switching mechanisms in mitochondria, the energy source for cellular activity. Cytochrome molecules are believed to be responsible for the light absorption in mitochondria. Cytochromes are synthesized from protoporphyrin IX and absorb wavelengths of light from 562 to 600 nm. It is believed that LED light absorption causes conformational changes in antenna molecules within the mitochondrial membrane. Proton translocation initiates a pump, which ultimately leads to energy for conversion of adenosine diphosphate (ADP) to adenosine triphosphate (ATP). This essentially recharges the "cell battery" and provides more energy for cellular activity.

Others have confirmed that mitochondrial ATP availability can influence cellular growth and reproduction, with lack of mitochondrial ATP associated with oxidative stress [37]. Cellular aging may be associated with decreased mitochondrial DNA activity [38]. It has been concluded that LED light represents a novel, non-invasive, therapeutic intervention for the treatment of numerous diseases linked to mitochondrial dysfunction [39].

Previous work has also demonstrated rapid ATP production within mitochondria of cultured fibroblasts exposed to 590–870 nm yellow/infrared LED light only with the proper pulsing sequence [9,40]. New ATP production occurs rapidly after LED photomodulation, triggering subsequent metabolic activity of fibroblasts [19]. There also appear to be receptor-like mechanisms, which result in modulation of the expression of gene activity producing upregulation or downregulation of gene activity as well as wide-ranging cell signaling pathway actions. It has also been shown that near IR light alters the mitochondrial biogenesis signalling in cell culture [41]. The choice of photomodulation parameters has a vital role in determining the overall pattern of gene upregulation and/or downregulation. In our experience, use of LED yellow/infrared light without the proper pulsing sequence leads to minimal or no consequences on mitochrondrial ATP production.

Conclusions

LED arrays for photomodulation are useful for collagen stimulation, textural smoothing, and reduction of inflammation. Pilot wound healing studies show slightly accelerated wound resolution. Cellular rescue from UV damage and other toxic insults has been shown in small studies. Thermal, non-ablative photorejuvenation and non-thermal LED photomodulation have a synergistic effect. LED photomodulation is delivered immediately subsequent to the thermal-based treatment for its anti-inflammatory effects, which may reduce the thermally induced erythema and edema of non-ablative treatments. Delivery of LED light immediately before and after UV or thermal injury appears to increase anti-inflammatory and protective effects.

As photomodulation gains in popularity, applications arise from expanding research. For example, treatment of hyperpigmentation with 830 and 850 nm LEDs demonstrate the ability to inhibit melanin synthesis *in vitro* as evidenced by decreased expression of the tyrosinase family of genes (i.e. TRP1 and TRP2) [42]. New data is being published on the beneficial effects of photomodulation on a monthly basis for applications like enhanced blood vessel growth, hair growth/alopecia improvement, and dopaminergic cell survival in the brain [43,44,45]. Currently LED photomodulation has been studied and shown to be effective extensively in skin [46], but continuing new research will only expand as the technology improves and allows photomodulation to reach areas that current therapies cannot.

References [CH3]

1 Weiss RA, Weiss MA, Beasley KL, Munavalli G. (2005) Our approach to non-ablative treatment of photoaging. *Lasers Surg Med* **37**, 2–8.

2 Munavalli GS, Weiss RA, Halder RM. (2005) Photoaging and nonablative photorejuvenation in ethnic skin. *Dermatol Surg* **31**, 1250–60.

3 Weiss RA, McDaniel DH, Geronemus RG. (2003) Review of nonablative photorejuvenation: reversal of the aging effects of the sun and environmental damage using laser and light sources. *Semin Cutan Med Surg* **22**, 93–106.

4 Weiss RA, Gold M, Bene N, Biron JA, Munavalli G, Weiss M, *et al.* (2006) Prospective clinical evaluation of 1440-nm laser delivered by microarray for treatment of photoaging and scars. *J Drugs Dermatol* **5**, 740–4.

5 Weiss RA, Goldman MP, Weiss MA. (2000) Treatment of poikiloderma of Civatte with an intense pulsed light source. *Dermatol Surg* **26**, 823–7.

6 Fatemi A, Weiss MA, Weiss RA. (2002) Short-term histologic effects of nonablative resurfacing: results with a dynamically cooled millisecond-domain 1320 nm Nd:YAG laser. *Dermatol Surg* **28**, 172–6.
7 Bogle MA. (2008) Fractionated mid-infrared resurfacing. *Semin Cutan Med Surg* **27**, 252–8.
8 Weiss RA, McDaniel DH, Geronemus RG. (2003) Review of nonablative photorejuvenation: reversal of the aging effects of the sun and environmental damage using laser and light sources. *Semin Cutan Med Surg* **22**, 93–106.
9 McDaniel DH, Weiss RA, Geronemus R, Ginn L, Newman J. (2002) Light-tissue interactions I: photothermolysis vs photomodulation laboratory findings. *Lasers Surg Med* **14**, 25.
10 McDaniel DH, Weiss RA, Geronemus R, *et al.* (2002) Light-tissue interactions II: photothermolysis vs photomodulation clinical applications. *Lasers Surg* Med 14, 25.
11 Whelan HT, Smits RL Jr, Buchman EV, *et al.* (2001) Effect of NASA light-emitting diode irradiation on wound healing. *J Clin Laser Med Surg* **19**, 305–14.
12 Whelan HT, Buchmann EV, Dhokalia A, *et al.* (2003) Effect of NASA light-emitting diode irradiation on molecular changes for wound healing in diabetic mice. *J Clin Laser Med Surg* **21**, 67–74.
13 Whelan HT, Connelly JF, Hodgson BD, *et al.* (2002) NASA light-emitting diodes for the prevention of oral mucositis in pediatric bone marrow transplant patients. *J Clin Laser Med Surg* **20**, 319–24.
14 Walker MD, Rumpf S, Baxter GD, *et al.* (2000) Effect of low-intensity laser irradiation (660 nm) on a radiation-impaired wound-healing model in murine skin. *Lasers Surg Med* **26**, 41–7.
15 Lowe AS, Walker MD, O'Byrne M, *et al.* (1998) Effect of low intensity monochromatic light therapy (890 nm) on a radiation-impaired, wound-healing model in murine skin. *Lasers Surg Med* **23**, 291–8.
16 Weiss RA, McDaniel DH, Geronemus RG, *et al.* (2005) Clinical experience with light-emitting diode (LED) photomodulation. *Dermatol Surg* **31**, 1199–205.
17 Weiss RA, McDaniel DH, Geronemus RG, Weiss MA. (2005) Clinical trial of a novel non-thermal LED array for reversal of photoaging: clinical, histologic, and surface profilometric results. *Lasers Surg Med* **36**, 85–91.
18 McDaniel DH, Newman J, Geronemus R, *et al.* (2003) Non-ablative non-thermal LED photomodulation: a multicenter clinical photoaging trial. *Lasers Surg Med* **15**, 22.
19 Geronemus R, Weiss RA, Weiss MA, *et al.* (2003) Non-ablative LED photomodulation: light activated fibroblast stimulation clinical trial. *Lasers Surg Med* **25**, 22.
20 Weiss RA, McDaniel DH, Geronemus R, *et al.* (2004) Non-ablative, non-thermal light emitting diode (LED) phototherapy of photoaged skin. *Lasers Surg Med* **16**, 31.
21 Weiss RA, Weiss MA, Geronemus RG, McDaniel DH. (2004) A novel non-thermal non-ablative full panel led photomodulation device for reversal of photoaging: digital microscopic and clinical results in various skin types. *J Drugs Dermatol* **3**, 605–10.
22 Goldberg DJ, Amin S, Russell BA, *et al.* (2006) Combined 633-nm and 830-nm led treatment of photoaging skin. *J Drugs Dermatol* **5**, 748–53.
23 Russell BA, Kellett N, Reilly LR. (2005) A study to determine the efficacy of combination LED light therapy (633 nm and 830 nm) in facial skin rejuvenation. *J Cosmet Laser Ther* **7**, 196–200.
24 Weiss RA, McDaniel DH, Geronemus RG, Weiss MA. (2005) Clinical trial of a novel non-thermal LED array for reversal of photoaging: clinical, histologic, and surface profilometric results. *Lasers Surg Med* **36**, 85–91.
25 Khoury JG, Goldman MP. (2008) Use of light-emitting diode photomodulation to reduce erythema and discomfort after intense pulsed light treatment of photodamage. *J Cosmet Dermatol* **7**, 30–4.
26 DeLand MM, Weiss RA, McDaniel DH, Geronemus RG. (2007) Treatment of radiation-induced dermatitis with light-emitting diode (LED) photomodulation. *Lasers Surg Med* **39**, 164–8.
27 Choi M, Kim JE, Cho KH, Lee JH. (2013) In vivo and in vitro analysis of low level light therapy: a useful therapeutic approach for sensitive skin. *Lasers Med Sci.* **28**, 1573–9.
28 Gupta A, Dai T, Hamblin MR. (2013) Effect of red and near-infrared wavelengths on low level laser (light) therapy-induced healing of partial-thickness dermal abrasion in mice. Epub ahead of print.
29 Dougal G, Lee SY. (2013) Evaluation of the efficacy of low-level light therapy using 1072nm infrared light for the treatment of herpes simplex labialis. *Clin Exp Dermatol.* **38**, 713–8.
30 Eells JT, Henry MM, Summerfelt P, *et al.* (2003) Therapeutic photobiomodulation for methanol-induced retinal toxicity. *Proc Natl Acad Sci USA* **100**, 3439–44.
31 Eells JT, Henry MM, Summerfelt P, *et al.* (2003) Therapeutic photobiomodulation for methanol-induced retinal toxicity. *Proc Natl Acad Sci U S A* **100**, 3439–44.
32 McDaniel DH, Weiss RA, Geronemus R, Weiss MA. (2006) LED photomodulation 'reverses' acute retinal injury. Annual meeting of the American Society for Laser Medicine and Surgery, Boston, MA, April 6, 2006.
33 Tang J, Du Y, Lee CA, *et al.* (2013) Low-intensity far-red light inhibits early lesions that contribute to diabetic retinopathy in vivo and in vitro. *Invest Opthalmol Vis Sci.* **54**, 3681–90.
34 Naroli R, Valter K, Barbosa M, *et al.* (2013) 670nm photobiomodulation as a novel protection against retinopathy of prematurity: evidence from oxygen induced retinopathy models. *PLoS One* **8**, e72135.
35 Kim CH, Cheong KA, Lee AY. (2013) 850nm light-emitting-diode phototherapy plus low-dose tacrolimus (FK-506) as combination therapy in the treatment of dermatophagoides farina-induced atopic dermatitis-like skin lesions in NC/Nga mice. **72**, 142–8.
36 Tarstedt M, Rosdahl I, Berne B, *et al.* (2005) A randomized multicenter study to compare two treatment regimens of topical methyl aminolevulinate (Metvix)-PDT in actinic keratosis of the face and scalp. *Acta Derm Venereol* **85**, 424–8.
37 Chen HM, Yu CH, Tu PC, *et al.* (2005) Successful treatment of oral verrucous hyperplasia and oral leukoplakia with topical 5-aminolevulinic acid-mediated photodynamic therapy. *Lasers Surg Med* **37**, 114–22.
38 Weiss RA, McDaniel DH, Geronemus RG, *et al.* (2005) Clinical experience with light-emitting diode (LED) photomodulation. *Dermatol Surg* **31**, 1199–205.
39 Zhang X, Wu XQ, Lu S, *et al.* (2006) Deficit of mitochondria-derived ATP during oxidative stress impairs mouse MII oocyte spindles. *Cell Res* **16**, 841–50.
40 Sorensen M, Sanz A, Gomez J, *et al.* (2006) Effects of fasting on oxidative stress in rat liver mitochondria. *Free Radic Res* **40**, 339–47.
41 Desmet KD, Paz DA, Corry JJ, *et al.* (2006) Clinical and experimental applications of NIR-LED photobiomodulation. *Photomed Laser Surg* **24**, 121–8.
42 Weiss RA, Weiss MA, McDaniel DH, *et al.* (2003) Comparison of non-ablative fibroblast photoactivation with and without application of topical cosmeceutical agents. *Lasers Surg Med* **15**, 23.

43 Nguyen LM, Malamo AG, Larkin-Kaiser KA, *et al.* (2013) Effect of near-infrared light exposure on mitochondrial signalling in C2C12 muscle cells. Mitochondrion Epub ahead of print.

44 Kim JM, Kim NH, Tian YS, Lee AY. (2012) Light-emitting diodes at 830 and 850 nm inhibit melanin synthesis in vitro. *Acta Derm Venereol* **92**, 675–80.

45 Zaidi M, Krolikowki JG, Jones DW, *et al.* (2013) Transient repetitive exposure to low level light therapy enhances collateral blood vessel growth in the ischemic hindlimb of the tight skin mouse. *Photochem Photobiol* **89**, 709–13.

46 Lanzafame RJ, Blanche RR, Bodian AB, *et al.* (2013) The growth of human scalp hair mediated by visible red laser and LED sources in males. *Lasers Surg Med* **45**, 487–95.

47 Moro C, Massari NE, Torres N, *et al.* Photobiomodulation inside the brain: a novel method of applying near-infrared light intracranially and its impact on dopaminergic cell survival in MPTP-treated mice. *J Neurosurg* Epub ahead of print.

48 Avci P, Gupta A, Sadasivam M, *et al.* (2013) Low-level laser (light) therapy (LLLT) in skin: stimulating, healing, restoring. *Semin Cutan Med Surg* **32**, 41–52.

SECTION 5 Skin Contouring Techniques

CHAPTER 53
Liposuction: Manual, Mechanical, and Laser Assisted

Anne Goldsberry,[1] Emily Tierney,[2] and C. William Hanke[1]
[1]Laser and Skin Surgery Center of Indiana, Carmel, IN, USA
[2]Department of Dermatology, Tufts University School of Medicine, Boston, MA, USA

BASIC CONCEPTS

- The safety profile for liposuction is significantly improved when tumescent local anesthesia is employed.
- Tumescent local anesthesia utilizing lidocaine with epinephrine allows for the removal of large volumes of fat with minimal associated blood loss and postoperative morbidity.
- Liposuction is a procedure for patients who are either at or approaching their goal weight, to achieve a more esthetic figure, contour, and shape in conjunction with a diet and exercise regimen.
- Preoperative consultation, setting realistic patient expectations for improvement, establishing patients' overall health status and past medical history and discussion of risks and benefits of the procedure are critical to the success of the procedure.
- Laser-assisted tumescent liposuction has been purported to result in mechanical cavitation of fat, resulting in greater ease of suction and greater skin retraction; however, additional studies are needed to confirm these results.

Introduction: history of liposuction with tumescent local anesthesia

The early history of liposuction begins with Fischer's description of hollow cannula liposuction in 1976 [1]. Shortly thereafter, Ilouz, a Frenchman trained in obstetrics and gynecology, and Fournier, a general surgeon, began practicing liposuction using the "wet technique," involving injection of hypotonic saline and hyaluronic acid into the fat prior to suction [2]. Fournier pioneered the "criss-cross" technique and syringe liposuction and became a teacher of the technique [3].

In the early 1980s, Saul Asken, Sam Stegman, Ted Tromovitch and several other American dermatologists began utilizing local anesthesia for liposuction [4]. Asken published two complete textbooks describing his techniques.[5,6] Jeffrey Klein, another American dermatologist, first described his "Tumescent Technique" for liposuction in 1987 [7].

In 1988, Hanke and Bernstein published a report on the safety of the TLA technique for liposuction, reporting the results of 9,478 patients treated by dermatologists [8]. Shortly after attending Fournier's liposuction course in Paris, William Hanke, the editor-in-chief of the *Journal of Dermatologic Surgery and Oncology*, commissioned an issue of the journal dedicated to liposuction. Further innovations to the field evolved with the publication by Hanke and colleagues documenting the safety of TLA in 15,336 patients in 1995 [9]. Additionally, while initial reports by Klein established the safety of tumescent liposuction using a lidocaine dose of 35 mg/kg in 1990 [10]., Ostad et al. [11]. reported the safety of lidocaine dosage up to 55 mg/kg. In 2000, Klein published a book entitled *Tumescent Technique* [12], highlighting many of his important contributions to the field including: the Klein microcannula, Klein infiltration pumps, multihole Klein Capistrano cannulas, and specific techniques for treating all body areas.

A textbook on liposuction published initially in German in 1999, first mentioned the term "tumescent local anesthesia."[13]. The book was republished in English in 2001 [14]. Klein's full text on Tumescent Technique, published in 2000, is currently out of print [15]. Other books on liposuction have been written by dermatologists in recent years [16,17,18].

Since Klein's introduction of the technique of TLA for liposuction in 1987, it has revolutionized the technique among dermatologic surgeons and surgeons of all specialties performing the procedure. Liposuction with TLA facilitates the removal of large volumes of fat with minimal blood loss or postoperative morbidity, excellent aesthetic results, and a remarkably superior safety profile to general anesthesia.

Cosmetic Dermatology: Products and Procedures, Second Edition. Edited by Zoe Diana Draelos.
© 2016 John Wiley & Sons, Ltd. Published 2016 by John Wiley & Sons, Ltd.

464 ANTI-AGING Skin Contouring Techniques

Table 53.1 Appropriate liposuction candidate selection.

Does the patient have realistic expectations of the procedure?
Is the patient at or near goal body weight?
Is the patient in good health in the absence of anticoagulant therapy?
Does the patient have localized fat deposits on the body that are diet and exercise resistant for which they are seeking treatment?
Does the patient have good or adequate skin tone?

Physiology: what skin contour problem does the procedure address and how does this procedure alter the contour problem?

Liposuction is a procedure that can assist patients who want to achieve a more idealized and balanced body contour (Table 53.1) [19–22]. It is designed for individuals at their ideal body weight who seek correction of single or multiple anatomic sites with focal excess adiposity and laxity [19–22]. The ideal liposuction patient is a patient of ideal body weight with focal disproportionate adiposity, resulting in contour deformity [19–22]. Importantly, liposuction is not a weight loss procedure, and it should be emphasized that patients seeking the goal of weight loss are not good candidates for the procedure (Table 53.1) [19–22]. In initial patient consultations, it is important to set realistic patient expectations for the results of the procedure. The results of liposuction in all anatomic sites are limited by the existing bony structure, the texture and quality of the skin, the tone and build of muscle, and the pre-existing adiposity in areas not amenable to liposuction.

Liposuction can help to achieve a more idealized and balanced body contour, and patients will largely vary in seeking correction of a single area or multiple anatomic sites to achieve their own personal optimal correction.

Advantages and disadvantages

Liposuction with TLA allows the removal of large volumes of fat with minimal blood loss or postoperative morbidity, excellent cosmesis, and a remarkable safety profile. TLA technique with the use of a dilute epinephrine and anesthetic achieves the aims of hemostasis and anesthesia at the surgical site [23–27]. The advantages of the technique include improved safety, precision, and patient convenience [23–27]. These advances have contributed to the enhanced safety profile and widespread growth in the popularity of the liposuction technique [23–27]. TLA can be utilized for any anatomic site treated with liposuction, from the neck to the ankles.

Advantages of the TLA technique include a significant reduction in blood loss attributed to the vasoconstrictive effects of epinephrine. This can be quantified by comparing the aspirate from TLA (containing 1–3% whole blood) with that from the procedure performed under general anesthesia (40% whole blood) [25]. Improved hemostasis results in both decreased blood loss as well as decreased bruising and discomfort for the patient in the postoperative phase [25]. In addition, the anesthetic and vasoconstrictive effects of the TLA create a reservoir effect, resulting in prolonged anesthesia of several hours' duration in the treated area [22–25]. Consequently, patients have a decreased reliance upon postoperative narcotics.

The TLA solution also results in a hydrodissection effect, whereby the pressure of the solution facilitates easier and more uniform penetration and removal of adipose tissue by the cannula (Figures >–53.1 and 53.2) [8–12,22–25]. Tumescent fluid enlarges, magnifies, and lifts targeted fat, allowing for more precise removal of fat [8–12,22–25].

With proper technique for infusion of the tumescent fluid, TLA can be performed without ancillary sedation and intravenous or general anesthesia [24,25]. With TLA, patient convenience is significantly enhanced during the perioperative recovery period where there is more rapid recovery [24–34]. In contrast, the recovery is much more prolonged after general anesthesia, both as a result of the after-effects of the anesthetic and from the increased bruising and discomfort associated with the procedure [24–34].

Complications with the TLA technique include discomfort, swelling, bruising, temporary loss of sensation, post-inflammatory hyperpigmentation, and minimal scarring at the incision sites. However, these complications are significantly less than those associated with the procedure performed under general anesthesia [24–34]. Potential risks of liposuction under general anesthesia include deep venous thrombosis, pulmonary embolus, abdominal or other organ perforation, infection, and bleeding [31,33].

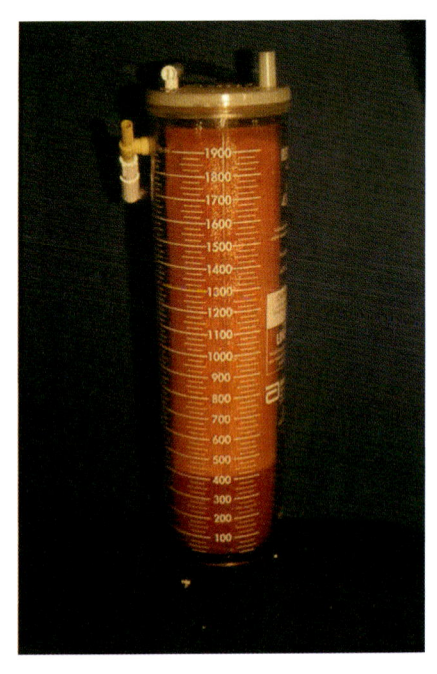

Figure 53.1 A 2-L liposuction canister filled with liposuction aspirate.

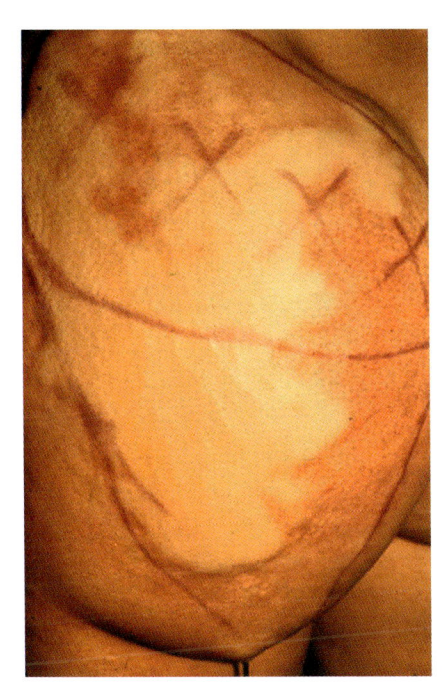

Figure 53.2 Blanching of skin visible after infusion of tumescent anesthesia with tumescent local anesthesia (TLA) technique.

Indications for tumescent liposuction, by anatomic site

Abdomen

Patient selection has a significant role in liposuction surgery of the abdomen. Patients should be within 10–25 lb. (5–12 kg) of their ideal body weight and should have good to excellent skin tone which will assist with skin contraction after the procedure [35].

Table 53.2 Five groups of patients: abdominal liposuction.

Liposuction: lower abdomen
Liposuction: upper and lower abdomen
Liposuction: hourglass abdomen; upper and lower abdomen, hips, waist, and back
Liposuction and skin excision: mini-abdominoplasty with or without umbilical translocation
Complete abdominoplasty

The overall body shape of the patient should be examined during the preoperative physician examination [35]. The patient should be marked while standing to identify the larger areas of fatty deposition in the abdomen [35]. Incision sites are made in the following locations: two to three in the suprapubic region, one at the umbilicus, and two on the lateral portions of the umbilical fat depositions [35]. The patient should be lying on his or her back for the procedure; however, towards the end of the procedure, it is helpful if the patient lies in both lateral decubitus positions to identify pockets of fat as they fall away from the rectus muscle [35]. The goal of abdominal liposuction should be to reduce the deeper fatty layers while preserving a superficial, even layer of fat attached to the skin [35]. Over suction can lead to dimpling of the skin, uneven fat deposits, and dermal necrosis [35].

Patients in group 1 (Table 53.2), lower abdomen only, are typically thin patients with a localized fatty deposition in the lower abdomen alone (Figure 53.3) [35]. These patients tend to respond very well to liposuction with high patient satisfaction.

Patients in group 2 (Table 53.2), requiring liposuction of both the upper and lower abdomen, must be carefully evaluated (Figure 53.4) [35]. This group may also be relatively thin; however, if suction of the lower abdomen alone is performed, they may

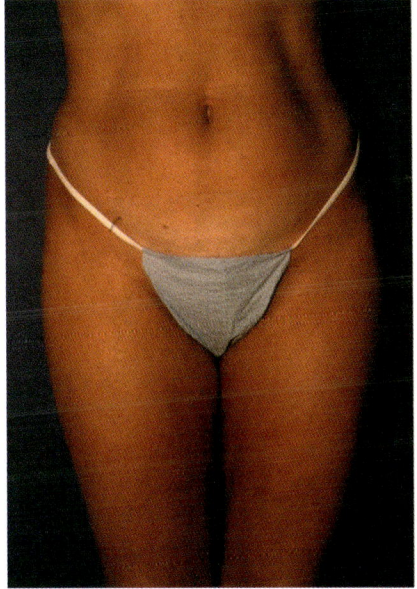

Figure 53.3 Lower abdomen, anterior view: (a) pretreatment; (b) post-treatment.

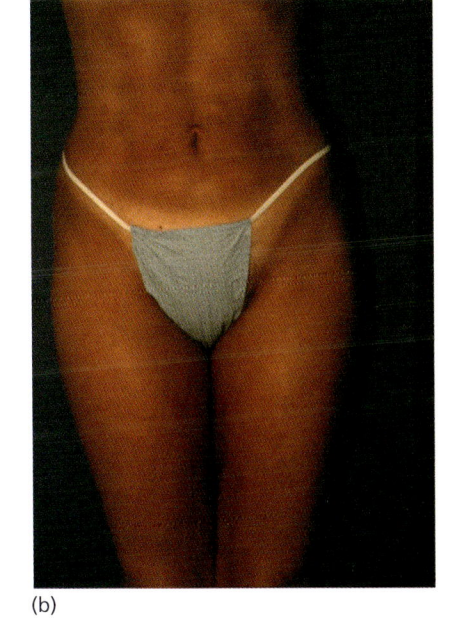

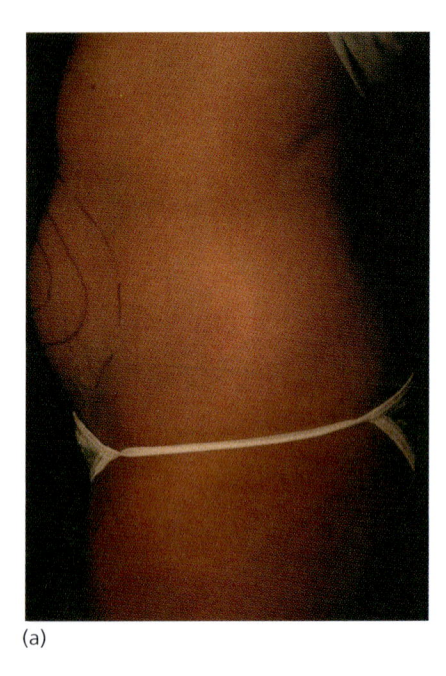

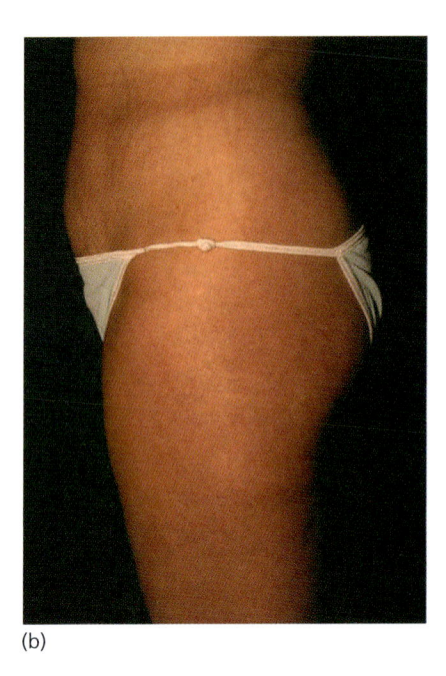

Figure 53.4 Lower abdomen and hips liposuction, lateral view: (a) pretreatment; (b) post-treatment.

have a protuberant overhanging upper abdomen [35]. Therefore, it is important to perform liposuction on both segments of the abdomen to ensure a proportionate appearance.

Patients requiring liposuction of the upper and lower abdomen in addition to the hips, waist, and back (group 3; Table 53.2; Figure 53.5) tend to be older postmenopausal women or those on hormone replacement therapy with a history of weight gain [35].

Men requesting liposuction of the abdomen may require more widespread liposuction to ensure a proportionate appearance as fat deposits in men in the abdomen are usually accompanied by excess fat on the chest, flanks, and back [35]. Many men are not good candidates for abdominal liposuction as much of the fat deposits are behind the rectus abdominis and thus are not accessible to suction during the liposuction procedure [35].

The fourth group of patients (Table 53.2) demonstrate atrophic, stretched skin from pregnancy, advancing age, and rapid fluctuations changes in weight [35]. More extensive liposuction is needed in these patients and liposuction alone is often not

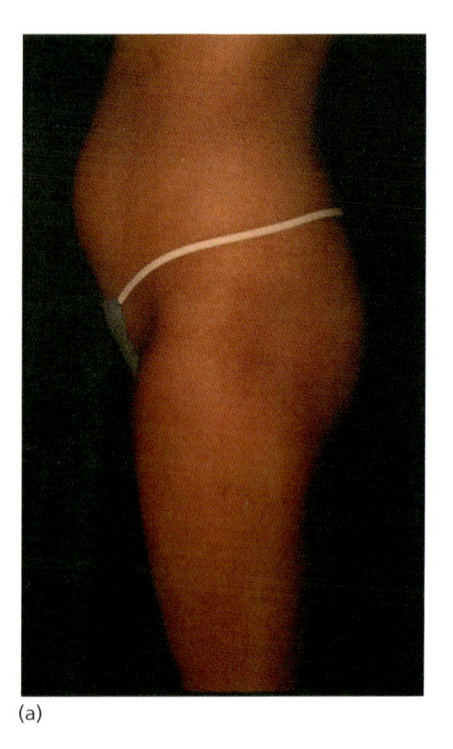

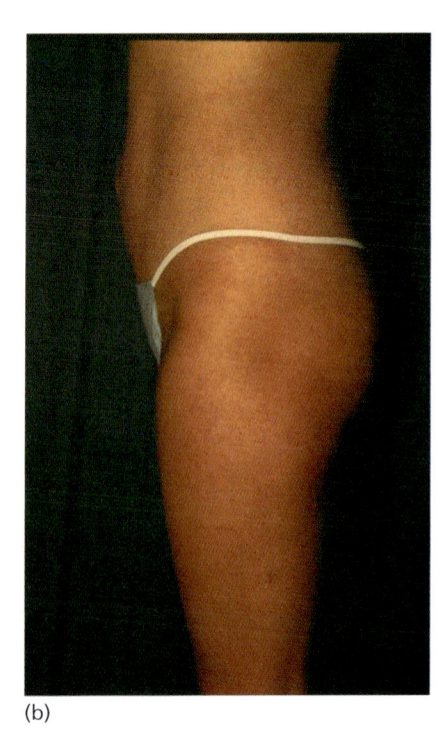

Figure 53.5 Lower abdomen, hips, and lateral thigh liposuction, lateral view: (a) pretreatment; (b) post-treatment.

satisfactory. Waiting 3–4 months after the procedure will allow the physician to assess if liposuction alone is sufficient or if the patient will require an abdominoplasty procedure to address skin redundancy [35].

Hips, outer thighs, and buttocks

Evaluation of patients for liposuction in these anatomic sites requires a three-dimensional and universal approach to all anatomic sites; otherwise a disproportionate appearance can result with more noticeable enlargement in the unsuctioned areas after suction of localized fat deposits. For the hips, outer thighs, and buttocks, it is important to observe and review carefully with the patient all changes in underlying musculature, cellulite, and inelastic skin, none of which can be improved with liposuction. For the hips, the patient should be placed in the lateral decubitus position. For the thighs, the patient should also be in the lateral decubitus position with a pillow placed between the legs, which mimics the standing position and allows the femur to be directed anteriomedially [30].

The end result of suctioning should be that a region is flat, not concave [35]. Suctioning should also be equal on both sides and careful steps should be taken to monitor that relatively equivalent amounts of fat are removed from either side [35].

Liposuction of the buttocks must be performed carefully, with special consideration to the inferolateral gluteal crease, where a banana roll, comprised of a defined infragluteal fat pocket, may worsen or lead to an atrophic buttock in the event of over suction [35]. Physical examination must focus on bony and muscular prominences and asymmetry. Realistic expectations must be established with the patient as liposuction will not assist with underlying bony asymmetry, the presence of large or asymmetrical muscle masses, or skin laxity. Conservative buttock suction is recommended with removal of no more than 30–50% of fat from the middle and deep fat layers [35]. Superficial suctioning of the buttocks should be avoided as it is likely to result in undesirable dimpling.

Arms

Liposuction of the arms is performed in women with laxity of the proximal arm musculature and who have a pendulous fatty protuberance of the posterior, lateral, or anterior upper arm (Figure 53.6). The fat distribution in the arms is best visualized when the arms are extended at 90° from the body. Avoiding over suctioning is critical for the arms and gentle liposuction should only be performed in the medial and posterior (extensor arms). As skin redundancy often contributes significantly to laxity of the arms, patients need to be advised that the goal is to decrease the convexity of the arms as opposed to complete removal of all redundancy of skin and soft tissue.

Excessive tumescent solution should be avoided in the upper arm region as there is a small risk for creation of "compartment syndrome" whereby a functional tourniquet develops distal to the infused region, brought about by fluid-induced compression of neural, vascular, and lymphatic structures in the area.

One position for the procedure is to lay the patient's arms entirely flat with palms facing down over the hips with the body in a lateral decubitus position, which will serve to maximally expose the posterior portion of the arm. The other position that is helpful is for the patient to be in a supine or lateral decubitus position with a hand brought behind the head, forearm flexed, and elbow pointing out, which also exposes the posterior portion of the arm. Liposuction to the axilla should be avoided given the risks of damage to the branches of the brachial plexus in this area.

Neck and jowls

The goal of liposuction of the neck and jowls is to give improved definition of the cervicomental angle and jawline [36–39]. Aging in this region can be caused by a multitude of factors, including ptosis of fatty tissue and decreased elastic tissue. These changes in the subcutaneous tissue of the neck allow the anterior margins of the platysma to slide forward and result in protrusion of the submental and submandibular fat [36–39]. Patients with excess laxity in this area may benefit from a spectrum of procedures, including facelifts, chin implants, platysmal plication, and CO_2 laser resurfacing. Careful selection of patients who will benefit from liposuction in this area is critical (Figure 53.7) [36–39].

Fullness in the neck and jowls can be attributed to a variety of factors, including redundant skin, muscle, or a low or anteriorly positioned hyoid bone (creating an obtuse cervicomental angle) [36–39]. Patients with low set or anteriorly placed hyoid bones are unlikely to benefit from liposuction alone. The ideal candidate should have a hyoid positioned at the level of the C3–C4

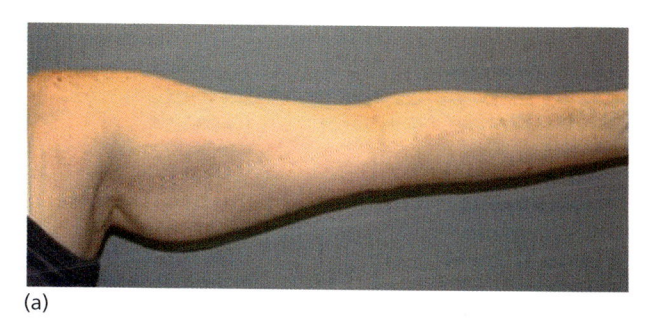

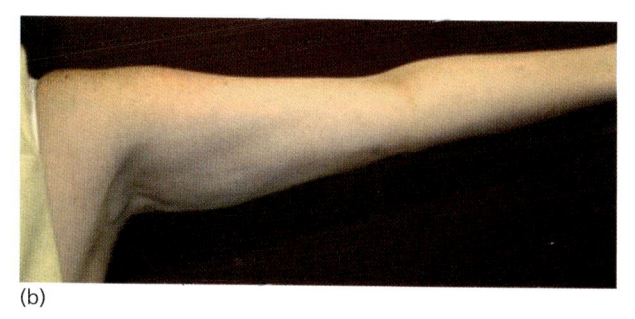

Figure 53.6 Arm, anterior view: (a) pretreatment; (b) post-treatment.

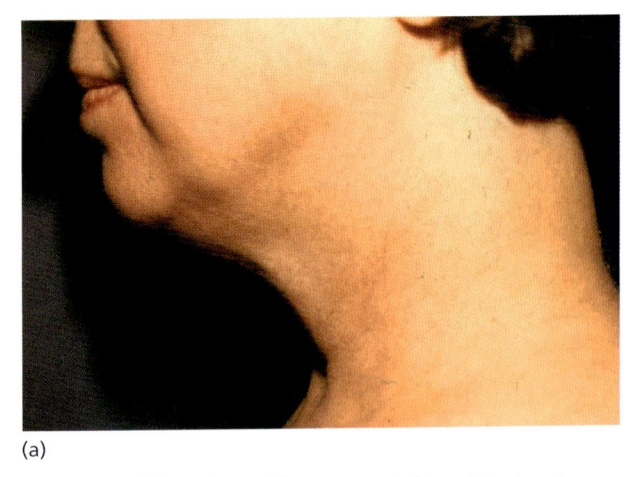

Figure 53.7 Neck, lateral view: (a) pretreatment; (b) post-treatment.

vertebrae, excellent skin elasticity, and a palpable submental fat pad [36–39].

In order to mark the neck liposuction patient, the anatomic boundaries must be distinguished, including the mandibular border, jowls, submental fat pad, anterior borders of the sternocleidomastoid, platsyma band, and thyroid cartilage (Figure 53.8) [36–39]. The patient should be seated with the head gently extended posteriorly and the chin raised with the small supportive pillow for neck support [36–39].

For liposuction of the neck and jowls, entry points should be along the submental crease, just below or lateral to the jowls [36–39]. If extensive lateral neck fat is present, additional insertion sites can be made in a neck fold behind the earlobes [36–39]. The suctioning plane should begin just above the platysma muscle, with subsequent suction with small (1.5–2 mm) cannulae [36–39]. The cannula should be delicately applied in this area to suction above the platsyma in order to avoid placing the cannula through the platysma [36–39]. In addition, the marginal mandibular branch of the facial nerve is located in this area (below the angle of the mandible at the anterior border of the masseter muscle), and care must be taken to avoid trauma to the nerve [36–39]. The nerve becomes increasingly superficial and more likely to be injured along or posterior (up to two fingerbreadths) to the posterior border of the sternocleidomastoid muscle [36–39]. The cannula can be used to elevate the subcutaneous fat away from the underlying structures in these areas to avoid injury to underlying structures [26–30]. Also, it is important to avoid over suctioning cheeks and along the jowl–cheek margin, as an undesirable hollowed appearance results from over suctioning in this area [36–39].

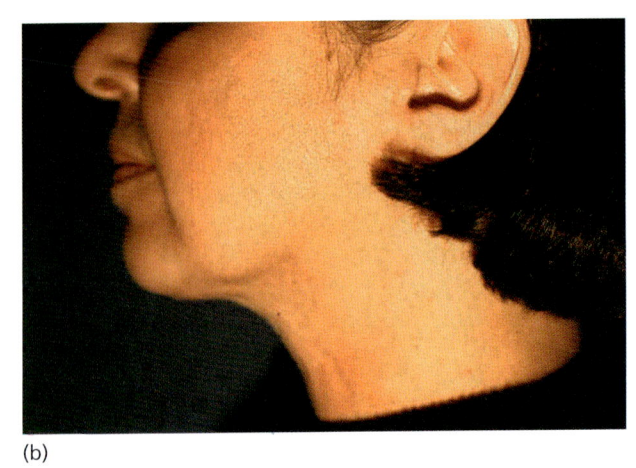

Female breast

Traditional breast reduction in women, reduction mammoplasty, requires general anesthesia with significant associated risks, including, seroma, hematoma, scarring, skin loss, and fat necrosis [40,41]. The procedure involves making a T-shaped incision extending from the areola to the inframammary folds, which in the majority of cases leaves an unattractive scar [40,41].

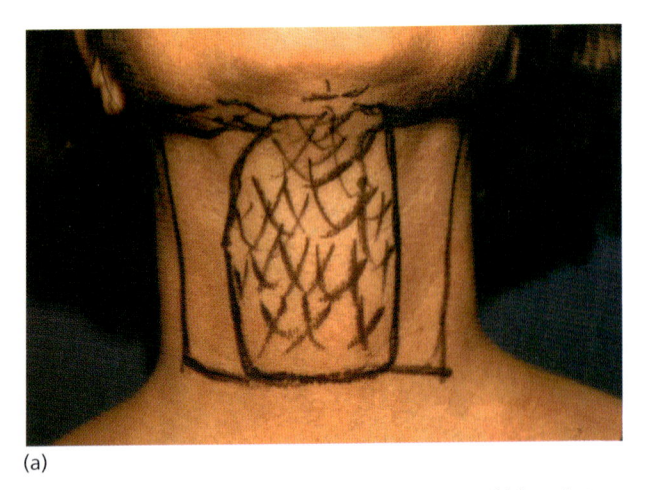

Figure 53.8 Neck liposuction markings: (a) anterior view; (b) lateral view.

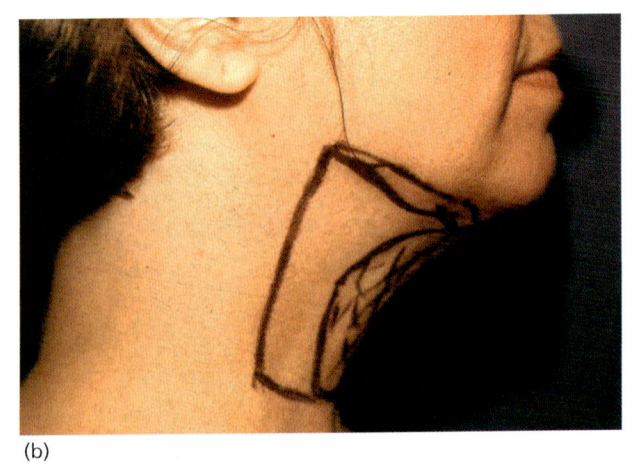

Liposuction as a means to decrease breast size is a relatively new procedure and has only been described in the literature in a handful of cases [40,41]. For women with moderate to severe breast enlargement, liposuction may not be sufficient given that it may not address issues of excess skin and soft tissue [40,41]. A preoperative breast weight should be taken to establish the optimal amount of fat reduction and to provide baseline to calculate the postoperative percent fat reduction [40,41]. Breast volume is often determined using a water displacement methodology. The breast is immersed into a five liter beaker filled with water, and the displaced water volume is measured in order to estimate the breast volume [42].

The patient should be positioned supine with the ipsilateral arm behind the head or with the arm posteriorly displaced in order to bring the breast flat against the chest wall [40,41]. Two incisions for suctioning should be made, one in the lateral and one in the medial inframammary crease [42]. Initially, it was thought that suctioning should focus in the mid to deep plane of the lateral and inferior quadrants of the breast [40,41]. However, Habbema advocates for a fan like pattern throughout the layers of the tissue for optimal contraction [42]. Subareolar and upper lateral quadrants, those areas with the highest concentration of glandular tissue, are spared from aggressive suction.[42]. It is less desirable for suction in the superior quadrant to preserve the natural contour of the breast, as the upper quadrants typically flatten with age [40,41]. The surgeon determines the amount of fat removed, calculated as a percentage of total fat, based upon preoperative measurement [40,41].

It was initially recommended that less than one-third of the measured total breast volume be removed in one session [40,41]; however more recent reports of up to 87% reduction suggest it might be useful for larger scale reduction [42]. Habbema reported a series of 151 women who underwent liposuction of the breasts [42]. Preoperative breast volume ranged from 175–4000 mL with an average of 1005 mL [42]. The breast volume removed ranged from 24–87% with an average of 53%. Preoperative breast ptosis ranged from 0.8–13 cm with an average of 6.5 cm. The average ptosis reduction was 50.2%. Furthermore, 77.5% and 21.8% of patients reported being very or mostly satisfied, respectively [42]. From the study, Habbema recommended the following selection criteria for breast reduction using liposuction with TLA: patients who decline traditional reduction mammoplasty, patients interested in a reduction of 50% or less, women 45 years-old or older, un-operated large breasts, asymmetry in breast volume, and patients who are poor candidates for general anesthesia [42].

Breast reduction in female breasts by liposuction alone represents a promising new application of this technology and presents significant advantages relative to traditional reduction mammoplasties, including less risk associated with general anesthesia, as well as benefits of decreased infection and scarring risks. Analysis of breast liposuction aspirate in 61 patients revealed that less than 15% had any evidence of glandular tissue. None of the aspirate specimens revealed any large glands [43].

This suggests that, unlike reduction mammoplasty, liposuction of the breast does not pose a risk to future lactation [43].

Male chest

A careful history and physician examination should be performed in men before attempting liposuction in the male chest, with specific attention to the palpation of the gynecomastia and regional lymph nodes [40,41,44]. Several authors also recommend palpation of the testes to evaluate for testicular tumors [40,41]. While rare, breast tumors do occur in men and thus all masses with suspicion for malignancy (asymmetry, firm, or fixed) should undergo mammogram, ultrasound, and/or biopsy [40,41]. Etiologies for male breast enlargement include fatty deposition, glandular deposition, medications (estrogen, spironolactone, digitalis, diazepam, phenytoin and clomiphene), alcoholism, hypogonadism, and hormone-secreting tumors of the pituitary, adrenal gland, and testis [40,41].

As the male breast is one of the most vascular sites for TLA, care must be taken to ensure the vasoconstrictive effect of epinephrine has taken effect prior to the procedure and that the pectoralis muscle is not traumatized during the anesthesia infusion or liposuction [40,41]. The male breast is also one of the most fibrous sites in which liposuction is performed, with significant variability in the content of glandular and fatty tissue present [40,41].

Incision sites for the liposuction cannula are placed along the periphery of the breast and in the inframammary crease to allow for complete infiltration and criss-cross suction of adipose tissue [40,41]. Suction is started with microcannula, allowing for easier tissue penetration, such as the 16-gauge Capistrano cannula for initial tunneling with transition to a larger 14-gauge cannula [40,41]. The subareolar breast tissue can be gently suctioned with the use of a 16-gauge short (5 or 7 cm) Capistrano cannula [40,41].

Anesthesia technique

Tumescent solution should be prepared on the day of the procedure utilizing 0.9% sodium chloride solution (normal saline) [8–12,19]. The anesthetic is lidocaine, available in 1% or 2% solution. Epinephrine and sodium bicarbonate are added to aid in vasoconstriction and buffering, respectively [8–12,19]. The doses utilized for TLA range from conservative doses of 30–35 mg/kg to as high as 55 mg/kg [8–12,19]. Doses at the lower end of the range can be utilized when patients are taking medications that inhibit cytochrome P450, specifically the CYP3A4 isoenzyme, responsible for the clearance of lidocaine [8–12,19]. In particularly smaller individuals, lidocaine concentrations should be limited to 0.05–0.075% as the total dose is limited by weight [8–12,19]. Recent studies show that a lidocaine concentration as low as 0.04% can provide adequate anesthesia [45]. Higher concentrations are generally advised in more sensitive areas, such as the chest, waist, and periumbilical area [8–12,19,45]. Epinephrine is added to the solution at a concentration of 1:1,000,000 (1 mg 1:1000 epinephrine in 1 L solution of saline) [8–12,19]. Finally, bicarbonate is added in the amount of 10 mEq in 1 L [8–12,19]. Before mixing, the saline should be warmed to enhance the comfort of the patient during the infiltration process [8–12,19].

TLA should be administered once the patient has been comfortably positioned for the procedure. Insertion sites should be anesthetized with 1% lidocaine with epinephrine (usually at a dilution of 1:100,000) [8–12,19]. The incisions are created using a No. 11 blade through the dermis to allow entry of the blunt-tipped infiltration cannula into the subcutaneous tissue [8–12,19]. The infiltration cannula should be inserted and the infiltration rate should be appropriately adjusted for the anatomic site [8–12,19]. The infiltration rates should be less than 100 mL per minute to minimize patient discomfort [8–12,19]. Gentle advancement of the cannula should occur prior to infiltration of the tumescent solution [8–12,19]. Anesthesia should be performed using a fanned approach from the entry site with care taken not to put excessive strain on the entry site [8–12,19]. If the patient experiences excessive pain, slowing the rate of infiltration can improve patient comfort [8–12,19]. The infiltration endpoint is reached when the edges of the field become firm and indurated and the area of infiltration is blanched (secondary to vasoconstriction effect of epinephrine) [8–12,19].

Standard and advanced operating technique

After infiltration of the TLA is complete and after allowing 15–20 minutes for full epinephrine effect to occur, fat suction can begin [8–12,19]. Suction can be performed through the same sites of insertion of the TLA [8–12,19]. More aggressive thinner cannulas should be used first to break up the fibrous septae and to create tunnels for subsequent removal of fat with larger (3 mm), less aggressive cannulae [8–12,19]. Suction movement should proceed in a linear and vertical fashion, with little horizontal movement, in the creation of subcutaneous tunnels [8–12,19]. The cannula should be directed so that the aperture is facing downwards or opposite the dermis [8–12,19]. Both deep and superficial tunneling should be performed so that the physician's free or "smart hand" monitors the motion and position of the cannula tip [8–12,19].

Initially during the suctioning, the area is tense from the infiltration of TLA; however, as the suctioning proceeds, the area becomes more flaccid and techniques are needed to maintain the cannula in a uniform plane to ensure uniform suctioning [8–12,19]. One helpful technique is to have the assistant gently grasp the flaccid skin adjacent to the suction area and roll in such a way to flatten the suctioned area [8–12,19]. Another helpful technique is to have an assistant flatten the region by placing counter traction of the skin while the surgeon continues suction guided by their "smart hand" [8–12,19].

The endpoint of fat suction is determined by a number of factors, such as the observation that the aspirate has become increasingly bloody and devoid of suctionable fat and palpation of the area revealing minimal persistence of fat pockets and even distribution of the remaining fat [8–12,19]. When this occurs, suctioning should stop in this area, and the cannula should be repositioned. Localized pockets of fat should be sought out and removed by placing the cannula (with the suction apparatus off) into tunnels and gently pulling back and up against the dermis. Pockets of fat may become more pronounced with this maneuver and further suctioning of these well-defined areas helps create a more even result. The total volume of fat removed in a single procedure should not exceed 4500 mL. This equates to 6000–8000 mL of total aspirate, assuming 50–60% of the aspirate of fat. If the patient possesses areas of fat where the estimated loss is greater than 4500 mL, treatments should be planned over multiple sessions [8–12,19].

Equipment

The fundamental equipment needed to perform liposuction includes an aspiration pump, liposuction cannulae, the infiltration pump, a sterile field, syringes with 1% lidocaine with or without epinephrine (to anesthetize the cannula insertion sites), a No. 11 blade, gauze, and clamps to secure tubing and drapes in place [46].

Various infiltration pumps for administration of the tumescent solution are available, the most optimal of which allow adjustment of the rate of administration of the TLA solution [46]. The infiltration pump is connected directly to the tumescent solution via intravenous tubing which is threaded through the power pump and connected directly to the tumescent solution through an infiltration cannula or needle [46].

The aspiration pump is an electrically powered device which is designed to create negative pressure and collect fatty tissue throughout the procedure [46]. There are a variety of machines available, the ideal of which are those with a closed collection system, overflow trap, and disposable air filter with efficient and uninterrupted suction [46].

The liposuction cannulae are comprised of stainless steel, aluminum, deldrin, or brass [46]. The shape, diameter, hole placement, and size determine the ease of fat removal as well as the relative injury to the tissue [46]. Easier fat removal is achieved with cannulae with several holes and a large-diameter tapered end (usually 3 mm), where the holes are located distally on the tip (e.g. Capistrano, Pinto, Cobra, Becker, and Eliminator cannulae; Wells Johnson Company, Tucson, AZ, USA) [46]. Cannulae with smaller diameters (less than 3 mm), blunted ends, fewer holes, or holes placed more proximally relative to the tip are less aggressive and gentler to the tissue (e.g. Klein, Fournier, Standard cannulae; Wells Johnson Company, Tucson, AZ, USA) [46].

In fibrous tissue, it is best to begin with a cannula with an aggressive tip and a small diameter [46]. As the fibrous tissue is diminished, a less aggressive cannula with a larger diameter tip can be utilized [46]. In areas where the fat is soft, such as the inner thigh, smaller cannulae can be utilized to avoid over suction. Per the guidelines of the American Academy of Dermatology regarding liposuction, the cannula diameter should be no greater than 4.5 mm in diameter.[46]. As most liposuction cannula utilized are between 2 and 3 mm in size, they comply with this recommendation [46].

Ultrasound assisted liposuction was introduced in the late 1990s and is associated with increased complications and is not recommended. Studies have shown an increased risk of blistering, seromas, dermal necrosis and burns [47–49].

Complications

Long-term experience has shown that the complications associated with liposuction under the TLA technique are minor and significantly less than those associated with complications with liposuction performed under intravenous or general anesthesia [28–34]. The most common complications of liposuction using TLA include bruising, swelling, soreness, inflammation of the incision sites, and postoperative fatigue [28–34].

Preoperative phase
Obtaining informed consent from each patient prior to the procedure and reviewing the risks of the procedure, especially of skin contour abnormalities in areas of poor skin elasticity, will allow the patient to be more accepting of the final results [26]. It should be emphasized that there are limitations to the procedure. Safety dictates the amount of fat that can be removed [26]. Additionally, as a body contouring procedure, liposuction will not improve pre-existing scars, pigmentary variation, cellulite, indentations, and skin textural changes [26]. Finally, it should be emphasized to the patient that adoption and/or continuing a regular exercise routine will assist with skin contraction and maintenance of results [26].

Preoperative assessment should also include a physical exam for possible abdominal wall hernias [26]. Blood tests should be performed to ensure the patient does not have an underlying bleeding tendency or liver transaminitis, which could also potentially be a sign of impaired clotting factor synthesis [26]. At a minimum, a full blood count with platelets, liver function tests, and a prothrombin time/partial thromboplastin time (PT/PTT) should be checked [26]. Detailed questions regarding bleeding complications with prior deliveries or surgeries may elicit a history of bleeding which gives an indication for further work-up [26]. This additional workup may include: bleeding time, von Willebrand's factor, factor V Leiden level, or hemophilia screen [26].

A review of medication intake, both prescription and over-the-counter, is essential to the safety and success of the TLA procedure [26]. Intake of aspirin and other non-steroidal anti-inflammatory drugs (NSAIDs) is contraindicated before surgery, because of inhibition of platelet activity and subsequent increased perioperative bleeding [26]. Aspirin should be discontinued 7–10 days prior to surgery [26]. Ibuprofen and other NSAIDs should be discontinued 4–7 days prior to surgery [26]. The discontinuation of vitamins and herbal supplements, such as vitamin E, chondroitin, glucosamine, Ginkgo biloba, ginseng and fish oil is encouraged because of the anticoagulant effects of these agents [26].

Intraoperative phase
The key to achieving a smooth end result with liposuction involves performing the suction from multiple angles and directions in a criss-cross motion.

During the procedure, sterile technique must be emphasized, with the use of antiseptic washes to the area the night before and immediately prior to the surgery. Superficial infections, usually around incision sites, are typically culture positive for *staphylococcus* and *streptococcus*. However, deeper infections which occur in a delayed fashion several months after the procedure occur with atypical mycobacterial species (Mycobacterium abscessus, M. chelonae, M. fortuitum) and have been associated with improper cleaning and sterilization of surgical instruments.

During liposuction, the surgeon should always use the non-dominant hand or "smart hand" to assess the position of the liposuction cannula at all times. Elevating the skin with the "smart hand" and then passing the cannula along the adipose tissue horizontally will preserve the integrity of the abdominal wall. Superficial placement of the cannula in this area is recommended to maximize the amount of fat removed, induce skin contraction, and allow a safe layered approach to fat removal.

One of the significant advantages of liposuction using the TLA technique is that it minimizes blood loss. However, often surgeons will fail to wait long enough after infiltration of the TLA solution until the vasoconstrictive effects of epinephrine (15–20 minutes after infiltration of TLA solution) have taken effect. During the procedure, the surgeons should keep a close eye on the aspirate, directing the cannula away from areas where there are greater volumes of blood relative to fat in the aspirate. Selecting the appropriate cannula size (4 mm should be the largest utilized) and blunt tip style will have a significant role in the decreased tendency for bleeding and hematoma formation. To decrease the risk of bleeding and hematoma formation, larger procedures such as high volume abdominal liposuction, should be considered in two stages.

During TLA, the maximum dosage of lidocaine used should be 55 mg/kg [10]. The lowest dose of lidocaine that provides complete local anesthesia should be utilized. The normal saline utilized should contain lidocaine in concentrations of 0.05–0.1% [10]. The peak plasma concentration of lidocaine occurs 12–18 hours postoperatively, given the slow systemic absorption of lidocaine from the adipose tissue [10]. Patients, family, and staff taking care of the patient should be aware of the symptoms and signs of lidocaine toxicity.

Postoperative phase

Postoperative compression garments will both enhance skin contraction and assist with more rapid removal of local tumescent solution. The compression garment is also critical in order to minimize or eliminate bleeding, hematoma and seroma formation, and to speed wound healing. Patient comfort after the procedure is also greatly improved by wearing compression garments. In general, it is recommended that the garment be worn around the clock for the first week and be worn half-time for the subsequent 2–3 weeks.

Any signs of infection should be evaluated and cultured as soon as possible. With atypical mycobacterial infections, it is important to obtain the culture medium requirements of the laboratory and to notify the laboratory that special processing of the specimen is needed. A rare case of necrotizing fasciitis has been reported with liposuction and thus any patient presenting with severe pain out of proportion to examination, surface blistering, and tenderness should be promptly evaluated for possible débridement and started immediately on broad-spectrum antibiotics and supportive care.

Lidocaine, epinephrine, and bicarbonate utilized in the tumescent solution have all been proven to have antimicrobial effects on a diverse range of pathogens (bacteria, fungi, viruses) and thus the large dilute volume of anesthetic solution with the tumescent technique may further have a role in the low rates of infection associated with this procedure. In addition, using fine cannulas (4 mm or less) will minimize deep bruising and seroma formation and infection risk.

Leaving the cannula sites open to drain leads to decreased hematoma and seroma formation. If significant hematomas form, they will usually spontaneously resolve or can be evacuated once they have liquefied. Large hematomas can be very uncomfortable for the patient and can prevent him or her from returning quickly to usual routines. Seromas need to be drained, sometimes repeatedly with recurrence, with subsequent compression applied to the area (Figure 53.9).

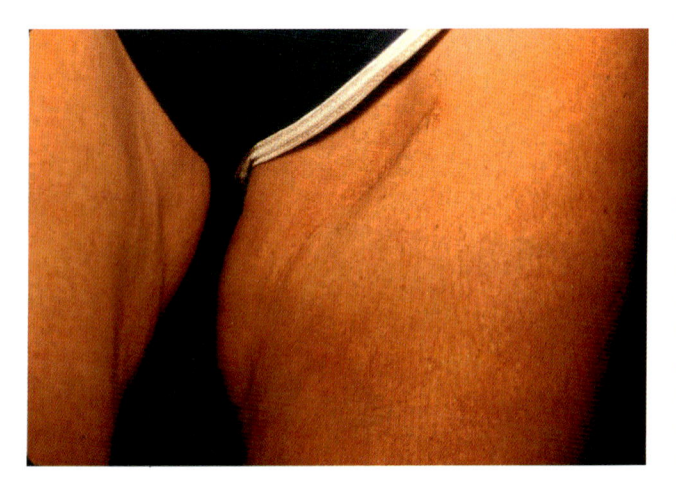

Figure 53.9 Adverse complication of liposuction: skin dimpling and scarring in medial thighs after overly aggressive liposuction procedure.

Conclusions and future directions

Liposuction with local TLA is a procedure that was designed and developed by dermatologic surgeons. It is a procedure with a documented safety record, longevity of results, and high levels of patient satisfaction. Liposuction using TLA in the office setting has a superior safety profile which has been documented in a number of studies in the dermatologic surgery literature by Bernstein, Hanke, Habbema, and Housman (Table 53.3).

Several of largest studies to date, the first by Hanke et al. in 1995 [9], reported data on 44,014 body areas treated with liposuction. There were no serious complications such as death, emboli, hypovolemic shock, perforation of thorax or peritoneum, thrombophlebitis, seizures, or toxic reactions to drugs. Subsequently, in 2002, Housman et al. [34] reported data on 66,570 liposuction procedures. No deaths were reported and the serious adverse event ratio was low at 0.68 per 1000. In 2004, Hanke surveyed 39 tumescent liposuction centers and 688 patients treated with the tumescent technique to examine liposuction practice and safety [50]. The overall complication rate was 0.7%, with a minor complication rate of 0.57% and a major complication rate of 0.14% (1/688 patients). Patient satisfaction was very high among the surveyed population, where 91% of patients surveyed were positive about their decision to have liposuction. Habbema in 2010 [45] reported 3430 procedures in which he gradually decreased the concentration of lidocaine in the TLA in order to identify the minimum concentration required for anesthesia. He reported that 400 mg/L in most body areas, and 500 mg/L for more sensitive areas, provided adequate anesthesia [45]. Use of this dilute concentration further lowers the risk of lidocaine toxicity with TLA.

In contrast, in the plastic surgery literature (Table 53.3) the case fatality and complication rates were significantly higher for liposuction. In the largest study to date among plastic surgeons by Grazer and de Jong in 2000 [51]. evaluating data on 496,245 procedures, the fatality rate was 19.1/100,000; where the most common causes of death included thromboembolism (23.1%), abdomen/viscous perforation (14.6%), anesthesia/sedation/medication (10%), fat embolism (8.5%), cardiorespiratory failure (5.4%), massive infection (5.4%), and hemorrhage (4.6%).

Laser-assisted liposuction

Current studies are undergoing evaluating the ability to liquefy or rupture fat cells using various lasers [52–58]. The laser devices most widely utilized to assist with liposuction include a helium-neon laser (635 nm), a diode laser (600–800 nm), and, most recently, a 1064 nm neodymium:yttrium aluminum garnet (Nd:YAG) laser [52–58]. The studies with a 635 nm diode laser utilized to release fat from adipocytes demonstrated changes in the adipose structure utilizing electron microscopy and magnetic resonance imaging (MRI) [52–59]. Six minutes of exposure to the 635 nm diode laser at 1.2 J/cm2 resulted in a transitory pore

Table 53.3 Liposuction safety studies.

Study/author	Year	Number of procedures	Specialty	Number of fatalities	Fatality rate
Hughes [68].	2001	94,159	Plastic surgery	Not stated	1/47, 415 (lipo only) 1/7,314 (lipo and other procedures) 1/3,281 (lipo and abdominoplasty
Jackson, Dolsky [67].	1997	200,000	Cosmetic surgery (derm, ENT, etc.)	1	2.4/100,000
ASPRS Task Force on Liposuction [66].	1998	24,295	Plastic surgery	5	20.6/100,000
Dillerud [65].	1991	3,511	Plastic surgery	0	0
Temourian, Rogers [64].	1991	112,756	Plastic surgery	15	12.7/100,000
Newman, Dolsky [63].	1984	5,458	Cosmetic surgery(derm, ENT, etc.)	0	1/38,426
Grazer, De Jong [51].	2000	496,245	Plastic surgery	95	19.1/100,000
Hanke et al. [50].	2004	688	Dermatologic surgery	0	0
Habbema [45].	2010	3,430	Dermatologic surgery	0	0
Housman et al. [34].	2002	66,570	Dermatologic surgery	0	0
Hanke et al. [9].	1995	15,336	Dermatologic surgery	0	0
Bernstein, Hanke [8].	1988	9,478	Dermatologic surgery	0	0

in the cell membrane with resultant release of the fat into the interstitial space [52–59].

Recent studies have evaluated both the clinical and histopathologic effects of the 1064 nm Nd:YAG laser and 980 nm diode laser in laser-assisted lipolysis [52–59]. A recent study by Mordon et al. [52] demonstrated both enhanced lipolysis and skin contraction with the laser-assisted devices. Using an optimal thermal modeling approach, the authors demonstrated that increased heat generated by the laser in the deep reticular dermis may result in collagen and elastin synthesis and resultant skin tightening which they observed clinically after laser lipolysis. Goldman demonstrated skin contraction and enhanced lipolysis with the use of the 1064 nm Nd:YAG laser for submental liposuction [53]. Clinical results of tissue tightening were correlated with histologic analysis confirming laser-induced rupture of the adipocyte membrane. Kim et al. [54] reported the results of 29 patients treated with laser lipolysis with the 1064 nm Nd:YAG device and demonstrated clinical improvement (at 3 months, average of 37%) as well as decreased adiposity as measured by MRI (average of 17% reduction in volume). Greater improvement was noted in smaller volume areas, such as the submentum, in both clinical outcome and dermal tightening. However, several other recent comparative trials evaluating laser-assisted liposuction with the 1064 nm Nd:YAG laser have shown equivocal results with laser-assisted liposuction relative to liposuction alone [57–59].

Laser-assisted liposuction has been purported to result in both mechanical cavitation of fat resulting in greater ease of suction and greater skin retraction after the procedure resulting in enhanced tightening. However, further studies are highly needed to evaluate scientifically the benefits of pretreatment with lasers for ease of adipose removal and enhanced cosmesis [52–58].

Liposuction with TLA for lipedema

Lipedema, or adipositas dolorosa, is a painful, hereditary disorder affecting women that involves accumulation of excess fatty tissue on the lower extremities [60–62]. The enlargement of the lower extremities is disproportionate to the trunk, upper extremities, neck and face [60–62]. Patients experience pain, sensitivity to touch and pressure, and bruise easily after minor trauma [60–62]. Medical histories on lipedema patients reveal that diet and exercise may not improve the affected area [60–62]. Physical exam reveals normal appearing feet with enlarged calves above the malleoli. This sharp demarcation at the ankle is known as the cuff sign of lipedema [60–62]. Approximately 30% of patients have upper extremity involvement, which similarly shows an abrupt transition at the wrists, sparing the hands [60–62]. Morbidity results from both the cosmetic and physical limitations of the disease.

Liposuction with TLA is a safe and highly effective treatment for lipedema. In 2010, Rapprich and Dingler [61] reported a series of 25 women with lipedema treated with liposuction. On average, the volume of the legs was reduced by approximately 7%. Patients also reported a statistically and clinically significant reduction in pain and psychological strain. In 2011, Schmeller *et al.* [62] reported survey results of 112 women with lipedema treated with liposuction. All patients noted improved shape and body proportions. Patients similarly noted symptom improvement including decreased spontaneous pain, sensitivity to pressure, edema, and bruising. Patients experienced improved movement, cosmesis, and quality of life.

All of the illustrations in the chapter are provided courtesy of C. William Hanke, MD.

References

1. Fischer G. (1990) Liposculpture: the "correct" history of liposuction. Part I. *J Dermatol Surg Oncol* **16**, 1087–9.
2. Illouz YG. (1983) Body contouring by lipolysis: a 5-year experience with over 3000 cases. *Plast Reconstr Surg* **72**, 591–7.
3. Fournier P. (1987) *Body Sculpting Through Syringe Liposuction and Autologous Fat Re-injection*. Corona del Mar: Samuel Rolf International.
4. Hanke CW, Moy RL, Roenigk RK, Roenigk HH, Jr., Spencer JM, Tierney EP, *et al.* (2013) Current status of surgery in dermatology. *J Am Acad Dermatol* **69**, 972–1001.
5. Asken S. (1988) *Liposuction Surgery and Autologous Fat Transplantation*. Norwalk, CT: Appleton and Lange.
6. Asken S. (1986) *Manual of Liposuction Surgery and Autologous Fat Transplantation under Local Anesthesia*. Irvine, CA: Terry and Associates.
7. Klein JA. (1987) The tumescent technique for liposuction surgery. *Am J Cosmet Surg* **4**:263–7.
8. Bernstein G, Hanke CW. (1988) Safety of liposuction: a review of 9478 cases performed by dermatologists. *J Dermatol Surg Oncol* **14**, 1112–4.
9. Hanke CW, Bernstein G, Bullock S. (1995) Safety of tumescent liposuction in 15,336 patients. National survey results. *Dermatol Surg* **21**, 459–62.
10. Klein JA. (1990) Tumescent technique for regional anesthesia permits lidocaine doses of 35 mg/kg for liposuction. *J Dermatol Surg Oncol* **16**, 248–63.
11. Ostad A, Kageyama N, Moy RL. (1996) Tumescent anesthesia with a lidocaine dose of 55 mg/kg is safe for liposuction. *Dermatol Surg* **22**, 921–7.
12. Klein J. (2000) *Tumescent Technique: TLA and Microcannular Liposuction*. St Louis, MO: Mosby.
13. Sommer B, Sattler G, Hanke C, eds. (1999) *Tumescenz Lokalanasthesie*. Berlin (Germany): Springer.
14. Hanke C, Sommer B, Sattler G, eds. (2001) *Tumescent local anesthesia*. Berlin (Germany): Springer.
15. Klein JA. (2000) *Tumescent Technique: Tumescent Anesthesia and Microcannular Liposcution*. St Louis, MO: Mosby.
16. Hanke CW, Sattler G. (2005) *Liposuction Procedures in Cosmetic Dermatology Series*. Philadelphia, PA: Elsevier.
17. Hanke CW, Sattler S, Sommer B. (2007) *Textbook of Liposuction*. Abingdon, United Kingdom: Informa Healthcare.
18. Narins RS. (2003) *Safe Liposuction and Fat Transfer*. New York: Marcel Dekker.
19. Hanke CW. (1999) State-of-the-art liposculpture in the new millennium. *J Cutan Med Surg* **3** Suppl **4**, S36–42.
20. Pasman WJ, Saris WH, Westerterp-Plantenga MS. (1999) Predictors of weight maintenance. *Obesity Research* **7**, 43–50.
21. Brownell KD, Rodin J. (1994) Medical, metabolic, and psychological effects of weight cycling. *Arch Intern Med* **154**, 1325–30.
22. Ozgur F, Tuncali D, Guler Gursu K. (1998) Life satisfaction, self-esteem, and body image: a psychosocial evaluation of aesthetic and reconstructive surgery candidates. *Aesthetic Plast Surg* **22**, 412–9.
23. Mann MW, Palm MD, Sengelmann RD. (2008) New advances in liposuction technology. *Semin Cutan Med Surg* **27**, 72–82.
24. Hanke CW. (1989) Liposuction under local anesthesia. *J Dermatol Surg Oncol* **15**, 12.
25. Lillis PJ. (1988) Liposuction surgery under local anesthesia: limited blood loss and minimal lidocaine absorption. *J Dermatol Surg Oncol* **14**, 1145–8.
26. Butterwick Kaminer MS. (2003) Liposuction consultation and preoperative considerations. In: NarisRS, ed. *Safe Liposuction and Fat Transfer*. New York: Marcel Dekker.
27. Jacob CI KM. (2003) Tumescent anesthesia. In: Narins RS, ed. *Safe Liposuction and Fat Transfer*. New York: Marcel Dekker;.
28. Hanke CW, Coleman WP, 3rd. (1999) Morbidity and mortality related to liposuction. Questions and answers. *Dermatol Clin* **17**,899–902, viii.
29. Coleman IW, Hanke CW, Lillis P, Bernstein G, Narins R. (1999) Does the location of the surgery or the specialty of the physician affect malpractice claims in liposuction? *Dermatol Surg* **25**, 343–7.
30. Landry GL, Gomez JE. (1991) Management of soft tissue injuries. *Adolescent Medicine* (Philadelphia, Pa) **2**, 125–40.
31. Klein J. (2000) Miscellaneous complications. In: Klein JA, ed. *Tumescent Technique, Tumescent Anesthesia and Microcannular Liposuction*. St. Louis, MO: Mosby.
32. Narins RS, Coleman WP, 3rd. (1997) Minimizing pain for liposuction anesthesia. *Dermatol Surg* **23**, 1137–40.
33. Klein J. Thrombosis and embolism. (2000) In: Klein JA, ed. *Tumescent Technique, Tumescent Anesthesia and Microcannular Liposuction*. St. Louis: Mosby.
34. Housman TS, Lawrence N, Mellen BG, *et al.* (2002) The safety of liposuction: results of a national survey. *Dermatol Surg* **28**, 971–8.
35. Narins RS. (2003) Abdomen, hourglass abdomen, flanks and modified abdominoplasty. In: Naris RS, ed. *Safe Liposuction and Fat Transfer*. New York: Marcel Dekker.
36. Jacob C, Kaminer MS. (2003) Surgical approaches to the aging neck. In: Narins RS, ed. *Safe Liposuction and Fat Transfer*. New York: Marcel Dekker.
37. Goddio AS. (1992) Suction lipectomy: the gold triangle at the neck. *Aesthetic Plast Surg.* **16**, 27–32.
38. Kamer FM, Minoli JJ. (1993) Postoperative platysmal band deformity. A pitfall of submental liposuction. *Arch Otolaryngol Head Neck Surg* **119**, 193–6.
39. Key D. (2008) Efficacy of skin tightening and contour correction of the lower face and jowl using 1320 nm laser lipolysis: a comparison evaluation of lipolysis without aspiration, lipolysis with aspiration and aspiration without lipolysis. *American Society of Laser Medicine and Surgery Conference*; Kissimmee, FL.
40. Samdal F, Kleppe G, Amland PF, Abyholm F. (1994) Surgical treatment of gynaecomastia. Five years' experience with liposuction. *Scan J Plast Recontstru Hand Surg* **28**, 123–30.
41. Matarasso A, Courtiss EH. (1991) Suction mammaplasty: the use of suction lipectomy to reduce large breasts. *Plast Reconstr Surg* **87**, 709–17.
42. Habbema L. (2009) Breast reduction using liposuction with tumescent local anesthesia and powered cannulas. *Dermatol Surg* **35**, 41–50; discussion – 2.

43 Habbema L, Alons JJ. (2010) Liposuction of the female breast: a histologic study of the aspirate. *Dermatol Surg* **36**, 1406–11.
44 Gray LN. (1998) Liposuction breast reduction. *Aesthetic Plast Surg* **22**, 159–62.
45 Habbema L. (2010) Efficacy of tumescent local anesthesia with variable lidocaine concentration in 3430 consecutive cases of liposuction. *J Am Acad Dermatol* **62**, 988–94.
46 Bernstein G. (1999) Instrumentation for liposuction. *Dermatol Clin* **17**, 735–49, v.
47 Fodor PB, Watson J. (1998) Personal experience with ultrasound-assisted lipoplasty: a pilot study comparing ultrasound-assisted lipoplasty with traditional lipoplasty. *Plast Reconstr Surg* **101**, 1103–16; discussion 17–9.
48 Maxwell GP, Gingrass MK. (1998) Ultrasound-assisted lipoplasty: a clinical study of 250 consecutive patients. *Plast Reconstr Surg* **101**, 189–202; discussion 3–4.
49 Klein JA. (2000) Critique of ultrasonic liposuction. In: Klein JA, ed. *Tumescent Technique, Tumescent Anesthesia and Microcannular Liposuction*. St. Louis: Mosby.
50 Hanke W, Cox SE, Kuznets N, Coleman WP, 3rd. (2004) Tumescent liposuction report performance measurement initiative: national survey results. *Dermatol Surg* **30**, 967–77; discussion 78.
51 Grazer FM, de Jong RH. (2000) Fatal outcomes from liposuction: census survey of cosmetic surgeons. *Plast Reconstr Surg* **105**, 436–46; discussion 47–8.
52 Mordon SR, Wassmer B, Reynaud JP, Zemmouri J. (2008) Mathematical modeling of laser lipolysis. *Biomed Eng Online* **7**:10.
53 Goldman A. (2006) Submental Nd:Yag laser-assisted liposuction. *Lasers Surg Med* **38**, 181–4.
54 Kim KH, Geronemus RG. (2006) Laser lipolysis using a novel 1,064 nm Nd:YAG Laser. *Dermatol Surg* **32**, 241–48; discussion 7.
55 Ichikawa K, Miyasaka M, Tanaka R, et al. (2005) Histologic evaluation of the pulsed Nd:YAG laser for laser lipolysis. *Lasers Surg Med* **36**, 43–6.
56 Morton S WB, Reynaud P, Zemmouri J. (2008) Mathematical modeling of laser lipolysis. *Abstract presented at American Society of Laser Medicine and Surgery Conference*; Kissimmee, FL.
57 Dressel TZB. (2008) Laser liposuction a work in progress. *Abstract presented at American Society of Laser Medicine and Surgery Conference*; Kissimmee, FL.
58 Weiss R WM, Beasley K. (2008) Laser lipolysis: skin contraction effect of 1320 nm. *Abstract presented at American Society of Laser Medicine and Surgery Conference*; Kissimmee, FL.
59 DiBernardo B GM, Saluja R, Woodhall K, Reyes J. (2008) Mulicenter study evaluation of sequential emission of lasers for the treatment of fat with laser assisted lipolysis. *Abstract presented at American Society of Laser Medicine and Surgery Conference*; Kissimmee, FL.
60 Langendoen SI, Habbema L, Nijsten TE, Neumann HA. (2009) Lipoedema: from clinical presentation to therapy. A review of the literature. *Br J Dermatol* **161**, 980–6.
61 Rapprich S, Dingler A, Podda M. (2011) Liposuction is an effective treatment for lipedema – results of a study with 25 patients. *J Dtsch Dermatol Ges* **9**, 33–40.
62 Schmeller W, Hueppe M, Meier-Vollrath I. (2012) Tumescent liposuction in lipoedema yields good long-term results. *Br J Dermatol* **166**, 161–8.
63 Dolsky RL, Newman J, Fetzek JR, Anderson RW. (1987) Liposuction. History, techniques, and complications. *Dermatol Clin* **5**, 313–33.
64 Teimourian B, Rogers WB, 3rd. (1989) A national survey of complications associated with suction lipectomy: a comparative study. *Plast Reconstr Surg* **84**, 628–31.
65 Dillerud E, Haheim LL. (1993) Long-term results of blunt suction lipectomy assessed by a patient questionnaire survey. *Plast Reconstr Surg* **92**, 35–42.
66 ASPRS Task Force on Liposuction [August 2, 2009]. Available from: www.plasticsurgery.org/Medical_Professionals/Publications/PSN_News_Bulletins/ASPS_urges_members_to_exercise_caution_in_lipoplasty_procedures_Task_Force_report_calls_for_scrutiny_of_training_large_volume_removals.html.
67 Dolsky RL. (1997) State of the art in liposuction. *Dermatol Surg* **23**, 1192–3.
68 Hughes CE, 3rd. (1999) Patient selection, planning, and marking in ultrasound-assisted lipoplasty. *Clin Plast Surg* **26**, 279–82; ix.

CHAPTER 54
Liposuction of the Neck

Kimberly J. Butterwick
Cosmetic Laser Dermatology, San Diego, CA, USA

> **BASIC CONCEPTS**
> - Neck liposuction is used to remove excess fat from the neck area and minimize skin sagging.
> - Small cannulas and multiple entry sites are necessary to achieve even fat removal without ridging or deformity.
> - Tumescent anesthesia is key to reducing pain and bruising while facilitating fat removal.
> - Proper selection of patients with fat in front of the platysma muscle can ensure a successful outcome.
> - Overremoval of fat on the lower neck should be avoided.

Introduction

One of the first signs of aging that prompts patients to seek cosmetic treatment is the sagging neck. Tumescent liposuction of this area often dramatically rejuvenates the neckline and is one of the most common body areas treated with this modality. Although this area may seem complicated to the novice surgeon, liposuction of the neck is relatively quick, safe, and readily learned. It is also well tolerated by patients with rapid healing in 3–4 days. With careful selection of patients and good technique, this is a very rewarding area for patients and surgeon alike.

Anatomy

The primary goal of liposuction of the neck is restoration of the cervicomental angle (CMA). This is the angle formed by the horizontal plane of the submental region and the vertical plane of the neck (Figure 54.1) [1]. The ideal angle is generally considered to be 90–100° or more, up to 135° [1-3]. Other anatomic features of a youthful neck include definition of the inferior mandibular border, subthyroid depression, a thyroid notch visible as a gentle indentation, and a visible anterior border of the sternocleidomastoid muscle [1]. The face should be distinct from the neck such that a shadow should be cast on to the upper neck by the mandible. With aging and/or genetics, there may be accumulation of submental fat leading to blunting of the CMA or a "double chin." Other anatomic factors may also contribute to an obtuse CMA such as a low-lying hyoid bone, microgenia, or retrognathia. Ideally, the hyoid bone should be positioned at the C3–C4 level [4]. Lateral to the submental region, there may be loss of definition of the submandibular region leading to an unattractive continuum between the face and the neck. Further contributing to fullness in this area may be ptotic submandibular glands located along the inferior midportion of the mandibular ramus. Other stigmata of aging in the lower third of the face may need to be addressed such as the presence of jowls and the development of a depression just medial to the jowl called the prejowl sulcus [5].

The platysma muscle is the thin layer of muscle just deep to the submental fat pad arising from the cervicopectoral fascia inferiorly and attaching to the depressor anguli oris, risorius, and mentalis muscles superiorly with a varying degree of decussation at the midline [6]. Approximately 75% of the time, the fibers interlace 1–2 cm below the chin but separate in the suprahyoid region. Less often, the fibers decussate all the way down to the thyroid cartilage or not at all [7]. With aging, the medial fibers of the platysma muscle may hypertrophy into thick visible bands. Deep to the platysma, there may be a collection of fat that is midline and submental. While the preplatysmal fat pad is accessible to tumescent liposuction, the retroplatysmal fat pad is not and requires direct excision for removal. Having the patient clench his or her teeth tightens the platysma and aides in distinguishing pre- or retroplatysmal fat [3]. The amount of submental retroplatysmal fat has been estimated to vary between 30% and 57% of the total amount [8].

Also deep to the platysma is the marginal mandibular branch of the facial nerve, which is vulnerable to trauma during liposuction of this area. This motor nerve runs along the mandible, parallel to the ramus and is typically most superficial at the anterior border of the masseter muscle (Figure 54.2). However, the position of this nerve is variable, and it can be found 3–4 cm inferior to the ramus. Caution must be exercised when suctioning this region because repeated pressure and rubbing

---

Cosmetic Dermatology: Products and Procedures, Second Edition. Edited by Zoe Diana Draelos.
© 2016 John Wiley & Sons, Ltd. Published 2016 by John Wiley & Sons, Ltd.

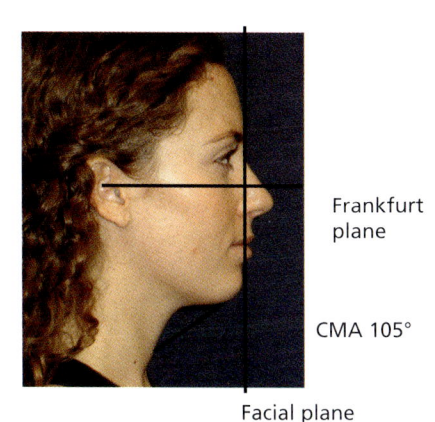

Figure 54.1 The youthful neck with a cervicomental angle of 100°. The facial and Frankfurt plane are shown with glabella, subnasale, and chin in alignment.

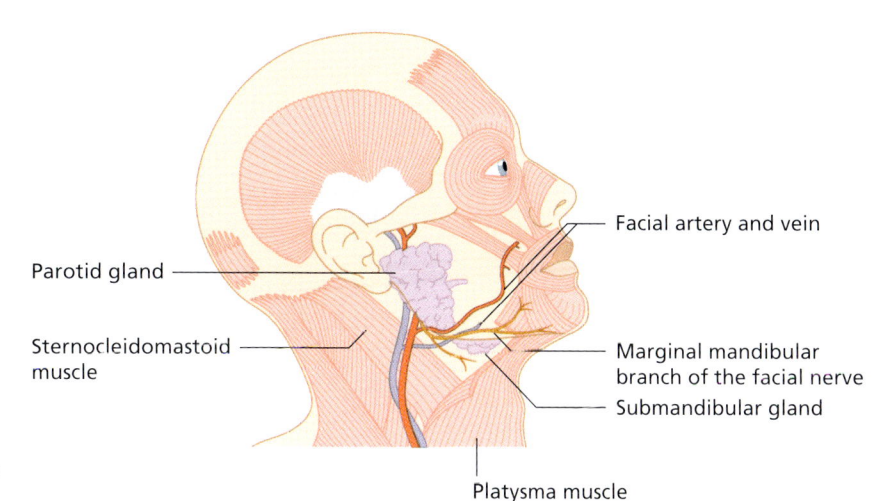

Figure 54.2 Marginal mandibular branch of the facial nerve and other relevant anatomy.

from the cannula may result in temporary neuropraxis. While this typically lasts only 4–6 weeks, the distorted appearance is very distressing to the patient. To minimize injury to this nerve, patients should be asked to clench their teeth and the anterior edge of the masseter should be marked where the nerve is likely to be found, at or just below the level of the ramus. Other techniques to minimize potential injury to this nerve are described below. Another structure less vulnerable to injury is the external jugular vein which passes over the sternocleidomastoid muscle. The vessel could be injured from inadvertent deep penetration by the cannula from a lateral position.

Aesthetic considerations

To the novice surgeon, liposuction of the neck entails simply removing fat in the submental area. However, there are some aesthetic principles and proportions that should be considered for optimal aesthetic results (Figure 54.1) [9,10]. When evaluating the cervicomental angle, one should evaluate the entire profile of the head and neck. The ideal profile should be viewed with the head held in the Frankfurt horizontal plane. This is the horizontal plane, parallel to the floor, in which a horizontal line can be drawn through the highest point of the ear canal meatus and the lowest point of the orbital rim [10]. In this position, the chin is at the proper level for assessing the CMA and for uniformity of preoperative and postoperative photographs. It is said that in this position, the glabella, nasal root, lip projection, and mentum should ideally align in a vertical facial plane. Utilizing this proportion enables the surgeon to assess the relative strength of the chin and the adequacy of volume in the face. The face should be divisible by thirds from the midline frontal scalp to glabella, the glabella to the infranasal area, and the infranasal area to the mentum. Often, the lower third of the face is reduced in volume because of bone loss, aging, genetics, or other factors.

Patient selection

Potential candidates for submental liposuction fall into three groups: correction of genetic traits, rejuvenation for mild to moderate aging, and restoration of more advanced aging. The latter two groups may also have some pre-existing hereditary factors. All groups should be assessed systematically and all determinates to the aging neck evaluated (Table 54.1).

478 ANTI-AGING Skin Contouring Techniques

Table 54.1 Preoperative assessment.

1	Cervicomental angle
2	Degree of submental fat
3	Platysma banding
4	Degree of subplatysma fat
5	Hyoid position
6	Presence of jowls
7	Position of submandibular glands
8	Adequacy of chin profile
9	Skin thickness
10	Skin laxity

The first group of patients tends to be relatively young, typically less than 30 years, and usually of normal weight, although this deposit makes them look heavier or older than they are. Although the skin quality is excellent, the profile is obscured by submental fat. There are often contributing factors to the obtuse CMA, such as microgenia or a low-lying hyoid bone. These limitations should be addressed at the time of the consultation. Patients in this age group may also have quite full cheeks, but with age cheek hollows often become more marked. Removal of fat in the cheeks may cause the patient to look older and gaunt years later.

The next group of patients is typically 35–50 years old with some skin laxity brought about by photoaging, facial volume loss, and a genetic tendency towards submental fat accumulation. They are often mildly overweight, but even at ideal weight, the problem persists.

The last group is over 55 years old and has submental fat but in addition significant skin redundancy, bone and volume loss, platysma banding, and photoaging. Many in this group would fare better with reconstructive surgery, but at times the risk:benefit ratio – that is, the improvement offered by liposuction alone – will satisfy those wishing to avoid the risks of a more invasive surgical procedure. These patients should be carefully assessed, as liposuction alone could significantly worsen the appearance of the skin, platysma bands, or expose ptotic submandibular glands.

In all three groups, males may show relatively less improvement than females. Their thickened, bearded skin retracts less readily than that of females. Even thinner females with little submental fat often show good benefit because of marked skin retraction after liposuction.

Consultation and physical examination

The consultation is a key step in communicating expected risks and benefits. In our practice, patients initially voice their concerns to a practice consultant. The consultant reviews treatment options and helps patients develop and prioritize their beauty wish list. Patients often pull back the neck tightly and, in the same breath, state they would never want a facelift. If liposuction

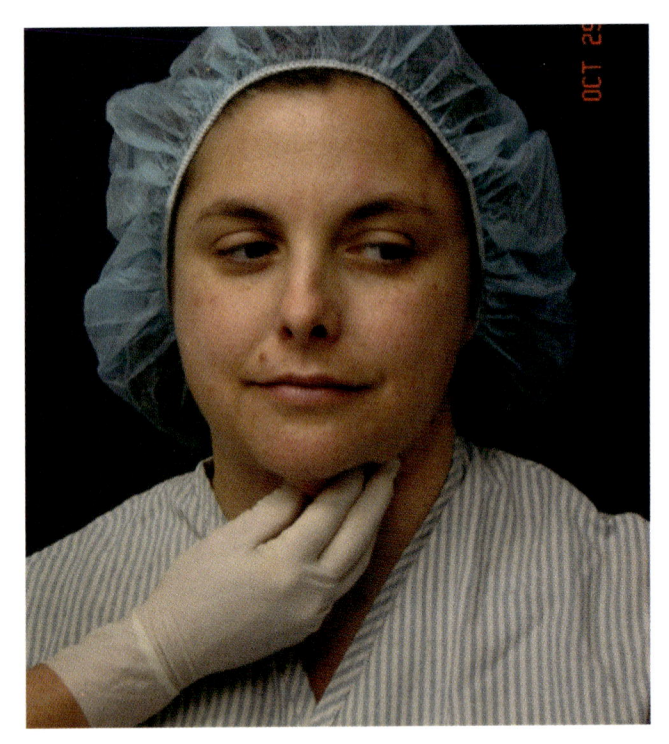

Figure 54.3 Grasping and tucking the submental fat to demonstrate expected results of submental liposuction without upward posterior retraction seen in rhytidectomy.

alone is being considered, it is helpful to grasp the submental fat and tuck it up under the chin. This maneuver essentially "removes" the fat from view without pulling up on the jowls (Figure 54.3). If the patient has lax, photoaged skin, the surgeon should bunch it up a little and show the patient that it could look more wrinkled after the procedure. The surgeon should pull the skin back and demonstrate the probable result of a rhytidectomy to help the patient visualize the different results of different procedures. Any contributing factors to the blunted neck angle are reviewed with the patient at this point and additional corrective measures and alternative treatments are discussed. Platysma bands can be identified by having the patient grimace. An overview of the risks is also part of the consultation.

At this point, the surgeon typically leaves the room, and the consultant answers additional questions, reviews the fee quote, and offers to schedule the procedure. Should the patient decide to proceed, he or she returns for a second visit for a preoperative examination. At this visit, the patient has a physical examination, reads and signs consents forms, and is given written preoperative and postoperative instructions. Preoperative laboratory studies and photographs are completed. Typical preoperative laboratory studies include: full blood count, chemistry panel, prothrombin time/partial thromboplastin time (PT/PTT), international normalized ratio, and viral titers to screen for hepatitis and HIV infection. A prescription for preoperative antibiotics is given to start the night before surgery for a total of 10 days.

Procedure

Markings

The preoperative markings are summarized in Table 54.2. With the patient in an upright position, the edge of the mandible is outlined and a circle is drawn around the perimeter of the main accumulation of fat in the submental area (Figure 54.4). An "X" is then marked on the most visible mound within that circle. An additional circle may be drawn just inferior to the submental area if indicated, or concentric circles may be drawn around the main deposit of fat. The jowls are outlined as they extend both superior and inferior to the mandibular border. Again, the fullest aspects of the jowl are marked with an "X." Laterally, fullness superior to the mandible is outlined. Inferior to the mandible, small "X's" or a line should be drawn where maximum definition is desired. This is the area where a linear shadow should be cast.

The patient is then instructed to clamp down on the back teeth. The edge of the masseter is then palpated and an "X" is placed at the probable location of the marginal mandibular nerve, preferably in a different color. The platysma is assessed during this maneuver and the bands may be outlined in another color. Other landmarks that may be highlighted include the anterior border of the sternocleidomastoid muscle, the hyoid bone, and the inferior border of the neck.

Table 54.2 Preoperative marking.

Mark border of mandible
Encircle submental fat and place "X" on apex
If present, outline jowl and excess fat in lower lateral cheek
Make a line or "X's" where submandibular concavity desired
Mark likely position of marginal mandibular nerve
Dot in platysma bands if indicated
Draw parallel vertical lines to base of neck

Parallel vertical lines are drawn from the immediate submental area down the remainder of the neck to the base of the neck. Fat is rarely removed from the lower two-thirds of the neck because the skin here is often so thin that it will look more aged and wrinkled if underlying fat is removed. The long vertical lines remind the surgeon not to remove fat but rather to tunnel through, without suction. Tunneling is thought to create tissue injury that will then stimulate some neocollagenesis and perhaps thicken or tighten the skin to some degree. On rare occasion if the patient has horizontal rhytids of the lower two-thirds of the neck and excessive fat, very conservative liposuction of the lower neck will significantly improve fat bulges and horizontal furrows.

Anesthesia and infiltration

Patients undergoing liposuction of the neck do not require general anesthesia and many of them could undergo the procedure without any sedation at all. However, most patients prefer to have some anxiolysis and are typically given 1 mg lorazepam p.o. prior to the procedure. Alternatively, if a surgicenter is utilized, an intravenous line may be started and the patient given 1.0 mg midazolam IV along with 25 μg fentanyl IV as a one-time dose. Intravenous medications are often preferred because the patient will feel instantly relaxed and will be nearly fully awake when the procedure is over. One must be careful with intravenous medications to avoid excessive sedation and apnea; however, the low doses utilized above result in mild sedation with appropriate responsiveness.

The patient is then positioned in a supine position with a neck roll partially under the shoulders so that the head rolls back comfortably in an extended position. After prepping with benzalkonium chloride antiseptic (Med Chem, Torrance, CA, USA), the patient is draped with sterile towels, including a sterile turban (Figure 54.5). A lap sponge is placed over the patient's eyes for comfort and protection.

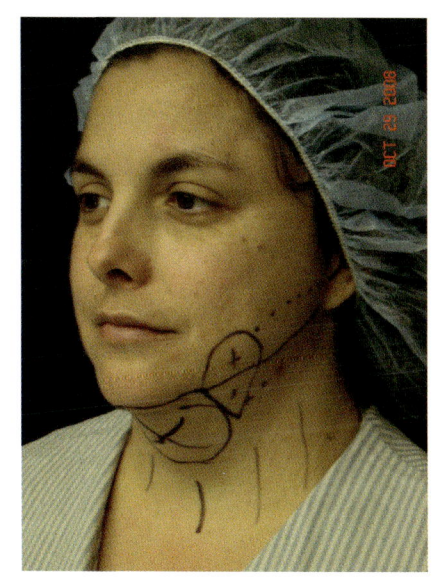

Figure 54.4 Preoperative markings.

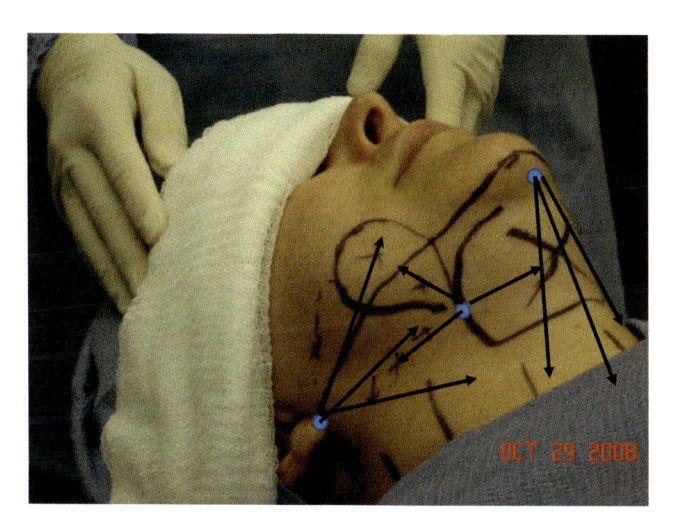

Figure 54.5 Operative position with chin extended. Three of the five entry sites are denoted with circles and typical fanning pattern shown.

Tumescent anesthesia of the neck is the next step. Superficial blebs of tumescent lidocaine are first made in five sites, corresponding to the entry sites for the cannula. Dilute lidocaine consisting of Klein's standard formula with lidocaine 0.1% is infiltrated into the subcutaneous space with the aid of an infusion pump [11]. A 25-gauge spinal needle is used initially in a fan-like motion, introduced through five blebs, until the entire surgical field has been partially infused. The tumescent fluid is warmed, the infusion rate is low, and the needle gauge is small, assuring that there is minimal discomfort for the patient. Approximately 50–100 mL is utilized at this point. The spinal needle is then changed to 20-gauge, at a faster infusion rate, so that very quickly, within 5–15 minutes, the entire surgical field is tumesced. The patient may feel a bit anxious at this point because the neck will feel taut. Reassure patients that they can still breathe and swallow and that the tightness will loosen within a few minutes of starting the liposuction. It should be noted that it is not necessary to infiltrate the lower half of the neck. While the procedure is underway, the solution will drift inferiorly to the sternal notch, so that at the end of the procedure, when tunneling the lower neck may be desired, the lower neck will have adequate anesthesia. Typical volumes of infiltrated solution are 400–500 mL.

Liposuction: standard operative techniques

The standard liposuction procedure utilizes five entry sites and a thorough suction with small cannulae (Table 54.3). The submental area is approached through three small stab incisions with an 11 blade. Although it may be tempting to perform the entire procedure through one site, the most thorough and smooth result requires criss-crossing through multiple sites. In addition, one avoids a depression which is commonly seen under a single incision site. Only small cannulae are utilized, such as the Klein 14 and 16 gauge Finesse, to avoid ridges or troughs in thin-skinned patients. In patients with thicker skin, a slightly more aggressive cannula is sometimes needed such as a 12-gauge Klein Finesse or the multi-holed Klein Capistrano, gauge 14. These smaller cannulas also preserve connective tissue strands throughout the fat and are thought to maximize retraction of the skin.

A thorough fanning technique is utilized through all three incisions with the cannula attached to the suction device. An assistant may anchor the skin at the entry site and elsewhere to minimize skin buckling, thereby facilitating long smooth strokes of the cannula. This is the area to be aggressive, from the submental crease to the superior edge of the thyroid cartilage, approximately 8–9 cm caudal to the submental crease. The end point in this area is a thin pinch of the skin. When lifting up a cannula under the skin, the overlying skin should be palpated and free of lumps. A thin layer of fat, approximately 3–5 mm in thickness should be left to prevent surface irregularities [12]. The cannula may be visible beneath the skin.

The patient's head is then turned to the side and a fourth incision site is made. If indicated by the preoperative examination, very conservative liposuction of the lower cheek is performed. Usually, less than 10 strokes of the cannula are needed in order to taper the face. One must be careful not to overresect this area and to feather (tunnel without suction) into the cheek immediately superior to the treated area in order to avoid a shelf or step-off. It is also important that fat is left behind. A strong, smooth, mandibular border is a youthful feature so it is rarely necessary to remove fat immediately overlying the mandible. The cannula is then directed approximately 3–4 cm below the ramus. This is a key area for removing fat to optimize definition between the head and the neck. Thorough removal is performed along this region. The surgeon must be mindful not to rasp against the ramus while performing liposuction with the head turned because of the proximity of the marginal mandibular nerve. In this position, the nerve may be located 3–4 cm below the mandible and become more superficial. Although it is deep to the platysma, this muscle is very thin and could be punctured by a small cannula [13]. If liposuction is needed near the ramus, one should pinch up the skin off the ramus and avoid deep fat.

Special attention is then directed toward the jowl. If the jowl is large, a separate stab incision is made with an 18-gauge No-Kor needle, at the most caudal extension of the jowl (Figure 54.6). A 16-gauge Klein Finesse cannula is then utilized to very conservatively remove less than 30% of the fat. Excessive

Table 54.3 Standard technique.

Debulk in midline submental region from three entry sites
Turn head laterally, suction lateral cheek/submandibular region
Avoid rasping mandible
Conservative suction of the jowl
Repeat steps 2 and 3 on contralateral side
Return head to central position. Tunnel inferiorly
Palpate all areas for smoothness
Apply microfoam tape and dressings

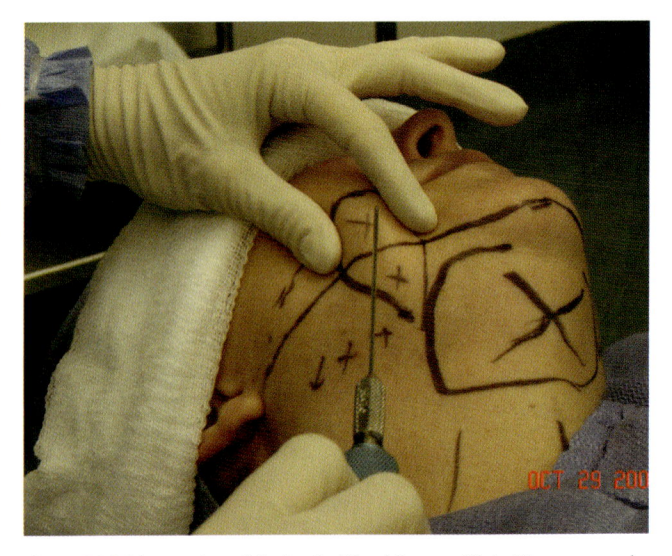

Figure 54.6 Liposuction of the jowl with a 16-gauge Klein Finesse cannula. The skin is pinched up by the non-dominant hand to avoid rasping the cannula against the mandible.

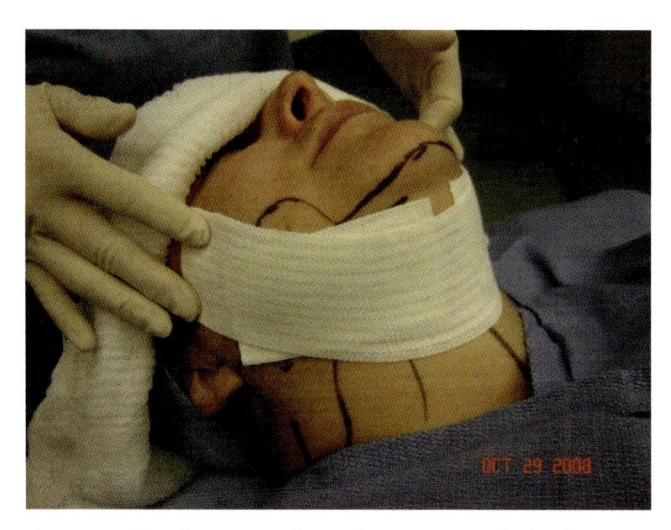

Figure 54.7 Microfoam tape with two shorter pieces applied with traction to the midline and a third piece across entire area. This helps to decrease central pooling.

removal in this area is not necessary as the skin will redrape nicely and overresection will result in deepening of the adjacent marionette fold. These same steps are then repeated on the contralateral side.

After liposuction of both sides, the head is then returned to a central position. A 14-gauge Klein Finesse cannula is passed through the three central incisions sites to check for remaining fat deposits.

Sometimes there are stubborn deposits inferior to the lowermost extension of the jowls and this area is specifically checked. Tunneling or feathering without suction is then performed with the cannula passing through the entire surgical field, down to the sternal notch without suction. Some surgeons recommend "windshield wiping" at this point in order to gain maximal skin retraction. In the author's opinion this is not necessary and may have a negative effect in the development of delayed and unattractive adherence of the skin to underlying fascia. If platysma bands were visible at the preoperative examination, it may be helpful to take a spatula-tipped cannula and tunnel underneath them to reduce cutaneous attachments. Others prefer a closed neck V-shaped neck dissector to release tethering fibrous bands [14].

At the end of the procedure, three pieces of microfoam tape (3M, St. Paul, MN, USA) are applied as shown in Figure 54.7. This helps to minimize pooling of tumescent fluid and free floating adipocytes in the submental area and minimizes postoperative bruising. It is removed 23–48 hours after the procedure.

Postoperative course

In addition to microfoam tape, patients wear a chin strap 24 hours a day for 3–4 days. The strap is then worn 2–4 hours per day for another 3 weeks. Immediately after the procedure, patients experience minimal to no discomfort. Mild discomfort may last 2–4 days. Patients may return to work after the initial few days at home. Purpura is typically minimal. If it develops, it tends to drift below the collar line and can be covered with clothing or scarves. During the first 2 weeks postoperatively, the submental area swells and patients will note increasing induration. There may be small focal areas of induration appearing as lumps or areas of stiff skin that crease unnaturally with movement. Patients should be advised ahead of time because induration always develops as an expected, temporary condition that resolves over a period of 4–8 weeks. Lymphatic massage may be helpful as the induration most likely represents a localized interstitial edema. Rarely, a larger nodule develops that is unsightly. Low doses of 2.5 mg/mL Kenalog (Bristol-Myers Squibb Princeton, NJ, USA) may be injected to reduce the edema more quickly.

After the healing process, expected benefits of liposuction of the neck and jowls include reduction of adipocities, and skin retraction leading to elevation of the submental area, flattening of the jowls, and a reduced cervicomental angle (Figure 54.8 and 54.9). The

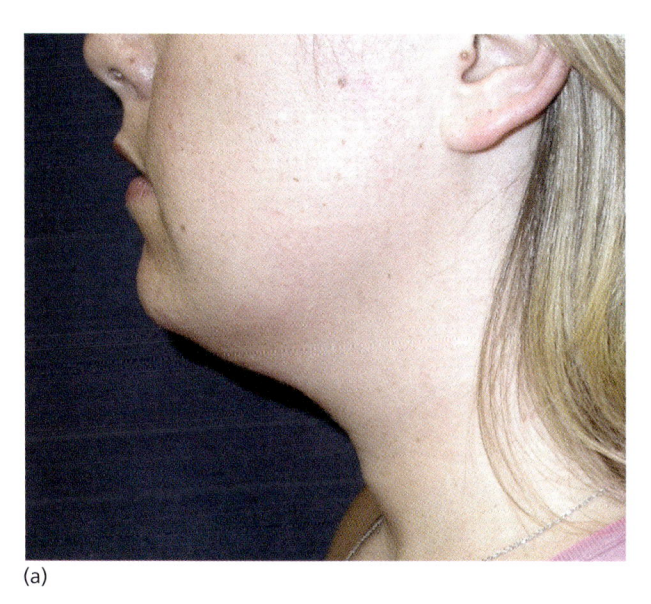

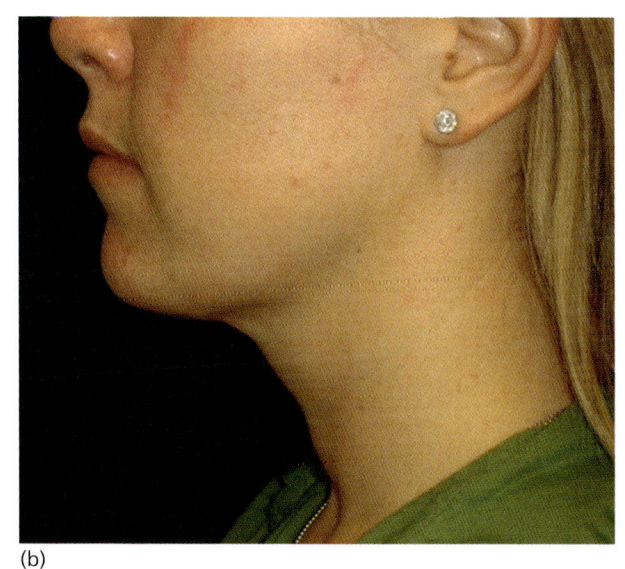

Figure 54.8 Before (a) and 3 years after (b) removal of 50 mL of supranatant fat.

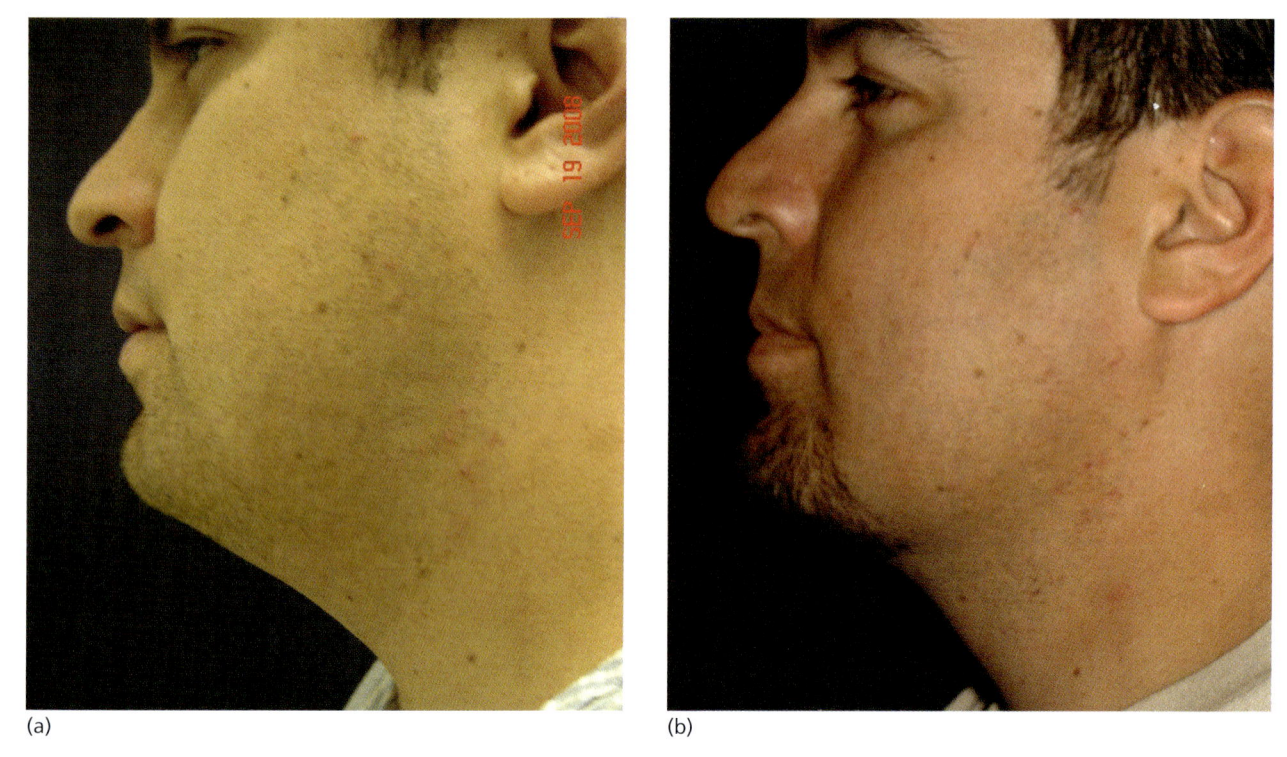

Figure 54.9 Before (a) and 1 month after (b) removal of 100 mL of supranatant fat. CoolLipo laser applied at 15 W, 40 Hz for 625 pulses with simultaneous suction. After suction, skin tightening was performed at 5 W, 50 Hz for 93 pulses.

capacity of the skin of the neck to retract and redrape in this area is outstanding and remarkable even compared to liposuction in other areas [15]. The very small incision sites (3 mm or less) heal readily and essentially ensure a scarless procedure. Avoiding both surgical scars and general anesthesia are key aspects of this procedure that factor into the patient's choice over more invasive options.

Complications

Submental liposuction has a very low rate of complications with proper careful technique. Immediate potential complications include bleeding or hematoma. With tumescent liposuction and blunt-tipped cannulas the risk of significant bleeding is very low. Postoperative compression further minimizes this risk.

Temporary injury to the marginal mandibular nerve is probably the most common complication. It is important to be aware of the likely position of this nerve, anterior to the masseter muscle and at the level of the ramus or 3–4 cm inferior to the border. The nerve is most vulnerable when the head is turned to the side. It is also prone to injury if one attempts to treat the jowl from a medial, submental incision site. Avoidance of brushing against the mandible in any position and avoidance of penetrating the thin platysma muscle is essential. In addition, approaching the jowl from the previously described inferior position should nearly eliminate this potential risk. If paresis develops, it presents not as ipsilateral weakness, but rather hyperkinesis of the contralateral side.

This side effect is temporary, rarely lasting beyond a few weeks, but it may last for 2–3 months. If troublesome to the patient, a few units of botulinum toxin may be placed in the contralateral, hyperkinetic, depressor labii inferioris. Permanent injury to the marginal mandibular nerve has not been reported after tumescent liposuction because there is no sharp instrumentation. Sensory nerves may also be temporarily affected. Reassurance that the numb feeling will resolve within 4–6 weeks generally consoles the patient. Postoperative edema has been mentioned previously.

One more troubling aspect of this is the development of a submental fold. This is most likely caused by the compression garment loosening in this area. Patients with larger necks, low hyoid bones, and who frequently flex their neck for work or hobbies (i.e. needlepoint) seem to be at risk for this complication, which presents as a ridge, just posterior to the submental crease. Careful taping with microfoam tape and admonition to elevate the chin regularly will mitigate this risk.

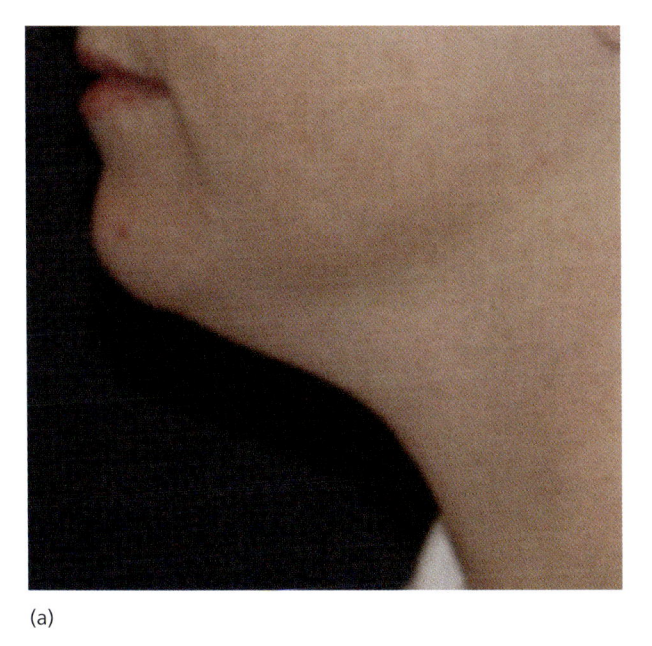

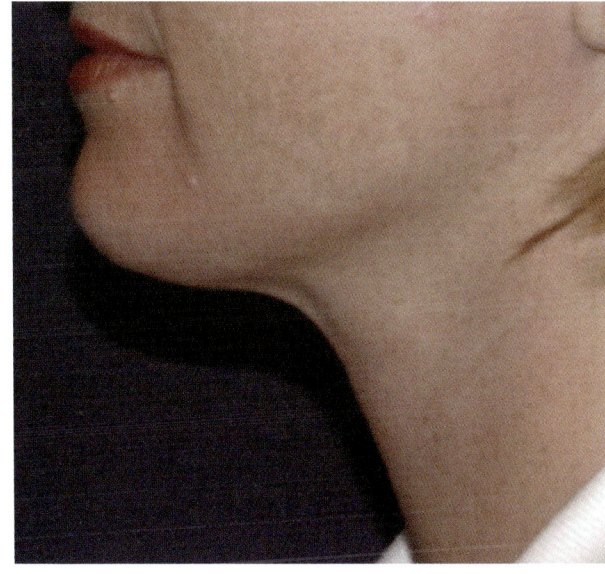

Figure 54.10 Small platysma bands unmasked after submental liposuction (b).

Overresection is an avoidable complication. Overresection in the submental area leads to a "cobra" neck in which there is an actual depression under the chin with flaring of the sides because of the relative overabundance of adjacent fat [16]. The jowls are another danger zone in which the surgeon may be overly aggressive and cause a depressed, aged appearance. If patients are thin-skinned and/or elderly, overresection will lead to increased wrinkling of the skin. Conservative liposuction, leaving a thin blanket of fat, is best in these patients.

Although it may not be a result of overresection, performing liposuction of the neck may unmask platysma bands and ptotic submandibular glands (Figure 54.10). A thorough preoperative examination should help to detect these patients. In one study of 301 patients, submental obesity and the anatomic pattern non-decussating platysma fibers were found to be significant correlates in the development of the postoperative platysmal banding [17]. The bands may be treated with botulinum toxin A (Allergan, Inc., Irvine, CA, USA) after surgery or adjuvant procedures such as platysmaplasty at the time of surgery.

Excessive defatting in a patient with a round face, without tapering the lower face, can result in a "lollipop" appearance. Tapering of the lower face will prevent this appearance; however, care must be given to feather superiorly to avoid a shelf or step off. Infection is very rare with tumescent liposuction of any area. Patients are advised of this low risk, which is further reduced by preoperative antibiotics, and sterile procedures during surgery.

Advanced and ancillary operating techniques

Submental liposuction is an excellent stand-alone procedure but it also lends itself to the addition of other procedures. At times, these procedures are essential for an acceptable outcome. Examples include platysmaplasty for thick, pronounced platysma bands that are present at rest or with mild animation [14,18]. A mini or full rhytidectomy may be added for excessively lax skin and jowls [11]. The use of various lasers and devices to melt fat and/or tighten skin has been touted by some, but at this point, clinical data are lacking. At other times, procedures may be added to enhance an otherwise good outcome. With photoaged skin, for example, one may perform a resurfacing procedure to the face and neck immediately following the liposuction procedure. A typical procedure would add a fractionated laser versus a more invasive laser to avoid the oozing and discomfort from more aggressive laser procedures while wearing the chin strap. If the chin is recessed and/or the chin height short, chin implants may be inserted through a submental incision [19]. Alternatively, autologous fat transfer may be easily added to the procedure (Figure 54.11) [20]. Fat may be utilized from the neck, but it is usually difficult to obtain enough fat through a hand-held syringe, particularly if the fat is to be centrifuged as well. Another donor site may be necessary. Other areas of the face in which volume restoration will enhance the neckline include the prejowl sulcus, marionette fold, or mandibular border. Full-face volume restoration if indicated will elevate the cheeks and jowls and often lift the submental area.

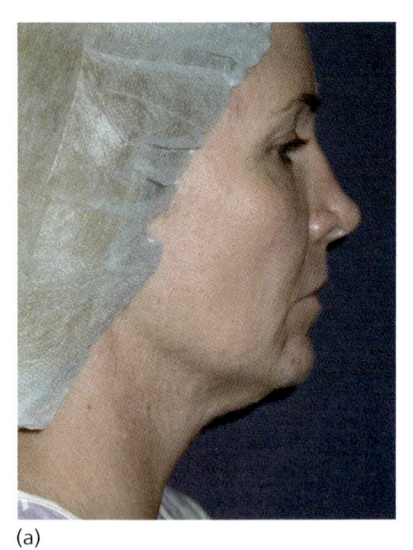

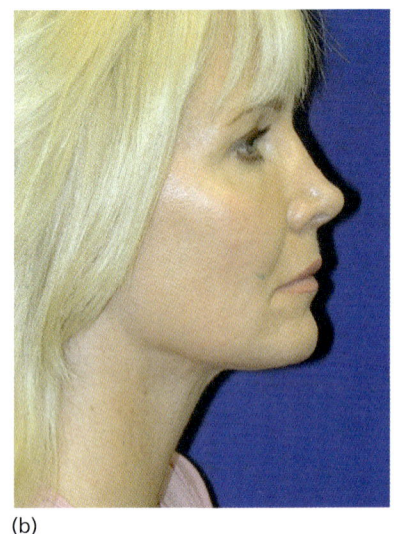

Figure 54.11 Before (a) and 6 months after (b) submental liposuction (25 mL) combined with fat augmentation to cheeks and chin (21 mL).

Conclusions

Liposuction of the neck is a procedure that is straightforward, takes 1 hour or less, and is rapidly healing with few complications. It is often a stand-alone procedure or it can be combined with other procedures that may be indicated in the aging patient or those with pre-existing anatomic factors. Proper patient selection and good technique that avoids overresection are key elements for achieving optimal results. Because aging of the neckline and drooping jowls are often the first major complaint of the aging patient, it is incumbent of the dermatologic surgeon to achieve mastery of this technique as it is likely to become one of his or her favorite procedures to perform.

References

1 Prendiville S, Kohoska MS, Hollenbeak CS, et al. (2002) A comparative study of surgical techniques on the cervicomental angle in human cadavers. *Arch Facial Plast Surg* **4**, 236–42.
2 Ellenbogen R, Karlin J. (1980) Visual criteria for success in restoring the youthful neck. *Plast Reconstr Surg* **66**, 826.
3 Jacob CI, Berkes BJ, Kaminer MS. (2000) Liposuction and surgical recontouring of the neck: a retrospective analysis. *Dermatol Surg* **26**, 635–2.
4 Moreno A, Bell WH, Zhi-Hao Y. (1994) Esthetic contour analysis of the submental cervical region. *J Oral Maxillofac Surg* **52**, 704–13.
5 Mittelman H. (1994) The anatomy of the aging mandible and its importance to facelift surgery. *Facial Plast Surg Clin N Am* **2**, 301–10.
6 de Castro CC. (1980) The anatomy of the platysma muscle. *Plast Reconstr Surg* **66**, 680–3.
7 Hoefflin SM. (1998) Anatomy of the platysma and lip depressor muscles: a simplified mnemonic approach. *Dermatol Surg* **24**, 1225–31.
8 Lambros V. (1992) Fat contouring in the face and neck. *Clin Plast Surg* **19**, 401–14.
9 Powell N, Humphreys B. (1984) *Proportions of the Aesthetic Face.* New York: Thieme-Stratton.
10 Farkas LG, Sohm P, Kolar JC, Katic MJ, Munro IR. (1985) Inclination of the facial profile: art versus reality. *Plast Reconstr Surg* **75**, 509–19.
11 Klein JA. (1990) Tumescent technique for regional anesthesia permits lidocaine doses of 35 mg/kg for liposuction. *J Dermatol Surg Oncol* **16**, 248–63.
12 Watson D. (2005) Submentoplasty. *Facial Plast Surg Clin N Am* **13**, 459–67.
13 Langdon RC. (2000) Liposuction of neck and jowls: five-incision method combining machine-assisted and syringe aspiration. *Dermatol Surg* **26**, 388–91.
14 Jacob CI, Kaminer MS. (2002) The corset platysma repair: a technique revisited. *Dermatol Surg* **28**, 257–62.
15 Goddio AS. (1992) Suction lipectomy: the gold triangle at the neck. *Aesth Plast Surg* **16**, 27–32.
16 Fattahi TT. (2004) Management of isolated neck deformity. *Atlas Oral Maxillofacial Surg Clin N Am* **12**, 261–70.
17 Kamer FM, Minoli JJ. (1993) Postoperative platysmal band deformity. *Arch Otolaryngol Head Neck Surg* **119**, 193–6.
18 Knipper P, Mitz V, Maladry D, Saad G. (1997) Is it necessary to suture the platysma muscles on the midline to improve the cervical profile? An anatomic study using 20 cadavers. *Ann Plast Surg* **39**, 566–71.
19 Newman J, Dolsky RL, Mai ST. (1984) Submental liposuction extraction with hard chin augmentation. *Arch Otolaryngol* **110**, 445–54.
20 Butterwick KJ. (2003) Enhancement of the results of neck liposuction with the FAMI technique. *J Drug Dermatol* **2**, 487–93.

CHAPTER 55

Hand Recontouring with Calcium Hydroxylapatite

Kenneth L. Edelson
Icahn School of Medicine at Mount Sinai and Private Practice, New York, NY, USA

> **BASIC CONCEPTS**
> - The aging hand is a common area of concern for patients.
> - Adequate treatment solutions were hampered by injection pain and the absence of treatment longevity.
> - The soft tissue filler calcium hydroxylapatite is effective for rejuvenating aging hands.
> - Calcium hydroxylapatite combined with lidocaine reduces pain of injection, improves product rheology of the procedure, and deposits the product in the correct metacarpal spaces.
> - The volume of injected calcium hydroxylapatite varies with physician preference.

Introduction

This chapter begins with a description of the aging hand, then identifies various cosmetic hand treatment products used by physicians for the past 20 years. Calcium hydroxylapatite is then introduced as an alternative to past dermal fillers. A discussion of how to add anesthesia to the calcium hydroxylapatite follows. The author then leads the reader through a step-by-step instruction of injection of the product into the aging hand. The chapter closes with a summary and a discussion of the various volumes of product and possible durability effects that have been used by various physicians.

Physiology of the hand

The great Irish playwright Oscar Wilde once said that "a woman who tells you her age will tell you anything." Well, in his day she did not have to; one could just examine her hands. Today, with the technology of hand recontouring, her secret is safe.

The hands have always been problem areas for physicians to rejuvenate and a myriad of applications and techniques have been used, both surgical and non-surgical with limited success. Until recently, no gratifying procedure has been successful in producing the effect of Botox on wrinkles or intense pulsed light (IPL) and lasers on vessels.

Signs of the aging hand include: a textural, crepe-like appearance, dryness, dyschromia, increased skin laxity, and volume loss giving the sunken appearance highlighting bones, tendons, and veins. A combination of both fractional non-ablative, or ablative laser resurfacing to address the epidermal defects, and the ideal subdermal filling agent to correct the loss of skin elasticity, volume, and wrinkling, is needed to address the aging hand. Both men and women can benefit from volume restoration and can attain a plumper, more youthful hand appearance with the proper technique and product.

A panoply of dermal fillers exists in the aesthetic marketplace. These have been well described in the 2008 American Society for Dermatologic Surgery (ASDS) guidelines publication [1]. Zyderm® collagen (Collagen Corp., Palo Alto, CA, USA), the original filler since 1982 and the gold standard for more than two decades, and Zyplast® (Collagen Corp., Palo Alto, CA, USA), followed by Cosmoderm® and Cosmoplast® (Allergan, Irvine, CA, USA) did not produce optimal results because of its consistency and flow characteristics, as well as lack of longevity. The filler was injected into the atrophic area, but did not cover objectionable structures. Collagen and hyaluronic acid fillers also did not flow well, yielding lumps and bumps.

Harvested fat has also been used by some physicians. However, the large-bore needles required for injection often leave unsightly puncture marks. More importantly, the results were modest at best, and short-lived, requiring a second surgical procedure to harvest the fat.

Advantages of calcium hydroxylapatite for treatment of the aging hand

In 2007, Florida dermatologists Mariano Busso (Coconut Grove) and David Applebaum (Boca Raton) reported off-label clinical experiences using calcium hydroxylapatite (CaHA;

Cosmetic Dermatology: Products and Procedures, Second Edition. Edited by Zoe Diana Draelos.
© 2016 John Wiley & Sons, Ltd. Published 2016 by John Wiley & Sons, Ltd.

Table 55.1 Representative treatment products for the aging hand.

Product category	Duration of effect*†	Advantages	Disadvantages
Autologous fat	Widely variable, from 4 months to more than 12 months	Biocompatibility, potential neovascularization	Harvesting required, not amenable to patients with lipodystrophy, does not conceal structures
Calcium hydroxylapatite (Radiesse®)	Approximately 12–15 months	Biocompatibility, collagen proliferation, immediate correction, no overcorrection needed, minimal pain	Time required for mixing with lidocaine
Collagen [bovine] (Zyderm®, Zyplast®) CosmoDerm®, CosmoPlast® (human)	Approximately 2–3 months	Long history of use in US aesthetics. No testing required	Skin testing for hypersensitivity reactions, does not conceal structures
Hyaluronic acids (Juvederm™, Restylane®, Perlane®)	Approximately 6–9 months	Wide variety of products available	Visibility of papules, color not easily blended into skin of dorsum, tindall effect, does not conceal structures
Poly-L-lactic acid (Sculptra®)	Approximately 18–24 months	Sustained collagenesis after a few weeks post-injection	Multiple treatments often necessary, does not conceal structures

*Facial areas (scant literature on longevity in hand).
†ASDS Guidelines.

Radiesse, BioForm Medical, San Mateo, CA, USA) for hand recontouring [2]. Their idea involved addition of lidocaine to the existing Radiesse compound. (Radiesse was approved in later 2006 for treatment of severe lines and wrinkles of the face such as nasolabial folds as well as treatment for HIV-associated facial lipoatrophy.) As a result, pain of treatment was reduced to nearly none, with immediately pleasing results to patients in one treatment session.

Radiesse consists of CaHA microspheres, 25 μm to 45 μm in diameter, in a carboxymethyl cellulose carrier gel. The CaHA is identical to the component found in human bone. The carrier gel disperses within weeks, leaving behind the calcium microspheres. It does not induce osteogenesis when placed in tissue but laboratory studies show neocollagenesis extending out to 72 weeks [3]. Hand recontouring required a substance that could not only fill atrophic areas of the dorsal hand, but could also conceal the vein and tendon color. Radiesse is white, opaque, possesses the proper viscosity, and flows smoothly with a low extrusion force (Table 55.1).

Technique of injection of CaHA into the hand

Contrary to the technique developed for collagen injection in 1982, CaHA hand recontouring requires a different injection technique: bolus injection, followed by vigorous massage, allowing the CaHA to fill where needed. It is a new technique, not predicated on line filling, but rather on steady vigorous massage to deliver the material to required atrophic areas (Table 55.2).

Table 55.2 Steps of in-office procedure for treatment of the aging hand.

1. Combine Radiesse with lidocaine, using a Luer-Lok connector for the Radiesse syringe and a 3-mL syringe containing 0.5 mL of 2% plain lidocaine.
2. Identify the areas of treatment, usually between the second and fifth metacarpals, from the dorsal crease of the wrist to the metacarpophalangeal joints.
3. Isolate the area of treatment with skin tenting between thumb and forefinger of non-injecting hand, or forceps.
4. Using a 27-gauge, 0.5-inch needle, inject the boluses of CaHA-lidocaine mixture into the areolar plane between the subcutaneous layer and superficial fascia of the hand as needed.
5. Have the patient make a fist of the injected hand, then firmly massage mixture to disperse.
6. Schedule follow-up with patient in 2–4 weeks; repeat treatment for any areas missed during initial visit.

Source: Busso & Applebaum, 2007 [Dermatol Ther 20, 385–87]. Adapted with permission of John Wiley & Sons

Preparing the Radiesse-lidocaine mixture

Prior to injecting CaHA into the hands, it is homogenized with 0.5 mL of 2% plain lidocaine. The 1.5 mL CaHA Luer-Lok syringe is attached via the connector included in the package, to the 3-mL Luer-Lok syringe, (also included in the package) containing 0.5 mL lidocaine (Figure 55.1) The use of a 3-mL Luer-Lok syringe is ideal for the homogenization process, because a high extrusion pressure is generated to mix the two liquids. The connector should be filled with lidocaine prior to making the connection, otherwise the CaHA will not flow. Instead, the plunger will move down without product emerging from the needle tip, the result of air in the mixture. The CaHA is first injected into the syringe containing the lidocaine and mixed slowly back and forth for 10 passes until the filler–lidocaine mixture is smooth and without bubbles (Figure 55.2) [4]. The

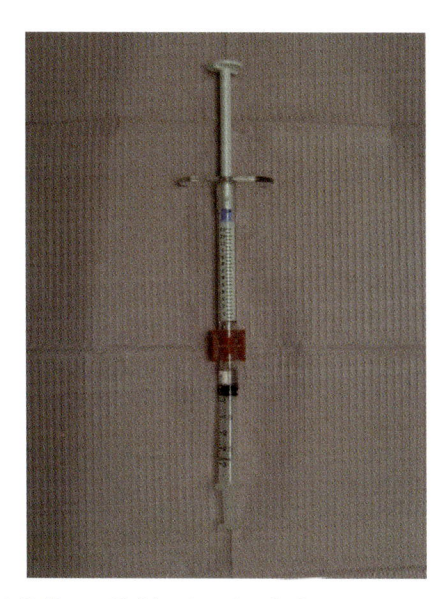

Figure 55.1 Radiesse with lidocaine using the Baxa connector.

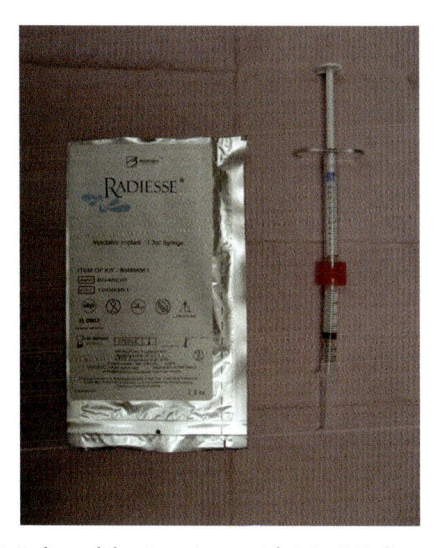

Figure 55.2 Radiesse–lidocaine mixture with 1.5 mL Radiesse and 0.5 mL 2% plain lidocaine.

addition of the anesthetic changes the viscosity and filler extrusion force, delivering a more malleable mixture which is less viscous and therefore requires a smaller extrusion force.

After this textbook was sent to the printer (which unfortunately is often the case in publishing), Merz received FDA approval in March 2015 for a new Radiesse (+) with Integral 0.3% Lidocaine mixed into the syringe. This will obviate the need for the mixing process, but for those of you who have the original Radiesse, follow the chapter instructions. The new Radiesse + also comes in the original volumes of 0.8cc and 1.5cc's.

Where to inject

Careful injection site selection can considerably limit the amount of bruising. Before injecting, carefully examine the hand to ensure selection of an area devoid of veins or tendons. The imaginary line of bolus injection(s) is midway between the dorsal crease of the wrist and the metacarpophalangeal joints, bound laterally by the fifth metacarpal and medially by the second metacarpal. This boundary can be modified depending on the injector's judgment regarding the location of the defects to be filled.

How to inject

The patient should be comfortably seated on an examination table with the hands extended in front of them, preferably resting on a Mayo stand covered with a soft pillow, adjusted to the height of the patient's knees, allowing gravity to have the desired effect on the defects to be corrected. The skin must be tented in order to separate it from the underlying veins and tendons (Figure 55.2). Entry is into the areolar plane, which is located between the superficial fascia and the subcutaneous fat. The thumb and forefinger of the non-injecting hand are used to lift the skin and create the entry point in the center of the tent (Figure 55.3). With a 27-gauge by 0.5 inch needle (or the new 28-gauge with 27-gauge inner lumen) attached to the prefilled CaHA syringe, inject 2–4 boluses of product across the previously described area of the dorsum of the hand, refilling the syringe when necessary. The average bolus amount is about 0.2–0.5 mL CaHA emulsion (Figure55.4, Figure 55.5, and Figure 55.6).

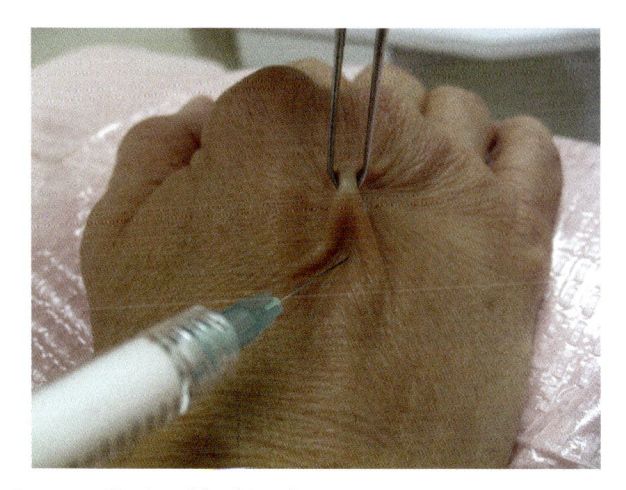

Figure 55.3 Tenting of the skin technique.

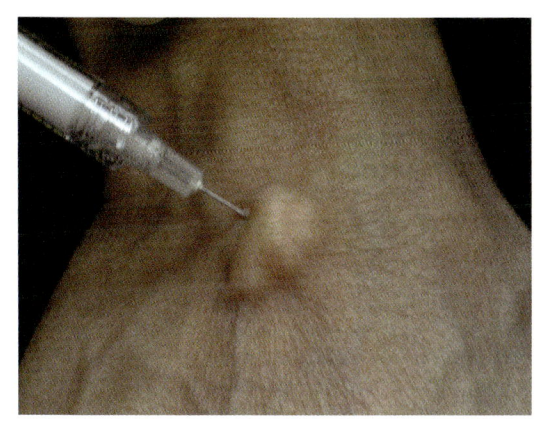

Figure 55.4 Injecting and forming bolus of Radiesse mixture (0.5 mL bolus) in the areolar plane.

488 **ANTI-AGING** Skin Contouring Techniques

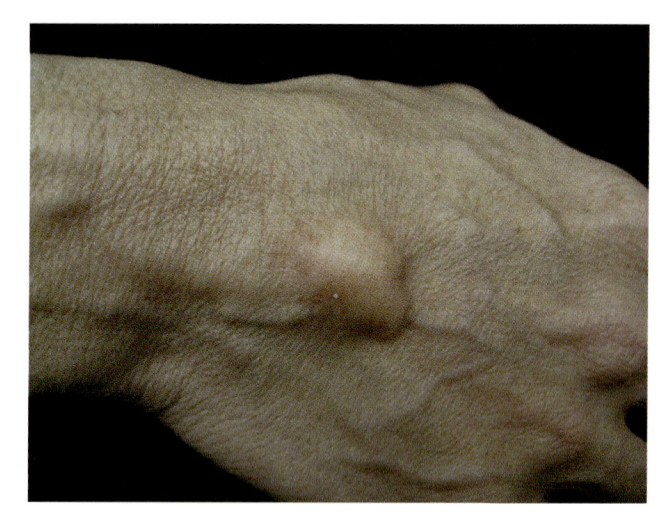

Figure 55.5 Injected bolus prior to closed-fist massage.

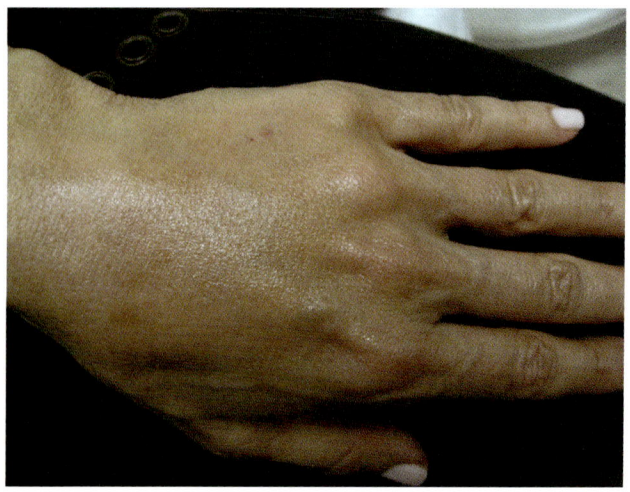

Figure 55.7 Partial massage of bolus into the dorsum.

Post-injection hand massage

At this point, massaging – the quintessential element of relocating the CaHA – is begun (Figure 55.7). Have the patient make a tight fist. To relieve friction and enhance the process, apply a liberal amount of Aquaphor (Beiersdorf Inc., Wilton, CT, USA) or white petrolatum to the dorsum. Begin pushing the boluses, one at a time, distally, laterally and medially, so that the bolus is flattened and spread as far as possible. Care should be taken not to encroach upon the metacarpophalangeal joints or the medial and lateral dorso-palmar junctions; product is not intended for these areas. After completing treatment of the first hand, have the patient sit on that hand while you treat the other hand. It will help in the smoothing out process as well as add to hemostasis if needed. In the event of a hematoma, have the patient hold pressure firmly for 5–10 minutes, and proceed to begin treating the contralateral hand. When the other hand is completed, go back and complete the "bruised" hand. Each hand usually requires between one and two 1.5-mL syringes. CaHA is also available in 0.3 mL and 0.8 mL syringes, should a full 1.5-mL syringe not be needed for the second syringe.

Post-treatment care

After treatment is completed apply ice packs to the hands. The patient leaves the office with the disposable pack, using it for as long as it stays cool. Use of the ice pack will help reduce some of the possible swelling. The patient should be told to carry on with normal activities beginning the following day. Schedule the patient for follow-up in 2 weeks, and if at this time there are skip areas noticed, fill them in using the 0.3-mL CaHA syringe mixed with 0.12 mL of 2% lidocaine.

Adverse events

Because it is a compound identical to that found in bone, CaHA has high biocompatibility and low adverse event risks. Adverse events in published studies have been few and of short duration [5-8]. They include ecchymosis, erythema, and occasional edema, when used in facial applications other than the lips. In general, the diluted product described for off-label use in the hands is even more forgiving. Clinical experiences with treatment of the aging hand suggest that adverse events in this area are infrequent and not severe. Anecdotal reports, however, have noted hand edema persist for 5–7 days post injection.

Results

Figures 55.8, Figure 55.9, Figure 55.10, and Figure 55.11 represent a 45-year-old female patient who received 1.5 mL CaHA mixture per hand during the initial visit, and did not have a touch-up performed. Figure55.12, Figure 55.13, Figure 55.14, Figure 55.15, and Figure 55.16 represent a 58-year-old female patient who also received 1.5 mL of CaHA mixture in each hand, and returned for a touch-up of the left hand only with 0.3 mL CaHA at week 8.

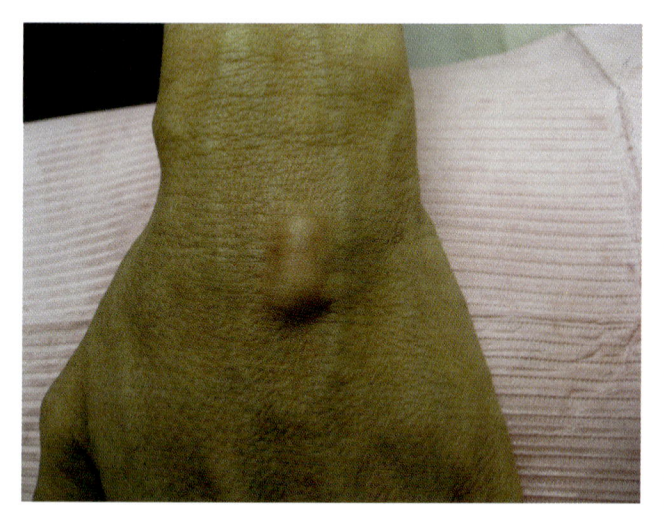

Figure 55.6 Injected bolus prior to closed-fist massage.

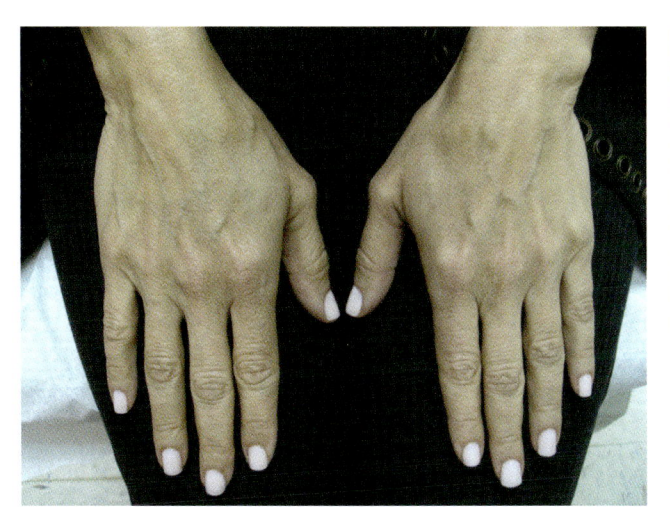

55. Hand Recontouring with Calcium Hydroxylapatite   489

Figure 55.8 45-year-old female patient prior to treatment.

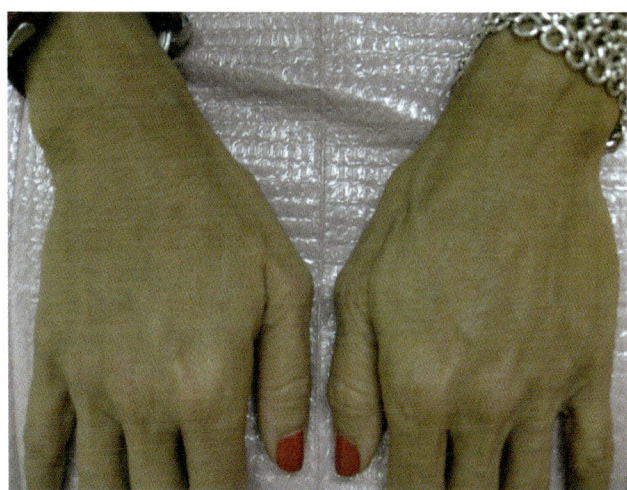

Figure 55.11 Same patient 12 weeks post-treatment.

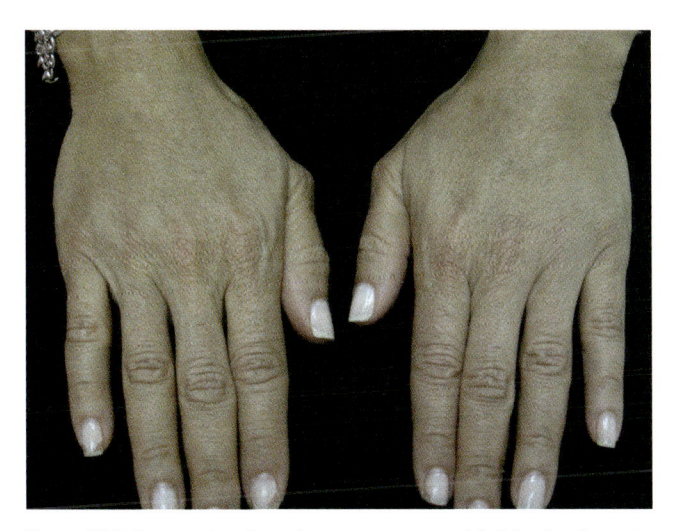

Figure 55.9 Same patient 2 weeks post-treatment with 1.5 mL mixture in each hand.

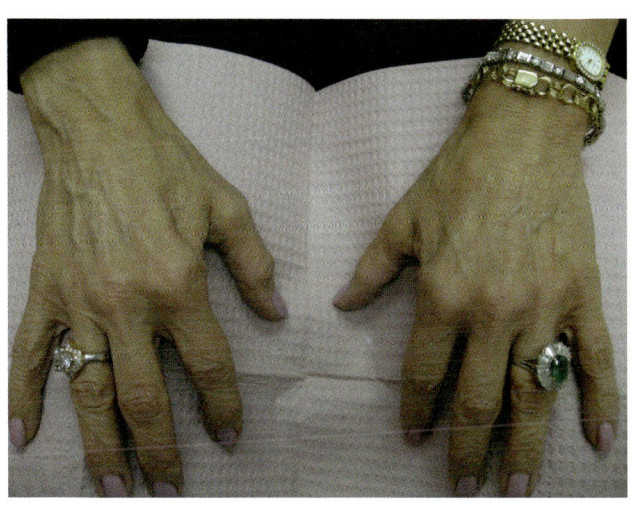

Figure 55.12 58-year-old female patient pretreatment (pianist).

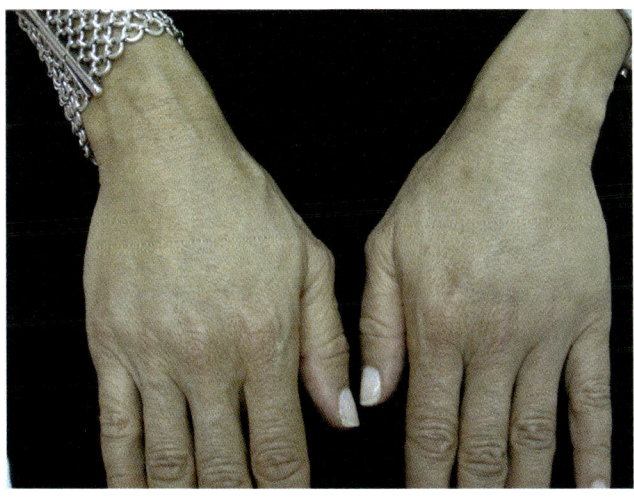

Figure 55.10 Same patient 8 weeks post-treatment.

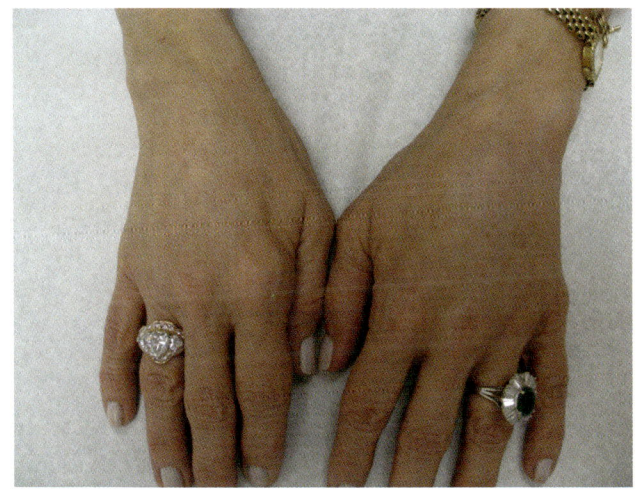

Figure 55.13 Same patient 2 weeks post-treatment with 1.5 mL Radiesse mixture for each hand.

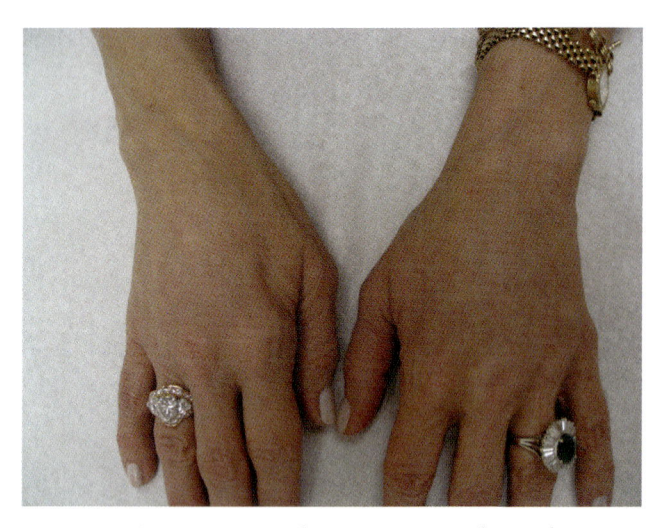

Figure 55.14 Same patient 8 weeks post-treatment with a touch-up using 0.3 mL Radiesse mixture for only left hand performed at 4 weeks after initial treatment.

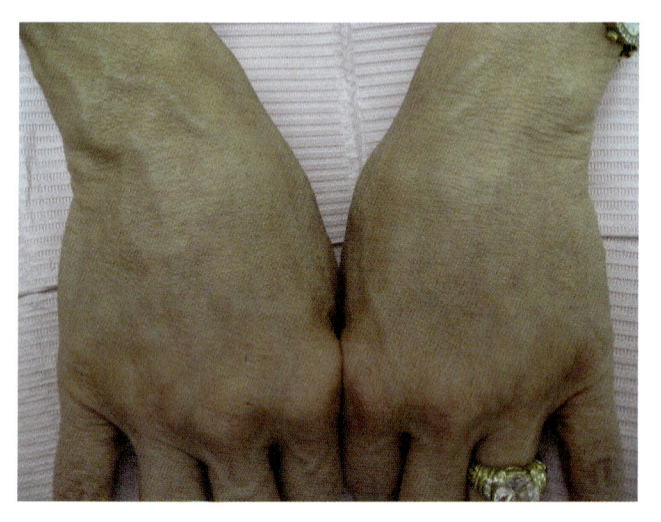

Figure 55.15 Same patient at 20 weeks after initial treatment.

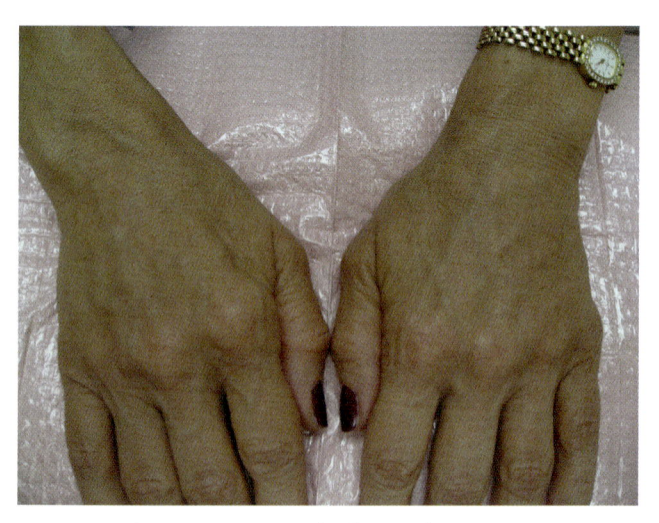

Figure 55.16 Same patient at 28 weeks after initial treatment.

Discussion

As with every new technique in surgery, refinements and modifications are the rule as time goes on. New approaches to the same technique give rise to slight revisions and adjustments leading to a better outcome. The original technique described by Busso was a single, voluminous bolus of an entire syringe of Radiesse and lidocaine, which was then spread out over the hand. Some physicians prefer the large-volume bolus approach; others believe it is less advantageous than the multiple, smaller-volume bolus approach.

The volume of lidocaine remains an open question. The original volumes of lidocaine with the single bolus injection were much smaller (0.10 mL per 1.5 mL CaHA) than the volumes found in many clinical settings today (0.23–2.0 mL per syringe). In many personal communications, the author has determined that a larger volume of lidocaine is preferred for optimum results. These volumes have ranged 0.12–2.0 mL lidocaine per 1.5-mL syringe of CaHA. A mixture of 0.5 mL of 2% lidocaine per 1.5-mL CaHA syringe and 0.12 mL for the 0.3-mL CaHA syringe appear optimal. There are several reasons why these two volumes are the volumes of choice. In the first place, considerably less hand swelling occurs when 0.5 mL lidocaine is used than using 2.0 mL. In addition, this volume enhances product flow and makes massage of injected mixture relatively easy. However, the most important reason is longevity and the convenience issue for the patient. Much less product is used with higher dilutions, and therefore the correction may not endure as long as with smaller dilutions. Busso's recent paper states "physicians have reported that they see no significant decrease in durability for media diluted with lidocaine" [4]. At this point, controlled clinical trials are needed to determine that dilution with lidocaine does not negatively affect longevity of CaHA correction, not only in the hands, but for all applications.

This issue of higher dilutions and possible decreased durability can easily be addressed, but it means more procedures at the 2-week follow-up than necessary. Follow-up sessions should address the missed areas that are inevitable, not retreating areas where the "excess" lidocaine has been absorbed. Another refinement that is helpful is the use of a smooth forceps to create the subsequent tents that might be needed. Once the emollient has been applied to the skin, a gloved hand on greasy skin will not be able to create the tent.

Conclusions

Past experiences with products for treating the aging hand have met with limited success. These products – harvested fat, collagen, and hyaluronic acids – have disadvantages for placement in the hands for contouring enhancements. Foremost among these is the short duration, usually less than 3 months, and the inability of all of the other fillers to conceal the objectionable structures of the aging hand. CaHA appears well-suited for consideration as a product for recontouring of the hand, with a duration of effect of 6 months or longer. Unlike other areas, where there is not a lot of muscle activity, the hand's muscles and tendons are constantly moving, creating the friction that accelerates product breakdown. This is in contrast to more static treatment areas where there is greater longevity of correction. Perhaps the single most important and unique characteristic of CaHA that makes it ideal for hand recontouring is its opacity, the trait that enables the concealment of the undesirable structures of the aging hand. CaHA is also clinically unchanged by the addition of lidocaine, enabling painless treatment.

It was been five years since the first edition of "Cosmetic Dermatology", was published, and I am pleased to report that the adverse events and longevity of correction have remained as stated in the original chapter in 2009.

References

1 Alam M, Gladstone H, Kramer EM, *et al.* Guidelines Task Force. (2008) American Society for Dermatologic Surgery (ASDS) Guidelines of Care: Injectable Fillers. *Dermatol Surg* **34**, 115–48.
2 Busso M, Applebaum D. (2007) Hand augmentation with Radiesse® (calcium hydroxylapatite). *Dermatol Ther* **20**, 315–7.
3 Berlin AL, Hussain M, Goldberg DJ. (2008) Calcium hydroxylapatite for facial filler rejuvenation: a histologic and immunohistochemical analysis. *Dermatol Surg* **34**, 64–S67.
4 Busso M, Voigts R. (2008) An investigation of changes in physical properties of injectable calcium hydroxylapatite in a carrier gel when mixed with lidocaine and with lidocaine/epinephrine. *Dermatol Surg* **34**, 16–24.
5 Tzikas TL. (2008) A 52-month summary of results using calcium hydroxylapatite for facial soft tissue augmentation. *Dermatol Surg* **34**, 9–15.
6 Carruthers A, Liebeskind M, Carruthers J, Forster BB. (2008) Radiographic and computed tomographic studies of calcium hydroxylapatite for treatment of HIV-associated facial lipoatrophy and correction of nasolabial folds. *Dermatol Surg* **34**, 78–84.
7 Moers-Carpi M, Vogt S, Martinez Santos B, *et al.* (2007) A multicenter, randomized trial comparing calcium hydroxyalaptite to two hyaluronic acids for treatment of nasolabial folds. *Dermatol Surg* **33**, 144–51.
8 Sadick NS, Katz BE, Roy D. (2007) A multicenter, 47-month study of safety and efficacy of calcium hydroxylapatite for soft tissue augmentation of nasolabial folds and other areas of the face. *Dermatol Surg* **33**, 122–7.

SECTION 6 Implementation of Cosmetic Dermatology into Therapeutics

CHAPTER 56
Anti-aging Regimens

Karen E. Burke
The Mount Sinai Medical Center, New York, NY, USA

> **BASIC CONCEPTS**
> - The appearance of aging skin can indeed be reversed without invasive treatments by daily skin care using scientifically proven techniques and products.
> - Proper cleansing and exfoliation smooth the skin's surface to decrease pore size and wrinkles within days.
> - Sun protection by application of ample amounts of high-SPF, UVA-protective, highly water-resistant sunscreen is essential to protect from photoaging and to enhance natural repair.
> - Topical retinoids as well as topical antioxidants such as vitamins C and E, selenium, genestein, and coenzyme Q10 not only protect from but also reverse photoaging if the correct molecular forms and concentrations are applied.

Introduction

In her book, *Survival of the Prettiest*, Etcoff [1] synthesizes literature and research from anthropology, biology, psychology, and archeology to show that indeed appreciation of one's own and others' beauty is hard-wired in human brains. Etcoff concludes, "Flawless skin is the most universally desired feature of beauty." This chapter presents a basic skin regimen to protect from photodamage and reverse the appearance of aging. The four necessary steps are cleansing, exfoliation, protection, and treatment. Helpful techniques and scientific research proving efficacy of specific ingredients are presented.

Cleansing

Proper cleansing is an essential component of skincare. The face accumulates endogenous and exogenous soils. Sebaceous gland size and density are greatest on the face, upper back, and chest. The natural oils, sweat, and sebum secretions create a hydrolipid film on the skin surface that, in addition to applied cosmetics, traps and accumulates environmental pollutants such as dust, airborne irritants, and compounds from cigarette smoke. Care must be taken to accomplish thorough cleansing without irritation or drying.

Therefore, a gentle, effective cleanser is of utmost importance. Surfactants are the ingredients that bind to dirt and oil for removal. These surfactants are classified by their charge on the surface-active moiety as anionic (negatively charged, for good foaming and lathering), cationic (positively charged), amphoteric (both positive and negative, considered to "condition" skin while helping to foam), and non-ionic (which are used in baby products to suppress foam) [2]. Components of surfactants can bind to the stratum corneum proteins, decreasing the skin's ability to bind and hold water. With continued, frequent use, surfactants can damage the skin barrier. New synthetic surfactants improve cleansing with less irritation.

Other components of cleansers include polypeptides and synthetic polymers to make the product smooth and to soften skin, polymers to moisturize, preservatives, opacifying agents, and fragrance. With frequent washing, these ingredients can cause sensitivities or contact allergy in certain individuals. Because cleansers are rinsed off, their contact time with the skin is reduced causing less contact allergy. Newer cleansers are less alkaline than older formulations, so they are less drying.

In recent years, antibacterial agents (e.g. triclosan and triclocarban) have been added to hand cleansers. Surprisingly, these agents are rarely skin irritants. However, some physicians voice concern, fearing development of bacterial resistance to these antibiotics with frequent use. Originally, triclosan was thought to kill

---

Cosmetic Dermatology: Products and Procedures, Second Edition. Edited by Zoe Diana Draelos.
© 2016 John Wiley & Sons, Ltd. Published 2016 by John Wiley & Sons, Ltd.

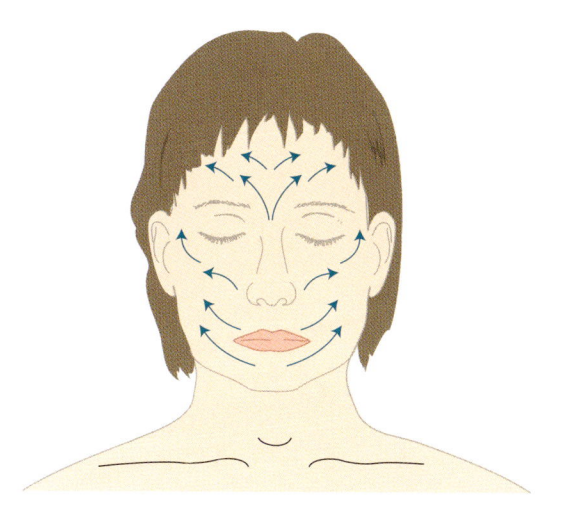

Figure 56.1 To treat wrinkles while washing, gently rub upward horizontally across the upper lip and "up and out" on the rest of the face – perpendicular to the direction of wrinkles.

bacteria by a "broad-based" mechanism, similar to alcohol and peroxide. However, recent research demonstrated that triclosan acts at a specific gene site in *Escherichia coli* to inhibit replication, so resistant strains could evolve [3]. Thorough washing with gentle cleansers removes dirt and has been shown to be as effective as using these antibacterial compounds.

Cleansing the face should be accomplished with lukewarm water and the fingertips. The face and neck should be washed with upward, outward motions. On the face, one should always rub perpendicular to the direction of those wrinkles that could develop later. On the forehead, cheeks, chin and neck, rub up and out; above the upper lip and under the eyes, the strokes should be first horizontal, then upward at the edges, as illustrated in Figure 56.1. Sunscreen, moisturizer, or other treatments should be applied immediately after gently towel-drying to seal in the water remaining on the skin's surface.

Exfoliation

Exfoliation is the rejuvenation treatment providing the most immediate improvement in appearance. Exfoliation removes the outer layers of stratum corneum, and thus treats the hyperkeratosis of dry skin. Exfoliative rubbing perpendicular to the direction of wrinkles (with upward, outward strokes) minimizes small wrinkles because the surface is smoothed (Figure 56.1).

Exfoliation can be chemical or mechanical. Chemical exfoliants such as hydroxyacids and retinoic acid remove dead surface cells by keratolysis. Mechanical exfoliants include cleansing grains, waxy creams that adhere to the surface cells, as well as slightly abrasive terry washcloths, non-woven polyester polishing pads, brushes, loofas, or mechanical brushes – all of which physically "sand" the skin surface by rubbing. Grainy exfoliants with aluminum oxide crystals can be effective, but the user must be careful not to get the grains into the eyes. Exfoliants to be avoided are those with apricot or almond kernels, walnut shells, and pumice – all of which have irregularly shaped particles with sharp edges which can be too rough for delicate skin and dangerous if they get into the eyes. The immediate improvement in small wrinkles by gentle exfoliation can be appreciated in Figure 56.2.

Masks are among the oldest face mechanical exfoliants. Masks can "wash off" or "peel off." Some "wash off" masks are made of clay, which harden and are removed with water rinsing. "Peel-off" masks contain synthetic polymers that are quite safe and effective. Some masks may irritate the skin; it is advisable to test on the inner wrist before treating the face.

Protection

The single most effective therapy for aging skin is sun protection [4]. Avoid sun exposure between 10am and 4pm, and beware of "hidden sun": UVA is not filtered by glass and neither UVA or UVB are filtered by clouds. People get their worst burns on cloudy days, especially when skiing or when on the beach or in the water when reflected rays double exposure. If one's indoor workspace is in direct sun, that person can become sun-burned through the window and suffer severe photoaging, as seen in Figure 56.3. Sunscreen should be applied often and generously every 90 minutes. Frequently missed areas with sunscreen application are just in front of the ears, around the eyes, above the lip, fingertips, and the scalp under thinning hair.

Sunscreens are classified as organic filters (which absorb photons of UV light) or inorganic filters (which reflect or scatter UV radiation) [5]. As shown in Figure 56.4, some organic sunscreen agents block only UVB (p-aminobenzoic acid [PABA] and its esters padamate A and O, the cinnamates, and salicylates); others absorb primarily UVB and some low wavelength UVA (octocrylene, benzophenones, anthranalides). Ecamsule, sold under the trade name Mexoryl™ XL or SL (Anthelios, La Roche-Posay, L'Oréal), blocks UVB as well as most UVA. The UVA absorbing sunscreen avobenzone (Parsol 1789) can degrade with exposure to UV [6], but stabilizing compounds (benzylidene camphor and diphenyl cyanoecrylate derivatives, both UVB filters) can be effectively added (Helioplex™, Neutrogena) [7]. The inorganic filters with microfine titanium dioxide and zinc oxide are total UVB blocks, titanium dioxide blocking low wavelength UVA and zinc oxide almost all UVA. Thus, zinc oxide provides better protection than titanium dioxide [8]. The new technology with microfine particles makes them non-opaque and cosmetically appealing. The concentration and the size of the microparticles determine SPF efficacy [5][1].

The ability of a sunscreen to prevent UVB-mediated erythema is measured by the internationally accepted standard sun protection factor (SPF), the ratio of equivalent exposure by

---

[1] A complete list of sunscreens with the Skin Cancer Foundation's Seal of Recommendation is available at www.skincancer.org

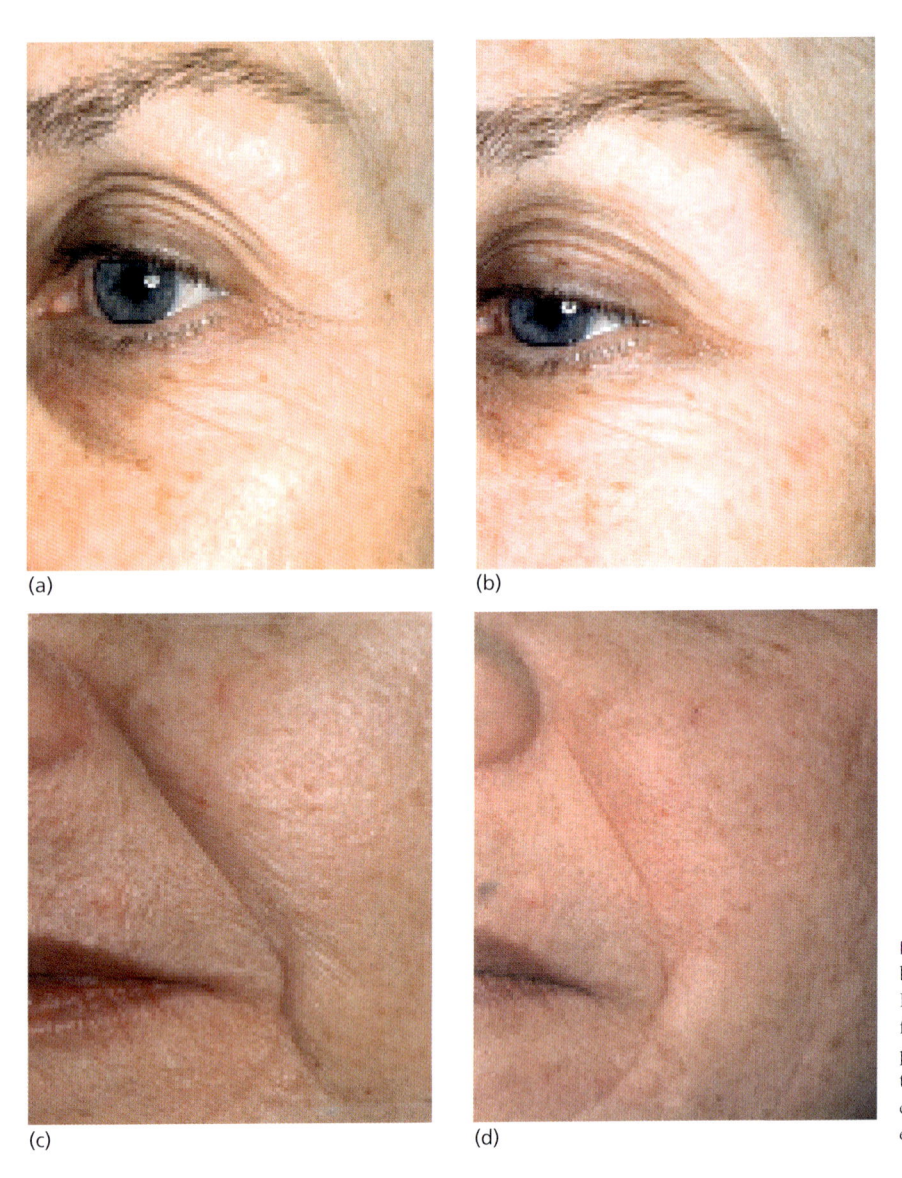

Figure 56.2 Tiny wrinkles and crepey skin can be treated immediately at home by exfoliation. Improvement is seen in this 60-year-old woman's face after she simply washed with a non-woven polyester polishing pad and used a waxy exfoliant that mechanically "sticks" and removes surface cells. (a) and (c), pre-exfoliation; (b) and (d), post-exfoliation.

UVB in sunscreen-protected compared with unprotected skin. (An SPF of 30 means that the amount of UB exposure in 10 minutes without sunscreen is equivalent to 10 minutes × 30 = 5 hours of exposure with sunscreen.) The SPF should be at least 30. Sunscreen labels may specify degree of UVB protection by stating the **SPF as 30+ or 50+**; higher SPFs may no longer be stated on the label. UVA protection is measured by degree of either *immediate pigment darkening* (dependent upon radiation-induced darkening of preformed melanin) or *persistent (delayed) pigment darkening* (as in a more complex response which induces production and transfer of melanin as well as proliferation of melanocytes). The latter assay is preferred in Europe and Japan. A sunscreen may be labelled "**Broad Spectrum**" only if the UVA critical wavelength (CW, the wavelength at which 90% of the UV above 320 nm is absorbed) is >370 nm. Only sunscreens of (1) SPF >15 and (2) broad spectrum can claim to protect against skin cancer and photoaging. If the SPF is <15, then the label must state specifically that this sunscreen protects only against sunburn, but not against skin cancer or photoaging.

After SPF, the second important criterion for a sunscreen is that it be "**highly water resistant**," meaning it is effective for about 80 minutes. (Labels read water resistant (40 minutes) or water resistant (80 minutes).) The terms "waterproof" and "sweat proof" may no longer be written on sunscreen labels, since these are considered to be "false promises." Many individuals prefer a different sunscreen for the face than for the body. These criteria are summarized in Table 56.1. This is particularly important for individuals with acne, since many ingredients that make a sunscreen formulation cosmetically smooth in texture or fragrant can be comedogenic).

56. Anti-aging Regimens 495

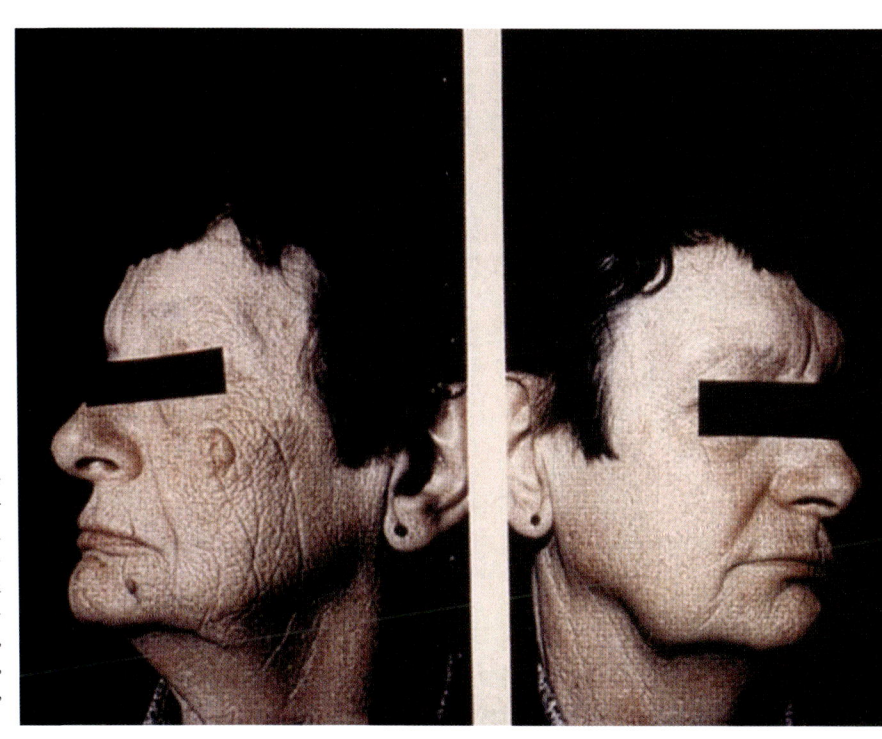

Figure 56.3 This secretary sat at the same desk for more than 30 years. Her left face which was exposed to UVA through the window shows severe photodamage, especially when compared with the less-exposed right side. Photograph courtesy of Michelle Verschoore, L'Oréal Advanced Research Laboratories, Clichy and Aulnay-Sous-Bois, France, and Pierre Moulin, Lyon, France.

Table 56.1 Criteria of a good sunscreen.

1. High SPF (SPF 30+ or preferably 50+)
2. Broad spectrum: Protection against UVA and UVB
3. Highly water resistant (80)
4. Non-comedogenic
5. Personally pleasing; lotion, gel or spray

SPF, sun protection factor.

Further protection with topical antioxidants and sun protective clothing, hats, and sunglasses are indicated. Sun protective clothing is rated using UV protective factor (UPF), measured by the amount of UV radiation transmitted through the fabric. A fabric with a UPF of 40–50 transmits only 2.6% of biologically effective radiation, in contrast with normal summer clothing that typically has a UPF of only 4–10, providing a maximum SPF of 30% but often only an SPF of about 2 if wet [9]. New products (such as SunGuard (2,2′-(1,2-ethenediyl)bis[5-[[4-(methylamino)-6[[4-(methylamino)catonyl]-phenyl]amino]-1,3,5-triazin-2-yl]amino]-, disodium salt)) have recently become available to be added when washing clothes to give a UPF of 30 that lasts 20 washes.

Treatment

There are several medical treatments for anti-aging purposes. These include retinoic acid, hydroxy acids, and topical antioxidants. Many products are advertised, but their efficacy may not have been demonstrated by rigorous placebo-controlled, double-blind clinical trials.

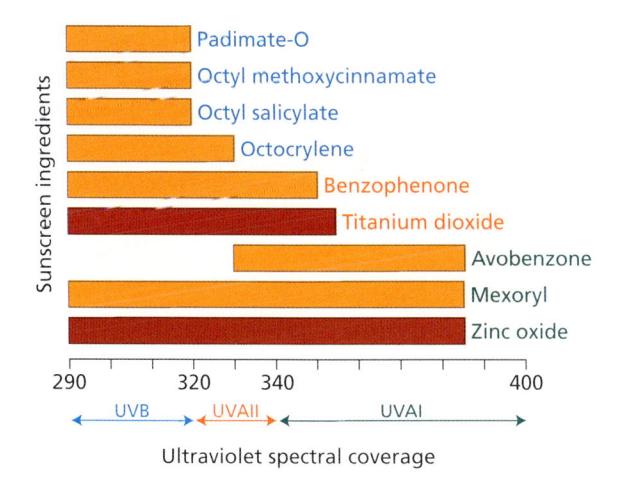

Figure 56.4 Ultraviolet spectral coverage of sunscreen ingredients.

Hydroxyacids

Hydroxyacids (HAs) have been used for centuries. Cleopatra routinely applied HAs and Marie Antoinette washed with red wine, benefitting from tartaric acid.

Hydroxyacids were reintroduced to dermatology in 1974 when Van Scott and Yu [10] reported improvement of severe hyperkeratosis and icthyosis. Hydroxyacids are classified by the position of the hydroxyl group attached to the acid moiety: α-hydroxyacids (AHAs) (glycolic acid, lactic acid, and citric acid), β-hydroxyacids (BHAs) (tropic acid, salicylic acid [SA] – called a BHA but actually an α-hydroxybenzoic acid), and the "new generation" polyhydroxy acids (PHAs) (gluconolactone or lactobionic acid – a naturally occurring component of skin). AHAs act rapidly (within 2 weeks) to smooth the surface skin by reducing epidermal corneocyte adhesion, first at the innermost level of the stratum corneum (just above the stratum granulosum) [11]. Epidermal damage of photoaging is corrected in 14–16 weeks, resulting in a thinned stratum corneum, epidermal acanthosis, and decreased melanogenesis [12]. An increase in epidermal intercellular hyaluronic acid improves surface moisturization by water retention.

An elegant study demonstrated that epidermal keratolysis is followed by dermal penetration which increases synthesis of glycosaminoglycans and increases fibroblast proliferation and production of collagen and elastin [13]. A 25% increase in skin thickness was measured after 6 months' treatment with 25% AHAs with no inflammation.

SA is unique among the hydroxyacids in that it is lipophilic and is particularly attracted to sebaceous orifices, thereby exhibiting its keratolytic properties not only to smooth surface wrinkles, but also to decrease pore size and prevent acne. As an excellent keratolytic agent, SA solubilizes intercellular cement by disrupting corneocyte adhesion layer by layer, from the surface downward. SA may also be directly bacteriostatic.

The PHAs have several advantages. They have larger molecules, so they penetrate the skin gradually and are therefore less irritating than AHAs or SA. PHAs are recommended for patients with sensitive skin, rosacea, or atopic dermatitis [12]. They can even be used in conjunction with retinoic acid without irritation. PHAs also give improved moisturization of the stratum corneum when compared with AHAs. PHAs have antiinflammatory and antioxidant activity, further enhancing repair of cutaneous photoaging [14].

Three key factors determine HA efficacy:

1. *Type of hydroxyacid* (described above).
2. *Concentration*: the higher the concentration, the more effective but the more possible irritation. Concentrations of 8–12% glycolic and lactic acids are available by prescription, as are concentrations of SA greater than 3%. Higher concentrations are used for medical chemical peels.
3. *pH (acidity)*: the amount of biologically free acid determines the clinical strength [13]. To be effective, the hydroxyacid must be acidic.

There is a delicate balance in attaining efficacy without irritation. For each type of hydroxyacid or mixture thereof, the concentration and pH determines the strength and the clinical benefits [13].

Retinoids

Retinoids are the "gold standard" for reversing photoaging of the skin. Retinoic acid (tretinoin) has been used for more than 35 years for the treatment of acne. In the late 1980s, the remarkable clinical improvement of wrinkles and solar lentigos after treatment with topical tretinoin was documented [15,16,17]. UV exposure leads to decreased expression of retinoic acid receptors (RAR) and retinoic X receptors (RXR) (in particular, RAR-α and RXR-γ, the two major nuclear receptors in keratinocytes) with subsequent activation of transcription factors (AP-1 and NF-IF) which increase proliferation and inflammation and activate the matrix metaloproteinases (MMPs) that break down extracellular matrix proteins [18]. By binding to these receptors, topical retinoids restore expression, thereby reversing UV-induced damage at all levels of the epidermis and dermis [19,20].

Retinoids increase epidermal proliferation causing epidermal thickening with compaction of the stratum corneum and deposition of glycosaminoglycans intercellularly; with epidermal proliferation, inhibition of excess melanogenesis and shedding of melanin-laden keratinocytes resolves mottled hyperpigmentation; and retinoids directly induce collagen synthesis and reduce collagen breakdown by inhibiting the UV-induced MMPs [21,22], thereby correcting wrinkles.

Topical tretinoin also reverses intrinsic aging, perhaps even more significantly in non-sun-exposed than in photoaged skin. A marked increase in epidermal thickness (with a more undulating dermoepidermal junction), in anchoring fibrils, and in dermal angiogenesis with new elastic fibers and glycosaminoglycans was observed [23].

Previously, topical tretinoin was postulated to make the skin more sensitive to UV exposure. Indeed, resolution of unattractive hyperkeratosis may allow more UV to penetrate deeper, but the inhibition of the UV-induced MMPs that break down collagen results in less UV damage with tretinoin treatment. Occasionally, irritation (retinoid dermatitis) can occur, especially when beginning treatment. This can usually be avoided by starting with lower concentrations (0.025% cream instead of 0.05% cream or 0.01% gel), other formulations (microsphere gels, new generic formulations, or different retinoids as described below), and less frequent application. Patients with sensitive skin should begin with a mild formulation, applying initially each 3 days and increasing to daily over several weeks or months. Most of the improvement occurs within the first year; improvement is maintained with continued use, as proven by up to 4-year histologic studies [22].

Other "second generation" retinoids have been proven effective in treating photodamage [22]. Retinaldehyde cream (0.05%) and retinol cream (up to 1.6%) are comparable to tretinoin in efficacy, but are more irritating. Tazarotene (0.5% and 0.1%) may give faster improvement but is also more irritating. Adapalene (0.1% cream and gel) is less irritating but probably less effective than tretinoin.

Antioxidants

The skin naturally uses nutritional antioxidants to protect itself from photodamage and topical application has been investigated. The challenge is to make topical antioxidant formulations that are stable and that give percutaneous absorption to deliver high concentrations of the active forms to the dermis as well as the epidermis. The advantage is that only once-per-day application of topical antioxidants provides a **reservoir of protection** that cannot be perspired or washed away, markedly enhancing sun protection.

Vitamin C

If the retinoids are the "gold standard," topical vitamin C is the "silver standard" for reversing photoaging of the skin. Vitamin C (L-ascorbic acid) is the body's major aqueous-phase antioxidant. Dietary vitamin C is absolutely required for life.

Environmental free-radical stress depletes vitamin C levels in the skin. UV exposure of 1.6 minimal erythema dose (MED) decreases vitamin C to 70% normal, and 10 MED to 54% [20]. Although vitamin C is itself not a sunscreen, topical vitamin C protects against solar damage. As an antioxidant, vitamin C deactivates the UV-induced free radicals, decreasing erythema and sunburn. This protection has been confirmed by histologically: treatment with topical 10% vitamin C decreases the number of abnormal "sunburn cells" by 40–60% and reduces the UV damage to DNA by 62% [24].

The main function of vitamin C is as the essential co-factor for collagen synthesis. When 10% vitamin C was added to in vitro elderly fibroblasts, collagen proliferation and synthesis increased by factors of 6 and 2, respectively [25]. With this enhancement of collagen synthesis, topical vitamin C (15%) is impressively effective in reducing wrinkles of photoaging. Although optimal efficacy is noted after 6 months, appreciable improvement of periorbital wrinkles can be seen after 3–4 months. This formulation also treats rosacea [26] by building firm collagen that constricts microvasculature and by its anti-inflammatory efficacy. Both of these activities enhance wound healing: When vitamin C was applied both before and after surgery, healing time was substantially shortened [27]. Vitamin C also inhibits tyrosinase, thereby lightening solar lentigos. In this author's experience, topical vitamin C (15%) is the most effective depigmenting agent currently available. Lightening of solar lentigos can be appreciated after only 1–2 months, while all other agents require at least 3–4 months before lightening is noted. Another important action of vitamin C on the skin is that topical vitamin C increases the synthesis of several specific lipids of the skin surface [28]. Not only does this mean that vitamin C helps the natural moisturization of the skin, but it also enhances the protective barrier function of the skin [29].

Formulation is key to optimizing percutaneous absorption of vitamin C. Because L-ascorbic acid is such an excellent antioxidant, it is inherently unstable when exposed to oxygen. Creating an effective topical delivery system is crucial and quite difficult. Many products contain stable derivatives, which are either (or both) not absorbed or not metabolized by the skin (such as ascorbyl-6-palmitate or magnesium ascorbyl phosphate) and therefore have no appreciable cutaneous activity [30]. Other formulations do not result in measurable absorption of vitamin C because they are not at the correct pH. Topical absorption of 10% vitamin C cream was proven by radioactive labeling studies in pigs. After treatment, 8.2% was found in the dermis, and 0.7% was in the blood [30]. The most effective concentration for topical delivery is 20%, giving maximal skin levels after 3 days.

Vitamin E (d-α-tocopherol)

Natural vitamin E is the most important lipid-soluble, membrane-bound antioxidant in the body. Natural dietary vitamin E can exist in four methylated forms (α, β, χ, δ); synthetic vitamin E is a mixture of eight (d,l) stereoisomers. The d-α-tocopherol isomer has the greatest biologic efficacy. In order to attain activity through cutaneous application, the natural non-esterified form must be applied in concentrations greater than 2% (5% is optimal) [31]. Most commercial products containing "vitamin E" contain a mixture of 32 synthetic isomers, esterified, and in quite low concentrations. Allergic contact dermatitis has been reported from such formulations, although no adverse reaction has ever been reported with the natural d-α-tocopherol.

In a mouse model, topical d-α-tocopherol has been shown to be impressively effective in protecting against all acute and chronic UV-induced damage, and far more effective than the esterified topical d α-tocopherol succinate [31]. Sunburn and tanning are markedly decreased, and the time of onset of skin cancer is delayed and the incidence is markedly decreased. In humans the minimal erythema dose (MED) of UVB is increased after treatment with topical d-α-tocopherol. Vitamin E has also been demonstrated to reverse photoaging dramatically. Figure 56.5 shows the impressive decrease in periorbital rhytides after 4 months of daily application of d-α-tocopherol (5%). Histology confirmed this improvement in a mouse model. The UV-induced epidermal hypertrophy and hyperkeratosis, the increased incidence of damaged "sunburn cells" in the basal layer, and the disruption of dermal collagen and elastin were all corrected after 8 weeks of topical treatment (KF Burke, L Riciotti, EG Gross, unpublished observations).

Topical d-α-tocopherol is also anti-inflammatory and accelerates healing. Frequent application is very effective in healing acute burns, and when applied after laser surgery, healing is accelerated. Many studies have demonstrated decreased hypertrophic scarring when vitamin E is applied throughout the healing process.

Vitamin C with vitamin E

In cells, vitamins C and E interact synergistically to provide antioxidant protection. In membranes, vitamin E is oxidized as it quenches peroxyl free radicals and intracellular vitamin C regenerates the vitamin E activity [32]. Oral vitamin C with E in high doses protects against UV-induced erythema in humans, whereas either vitamin alone is ineffective [33]. Compared to twofold protection for either vitamin alone, topical L-ascorbic acid (15%) with α-tocopherol (1%) gives fourfold protection against UV-induced erythema, decreasing the number of damaged "sunburn cells" seen histologically and decreasing thiamine dimer formation in porcine skin [34]. Fortunately, mixing these hydrophilic and lipophilic antioxidants in a topical formulation stabilizes each.

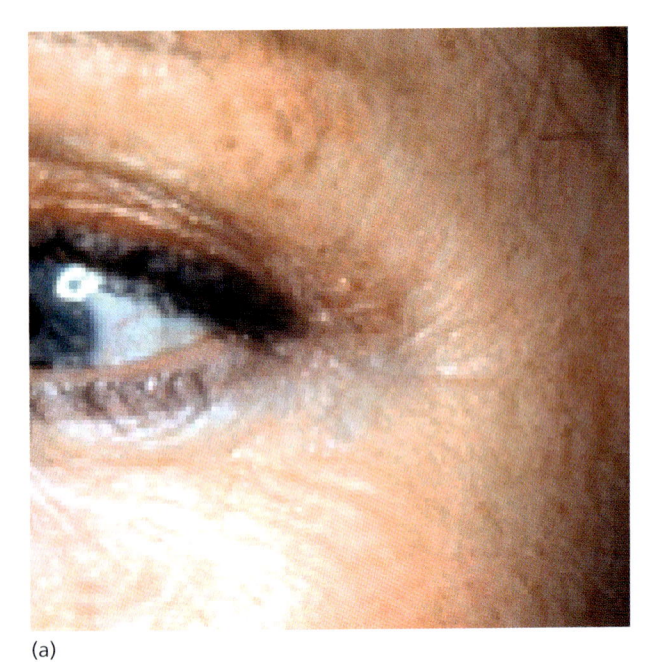

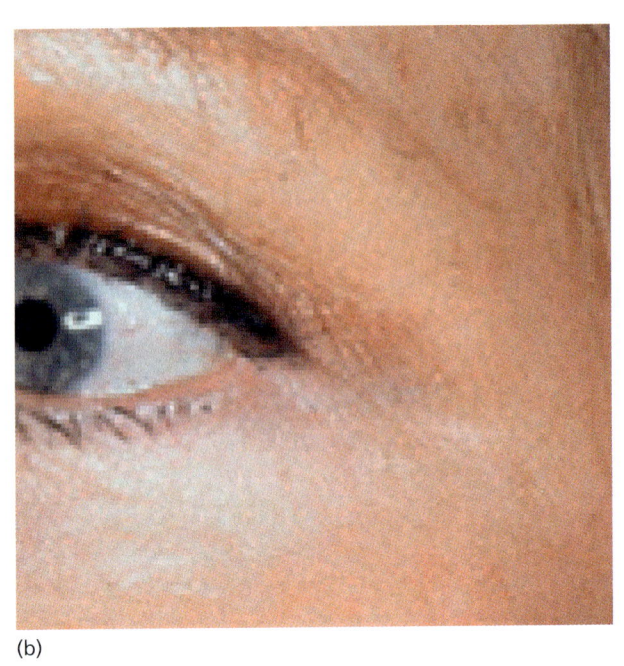

Figure 56.5 Correction of periorbital wrinkles after 4 months of once-daily treatment with 0.05% d-α-tocopherol cream. (a) Before. (b) After.

Vitamin C with vitamin E and ferulic acid

Ferulic acid is a potent antioxidant present in the cell walls of grains, fruits, and vegetables. Ferulic acid alone absorbs some UV and therefore is itself a weak sunscreen. When mixed with vitamins C and E, it further stabilizes the formulation and acts synergistically to double the photoprotection from fourfold to eightfold [35]. This triple antioxidant combination has been made into the SkinCeuticals product C E Ferulic (15% vitamin C, 1% vitamin E, and 0.5% ferulic acid).

Other antioxidants

Coenzyme Q10

Coenzyme Q10 (ubiquinone or CoQ10) is a component of the mitochondrial electron transport chain in all plant and animal cells, including human cells, especially in organs with high rates of metabolism such as the heart, liver, and kidney. In the skin, CoQ10 acts as an antioxidant, although the level is naturally relatively low, with 10 times more in the epidermis than the dermis [36]. CoQ10 has been shown to reverse natural intrinsic aging as an energy generator as well as an antioxidant and a regulator of gene induction. CoQ10 treatment increases rates of cell division as well as synthesis of natural hyaluronic acid and collagen type IV and elastin [37]. CoQ10 treatment also protects from UV-induced degradation of collagen. [38]. Decreased wrinkle depth was documented by optical profilometry using 0.3% ubiquinol cream for 6 months [39]. CoQ10 also suppresses UVA destruction of collagen [38]. CoQ10 further reverses the unattractive hyperpigmentation seen with photoaging by inhibiting tyrosinase activity, thereby decreasing synthesis of melanin [38].

Ongoing medical research continues to demonstrate the efficacy of CoQ10 in healing aging skin – both intrinsic and extrinsic. This will certainly become a more frequently used topical cosmeceutical.

α-Lipoic acid

α-Lipoic acid (αLA), made in cells of all plants and animals, has many impressive antioxidant properties and has been shown to retard aging in heart and brain cells in laboratory studies. However, the evidence for reversal of photoaging in the skin is scant: 33 women applied 5% αLA to half of their faces for 12 weeks and noted some decrease in wrinkles, skin roughness, and fading of dark spots [40].

Recent research does not confirm efficacy of αLA in protecting against sun damage. αLA provides little or no protection against UV irradiation [41]. Furthermore, αLA is not stable because of its low melting point and it decomposes when exposed to UVA [42]. Thus it is extremely difficult to make a product with enough stability to assure an effective shelf life.

Selenium

Selenium is a trace mineral essential to human life because it is the required co-factor for the intracellular antioxidant enzymes glutathione peroxidase and thiodoxin reductase. Topical L-selenomethionine (0.02–0.05%) has been shown to protect the skin from both acute and chronic UV damage [43]. In mice, topical L-selenomethionine completely stops sunburn, decreases tanning, and delays the onset and decreases the incidence of skin cancer [43]. Application increases MED in humans [44], even when MED is measured 24 hours after application, proving that

Table 56.2 Photoprotection and reversal of photoaging.

Treatment agent	Source	Photoprotection	Treatment of wrinkles	Treatment of solar lentigos
α-Hydroxy acids	Sugar cane, milk, fruits*	–	++	++
β-Hydroxy acids	Willow or sweet birch bark, wintergreen leaves*	–	++	++
Retinoic acid	Vitamin A*	Dermis only	++++	++++
Vitamin C	Citrus fruits, red peppers	+++	++++	++++
Vitamin E (d-α)	Sunflower oil	+++	++++	+++
Ferulic acid	Cell wall of fruits, grains, vegetables	++++	?	?
Coenzyme Q10 (ubiquinone)	Fish, shellfish, spinach, nuts	Dermis only	++	?
α-Lipoic acid	All plant and animal cells (including humans)*	–	+	+
L-selenomethionine	Grains, saltwater fish	++++	++++	++
Genistein	Soy	+++	?	?

+, Minimal effect noted in good studies; ++++, maximal effect (a "gold standard") ?, not studied.
* Produced synthetically for cosmetic products.

this antioxidant is absorbed, providing a reservoir of protection from UV. Furthermore, when applied to sun-damaged skin, topical L-selenomethionine was shown clinically and histologically to reverse photoaging as effectively if not even more effectively than retinoic acid – with a decrease in hyperkeratosis and regeneration of collagen and repair of elastic tissue [45]. Topical L-selenomethionine also accelerates wound healing.

Genistein

Genistein is a potent antioxidant isolated from soy, which has been proven to protect against UV-induced erythema and skin cancer [46]. As a phytoestrogen with an affinity for both α- and β-nuclear estrogen receptors, genistein confers the additional benefit of stimulating hyaluronic acid, collagen, and elastin synthesis and thus may prove to be an excellent treatment for wrinkles and for hydration of the skin.

In Table 56.2, this author has summarized her personal impressions of the clinical efficacy of well-researched topicals for photoprotection and reversal of photoaging. Others include niacinamide (smoothing texture, improving red blotchiness, and dark spots, decreasing yellowing, and improving fine lines, wrinkles, and elasticity – but is only about one-third to one-fifth as effective as retinoic acid), and kinetin (a synthetic plant growth hormone that retards senescence in plants, shown to reverse aging of skin cells in the laboratory, but in the author's experience only minimally helpful clinically in correcting wrinkles).

Conclusions

The appearance of aging skin can be treated non-invasively. Strategies include primary prevention (with changes in lifestyle by not smoking, avoiding excessive sun exposure, and assiduous protection when in the sun) and treatment. Some treatments improve the appearance immediately and others act physiologically to inhibit further photodamage and to reverse previous damage at a molecular level. New therapies for photoaging are promoted, but many have not been subjected to large, placebo-controlled, double-blind, clinical trials.

References

1. Etcoff N. (1999) *Survival of the Prettiest: The Science of Beauty*. New York: Anchor Books, Random House.
2. Rieger MM. (2000) Skin cleansing products. In: Rieger MM, ed. *Harry's Cosmeticology*. New York: Chemical Publishing Company, Inc., pp. 485–500.
3. Levy CW, Roujeinikova A, Sedelnikova S, Baker PJ, Stuitje AR, Slabas AR, et al. (1999) Molecular basis of triclosan activity. *Nature* **308**, 383–4.
4. Glaser DA. (2003) Anti-aging products and cosmeceuticals. *Facial Plast Surg Clin North Am* **11**, 219–27.
5. Forestier S. (2008) Rationale for sunscreen development. *J Am Acad Dermatol* **58**, S133–8.
6. Roscher NM, Lindeman MKO, Kong SB, et al. (1994) Photo-decomposition of several compounds commonly used as sunscreen agents. *J Photochem Photobiol A* **80**, 417–21.
7. Deflandre A, Forestier S, Lang G, et al., inventors; L'Oreal, assignee. (1997) Photostable cosmetic composition containing a UV-A screen and a UV-B screen and a process for stabilizing the UV-A screen with the UV-B screen. US patent US 5605680. February 25.
8. Pinnell SR, Fairhurst D, Gillies R, et al. (2000) Microfine zinc oxide is a superior sunscreen ingredient to microfine titanium dioxide. *Dermatol Surg* **26**, 309–14.
9. Diffey BL. (2001) Sun protection with clothing. *Br J Dermatol* **144**, 449–51.

10 Van Scott EJ, Yu RJ. (1974) Control of keratinization with the alpha hydroxy acids and related compounds. *Arch Dermatol* **110**, 586–90.
11 Van Scott EJ, Ditre CM, Yu RJ. (1996) Alpha-hydroxyacids in the treatment of signs of photoaging. *Clin Dermatol* **14**, 217–26.
12 Grimes PE, Green BA, Wildnauer RH, Edison BL. (2004) The use of polyhydroxy acids (PHAs) in photoaged skin. *Cutis* **73**, 3–13.
13 Ditre CM, Griffin TD, Murphy GF, et al. (1996) Effects of AHAs on photoaged skin: a pilot clinical, histological and ultra-structural study. *J Am Acad Dermatol* **34**, 187–95.
14 Green BA, Briden E. (2009) PHAs and bionic acids: next generation hydroxy acids. In: Draelos ZD, ed. *Cosmeceuticals.*, 2nd edn. The Netherlands: Elsevier Inc., 209–15.
15 Weiss JS, Ellis CN, Headington JT, et al. (1988) Topical tretinoin improves photodamaged skin: a double-blind, vehicle-controlled study. *JAMA* **259**, 527–32.
16 Kligman AM, Grove GL, Hirose R, Leyden JJ. (1986) Topical tretinoin for photoaged skin. *J Am Acad Dermatol* **15**, 836–56.
17 Burke KE, Graham GF. (1988) Tretinoin for photoaging skin: North Carolina vs. New York. *JAMA* **260**, 3130.
18 Fisher GJ, Wang ZQ, Datta SE. (1997) Pathophysiology of premature skin aging induced by ultraviolet radiation. *N Engl J Med* **337**, 1419–28.
19 Stratigos AJ, Katsambas AD. (2005) The role of topical retinoids in the treatment of photoaging. *Drugs* **65**, 1061–72.
20 Shindo Y, Wit E, Han D, Packer L. (1994) Dose–response effects of acute ultraviolet irradiation on antioxidants and molecular markers of oxidation in murine epidermis and dermis. *J Invest Dermatol* **23**, 470–5.
21 Wang Z, Boudjelal M, Kang S, et al. (1999) Ultraviolet irradiation of human skin causes functional vitamin A deficiency, preventable by all-trans retinoic acid pre-treatment. *Nat Med* **5**, 418–22.
22 Bhawan J, Olsen E, Lufrano L, et al. (1996) Histologic evaluation of the long-term effects of tretinoin on photoaged skin. *J Dermatol Sci* **11**, 177–82.
23 Kligman AM, Dogadkina D, Lauker RM. (1993) Effects of topical tretinoin on non-sun-exposed protected skin of the elderly. *J Am Acad Dermatol* **39**, 25–33.
24 Darr D, Combs S, Dunston S, et al. (1992) Topical vitamin C protects porcine skin from ultraviolet radiation-induced damage. *Br J Dermatol* **127**, 247–53.
25 Phillips CL, Combs SB, Pinnell SR. (1994) Effects of ascorbic acid on proliferation and collagen synthesis in relation to donor age of human dermal fibroblasts. *J Invest Derm* **103**, 228–32.
26 Bergfeld W, Pinnell S. (1996) Topical vitamin C. *Dialogues Dermatol Am Acad Derm* **38**, 1.
27 Alster TS, West TB. Effect of vitamin C on postoperative CO2 laser resurfacing erythema. *Dermatol Surg* **24**, 331–4.
28 Uchida Y, Behne M, Quiac D, et al. (2001) Vitamin stimulates sphingolipid production and markers of barrier formation in submerged human keratinocyte cultures. *J Invest Dermatol* **117**, 1307–13.
29 Catiel-Higournenc Farrais C, Guey C, Schmidt R, et al. Private communications: L'Oréal Advanced Research Laboratories, Clichy and Aulnay-sous-Bois, France.
30 Pinnell SR, Yang HS, Omar M, et al. (2001) Topical L-ascorbic acid: percutaneous absorption studies. *Dermatol Surg* **27**, 137–42.
31 Burke KE, Clive J, Combs GF Jr, et al. (2001) The effects of topical and oral vitamin E on pigmentation and skin cancer induced by ultraviolet irradiation in Skh:2 hairless mice. *J Nutr Cancer* **38**, 87–97.
32 Chan AC. (1993) Partners in defense, vitamin E and vitamin C. *Can J Physiol Pharmacol* **71**, 725–31.
33 Fuchs J, Kern H. (1998) Modulation of UV-light-induced skin inflammation by d-α-tocopherol and L-ascorbic acid: a clinical study using solar simulated radiation. *Free Radic Biol Med* **25**, 1006–12.
34 Lin JY, Selim MA, Shea CR, et al. (2003) UV photoprotection by combination topical antioxidants vitamin C and E. *J Am Acad Dermatol* **48**, 866–74.
35 Lin FH, Lin JY, Gupta RD, et al. (2005) Ferulic acid stabilizes a solution of vitamins C and E and doubles its photoprotection of skin. *J Invest Dermatol* **125**, 826–32.
36 Hoppe U, Bergemann J, Diembeck W, et al. (1999) Coenzyme Q10, a cutaneous antioxidant and energizer. *BioFactors* **9**, 371–8.
37 Blatt T, Littarru GP. (2011) Biochemical rationale and experimental data on the anti-aging properties of CoQ10 at skin level. *Biofactors* **37**, 381-5.
38 Zhang M, Dang L, Guo F, et al. (2012) Coenzyme Q10 enhances dermal elastin expression, inhibits IL-1α production and melanin synthesis in vitro. *International Journal of Cosmetic Science* **34**, 273–9.
39 Eucerin Q10 Anti-Wrinkle Sensitive Skin Crème. (2003) From Wrinkle Reduction Study 2003. In: Eucerin Q10 Product Compendium. Wilton, CT: Beiersdorf Inc., p. 11.
40 Beitner H. (2003) Randomized, placebo-controlled, double blind study on the clinical efficacy of a cream containing 5% alpha-lipoic acid related to photoaging of facial skin. *Br J Dermatol* **149**, 841–9.
41 Pinnell SR, Lin J-Y, Lin F-H, et al. (2004) Alpha lipoic acid is ineffective as a topical photoprotectant of skin. Poster presentation, 62nd Annual Meeting of the American Academy of Dermatology, Washington, DC.
42 Matsugo S, Bito T, Konishi T. (2011) Photochemical stability of lipoic acid and its impact on skin ageing. *Free Rad Res* **45**, 918–24.
43 Burke KE, Combs GF, Gross EG, et al. (1992) The effects of topical and oral L-selenomethionine on pigmentation and skin cancer induced by ultraviolet irradiation. *Nutr Cancer* **17**, 123–37.
44 Burke KE, Burford RG, Combs GR Jr, et al. (1992) The effect of topical L-selenomethionine on minimal erythema dose of ultraviolet irradiation in humans. *Photodermatol Photoimmun Photomed* **9**, 52–7.
45 Burke KE. (1994) Method for the prevention and reversal of the extrinsic aging of the skin by transdermal application of selenamino acids and compositions therefore. US Patent #5,330,757, July 19.
46 Wei H, Saladi R, Lu Y, Wang Y, et al. (2003) Isoflavone genistein: photoprotection and clinical implications in dermatology. *J Nutrition* **133**, 3811S–9S.

CHAPTER 57

Over-the-counter Acne Treatments

Emmy M. Graber[1] and Diane Thiboutot[2]
[1]Boston University School of Medicine, Boston, MA, USA
[2]Private Practice, Boston, MA, USA

> **BASIC CONCEPTS**
> - Over-the-counter cosmeceutical products are frequently used in the treatment of acne.
> - Topical benzoyl peroxide is one of the most effective over-the-counter acne treatments.
> - Other active agents in acne products include hydroxy acids, salicylic acid, sulfur, and retinol.
> - Leave-on products have a more profound effect on acne than cleansers.
> - Cleansing cloths and scrubs may be used for their sebum removal and keratolytic activity.

Introduction

Although acne is one of the most common conditions that a general dermatologist treats [1], most people with acne will first try to self-treat before seeking the assistance of a healthcare professional. A survey carried out in 2000 demonstrated that 75% of acne sufferers waited about 1 year prior to seeking the help of a healthcare professional [2]. Another study estimated that one-third of those battling acne will ever consult a physician regarding their condition [3]. Without the assistance of a physician, patients will often turn to the drugstore shelves to treat their acne.

A plethora of over-the-counter (OTC) modalities exists for treating acne. These modalities include topical cleansers, creams, lotions, gels, and masks as well as mechanical treatments, essential oils, and oral vitamins. The non-prescription acne market is one of the fastest growing segments of the dermatologic industry. This OTC market worldwide is estimated to be 2–4 times the size of the prescription market [4]. Estimates from 2001 revealed that consumers spend approximately $100 million per year on OTC anti-acne products [5].

The Food and Drug Administration (FDA) is the regulatory agency that presides over the marketing of non-prescription acne products. In the Final Acne Monograph, the FDA states that any product labeled as an "acne drug product" is defined as: "A drug product used to reduce the number of acne blemishes, acne pimples, blackheads and whiteheads." The FDA defines OTC products that fit this description to include: salicylic acid, sulfur, sulfur combined with resorcinol, and benzoyl peroxide [6]. Although products cannot be sold bearing an anti-acne label unless they contain one of the above approved ingredients, many other products are marketed towards the acne-prone consumer claiming to "heal," "purify," or "cleanse," the skin and pores.

In this chapter we address OTC products that are marketed for the treatment of acne, not just those products that the FDA defines as an "acne drug product." There are a multitude of OTC products with labeling that implies an acne efficacy. Some of these washes and leave-on products contain benzoyl peroxide, salicylic acid, alfa-hydroxy acids, polyhydroxy acids, retinol, or sulfur. Mechanical treatments exist as well and come in the form of cleansing brushes, adhesive pads, heating devices, and scrubs. Some patients may turn to homeopathic remedies such as tea tree oil or chamomile. Oral vitamins, such as vitamin A, zinc, or nicotinamide are also tried as an OTC acne fix.

Soaps and syndets

Studies show that over half of those with acne believe that their condition is caused by poor hygiene and dirt on the skin [7]. This belief often leads patients to alter both how they wash their face and their face washing frequency. While washing the face twice daily is more optimal then washing once or four times daily, the quantity of cleansings probably does not matter as much as the substance that is used to wash the face [8]. A multitude of cleansers exist and can be categorized as either soaps or syndets. Traditional soaps are made of fats and an alkali and have a basic pH of 9–10. This pH, which is higher than the skin's pH, disrupts the intercellular lipids that hold the stratum corneum together. The disintegration of the intercellular "cement"

Cosmetic Dermatology: Products and Procedures, Second Edition. Edited by Zoe Diana Draelos.
© 2016 John Wiley & Sons, Ltd. Published 2016 by John Wiley & Sons, Ltd.

causes skin irritation. Syndets are made of synthetic detergents and have a pH of 5.5–7, similar to the skin's natural pH. Because syndets only contain less than 10% soap, they are much less damaging to the stratum corneum [9]. The benefit of syndet cleansers specifically for acne patients has been demonstrated in studies.

One study, looking at 25 patients undergoing acne treatment, were randomized to cleanse with either a soap or a syndet. After 4 weeks, those using the syndet cleanser reported having significantly less acne and less oil. Both patients and dermatologists reported less irritation in those using the syndet cleanser [10]. Although not all-inclusive, some brands of syndet cleansers include Cetaphil, Aveeno, Purpose, Basis, Oil of Olay, and Dove. There are additional cleansers that are marketed specifically for acne use that contain an active anti-acne ingredient (e.g. benzoyl peroxide or salicylic acid).

Benzoyl peroxide

Benzoyl peroxide is commonly found in OTC anti-acne washes, creams, and lotions. In fact, 23% of people aged 13–27 have used an OTC benzoyl peroxide product [11]. Benzoyl peroxide was first utilized in 1917 to bleach flour. In the 1960s, benzoyl peroxide began to have medical applications for treating leg and decubitus ulcers. Several years later, in 1979, it was first used for treating acne. Benzoyl peroxide has antibacterial, anti-inflammatory, and comedolytic properties, which makes it effective in acne treatment. It has antimicrobial properties against *Propionibacterium acnes* and *Staphylococcal aureus*. One study demonstrated an almost 2-log10 decrease in *P. acnes* concentration just after 2 days of 5% benzoyl peroxide use [12]. Another study confirmed this fast-acting effect showing that *P. acnes* counts reduced by a mean of 2-log10 after applying 10% benzoyl peroxide cream for 3 days. After 7 days, there was no further decline in *P. acnes* levels [13]. Benzoyl peroxide has greater antimicrobial properties against *P. acnes* than any of the topical antibiotics alone. However, unlike the antibiotics, benzoyl peroxide will not induce bacterial resistance. Using a topical antibiotic with the addition of benzoyl peroxide will increase the bactericidal effect of the antibiotic (Figure 57.1) [14]. Furthermore, it will also prevent the development of *P. acnes* resistance when used in combination with a topical or oral antibiotic [15].

Benzoyl peroxide also acts as an anti-inflammatory agent by reducing oxygen free radicals and also by lessening *P. acnes* density. The reduction of *P. acnes* has a profound anti-inflammatory effect because the bacteria induce monocytes to produce tumor necrosis factor α (TNF-α), interleukin-1β, and interleukin-8 [16,17]. The strong anti-inflammatory and antibacterial effects of benzoyl peroxide can be parlayed into good clinical results, as shown in a large UK study. This study looked at five antimicrobial acne treatments over an 18-week period. Subjects used either oral oxytetracycline, oral minocycline, benzoyl peroxide, separate administration of topical erythromycin and benzoyl peroxide, or a combination product with containing both topical erythromycin and benzoyl peroxide. The 5% benzoyl peroxide used twice daily had similar efficacy to 100 mg minocycline once daily. This study also carried out a cost-effectiveness analysis and found that the least expensive treatment (benzoyl peroxide) was 12 times more cost-effective than minocycline [18].

Besides being an anti-inflammatory, benzoyl peroxide is also comedolytic. One study utilizing the rabbit ear comedogenicity assay showed a 10% reduction of comedones [19]. Another study compared 5% benzoyl peroxide twice daily with 0.05% tretinoin once daily for 8 weeks. Both treatments were "extremely effective" for all acneiform lesions but significantly reduced both open and closed comedones after only 2 weeks [20].

Benzoyl peroxide is available OTC in 2.5–10% strengths and as either washes or leave-on products (e.g. cream, lotion, gel). Leave-on products reduce *P. acnes* counts more than the washes, although both significantly reduce *P. acnes* on the skin [14]. There is some indication that gel formulations may be more stable and release benzoyl peroxide more consistently than creams and lotions [21]. Equal reductions of acneiform lesions are seen with benzoyl peroxide strengths of 2.5, 5, and 10%. Increasing the strength of benzoyl peroxide seems only to intensify the irritation [22]. Skin irritation to benzoyl peroxide is one of its greatest

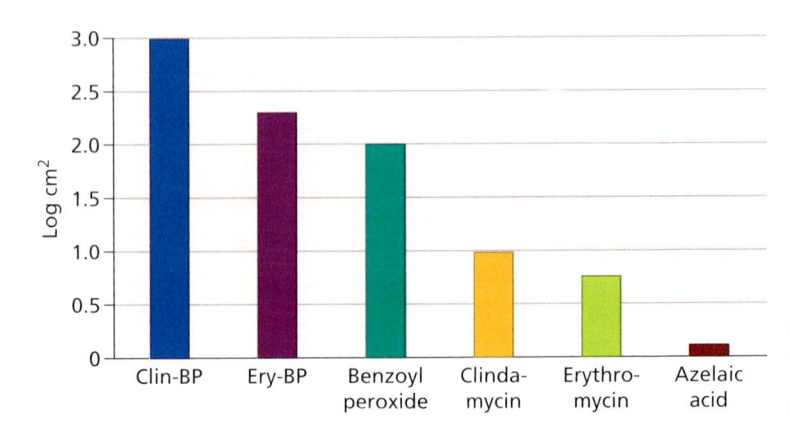

Figure 57.1 Reduction in *Propionibacterium acnes* with topical therapy. Clin-BP, clindamycin and benzoyl peroxide; Ery-BP, erythromycin and benzoyl peroxide. (Source: Leden, 2001 [*Semin Cutan Med Surg* **20**, 13943]. Reproduced with permission of Elsevier.)

barriers to use. Redness, stinging, and dryness may be manifestations of irritation. Many patients describe this as an "allergy" to benzoyl peroxide. However, true allergic contact dermatitis to benzoyl peroxide is estimated at only 1–2.5% of patients with acne [23,24]. Patients should be warned about irritation that may result and should also be told of the propensity for benzoyl peroxide to bleach fabrics and hair.

In addition to being available OTC, benzoyl peroxide is also available as a prescription. These prescription products may contain different formulations that may enhance penetration and decrease irritation, although no head-to-head trials exist comparing prescription with OTC benzoyl peroxide.

Since mouse studies have shown that benzoyl peroxide can produce DNA strand breaks, there has been some question to its carcinogenic potential. However, two case–control studies showed no correlation between benzoyl peroxide use and skin cancer. Additionally, 23 carcinogenicity studies in rodents produced negative results [11]. Epidemiologic evaluations have shown no association between benzoyl peroxide and malignant melanoma [25].

Alpha-hydroxy acids

The hydroxy acids are another common OTC anti-acne ingredient found in washes and leave-on products. There are two main classes of hydroxy acids that are used for treating acne: alpha-hydroxy acids and beta-hydroxy acids (Table 57.1). The alpha-hydroxy acids are water-soluble, penetrate the epidermis and even into the dermis at higher concentrations. They act by desquamating the stratum corneum (i.e. exfoliation). Specifically, alpha-hydroxy acids disrupt corneocyte adhesion in the upper stratum corneum, possible by chelating calcium [26]. This results clinically in a smoother appearance to the skin, and may also give the illusion of reducing pore size [27]. Alpha-hydroxy acids also promote epidermolysis, disperse basal layer melanin, and when strong enough to penetrate the dermis they may increase collagen synthesis [28]. These effects may make alpha-hydroxy acids helpful for acne prevention and treatment of postinflammatory hyperpigmentation. The most common OTC alpha-hydroxy acids are glycolic acid (derived from sugar cane) and lactic acid (from sour milk) and are found in less than 10% concentration.

Salicylic acid

The only beta-hydroxy acid used in dermatology is salicylic acid. Unlike the alpha-hydroxy acids, it is lipid-soluble allowing it to penetrate not only the epidermis but also the pilosebaceous unit. This added penetration makes it comedolytic, thus giving it superiority over the alfa-hydroxy acids in treating acne [29]. Salicylic acid also exerts anti-inflammatory effects by inhibiting arachidonic acid.

Multiple studies exist demonstrating the superiority of salicylic acid to placebo or to benzoyl peroxide. One study examined 49 patients who applied either 0.5% salicylic acid or placebo twice daily for 12 weeks. Those who applied the salicylic acid had significantly reduced inflammatory papules and open comedones, but closed comedones were not diminished [30]. One of the two studies submitted to the FDA during the OTC approval phase was a 12-week, double-blind investigation of 180 subjects. It compared the efficacy of 2% salicylic acid solution with a vehicle solution and 5% benzoyl peroxide. Of the subjects treated with the salicylic acid, 40% showed a good or excellent response versus 5% in the vehicle group and only 2% in the benzoyl peroxide group. Salicylic acid was better than either vehicle or benzoyl peroxide in improving total lesions, inflammatory lesions, and open comedones, but not closed comedones.

The second study submitted to the FDA involved 187 subjects and compared 0.5% and 2% salicylic acid solution with the vehicle solution. Both 0.5% and 2% salicylic acid were superior to the vehicle in reducing inflammatory lesions, open and closed comedones, and total lesions [31].

There are also several studies that demonstrate the efficacy of salicylic acid formulations other than solution. A cross-over study evaluating a 2% salicylic acid cleanser and a 10% benzoyl peroxide lotion in 30 patients found the salicylic acid cleanser to be superior at improving comedones [32]. Another study demonstrated the efficacy of a 2% salicylic acid scrub in reducing open comedones [33]. Based on these studies, many consider salicylic acid more effective than benzoyl peroxide in treating comedonal acne, but less effective than benzoyl peroxide in treating inflammatory acne [31]. Unlike benzoyl peroxide, salicylic acid does not have the ability to prevent resistance when used in combination with oral or topical antibiotics.

Table 57.1 Hydroxy acids

Hydroxy acid	Solubility	Source	Penetration	Action	Over-the-counter strength
Alph-hydroxy acids	Water soluble		Dermis (at high concentrations)	Exfoliative	Less than 10%
Glycolic acid		Sugar cane			
Lactic acid		Sour milk			
Beta-hydroxy acid	Lipid soluble		Epidermis and pilosebaceous unit	Exfoliative, comedolytic, anti-inflammatory	0.05–5%
Salicylic acid		Willow bark, wintergreen, sweet birch			

Polyhydroxy acids

A third class of hydroxy acids, polyhydroxy acids, is becoming more popular in OTC dermatologic formulations. Polyhydroxy acids have been shown to be less irritating than alpha-hydroxy acids, but their larger particle size may limit penetration [34]. Lactobionic acid and gluconolactone are polyhydroxy acids most often found in topicals marketed for anti-aging purposes but may someday also be found in OTC acne treatments.

Although very little of either the topical benzoyl peroxide or hydroxy acids is absorbed systemically, both of these OTC products are pregnancy category C. Like benzoyl peroxide, the hydroxy acids can cause skin irritation marked by dryness, erythema, and flaking. Use of the hydroxy acids can also lead to greater sun sensitivity. Although generally safe, toxic levels of salicylic acid (known as salicylism) can occur if salicylic acid is used on a large body surface area in patients with icthyosis or excoriations. Use of salicylic acid is contraindicated in any patient with an aspirin allergy [35].

Sulfur

Sulfur is a yellow, non-metallic element that has been used for centuries to treat various dermatologic conditions. A physician in Ancient Rome, Aulus Cornelius Celsus (ca 25 bc – ca 50 bc), *wrote De Medicina*, a medical text which includes the use of sulfur in mineral baths to treat acne [36]. Sulfur continues to be used today for a variety of conditions because of its antifungal and bacteriostatic properties [37]. It is believed by some to also have a keratolytic effect. Although the precise mechanism of action is not known, sulfur is thought to interact with cysteine in the stratum corneum causing a reduction in sulfur to hydrogen sulfide. Hydrogen sulfide in turn degrades keratin, producing the keratolytic effect of sulfur [38]. Although one study has shown sulfur to be comedogenic [39], further studies have not validated this claim [40]. Sulfur is available OTC in concentrations of 3–8% and is often found in combination with resorcinol or resorcinol monoacetate. The malodor and messiness of sulfur limits its use.

Triclosan and triclocarban

Triclosan and triclocarban are two antimicrobials that are found in cleansers marketed for acne treatment and are often labeled as "antibacterial" cleansers. Including having effects against P. acnes, both of these antimicrobials are effective against Gram-positive bacteria and triclocarban also is effective against Gram-negative bacteria. Studies are scant, but there is some evidence that these antimicrobials improve acne [41,42].

Retinols

Retinols are a group of vitamin A derivatives that are available topically OTC in various forms such as retinol, retinyl propionate, and retinyl palmitate. Both retinol and retinyl propionate are absorbed by keratinocytes where they are reversibly oxidized into retinaldehyde, whereas retinyl palmitate is inactive. Retinaldehyde is irreversibly converted into all-*trans* retinoic acid (i.e. tretinoin). Tretinoin is transported into the keratinocyte nucleus where it acts by binding to the hormone response elements. There are no large multicenter trials that evaluate the efficacy of the retinols. In general, the retinols are 20 times less potent than topical tretinoin but exhibit greater penetration than tretinoin [43]. 0.25% Topical retinol induces cellular and molecular changes similar to that observed with 0.025% tretinoin without causing the irritation typical of tretinoin. However, it should be noted that most OTC formulations of retinol come in only 0.04–0.07% [44].

Cleansing cloths

Cleansing cloths are disposable, dry towelettes that are impregnated with a cleanser and possibly an anti-acne ingredient. Just prior to use, most of them need to be moistened with water. They are manufactured by combining polyester, rayon, cotton, and cellulose fibers through a thermal process. Many cloths are impregnated with triclosan or a hydroxy acid. Their effect on the skin is determined in part by their ingredients but also by the type of weave. The cloths may be either open or closed weave. Cloths with an open weave have 2–3 mm between fibers. This relatively large spacing between the fibers decreases the cloth's contact area with the skin and in turn lessens irritancy. The closed weave cloths have less space between each individual fiber and are more irritating to the skin [45]. There are no known published trials evaluating the efficacy of cleansing cloths against acne.

Mechanical treatments

In addition to the above-described anti-acne ingredients, there are several OTC treatments designed to mechanically rid the skin of acne. Some of these treatments, such as scrubs and cleansing brushes, physically abrade the skin in an attempt to control acne. There are many abrasive scrubs available OTC that patients will often try to combat acne. Scrubs are topical agents that incorporate particles that mechanically abrade the skin and thin the stratum corneum. In general, three classes of scrubs exist. The most abrasive scrubs are made of aluminum oxide particles and ground fruit pits. These particles are the harshest on the skin, in part because of their irregular shape. The second, and milder, class of scrubs is made of polyethylene beads that are smooth and round particles. The mildest class of scrubs is composed of sodium tetraborate decahydrate granules, which soften and dissolve soon after application [45]. To our knowledge, there is only one published study looking at the effect of scrubs on acne. This study showed that scrubs did not improve comedones, but in fact worsened them. The abrasives also caused peeling and erythema. However, resorption of inflammatory lesions was somewhat augmented by the abrasives [46]. Some scrubs also include benzoyl peroxide or a hydroxy acid in order to target the consumer with acne.

In addition to scrubs, another cleansing method designed to thin the stratum corneum is the cleansing brush. Some cleansing brushes (e.g. Sonic™ Skin Care Brush [Pacific Bioscience Labs, Bellevue, MA, USA]) are handheld, battery operator devices with an oscillating brush head while others are simply handheld, coarse pads (Clean and Clear™ Blackhead Eraser [Johnson and Johnson, New Brunswick, NJ, USA]). There are no published trials evaluating the efficacy of either of these devices for removing acne. However, there is a small internally performed study by the makers of the Sonic™ Skin Care Brush demonstrating the brush to remove 2.34 times more foundation than traditional cleansing methods.

There are also adhesive pads (Biore™ [Kao Brands Co., Cincinnati, OH, USA]) on the market that are purported "to get rid of pore clogging buildup and blackheads" [47]. These disposable pads are applied to wet skin and left in place for 10 minutes, over which time the pad will stiffen. The active agent of these pads is polyquaternium 37, a cationic hydrocolloid substance that binds to the anionic component of comedonal plugs [48]. Although no studies exist evaluating the pads' efficacy in treating acne, there is a report of its success in treating trichostasis spinulosa [48].

Besides mechanical agents such as brushes and pads, there are also handheld devices that patients can purchase for home-use. One such heating device (Zeno™ [Zeno Corp., Houston, TX, USA]) is designed to speed the resolution of existing acne lesions. The user is directed to apply the device to individual acne lesions for 2.5 minutes, for 2–3 times a day. The device heats to 121°Fahrenheit, killing P. acnes. The exact mechanism by which the delivered heat kills this bacterium is unknown. Data from the manufacturer demonstrates that lesions treated with the Zeno device clear on average 1.3 days faster than those treated with a placebo [49].

There are several light emitting diode (LED) devices that are available over-the-counter that patients can purchase for use at home. LED is nonablative and athermal mode of treatment [50] that releases narrow bands of polychromatic, low-intensity light. The polychromatic light may include light in the blue, red, and/or near-infrared spectrum. Blue light may improve inflammatory acne by activating corproporphyrin III and protoporphyrin IX which can destroy P. acnes [51]. Blue light reduces the proliferative activity of keratinocytes and fibroblasts without increased cell death [52]. Red light may stimulate mitochondrial activity and modulate cytokine release from macrophages resulting in a reduced inflammatory response in inflammatory acne [51]. In non-inflammatory acne, LED may reduce sebum production and mean size of sebaceous glands [51]. Near-infrared light (830 nm) is absorbed in the cellular membrane and may enhance chemotaxis of neutrophils, macrophages, and fibroblasts to the treated area; increase cellular recruitment, metabolism, and mitosis; and, accelerate degranulation of mast cells [50]. TGF-beta I is overproduced and poorly regulated in scars, leading to fibroblastic proliferation; low-level light therapy with near-infrared light may also modulate TGF-beta I [53].

Several at home handheld LED devices are commercially available but studies evaluating their efficacy are limited and many of the existing studies lack scientific rigor. A randomized-controlled trial of a combination blue- and red- light LED device (OCimple Light Therapy System MP200) used in mild-to-moderate acne has shown to decrease both inflammatory and non-inflammatory acne lesions [51]. This study evaluated lesions on the forehead and cheeks of 35 subjects before and after serial application of 420-nm blue light and 660-nm red light for 2.5 minutes, twice daily for four weeks with resulting decrease in number of inflammatory lesion counts by 26.3% during the course of treatment, and further decrease by 76.8% at eight weeks after completion of treatment [51]. Non-inflammatory lesions decreased by 22.3% at 2 weeks of treatment and by 53.7% at 12 weeks after treatment [51]. Hematoxylin and eosin stains of 2mm punch biopsies taken at baseline and 12 weeks revealed a significant decrease in inflammatory lesions [51].

A prospective study evaluated a 405–460 nm blue-violet LED device (Silk'n Blue Device) two times weekly for four weeks for the treatment of mild to moderate inflammatory acne in 17 patients, with significant reduction in acne lesions by 35% at one month and by an additional 39% at three months after treatment [56]. However, this trial was neither blinded nor controlled. This study was not controlled for other topical or oral acne treatments simultaneously used by the study participants [56].

A prospective, single-center, open-label study was conducted to evaluate the efficacy of two fluences (A: 29 J/cm2/day vs. B: 2J/cm2/day) of 412 nm blue light (TRIA Beauty Blue Light Device) for the treatment of mild to moderate acne [57,58]. 32 subjects treated a 3 × 5cm area on one cheek with fluence A and contralateral cheek with fluence B [20]. Blue light at fluence A was associated with significant reductions from baseline to as early as Week 1 of treatment, while blue light at fluence B was showed this association by Week 3 [57,58]. Significant reductions in subject report of both the number and severity of flares and improvement in the skin's appearance [57,58]. 53% of subjects considered the treatment gentler than traditional acne treatments [57,58].

A prospective, randomized, self-control study evaluated the efficacy of an a home-use blue light device (Tanda Zap device) vs. a sham device applied on 30 subjects in office for 2 minutes twice daily for 2 days; revealing significant difference in the size and erythema of lesions [59]. While patients and physicians both agreed with the improvement, neither were blinded to the treatment [59].

Essential oils

Patients who are seeking a homeopathic approach to treating acne may seek out essential oils and oral vitamins. Two topical essential oils that can be used are tea tree oil and chamomile. Tea tree oil is derived from the Australian tree *Melaleuca alternifolia*. The oil contains several antimicrobial substances including terpinen-4-ol, alpha-terpineol, and alfa-pinene [62]. A comparative study of 5% tea tree oil versus 5% benzoyl peroxide showed that both substances significantly reduce acne. The tea tree oil had a slower onset but was less irritating than the benzoyl peroxide [61]. It should be noted that the majority of tea tree oil available OTC is no more than 1% concentration. Chamomile is derived from the German chamomile plant *Matricaria recutita*. The active ingredient is alfa bisabolol. One study demonstrated that alpha bisabolol has an anti-inflammatory effect in the skin equal to that of 0.25% hydrocortisone [62]. Because of this anti-inflammatory effect, some will try this homeopathic approach to treat their acne.

Oral vitamins

Oral vitamins that have been tried for the treatment of acne include zinc, nicotinamide, and vitamin A. Zinc sulfonate was first used as an acne treatment in 1970. Later, in the 1980s, a different formulation of zinc was developed – zinc gluconate. In patients with acne, zinc inhibits chemotaxis, is bacteriostatic against P. acnes, and reduces TNF-α production. *In vitro*, zinc inhibits type I 5-alpha reductase, a key enzyme in the hormonal impact on acne [63]. A randomized, double-blind study of 332 patients compared 30 mg/day zinc gluconate with 100 mg/day minocycline. At 90 days, patients treated with either medication had significant reductions of papules and pustules. However, minocycline-treated subjects had a 17% greater reduction in inflammatory lesions than those treated with zinc [64].

It should be noted that the recommended daily allowance of zinc is 15 mg, half the dose than is often used to treat acne. The most common side effect of zinc supplementation is gastrointestinal upset. Although generally safe at common doses (even safe in pregnancy), side effects can ensue when higher doses are used. In an anecdotal report, a desperate teenage boy with acne self-medicated with 300 mg/day zinc for 2 years. As a result, he developed severe anemia, leucopenia, and neutropenia, which improved upon cessation of the zinc [65].

Another oral vitamin often utilized for acne treatment is nicotinamide (also known as niacinamide), a water-soluble B vitamin. Nicotinamide can improve acne by both inhibiting white blood cell chemotaxis and by inhibiting the release of lysosomal enzymes by white blood cells which damage the follicular wall [66]. Although the recommended daily allowance of nicotinamide is 20 mg, studies showing its beneficial effect for acne have used 750–1000 mg/day [67]. Supplementation is safe up to 3000 mg/day, at which point it may induce reversible elevations of liver function tests. Oral nicotinamide is also available as a prescription in combination with zinc, copper, and folic acid in a product known as Nicomide (DUSA Pharmaceuticals, Inc., Wilmington, MA, USA) and has shown success in treating acne [68]. Topical nicotinamide has not shown benefit in treating acne [69].

Vitamin A is a fat-soluble vitamin that can be used in high doses to treat acne. Interestingly, those with acne tend to have lower plasma levels of vitamin A than controls [70,71]. Vitamin A binds to some of the same nuclear receptors as isotretinoin (13-cis retinoic acid). The recommended daily allowance of vitamin A is 50 000–100 000 IU. It is effective for acne at 300 000 IU/day in females and 400 000–500 000 IU/day in males [72]. At these high doses most patients experience similar side effects to those who are on isotretinoin (e.g. xerosis and cheilitis). High doses of vitamin A also have the potential to induce liver and kidney damage and to cause pseudotumor cerebri.

Conclusions

Because many patients will turn to OTC remedies to treat their acne, it is important that the physician understand what is available to patients. The ability of the physician to speak knowledgeably on OTC remedies instils patient confidence in the physician. Many of these OTC treatments may be used beneficially; however, it is helpful for the physician to advise the patient on both their advantages and shortcomings. Some OTC treatments may enhance the use of prescription medications while others may only cause further irritation. Ultimately, the physician should be educated on merging OTC and prescription acne medications to best help the patient with acne.

References

1 Feldman SR, Fleischer AB Jr. (2000) Role of the dermatologist in the delivery of dermatologic care. *Dermatol Clin* **18**, 223–7.
2 Woodard I. (2002) Adolescent acne: a stepwise approach to management. *Top Adv Nurs Pract J* **2**.
3 Malus M, LaChance PA, Lamy L, *et al.* (1987) Priorities in adolescent health care: the teenager's viewpoint. *J Fam Pract* **25**, 159–62.
4 Bowe WP, Shalita A. (2008) Effective over-the-counter acne treatments. *Semin Cutan Med Surg* **27**, 170–6.
5 Agency for Healthcare Research and Quality. (2001) *Management of Acne*. March 2001, Contract No. 01-E018.
6 21 CFR Part 333.350(b)(2), 21 CFR (1991).
7 Clearihan L. (2001) Acne: myths and management issues. *Aust Fam Physician* **30**, 1039–44.
8 Choi JM, Lew VK, Kimball AB. (2006) A single-blinded, randomized, controlled clinical trial evaluating the effect of face washing on acne vulgaris. *Pediatr Dermatol* **23**, 421–7.
9 Abbas S, Goldberg JW, Massaro M. (2004) Personal cleanser technology and clinical performance. *Dermatol Ther* **17** (Suppl 1), 35–42.

10 Subramanyan K. (2004) Role of mild cleansing in the management of patient skin. *Dermatol Ther* **17**, 26–34.
11 Kraus AL, Munro IC, Orr JC, *et al.* (1995) Benzoyl peroxide: an integrated human safety assessment for carcinogenicity. *Regul Toxicol Pharmacol* **21**, 87–107.
12 Bojar RA, Cunliffe WJ, Holland KT. (1995) Short-term treatment of acne vulgaris with benzoyl peroxide: effects on the surface and follicular cutaneous microflora. *Br J Dermatol* **132**, 204–8.
13 Pagnoni A, Kligman AM, Kollias N, *et al.* (1999) Digital fluorescence photography can assess the suppressive effect of benzoyl peroxide on Propionibacterium acnes. *J Am Acad Dermatol* **41**, 710–6.
14 Leyden JJ. (2001) Current issues in antimicrobial therapy for the treatment of acne. *J Eur Acad Dermatol Venereol* **15** (Suppl 3), 51–5.
15 Berson DS, Shalita AR. (1995) The treatment of acne: the role of combination therapies. *J Am Acad Dermatol* **32**, 31–41.
16 Kim J, Ochoa M, Krutzik S, *et al.* (2002) Activation of toll-like receptor 2 in acne triggers inflammatory cytokine responses. *J Immunol* **169**, 1535–41.
17 Vowels B, Yang S, Leyden J. (1995) Induction of proinflammatory cytokines by a soluble factor of Propionibacterium acnes: implications for chronic inflammatory acne. *Infect Immun* **63**, 3158–65.
18 Ozolins M, Eady EA, Avery AJ, *et al.* (2004) Comparison of five antimicrobial regimens for treatment of mild to moderate inflammatory facial acne vulgaris in the community: randomised controlled trial. *Lancet* **364**, 2188–95.
19 Tucker SB, Flannigan SA, Dunbar M Jr, Drotman RB. (1986) Development of an objective comedogenicity assay. *Arch Dermatol* **122**, 660–5.
20 Belknap BS. (1979) Treatment of acne with 5% benzoyl peroxide gel or 0.05% retinoic acid cream. *Cutis* **23**, 856–9.
21 Gollnick H, Cunliffe W, Berson D, *et al.* (2003) Management of acne: a report from a Global Alliance to Improve Outcomes in Acne. *J Am Acad Dermatol* **49** (Suppl), S1–37.
22 Mills OH Jr, Kligman AM, Pochi P, Comite H. (1986) Comparing 2.5%, 5%, and 10% benzoyl peroxide on inflammatory acne vulgaris. *Int J Dermatol* **25**, 664–7.
23 Balato N, Lembo G, Cuccurullo FM, *et al.* (1996) Acne and allergic contact dermatitis. *Contact Derm* **34**, 68–9.
24 Morelli R, Lanzarini M, Vincenzi C. (1989) Contact dermatitis due to benzoyl peroxide. *Contact Derm* **20**, 238–9.
25 Cartwright RA, Hughes BR, Cunliffe WJ. (1988) Malignant melanoma, benzoyl peroxide and acne: a pilot epidemiological case–control investigation. *Br J Dermatol* **118**, 239–42.
26 Berardesca E, Distante F, Vignoli GP, *et al.* (1997) Alpha hydroxyacids modulate stratum corneum barrier function. *Br J Dermatol* **137**, 934–8.
27 Bergfeld W, Tung R, Vidimos A, *et al.* (1997) Improving the cosmetic appearance of photoaged skin with glycolic acid. *J Am Acad Dermatol* **36**, 1011–3.
28 Tung RC, Bergfeld WF, Vidimos AT, Remzi BK. (2000) Alpha hydroxy acid-based cosmetic procedures: guidelines for patient management. *Am J Clin Dermatol* **1**, 81–8.
29 Kligman AM. (1997) A comparative evaluation of a novel low-strength salicylic acid cream and glycolic acid products on human skin. *Cosmet Dermatol* **11** (Suppl).
30 Shalita AR. (1981) Treatment of mild and moderate acne vulgaris with salicylic acid in an alcohol-detergent vehicle. *Cutis* **28**, 556–8.
31 Chen T, Appa Y. (2006) Over-the-counter acne medications. In: Draelos ZD, Thaman LA, eds. *Cosmetic Formulations of Skin Care Products*. New York: Taylor & Francis, pp. 251–71.
32 Shalita AR. (1989) Comparison of a salicylic acid cleanser and a benzoyl peroxide wash in the treatment of acne vulgaris. *Clin Ther* **11**, 264–7.
33 Pagnoni A, Chen T, Duong H, *et al.* (2004) Clinical evaluation of a salicylic acid containing scrub, toner, mask and regimen in reducing blackheads. 61st meeting, American Academy of Dermatology, February 2004, Poster 61.
34 Grimes PE, Green BA, Wildnauer RH, Edison BL. (2004) The use of polyhydroxy acids (PHAs) in photoaged skin. *Cutis* **73** (Suppl), 3–13.
35 Brubacher JR, Hoffman RS. (1996) Salicylism from topical salicylates: review of the literature. *J Toxicol Clin Toxicol* **34**, 431–6.
36 Thayer B. (2006) Celsus: De Medicina. Available from: http://penelope.uchicago.edu/Thayer/E/Roman/Texts/Celsus/home.html.
37 Gupta AK, Nicol K, Gupta AK, Nicol K. (2004) The use of sulfur in dermatology. *J Drugs Dermatol* **3**, 427–31.
38 Lin AN, Reimer RJ, Carter DM. (1988) Sulfur revisited [see comment]. *J Am Acad Dermatol* **18**, 553–8.
39 Mills OH Jr, Kligman AM. (1972) Is sulphur helpful or harmful in acne vulgaris? *Br J Dermatol* **86**, 620–7.
40 Fulton JE Jr, Pay SR, Fulton JE 3rd. (1984) Comedogenicity of current therapeutic products, cosmetics, and ingredients in the rabbit ear. *J Am Acad Dermatol* **10**, 96–105.
41 Franz E, Weidner-Strahl S. (1978) The effectiveness of topical antibacterials in acne: a double-blind clinical study. *J Intern Med Res* **6**, 72–7.
42 Lee TW, Kim JC, Hwang SJ. (2003) Hydrogel patches containing triclosan for acne treatment. *Eur J Pharm Biopharm* **56**, 407–12.
43 Duell EA, Kang S, Voorhees JJ. (1997) Unoccluded retinol penetrates human skin in vivo more effectively than unoccluded retinyl palmitate or retinoic acid. *J Invest Dermatol* **109**, 301–5.
44 Kang S, Leyden JJ, Lowe NJ, *et al.* (2001) Tazarotene cream for the treatment of facial photodamage: a multicenter, investigator-masked, randomized, vehicle-controlled, parallel comparison of 0.01%, 0.025%, 0.05%, and 0.1% tazarotene creams with 0.05% tretinoin emollient cream applied once daily for 24 weeks [see comment]. *Arch Dermatol* **137**, 1597–604.
45 Draelos Z. (2005) Reexamining methods of facial cleansing. *Cosmet Dermatol* **18**, 173–5.
46 Mills OH Jr, Kligman AM. (1979) Evaluation of abrasives in acne therapy. *Cutis* **23**, 704–5.
47 Available from: www.biore.com.
48 Elston DM. (2000) Treatment of trichostasis spinulosa with a hydroactive adhesive pad. *Cutis* **66**, 77–8.
49 Bruce S, Conrad C, Peterson RD, *et al.* Significant efficacy and safety of low level intermittent heat in patients with mild to moderate acne. www.myzenoeurope.com/doc/zenowhite.pdf.
50 Sadick NS. (2008) A study to determine the efficacy of a novel handheld light-emitting diode device in the treatment of photoaged skin. *J Cosmet Dermatol* **7**(4), 263–7.
51 Kwon HH, Lee JB, Yoon JY, *et al.* (2013) The clinical and histological effect of home-use, combination blue-red LED phototherapy for mild-to-moderate acne vulgaris in Korean patients: a double-blind, randomized controlled trial. *Br J Dermatol* **168**, 1088–94.
52 Weinstabl A, Hoff-Lesch S, Merk HF, von Felbert V. (2011) Prospective randomized study on the efficacy of blue light in the treatment of psoriasis vulgaris. *Dermatology* **223**, 251–9.
53 Barolet D, Boucher A. (2010) Prophylactic low-level light therapy for the treatment of hypertrophic scars and keloids: a case series. *Lasers Surg Med* **42**, 597–601.

54 Green J, Kaufman J. (2011) Home-use acne devices offer expanded options for patients. *Dermatology Times*.
55 Horfelt C, Stenquist B, Larko O, *et al.* (2007) Photodynamic therapy for acne vulgaris: a pilot study of the dose-response and mechanism of action. *Acta Dermato-venereol* **87**, 325–9.
56 Gold MH, Biron JA, Sensing W. (2013) Clinical and usability study to determine the safety and efficacy of the Silk'n Blue Device for the treatment of mild to moderate inflammatory acne vulgaris. *J Cosmet Laser Ther* **16**, 108–13.
57 Wheeland RG, Koreck A. (2012) Safety and Effectiveness of a New Blue Light Device for the Self-treatment of Mild-to-moderate Acne. *J Clin Aesthet Dermatol* **5**, 25–31.
58 Wheeland RG, Dhawan S. (2011) Evaluation of self-treatment of mild-to-moderate facial acne with a blue light treatment system. *J Drugs Dermatol* **10**, 596–602.
59 Gold MH, Sensing W, Biron JA. (2011) Clinical efficacy of home-use blue-light therapy for mild-to moderate acne. *J Cosmet Laser Ther* **13**, 308–314.
60 Raman A. (1995) Antimicrobial effects of tea-tree oil and its major components on Staphylococcus aureus, Staph. epidermidis and Propionibacterium acnes. *Lett Appl Microbiol* **21**, 242–5.
61 Bassett IB. (1990) A comparative study of tea-tree oil versus benzoyl peroxide in the treatment of acne. *Med J Aust* **153**, 455–8.
62 Brown DJ, Dattner AM. (1998) Phytotherapeutic approaches to common dermatological conditions. *Arch Dermatol* **134**, 1401–4.
63 Dreno B, Trossaert M, Boiteau HL, Litoux P. (1992) Zinc salts effects on granulocyte zinc concentration and chemotaxis in acne patients. *Acta Derm Venereol* **72**, 250–2.
64 Dreno B, Moyse D, Alirezai M, Amblard P, Auffret N, Beylot C, *et al.* (2001) Multicenter randomized comparative double-blind controlled clinical trial of the safety and efficacy of zinc gluconate versus minocycline hydrochloride in the treatment of inflammatory acne vulgaris. *Dermatology* **203**, 135–40.
65 Porea TJ, Belmont JW, Mahoney DH Jr. (2000) Zinc-induced anemia and neutropenia in an adolescent. *J Pediatr* **136**, 688–90.
66 Fivenson DP. (2006) The mechanisms of action of nicotinamide and zinc in inflammatory skin disease. *Cutis* **77** (Suppl), 5–10.
67 Niren NM. (2006) Pharmacologic doses of nicotinamide in the treatment of inflammatory skin conditions: a review. *Cutis* **77** (Suppl), 11–6.
68 Niren NM, Torok HM. (2006) The Nicomide Improvement in Clinical Outcomes Study (NICOS): results of an 8-week trial. *Cutis* **77** (Suppl), 17–28.
69 Shalita AR, Smith JG, Parish LC, Sofman MS, Chalker DK. (1995) Topical nicotinamide compared with clindamycin gel in the treatment of inflammatory acne vulgaris. *Int J Dermatol* **34**, 434–7.
70 Vahlquist A, Michaelsson G, Juhlin L. (1978) Acne treatment with oral zinc and vitamin A: effects on the serum levels of zinc and retinol binding protein (RBP). *Acta Derm Venereol* **58**, 437–42.
71 El-Akawi Z, Abdel-Latif N, Abdul-Razzak K. (2006) Does the plasma level of vitamins A and E affect acne condition? *Clin Exp Dermatol* **31**, 430–4.
72 Kligman AM, Mills OH Jr, Leyden JJ, Gross PR, Allen HB, Rudolph RI. (1981) Oral vitamin A in acne vulgaris. Preliminary report. *Int J Dermatol* **20**, 278–85.

CHAPTER 58
Rosacea Regimens

Joseph Bikowski
Bikowski Skin Care Center, Sewickley, PA, USA

> **BASIC CONCEPTS**
> - Rosacea is a chronic vascular disorder characterized by flushing, redness, telangiectases, and inflammatory skin lesions.
> - Skincare products and cosmetics can provide moisturization, support epidermal barrier function, and also camouflage underlying erythema.
> - Cleansers, moisturizers, and sunscreens can impact the appearance of rosacea; Sunscreens prevent against additional photodamage.
> - Skincare products can be used in conjunction with prescription medications for optimal symptom reduction. Light-based devices can treat telangiectases.

Introduction

Rosacea is a chronic vascular disorder affecting the facial skin and eyes that typically is characterized by a chronic cycle of remission and flare. Regardless of disease severity (Figure 58.1a–c), this disease has cosmetic consequences for the patient, including flushing, redness, telangiectasia, papules, and/or pustules. Current estimates suggest that 16 million or more people in the USA have rosacea [1,2]. Because there is no cure for the disease, management consists of the avoidance of disease triggers and the use of both prescription and over-the-counter (OTC) products that work in concert to achieve remission, prevent flares, reduce erythema, and camouflage disease manifestations, such as flushing and redness.

Physiology of rosacea

Rosacea is found most frequently in fair-skinned individuals with Fitzpatrick type I skin who tend to burn rather than tan. UV radiation damages blood vessels and supporting tissue. In fact, cumulative sun exposure is now considered a causative factor in the disease [3]. Rosacea is most often diagnosed in patients between the ages of 30 and 60 years [3], but it also can begin in adolescence – when it is often mistaken for acne vulgaris – or in individuals older than 60 years.

The etiology and pathogenesis of rosacea have not been established, nor are there any known histologic or serologic markers of the disease. However, rosacea is diagnosed by the presence of one or more primary disease features, including flushing (transient erythema), non-transient erythema, telangiectasia, papules, and pustules. Secondary diagnostic features include burning/stinging, plaque formation, dryness, edema, ocular manifestations, peripheral location, and/or phymatous changes [5].

Although these disease features often occur in various combinations, four rosacea subtypes have been classified and agreed upon to assist in the diagnosis and selection of appropriate treatment [5] (Figure 58.2a–d). Subtype 1 is erythematotelangiectatic rosacea (Figure 58.2a), which is characterized by flushing episodes lasting more than 10 minutes and persistent erythema of the central face. Telangiectases are often present. These patients may also complain of central facial edema, stinging and burning, roughness or scaling. A history of flushing alone is common.

Subtype 2 is papulopustular rosacea (Figure 58.2b), which is characterized by persistent erythema, with transient papules and/or pustules on the central face. Subtype 2 resembles acne, but without comedones; however, acne and papulopustular rosacea can occur simultaneously. Papules and pustules also can occur around the mouth, nose, or eyes, and some patients report burning and stinging.

Subtype 3 is phymatous rosacea (Figure 58.2c), which includes thickening skin and nodularities. Rhinophyma, nose involvement, is the most common presentation; however, ears, chin, and forehead may be involved. Patients may also have telangiectasias and/or patulous follicles in the phymatous area.

Cosmetic Dermatology: Products and Procedures, Second Edition. Edited by Zoe Diana Draelos.
© 2016 John Wiley & Sons, Ltd. Published 2016 by John Wiley & Sons, Ltd.

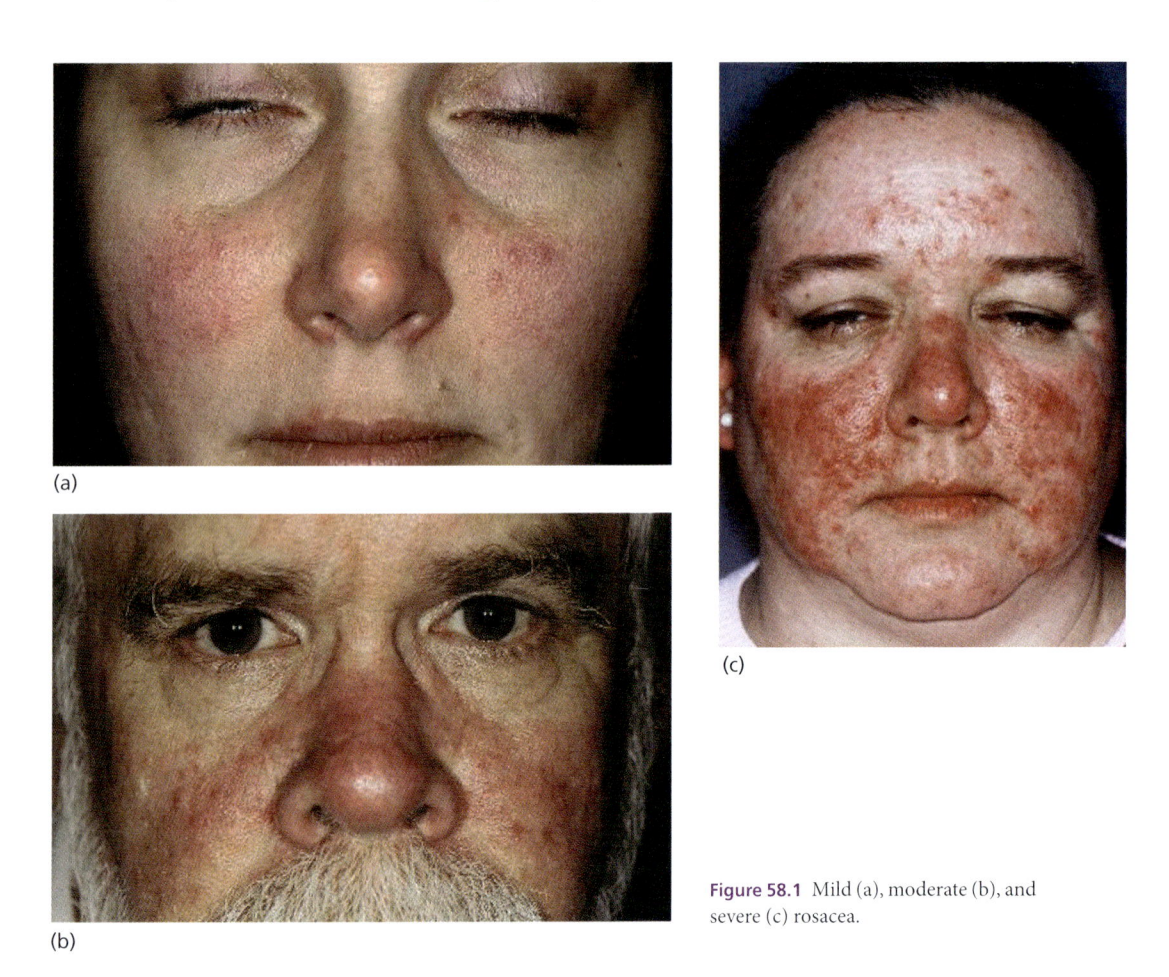

Figure 58.1 Mild (a), moderate (b), and severe (c) rosacea.

Subtype 4 is ocular rosacea (Figure 58.2d), which should be considered if the patient has one or more of the following ocular signs: watery or bloodshot eyes, foreign body sensation, burning or stinging, dryness, itching, light sensitivity, blurred vision, telangiectasia of the conjunctiva and lid margin, or lid and periocular erythema. Blepharitis and conjunctivitis are also found commonly in rosacea patients with ocular manifestations. Ocular rosacea can precede cutaneous signs by years, but it is found most frequently along with cutaneous disease.

Rosacea flare

Across the various subtypes and presentations, rosacea typically is characterized by a chronic cycle of remission and flare. Sun avoidance is crucial for every patient to minimize further cutaneous damage, prevent skin cancer, and avoid recurrent flares. There are, however, numerous other possible disease triggers. Table 58.1 is only a partial list of flare factors, but it is sufficient to illustrate how challenging flare avoidance is for patients and why it is nearly impossible for them to avoid triggers completely.

Because rosacea pathophysiology has not yet been fully described, treatment targets the signs and symptoms of the disease without a full understanding of disease mechanisms. Disease manifestations and treatment-related cosmetic sequelae necessitate the use of both OTC and prescription products for long-term treatment and to treat or camouflage skin redness, flushing, and blemishes.

Rosacea skincare: available OTC products

Rosacea patients often self-describe their skin as "sensitive". This is a non-specific, non-medical term that can vary in meaning from patient to patient. Therefore, patients should be encouraged to be specific about their skin symptoms. In general, patients with rosacea should be counseled to avoid astringents, soaps, fresheners, toners, facial scrubs, masks, and most OTC skincare "programs". However, even though the list of verboten agents is long, there are numerous safe and effective cleansers, moisturizers, sunscreens, and cosmetics available for rosacea patients. Disease management is aimed at achieving synergy between prescription and OTC products to ensure maximum efficacy of active drugs, extend remission, and conceal redness and blemishes. People with rosacea tend to have skin that is extremely sensitive to chemical irritants, so

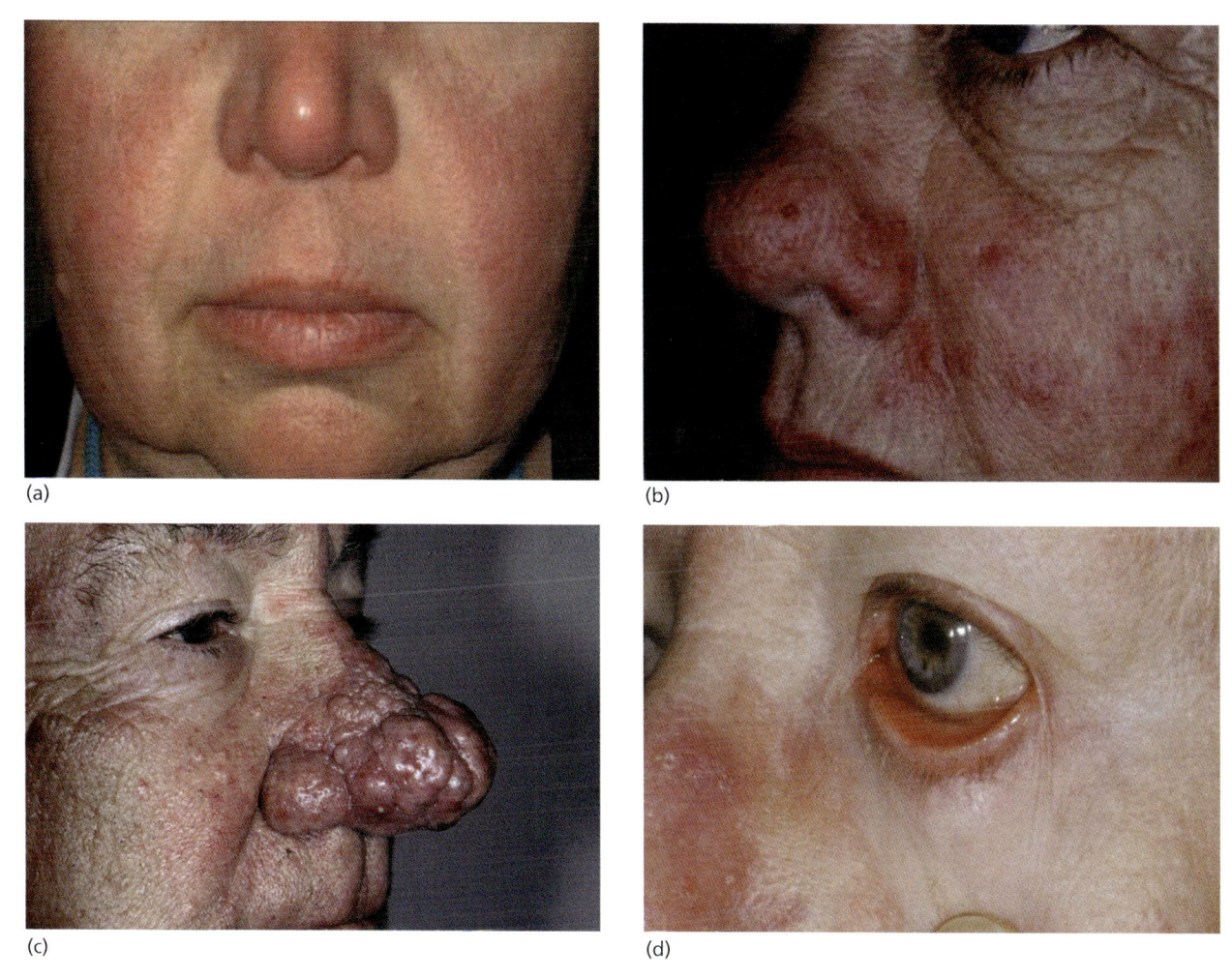

Figure 58.2 Rosacea clinical subtypes: (a) subtype 1; (b) subtype 2; (c) subtype 3; (d) subtype 4.

it is important that patients try to avoid all sources of irritation. Furthermore, the skin care regimen of a rosacea patient needs to be simple; the more the skin is specifically manipulated the more opportunity there is for unnecessary irritation. Additionally, simplified regimens are expected to encourage adherence.

Cleansing and moisturizing

A proper cleansing and moisturizing routine is an important part of rosacea management. Patients should be counseled that daily cleansing is important to rid the skin of surface dirt, makeup, dead skin, and excess oil, but they should avoid scrubbing the skin and wash with only cool water. The ideal cleanser for rosacea skin is a product that leaves minimal residue, is noncomedogenic and lipid free, and contains non-ionic surfactants with a neutral or slightly acidic pH [5]. Table 58.2 lists some recommended cleansers for rosacea patients.

Moisturizing is important in order to maintain the softness and elasticity of the skin, and therapeutic moisturizers devoid of irritants are important adjunctive therapy in rosacea management [6]. A large proportion of rosacea patients have clinically dry skin, and some topical rosacea medications (e.g. topical metronidazole) can cause further drying and irritation. Furthermore, there is increasing evidence that epidermal barrier dysfunction, which is associated with transepidermal water loss and contributes to skin dryness and inflammation, is linked with rosacea. Epidermal barrier dysfunction is associated with elevation of inflammatory serine proteases in various dermatoses, including atopic dermatitis and rosacea [7]. In rosacea specifically, epidermal barrier dysfunction has been identified, involving predominantly the central facial region in both inflammatory (papulopustular) and erythematotelangiectatic subtypes [8].

Use of moisturizers formulated with a combination of emollients and humectants is recommended to help keep the stratum corneum intact to either repair or prevent skin barrier

Table 58.1 Potential rosacea flare factors.

Factors	Percent affected
Sun exposure	81%
Emotional stress	79%
Hot weather	75%
Wind	57%
Heavy exercise	56%
Alcohol consumption	52%
Hot baths	51%
Cold weather	46%
Spicy foods	45%
Humidity	44%
Indoor heat	41%
Certain skin-care products	41%
Heated beverages	36%
Certain cosmetics	27%
Medications	15%
Medical conditions	15%
Certain fruits	13%
Marinated meats	10%
Certain vegetables	9%
Dairy products	8%
Other factors	24%

As reported by Members of the National Rosacea Society in its survey of members. National Rosacea Society website, National Rosacea Society. www.rosacea.org/patients/materials/triggersgraph.php. Accessed 29 June 2015.
Source: Rosacea Triggers Survey (www.rosacea.org/patients/materials/triggersgraph.php). Reproduced with permission of National Rosacea Society.

Table 58.2 Recommended over-the-counter cleansers for rosacea skincare.

Cleansers	Benefits
Avene® Extremely gentle cleanser lotion	No rinse, fragrance-free, paraben-free, non-comedogenic, non-irritating
Cetaphil® Gentle skin cleanser	Lipid-free, neutral pH, soap-free, non-comedogenic, fragrance-free, leaves no residue, non-irritating
CeraVe® Hydrating cleanser	Lipid-free, multi-vesicular emulsion, soap-free, non-comedogenic, hydrating, leaves no residue
Eucerin® Gentle hydrating cleanser	Lipid-free, soap-free, non-comedogenic, fragrance-free, leaves no residue, non-irritating
L'Oréal® Plénitude gentle foaming cleanser	Lipid-free, soap-free, non-comedogenic, leaves no residue, non-irritating
Purpose® Gentle cleansing wash	Lipid-free, soap-free, non-comedogenic, soap-free, non-irritating
Eucerin® Redness relief soothing cleanser	Soap-free gel, non-irritating, non-drying, fragrance-free, non-comedogenic, contains licochalcone A

All trademarks are property of their respective owner.

Table 58.3 Recommended over-the-counter moisturizers for rosacea skincare.

Moisturizers	Benefits
Cetaphil® Moisturizing cream	Non-greasy, cosmetically appealing, fragrance-free and non-comedogenic. Contains sweet almond oil, which is a source of essential fatty acids
CeraVe® Facial moisturizing lotion AM/PM	Ceramide-rich; contains niacinamide, which may reduce redness
Eucerin® Redness relief soothing moisture lotion SPF 15 or daily protecting lotion SPF 16	Contains licochalcone A; protects from UVA/UVB; fragrance-free, oil-free, non-irritating, non-comedogenic; daily protecting lotion contains green color neutralizers
Neutrogena® Oil-free moisture, various formulations	Oil-free, non-comedogenic, hypoallergenic, fragrance-free
Olay® Complete all-day moisturizer with sunscreen	Color and fragrance-free; contains vitamin E; SPF 15, protects against UVA and UVB
Rosaliac® Anti-redness moisturizer	Contains vita min C to reduce redness and green tint to conceal redness; Relatively expensive

All trademarks are property of their respective owner.

dysfunction. Furthermore, moisturizing dry skin lessens the itchiness and irritation that rosacea patients often experience as a part of their condition. Some OTC moisturizers are now available that incorporate high ratios of lipids and/or ceramides to support epidermal barrier function. Given the finding of epidermal barrier dysfunction in rosacea, the use of prescription barrier repair agents may be considered for some rosacea patients who do not respond to OTC moisturizers. Table 58.3 lists some OTC moisturizers that can be used as part of a rosacea skin care regimen.

Cosmetics

Until recently, there has been no medical treatment for the erythema of rosacea. Therapeutic options, including novel agents, are discussed below. Nonetheless, cosmetics are and will continue to be used to camouflage disease signs and symptoms, which is an important part of disease management. Rosacea patients should be counseled to avoid products containing menthol, camphor, or sodium lauryl sulfate, as these can be irritating. It is also recommended that rosacea patients avoid the use of waterproof cosmetics and heavy foundations because they are mechanically harder to apply, and their removal often requires the use of irritating solvents.

Mineral-based make-ups have become increasingly popular in recent years, and some products appear to be well-suited for use by rosacea patients because they contain all or mostly inert

Table 58.4 Recommended over-the-counter cosmetics for rosacea skincare.

Cosmetics	Benefits
DermaBlend® Cover crème foundation; smooth indulgence foundation/concealer	Allergy tested, non-comedogenic, fragrance-free, mineral-based
ColoreScience®	Contains pure, micronized minerals; offers UVA/UVB protection; waterproof
Eucerin® redness relief concealer	Smooth formula blends easily into the skin. Fragrance-free, oil-free, non-irritating, non-comedogenic, contains licochalcone A and has green color neutralizers
Cellex-C® Eye contour cream with a 5% L-ascorbic acid	Contains L-ascorbic acid and zinc; lightweight; expensive

All trademarks are property of their respective owner.

ingredients, including preservatives and fragrances. However, some mineral makeup formulations were found in a recent analysis to contain irritants and allergens [9].

Pigmentation irregularities can be camouflaged by applying foundations of complementary colors [7]. For example, red skin can be camouflaged by applying a green foundation, which is the complementary color to red; the combination of green and red creates a brown tone, and this can be covered further, if desired, by a light foundation that spreads easily. Furthermore, a yellow skin tone will turn brown when complemented with purple foundation. Figure 58.3 (a & b) shows how effective green-tinted makeup can be in camouflaging redness. Fortunately, there are an increasing number of tinted cosmetics and skincare products available to help camouflage rosacea redness, some of which are listed in Table 58.4.

Sunscreens

The daily, uninterrupted use of sunscreen is a cornerstone of the long-term management of rosacea. Sun exposure is the leading cause of rosacea flares, and patients should be advised to use a sunscreen daily, irrespective of cloud coverage, with a sun protection factor (SPF) of at least 30. However, patients should be advised that an appropriate sunscreen contains both UVB blockers (e.g. octyl methoxycinnamate, homosalate), as well as UVA blockers (e.g. avobenzone, ecamsule, titanium dioxide, oxybenzone, sulisobenzone, and zinc oxide) [7]. New FDA sunscreen labeling requirements have been met with mixed reactions by clinicians [10]. In light of label revisions, patients should be advised to select a formulation that confers broad-spectrum protection and to adhere to label instructions for frequency of reapplication.

It is also important that the sunscreen be non-irritating, and patients with rosacea may have better tolerance of products containing dimethicone or cyclomethicone [8]. Alternatively, patients may use formulations containing physical sunscreens – zinc oxide or titanium dioxide – only. Mineral make-ups often provide broad-spectrum protection against ultraviolet (UV) radiation and can be used as physical sunblocks [11]. Furthermore, green-tinted sunscreens have the additional benefit of camouflaging erythema. Examples of some recommended sunscreens for rosacea can be found in Table 58.5.

Cleansing, moisturizing, camouflaging, and using sunscreen are the primary elements of a rosacea skincare regimen. OTC products that have a green tint or that are cosmetically elegant can be applied during the day, and prescription products used to treat erythema and redness that are less cosmetically elegant can be applied at night. Patients with long-term rosacea often have sensitive skin and can be the most difficult to treat.

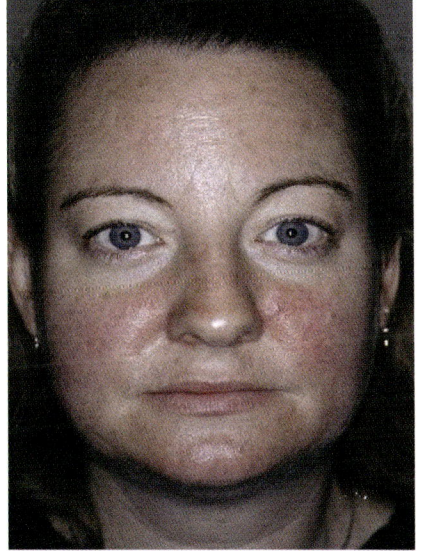

Figure 58.3 The effect of green-tinted makeup on reddened skin. (a) Patient with rosacea. (b) Camouflage of patient's rosacea using green-tinted makeup.

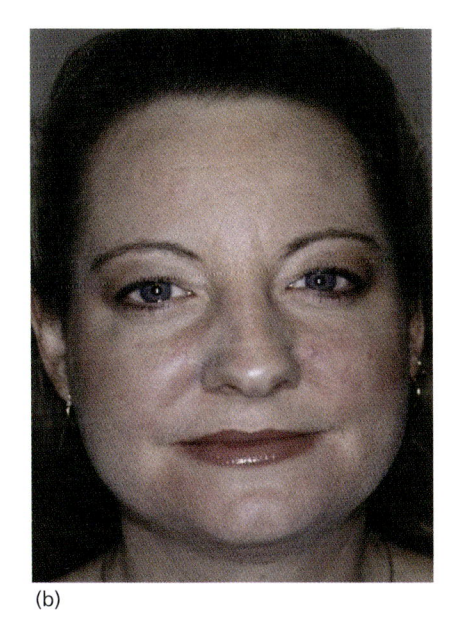

Table 58.5 Recommended over-the-counter sunscreens for rosacea skincare.

Sunscreens	Benefits
Aveeno daily moisturizing lotion with sunscreen	Contains colloidal oatmeal; fragrance free, non-greasy, and non-comedogenic
Avene® High protection mineral cream	100% mineral, broad-spectrum; developed for sensitive skin
Elat MD® UV clear	Broad spectrum; zinc oxide-based; Contains niacinamide; Fragrance-free, oil-free, paraben-free, sensitivity-free and non-comedogenic
L'Oréal®/La Roche-Posay® Anthelios®	Contains ecamsule; expensive
Neutrogena Helioplex™	Contains avobenzone; protects from UVA/UVB
Active photo barrier complex™	Contains avobenzone; protects from UVA
Titanium dioxide/zinc oxide formulations	Effective options for UVA protection. Older formulations made patients look pale, but newer manufacturing techniques have made these effective products cosmetically elegant
Vanicream® Sunscreen, sensitive skin	Broad spectrum; Free of any additives including dyes and masking fragrances, No parabens, formaldehyde, preservatives

All trademarks are property of their respective owner.

Available prescription agents

Oral and topical prescription agents are fundamental in the management of rosacea. Mild to moderate rosacea can be treated with topical monotherapy or topical combination therapy with or without an oral antibiotic. Moderate to severe rosacea necessitates the use of oral antibiotic therapy until remission is achieved, usually for 3–4 months. Remission can often be maintained by continuing the topical therapy alone or in combination with a low-dose oral antibiotic [2]. Because rosacea pathogenesis is so poorly understood, management is focused on treating disease endpoints rather than the underlying disease. In general, inflammation is treated with an anti-inflammatory agent, papules and pustules are treated with antibiotics (with no target organism), flushing is treated with vasoconstrictors, and telangiectasias are treated with light-based therapies.

Oral antibiotic therapy

Papular-pustular rosacea responds well to oral antibiotics, although their efficacy likely is brought about by their anti-inflammatory effects more than their antimicrobial effects [3]. Standard antibiotic agents include tetracyclines (tetracycline, doxycycline, and minocycline), erythromycin, and co-trimoxazole, although the latter is usually reserved for use in Gram-negative rosacea or for patients who have not responded to other therapies [12]. These agents have been used for decades and are associated with a relatively good safety profile [12].

Tetracyclines are the most commonly prescribed oral antibiotics for rosacea, but there is apprehension about antibiotic resistance with the long-term use of these and other antibiotic agents. In response to this concern, an anti-inflammatory dose formulation of doxycycline (40 mg delayed-release formulation) has been formulated for the treatment of rosacea. Long-term use of this delayed-release formulation did not alter bacterial susceptibility to antibiotics during a 9-month period [13]. Furthermore, a 16-week comparison study showed that both the 40-mg delayed-release and the 100-mg formulations in combination with 1% metronidazole topical gel are equally effective for the treatment of moderate to severe rosacea with a similar onset of action, and the delayed-release group had a superior side effect profile including fewer gastrointestinal effects [14].

Topical therapy

Topical therapy for rosacea reduces inflammatory lesions (papules and pustules), decreases erythema, improves pruritus, burning, and stinging, and reduces the incidence and intensity of flares [2]. Standard topical therapies include sulfacetamide 10%/sulfur 5%, metronidazole, and azelaic acid (AzA). Topical erythromycin and clindamycin are second-line agents, but data regarding their efficacy in rosacea treatment are limited [2].

Sulfacetamide-sulfur has anti-inflammatory properties, and the gel is available in a green-tinted formulation, which has the advantage of simultaneously treating inflammation and toning down redness. Sulfacetamide-sulfur also has been combined with avobenzone (UVA filter) and octinoxate (UVB filter) in an SPF 18 formulation, which has shown superior efficacy to topical metronidazole in investigator global severity scores, percent reductions in inflammatory lesions, and improvement in erythema [15]. Overall, these leave-on products have demonstrated favorable safety and tolerability profiles [2]. Furthermore, sulfacetamide-sulfur cleansers also have demonstrated efficacy as adjunctive therapy in combination with other topical and/or systemic agents [2].

Other treatment modalities

Flushing is a challenging aspect of rosacea management and a source of frustration for most patients. Low-dose beta-blockers, selective serotonin reuptake inhibitors, and clonidine have been used off-label to treat the flushing of rosacea [16].

New to the market is a topical prescription gel containing the alpha-agonist brimonidine tartrate 0.5%. Reduction in background erythema is evident as early as 30 minutes after application of the gel. Data from two identically designed randomized, double-blind, vehicle controlled Phase III trials showed that topical brimonidine gel applied once-daily was significantly more effective than vehicle gel throughout 12 hours. Evaluations included the Clinician's Erythema Assessment and Patient's Self-Assessment. Adverse events were mostly dermatological, mild, and transient, with a slightly higher incidence of adverse events in the active treatment group [17].

Light-based therapies

Many patients are frustrated with the poor efficacy of oral and topical therapies in resolving telangiectasia and persistent erythema. However, light-based and laser therapies have demonstrated efficacy in the improvement of vascular disease features. Potassium tytanil phosphate (KTP), pulsed dye lasers (PDL), neodymium:yttrium-aluminum-garnet (Nd:YAG), and intense pulsed light (IPL) have all been used for telangiectases, with PDL offering superior clearance rates compared with other sources [18].

Despite the efficacy of the pulsed dye laser in reducing telangiectasia, flushing, and erythema by eliminating hemoglobin within increased dilated vessels in rosacea skin, efficacy is inconsistent, and treatment can be limited by the frequent occurrence of purpura, which can be long-lasting and difficult to conceal [19].

More recently, intense pulsed light (IPL) therapy has been used with success to treat vascular symptoms of rosacea. IPL utilizes selective photothermolysis with a broad spectrum of light to destroy targeted vessels by coagulation while sparing surrounding tissue [2]. IPL is advantageous because it can penetrate the skin more effectively than lasers. Furthermore, variable light durations can target vessels of different sizes at multiple depths, IPL's increased spot size allows a larger treatment area, and sequential pulsing provides for epidermal cooling between pulses [18,19].

Natural actives

Cosmetic products with natural actives can be useful to soothe irritation associated with rosacea. Vitamin C is an antioxidant with numerous positive effects on the skin including collagen repair, normalization of photodamage, and anti-inflammatory properties. The use of a 5.0% vitamin C preparation demonstrated efficacy in objective and subjective improvement in erythema, which might be because of its anti-inflammatory effects [3]. There are currently three or four anti-redness products available, and the anti-redness moisturizer listed in Table 58.3 also has a green tint, which heals and conceals redness simultaneously.

Licochalcone A is a major phenolic constituent of the licorice species *Glycyrrhiza inflata* which exhibits anti-inflammatory and antimicrobial effects, and improves redness and irritation [20]. The Eucerin® Redness Relief line has an SPF lotion and spot concealer containing licochalcone A with a green-tinted base, which provides both an anti-inflammatory component and redness camouflage. A study assessing the efficacy of this product line in reducing irritation in patients with mild to moderate facial redness showed that a regimen of cleanser, SPF lotion, spot concealer, and night cream containing licochalcone A improved redness and was compatible with daily metronidazole treatment [21].

Chrysanthellum indicum is a plant-based extract containing phenylpropanoic acids, flavonoids, and saponosids with documented effects on vascular wall permeability and on the increase of the mechanical resistance of capillaries [22]. A cream containing *C. indicum* was recently evaluated in 246 patients with moderate rosacea. Results showed that 12-week, twice daily treatment with the *C. indicum* extract-based cream was significantly more effective than placebo in reducing erythema. Furthermore, this cream has vitamin P properties, which may be responsible for reducing or preventing microcirculation disorders involved in the erythema of rosacea [22].

Alfa-hydroxy acid-based cosmetic peels and at-home regimens also have shown promise for rosacea treatment. A regimen of a daytime cream containing SPF 15 and gluconolactone 8%, and an evening cream with gluconolactone 8% demonstrated significant improvement in texture, fine lines, photodamage, dryness, and erythema, and 80% of patients rated the cosmetic acceptability of these products as good to excellent [23]. A polyhydroxy acid skin care regimen (cleanser and moisturizer) also demonstrated good tolerability and efficacy in combination with AzA 15% in patients with sensitive skin conditions [24]. This regimen significantly added to the reduction of facial erythema, did not interfere with the efficacy of AzA 15%, and smoothed the skin, which could further enhance patient satisfaction with the products. Glycolic acid peels and topical glycolic acid products added to an antibacterial regimen also have demonstrated dramatic improvement in skin texture and follicular pores, and in the resolution of comedones, papules, and pustules [23]. An additional benefit of these products and procedures is that they provide a treatment option for pregnant women because glycolic acid products, as well as AzA 15%, are not contraindicated in pregnancy.

Conclusions

Management of rosacea requires avoidance of disease triggers, an appropriate skincare regimen – including moisturizers, and use of oral and topical prescription agents to address specific symptoms. While rosacea cannot be cured, treatment is aimed at achieving remission, maximizing time to flare, concealing redness, and now through the use of topical agents or light-based devices, treating redness and telangiectases. A non-irritating skincare regimen is essential for long-term disease management. A variety of OTC cleansers, moisturizers, sunscreens, and cosmetics are available to keep skin healthy, and an increasing number of OTC products are tinted and/or contain natural anti-redness actives, such as vitamin C and licochalcone A, which can be used in combination with prescription agents to maximize response. Prescription barrier repair agents may also be considered.

Although the pathogenesis of rosacea still has not been elucidated, there is hope that future rosacea therapies will target the disease at the genetic level, which is now common for other inflammatory skin disorders such as atopic dermatitis. There is ongoing research on vascular endothelial growth factor (VEGF) antagonists. It would appear that retinoids can modulate VEGF expression in the skin, and topical retinoic acid has demonstrated beneficial effects on vascular components of rosacea, specifically erythema and telangiectasia. Natural actives and botanicals will continue to be evaluated for their positive effects on the skin, and work remains to be done in optimizing light-based therapy in terms of clarifying treatment parameters, optimal treatment frequency, and the utility of adjuvant light-based therapies.

References

1 Del Rosso JQ. (2004) Medical treatment of rosacea with emphasis on topical therapies. *Expert Opin Pharmacother* **5**, 5–13.
2 Rosacea.org
3 Cohen AF, Tiemstra JD. (2002) Diagnosis and treatment of rosacea. *J Am Board Fam Pract* **15**, 214–7. Wilkin J, Dahl M, Detmar M, et al. (2002) Standard classification of rosacea: report of the National Rosacea Society Expert Committee on the Classification and Staging of Rosacea. *J Am Acad Dermatol* **46**, 584–7.
4 Bikowski J. (2001) The use of cleansers as therapeutic concomitants in various dermatologic disorders. *Cutis* **68** (Suppl), 12–9.
5 Bikowski J. (2001) The use of therapeutic moisturizers in various dermatologic disorders. *Cutis* **68** (Suppl), 3–11.
6 Draelos ZD. (2007) Cosmetics. Emedicine online journal. Available at: http://emedicine.com/derm/topic502.htm. Accessed 29 June 2015.
7 Nichols K, Desai N, Lebwohl MG. (1998) Effective sunscreen ingredients and cutaneous irritation in patients with rosacea. *Cutis* **61**, 344–6.
8 Dirschka T, Tronnier H, Fölster-Holst R. (2004) Epithelial barrier function and atopic diathesis in rosacea and perioral dermatitis. *Br J Dermatol* **150**, 1136–41.
9 Bi MY, Katta R. (2010) Mineral make-up and its potential utility in patients with contact dermatitis. *J Am Acad Dermatol* **62**(3), 519–22.
10 Pigeon, T. (2012) Update on sunscreen labeling and regulation. *Practical Dermatol* **9**, 27–30.
11 Sundaram H. (2010) Medical grade mineral cosmetics: their benefits and role in patient care. *Practical Dermatol* **7**, 50–52.
12 Del Rosso JQ. (2000) Systemic therapy for rosacea: focus on oral antibiotic therapy and safety. *Cutis* **66** (Suppl), 7–13.
13 Walker C, Webster G. (2007) *The effect of anti-inflammatory dose doxycycline 40 mg once-daily for 9 months on bacterial flora: Subset analysis from a multicenter, double-blind, randomized trial.* Poster presented at 26th Anniversary Fall Clinical Dermatology Conference; October 18–27, 2007, Las Vegas, Nevada.
14 Del Rosso JQ. (2008) *Comparison of anti-inflammatory dose doxycycline (40 mg delayed-release) vs doxycycline 100 mg in the treatment of rosacea.* Poster presented at 8th Annual Caribbean Dermatology Symposium, January 15–19, 2008; St. Thomas, US Virgin Islands.
15 Shalita AR, Dosik JS, Neumaier GJ, et al. (2003) A comparative efficacy study of Rosac® cream with sunscreens (sodium sulfacetamide 10% and sulfur 5%) and MetroCream® (metronidazole 0.75%) in the twice daily treatment of rosacea. *Skin Aging* Oct (Suppl), 17–22.
16 Baldwin HE. (2007) Systemic therapy for rosacea. *Skin Ther Lett* **12**, 1–5; 9.
17 Fowler J Jr, Jackson M, Moore A, et al. (2013) Efficacy and safety of once-daily topical brimonidine tartrate gel 0.5% for the treatment of moderate to severe facial erythema of rosacea: results of two randomized, double-blind, and vehicle-controlled pivotal studies. *J Drugs Dermatol* **12**, 650–56.
18 Bencini PL, Tourlaki A, De Giorgi V, Galimberti M. (2012) Laser use for cutaneous vascular alterations of cosmetic interest. *Dermatol Ther* **25**, 340–51.
19 Bikowski JB, Goldman MP. (2004) Rosacea: where are we now? *J Drugs Dermatol* **3**, 251–58.
20 Kolbe L, Immeyer J, Batzer J, Wensorra U, tom Dieke K, Mundt C, et al. (2006) Anti-inflammatory efficacy of licochalcone A: correlation of clinical potency and *in vitro* effects. *Arch Dermatol Res* **298**, 23–30.
21 Weber TM, Ceilley RI, Buerger A, Kolbe L, Trookman NS, Rizer RL, et al. (2006) Skin tolerance, efficacy, and quality of life of patients with red facial skin using a skin care regimen containing licochalcone A. *J Cosmet Dermatol* **5**, 227–32.
22 Rigopoulos D, Kalogeromitros D, Gregoriou S, Pacouret JM, Koch C, Fisher N, et al. (2005) Randomized placebo-controlled trial of a flavonoid-rich plant extract-based cream in the treatment of rosacea. *J Eur Acad Dermatol Venereol* **19**, 564–8.
23 Tung RC, Bergfeld WF, Vidimos AT, Remzi BK. (2000) Alpha-hydroxy acid-based cosmetic procedures: guidelines for patient management. *Am J Clin Dermatol* **1**, 81–8.
24 Draelos ZD, Green BA, Edison BL. (2006) An evaluation of a polyhydroxy acid skin care regimen in combination with azelaic acid 15% gel in rosacea patients. *J Cosmet Dermatol* 5, 23–9.

CHAPTER 59
Eczema Regimens

Zoe D. Draelos

Department of Dermatology, Duke University School of Medicine Durham, NC, USA

> **BASIC CONCEPTS**
> - Dry skin affected by eczema is characterized by loss of intercellular lipids which results in barrier deficits.
> - Moisturizers are an important part of eczema treatment as they provide an environment optimal for barrier repair.
> - Moisturizers function by impeding transepidermal water loss with oily occlusive substances, such as petrolatum, mineral oil, vegetable oils, and dimethicone, and by attracting water to the dehydrated stratum corneum and epidermis with humectants, such as glycerin, sodium PCA, propylene glycol, lactic acid, and urea.
> - Moisturizing ingredients can be delivered to the skin surface by emulsions, liposomes, and niosomes.
> - Careful moisturizer selection is key to the treatment and prevention of eczematous skin disease.

Introduction

Eczematous skin disease is one of the most commonly treated dermatologic conditions. While topical prescription corticosteroids and calcineurin inhibitors are the mainstay of therapy, cosmeceutical moisturizers are key to the treatment and prevention of disease. Moisturizers enhance the skin barrier, decreasing stinging and burning from a sensory standpoint and improving the look and feel of the skin. Moisturizers can also smooth desquamating corneocytes and fill corneocytes gaps to create the impression of tactile smoothness. This effect is temporary, of course, until the moisturizer is removed from the skin surface by wiping or cleansing. From a functional standpoint, moisturizers can create an optimal environment for healing and minimize the appearance of lines of dehydration by decreasing transepidermal water loss. Transepidermal water loss increases when the "brick and mortar" organization of the protein-rich corneocytes held together by intercellular lipids is damaged. A well-formulated cosmeceutical moisturizer can decrease the water loss until healing occurs.

Etiology

Eczema is characterized by barrier disruption, which is the most common cause of sensitive skin. The barrier can be disrupted chemically through the use of cleansers and cosmetics that remove intercellular lipids or physically through the use of abrasive substances that induce stratum corneum exfoliation. In some cases, the barrier may be defective because of insufficient sebum production, inadequate intercellular lipids, or abnormal keratinocyte organization. The end result is the induction of the inflammatory cascade accompanied by erythema, desquamation, itching, stinging, burning, and possibly pain. The immediate goal of treatment is to stop the inflammation through the use of topical, oral, or injectable corticosteroids, depending on the severity of the eczema and the percent body surface area involved. In dermatology, topical corticosteroids are most frequently employed with low potency corticosteroids (desonide) used on the face and intertrigenous areas, medium potency corticosteroids (triamcinolone) on the upper chest and arms, high potency corticosteroids (fluocinonide) on the legs and back, and ultra high potency corticosteroids (clobetasol) used on the hands and feet. Newer topical options for the treatment of eczema-induced sensitive skin include the calcineurin inhibitors, pimecrolimus, and tracrolimus.

However, the resolution of the inflammation is not sufficient for the treatment of eczema. Proper skin care must also be instituted to minimize the return of the conditions that led to the onset of eczema.

Moisturizer mechanism of action

Moisturizers are incorporated into eczema treatment regimens to reduce transepidermal water loss. There are three cosmeceutical ingredient categories that can reduce transepidermal water loss: occlusives, humectants, and hydrophilic matrices [1]. The

---

Cosmetic Dermatology: Products and Procedures, Second Edition. Edited by Zoe Diana Draelos.
© 2016 John Wiley & Sons, Ltd. Published 2016 by John Wiley & Sons, Ltd.

Table 59.1 Occlusive moisturizing ingredients to inhibit transepidermal water loss.

1. Hydrocarbon oils and waxes: petrolatum, mineral oil, paraffin, squalene
2. Silicone oils
3. Vegetable and animal fats
4. Fatty acids: lanolin acid, stearic acid
5. Fatty alcohol: lanolin alcohol, cetyl alcohol
6. Polyhydric alcohols: propylene glycol
7. Wax esters: lanolin, beeswax, stearyl stearate
8. Vegetable waxes: carnauba, candelilla
9. Phospholipids: lecithin
10. Sterols: cholesterol

most common method for reducing transepidermal water loss is the application of an occlusive ingredient to the skin surface. These are oily substances that create a barrier to water evaporation. The more commonly used occlusive ingredients in current formulations and their chemical category are listed in Table 59.1 [2].

The most popular and effective occlusive ingredient is time-tested petrolatum, which blocks 99% of water loss from the skin surface [3]. This remaining 1% transepidermal water loss is necessary to provide the cellular message for barrier repair initiation. If the transepidermal water loss is completely halted, the removal of the occlusion results in failure to repair the barrier and water loss quickly resumes at its preapplication level. Thus, the occlusion does not initiate barrier repair [4]. Petrolatum does not function as an impermeable barrier, rather it permeates throughout the interstices of the stratum corneum allowing barrier function to be re-established [5]. Moisturizers for eczematous disease must contain several occlusive moisturizing ingredients.

In addition to occlusive ingredients, a therapeutic moisturizer for eczema must contain humectants. Humectants are substances that attract water to the viable epidermis and stratum corneum from the dermis. They function as a sponge to hold and release water as necessary. Examples of humectants include glycerin, honey, sodium lactate, urea, propylene glycol, sorbitol, pyrrolidone carboxylic acid, gelatin, hyaluronic acid, vitamins, and some proteins [2,6].

Humectants only draw water from the environment when the ambient humidity exceeds 70%. In environmentally controlled spaces, this does not occur, thus humectants pull water from the deeper epidermal and dermal tissues to rehydrate the stratum corneum. A therapeutic moisturizer for eczema must trap the water in the skin with an occlusive film placed on top of the stratum corneum [7]. Humectants also allow the skin to feel smoother by filling holes in the stratum corneum through swelling [8,9]. Therefore, a moisturizer recommended for eczema must combine both occlusive and humectant ingredients for optimal efficacy and patient aesthetics. Occlusive and humectant moisturizers are the formulations most beneficial in the treatment of eczema and include the majority of those found in the dermatologic sample closet (Eucerin Cream and Lotion, Beiersdorf; Norwegian Formula Moisturizers, Neutrogena; Aveeno Cream and Lotion, Johnson & Johnson; Olay Daily Facial Moisturizer, Procter & Gamble, Plentitude, L'Oréal; Cetaphil Cream and Lotion, Galderma; CeraVe Cream and Lotion, Coria).

A third type of moisturizing formulation is known as the hydrophilic matrix. Hydrophilic matrices are large molecular weight substances that create a film over the skin surface thereby retarding water evaporation. The first hydrophilic matrix developed was an oatmeal bath (Aveeno Oatmeal Bath, Johnson & Johnson). The colloidal oatmeal created a film that prevented water from leaving the skin to enter the bath water. Newer hydrophilic matrices include peptides and proteins, but they do not provide meaningful skin moisturization in the eczema patient.

Moisturizer goals in eczema

The goal of all moisturizing emulsions is to accomplish skin remoisturization, which occurs in four steps: initiation of barrier repair, alteration of surface cutaneous moisture partition coefficient, onset of dermal–epidermal moisture diffusion, and synthesis of intercellular lipids [10]. These steps must occur sequentially in order for proper skin barrier repair. Once the barrier has repaired, there must be some substance that holds and regulates the skin water content. This substance has been termed the natural moisturizing factor (NMF). The constituents of the NMF consist of a mixture of amino acids, derivatives of amino acids, and salts (Figure 59.1). [11]. The NMF is actually derived from profillagrin in the living epidermis that is broken down into filaggrin. Filaggrin is responsible for the mechanical stability of the outer epidermis, but degrades with the help of proteases to become NMR, which is essential for skin water content maintenance. Persons with severe atopic dermatitis demonstrate genetic filaggrin deficiency. Ten percent of the dry weight of the stratum corneum cells is composed of NMF in well-hydrated skin [12]. Cosmeceutical moisturizing emulsions try to duplicate the effect of the NMF.

Another important structure in the maintenance of skin water content are the aquaporins, which are a family of 13 proteins found in the cell membranes that regulate water and glycerol passage in and out of cells (Figure 59.2). Aquaporins 1, 2, 4, 5, and 8 are water channels while aquaporins 3, 7, 9, and 10 are aquaglyceroporins. Aquaporins 6, 11, and 12 are "unorthodox" aquaporins. Of these, the most important in the skin is aquaporin 3. Glycerin is transported in aquaporin 3 channels to phospholipase D resulting in phosphatidylglycerol, a lipid that signals enzymes of cell differentiation. This discovery has led to a renewed interest in glycerin as a modulator of skin function in eczema patients.

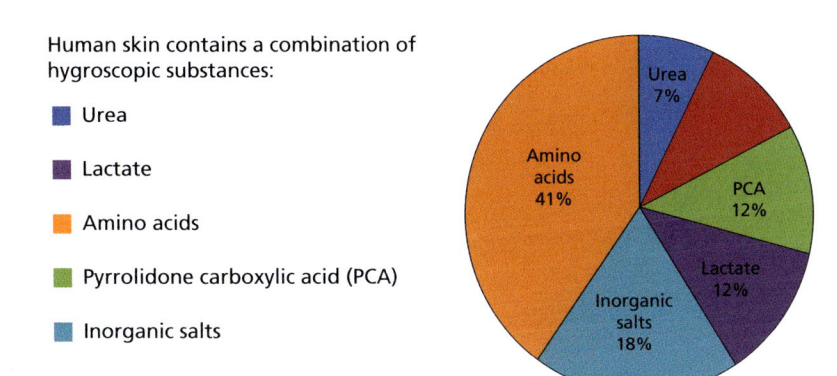

Human skin contains a combination of hygroscopic substances:

- Urea
- Lactate
- Amino acids
- Pyrrolidone carboxylic acid (PCA)
- Inorganic salts

Urea 7%
Amino acids 41%
PCA 12%
Lactate 12%
Inorganic salts 18%

Figure 59.1 The constituents of the natural moisturizing factor responsible for maintaining the water content of the skin.

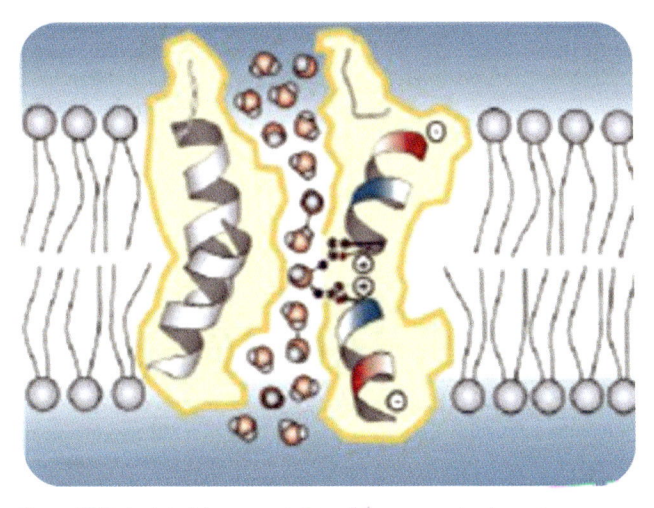

Figure 59.2 A pictorial representation of the aquaporin channels necessary to maintain cellular osmotic balance.

Moisturizer delivery systems

Another method for optimizing the ability of moisturizers to create an environment for healing in eczema patients is through novel delivery of the ingredients. This has led to the development of delivery systems that can time release substances onto the skin surface and improve product aesthetics. For example, petrolatum is the most effective ingredient for skin healing, yet it leaves an easily removed, sticky, greasy film on the skin surface. A delivery system could allow small amounts of petrolatum to be released onto the skin surface avoiding the aesthetic drawbacks. Examples of delivery systems relevant to eczema treatment include emulsions, serums, liposomes, niosomes, multivesicular emulsions, and nanoemulsions.

Moisturizing emulsions

Most moisturizers developed for the treatment of eczema are emulsions [13]. An emulsion is formed from oil and water mixed and held in solution by an emulsifier. Most emulsifiers are surfactants, or soaps, which dissolve the two non-miscible ingredients. The most common emulsions are oil-in-water, where the oil is dissolved in the water [14]. This emulsion is the most popular among patients because the water evaporates leaving behind a thin film of oily ingredients. If the emulsion can be poured from a bottle, it is considered a lotion. These moisturizing products are popular for eczema treatment, but may make the eczema worse as the repeated wetting and drying of the skin results in further maceration. Cream oil-in-water emulsions are preferred because the environment created for barrier repair is far superior.

Water-in-oil emulsions, where the water-soluble substances are dissolved in the oil-soluble substances, are less popular because of their greasy aesthetics. Most ointments are water-in-oil emulsions, but they leave the skin feeling warm and sticky. Ointments deliver higher levels of moisturization because the water phase is small, leaving behind a proportionately larger concentration of ingredients capable of retarding transepidermal water loss. Even though their efficacy is greater, most eczema patients prefer more aesthetic formulations.

Moisturizing serums

A specialized form of emulsion is a serum. Serums are usually low viscosity, oil-in-water emulsions that deliver of thin film of active ingredients to the skin surface. For example, a high concentration glycerin serum can be placed under a high concentration petrolatum oil-in-water emulsion to provide robust skin moisturization. Sometimes a serum will contain cosmeceutical barrier enhancing ingredients, such as ceramides, cholesterol, and free fatty acids.

Moisturizing liposomes and niosomes

Moisturizing ingredients can be incorporated into structures with unique physical properties on the skin, such as liposomes and niosomes (Table 59.2). Liposomes are spherical vesicles with a diameter 25–5000 nm formed from membranes consisting of bilayer amphiphilic molecules, which possess both polar and non-polar ends. The polar heads are directed toward the inside of the vesicle and toward its outer surface while the non-polar, or lipophilic tails, are directed toward the middle of the bilayer.

Liposomes are based on the natural structure of the cell membrane, which has been highly conserved through evolutionary change. The name is derived from the Greek word "lipid" meaning fat, and "soma" meaning body. Liposomes are primarily formed from phospholipids, such as phosphatidylcholine, but

Table 59.2 Special moisturizer delivery systems.

Delivery system	Structure	Advantages vs. disadvantages
Liposomes	Spherical vesicles consisting of bilayer amphiphilic molecules with polar and non-polar ends	Can deliver hydrophilic and hydrophobic substances to the skin surface without an emulsifier
Multivesicular emulsion (MVE)	Liposome within a liposome within a liposome to form concentric liposomes	Deliver multiple moisturizing ingredients (glycerin, dimethicone, sphingolipids, ceramides) simultaneously
Niosome	Liposome composed of non-ionic surfactants, such as ethoxylated fatty alcohols and synthetic polyglycerol ethers	Non-ionic surfactants do not moisturize the skin surface
Nanoemulsions	Emulsions with 20–300 nm droplets	Allow enhanced skin penetration due to small droplet size

may also be composed of surfactants, such as dioleoylphosphatidylethanolamine. Their functionality may be influenced by chemical composition, vesicle size, shape, surface charge, lamellarity, and homogeneity.

The liposome is an extremely versatile structure. It can contain aqueous substances in its core, or nothing at all. Hydrophobic substances can dissolve in the phospholipid bilayer shell, which allows liposomes to deliver both oil-soluble and water-soluble substances without need for an emulsifier. Thus, the internal moisturizer payload plus the phospholipid membrane can both function as moisturizers.

It is unlikely that liposomes diffuse across the stratum corneum barrier intact. The corneocytes are embedded in intercellular lipids, composed of ceramides, glycosylceramides, cholesterol, and fatty acids, which are structurally different from the phospholipids of the liposome. It is postulated that liposomes penetrate through the appendageal structures. They may also fuse with other bilayers, such as cell membranes, to release their ingredients. This is the mechanism by which liposomes can function as moisturizers, supplementing deficient intercellular lipids.

Niosomes are a specialized form of liposome composed of non-ionic surfactants. These are detergents, such as ethoxylated fatty alcohols and synthetic polyglycerol ethers (polyoxyethylene alkylester, polyoxyethylene alkylether). These liposomes do not deliver the moisturizing phospholipids to the skin surface.

Multivesicular emulsions

Another variant of the liposome is a multivesicular emulsion (MVE) (Figure 59.3). The MVE is created through a physical mixing technique, which makes them more stable, but also less expensive to produce. An MVE can be thought of as a liposome within a liposome within a liposome. Thus, with the release of each liposome, additional moisturizing ingredients can be deposited on the skin surface. MVEs can deliver glycerin, dimethicone, sphingolipids, and ceramides to the skin surface simultaneously.

Moisturizing nanoemulsions

Nanoemulsions are similar to regular emulsions with an oil-loving hydrophobic phase and a water-loving hydrophilic, except droplets in these emulsions are on the nano scale of 20–300 nm [15]. If the nano droplets are larger than 100 nm, the emulsion appears white, while nanoemulsions with droplets of 70 nm are transparent. Nanoemulsions offer the ability to deliver highly hydrophobic or lipophilic substances into the skin, which could not otherwise penetrate. The stratum corneum is an excellent barrier to lipophilic ingredients.

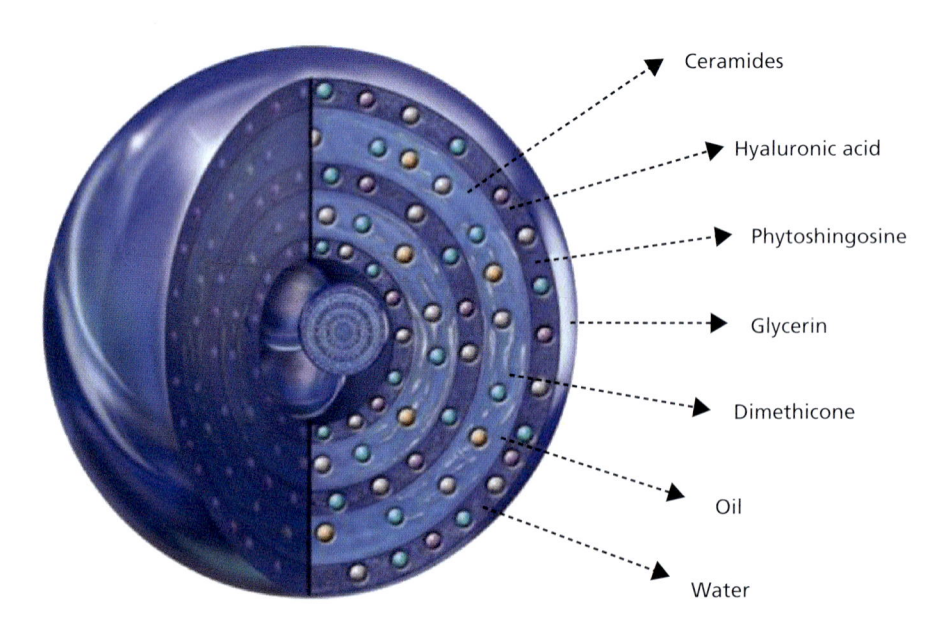

Figure 59.3 A multivesicular emulsion can dissolve many ingredients in the concentric liposomes.

For example, new nanoemulsions of ubiquinone have been developed. Ubiquinone, also known as coenzyme Q10, is an important antioxidant manufactured by the body and found in all skin cells. It is found in both hydrophilic and hydrophobic cellular compartments, but topical delivery has been challenging. Nanoemulsions have successfully delivered higher concentrations of ubiquinone into the skin with the goal of enhancing the skin's natural antioxidant capabilities, while leaving beyond a moisturizing film from the other ingredients in the emulsion.

Developing a moisturizer regimen

This chapter has discussed the goals of moisturization, the various types of moisturizers, and some of the unique moisturizer delivery systems. The biggest challenge for the clinician is adding moisturizers or combining moisturizers as part of a treatment regimen.

Patients with eczema require basic hygiene. The face and body must be cleansed. There is no doubt that the synthetic detergent cleansers, also known as syndets, provide the best skin cleansing while minimizing barrier damage. Bars based on sodium cocyl isethionate appear to perform the best (Dove, Unilever; Olay, Procter & Gamble). There are some patients, however, who only require the use of a facial syndet cleanser occasionally, because sebum production and physical activity are minimal. For these patients, a lipid-free cleanser is preferable because it can be used without water and wiped away (Cetaphil, Galderma; CerVe, Coria). These products may contain water, glycerin, cetyl alcohol, stearyl alcohol, sodium laurel sulfate, and occasionally propylene glycol. They leave behind a thin moisturizing film and can be used effectively in persons with excessively dry, sensitive, or dermatitic skin. They do not have strong antibacterial properties, however, and may not remove odor from the armpit or groin. Lipid-free cleansers are best used where minimal cleansing is desired.

After completing cleansing, the eczema patient requires moisturization. The moisturizer should create an optimal environment for barrier repair, while not inducing any type of skin reaction. For example, the product should not contain any mild irritants that may present as an acneiform eruption in the eczema patient because of the presence of follicular irritant contact dermatitis. The best moisturizers are simple oil-in-water emulsions. The morning moisturizer should provide SPF 30 photoprotection. A variety of sunscreen-containing moisturizers are on the market for this purpose (Olay Complete Defense SPF 30, Procter & Gamble; Neutrogena Daily Defense SPF 30, Johnson & Johnson). If additional hydration is required, a moisturizer can be applied to the face followed by a second sunscreen-containing moisturizer on top. It is possible to layer moisturizers for additive benefit. The sunscreen-containing moisturizer should be applied last, as it does not need to touch the skin to provide optimal photoprotection.

The evening moisturizer provides the best opportunity for barrier repair, because the body is at rest. The best ingredient for barrier repair is white petrolatum, but dimethicone and cyclomethicone are commonly added to decrease the greasiness of a simple petrolatum and water formulation. Basic night creams containing these ingredients, in addition to glycerin, are the mainstay of therapeutic eczema moisturizers. It is important to remember that fewer ingredients are preferred, because more ingredient exposure creates added opportunities for sensitization or an adverse event.

Conclusions

Eczema treatment requires the use of prescription medications in conjunction with skincare products. Both must be judiciously selected to insure optimal results. Thorough resolution of eczema requires alleviation of the disease, the treatment phase, and prevention of recurrence, the maintenance phase. This chapter has discussed those concepts that are key to designing a maintenance phase regimen for eczema patients.

References

1 Baker CG. (1987) Moisturization: new methods to support time proven ingredients. *Cosmet Toilet* **102**, 99–102.
2 De Groot AC, Weyland JW, Nater JP. (1994) *Unwanted Effects of Cosmetics and Drugs Used in Dermatology*, 3rd edn. Amsterdam: Elsevier, pp. 498–500.
3 Friberg SE, Ma Z. (1993) Stratum corneum lipids, petrolatum and white oils. *Cosmet Toilet* **107**, 55–9.
4 Grubauer G, Feingold KR, Elias PM. (1987) Relationship of epidermal lipogenesis to cutaneous barrier function. *J Lipid Res* **28**, 746–52.
5 Ghadially R, Halkier-Sorensen L, Elias PM. (1992) Effects of petrolatum on stratum corneum structure and function. *J Am Acad Dermatol* **26**, 387–96.
6 Spencer TS. (1988) Dry skin and skin moisturizers. *Clin Dermatol* **6**, 24–8.
7 Rieger MM, Deem DE. (1974) Skin moisturizers II. The effects of cosmetic ingredients on human stratum corneum. *J Soc Cosmet Chem* **25**, 253–59.
8 Robbins CR, Fernee KM. (1983) Some observations on the swelling of human epidermal membrane. *J Sos Cosmet Chem* **37**, 21–34.
9 Idson B. (1992) Dry skin: moisturizing and emolliency. *Cosmet Toilet* **107**, 69–78.
10 Jackson EM. (1992) Moisturizers: What's in them? How do they work? *Am J Contact Derm* **3**, 162–8.
11 Wehr RF, Krochmal L. (1987) Considerations in selecting a moisturizer. *Cutis* **39**, 512–5.
12 Rawlings AV, Scott IR, Harding CR, Bowser PA. (1994) Stratum corneum moisturization at the molecular level. *Prog Dermatol* **28**, 1–12.
13 Chanchal D, Swarnlata S. ((2008) Novel approaches in herbal cosmetics. *J Cosmet Dermatol* **7**, 89–95.
14 Carlotti ME, Gallarate M, Rossatto V. (2003) O/W microemulsions as a vehicle for sunscreen. *J Cosmet Sci* **54**, 451–59.
15 Kaur IP, Agrawal R. (2007) Nanotechnology: a new paradigm in cosmeceuticals. *Recent Pat Drug Deliv Formul* **1**, 171–82.

CHAPTER 60
Psoriasis Regimens*

Laura F. Sandoval, Karen E. Huang, and Steven R. Feldman
Center for Dermatology Research, Wake Forest University School of Medicine; Winston-Salem, NC, USA

> **BASIC CONCEPTS**
> - Psoriasis is a common condition that can be treated with a variety of over-the-counter skincare products.
> - Over-the-counter skincare products helpful for the treatment of psoriasis include moisturizers, keratolytics, tar, hydrocortisone, salicylic acid, and tanning booth radiation exposure.
> - Compliance is key in psoriasis therapy, which may be encouraged by over-the-counter skincare products.
> - Over-the-counter skincare products can be combined with prescription medications for optimal treatment.

Introduction

Psoriasis is a chronic inflammatory skin disease that affects an estimated 7.5 million people in the United States and 125 million worldwide, with about 30% of these patients also suffering from psoriatic arthritis. Men and women are affected equally. The disease may occur at any age, most frequently starts in the late teens and early 20s, and is most prevalent in the third through fifth decades of life. Caucasians are twice as likely as African-Americans to have been *diagnosed* with psoriasis, though this may not translate directly to prevalence in these populations [1]. The etiology of psoriasis is not yet fully characterized. There is tremendous variation in individuals' disease presentation and response to treatment, adding to the complexity of psoriasis treatment.

The majority of patients with psoriasis have limited, or so called "mild", disease, covering less than 3% of total body surface area [2]. However, the disease burden does not correlate closely with the extent of disease, and even patients with limited areas of psoriasis can suffer from significant psychosocial stress and depression [3,4]. Only about one in six people with psoriasis sees a doctor for their disease in any given year. The remaining psoriasis patients do not seek treatment by a dermatologist. They may be untreated, or they may self-treat with a variety of over-the-counter (OTC) medications.

Psoriasis has a significant impact on quality of life. A recent survey by the National Psoriasis Foundation found psoriasis has both an emotional impact and physical impact [5]. The poor quality of life seen in psoriasis patients is due in part to the cutaneous manifestations of the disease and the treatment regimens. Patients claim physical appearance to be a large negative factor in quality of life, and in addition to feeling embarrassed and self-conscious, the majority of patients experience anger, frustration, and helplessness [5]. The concern over physical appearance increases as the extent of disease spreads. The treatment regimens can also negatively impact quality of life, as they often require multiple daily applications, come in messy greasy vehicles, and can be very expensive.

This chapter focuses on the role of OTC medications in psoriasis and describes strengths and weaknesses of different OTC products. We will briefly discuss the role of OTC medications as part of a combination treatment regimen. Patient compliance is a major factor affecting the effectiveness of psoriasis treatments, and we discuss the future development of OTC medications.

Physiology

Psoriasis is a multifactorial, T-cell mediated autoimmune disease, involving genetics, immune system alterations, and environmental

---

* **Funding/Conflicts of interest:** The Center for Dermatology Research is supported by an unrestricted educational grant from Galderma Laboratories, L.P. Dr. Feldman is a consultant and speaker for Galderma, Stiefel/GlaxoSmithKline, Abbott Labs, Warner Chilcott, Janssen, Amgen, Photomedex, Genentech, BiogenIdec, and Bristol Myers Squibb. Dr. Feldman has received grants from Galderma, Astellas, Abbott Labs, Warner Chilcott, Janssen, Amgen, Photomedex, Genentech, BiogenIdec, Coria/Valeant, Pharmaderm, Ortho Pharmaceuticals, Aventis Pharmaceuticals, Roche Dermatology, 3M, Bristol Myers Squibb, Stiefel/GlaxoSmithKline, Novartis, Medicis, Leo, HanAll Pharmaceuticals, Celgene, Basilea, and Anacor and has received stock options from Photomedex. Dr. Feldman is the founder and holds stock in Causa Research.

Cosmetic Dermatology: Products and Procedures, Second Edition. Edited by Zoe Diana Draelos.
© 2016 John Wiley & Sons, Ltd. Published 2016 by John Wiley & Sons, Ltd.

factors. Normal keratinocytes remain in the epidermis for 300 hours, but psoriasis keratinocytes only remain in the epidermis for 36 hours. This shortening of the keratinocyte life cycle is associated with an increased proliferation of keratinocytes and subsequent plaque formation [6]. The pathophysiology behind the shortened keratinocyte life cycle is at least in part due to a complex immune reaction. Both the innate and adaptive immune systems play a role. This cascade is largely driven by dysregulation of helper T cells and their release of cytokines and TNF-α into the dermis. The presence of cytokines in the dermis triggers infiltration and activation of both polymorphonuclear and mononuclear leukocytes [7]. Many different proinflammatory cytokines, chemokines, and chemical mediators are present in the dermis and epidermis of psoriatic skin, including IL-4, IL-6, IL-12, IL-22, IL-23, IL-17, IFN-γ and TGF-β to name a few [6,8]. The roles of each of these cytokines have yet to be fully understood, however as their roles become better identified, they are increasingly being targeted in potential therapies.

Genetics impacts psoriasis, as up to 70% of identical twins both develop this disease [9]. Psoriasis has been associated with certain HLA genotypes, and psoriasis risk allele PSORS1 that codes for HLA-Cw6 genotype has been identified as a major risk allele [10]. However, no single allele can be called the "psoriasis gene" because there are multiple alleles that contribute to the inheritance and risk of developing psoriasis. There are at least nineteen other genetic loci that have also been identified as psoriasis risk alleles [11]. Complex inherited diseases such as psoriasis require large studies of many affected families in order to begin to identify all the possible genetic loci, a task that has been difficult to achieve, but considerable progress has been made in the last few years resulting in a significant increase in candidate genes.

A temporal relationship has been established between psychosocial stress and psoriasis flares [12]. At baseline, psoriasis patients have high stress levels and poor quality of life [13]. Up to 80% of psoriasis patients report that a stressful event triggered a psoriasis flare during the course of their disease. Most of these stress-related flares occur within two weeks of the stressful event [14]. Obesity is a risk factor both for developing psoriasis and for increased severity of psoriasis [15]. Streptococcal type A infections have also been reported to cause psoriasis outbreaks. The link between streptococcal infections and psoriasis has been extensively researched, but no single hypothesis has emerged. Some theories posit there exists molecular mimicry between streptococcal antigens and keratinocytes, while other theories blame bacterial superantigens [6].

These genetic, biologic, and environmental factors combine to create the "perfect storm" of psoriasis. The shortened keratinocyte life cycle results in thick scales that accumulate on the surface of the skin. The inflammatory infiltrates cause dysfunction of skin's natural barrier. Inflammatory cytokines cause vascular capillary dilatation which results in skin erythema and helps perpetuate the inflammatory process [16]. The end result is dry, cracked, inflamed plaques that can be both painful and pruritic.

Role of OTC medications

Psoriasis education

The first step in any psoriasis treatment regimen is education. Empowering patients with knowledge about their disease allows them to make informed decisions about their care and creates realistic expectations for treatment outcomes. The National Psoriasis Foundation is a great resource for patients, providing educational resources, as well as resources to help patients feel less isolated. Foundation members feel more satisfied with their treatment and have less disease burden. The Foundation's website has an OTC treatment guide that provides information on many OTC products commonly used for psoriasis (www.psoriasis.org/about-psoriasis/treatments/topicals/over-the-counter). The site also provides information to help patients screen out non-prescription remedies that are touted for their efficacy but which are at best unproven.

Role of self-treating

Patients who self-treat their psoriasis tend to have mild disease and can achieve a measure of control with over-the-counter medications alone. For these patients OTC medications provide symptom relief (reduced pruritus) or improve the skin's cosmetic appearance [17]. Based on their experiences, some dermatologists may feel OTC medications have little efficacy; such an impression may be based on seeing only the patients who have failed to adequately control their disease with OTC medications. People who do achieve adequate control with OTCs alone would be less likely to feel the need to visit a dermatologist. For those patients who do visit a dermatologist for prescription treatment, OTC medications may still play an important role in reducing symptoms and improving appearance. Additionally, OTC medications like moisturizers and keratolytics can serve to increase the efficacy of prescription topical corticosteroids and phototherapy.

OTC products recommended by physicians

The National Ambulatory Care Survey (NAMCS) provides a representative snapshot of psoriasis treatment in the United States [18]. Through this survey, the estimated frequency of prescription and OTC medications prescribed by dermatologists and non-dermatologists are tabulated each year. OTC treatment options for psoriasis are estimated to cost $500 million and to account for 40% of all psoriasis-related expenditures [19]. The NAMCS provides data on the OTC psoriasis treatments most commonly recommended by physicians. We looked at NAMCS data from 1996–2010 and identified the most common OTC prescriptions for psoriasis in each of three five-year periods.

Since 1996, keratolytics have been the leading OTC medication for psoriasis, while hydrocortisone, moisturizers, and tar are comparable in their prescribing patterns. (Figure 60.1). When the keratolytics were broken down into individual types, salicylic acid, lactic acid, and urea were the three most commonly prescribed keratolytics, with salicylic acid most frequently prescribed (Figure 60.2). The prescribing of salicylic

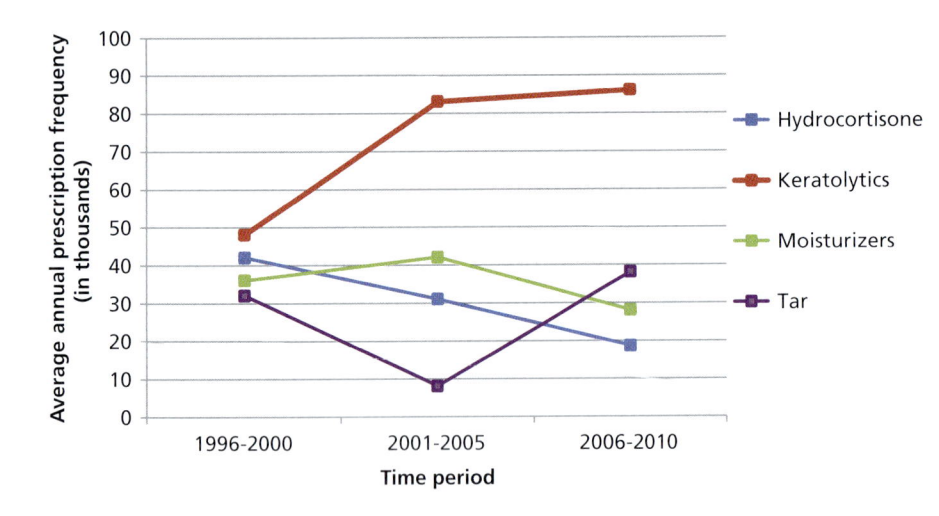

Figure 60.1 OTC psoriasis medications prescribed by physicians from 1996–2010. NAMCS data was used to find the prescription frequency of OTC medications prescribed by both dermatologists and non-dermatologists. Yearly data was then grouped in three five-year time periods. OTC medications were grouped in hydrocortisone, keratolytics, moisturizers, and tar preparations.

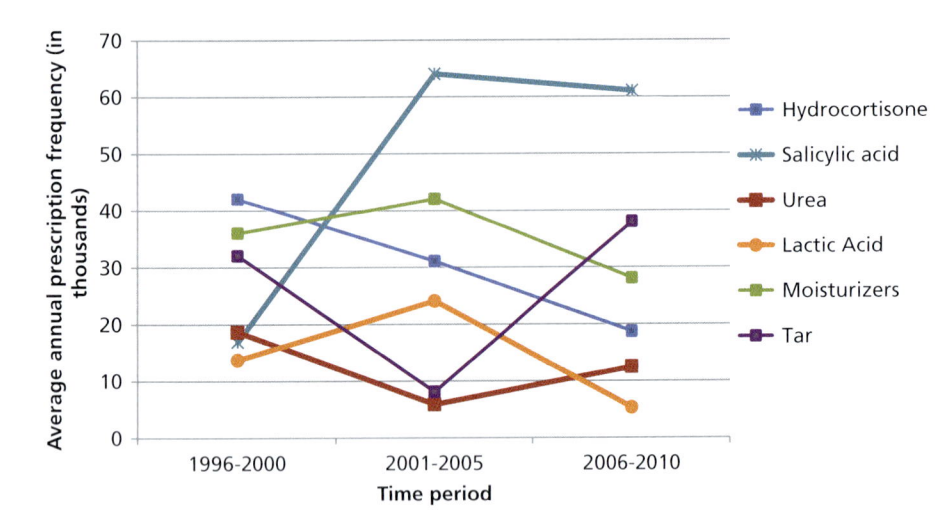

Figure 60.2 OTC psoriasis medications prescribed by physicians from 1996–2010. NAMCS data was used to find the prescription frequency of OTC medications prescribed by both dermatologists and non-dermatologists. Yearly data was then grouped in three five-year time periods. OTC medications analyzed included hydrocortisone, salicylic acid, lactic acid, urea, moisturizers, and tar preparations.

acid has increased over time, while the prescribing of hydrocortisone has steadily declined.

Compliance in psoriasis treatment

Psoriasis patients are among the worst in terms of compliance with treatment regimens [20]. Psoriasis patients have levels of depression and anxiety that are higher than other dermatologic disease patients [3]. Depression and disease burden can negatively affect the patients' ability to adhere to treatment [21]. Adherence to topical medications is worse than adherence to oral medications, with the number of daily applications, the chronicity of treatment and the complexity of the treatment regimen affecting overall compliance [22].

Topicals have traditionally been messy, greasy, and generally unappealing from a cosmetic perspective. When choosing a topical preparation for a patient, that particular patient's preferences are critical to consider. While ointments may be said to be more efficacious for psoriasis, they will not be efficacious for patients who find them too messy to use.

OTC medications allow patients access to a wide variety of treatment options at relatively low cost. Patients can try out different vehicles and different combinations of products to achieve the best improvement. OTC products give patients the independence to experiment with products until they find one they prefer, rather than having to go through a dermatologist every time they want to switch products or try something new.

Moisturizers and keratolytics

Dry skin is often a sign of poor barrier function, as is the case in psoriasis. Symptoms of psoriasis include scaling, itching, and increased sensitivity. Moisturizers can improve the skin's hydration in two ways. First, the hydrophobic emollients like petrolatum provide occlusive benefits, meaning they create a physical layer of protection on the surface of the skin that acts to slow epidermal water loss. Second, hydrophilic emollients like glycerine provide humectant benefits, meaning they attract moisture from the air and help skin preserve its water content. Some moisturizers only contain either hydrophobic or hydrophilic elements, but most contain both compounds. The net effect of this increase in moisture on psoriatic skin is a decrease in appearance of scale. Factors such as number of applications and thickness of the applied layer impact success. Moisturizers can often make scale completely invisible by changing the refractive index of scale so less light is reflected. Several skin care lines such as Cetaphil® and Accent® have moisturizers and cleansers that they recommend for psoriasis. While these may be popular choices amongst dermatologist in general for sensitive skin and skin diseases, these moisturizers are not specifically formulated for psoriasis treatment and we are unaware of evidence showing that they are any better or worse than other moisturizers. Interesting, the National Psoriasis foundation suggests that even cooking oils and shortening can be as effective and an economic alternative to often pricey commercial moisturizers [1].

Keratolytics differ from moisturizers in that they actually dissolve the scales on the skin's surface. Keratolytics help decrease the thickness of the hyperkeratotic plaque from the top surface inward by softening the scaly layers allowing for easy removal [23]. Salicylic acid comes in a wide variety of vehicles from shampoo to gels to creams. OTC concentrations approved for psoriasis use range from 1–3%. OTC concentrations exist up to 6%, but concentrations above 3% have not been FDA approved for psoriasis [24]. OTC lactic acid products come in 5–12% concentrations. Other OTC keratolytics include phenol (which is often used in scalp preparations) and urea products. OTC urea preparations range from 10–25% concentrations and typically are sold as lotions or creams [24]. Keratolytics such as these can be found OTC in single preparations or in OTC combinations with a moisturizer. Combination products allow the scale to be camouflaged by moisturizer as the keratolytics gradually thin the psoriatic plaques. Keratolytics can cause irritant contact dermatitis secondary to their acidic nature. Therefore it is important for patients to find a keratolytic product with a potency that is effective but minimizes irritation.

Tar

Tar is one of the oldest treatments for psoriasis, but its exact mechanism of action remains unknown. Tar is believed to reduce epidermal hyperproliferation and exert anti-inflammatory effects on psoriasis skin. It also has anti-pruritic effects that can provide a great deal of symptom relief [25]. Tar is developed from coal or wood and can be sold as crude or refined tar products. Most tar products for psoriasis treatment are coal tar products, and are available OTC in concentrations of 0.5–5%. OTC formulations are varied and include shampoos, soaps, lotions, creams, and ointments [24]. Tar shampoos and ointments can be very helpful in the treatment of scalp psoriasis [26].

There are several downsides to tar products that prevent them from being used more commonly to treat psoriasis. Traditional tar preparations have been messy, malodorous and stain skin and clothing. This is especially true of crude tar products. Newer products that use refined tar have tried to minimize these unwanted side effects, increasing the aesthetic appeal of tar topicals while maintaining the desired efficacy [26,27]. Despite improvements in the vehicle and odor, patient compliance with tar products may be poor. Tar can also cause unwanted skin reactions like contact irritation and folliculitis, further decreasing patient compliance. Another component of tar therapy that affects both patient use and physician prescribing is the fear of its carcinogenic properties. While there is no clear evidence showing an increased risk of cancer in humans, and while a large cohort study found that coal tar did not increase risk for non-skin malignancies or skin cancers, several animal studies have demonstrated an increased risk of cancer with topical tar application [28,29].

All OTC tar products are covered by an FDA monograph that permits marketing and sales of tar products of certain concentrations for an indication of psoriasis [30]. Other ingredients that are generally regarded as safe may also be in the product. Thus, companies can create and market many different products and claim they are effective for psoriasis as long as the product contains the appropriate concentration of tar. Companies can create all manners of fruit and vegetable extracts and claim their product is FDA approved for the treatment of psoriasis by incorporating tar into the product.

Hydrocortisone

Topical hydrocortisone cream is available OTC in 0.5% and 1% concentrations and is a low-potency corticosteroid with anti-inflammatory and anti-itch properties. In a survey conducted by the National Psoriasis Foundation, psoriasis patients named "scaling", "itching", and "skin redness" as their most common symptoms [31]. Topical corticosteroids help relieve these symptoms. Despite their low potency, OTC hydrocortisone treatments can play an important role in psoriasis management. A benefit of low-potency OTC hydrocortisone is that psoriasis patients can use this corticosteroid to self-treat more sensitive areas of their skin, such as the face, axilla, and genital area.

Other OTC products

While many of the OTC psoriasis products are likely to contain one of the above commonly used drugs as the active ingredient, there are many other agents that are used in psoriasis treatment. The National Psoriasis Foundation is a great resource for recommendations, and list agents such as aloe vera, jojoba, zinc pyrithione, and capsaicin, however, adding that the effectiveness of these may not be known and warning of potential adverse effects such as irritation [1]. Zinc pyrithione, specifically, has conflicting data on its effectiveness for psoriasis [32,33].

Castederm, a product containing phenol, is recommended for inverse psoriasis. To help remove scale, the Foundation suggests adding oil, oatmeal, Epson salts, or Dead Sea salts to the bath. In addition, products containing camphor, diphenhydramine hydrochloride (HCl), benzocaine and menthol are recommended for itch.

Ultraviolet light (UV) therapy

Phototherapy has been a mainstay treatment for psoriasis for millennia. Up until the 1990s, broad spectrum UVB was the treatment of choice. More recently, narrowband (300–313 nm) UVB boxes were introduced, as well as devices designed to provide localized therapy to individual lesions [34]. The addition of PUVA therapy for severe psoriasis in the 1990's further expanded the use of phototherapy for psoriasis [35]. Many psoriasis patients realize the benefit of UV exposure before any prescription phototherapy is used through the seasonal variation in their psoriasis and the beneficial effect of outdoor (and sometimes indoor) tanning on their disease. Benefits of non-prescription phototherapy over prescription phototherapy include greater convenience and lower cost, albeit at the expense of less control over dosimetry. Prescription phototherapy requires patients to travel to the dermatologist's office anywhere from three to five times a week to receive UV treatments. This can be costly and inconvenient to patients, which compromises the overall benefit and accessibility of the treatment. Home light units are also an option that can be cost-effective, convenient, and result in good patient adherence.

Sun exposure is the least costly way to obtain phototherapy for psoriasis, though it may be inconvenient or inaccessible (depending on geography). Dosimetry is difficult to control. Commercial tanning beds provide another phototherapy option. Although these devices radiate mostly UVA light, the most widely used commercial tanning bulbs have about 5% of the output that is in the UVB range and this may contribute to tanning bed efficacy. Some dermatologists discourage use of tanning beds for treating psoriasis because of the potential and poorly defined risk of skin cancer and premature aging. However, tanning beds can be an option for psoriasis patients who cannot afford or who do not have access to home or dermatologist-administered UVB therapies. Some dermatologists may not think tanning beds are effective based on their experiences seeing patients who have tried tanning and saw no benefit. Dermatologists should keep in mind that the people who tried tanning and did find it to be effective for clearing their psoriasis may not come to the dermatologist.

If tanning bed use is recommended by a dermatologist for a particular patient, patient education and guidance for use should be provided and realistic expectations about length of time until improvement should be set. Most patients will require multiple tanning sessions over several weeks before seeing improvement in their skin. To help control the dosimetry, patients should use the same tanning bed for each exposure (not switching between tanning establishments or between beds within a single establishment). Tanning bed operators are familiar with their equipment and will likely recommend a safe starting dose, but starting with half that dose may provide a greater degree of safety, particularly if the tanning bed is used in conjunction with oral retinoid treatment (tanning beds should not be used in conjunction with psoralen as life-threatening burns may result). Sunscreen or protective clothing can be recommended to protect unaffected skin, and eye protection should be worn. These measures help patients avoid burning their skin and minimize the risk of developing skin cancer or cataracts [1].

Psoriasis patients may inquire if OTC tanning is safe to use with other psoriasis medications. Topical corticosteroids are safe to use with phototherapy and may even enhance the UV light's effect by thinning the psoriatic plaques, though there is concern that corticosteroids reduce the remission periods associated with phototherapy. Topical vitamin D analogues are effective in combination with UV therapy, however the light may inactivate vitamin D analogues, so it is recommended for patients to apply the topical after or a minimum of 2 hours prior to phototherapy sessions [36]. Coal tar can also be used in combination with phototherapy, but should be removed from the body prior to treatment since it can act as a physical blocker reducing the light exposure [37]. The Goeckerman treatment, which combines topical crude coal tar and UVB phototherapy, is a classic, yet often forgotten, psoriasis therapy. This combination's success was first described by Dr. Goeckerman in 1925, and continues to be one of the most effective psoriasis treatments in use today. The Goeckerman treatment can induce remission even when the most technologically advanced regimens like biologics fail [38,39]. Goeckerman treatment is typically administered by a dermatologist in the inpatient or specialized outpatient psoriasis treatment center. Patients can attempt to mimic the effects of Goeckerman by using outdoor or indoor UV therapy followed by prolonged OTC tar ointment used under plastic wrap or sauna suit occlusion.

In terms of systemic therapies, oral retinoids are not only safe to use with phototherapy, they are frequently prescribed in combination with phototherapy because they can improve the phototherapy's efficacy [40]. While methotrexate is safe to use with phototherapy, cyclosporine should not be used with UVB therapy because of concerns for increased risk of skin cancer [41].

Combination regimens

Most psoriasis treatment regimens do not rely on only one drug to effectively treat psoriasis. Specific combinations of therapies often produce the best results with the least amount of side effects. The caution with combination treatment regimens is that overly complex regimens can confuse and discourage patients and negatively affect treatment adherence. The goal of a dermatologist should be to develop a streamlined regimen that focuses on the individual patient's treatment goals and lifestyle.

OTC medications play a large role in combination psoriasis therapies. Keratolytics are used to enhance the ability of topical corticosteroids to penetrate the epidermis and target dermal inflammation. Topical corticosteroids can penetrate skin two to three times better with keratolytics than without. This results in better relief of symptoms like scaling and pruritus [23]. Keratolytics have similar effects with tar products and UV phototherapy. Moisturizers can also enhance the efficacy of topical corticosteroids [42]. When prescribing such combination regimens, however, it is essential to consider that complicating the regimen may reduce treatment adherence, resulting in the loss of any potential gains expected from increased penetration.

Summary

OTC medications play a large role in the treatment regimen of self-treating patients and those managed by a dermatologist. For the vast majority of people with psoriasis who choose to self-treat their disease, OTC medications provide relief of symptoms like pruritus, erythema, and dry skin as well as effectively controlling plaque formation. For the minority of patients who require a dermatologist, OTC medications still provide a degree of symptom relief, and are commonly used in combination with prescription medications. The NAMCS data show that dermatologists prescribe OTC hydrocortisone, keratolytics, tar, and moisturizers to supplement prescription psoriasis therapies. The large percentage of psoriasis patients who rely on OTC medications continues to drive the production of new and improved OTC products. New moisturizers are constantly being developed to increase skin's hydration, and new keratolytics seek to improve the appearance of hyperkeratotic plaques while minimizing skin irritation. Improved vehicles like foams and sprays for OTC corticosteroids are being developed to increase efficacy and make them more attractive to patients. New tar extracts and derivatives are designed to be less messy and smelly than their older counterparts; by increasing patient adherence, such treatments may offer improved efficacy outcomes.

Future trends in OTC psoriasis medications can be considered in two different populations. In those people who entirely self-treat and do not see a dermatologist, there will probably be a continued increase in the use of products like moisturizers, keratolytics, and tar as the products continue to improve. In patients who see a dermatologist, there may be a decrease in some OTC use of medications like keratolytics as more and more topical prescriptions are switching to combination topical products that contain a prescription drug along with an OTC drug. An example of this would be a high-potency topical corticosteroid ointment that also contains salicylic acid. Prescription topicals are now available in new vehicles like foams and sprays that reduce the messy application process. This movement towards multiple therapies in one product and improved prescription vehicles may result in a decrease in the prescription of OTC topical medications. Biologic agents have revolutionized treatment in a small population of psoriasis patients, inducing rapid and complete remission and thereby reducing their need for complicated combination regimens.

References

1. National Psoriasis Foundation. www.psoriasis.org. Accessed 29 June 2015.
2. Stern RS, Nijsten T, Feldman SR, et al. (2004) Psoriasis is common, carries a substantial burden even when not extensive, and is associated with widespread treatment dissatisfaction. *J Investig Dermatol Symp Proc* **9**, 136–9.
3. Evers AWM, Lu Y, Duller P, et al. (2005) Common burden of chronic skin diseases? Contributors to psychological distress in adults with psoriasis and atopic dermatitis. *Br J Dermatol* **152**, 1275–81.
4. Gupta MA, Gupta AK. (1998) Depression and suicidal ideation in dermatology patients with acne, alopecia areata, atopic dermatitis and psoriasis. *Br J Dermatol* **139**, 846–50.
5. Armstrong AW, Schupp C, Wu J, et al. (2012) Quality of life and work productivity impairment among psoriasis patients: findings from the National Psoriasis Foundation survey data 2003–2011. *PLoS One* **7**, e52935.
6. Nickoloff BJ, Qin JZ, Nestle FO. (2007) Immunopathogenesis of psoriasis. *Clin Rev Allergy Immunol* **33**, 45–56.
7. Linden KG, Weinstein GD. (1999) Psoriasis: current perspectives with an emphasis on treatment. *Am J Med* **107**, 595–605.
8. Mudigonda P, Mudigonda T, Feneran AN, et al. (2012) Interleukin-23 and interleukin-17: importance in pathogenesis and therapy of psoriasis. *Dermatol Online J* **18**, 1.
9. Valdimarsson H. (2007) The genetic basis of psoriasis. *Clin Dermatol* **25**, 563–7.
10. Nair RP, Stuart PE, Nister I, et al. (2006) Sequence and haplotype analysis supports HLA-C as the psoriasis susceptibility 1 gene. *Am J Hum Genet* **78**, 827–51.
11. Rahman M, Alam K, Ahmad MZ, et al. (2012) Classical to current approach for treatment of psoriasis: a review. *Endocr Metab Immune Disord Drug Targets* **12**, 287–302.
12. Hunter HJ, Griffiths CE, Kleyn CE. (2013) Does psychosocial stress play a role in the exacerbation of psoriasis? *Br J Dermatol* **169**, 965–74.
13. Misery L, Thomas L, Jullien D, et al. (2008) Comparative study of stress and quality of life in outpatients consulting for different dermatoses in 5 academic departments of dermatology. *Eur J Dermatol* **18**, 412–5.
14. Kimyai-Asadi A, Usman A. (2001) The role of psychological stress in skin disease. *J Cutan Med Surg* **5**, 140–45.
15. Azfar RS, Gelfand JM. (2008) Psoriasis and metabolic disease: epidemiology and pathophysiology. *Curr Opin Rheumatol* **20**, 416–22.
16. Joshi R. (2004) Immunopathogenesis of psoriasis. *Indian J Dermatol Venereol Leprol* **70**, 10–12.
17. Proksch E. (2008) The role of emollients in the management of diseases with chronic dry skin. *Skin Pharmacol Physiol* **21**, 75–80.
18. National Center for Health Statistics (2010) National Ambulatory Medical Care Survey (NAMCS) and National Hospital Ambulatory Medical Care Survey (NHAMCS). www.cdc.gov/nchs/about/major/ahcd/ahcd1.htm. Assessed 29 June 2015.

19. Bickers DR, Lim HW, Margolis D, et al. (2004) *Burden of Skin Diseases*. Located online at www.sidnet.org/pdfs/Burden%20of%20Skin%20Diseases%202004.pdf.
20. Storm A, Andersen SE, Benfeldt E, et al. (2008) One in 3 prescriptions are never redeemed: primary nonadherence in an outpatient clinic. *J Am Acad Dermatol* **59**, 27–33.
21. Sundbom LT, Bingefors K. (2013) The influence of symptoms of anxiety and depression on medication nonadherence and its causes: a population based survey of prescription drug users in Sweden. *Patient Prefer Adherence* **7**, 805–11.
22. Carroll CL, Feldman SR, Camacho FT, et al. (2004) Adherence to topical therapy decreases during the course of an 8-week psoriasis clinical trial: Commonly used methods of measuring adherence to topical therapy overestimate actual use. *J Am Acad Dermatol* **51**, 212–6.
23. Koo J, Cuffie CA, Tanner DJ, et al. (1998) Mometasone furoate 0.1%-salicylic acid 5% ointment versus mometasone furoate 0.1% ointment in the treatment of moderate-to-severe psoriasis: a multicenter study. *Clin Ther* **20**, 283–91.
24. National Psoriasis Foundation Treatment Guide. http://psoriasis.org/treatment/guide/otc/. Accessed 29 June 2015.
25. Roelofzen JH, Aben KK, van der Valk PG, et al. (2007) Coal tar in dermatology. *J Dermatolog Treat* **18**, 329–34.
26. Dodd WA. (1993) TARS. Their role in the treatment of psoriasis. *Dermatol Clin* **11**, 131–5.
27. Mefford L. (2008) NeoStrata(R) Announces the Launch of PSORENT(TM) Psoriasis Topical Treatment. www.reuters.com/article/pressRelease/idUS169492+04-Feb-2008+PRN20080204. Accessed 29 June 2015.
28. van Schooten FJ, Godschalk R. (1996) Coal tar therapy. Is it carcinogenic? *Drug Saf* **15**, 374–7.
29. Roelofzen JH, Aben KK, Oldenhof UT, et al. (2010) No increased risk of cancer after coal tar treatment in patients with psoriasis or eczema. *J Invest Dermatol* **130**, 953–61.
30. Kessler DA. (1991) Food and Drug Administration: Dandruff, seborrheic dermatitis, and psoriasis drug products for over-the-counter human use; Final Monograph. *Federal Register* **56**, 63554–69. Found online at www.fda.gov/cder/otcmonographs/Dandruff&Seborrheic_Dermatitis&Psoriasis/dandruff_seborrheic_dermatitis_psoriasis_FR_19911204.pdf.
31. Krueger G, Koo J, Lebwohl M, et al. (2001) The impact of psoriasis on quality of life: results of a 1998 National Psoriasis Foundation patient-membership survey. *Arch Dermatol* **137**, 280–84.
32. Housman TS, Keil KA, Mellen BG, et al. (2003) The use of 0.25% zinc pyrithione spray does not enhance the efficacy of clobetasol propionate 0.05% foam in the treatment of psoriasis. *J Am Acad Dermatol* **49**, 79–82.
33. Sadeghian G, Ziaei H, Nilforoushzadeh MA. (2011) Treatment of localized psoriasis with a topical formulation of zinc pyrithione. *Acta Dermatovenerol Alp Panonica Adriat* **20**, 187–90.
34. Stein KR, Pearce DJ, Feldman SR. (2008) Targeted UV therapy in the treatment of psoriasis. *J Dermatolog Treat* **19**, 141–5.
35. Kostović K, Pasić A. (2004) Phototherapy of psoriasis: review and update. *Acta Dermatovenerol Croat* **12**, 42–50.
36. Lapolla W, Yentzer BA, Bagel J, et al. (2011) A review of phototherapy protocols for psoriasis treatment. *J Am Acad Dermatol* **64**, 936–49.
37. Paghdal KV, Schwartz RA. (2009) Topical tar: back to the future. *J Am Acad Dermatol* **61**, 294–302.
38. Fitzmaurice S, Bhutani T, Koo J. (2013) Goeckerman regimen for management of psoriasis refractory to biologic therapy: the University of California San Francisco experience. *J Am Acad Dermatol* **69**, 648–49.
39. Serrao R, Davis MD. (2009) Goeckerman treatment for remission of psoriasis refractory to biologic therapy. *J Am Acad Dermatol* **60**, 348–9.
40. Carlin CS, Callis KP, Krueger GG. (2003) Efficacy of acitretin and commercial tanning bed therapy for psoriasis. *Arch Dermatol* **139**, 436–42.
41. Zanolli, MM (2004) Phototherapy arsenal in the treatment of psoriasis. *Dermatol Clin* **22**, 397–406.
42. Ghali FE. (2005) Improved clinical outcomes with moisturization in dermatologic disease. *Cutis* **76**(6 Suppl), 13–8.

Index

Page numbers in *italic* refer to figures.
Page numbers in **bold** refer to tables.

A

abdomen, liposuction, 465–467
abscesses, from filler injection, 377
absorption promoters, 68
accelerants, 68
Accent Device (radiofrequency device), 434
acetic acid, after peels, 407
acetone, 223, 405
N-acetyl-Glu-Glu-Met-Gln-Arg-Arg-NH2 (hexapeptide), 313
acetyl-Ser-Asp-Lys-Pro (tetrapeptide), 311
acetyl-tetrapeptide 2, 314
N-acetyl-Tyr-Arg-hexadecylester, 313
acidic permanent waves, 258
acidity, stratum corneum, 9
acne
 autologous fibroblast cell therapy, 387
 camouflage, *191*
 cross-polarized light photography, 45
 dermabrasion, 438, 440, 442
 diode laser, 433
 dry ice, 398
 glycolic acid peels, *354*
 hydroxyacids, 354, 503
 isotretinoin, 328
 mildness of cleansing, 93, *94*
 Nd:YAG lasers, 432
  Q-switched, 432
 oats for, 290
 over-the-counter treatments, 501–508
 peels, 400–401
 postinflammatory hyperpigmentation, 25
 sunscreens, 494
 UV fluorescence photography, 46
acrylates
 contact dermatitis, 214
 nail lacquers, 219
acrylics, 77
 allergy, 58
 artificial nail enhancements, 226–228
actinic keratosis, medium depth peels, 404, *410*
activator protein-1 (AP-1), 15, 318–319
 corticosteroids on, 301–302
 retinoic acid on, 18
 UV radiation on, 16

Active FX-Lumenis laser, 415–419, *420*, 427
Active photo barrier complex™, **514**
acyclovir, 405
acyl isethionate bars, 85, 86, 87, *89*, 90–92
adapalene, 496
Aδ nociceptors, 37
adhesion molecules, 298–299, 305
adhesion promoters, artificial nail enhancements, 228
adhesive pads, acne, 505
adipose-derived stem cells, 323, 388
advanced glycation end products, 296–297, 349, 361
adverse effects, 52–64, *see also* contact dermatitis
 adipose-derived stem cells, 388
 antiperspirants, 164
 artificial nail enhancements, 231–232
 autologous fibroblast cell therapy, 388
 botulinum toxins, 372
 collagen, 387
 cosmeceuticals, 284–285
 laser therapy, 412
 panthenol relieving, 342
 permanent waves, 259–260
 platelet-rich plasma, 386–387
aerosol hairsprays, 273–274, 276
African-American skin, *see also* ashy skin; ethnic skin
 photoaging, 17, 29
African hair, 29–31
 styling aids, 276–278
age-spots, 314
 vitamin C on, 497
aging, *see also* photoaging
 ethnic skin, 27–28
 face, 27–28, 375, 380
 hair, 253
 hands, 485, **486**
 inflammation, 299
 lips, 194–195
 microvasculature, 15, 195
 neck, 28
  nonablative lasers on, 434–435
 nutrients for, 360
 vs photoaging, 13–14
 reactive oxygen species, 296–297

alcohol
 as penetration enhancer, **68**
 for percutaneous delivery, **67**
 as solvent, 105
 in sunless tanning agents, 151
 TFM rating, 114
 toners, 106
alcohol-based hand sanitizers, 113–114, 117–118
 guidelines, 112
 organisms not affected, 118
 safety, 119
 soaps *vs*, 119
aldobionic acids *see* bionic acids
alexandrite laser, 447–448
alkaline perms, 258
alkalizers
 hair dyes, 240
 perming lotions, 256
alkyl sulfates, 97
allergens
 balsam of Peru as, 55
 hair dyes, 246
allergic contact dermatitis, 53
 fragrances, 55
 preservatives, 55–56
 tattooing, 59
allergic reactions, 11, 57–60
 autologous fibroblast cell therapy, 388
 botanicals, 285
  papaya, 290
 formalin, 222
 hair dyes, 244, 245, 246–248
 hair styling aids, 278
 nail cosmetics, 213–214
 UV gel nail polish, 223
Allergy Alert Test, hair dyes, 245, 247, 248
all-*trans*-retinoic acid (tRA), 18
aloe, 287–288
alpha bisobolol, 506
α-hydroxyacids, 346–347, 351, 495–496, **499**
 acne, 503
 as peeling agents, 353, 395–396
 rosacea, 515
α-lipoic acid, **358**, 498, **499**
α-tocopherol acetate, 343, *see also* d-α-tocopherol
aluminum salts, 163, 164

Cosmetic Dermatology: Products and Procedures, Second Edition. Edited by Zoe Diana Draelos.
© 2016 John Wiley & Sons, Ltd. Published 2016 by John Wiley & Sons, Ltd.

Alzheimer disease, aluminum and, 164
Amedori products, 340
American Society of Testing and Materials, protocol E 1174, 115
amino acetates, **68**
amino acids, 308–309
    dihydroacetone on, 149
    glycation, 296
    hair, 253, 254
        ethnicity, 30
    in sunless tanning agents, 149
aminoglycosides, **366**
aminolevulinic acid
    hair removal, 449
    IPL with, 432
    PDL laser with, 431
ammonium persulfate, 58
ammonium thioglycolate, 58, 259–260, 264, *see also* thiol procedure
amphoteric surfactants, 104, 125, 237, 492
a-MSH (peptide), analogs, 314
anagen, hair growth, 167, 252, 446
    eyelashes, 200
anaphylaxis, herbs causing, 285
angiogenesis
    retinoids on, 18
    UV radiation causing, 15
anhydrous formulations
    antiperspirants, 163
    mascara, 201, 205
anionic surfactants, 104, 237, 492
anthralin, antioxidant testing, 348
antibacterials
    benzoyl peroxide as, 502
    in hand cleansers, 492–493, *see also* antimicrobial handwashes
    hydroxyacids with, 354
    for liposuction, 478
    odor neutralization, 163
    rosacea, 514
antibacterial soaps, 85
antibiotic-resistant infections, 110
anticholinergics, 165
anticoagulants
    botulinum toxin treatment and, 372
    liposuction and, 471
antifungals
    nail lacquers, 220
    shampoos, 127, 128
antigen-presenting cells, 53, 299
anti-inflammatories, 295, 301–305
    antioxidants as, 297–298, 299, 300
    benzoyl peroxide as, 502
    efficacy, 303–304
    herbs, 287, 299–300, 303–304
    topical formulations, 304–305
anti-inflammatory effects, LED photomodulation, 458–460
antimicrobial barrier, 6
antimicrobial handwashes, 113–114
    efficacy, 114–118
antioxidants, 19, 295–301, **358**, 359, 496–499
    chemistry, 297

depletion, 8
freshness, 286
hydroxyacids as, 348–349
lipsticks, 197
natural ointments, 78
non-invasive assessment, 48
peptides, 310–312
Pinnell formulation, 48
protective factor, 48, **49**
retinoids as, 329, 330
topical formulations, 300–301, 303–305
vitamin E as, 297, **358**
antiperspirants, 160–165
antiplatelet drugs
    botulinum toxin treatment and, 372
    liposuction and, 471
apocrine glands, 160, *161*, 162
apples, 292
application devices, allergy, 58
aquaporins, 6–7, 135, 144–146, 518
aqueous roll-ons, antiperspirants, 163
Arg-Gly-Asp-Ser (tetrapeptide), 311
arginine, dihydroacetone on, 149
arm
    liposuction, 467
    nonablative rejuvenation systems, 435
aromatic hydroxyacids, 347–348
arrector pili, 167
artificial nail enhancements, 226–233
    removal, 230
ascorbates *see* vitamin C
ashy skin
    body washes on, 100–101
    mildness of cleansing, 91–92
Asia, hair straightening, 265
aspirin
    botulinum toxin treatment and, 372
    liposuction and, 471
astaxanthin, **358**, 360
ASTM protocol E 1174, 115
asymetic effects
    botulinum toxin treatment, 372–373
    filler injection, 377
atopic dermatitis, *see also* eczema
    body washes, 101
    facial moisturizers for, 136–137
    formaldehyde releasers, 56
    LED light with tacrolimus, 460
    LED photomodulation on, 458
    microbiota, 111–112
    mildness of cleansing, 92–93
    urea deficiency, 142
ATP, LED light on, 460
Australia, approved sunscreens, 154
autologous fat transplantation, 388, 483, **486**
autologous fillers, 385–389
automated applicators, mascara, 206
auto-oxidation, botanicals, 286
Aveeno moisturizer, **514**
Avene® Extremely Gentle, **512**
Avene® High Protection, **514**
avobenzone, 155, 493
axilla, liposuction and, 467

axons, somatosensory, 33, 34–36
azelaic acid
    gluconolactone with, 354
    rosacea, 515
azeloyl tetrapeptide 23, 311
Azfibrocel-T, 387
azone, **68**

B
bacteria, 6, *see also* microbiota
    biofilms, 377–378
    fillers made from, 375–376
    retinaldehyde on, 328–329, 330
baked eyeshadows, 204
balsam of Peru, as allergen, 55
banana peel, antioxidant testing, 348
bandages, after dermabrasion, 442
barbershops, 166
bar cleansers, 83–95
    effects on skin, 85–90
    manufacture, 84
barrier functions of epidermis, 5–8
    eczema, 517
    niacinamide on, 339–340
    panthenol on, 342
    rosacea, 511
    tests, 136
basal layer, UV filtration, 25
basecoats, nails, 217, **218**
basic soaps, 84
basophilic degeneration, 14
beads
    body washes, 97–98
    scrubs, 106
beard, 168
    pseudofolliculitis barbae, 172
    stubble recreation, 188
beeswax, **196**
Belotero (hyaluronic acid product), 376
Belotero Balance, 376, 377
benefit agents, body washes, 97–98
benzoic acid, 347–348
benzophenones, 155
benzoyl peroxide, 502–503
    salicylic acid *vs*, 503
    tea tree oil *vs*, 506
bergamot oil, 57
β-carotene, 18, **358**
β-hydroxyacids, 347, **499**, **503**
bicarbonate, tumescent local anesthesia, 470
Bimatoprost, 203
binders, compact powders, 180
bio-availability
    actives in shampoo, 127–128
    zinc pyrithione, 129
biofilms, filler injection, 377–378
bioinstrumentation, 42, 43
biologics, 303, 305, 527
bionic acids, 347, 348
    for dry skin, 352
    on glycation, 349–350
    on matrix metalloproteinases, 351

biopsy, for autologous fibroblast cell therapy, 387
Bio-Restorative Skin Cream, 321
biotin, 213
biotinyl-GHK, 312
bipolar radiofrequency devices, 451, 453–454
bite force, botulinum toxin on, 372
black henna tattoos, pPD in, 247
blade shaving, 166–173
bleaching agents
    allergy, 57
    for hair, 58, 240, 241, 242
    ultrasound with, 70
blepharopigmentation, 203
blinded trials, *see also* randomized trials
    botanicals, 285
blindness, from polylactic acid therapy, 393
blistering, after hair removal, *449*
blood, platelet-rich plasma preparation, 385–386
blood flow, nicotinic acid on, 340, 341
blood loss, liposuction, 464, 471
blood vessels, *see also* microvasculature
    filler injection, 377
blue light, acne, 505
Blue Peel, 400
BMDM (butyl methoxy dibenzoyl methane), 155, 493
body washes, 96–102
BoNTA, 364, 365, *see also* botulinum toxins
    with fillers, 372
    topical formulation, 373
botanicals, 283–294
    allergy, 57, 285
    anti-inflammatories, 299–300, 303–304
    clinical studies, 292–293
    efficacy, 285
    evaluation, 285–286
    factors on quality, 284
    rosacea, 515
Botox®, 364, 365, *see also* botulinum toxins
    low-protein formulation, 372
botulinum toxins, 364–374
    after laser treatment, 427
    allergy, 59
    complications, 372–373
    contraindications, **366**
    fillers with, 372
    hyperhidrosis, 165
    laser therapy with, 413
    before laser treatment, 426–427
    marginal mandibular branch of facial nerve, 482
    before medium depth peels, 405
    platysma bands, 483
bovine collagen, 60
    aging hand, **486**
    intradermal challenge, 60
brain, somatosensory system, 39–40
Brazil, hair straightening, 265
breast, liposuction, 468–469
breast cancer
    antiperspirants and, 164
    male, 469
    radiation dermatitis, LED photomodulation on, 459
brilliances, lips, 197
brimonidine tartrate, 514–515
bristles, mascara brushes, 202
brittle nails, 209, 210, *211*, 213, *222*
broadspectrum sunscreens, 18, 158, 494
bromates, perming lotions, 258
bromelain, 290–291
brow ptosis, 27
bruising
    filler injection, 377
    platelet-rich plasma, 387
    polylactic acid therapy, 391
brushes
    for cleansing, 505
    dermabrasion, 440, 441, 442
    mascara, 201–202, *203*
buffering, *see also* pH
    antiperspirants, 163
buffer salts, perming lotions, 257
bunny lines, botulinum toxin treatment, 370
burning sensation, trichloroacetic acid, 407
buttocks, liposuction, 467
butyl methoxy dibenzoyl methane, 155, 493

C

Cade test, 116
caffeine, 19, 288
calcineurin, 303
calcium
    on corneocytes, 8, 9
    nail plate, 209
calcium hydroxylapatite, 60, 380–384, 485–491
California, regulations on solvents, 223–224
camouflage, 186–192
    rosacea, 512–513
Camptotheca acuminata (happy tree), 286
Canada, antiperspirants, regulations, 162
cancer, *see also* breast cancer
    adipose-derived stem cells, 388
    benzoyl peroxide and, 503
    growth factors and, 322
    hair dyes, 248
    PGE-2, 305
    tar, 525
    trichloroacetic acid and, 409
    vitamin A deficiency, 326
candelilla wax, **196**
Canfield VISIA camera systems, 44
cannulas
    liposuction, 470–471, 480
    for polylactic acid, 391
capacitance, 9–10
capillaries *see* microvasculature
carbohydrates, excess, **358**
carbomers, 77
Carbon Black, 205
carbon dioxide, solid, **396**, 398, 402
carbon dioxide lasers, 412–428
    complications, 427
    dermabrasion *vs*, 439
    on PGE-2 levels, 305
    postoperative care, 427
        LED photomodulation, 459
    techniques, 426–427
carnosine, 310, 311, 361
carnuba wax, **196**
β-carotene, 18, **358**
carotenoids, 359
carriers, perming lotions, 257
Carruthers, A. and J., studies of BoNTA, 365
Castederm, 526
castor oil, 196
catagen, hair growth, 167, 252, 446
catalase, 315
cathelin-related antimicrobial peptide, 6
cathepsins, 17, 26
cationic emulsifiers, 76, 104, 492
cationic polymers, shampoos, 126
CCM Complex (Histogen), 321, 323
CD44, 330
CD44v3, 328
C E Ferulic (SkinCeuticals), 498
celecoxib, 303
cell conditioned media (CCM), 321, 323
cell cultures
    fibroblasts, 387
    growth factors from, 323
Cellex-C® Eye contour cream, **513**
cellular growth factors, 318–324
Centers for Disease Control, on hand hygiene, 112
central projections, sensory nervous system, 38–40
central venous catheters, colonizations, antimicrobial handwashes and, 117
centrifugation, platelet-rich plasma preparation, 386
ceramides, 5, 8, 26
CeraVe® Facial moisturizer, **512**
CeraVe® Hydrating cleanser, **512**
cerebral cortex, somatosensory system, 40
ceruse, 178
cervicomental angle, 476, 477, 478
Cetaphil® Gentle skin cleanser, **512**
Cetaphil® Moisturizing cream, **512**
chamomile, 289, 506
charentais cantaloupe, 288
charge (electrical), effect of pH, 87
cheek, liposuction, 480
cheilitis, 195
cheiloscopy, 194
chelating agents, *see also* neutralization
    hair dyes, 246
chemical bio-availability, zinc pyrithione, 129
chemical penetration enhancers, 68
chemical reconstruction of skin scars (CROSS), 400
chemical reduction
    hair straightening, 264–265
    permanent waves, 251, 254, 256

chemistry
	antioxidants, 297
	antiperspirants, 163
	hair, 253–254
	UV radiation, 155
chest (male), liposuction, 469
children
	hair dye allergy, 247
	MRSA, hand hygiene, 118
chin, dimpled, 371
Chinese herbals, toxicity, 285
chin rests, photography, 44
chlorides, aluminum, 163
cholesterol, 8
chroma (color coordinate), 188
Chromasphere™, *183*, 184
chromophores, 155
	laser hair removal, 446
Chrysanthellum indicum, 515
CIELAB, L*a*b* standard, 151
cineole, **68**
cinnamaldehyde, 55
CI numbers (Color Index numbers), 219–220
circadian rhythm, 8
citric acid, 347, 395–396
c-Jun protein, 18
classifications
	hair curliness, 262, *263*
	photoaging, **403**
	rosacea, 509–510
	sunscreens, 154
cleansing agents, 492–493, *see also* bar cleansers; hand sanitizers
	acne, 501–502
	adverse skin reactions, 55, 57
	body washes, 96–102
	eczema, 521
	face, 103–109
	rosacea, 511, **512**
cleansing brushes, 505
cleansing cloths, **105**, 106–107, 108
	acne, 504
cleansing devices, 107
climate, dry skin, 89, 90
climbazole, 127
clinical studies, *see also* blinded trials; randomized trials
	antioxidants, 304
	hand microbiota removal, 116–117
	herbs, 292–293
clinics, camouflage, 191
clockwise rotation, wire brushes, 441, 442
clogging, polylactic acid, 391
clostridial proteins, 365, *see also* botulinum toxins
clothing, UV protection factor ratings, 18, 495
C-mechano-heat nociceptors, 37
CO₂RE laser, 424
coacervates, 126–127, 129, 130
coal tar, 127, 525, 526
cobra neck, 483
coenzyme Q10, **358**, 361, 498, **499**
	nanoemulsions, 521

co-factors for enzymes
	vitamin B3 derivatives, 339–340
	vitamin C, 342
coffee, 288
coffeeberry extract, 288
cold air cooling, laser therapy, 427
cold sense, 36, *37*
cold therapy, forehead, 373
collagen, 15, 27
	aging hand, **486**
	fillers, 60, 376, 387
	glycation, 296
	hyaluronic acid fillers on, 378
	low energy light on synthesis, 457
	nonablative rejuvenation systems on, 429
	photoaging, 14, 15, 16
	radiofrequency devices on, 433, 434
	vitamin C for synthesis, 497
	wound healing, 437
collagen (bovine) *see* bovine collagen
color additives, sunless tanning agents as, 150
coloration of skin, sunless tanning agents, 150
ColoreScience®, **513**
Color Index numbers (CI numbers), 219–220
color measurement, 151, 187–188
color rinses, 240
colors (pigments)
	body washes, 98
	camouflage, 187, 513
	eyelashes, 203
	facial foundation, 181, 182
		testing, 183–184
	hair *see* hair dyes
	L*a*b* standard, CIE, 151
	lipsticks, 196–197
	nail cosmetics, 217, 219–220
		UV-curable, 222–223
color standard chips, digital photography, 43
combination regimens, psoriasis, 526–527
combs, hair straightening, 263, 266
comedolytics
	benzoyl peroxide as, 502
	salicylic acid as, 503
Commission Internationale d'Eclairage, L*a*b* standard, 151
community setting, hand hygiene, 118
compact foundations, 178, 179–182
compartment syndrome, 467
complexing agents, perming lotions, 257
complexion makeup *see* makeup
compliance
	handwashing guidelines, 113
	psoriasis treatment, 524
compression garments, liposuction, 472
conditioners
	after hair straightening, 268
	eyelashes, 206
	perming, **256**, 257, 258
	rinse-off, 130
	shampoos, 126, 237–238
		for colored hair, 246

conductance, 26, 136
confocal laser scanning microscope, 50
confocal Raman microspectrometry, 72
congenital anomalies, from botanicals, 285
consent
	botulinum toxin treatment, 366
	liposuction, 471
	medium depth peels, 405
consort dermatitis, 58
consultations
	dermabrasion, 439–440
	hair styling, 278
	laser hair removal, 446
	liposuction, 471, 478
	radiofrequency therapy, 452
consumer research
	body washes, 98–99
	facial moisturizers, 136
contact dermatitis, 26, 52–64
	diagnosis and treatment, 60
	nail cosmetics, 213–214
contact lens solutions, allergy, 56
contact urticaria, 53
continuous process manufacture, bar cleansers, 84
contouring, 186, 188
controlled application tests
	body washes, 99
	soaps *vs* syndets, 90, 91
Controlled Chaos Technology™, 422
cooling
	laser therapy, 427
	radiofrequency therapy, 452
Cool Scan setting, laser therapy, 427
copper, **358**, 360
coQ10 *see* coenzyme Q10
corneocytes, 3–4, 8, 25, 132–133
	build-up, 86
	lips, 194, 195
corneodesmosomes, 5
Corneometer®, 9–10
corneometry (conductance), 26, 136
cornified cell envelope, 4–5, 6
corrective makeup *see* camouflage
corrugator supercilii, 368
cortex, hair shaft, 167, 235, 251, 262
	relaxers on, 268
cortical cells, hair, 251, *252*
corticosteroids, 301–302
	after laser therapy, 427
	allergy, 57–58
	body washes sparing, 101
	eczema, 517
	hydrocortisone, 525
	psoriasis, 526, 527
cosmetical optimization, 129, 130
Cosmetic Ingredient Review (CTFA), 52
cosmetic intolerance syndrome *see* sensitive skin
costs
	peptides, 310
	psoriasis, 523
	Sculptra®, 391

counseling, laser hair removal, 446
counter-clockwise rotation, wire brushes, 441
couplers, hair dyes, 242, **243**
covalent bonds, hair, 262
creams, 75–77
　hair styling aids, 275
　sunless tanning agents, 149–150
critical micelle concentration, 104
critical wavelength values, UVA protection measurements, 158
criticisms, antimicrobial handwash standards, 115
CROSS (chemical reconstruction of skin scars), 400
cross-linking
　collagen, 15, 16
　hyaluronic acid, 376
　proteins, 6
　　glycation, 361
　　hair, 253
　　with lipids, 5
cross-polarized light photography, 45
cross-reactions
　botanicals, 285
　hair dye allergy, 248
crow's feet, botulinum toxin treatment, 368–369
cryogen sprays, *see also* refrigerant sprays
　radiofrequency therapy, 452
'crystal' products, 163
C-tactile afferents, 38
cucumber, 288–289
cuff sign, lipedema, 473
cuneate fasciculus, 38
Cupidon arch, 194
curcumin, 291, 299, *300*
curlers, 255
curliness of hair, 29–30, 251, 262, *263*, *see also* permanent waves
cuticle
　hair, 30–31, 167, 234–235, 251, *252*
　　relaxers on, 267–268
　nails, **215**
cutting edges, razor blades, 169–171
cyanoacrylates, nail wraps, 229–230
cyclooxygenases, 302, 305
cyclosporine, 303
　botulinum toxins and, **366**
　phototherapy and, 526
cysteamine, 58, 256
cysteine, in melanogenesis, 24
cysteine proteases, 7
L-cystine, hair, 253, *254*
cytochrome P450 inhibitors, lidocaine doses and, 469
cytochromes, LED light on, 460
cytokeratins, lips, 194
cytokines, 9, 24
　corticosteroids on, 301
　cosmeceuticals, 320–321
　inflammation, 298, 299, 305
　psoriasis, 523
　wound healing, 319

D

daily use moisturizers, sunless tanning agents, 151
d-α-tocopherol, 497, *498*, *499*, *see also* vitamin E
dandruff, 124, *125*, 130
dappen dishes, 226–227
date palm fruit, 292
death
　from botanicals, 285, 288
　　oleander, 290
　rates, liposuction, 472, **473**
decalcification *see* neutralization
decussations, sensory projections, 38
Deep FX-Lumenis laser, 415–419, *420*, 427
defatting, 398
　medium depth peels, 405
degradable polymer gels, allergy, 59
degreasing *see* defatting
dehydrators, nails, 228
dehydroalanine, 266
dehydrocholesterol, 343
delayed hypersensitivity, hair dyes, 246
ΔE (Euclidean distance), 151
δ-tocopherylglucopyranoside, 330, 331
demi-permanent hair dyes, 240–241
denaturation, hair proteins, 263–264
dendritic cells, 299
denervation, botulinum toxins, 365
deodorants, 160–165
　soaps, 85
depigmentation
　Kligman and Willis formula, 329
　serine protease inhibitors, 24
depressor anguli oris, 371, 373
depressor labii inferioris, paralysis, 373
depressor supercilii, 368
depth controlled peels, trichloroacetic acid, 400
DermaBlend® Cover, **513**
dermabrasion, 437–444
dermatoporosis, 326, 330
dermis
　alpha-hydroxyacids on, 351–352
　lips, 194
　melanin color, 25
　nonablative rejuvenation systems on, 429
　peels, 395
　photoaging, 13, 14, 28–29
　　microvasculature, 15
　retinoids on, 337
　skin of color, 27
　thickness, 34
dermoepidermal junction, 27, 28
desmosomes, 5, 90
desquamation, 5, 6, 7, 8
　by alpha-hydroxyacids, 351, 353
　glycerol on, 135
　hydration on, 133
　tests, 9
detergents, *see also* syndets
　bar cleansers, 83, 86
　shampoos, 237
developers, hair dyes, 243

DHHB (diethylamino hydroxybenzoyl hexyl benzoate), 155
diabetes mellitus
　feet, moisturizers, 143, *145*
　LED photomodulation on retinopathy, 459
diamond fraises, 440
dibutyl phthalate, 219
diclofenac, 302, 303
dietary nutrients, 357–363
diethylamino hydroxybenzoyl hexyl benzoate, 155
diffusion, 66
digital photography, 42, 43–46
dihydroacetone, 148–149, 188
di-isostearylmalate, **196**
dimethicone, shampoos, 237
dimethyl urea, 221
dimpled chin, 371
diode laser, 433
　hair removal, 448
　liposuction, 472–473
discoloration of nails, **208**, **215**
disinfection, schools, 118
disodium phenyl dibenzimidazole tetrasulfonate, 156
distal phalanx, 209
disulfide bonds, hair proteins, 253, 254, 255
DNA, UV radiation on, 14–15, 16, 53
docosahexaenoic acid, **358**
dopaquinone, 24
dorsal horn, 38
double chin, 28, 476
double edge razors, 169
double-sided mascara products, 201
Dove bar, 85, 90
downturned smile, 371, 373
doxycycline, rosacea, 514
DPDT (disodium phenyl dibenzimidazole tetrasulfonate), 156
dressings
　after dermabrasion, 442
　after liposuction, 481
driving, occupational, 15
drometrizole trisiloxane, 155–156
drooling, from botulinum toxin treatment, 373
drug history, liposuction, 471
dry cleansing cloths, **105**, 107
dry-hair shampoos, 237
dry ice *see* carbon dioxide
dry skin, 88–90
　body washes, performance, 98–100
　face, 132–133
　facial cleansers, 109
　genetics, 93–94
　hand moisturizers on, 143, *144*
　lips, 195
　pigmentation and, 26
　rosacea, 511
　soaps, 85
　syndet bars, 87
　water paradox, 86, *88*, 89–90
D-squames, 136
DTS (drometrizole trisiloxane), 155–156

dyes *see* colors; hair dyes
dyschromia, **208**
dysphagia, from botulinum toxin treatment, 371, 373
Dysport®, 364, 365–366

E
East Asians, photoaging, 17
ecamsule, 493
eccrine glands, 160, *161*, 162
ectropion, **200**
eczema, 517–521, *see also* atopic dermatitis; inflammatory skin diseases; *specific diseases*
    facial moisturizers for, 137
    hand moisturizers on, 143, *144*
    occupational, 58
eczema area severity index, mildness of cleansing, 93
edema, after liposuction, 481
education, nail care practitioners, 232
eicosapentaenoic acid, **358**
elastic fibers, photoaging, 28
elasticity, 27
    niacinamide on, 340
    nutrients for, 361
    peptides for, 313–314
elastic recovery, 27
elastin promoter gene, antioxidant testing, 348
elastosis, 13, 14, 28, 319
    antioxidant testing, 348
    cathepsins, 17
Elat MD® UV Clear, **514**
electric brushes, 505
electric razors, 167
electron microscopy, 10
    African hair, 30–31
    effect of moisturizers, 142
electro-optical synergy, hair removal, 448
electrostatic salt links, hair shaft keratin, 235, 262
embolization, from polylactic acid therapy, 393
emollients, 10, 76
    antimicrobial handwashes, 113
    cleansers, **105**, 106
    hair styling aids, 270, 272, 273, **274**
    moisturizers, **134**, 135
    for percutaneous delivery, **67**
    sunless tanning agents, 150
emotive ingredients, bar cleansers, 84
emulsifiers, 76, 140
    facial foundation, 179
    moisturizers, **134**
    sunless tanning agents, 150
emulsions, 75–76, 77, **78**, 104
    facial foundation, 179
    hair styling aids, 275, **276**
    moisturizers, 140, 519, 520, 521
    for percutaneous delivery, 66
    phase separation, body washes, 97
EN 1499 and EN 1500 (protocols), 115
endocuticle, African hair, 31
endpapers, perming, **256**

enhanced glycerol derivative (EGD), 145
enkephalin, 312
entropion, **200**
enzymes, 314–315
    co-factors
        vitamin B3 derivatives, 339–340
        vitamin C, 342
    lip skin surface, 194, 195
    proteolytic, 7, 314
epidermal growth factor receptor, curcumin on, 299
epidermis, 3–12, *see also* barrier functions of epidermis; transepidermal delivery; transepidermal water loss
    alpha-hydroxyacids on, 351
    labial, 194
    melanin color, 25
    photoaging, 13, 14, 28
    skin of color, 25–26
epinephrine, tumescent local anesthesia, 469
erbium:glass lasers, 432–433
erbium:YAG lasers, 412, 413, *414*, 419–420, 424, 425
erythema
    after peels, 407
    antioxidant assessment, 48
    body washes on, 100
    camouflage, 191
    LED photomodulation on, 458–459
    rosacea, 514–515
erythematotelangiectatic rosacea, 509, *511*
erythrulose, 149
essences, facial foundation, 179
essential oils
    acne, 506
    for percutaneous delivery, **68**
estradiol, percutaneous delivery, 73
Etcoff, N., *Survival of the Prettiest*, 492
ethnic skin, 23–32, *see also* ashy skin
    facial foundation, 182
    photoaging, 17–18, 25, 28–29
    polylactic acid therapy, 392
ethyl acetate, 223–224
ethyl acrylate, *227*
N,N'-ethylenediamine disuccinic acid, 246
Eucerin® Redness (products), **512**, **513**, 515
Euclidean distance, color evaluation, 151
EU Cosmetics Directive, 259
eudermatrophic agents, hydroxyacids as, 351, 353
eugenol, **68**
eumelanin, 7, 23, 241
Europe
    antimicrobial handwashes, assessment protocols, 115
    UVA protection measurements, 158
European baseline series, fragrances, 55, **56**
eutectic blends, 67
evaporimeters, 9, 136
excimer laser, for hypopigmentation, 442
excipients, skin penetration, 66–67
exfoliation, 493, *494*
    cleansers for, 108

exocuticle, African hair, 31
extensibility of skin, 27
extensions
    eyelashes, 203
    nails, 211, **215**
external jugular vein, 477
extracellular matrix, glycation, 296
extracellular signal-related kinases, 18
extremozymes, 315
eye(s), *see also* retina
    cosmetics, 199–206
    ocular rosacea, 510, *511*
    protection from lasers, 446
eyebrows, 203
    lateral brow lift, 370
    ptosis, 27, 372
    unilateral raised, 372–373
eyelashes, 200
    conditioners, 206
    cosmetics, 199, 201–203
    extensions, 203
eyelids
    aging, 27
    cucumber, 288
    dermatitis, 56, 58
    jelly rolls, 369
    ptosis, 368, 373
    radiofrequency therapy, 453
    tattooing, 203
    trichloroacetic acid, 406
eyeliners, 199, 204
eyeshadow, 199, 204

F
face, *see also specific resurfacing techniques*
    aging, 27–28, 375, 380
    botulinum toxin treatment, 366–373
    cleansers, 103–109
        selection guide, 107–109
    fillers, 375
    foundations, 177–185, *see also* makeup
    rosacea, 512–513
    moisturizers, 132–138
    sensory perception, 33, 39
    washing, 493
facial nerve, liposuction and, 468, 476–477, 480, 482
Fair Packaging and Labeling Act, 52
false eyelashes, 202–203
famciclovir, 405
farnesol, **68**
fats, dietary excess, **358**
fat transplantation, 388, 483, **486**
fatty acids, **68**
    free, 8
    Malassezia yeasts on, 124
    omega-3, **358**, 360, 361
    peroxidation, 296
    soaps, 84, 97
    volatile, 160
        neutralization, 163
Federal Food, Drug and Cosmetic Act, 52
feedback, radiofrequency therapy, 452

feel modifiers, body washes, 98
feet
   moisturizers, 143–144, *145*
   skin, 139
ferulic acid, 498, **499**
feverfew, 289
fibers
   cleansing cloths, 106–107
   in mascaras, 201
fibroblast growth factors, **320**, 321
fibroblasts, 16–17
   aged, 17
   autologous cell therapy, 387–388
   hyaluronic acid fillers on, 378
   low energy light on, 456–457
   Nd:YAG laser on, 432
   skin of color, 27
   vitamin C on, 497
Fibrocell Science, Inc., 387
fibroplastic response, calcium hydroxylapatite, 380
fibrous tissue, liposuction, 470–471
Fick's law, 66
fig leaves, 57
filaggrin, 5, 6, 9, 53, 93–94, 140, 518
filing, nails, 212, 228, 232
Filipino hair, thiol procedure, **265**
fillers, *see also under* hyaluronic acid
   adverse skin reactions, 53, 59
   autologous, 385–389
   botulinum toxin with, 372
   calcium hydroxylapatite, 60, 380–384, 485–491
   collagen, 60, 376, 387
   hands, 485, **486**
   polylactic acid, 390–394, **486**
   powders, 180, 181
   radiofrequency and nonablative therapy, 453
film-forming polymers, 272
filters, UV radiation, 154–155, *see also* sunscreens
fingerpad method, antimicrobial handwash assessment, 115
finishing powders, 180
firmness of skin, tests, 183
fish oils, **358**, 360
Fitzpatrick skin types
   dermabrasion, 440
   peels, 404
   photoaging, 17, 25
fixing lotions, permanent waves, 254
flaking
   scalp, 124, *125*
   skin, 90
flares
   psoriasis, 523
   rosacea, 510, **512**
flat irons, 264
flavonoids, **358**, 359
   licorice, 289–290
   vitamin P, 343
flaxseed, 292
f-layer, hair epicuticle, 235, 245, 251

flexibility, nails, 210
flora *see* bacteria; microbiota
fluorescence photography, 46
fluorescent UV nail lamps, 228
fluor-hydroxy pulse peel, 400
flushing
   nicotinic acid, 341
   rosacea, 514–515
folliculitis barbae, 172
food allergies, 55
Food and Drug Administration
   on acne drug products, 501
   on antifungals, 220
   approved fillers, **376**
   Food Code, on hand hygiene, 112
   on handwashes, 113, 115
   permanent hair reduction (term), 445, 450
   regulations, 52
      antimicrobial handwashes, 114
      cosmeceuticals, 284
      medical devices, 70
      stability testing of ointments, 79
   on sunless tanning agents, 150
   sunscreens, 154, 156–157, 158
   tar products, 525
Food Drugs & Cosmetic Act, 284
food handling, hand sanitizers and, 113
food supplements *see* oral supplements
forceps, for calcium hydroxylapatite treatment, 490
forehead, botulinum toxin treatment, 367–368, 372–373
foreign body reactions, fillers, 53–54, 59–60
forensic medicine, lip topology, 194
formaldehyde, 222
formaldehyde releasers, 56
formalin, 222
   as nail hardener, 221
formulations
   antiperspirants, 163, *164*
   hair dyes, 242–243
   hair styling aids, 272–273
   peeling agents, 395–398, 402–403
   perm lotions, 255–258
   retinoids, 338–339
   for skin penetration, 66–67
   sunscreens, 156
   topical antioxidants, 300–301, 303–305
   vitamin B3, 341
   vitamin C, 343, 497
foundations (face), 177–185, 512–513
fractionated CO_2 laser resurfacing, 414–426
fragrances
   allergy, 55
   body washes, 98
   labeling, 52, 55, **56**
   moisturizers, 135
Frankfurt plane, 477
Franz cells, 71–72
Fraxel Re:Pair laser, 417–420
freckles, lasers compared, 430
free fatty acids, 8
free nerve endings, 37

free radicals, 16, 295–296
   retinoids on, 329
   on vitamin C, 497
friction, cleaning, 105
Frigiderm, 441
frontalis, 370
   botulinum toxin treatment, 367–368, 372–373
frosting
   levels, 406
   trichloroacetic acid, 396, *397*, 406
fruit seeds
   body washes, 98
   scrubs, 106
functional MRI, 40

G

GAGs *see* glycosaminoglycans
G.A. Morgan Hair Refining Cream, 265
gastrointestinal infections, hand hygiene, 118
gelees, sunless tanning agents, 150
gel hardness, hyaluronic acid product, 376
gel matrices, bionic acids, 348
gel polish, nail coatings, 230–231
gels
   hair styling aids, 275, **276**
   sunless tanning agents, 150
general anesthesia, liposuction, 464
genetics
   dry skin, 93–94
   melanogenesis, 24
   photoaging, 17
   psoriasis, 523
genistein, 300, 499
Gentlewaves®, 457, *458*
German chamomile, 289, 506
Gillette safety razor, 166
glabella
   botulinum toxin treatment, 368
   calcium hydroxylapatite and, 383
glabridin, 290
glabrous skin, 34, *35*
   sensory perception, 34, *36*
Glogau's classification, photoaging, **403**
glosses, lips, 197
glow moisturizers, sunless tanning agents, 151
glucocorticoid receptors, 301, 302
gluconolactone, 347, 348, 495–496
   with azelaic acid, 354
   rosacea, 515
   on sun sensitivity, 350
glutathione, 297, 310–311
glycation, 149, 296–297, 361
   hydroxyacids on, 349–350
   niacinamide on, 340
glycerides, **68**
glycerol, 6–7, 134–135, 137, 518
   enhanced derivatives, 145
glyceryl monothioglycolate, 58, 256, 258
glycolic acid
   acne, 503
   on dermis, 352
   fluor-hydroxy pulse peel, 400

glycolic acid (*continued*)
    before medium depth peel, 403
    as peeling agent, 353, *354*, 395–396
    on sunburn cells, 350
glycols, **68**, 77
glycosaminoglycans
    alpha-hydroxyacids on, 351–352
    hyaluronic acid as, 375
    niacinamide on, 340
    retinoids on, 337
glycylglycine oleamide (OGG), *327*, 331
Gly-His-Lys (tripeptide), 312
glyoxal, 221–222
Goeckerman treatment, 526
golden fern, 289
G prime, hyaluronic acid product, 376
gracile fasciculus, 38
grading, skin response, 42
grafts, camouflage, 188
granulomatous reactions, 54, 59, 60
grape extract, 289
grape seed extract, **358**
graying of hair, 241, 244–245
    setting lotions, 274
green tea, 19, 289, **358**, 360
green tints, rosacea camouflage, 513
grenz zone, 28
grooming, 40
    nails, 210–215
ground substance *see* glycosaminoglycans
growers, eyelashes, 206
growth factors
    after laser therapy, 427
    assays, 322–323
    cellular, 318–324
    from platelets, 385, **386**
GSH (glutathione), 297, 310–311
guanidine relaxers, 266, 268
guidelines, hand hygiene, 112
guide photographs, 46
gummy smile, 370

H
H1N1 influenza, efficacy of handwashes, 116–117
hair, 29, 167–169, 234–238, 251–252, 270–272, *see also* African hair; permanent waves
    biotinyl-GHK on growth, 312
    chemistry, 253–254
    damage
        from permanent waving, 259, **260**
        protection by styling aids, 278
    dyes on, 244, 245–246
    ethnic differences, 29–31
    eyelashes, 200
    growth cycle, 167–168, 446
    hydration, 168, 171
    mimicking for camouflage, 188
    pH, 253, 256
    platelet-rich plasma therapy, 385
    relaxers on, 267–268
    removal, 166, 191, 445–450
        blade shaving, 166–173

    scalp, 124, 168
    shampoo benefits, 130–131
    shaving action, 169
    straightening, 262–269
        technique, 266–267, 268–269
    styling, 270–279
    water and, 252–253, **256**, 271–272
hair dyes, 239–250
    allergy, 58, 246
    oxidation to form, 242
hair follicles, 29, 167, 234, 445–446
    eyelashes, 200
    nerve supply, 168
    transplantation, 203
    zinc pyrithione bio-availability, 129
hair matrix, 445
hair shaft, 234–235, *see also* cortex
    cross-section shape, 29, *30*, 252, 277
    medulla, 167, 235, 251
hairsprays, 273–274, **276**
    silicones, 276
hairy skin, 35
halogenation, corticosteroids, 57–58
hand, 139
    aging, 485, **486**
    calcium hydroxylapatite, 383, 485–491
    hygiene, 112–113
    moisturizers, 142–143, *144*
    occupational eczema, 58
    polylactic acid therapy, 393
hand sanitizers, 110–123
    antibacterials in, 492–493, *see also* antimicrobial handwashes
    efficacy, 114–118
    safety, 118–119
handwashing technique, 112–113
    on microbiota, 111, 113
happy tree (*Camptotheca acuminata*), 286
haptens, 53
hardeners, nails, 217, **218**, 220–222, **223**
    allergy, 58
headache, from BoNTA treatment, 372
healthcare-associated infections, 110, 117–118
heat
    on hair, 253, 278, *see also* thermal processing
    pain sense, 37
    photoaging, 29
    from radiofrequency devices, 433, 451–452
    with thiol procedure, 264–265, 268–269
heating devices, acne, 505
heel skin, 143, *145*
hematomas
    calcium hydroxylapatite to hands, 488
    liposuction, 472
hemoglobin, laser wavelengths targeting, 430
Henle's layer, hair follicles, 234
henna, 59
heparin binding-epidermal growth factor, 328
herbal ingredients *see* botanicals
herpes simplex
    after peels, 407
    dermabrasion and, 440, 442, **443**

        LED photomodulation on lesions, 459
        before peels, 404, 405
high performance liquid chromatography, sunless tanning agents, 149
hips, liposuction, 467
histamine, 37
histopathology, photoaging, 28–29
historical aspects
    bar cleansers, 83
    complexion makeup, 177–178
    dermabrasion, 437
    eye cosmetics, 199–200
    facial cleansing, 103
    hair removal, 166
    lip cosmetics, 195
    liposuction, 463
    nail cosmetics, 217
    soaps, 96
HIV-associated lipoatrophy, polylactic acid therapy, 392
home hand hygiene, 118
homunculus, somatosensory, *39*
hormones, 8–9, 309
hospital infections, handwashes and, 117–118
hot combs, 263
households, hand hygiene, 118
hue, 187
human albumin, allergy, 59
human oligopeptides, **323**
humectants, 6–7, 10, 77
    in alcohol-based hand rubs, 114
    in moisturizers, 134–135, 140, **141**, 142, 518
    psoriasis, 524–525
humidity, 8, 9, *see also* water
Hutchinson–Gilford progeria syndrome, 17
Huxley's layer, hair follicles, 234
hyaluronan, 328, 329–330, 331
hyaluronic acid
    alpha-hydroxyacids on, 351–352
    fillers, 59, 375–379
        aging hand, **486**
        botulinum toxin with, 372
hyaluronidase, 59
hydration, 6–7, 9, 10
    on desquamation, 133
    of hair, 168, 171
    measurement, 9–10, 26
    nutrients for, 361
    panthenol, 342
    for percutaneous delivery, 67
hydrocarbons, hair straightening, 264
hydrocortisone, 525
hydrodissection, 464
hydrogel dressings, 442
hydrogen bonds, hair, 262, 271–272
hydrogen peroxide
    hair bleaches, 58
    hair dyes, 240, 242, 243, 244, 245
    perming lotions, 257
    regulations, 258
hydrolyzed proteins
    nail cosmetics, **223**
    shampoos, 237

hydrophilic matrices, 518
hydroquinone
 antioxidant testing, 348
 priming for peeling, 398
hydroquinone derivatives, 57
hydroxide straighteners, 265–268
hydroxyacids, 346–356, 495–496, **499**
 acne, 354, 503
 peels, 353, *354*, 395–396
  rosacea, 515
 synergy with drugs, 353–354
hydroxyethyl-p-phenylenediamine, 247–248
hyoid bone, 467–468, 476
hyperalgesia, 37
hyperhidrosis, 164–165
hyperkeratosis, hydroxyacids for, 352–353
hyperpigmentation, 25, *see also* postinflammatory hyperpigmentation
 after dermabrasion, 442, **443**
 camouflage, *189*
 LED light on, 460
 licorice for, 290
 niacinamide on, 340, 341
 from peels, 407
 retinoids on, 329, 338
 UV reflectance photography, 45–46
hyponychium, 208
hypopigmentation, 25
 after dermabrasion, 442, **443**
 after hair removal, 449
hypotrichosis, **200**

I

ice packs
 for botulinum toxin treatment, 366
 calcium hydroxylapatite to hands, 488
ID reaction, tattooing, 59
IκK, corticosteroids on, 301
image analysis, 42, 48, 49
imaging techniques, 10, 50
imbalance *see* asymetic effects
imbibing times, Sculptra®, 390
imines, hair dyes, 242
immune function, 6
 psoriasis, 523
immunogenicity, botulinum toxins, 372
immunohistochemistry, 10
immunomodulators, 303
immunosuppression
 corticosteroids, 302
 by UV radiation, 19
indomethacin, nanocapsules, 69, *70*
induration, after liposuction, 481
infections, 110, 117–118, *see also* viral infections
 after dermabrasion, 442, **443**
  staff, **443**
 after liposuction, 471, 472
 nail care, 217, *219*, 232
 from peels, 407
 psoriasis, 523
 retinaldehyde on, 328–329
 surrogate models, 118

infiltration pumps, liposuction, 470
infiltration rates, tumescent local anesthesia, 470
inflammation, 8, 298–300, *see also* cytokines
 antioxidants on, 297–298
 dyspigmentation, 25
 eczema, 517
 from filler injection, 54, 377
 hyperalgesia, 37
 LED photomodulation on, 458–460
 photoaging, 14, 299
 from protease-activated receptor 2, 24
 scalp, 124
 wound healing, 318–319
inflammatory skin diseases, *see also specific diseases*
 facial moisturizers for, 136–137
influenza (H1N1), efficacy of handwashes, 116–117
infrared light devices, 433
injectables *see* fillers
injection
 adipose-derived stem cells, 388
 autologous fibroblast cell therapy, 387
 botulinum toxins, 366–372
 fillers, 377, 391–393
  calcium hydroxylapatite, 380–381, 487
 micro-injection, 324
 platelet-rich plasma, 386
injuries, *see also* wound healing
 camouflage, 188–190
inorganic UV filters, 155, 493
intense pulsed light system, 431–432
 erythema, LED photomodulation on, 458–459
 hair removal, 448, *449*
 rosacea, 515
intensity (color coordinate), 188
intensity-modulated radiation treatments, dermatitis, LED photomodulation on, 459
intensive care units, hand cleansing, 117
interference pigments, lipsticks, 197
interleukin 1, 305
intermediate size HA fragments (HAFi), 330, 331
interneurons, 38
intracrine concept, 326–328
intraoral approach, calcium hydroxylapatite, 383
intrinsic point of neutrality, hair, 253
in vitro assays, antimicrobial handwashes, 114
in vitro models
 lipid peroxidation, 349
 photoaging, antioxidant testing, 348
in vivo and *in vitro* assessment, percutaneous delivery, 71–72, **73**
in vivo models
 resident microbiota, 116
 transient microbiota, 114–116
involucrin, lips, 194
ionization, skin penetration and, 66
iontophoresis, 71
 hyperhidrosis, 165

Iopidine, for eyelid ptosis, 373
iovera (cold therapy device), 373
IPL *see* intense pulsed light system
iron oxides, facial foundation, 181
irons, 264
irritant contact dermatitis, 52–53
irritants, 54–55
 barrier function testing, 136
irritation, 26, 54–55
 antiperspirants, 164
 benzoyl peroxide, 502–503
 from cosmetics, 11
 dandruff, shampoos on, 130
 hair dyes, 244
 hair styling aids, 275
 hand moisturizers on, 143
 handwashing, 118–119
 lack of, hydroxyacids, 350–351
 nail cosmetics, 214
 nociception, 37
 perming lotions, 260
 retinoids, 54, 326, 496
 shaving, 168–169
isethionate syndet bars, 85, 86, 87, 89, 90–92
ISO 24444, sunscreens, 156
isoionic point, hair, 253
isopropanol, 114
isopropyl myristate, 55
isotretinoin, 328
 dermabrasion and, 440
 medium depth peels after, 404
itch sense, 37–38

J

Japan
 approved sunscreens, 154
 regulations, perming lotions, 258
 thiol procedure, **265**
 UVA protection measurements, 158
jaw line, 28
 liposuction, 467, 468, 480–481
 polylactic acid therapy, 392
jelly rolls, eyelids, 369
Jessner's solution, 396, 402, 403–405, *408*, *409*, *410*
 before medium depth peels, 406
jowling, 28
 liposuction, 467, 468, 476, 480–481
Juvederm, hyaluronic acid products, 376

K

K38 patterns, hair curl, 30
keratin granulations, nails, 214
keratinocytes, 3–4
 melanosome transfer to, 23, 24
 psoriasis, 523
 UV radiation on, 24
keratins
 hair, 235–237
 hair follicles, 234
 hair shafts, 235, 262
keratohyalin granules, 5
keratolytics, psoriasis, 523–524, 525, 527
ketoamines, 296

ketoconazole, 127
ketones, 219, 223
kinetin, 323, 499
Kligman and Willis formula, depigmentation, 329
KTP laser, 430
kwashiorkor, nail plate, 209
kyotorphine, 312, *313*

L
labeling of products, 52
　colors, 219–220
　fragrances, 55, **56**
　mislabeling, 284
　nail lacquers, 217
　sunless tanning agents, 150, 151
　sunscreens, 157, 494
laboratory tests, liposuction, 471, 472, 478
L*a*b* standard, Commission Internationale d'Eclairage, 151
lacquers, nails, 217–221
　photoinitiators, **221**, **222**, **223**
　removers, 223–224
lactates, 142
lactic acid
　acne, 503
　as peeling agent, 353, 395–396
lactobionic acid, 349, 351
lake form, colors, 219
lamellar granules, 5
lamina propria, lips, 194
Langerhans cells, 299
　lips, 194
lanolin, 135
　allergy, 57
lanthionine, 266
large body areas, radiofrequency therapy, 453
lasers, 413–414, *see also* carbon dioxide lasers
　hair removal, 445–450
　　camouflaging erythema, 191
　for hypopigmentation, 442
　liposuction, 472–473
　nonablative, 429–436
　rosacea, 515
　safety, 446
lateral brow lift, 370
latex allergy, 58
lathering cleansers, 105–106, 107
Latisse, 203
laxity of skin, *see also* ptosis
　infrared light devices, 433
　radiofrequency devices, 451–455
LD50, botulinum toxins
　humans, 366
　mice, 365
leave-on products
　bergamot oil, 57
　hand sanitizers as, 114
　moisturizers, 97, 99, 100
lecithin, 76
legal medicine, lip topology, 194
legislation, 52, *see also* regulations
　fragrances, 55, **56**

lentigines, *see also* age-spots
　lasers compared, 430
leukocytes, inflammation, 298–299
leukotriene-C4, 25
levator labii superioris alaeque nasi, 370
levulinic acid, photodynamic therapy, 459–460
licochalcone A, 515
licorice, 289–290
lidocaine
　mixing with calcium hydroxylapatite, 383, 486–487, 490
　Sculptra®, 390
　tumescent local anesthesia, 469, 471
light-emitting diodes
　acne treatment devices, 505
　photomodulation, 456–462
　UV radiation, 223, 228
light energy devices, *see also* intense pulsed light system
　skin tightening, 453–454
lighteners/brighteners (herbs), 287
lightening products *see* bleaching agents
lighting
　photography, 44
　raking light optical profilometry, 47
linolenic acid, 292
linseed, 292
lipedema, liposuction for, 473–474
lipid-free cleansers, 521
lipids, 8
　cleansing agents on, 85, 89
　in cosmetics, 10
　　solid lipid nanoparticles, 69
　as emollients, 135
　emulsifiers on, 76, 104
　ethnic skin, 26
　inter-corneocyte, 3, 5
　lutein/zeaxanthin on, 361
　Malassezia yeasts on, 124
　nail plate, 209–210
　oral, 360
　permeability barrier, 5
　peroxidation, 16, 295–296
　　carotenoids on, 359
　　in vitro model, 349
　pH on, 86
　vitamin C on synthesis, 497
　vitamin E on, 297
lipoatrophy, 380
　polylactic acid therapy, 392, 393
lipolysis, lasers, 473
liporeceptors, 8–9
liposomes, 69, 519–520
liposuction, 463–475
　neck, 467–468, 476–484
　technique, 470, 471, 479–482
　volume removed, 470
lip prints, 194
lips, 193–195
　botulinum toxin treatment, 371
　glosses and brilliances, 197
　LED photomodulation on HSV lesions, 459

lipsticks, 193, 195–197
　actives, 197
liquid cleansers, 93
　lathering cleansers, 105–106, 107
liquid crystal emulsifiers, 76
liquid eyeliners, 204
liquid nitrogen, 398, 441
liquid systems, artificial nail enhancements, 226–228, 232
liver X receptor, 9
local anesthesia, *see also* topical anesthesia; tumescent local anesthesia
　adverse reactions, 59
　dermabrasion, 441, 442
　Sculptra®, 390
log P (partition coefficient), 301
lollipop appearance, 483
Londinium ointment can, 178
long pulsed lasers
　dye lasers, 431
　hair removal, 447–448
　Nd:YAG lasers, collagen synthesis, 429
long wear eye cosmetics, 205
loose powders, facial foundation, 180
L'Oréal Curl Classification, 262, *263*
L'Oréal/La Roche-Posay® Anthelios®, **514**
L'Oréal Plénitude cleanser, **512**
lotions, 75–76, 519
　hair styling aids, 277–278
　　perming lotions, 254
　　setting lotions, 274
low energy light therapy, 456–457, 505
lower face, aging, 28
low threshold mechanoreceptors, 34
lubricating strips, razors, *170*, 171
lunula, 207
lutein, **358**, 359, 361
luteolin, 300
Lux 2940 laser, 425, *426*
lycopene, **358**, 359
lye relaxers, 265–268
lymph drainage, lips, 194
lysine, dihydroacetone on, 149

M
macular lesions, camouflage, 188
madarosis, **200**
Maillard reaction, 349
maitake mushroom, 290
makeup, 177–185, *see also* camouflage; lipsticks
　after laser therapy, 427
　body wash testing, 98
　cleansers to remove, 108
　removal for BoNTA treatment, 372
　rosacea, 512–513
　wet cleansing cloths as removers, 107
malar soft tissue, aging, 28
Malassezia yeasts, 124
　antifungals *vs*, 127
male chest, liposuction, 469
male consumer needs, body washes, 99
malic acid, 347, 395–396
malpighian layer, UV filtration, 25

maltobionic acid
  gel matrix, 348
  on glycation, 350
  on matrix metalloproteinases, 351
  on wrinkles, *353*
mammoplasty (reduction), 468
mandible, *see also* jaw line
  Nefertiti lift, 371
manicures, 210–215
  UV gels, 230–231
manufacture, bar cleansers, 84
marginal mandibular branch, facial nerve, 468, 476–477, 480, 482
market share, bar cleansers, 83
markings, neck liposuction, 479
mascara, 199–200, 201–202, 205
  applicators, 201–202, *203*, 205–206
masking of odors, 163
masks, 493
massage
  calcium hydroxylapatite, 486, 488
  polylactic acid therapy, 391
masseter, hypertrophy, 372
mast cells, ethnicity, 26
matrikines, 311
matrix delivery systems, antiperspirants, 163, *164*
matrix metalloproteinases, 318
  bionic acids on, 351
  chronic inflammation, 299
  low energy light on, 457
  retinoids on, 496
  UV-induced, 16, 136
matrix proteins, hair, 254
matt finish, tests, 184
meadowfoam, *292*
mechanical factors, irritation, 54–55
mechanical tension, on fibroblasts, 16–17
medial lemniscus, 38
medication history, liposuction, 471
medulla, hair shaft, 167, 235, 251
Meissner corpuscles, 34
meladine, 449
melanin, 7, 17–18, 23
  bleaching, 242
  dermis *vs* epidermis, 25
  hair, 241
  hydroxyacids on, 353
  laser hair removal, 446
  LED light on synthesis, 460
  lips, 194, 195
  retinaldehyde on, 330
  synthesis, *24*
    peptides affecting, 314
melanocortin-1 receptor, 24
melanocytes, 23–25, 241
  behavior modulation, 248–249
  retinaldehyde on, 330
melanosomes, 23, 24, 29
melasma
  camouflage, *190*
  peels, 401
  pycnogenol for, 291

melt cast manufacture, bar cleansers, 84
melting points, eutectic blends, 67
men *see* male consumer needs
mentalis, 371
menthol, **68**
mercury, 57
Merkel disks, 34
mesocortical cells, hair, 29–30
mesotherapy, 324
metal ions, tap water, 245–246
metal oxides, *see also* titanium dioxide; zinc oxide
  nanoparticles, 155
methacrylates, 60, 226, *227*, 232
methacrylic acid, 228
methicillin-resistant *S. aureus*, hand hygiene, 117, 118
methionine sulfoxide reductases, 312
methotrexate, phototherapy and, 526
2-methoxymethyl-p-phenylenediamine, 248
methyl acetate, 224
methylchloroisothiazolinone, 56
methylene glycol, 222
methyl ethyl ketone, 223–224
methylisothiazolinone, 56
methyl methacrylate, 232
metronidazole, rosacea, 514
Mexoryl SX™ (UV filter), 155
Mexoryl XL™, 155–156
micelles, 104
microbeams, Pixel 2940 laser, 424
microbiota
  hands, 110–112
  resistance to antimicrobials, 119
  skin damage, 119
  in vivo models, 114–116
microdialysis, 72
micro fibrils, hair, 254
microfine particles, *see also* nanoparticles
  sunscreens, 493
microfins, razors, 171
microflora *see* bacteria; microbiota
micro-injection, 324
microneedles, 70–71
microneurography, 36, 40
microspheres, calcium hydroxylapatite, 380, *381*
microvasculature, *see also* blood flow
  aging, 15, 195
  lips, 194, 195
  nail bed, 208–209
  superficial vascular plexus, 28
midface, aging, 28
mildness
  bar cleansers, 85, 86, 90–93, *94*
  facial cleansers, 108–109
milia, 442, **443**
milks, **105**, 106
milk thistle, 290
mineral makeups, rosacea, 512–513
minimal erythema dose, UV radiation, 48
minocycline
  benzoyl peroxide *vs*, 502
  zinc gluconate *vs*, 506

mislabeling, 284
mitochondria, LED light on, 459, 460
mitochondrial DNA
  herbs protecting, 286
  UV radiation on, 16
mitogen activated protein kinases, 296, 297
MiXto SX laser, 420–421
Mohs surgery, dermabrasion after, *438*, 439
moisturization, 6–7
moisturizers, 10
  after shaving, 172
  allergy, 57
  body washes, 96–97, 98–100
  definition, 133
  delivery systems, 519–521
  dry cleansing cloths, 107
  eczema, 517–521
  facial, 132–138
  hands and feet, 139–147
  panthenol as, 342
  psoriasis, 524–525, 527
  regimens, 521
  rosacea, 511–512
  in sunless tanning agents, 151
  tests, 183
molded applicators, mascara, 202, *203*, 205–206
molecular biology, photoaging, 15–17
molecular weight, for skin penetration, 66
monographs
  antiperspirants, 162
  sunscreens, 154, 156–157
monopolar radiofrequency devices, 451–453
Morgan, Garrett A., 265
Mosaic eCO$_2$™ laser, 421–422, *423*
mountain rose, 292
mousses, hair styling aids, 275, **276**
MSH cell surface receptor gene, 24
mucosa, labial, 193
multi-blade razors, 167, 169–170
multivesicular emulsions, 520
murine β-defensins, 6
mushrooms, 290
myelination, sensory axons, 34
Myobloc®, 364
myristoyl-nicotinate, 341

N
NAD+ (nicotinamide adenine dinucleotide), 339
nail bed, 208–209
nail folds, 207–208
nail matrix, 207
nail plate, 207, 209–210
  thickness, 210
nails, 207–225
  artificial enhancements, 226–233
    removal, 230
  colored cosmetics, 217, 219–220
    UV-curable, 222–223
  damage, 232
  growth, 209
  hardeners, 217, **218**, 220–222, **223**
    allergy, 58

nails (*continued*)
    polishes, 212–214, 217, *see also* UV gels
        allergy, 58
nanocapsules, 69, *70*
nanoemulsions, 520–521
nanoparticles, *see also* microfine particles
    lipids, 69
    metal oxides, 155
Naphcon, for eyelid ptosis, 373
nasalis, 370
nasolabial fold, 370, 378, 383
National Ambulatory Care Survey, psoriasis, 523, *524*
National Psoriasis Foundation, 523
natural (term), 284
natural moisturizing factors (NMF), 6–7, 10, 140–142, 308, 518, *519*
    from filaggrin, 5
    soaps on, 85–86
    water on, 89–90
natural ointments, 78
near-infrared light, acne, 505
neck
    aging, 28
        nonablative lasers on, 434–435
    liposuction, 467–468, 476–484
    washing, 493
necrosis
    from laser therapy, 413
    from polylactic acid therapy, 393
necrotizing fasciitis, 472
Nefertiti lift, 371
neodymium:YAG lasers, 432–433
    collagen synthesis, 429
    hair removal, 448
    liposuction, 473
Neo-Heliopan AP®, 156
neonatal intensive care units, antimicrobial handwashes, 117
nerve supply
    hair follicles, 168
    lips, 194
    skin, 33–41
neurons
    central projections, 38–39
    somatosensory, 33, 34–36
neuropeptides, 312–313
neutralization
    after hair straightening, 267, 269
    alpha-hydroxyacids, 353
    camouflage, 188
    odors, 163
    perming, **256**, 257–258
neutral permanent waves, 258
Neutrogena®, soap bars, 84–85
Neutrogena Helioplex™, **514**
Neutrogena® Oil-free, **512**
New Drug Applications, sunscreens, 154
niacinamide, 339–341, 344, 499, 506
Nicomide, 506
nicotinamide adenine dinucleotide, 339
nicotinate esters, formulations, 341
nicotinic acid, on blood flow, 340, 341

niosomes, 69, 520
nitric oxide, 16
nitro-dyes, 240
nitrogen compounds, in sunless tanning agents, 149
no-base relaxers, 265
nociception, 37
nodules, Sculptra®, 59, 393
no-light gels, 230
no-lye relaxers, 266, 268
nonablative rejuvenation systems, 429–436
    radiofrequency devices with, 434, 453
non-invasive techniques, skin assessment, 42–51
non-ionic surfactants, 104, 125, 492
non-polar solvents, 105
non-steroidal anti-inflammatory drugs, 302–303, 471
non-thermal photomodulation, 456
non-transfer facial foundation, 179
norovirus, hand sanitizers and, 113, 118
no-rub mists, sunless tanning agents, 151
Norwalk virus, 118
nosocomial infections, handwashes and, 117–118
NSAIDs, 302–303, 471
nuclear factor kappa-B, 297, 299
    corticosteroids on, 301, 302
nuclear factor of activated T cells, 303
nuclear hormone receptors, 8–9
nucleic acids
    herbs modifying, **288**, *see also* mitochondrial DNA
nurses, camouflage, 192
nutrients, dietary, 357–363

O

oatmeal, 290, 518
occlusion, for percutaneous delivery, 67
occlusives, in moisturizers, **134**, 135, 140, **141**, 518
occupations
    formaldehyde allergy, 56
    hand eczema, 58
    sun exposure, 15, 493, *495*
OCimple Light Therapy System MP200, 505
octopirox, 127
ocular rosacea, 510, *511*
odors, prevention, 163
off-axis lighting, 44, 47
off-label uses
    botulinum toxins, 364, 365
    calcium hydroxylapatite, 383
OGG (glycylglycine oleamide), *327*, 331
oil-in-water emulsions, 75, 76, 77, 179, 519
oils, lipsticks, 196
oily cleansers, 105
oily skin, facial cleansers, 108
ointments, 76–79, 519, 524
Olay® Complete, **512**
Olay® Daily Facials, 107
oleander, 290
oligopeptides, definition, 309

omega-3 fatty acids, **358**, 360, 361
OMNIFIT handpiece, Pixel CO$_2$ laser, 423
Omnilux™, 458
onychocytes, 207
onycholysis, 208, 209, 215
onychomycosis, *213*
onychorrhexis, **208**
onychoschizia, **208**, 210, *211*
opacifiers, perming lotions, 257
ophthalmic products, allergy, 56
optical coherence tomography, 50
optical energy devices *see* light energy devices
optical profilometry, 46–47, *48*
ORAC assays, 297
oral supplements, 357–363
    vitamins, acne, 506
orbicularis oculi, 367, 368, 369, 370
orbicularis oris, 193
    complications of botulinum toxin treatment, 373
organic (term), 284
organic UV filters, 155, 493
orthocortical cells, hair, 29–30
overresection, neck liposuction, 483
over-the-counter treatments
    acne, 501–508
    antiperspirants as, 162
    psoriasis, 523–526, 527
    rosacea, 510–511, **512**, **513**
oxalic acid, 395–396
oxazolidinones, **68**
oxidation, *see also* auto-oxidation; peroxidation of lipids
    dye formation, 242
    hair straightening, 264
    prevention *see* antioxidants
oxidative stress, 296, 329
    niacinamide on, 339
    from UV radiation, 7–8, 14, 16
    on vitamin C, 497
oxidizing agents, hair bleaches, 58, 240
oxoretinoids, 325, *327*
oxygen inhibition layers, UV-curable artificial nails, 229, 232
oxytalan fibers, 28
ozokerite, **196**

P

Pacinian corpuscles, 34
pain sense, 37
painting of nails, 212–213, 217, *218*
Pal-GHK, 312
Pal-GQPR, 311, 312
Pal-KTTKS (matrikine), 311
Palomar StarLux 500, 425, *426*
p-aminobenzoic acid, 493
panthenol, 341–342
papaya, 290
papillary dermis, 27
    alpha-hydroxyacids on, 352
papules, Sculptra®, 59, 393
papulonodular lesions, camouflage, 188
papulopustular rosacea, 509, *511*

parabens, 56
paracortical cells, hair, 29
paraffin wax, **196**
parallel-polarized light photography, 45
para-phenylenediamine, 246, 247
para-toluenediamine, 246
paronychia, 208, 215
parthenolide, 289
particulates, *see also* nanoparticles
    body washes, 97–98
    exfoliants, 493
    scrubs, 106, 504–505
    zinc pyrithione as, 128
partition coefficients, skin penetration and, 66, 300–301
patches, transdermal, 70
patch testing, 60
    corticosteroids, 58
    fragrances, 55
    local anesthetics, 59
patting, camouflage, 188
Pears soap, 84
pedicures, 210–215
peels
    hydroxyacids, 353, *354*, 395–396
        rosacea, 515
    irritants used, 54
    medium depth, 402–411
        complications, 407–409
        contraindications, 404
    superficial, 395–401
pencils, eyeliners, 204
penetration enhancement vectors, 69
penetration enhancers, 67–69
penetration of skin, 7, 66–71
    devices enhancing, 70–71
    niacinamide, 341
    partition coefficients and, 66, 300–301
    peptides, 310
penicillamine, **366**
peptides, 308–314
    analysis, 310
    definition, 309
percutaneous delivery, 65–74
perfume, lipsticks, 197
perioral area, botulinum toxin treatment, 371–372
periorbital treatment, botulinum toxins, 368–370
permanent dyes, hair, 58, 239, 240–241, 242–243
permanent hair reduction (term), 445, 450
permanent waves, 58, 251–261
    technique, **256**, 258
permeability barrier, 5
    drug routes across, 7
perming, eyelashes, 203
perming lotions, 254
peroxidation of lipids, 16, 295–296
    carotenoids on, 359
    in vitro model, 349
peroxisome proliferator activator receptor, 9
persistent pigment darkening methods, 158

petrolatum, 77, **78**, 135, 518
    body washes depositing, 98, 100–101
    cleansing cloths, 107
pH, *see also* buffering
    antimicrobial handwashes, 114
    bar cleansers, 86–88, *89*
    hair, 253, 256
    neutralizing shampoos, 267
    skin penetration and, 66
    soaps, 84, 85, 86–88
    stratum corneum, 9
    sulfites, 265
    sunless tanning agents, 149
    surfactants, 104
phase separation, body washes, 97
phenol, 353
phenylmercuric acetate, 56
phenyl side chain, alpha-hydroxyacids, 346–347
pheomelanin, 7, 23, 241
phosphatidylglycerol, 518
photoaging, 13–22, 493, *495*
    ethnic skin, 17–18, 25, 28–29
    face, 27
    Glogau's classification, **403**
    hands, polylactic acid therapy, 393
    herbs for, 286–287
    hydroxyacids on, 353
    inflammation, 14, 299
    medium depth peels, 403
    nonablative rejuvenation systems, 434
    prevention, 18–19, 493
    retinoids, 496
    in vitro model, antioxidant testing, 348
photobiology, retinoids, 328
photodamage
    mildness of cleansing, 92
    nutrients for, 360, 497, **499**
photodynamic therapy
    hair removal, 449
    LED light, 459–460
photoepilation, 445–450
photography, digital, 42, 43–46
photoinitiators, nail lacquers, **221**, 222, **223**
photomodulation, by light-emitting diodes, 456–462
photoprotection, *see also* sunscreens
    golden fern, 289
    herbs for, 287
photoreactivity, 155
photo-stabilizers, 155
phototherapy, psoriasis, 526
phototoxic dermatitis, 53
phrynoderma, 326, 328
phymatous rosacea, 509, *511*
physical cleaning, 105, 108
physical penetration enhancers, 69
phytokinins, 323
phytophotodermatitis, 53, 57
pigmentation, 23–32
    hair, 241–242
    hydroxyacids on, 353
    lips, defects, 195

    niacinamide on, 340, 341
    from peels, 407
    retinoids on, 329, 338
pigments *see* colors
pilosebaceous units, 167
pimecrolimus, 303
pineapple, 290–291
Pinnell formulation, antioxidant, 48
Pixel 2940 (Er:YAG laser), 424
Pixel CO$_2$ laser, 423
PKEK (Pro-Lys-Glu-Lys), 314
plants, *see also* botanicals
    phytophotodermatitis from, 53
plasticizers
    nail lacquers, 219, **221**, **223**
    nails, 210
platelet morphology, zinc pyrithione, 128
platelet-rich plasma, 385–387
platysma, 476, 480
    aging, 28
    bands, 371–372, 373, 483
pleasure sense, 38
plugging effect, antiperspirants, 162
polarized light photography, 45
polar solvents, 105
poliosis, **200**
polishes, nails, 212–214, 217, *see also* UV gels
    allergy, 58
polybutene, **196**
polydensification, Belotero, 376
polydimethylsiloxanes, 60
polyglyceryl-2 triisostearate, **196**
polyhydroxy acids (PHAs), 347, 348, 495–496
    acne, 504
    for dry skin, 352
    on glycation, 349–350
    rosacea, 515
polylactic acid fillers, 390–394, **486**
polymerization, artificial nail enhancements, 227
polymers, 492
    allergy, 59
    hair styling aids, 270, 272, **273**
        overuse, 278
    mascara, 201, 205
    shampoos, 126
polymethylmethacrylate, 60
polymodal nociceptors, 37
polyphenols, **358**
polyquaternium 37, 505
pomades, 275
pomegranate, 291
postinflammatory hyperpigmentation, 25
    laser therapy, 412
    peels, 401
postinflammatory hypopigmentation, 25
potassium alum, 163
potassium titanyl phosphate laser, 430
powders
    facial foundation, 180–181
    setting camouflage, 188
powder systems, artificial nail enhancements, 226–228, 232

p-phenylenediamine, 58
pregnancy *see* congenital anomalies
prejowl sulcus, 476
preservatives
 allergy, 55–56
 facial foundation, 182
 lipsticks, 197
 moisturizers, 134, 136
 sunless tanning agents, 150
presurgical hand antisepsis, standards, 115
pre-test, hair dyes, 245, 247, 248
prevalence, hair dye allergy, 246–247
primary afferents, 33
primary intermediates, hair dyes, 242
primary sunscreens, 153
priming, for peeling, 398
probability, efficacy, 285
procerus, 368
procollagen, 15, 16
ProFractional lasers (Sciton), 424, *425*
progerin, 17
pro-ligands, 326–328
Pro-Lys-Glu-Lys (tetrapeptide), 314
propellants, hairsprays, 273–274
Propionibacterium acnes, 111
 benzoyl peroxide on, 502
 UV fluorescence photography, 46
proprioception, 33
propylene glycol, for percutaneous delivery, **67**
4-propyl guaiacol, 301
prostaglandin analogs, eyelash growth, 203
prostaglandin E-2, 298, 299, 305
 NSAIDs on, 303
prostheses *see* artificial nail enhancements
protease-activated receptor 2 (PAR-2), 24–25
protease inhibitors, 7, 8
proteases, 136
protective factor (PF)
 antioxidants, 48, **49**
 sunlight, 25
protein binding, cleansing agents, 85
proteins, 314–315, *see also* hydrolyzed proteins
 antimicrobial, 6
 cornified cell envelope, 4–5, 6
 cross-links with lipids, 5
 definition, 309
 desmosomes, 5
 glycation, 361
 hair, 253–254
  denaturation, 263–264
  disulfide bonds, *253*, 254, 255
proteolytic enzymes, 7, 314
provisional matrix, foreign body reactions, 54
pseudofolliculitis barbae, 172
pseudohypopigmentation, after dermabrasion, **443**
Pseudomonas, nail discoloration, **208**, *215*
psoralen, tanning beds and, 526
psoriasis, 522–528
 hydroxyacids for, 352–353
 nails, *213*
 urea deficiency, 142
PSP (Neocutis), 323

psychological effects, hair dyes, 244
psychophysical channels, sensory perception, 34
psychosocial stress, psoriasis, 523
ptosis
 breast, 469
 eyebrows, 27, 372
 eyelids, 368, 373
 infrared light devices, 433
 peptides for, 313–314
 submandibular glands, 483
pulse dye lasers, 430–431
 collagen synthesis, 429
 rosacea, 515
pump hairsprays, 273, 276
pumpkin, 291
Purpose® Gentle, **512**
purpura, after liposuction, 481
p values, efficacy, 285
pycnogenol, 291, **358**, 361
pyrrolidones, **68**
pyruvic acid, 396

Q
Q-switched lasers, 413
Q-switched Nd:YAG lasers, 432
 collagen synthesis, 429
quality of life
 camouflage, 192
 psoriasis, 522
Quantitative Risk Assessment, hair dyes, 246

R
RAB27A (gene), 24
radiance, skin, 50
radiation dermatitis, LED photomodulation on, 459
Radiesse, 383, 486
radiofrequency devices
 hair removal, 448
 rejuvenation systems, 429, 433–434, 451–455
raking light optical profilometry, 46–47, 48
raking light photography, 44, *45*
Raman microspectrometry, confocal, 72
randomized trials, *see also* blinded trials
 hand hygiene, 117
RAR ligands, 325, 328, 496
razors, 166–167, 169–172
reactive oxygen species, 16, 295–297, 318
rebalancing, artificial nail enhancements, 228
receptive fields, low threshold mechanoreceptors, 34
receptor for advanced glycation end products (RAGE), 297
re-coloring, hair, 246
recombinant growth factors, 323
reconstitution
 botulinum toxins, 366
 Sculptra®, 390
red light, acne, 505
reducing sugars, as sunless tanning agents, 149
reduction (chemical)

 hair straightening, 264–265
 permanent waves, 251, 254, 256
reduction mammoplasty, 468
red wine, 289
reflectance confocal microscopy, 26
refrigerant sprays, *see also* cryogen sprays
 dermabrasion, 441
regulations, *see also* Food and Drug Administration
 antiperspirants, 162
 botanicals, 283–284
 eye cosmetics, 204–205
 hairsprays, 273–274
 lipstick colors, 196
 medical devices, 70
 nail lacquer removers, 223–224
 permanent waves, 258, 259
 sunless tanning agents, 150, 151
 sunscreens, 153–155, 156–158
relaxers, hair straightening, 265–268
removers
 camouflage, 188
 nail lacquers, 223–224
 wet cleansing cloths as, 107
Repeat Insult Patch Test, 285
resident microbiota, 111
 in vivo models, 116
resins, nail cosmetics, 213–214, 219, **221**, 222, *223*, **223**
resorcinol, **396**, 397–398
respiratory infections, hand hygiene, 118
Restylane (hyaluronic acid product), 376
resurfacing, *see also* nonablative rejuvenation systems; peels
 with carbon dioxide lasers, 412–428
 dermabrasion, 437–444
resveratrol, 19, **358**
reticular dermis, 27
Retin A®, 359
retina, protection by LED photomodulation, 459
retinaldehyde, 328–329, 330, 338, 496
retinoic acid, **499**, *see also* all-*trans*-retinoic acid
retinoids, 18, 325–335, 336–339, 359, 496
 dermabrasion and, 440
 irritation, 54, 326, 496
 before medium depth peels, 405
 phototherapy and, 526
 rosacea, 516
retinol, 330–331, 496, 504
retinyl esters, 329, 330–331, 338, 504
retraction, for dermabrasion, 441
rheology modifiers, hair styling aids, 272
rhinophyma
 dermabrasion for, 438
 phymatous rosacea, 509, *511*
rhinovirus, efficacy of handwashes, 116
rhytides
 application of trichloroacetic acid, 406
 bipolar RF and light, 454
 botulinum toxin treatment, 365, 368–369
 dermabrasion for, 438

fractionated CO$_2$ laser resurfacing, 415, 419–420
   glycolic acid peels, *354*
   nonablative lasers, 429–436
riboflavin, 357
ridging, nail plate, 207
ringing gels, 275
rinse-off conditioners, 130
ritual preference, facial cleansers, 108
roll-ons, antiperspirants, 163
rosacea, 509–516
   glycolic acid peels, *354*
   medium depth peels and, 404
   mildness of cleansing, 93, *94*
   vitamin C on, 497, 515
Rosaliac® Anti-redness, **512**
rosemary, 291
ruby laser, hair removal, 447
Ruffini endings, 34
RXR ligands, 325, 328, 496

S

Safe Cosmetics and Personal Care Products Act, 52
safety
   botulinum toxins, 366
   cosmeceuticals, 284–285
   dermabrasion, **443**
   eye cosmetics, 204–205
   facial foundation, 182
   hair dyes, 246–248
   hairsprays, 274
   hand cleansers, 118–119
   lasers, 446
   nail cosmetics, 215
   peels, 398, 400
   peptides, 310
   permanent waves, 258, 259–260
   tanning beds, 526
   UV lamps, 233
safety razors, 166
safflower, 292
sage, 291
sagging *see* ptosis
salicylic acid (SA), 347–348, 496
   acne, 503
   as peeling agent, 353, **396**
   psoriasis, 523–524, *525*
   for scalp, 127
   technique, 397
sallowness, hydroxyacids on, 349
salt links, hair shaft keratin, 235, 262
saturation (color coordinate), 188
SCAAR FX laser treatment, 416
scalp, 124, *125*
   hair, 124, 168
   perming lotions on, 260
scanning CO$_2$ lasers, 412, 415
scarring, *see also* acne
   after dermabrasion, 443, **443**
   after peels, 407–409
   camouflage, 188
   dermabrasion for, 438

scents *see* fragrances
Schiff bases, 296
schools, hand hygiene, 118
Sciton ProFractional lasers, 424, *425*
screening, fragrances, 55
scrubbing, 53
scrubs, **105**, 106, 504–505
scrubs (surgical), standards, 115
sculpting, nails, 227
Sculptra®, 59, 390–394
sebaceous glands, 167
sebaceous oil
   facial cleansers to remove, 108
   scalp, 124
seborrheic dermatitis, 124, *125*
sebum, 167
   niacinamide on, 339, **340**
secondary metabolites (SM), 284, 285
secondary sunscreens, 153–154
sedation
   dermabrasion, 442
   liposuction, 479
   medium depth peels, 405
seeds *see* fruit seeds
selective photothermolysis, 446
selenium, **358**, 360, 498–499
selenium sulfide, 127
L-selenomethionine, 498–499
self-tanners *see* sunless tanning products
semi-permanent hair dyes, 58, 240
semi-permanent mascaras, 205
semi-permeable hydrogel dressings, 442
sensitive skin, 11, 55
   hydroxyacids on, 351
   LED photomodulation on, 459
   retinoids, 496
   rosacea, 510–511
   shaving, 172
sensitization, 53
sensory perception, 33–41
   irritation, 55
   lips, 194
   skin of color, 27
serine protease inhibitors, 24
serine proteases, 7, 24
seromas, liposuction, 472
serums
   hair styling aids, 276
   moisturizers, 519
setting lotions, 274
setting powders, camouflage, 188
shade guides, hair dyes, 245
shampoos, 124–131, 237–238
   allergy, 57
   for colored hair, 246
   neutralizing, 267
sharpness, razor blades, 169–170, *171*
shaving, 166–173
shellac, 212–213
shiitake mushroom, 290
SIAScope, 49
signaling pathways
   antioxidants on, 297–298

   calcineurin, 303
   corticosteroids on, 301–302
   reactive oxygen species on, 296, 297
silicone oils, facial foundation, 179
silicones, *see also* bovine collagen
   artificial, 135
   granulomatous reactions, 60
   hair straightening, 264
   hair styling aids, 276
   shampoos, 237, 238
   sunless tanning agents, 150
Silk'n Blue Device, 505
silymarin, 290
skin benefit agents, body washes, 97–98
SkinChip®, 10
skin diseases, *see also specific diseases*
   dermabrasion and, 440
   medium depth peels and, 404
skin-friendly emulsifiers, 76
skin type, *see also* Fitzpatrick skin types
   facial cleansers, **105**, 107–108
Smad complex, 15, 16
SmartSkin laser, 424
SmartXide DOT (laser), 423–424
smile
   downturned, 371, *373*
   gummy, 370
soaps, 83, 84, 96
   acne, 501–502
   alcohol-based hand sanitizers *vs*, 119
   bar cleansers, 84–85, *88*
   body washes, 97
   irritation, 55
   pH, 84, 85, 86–88
   superfatted, 84, 86
   syndets *vs*, 90–94
sodium acyl isethionate *see* syndets
sodium hydroxide, straighteners, 265–268
sodium lauryl sulfate, 55, 136
soft tissue augmentation *see* fillers
soil models
   antimicrobial handwash standards, 115
   body wash testing, 98
Solaraze®, 302, 303
solar radiation *see* UV radiation
solid lipid nanoparticles, 69
solubility, for percutaneous delivery, 67
solubilizing agents, perming lotions, 257
solvents, 55, 105
   brittle nails, 213
   nail lacquers, 219, **221**, **223**
      removers, 223–224
   for percutaneous delivery, 68
   toners, 106
somatosensory system, 33–41
Sonic™ Skin Care Brush, 505
sorbic acid, 55
South-East Asians, photoaging, 17
soy, 291
spatial distribution, actives from shampoo, 128–129
spectrophotometry, sunless tanning agents, 151
spectroradiometers, *183*

speech, botulinum toxin complications, 373
spinal cord, 38–39
spinal nucleus of V, 39
spinothalamic tract, 38–39
split-face tests, bar cleansers, 92
spoolies (brushes), 203
spray booths, sunless tanning, 151
spray gels, hair styling aids, 275
sprays *see* hairsprays
stability
    botulinum toxins, 365–366
    growth factors, 322
    ointments, 78–79
    peptides, 310
    retinoids, 339
    vitamin C, 343
staining, nail colors, 220
Staphylococcus aureus, 111–112
    methicillin-resistant, hand hygiene, 117, 118
Staphylococcus epidermidis, 111
statistical significance, efficacy, 285
stearic acid
    acyl isethionate bars, 86
    Dove bar, 85
stem cells, 323
    adipose-derived, 323, 388
    hair follicles, 234
Stephens & Associates, Inc., photographic studios, 44
Stephens Wrinkle Imaging using Raking Light (SWIRL), 47–48
sterility, liposuction, 479
storage
    growth factors, 322
    retinoids, 339
    sunless tanning agents, 149
straightening of hair, 262–269
    technique, 266–267, 268–269
strand tests
    hair dyes, 245
    thiol procedure, 268
stratum corneum, 3–8, 65, 132–133
    alpha-hydroxyacids on, 351
    cleansing agents on, 85–86
    pH, 9
    shaving on, 171
    skin of color, 25
    surfactants on, 87, *89*
    swelling, 86, *87*
    urea on, 142
    UV filtration, 25
stratum lucidum, photoaging, 28
streptococcal infections, psoriasis, 523
stress, 8
    psoriasis, 523
stubble recreation, beards, 188
styes, **200**
subcutaneous papules, Sculptra®, 59, 393
subdermal radiofrequency probes, 454
subepidermal low echogenic band, 312
submandibular glands, ptosis, 483
submental fat, 478
submental fold, after liposuction, 482

submicron delivery systems, 69
substrate cleansers *see* cleansing cloths
sugars
    in diet, 361
    hair straightening, 264
    as sunless tanning agents, 149
sulfacetamide-sulfur, 514
sulfite perms, 258
sulfites, hair straightening, 265
sulfoxidized methionine, 312
sulfur, 127
    acne, 504
    nail plate, 209
sulfur bridges, hair proteins, *253, 254*, 255
sunburn
    Solareze® for, 303
    studies, 304
sunburn cells, glycolic acid on, 350
SunGuard, 495
sunless tanning products, 148–152
    acetyl pentapeptide, 314
sunlight *see* UV radiation
sun protection factor, 18, 493–494
    measurement, 156–157
    skin of color, 25
    UVA protection factor *vs*, 156
sunscreens, 18, 153–159, 493–495
    after laser therapy, 427
    criteria, 155, **157**
    evaluation, 156–158
    in facial moisturizers, 136, 521
    in nail lacquers, 220, **221**
    retinoids as, 328
    rosacea, 513, **514**
    in sunless tanning agents, 149, 151
    tests, 156–158
    UV fluorescence photography, 46
supercontraction, hair straightening, 266
superfatted soaps, 84, 86
superficial musculoaponeurotic system, 28
superficial peels, 395–401
superficial vascular plexus, photoaging, 28
superoxide dismutase, 315
supersaturation, 67
supplements *see* oral supplements
surfactants, 492, *see also* detergents
    on antiseptics, 114
    bar cleansers, 83–84
    body washes, 97, 98
    cleansing cloths, 107
    cleansing effect, 104
    lathering cleansers, 105–106
    for percutaneous delivery, **67, 68**
    perming lotions, 257
    shampoos, 125–126
    shave gels, 171
    on skin barrier, 10
    on stratum corneum, 87, *89*
surgery (cosmetic), lips, 195
surrogate models, infections, 118
Survival of the Prettiest (Etcoff), 492
sweating, 160–162, 164–165
swelling

    after dermabrasion, 442
    filler injection, 377
    stratum corneum, 86, *87*
swine flu, efficacy of handwashes, 116–117
SWIRL (Stephens Wrinkle Imaging using Raking Light), 47–48
Swiss apple, 291
sympathetic nerves, 38
synapses, central projections, 38
syndets, 84
    acne, 502
    bar cleansers, 85, 86, 87, *88*
    body washes, 97
    eczema, 521
    soaps *vs*, 90–94
synthetic growth factors, 323

T

T4 endonuclease V, 314–315
tacrolimus, 303
    LED light with, 460
talc, 181
tamarind, 291
tanning beds, psoriasis, 526
tanning products (sunless), 148–152
    acetyl pentapeptide, 314
tape stripping, 9
    percutaneous delivery assessment, 72
tap water, metal ions, 245–246
tar
    psoriasis, 525, 526
    scalp care, 127
tartaric acid, 395–396
tattooing
    adverse skin reactions, 58–59
    black henna tattoos, pPD in, 247
    eyelids, 203
    mimicking hair, 188
tazarotene cream, 18–19, 496
TCA Blue Peel, 400
TDSA (UV filter), 155
tea, 289
tear troughs, polylactic acid therapy, 392–393
tea tree oil, acne, 506
telangiectasia, camouflage, *191*
telogen, hair growth, 167–168, 252, 446
    eyelashes, 200
telomerase, happy tree on, 286
temperature sense, 36, *37*
temporal fusion plane, 370
temporal wasting, polylactic acid therapy, 392
temporary hair dyes, 240
Tentative Final Monograph (FDA 1994), on handwashes, 113–114, 115
tenting technique, calcium hydroxylapatite to hands, 487, 490
teratogenesis, botanicals, 285
terminal hair, 29, 167, 446
terpenes, **68**
terpenoids, **68**
terphthalilydine dicamphor sulfonic acid, approval, 154
tetracyclines, rosacea, 514

tetrapeptides, tissue repair, 311
texturing agents
    lipsticks, 196
    relaxers, **266**
thalamocortical afferents, 39–40
therapeutic shampoos, 124, 125, 126–127
therapists, camouflage, 192
Thermacool RF device, 433–434, 452
Thermafrax, 453
thermal coagulation, ProFractional-XC laser, 424
thermal damage, lasers, 412, 413
thermal processing, hair straightening, 263–265
thermal waves, 258
thickeners, 77
    for ascorbyl phosphates, 343
    hair styling aids, 275
    perming lotions, 257
    sunless tanning agents, 150
thighs, liposuction, 467
thioglycolate *see* ammonium thioglycolate
thioglycolic acid, 256
    regulations, 258
thiolactic acid, 256
thiol procedure, 264–265, 268–269
thixotropic agents, nail lacquers, 220, **221**
threading, eyebrows, 203
3D imaging systems, 50
Tierney, E.P., on SmartXide DOT (laser), 423–424
tighteners (herbs), 287, **288**
tightening *see* laxity of skin
Time and Extent Applications (FDA), sunscreens, 154
tinting
    eyelashes, 203
    rosacea camouflage, 513
tip and overlay technique, artificial nail enhancements, 227
tissue dwell times, carbon dioxide lasers, 412
tissue remodeling, 319
tissue repair peptides, 311–313
titanium dioxide, 155, 493
    facial foundation, 181
    rosacea, **514**
T lymphocytes, 53, 299
TNS Essential Serum, after laser therapy, 427
TNS Recovery Complex, 321, *322*, 323
tocopherol, *see also* vitamin E
    α-tocopherol acetate, 343
    d-α-tocopherol, 497, *498*, **499**
δ-tocopherylglucopyranoside, 330, 331
toluene, 219
tomato paste, 359
toners, **105**, 106
topcoats, nails, 217, **218**, 220
topical anesthesia
    autologous fibroblast cell therapy, 387
    calcium hydroxylapatite injection, 383
    laser therapy, 427
tosylamide-formaldehyde resin, 213–214, 219, 222, *223*
touch, 34–36

toxic substances, protection from, 7
Trac II (multi-blade razor), 167
training, nail care practitioners, 232
transdermal patches, 70
transepidermal delivery, 65, *see also* percutaneous delivery
transepidermal water loss, 9
    blockade, 518
    body washes on, 100
    rosacea, 511
    by site, 132, *133*
    skin of color, 26
    soaps *vs* syndets, 90
    tests, 136
transforming growth factor α, 25
transforming growth factor β, 15, 16
transglutaminases, 5, 6
transient microbiota, 111
    in vivo models, 114–116
transparency, facial foundation, 179
transparent soaps, 84–85
transplantation, autologous fat, 388, 483, **486**
transplants, eyelashes, 203
trans-urocanic acid, 7
tretinoin, 18–19, **396**, 397, 496
    acne, 504
    benzoyl peroxide *vs*, 502
    before medium depth peels, 405
triamcinolone, for PLLA nodules, 393
trichiasis, **200**
trichloroacetic acid (TCA), 353, 396–397, 402–405, 406, *408*, *409*, *410*
    burning sensation, 407
    depth controlled peels, 400
triclocarbon, 504
triclosan
    acne, 504
    on *E. coli*, 492–493
    on MRSA, 117
    odor neutralization, 163
    tests for resistance, 119
triethanolamine soap, 85
trigeminal nerve, 39
trimethylpropane triisostearate, **196**
trimming, nails, 212
tripeptides, 309
tryptase reactivity, mast cells, ethnicity, 26
tumescent local anesthesia, 464, 469–470
    historical aspects, 463
    lidocaine dosage, 471
    neck, 480
tumor necrosis factor (TNF), 305
    feverfew on release, 289
Tunable Resurfacing Laser, 413
turmeric, 291–292
two-phase toners, 106
two-way cakes, powders, 180
Tyndall effect, 376–377
type IV reactions, hair dyes, 246
Tyr-Arg (dipeptide), 312, *313*
tyrosinase
    LED light on, 460
    in melanogenesis, 24
tyrosinase-related proteins, 24

U
ubiquinone *see* coenzyme Q10
Ultrapulse CO$_2$ laser, 412, *414*, 415, 427
ultrasound
    liposuction and, 471
    for penetration enhancement, 70
ultraviolet radiation *see* UV radiation
unevenness *see* asymetric effects
units, botulinum toxin quantities, 365
urea, **68**, 140, 141–143, 145–146, 525
urticaria, 53
UV fluorescence photography, 46
UV gels
    artificial nail enhancements, **227**, 228–229
    manicures, 230–231
    nail polish, 222–223, **227**
UV lamps
    nail care, 223, *224*, 232, 233
    safety, 233
UV protection factor ratings, 18, 156–157, 495
UV radiation, 14–15, 153, *see also* photoaging; photodamage
    absorption by retinoids, 328, 330, 331
    on African-American skin, 17
    on colored hair, 246
    for curing nail polish, 223, *224*
    elastosis, 319
    erythema, LED photomodulation on, 459
    on face, 132
    filters, *see also* sunscreens
        approved, 154–155
    hydroxyacids on sensitivity, 350
    lips, 194
    minimal erythema dose, 48
    on molecules, 155
    in nail care, 213, **218**, 223, *224*, 232, 233
    phytophotodermatitis, 53
    pigmentation, 24–25
    protection from, 18
        extremozymes, 315
        niacinamide on, 340
        nutrients, 357–360
        vitamin E, 343
    protective factor, 25
    for psoriasis, 526
    rosacea, 509, 513
    skin barrier, 7–8
    UVA protection criteria, 158
    on vitamin C, 297
UV reflectance photography, 45–46

V
vacuum, bipolar RF and, 454
valacyclovir, 405, 440, 442, **443**
value (color coordinate), 187
Vanicream® Sunscreen, **514**
vascular complications, filler injection, 377
vascular endothelial growth factor
    retinoids on, 18
    UV radiation and, 15
vascular malformations, camouflage, *190*
vasculature *see* microvasculature
vectors, penetration enhancement, 69

vehicle controlled studies, 321
vehicle effect, skin penetration, 66–67
vellus hair, 29, 167, 446
vermilion border, 193, 194
vesicles (penetration enhancement vectors), 69
vibrations, sensory testing, 34
viral infections, 110, 113, 116, 118, *see also* herpes simplex; HIV-associated lipoatrophy
viscosity, ingredients altering, 98
VISIA camera systems (Canfield), 44
visible light photography, 44
vitamin(s)
  oral, acne, 506
  topical, 336–345
vitamin A, 325–326, 328, 336–339, 359
  acne, 506
vitamin B3, 339–341, 344
vitamin B5, 341–342
vitamin C, 342–343, 357, **358**
  as anti-inflammatory, 299
  as antioxidant, 297
  on photodamage, 19, 360, 497, **499**
  rosacea, 497, 515
  vitamin E with, 359–360, 497, 498
vitamin D, 343, **358**
  phototherapy and, 526
vitamin E, 343, **358**, 497, **499**
  as antioxidant, 297, **358**
  UV protection, 299
  with vitamin C, 359–360, 497, 498
  wound healing, **358**, 361
vitamin K, 343
vitamin P, 343
vitiligo, camouflage, 188, *189*
VivaScope, confocal laser scanning microscope, 50
VivoSight, optical coherence tomography, 50
volatile fatty acids, 160
  neutralization, 163
volatile oils, facial foundation, 179

W

warm sense, 36
washing, *see also* handwashing technique
  face and neck, 493
water, *see also* tap water
  binding by hydroxyacids, 348
  body washes, 97
  on colored hair, 246
  dry skin paradox, 86, *88*, 89–90
  hair and, 252–253, **256**, 271–272
  nail plate content, 209
  resistance, sunscreens, 494
  for Sculptra®, 390
water-based nail cosmetics, 219
water displacement, breast volume, 469
water evaporation barrier *see* permeability barrier; transepidermal water loss
water-in-oil emulsions, 75–76, 77, **78**, 179, 519
waterpacts, 180
waterproof mascaras, 201, 205
waxes
  hair styling aids, 270, 272, 273, **274**, 275–276
  lipsticks, 195, **196**
  mascara, 201
waxy pastes, lipsticks, 196
weight reduction, liposuction *vs*, 464
wet cleansing cloths, **105**, 107
wetness control, antiperspirants, 162–163
wet work, irritation, 55
whitening (historical), 177–178
white skin roll, lips, 194
white spots, nail cosmetic removal, 230–231
Whitfield's ointment, 348
windshield wiping technique, liposuction, 481
wine, 289
wire brushes, dermabrasion, 440, 441, 442
women, shaving, 167, 172
wood pencils, eyeliners, 204
Wood's lamp examination
  melanin, 25
  melasma, 401
World Health Organization, on hand hygiene, 112
wound care, after dermabrasion, 442–443
wound healing, 318–320
  after dermabrasion, 437
  after laser therapy, 413–414
  after medium depth peels, 407
  LED photomodulation on, 459
  nutrients for, 361
  tissue repair peptides, 311–313
  vitamin C on, 497
  vitamin E, **358**, 361
wraps, nails, **227**, 229–230
wrinkles
  hydroxyacids on, 353
  LED photomodulation, 457–458
  maltobionic acid on, *353*
  nonablative lasers, 431–435
  nutrients for, 360, 361
  photoaging, 29
  raking light optical profilometry, 46–47
  soaps *vs* syndets, 92
  3D imaging systems, 50
  tissue repair peptides, 311–313
  vitamin C on, 497

X

xenon lightbulbs, 448
Xeomin®, 364, 365
Xeo Pearl Fractionated laser, 426

Y

yellowing, niacinamide on, 340

Z

zeaxanthin, **358**, 359, 361
Zeno™ heating device, 505
zinc, **358**, 360
  acne, 506
  deficiency, 357
  toxicity, 506
zinc oxide, 155, 493
  rosacea, **514**
zinc pyrithione, 127–129, 130, 525
zirconium salts, 163
zoning, cleansing cloths, 107
zwitterionic (amphoteric) surfactants, 104, 125, 237, 492